Kidney Transplantation

Matthew R. Weir • Edgar V. Lerma
Editors

Kidney Transplantation

Practical Guide to Management

Springer

Editors
Matthew R. Weir
Department of Nephrology
University of Maryland School of Medicine
Baltimore, MD, USA

Edgar V. Lerma
Department of Nephrology
University of Illinois
Berwyn, IL, USA

ISBN 978-1-4939-0341-2 ISBN 978-1-4939-0342-9 (eBook)
DOI 10.1007/978-1-4939-0342-9
Springer New York Heidelberg Dordrecht London

Library of Congress Control Number: 2014932830

Printed on acid-free paper

Springer is part of Springer Science+Business Media (www.springer.com)

To my wonderful wife Duffy, and my three great children Ryan, Courtney, and Kerry, I thank you for the time to allow me to pursue my educational interests and my passion for patient care.
To all my patients with whom I have developed wonderful long-term relationships over my many years in clinical practice, I thank for the opportunity to improve your quality of life.
Thank you,

Matthew R. Weir

To all my mentors and friends at the University of Santo Tomas Faculty of Medicine and Surgery in Manila, Philippines, and Northwestern University Feinberg School of Medicine in Chicago, IL, who have, in one way or another, influenced and guided me to become the physician that I am.
To all the medical students, interns, and residents at Advocate Christ Medical Center whom I have taught or learned from, especially those who eventually decided to pursue nephrology as a career.
To my parents and my brothers, without whose unwavering love and support through the good and bad times, I would not have persevered and reached my goals in life.
Most especially, to my two lovely and precious daughters, Anastasia Zofia and Isabella Ann, whose smiles and laughter constantly provide me unparalleled joy and happiness, and my very loving and understanding wife, Michelle, who has always been supportive of my endeavors, both personally and professionally, and who sacrificed a lot of time and exhibited unwavering patience as I devoted a significant amount of time and effort to this project. Truly, they provide me with motivation and inspiration.

Edgar V. Lerma

Preface

Kidney transplantation is commonplace today. Many transplant recipients are being cared for in a variety of clinical practice situations which are often outside the transplant center. The purpose of this book is to provide the reader with an update of the main understandings that are important for the optimal management of medical and surgical issues in transplantation recipients. We have sought out the expertise of many key opinion leaders in the different areas of transplantation practice. Many of the authors are members of the organ transplantation program at the University of Maryland School of Medicine in Baltimore. This center with its large clinical practice has provided substantial experience in many of the clinical areas that are covered in this book. Hopefully, this compendium of new information will serve as an important resource in your practice to provide the best possible care for your transplant patients.

Baltimore, MD, USA — Matthew R. Weir
Berwyn, IL, USA — Edgar V. Lerma

Contents

Contributors

Kevin C. Abbott Nephrology Service, Department of Medicine, Walter Reed National Military Medical Center, Bethesda, MD, USA

Deborah B. Adey University of California, Davis, Sacramento, CA, USA

Ayub Akbari Clinical Epidemiology Program, Ottawa Hospital Research Institute, Ottawa, ON, Canada

Hala M. Alshayeb Department of Internal Medicine—Nephrology, Joan C. Edwards School of Medicine, Marshall University, Huntington, WV, USA

Baris Ata Kellogg School of Management, Northwestern University, Evanston, IL, USA

Roy D. Bloom Department of Medicine, Perelman School of Medicine, University of Pennsylvania, Philadelphia, PA, USA

Boonsong Kiangkitiwan Division of Nephrology, University of Maryland School of Medicine, Baltimore, MD, USA

Daniel C. Brennan Washington University in St. Louis, St. Louis, MO, USA

Marissa M. Brokhof Solid Organ Transplantation, University of Wisconsin Hospital and Clinics, Madison, WI, USA

Jonathan S. Bromberg Division of Transplantation, Department of Surgery, University of Maryland School of Medicine, Baltimore, MD, USA

Richard Bryson University of Maryland School of Medicine, Baltimore, MD, USA

Charles Cangro University of Maryland School of Medicine, Baltimore, MD, USA

Andres F. Carrion Division of Gastroenterology, University of Miami Miller School of Medicine, Miami, FL, USA

Nadia Chaudhri Division of Nephrology, Department of Medicine, University of Maryland, Baltimore, MD, USA

Darshika Chhabra Kidney Transplant Program, Advocate Christ Medical Center, Oak Lawn, IL, USA

David J. Cohen Division of Nephrology, Columbia University Medical Center, New York, NY, USA

Edward H. Cole Division of Nephrology, Department of Medicine, University of Toronto, Toronto, ON, Canada

James E. Cooper Division of Renal Diseases and Hypertension, Transplant Center, University of Colorado, Denver, CO, USA

Matthew Cooper Georgetown University School of Medicine, Kidney and Pancreas Transplantation, MedStar Georgetown Transplant Institute, Washington, DC, USA

Salvatore P. Costa Cardiology Section, Department of Medicine, Dartmouth Hitchcock Medical Center, Hanover, NH, USA

Francis L. Delmonico Department of Surgery, Harvard Medical School, Massachusetts General Hospital, Boston, MA, USA

Rowena Delos Santos Washington University School in St. Louis of Medicine, St. Louis, MO, USA

Arjang Djamali Division of Nephrology, University of Wisconsin, Madison, WI, USA

Anil Vamsi Doppalapudi Internal Medicine, Northwestern University, Chicago, IL, USA

Cinthia B. Drachenberg Department of Pathology, University of Maryland School of Medicine, Baltimore, MD, USA

Geoffrey K. Dube Division of Nephrology, Columbia University Medical Center, New York, NY, USA

Fabrizio Fabrizi Division of Nephrology and Dialysis, Maggiore Hospital, IRCCS Foundation, Milan, Italy

John J. Friedewald Nephrology and Organ Transplantation, Northwestern University Feinberg School of Medicine, Chicago, IL, USA

David R. Hager University of Wisconsin Hospital and Clinics, Madison, WI, USA

Abdolreza Haririan Division of Nephrology, Department of Medicine, University of Maryland School of Medicine, Baltimore, MD, USA

Hassan N. Ibrahim Division of Renal Diseases and Hypertension, University of Minnesota, Minneapolis, MN, USA

Michelle A. Josephson Department of Medicine, Section of Nephrology, University of Chicago Medicine, Chicago, IL, USA

Ahmed I. Kamal Department of Medicine and Transplantation, Mansoura University, Mansoura, Egypt

Bruce Kaplan Division of Transplant Medicine, Department of Medicine, University of Arizona College of Medicine, Tucson, AZ, USA

Sabine Karam Department of Clinical Medicine, Balamand University School of Medicine, Beirut, Lebanon

Sunil S. Karhadkar University of Maryland Medical Center, Baltimore, MD, USA

Eliyahu V. Khankin Beth Israel Deaconess Medical Center, Boston, MA, USA

S. Joseph Kim Faculty of Medicine, Institute for Health Policy, Management, and Evaluation, University of Toronto, Toronto, ON, Canada

David K. Klassen Division of Nephrology, Department of Medicine, University of Maryland School of Medicine, Baltimore, MD, USA

Greg A. Knoll Division of Nephrology, Kidney Research Centre, Ottawa Hospital Research Institute, Ottawa, ON, Canada

Andrew Kramer University of Maryland School of Medicine, Baltimore, MD, USA

Anurag Kumbham Internal Medicine, Southwest Georgia Healthcare Inc., Richland, GA, USA

Eric D. Langewisch Oregon Health and Science University, Portland, OR, USA

Sabrina Lee Department of Transplant, Keck Medical Center of USC, Los Angeles, CA, USA

David B. Leeser Kidney and Pancreas Transplantation, University of Maryland Medical Center, Baltimore, MD, USA

Krista L. Lentine Center for Outcomes Research, Abdominal Transplant Program, Saint Louis University School of Medicine, St. Louis, MO, USA

Edgar V. Lerma Department of Nephrology, University of Illinois at Chicago, Berwyn, IL, USA

Machaiah M. Madhrira Division of Nephrology, Department of Medicine, University of Arizona College of Medicine, Tucson, AZ, USA

Didier A. Mandelbrot Beth Israel Deaconess Medical Center, Boston, MA, USA

Wana Manitpisitkul Department of Pharmacy, University of Maryland Medical Center, Baltimore, MD, USA

Maria Manning University of Maryland Medical Center, Baltimore, MD, USA

Roslyn B. Mannon Division of Nephrology, Department of Medicine, University of Alabama at Birmingham, Birmingham, AL, USA

Dominique E. Martin Centre for Health and Society, School of Population Health, The University of Melbourne, Parkville, VIC, Australia

Paul Martin Division of Hepatology, University of Miami Miller School of Medicine, Miami, FL, USA

Arthur Matas Department of Surgery, University of Minnesota, Minneapolis, MN, USA

Dianne B. McKay University of California, San Diego, La Jolla, CA, USA

Charles Moussallem Department of Medicine, Perelman School of Medicine, University of Pennsylvania, Philadelphia, PA, USA

Joseph M. Nogueira Division of Nephrology, Department of Medicine, University of Maryland, Baltimore, MD, USA

Douglas J. Norman Oregon Health and Science University, Portland, OR, USA

John C. Papadimitriou Department of Pathology, University of Maryland School of Medicine, Baltimore, MD, USA

Todd E. Pesavento Comprehensive Transplant Center, Ohio State University, Columbus, OH, USA

Michael Phelan University of Maryland School of Medicine, Baltimore, MD, USA

Mihaela Popescu Department of Surgery, University of Maryland School of Medicine, Baltimore, MD, USA

Scott Reule Division of Renal Diseases and Hypertension, University of Minnesota, Minneapolis, MN, USA

Joseph Scalea Department of Surgery, University of Maryland School of Medicine, Baltimore, MD, USA

Sunita K. Singh Faculty of Medicine, Institute for Health Policy, Management, and Evaluation, University of Toronto, Toronto, ON, Canada

Stuart M. Sprague Department of Medicine, Section of Nephrology and Hypertension, NorthShore University Health System, Evanston, IL, USA

Stephen C. Textor Division of Nephrology and Hypertension, Department of Medicine, Mayo Clinic College of Medicine, Rochester, MN, USA

Richard Ugarte Division of Nephrology, Department of Medicine, University of Maryland School of Medicine, Baltimore, MD, USA

Jennifer E. Verbesey Georgetown University School of Medicine, Kidney and Pancreas Transplant Surgeon, MedStar Georgetown Transplant Institute, Washington, DC, USA

Vijay Vidyasagar Division of Nephrology, University of Wisconsin, Madison, WI, USA

Todd C. Villines Cardiology Service, Department of Medicine, Walter Reed National Military Medical Center, Bethesda, MD, USA

Hani M. Wadei Department of Transplantation, Mayo Clinic College of Medicine, Jacksonville, FL, USA

Ravinder Wali University of Maryland School of Medicine, Baltimore, MD, USA

Matthew R. Weir Department of Nephrology, University of Maryland School of Medicine, Baltimore, MD, USA

Adam Weltz Department of Surgery, University of Maryland School of Medicine, Baltimore, MD, USA

Nikita S. Wilson Vanderbilt Transplant Center, Vanderbilt University Medical Center, Nashville, TN, USA

Alexander C. Wiseman Division of Renal Diseases and Hypertension, Transplant Center, University of Colorado, Denver, CO, USA

Karl L. Womer Johns Hopkins University School of Medicine, Baltimore, MD, USA

Jade Wong-You-Cheong Department of Diagnostic Radiology, University of Maryland Medical Center, Baltimore, MD, USA

Jiangnan Xu Department of Surgery, University of Maryland School of Medicine, Baltimore, MD, USA

Part I

Graft and Patient Survival

1

Machaiah M. Madhrira, Karl L. Womer, and Bruce Kaplan

Introduction

Patient Survival

Kidney transplantation is agreed upon as the best treatment available for most patients with end-stage renal disease (ESRD). It not only improves quality of life [1–4] of our patients and reduces medical expense [2, 5] but also has shown to be a life-prolonging procedure. Multiple studies using renal transplant recipients with dialysis patients have found that patient survival is clearly better with renal transplantation than with dialysis [6–9]. However, randomized trials comparing survival between these two groups are neither feasible nor ethical. The reasons for improved survival are unclear, while one can postulate that transplant recipients are derived from a highly selected subgroup of patients on dialysis who are on average younger and healthier and of higher socioeconomic status than those dialysis patients not selected for transplantation. However, to negate this selection bias, Wolf et al. [10] merged data from the US Renal Data System (USRDS) with information about the renal transplantation waiting list from the Scientific Renal Transplant Registry (SRTR) operated by UNOS and showed large long-term benefits for cadaveric transplantation vs. maintenance dialysis, despite the increased short-term risk of death after transplantation (Fig. 1.1). There was improved survival with transplantation in both men and women, more profound in diabetics, and in all age groups, including those 60–74 years old. The long-term relative risk of death was lower among transplant recipients compared with waiting-list patients. When the results were analyzed according to race, transplantation reduced the long-term relative risk (RR) of death more among Asians and whites than among Native Americans and blacks. However, in all four racial groups, transplantation significantly reduced the long-term risk of death. In the last decade, studies have elucidated that the reduction in mortality among transplant recipients compared to dialysis patients is due in part to a decrease in cardiovascular events, especially among diabetic patients [11–13].

Graft Survival

Kidney transplantation has made dramatic strides in the last 50 years since the discovery of azathioprine as an immunosuppressive drug. One-year cadaveric renal allograft survival, previously zero, was increased by the combination of prednisone and azathioprine to 45–50 %. As technical and pharmacological advancements were made in the field of kidney transplantation, it became clear in the 1970s that transplantation of kidneys from living donors resulted in better initial and long-term graft survival rates than those of kidneys from cadaveric donors. By the mid-1990s, Hariharan et al. [14] using the Scientific Registry of Transplant Recipients (SRTR) data showed significant improvement in 1-year kidney allograft survival over a 7-year period (Table 1.1). This improvement in part may be due to a marked decrease in the incidence of acute rejection [15] though this data preceded the introduction of newer immunosuppressive drugs, as it took place in the era of treatment with cyclosporine (CsA) [16], muromonab-CD3 [17], azathioprine, and prednisone. Despite reductions in acute rejection rates and improvements in first-year survival, there was no improvement in long-term

M.M. Madhrira
Division of Nephrology, Department of Medicine, University of Arizona College of Medicine, 1501 N Campbell Avenue, Tucson, AZ 85724-5022, USA
e-mail: mmadhrira@deptofmed.arizona.edu

K.L. Womer
Johns Hopkins University School of Medicine, 1830 E Monument Street, Suite 416, Baltimore, MD 21287, USA
e-mail: Kwomer1@jhmi.edu

B. Kaplan (✉)
Division of Transplant Medicine, Department of Medicine, University of Arizona College of Medicine, 1501 N Campbell Avenue, Tucson, AZ 85724-5022, USA
e-mail: bkaplan@deptofmed.arizona.edu

M.R. Weir and E.V. Lerma (eds.), *Kidney Transplantation: Practical Guide to Management*,
DOI 10.1007/978-1-4939-0342-9_1,

graft survival [18]. As it became clear that non-immunologic factors [19] were important in long-term graft survival, efforts are being made to improve long-term outcomes through prevention of late allograft loss by targeting such factors. Using the SRTR, Lamb et al. [20] analyzed 252,910 adult kidney recipients transplanted between 1989 and 2005 and reported that renal allograft half-lives for deceased donor improved from 6.6 years in 1989 to 8.2 years in 2000 and a continued improvement to a projected 8.8 years in 2005. According to the 2008 Organ Procurement and Transplantation Network (OPTN)/Scientific Registry of Transplant Recipients (SRTR) Annual Report [21], the 1- and 5-year patient survival rates for recipients of living donor kidney transplants to recipients of cadaveric kidney transplants were 98.0 % vs. 96.0 % and 91.0 % vs. 83.0 %, respectively. In comparison the 1- and 5-year graft survival rates for recipients of living donor kidney transplants to recipients of cadaveric kidney transplants were 96.0 % vs. 92.0 % and 81.0 % vs. 71.0 %, respectively. These patient and graft survival rates have not changed much according to the most recent OPTN/SRTR reports.

The significant progress that has occurred over the last 2 decades in renal transplantation and the slow improvement in long-term attrition rate gives hope for bigger advances in the future to improve long-term graft and patient survival. This chapter will focus on the pre- and posttransplant donor and recipient risk factors important to graft and patient survival as well as effects of pharmacological advances on these outcome measures.

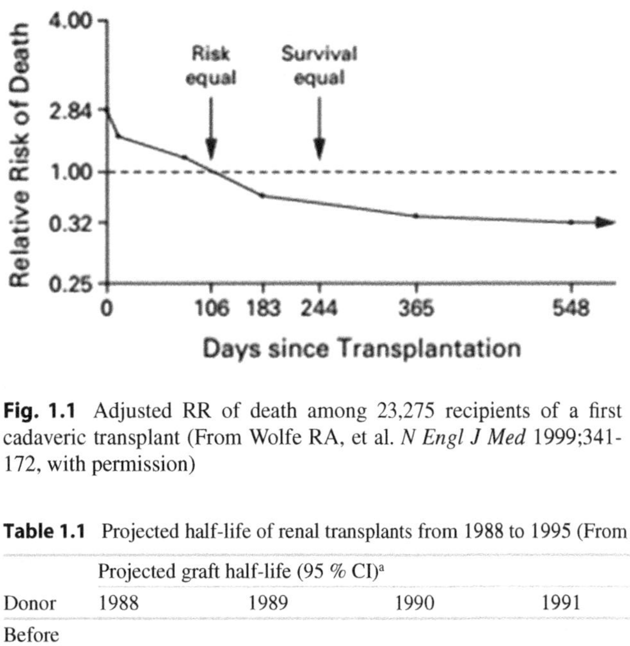

Fig. 1.1 Adjusted RR of death among 23,275 recipients of a first cadaveric transplant (From Wolfe RA, et al. *N Engl J Med* 1999;341-172, with permission)

Causes of Graft Loss: Major Etiologies

The most common causes of renal allograft loss are primary nonfunction of the allograft, death with a functioning graft, antibody-mediated rejection/interstitial fibrosis and tubular atrophy (IF/TA), and recurrent glomerular disease. However, the relative importance of these etiologies operates differentially over time. In the early posttransplantation period, primary nonfunction, technical complications, and antibody-mediated rejection (in sensitized individuals) remain the leading causes of graft loss. However, for the purposes of the chapter, only those etiologies responsible for late allograft loss will be reviewed.

Death with a Functioning Allograft

With the change in practice pattern in many centers and transplantation of older and sicker patient's data regarding the importance of death with a functioning allograft (9–38 %) has emerged as a major contributor to late allograft loss [22–27]. Depending on the age and comorbidities of the patient population, the transplant era, and the posttransplant interval being studied, death with a functioning allograft ranks as first or second among the leading causes of allograft loss [22–24, 28]. Recently El-Zoghby et al. [29] reported death with functioning allograft as the most commonly observed cause of graft loss accounting for 10.4 % of the study cohort. The underlying comorbidities mainly cardiovascular disease, infections, and cancer may be the reasons for death with graft function. Attention to cardiovascular risk factors along with prevention and prompt treatment of infection, tailoring of immunosuppressive medications by the level of renal function maintained by the graft would offer the greatest potential to improve the chance of living longer with functioning graft. General guidelines for cancer screening are usually followed.

Table 1.1 Projected half-life of renal transplants from 1988 to 1995 (From Hariharan S, et al. *N Engl J Med* 2000;342:605, with permission)

	Projected graft half-life (95 % CI)[a]							
Donor	1988	1989	1990	1991	1992	1993	1994	1995
Before censoring								
Living	12.7 (11.5–13.9)	15.0 (13.5–16.5)	14.8 (13.3–16.4)	14.8 (13.3–16.4)	16.9 (14.8–18.9)	16.7 (14.5–19.0)	21.8 (17.7–26.0)	21.6 (13.8–29.3)
Cadaveric	7.9 (7.6–8.3)	8.7 (8.3–9.0)	8.8 (8.4–9.2)	9.7 (9.2–10.1)	9.6 (9.1–10.1)	10.3 (9.7–11.0)	11.0 (10.1–11.9)	13.8 (11.2–16.4)
After censoring								
Living	16.9 (15.1–18.7)	20.8 (18.3–23.2)	19.9 (17.5–24.1)	21.5 (18.8–24.1)	21.9 (18.9–24.9)	22.9 (19.3–26.5)	35.0 (26.5–43.5)	35.9 (19.3–52.5)
Cadaveric	11.0 (10.5–11.5)	12.0 (11.4–12.6)	12.5 (11.8–13.2)	14.5 (13.6–15.4)	14.2 (13.2–15.1)	15.1 (13.9–16.3)	17.4 (15.5–19.3)	19.5 (15.1–23.8)

[a]CI denotes confidence interval

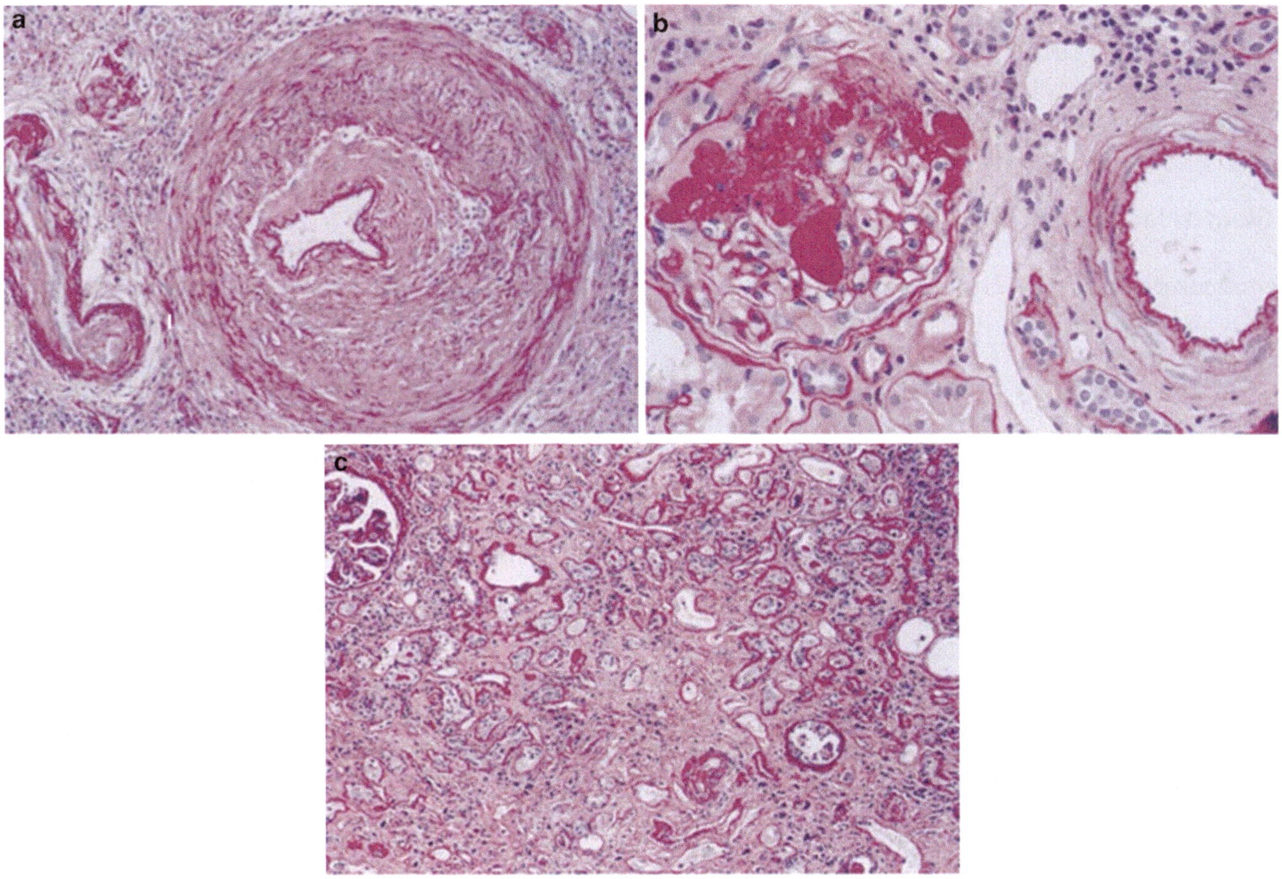

Fig. 1.2 Characteristic histopathologic findings in CAN: (**a**) glomerulosclerosis, (**b**) interstitial fibrosis, (**c**) obliterative vasculopathy, (From Sayegh MH. *Kidney Int* 1999;56:1967, with permission)

Interstitial Fibrosis and Tubular Atrophy

Late allograft failure was often labeled as chronic allograft nephropathy. More recently the terminology interstitial fibrosis and tubular atrophy (IF/TA), with no evidence of any specific etiology, has been used [30]. CAN is a poorly defined clinical-pathologic entity manifested clinically by a gradual decrease in renal function over months to years after transplantation, coupled with a variety of pathologic lesions [31]. Histopathologic findings include widespread obliterative vasculopathy, glomerulosclerosis, and interstitial fibrosis and tubular atrophy (Fig. 1.2). However, these changes overlap those of human aging and age-related diseases in native kidneys. The studies by El-Zoghby et al. [29] and the preliminary data by the Long-Term Deterioration of Kidney Allograft Function (DeKAF) [32] highlight the fact that the term IF/TA should not be used as a diagnostic term to explain kidney graft loss as inflammation in areas of tubular atrophy may be a potent predictor of allograft failure [33]. Both immunologic and non-immunologic factors have been shown to contribute to IF/TA [34], although these factors should be considered mutually exclusive.

Of the immunologic factors, antibody-mediated rejection is an important risk factor for the development of allograft loss. Further evidence for immunologic mechanisms stems from observations that the half-life of cadaveric renal allografts is longer when donated from human leukocyte antigen (HLA)-matched vs. HLA-mismatched donors [35]. Moreover, in a study by Legendre et al. [36], 2-year protocol biopsies on HLA-identical transplants who did not have episodes of AR or acute renal failure (ARF) showed no histopathologic findings of IF/TA. Both cellular [37–40] and humoral [41, 42] mechanisms likely play a role in the pathogenesis of IF/TA, although the relative contribution of each is the subject of intense debate. Non-immunologic factors include brain death in the donor, ischemia-reperfusion injury, inadequate donor kidney nephron mass, calcineurin inhibitor toxicity, hypertension, hyperlipidemia, cytomegalovirus (CMV) infection, and polyoma virus nephropathy.

To date, there have been no convincing studies to demonstrate that secondary intervention is effective in reducing the rate of graft loss. The ultimate goal in transplantation is to achieve a state of tolerance [43], which would ideally eliminate the immunologic factors, but which may also serve to attenuate the effects of the non-immunologic factors [44]. It is clear that any successful strategy will need to be broad based to account for the immunologic, physiologic, infectious, and metabolic aspects of this difficult problem.

Glomerular Disease

Glomerulonephritis (GN) is a major cause of ESRD and is the primary disease in roughly 30–50 % of patients undergoing renal transplantation [28, 45]. Recurrent disease, transplant glomerulopathy, and de novo glomerular disease account for the glomerular disease posttransplantation. Since it is not a common occurrence, accurate estimates of the rates of occurrence of different forms of GN may be difficult. Results from small studies should be interpreted with caution, and although reports from data registries give good estimates of rates of graft loss, they often lack information on recurrent rates and clinical outcomes. Recurrence has been reported in 6.0–19.4 % of renal allograft recipients, and the prevalence increases with the duration of follow-up [28, 46–49]. Previous studies have reported recurrent GN as the cause of graft loss in 1.1–8.4 % of transplant recipients [28, 46–50] with the most recent report by El-Zoghby et al. being 14.3 % [29].

The definition of recurrent GN requires an accurate histological diagnosis of both the pre- and posttransplant diseases. However, in many chronic GN patients with ESRD, a previous renal biopsy is not available. In posttransplantation also, renal biopsy may not be performed in cases of mild proteinuria. Secondly, the lack of specificity in the pathologic features of some conditions often leads to errors in diagnosis. Chronic transplant glomerulopathy may be mistaken for membranoproliferative GN and vice versa. Diagnostic dilemma between hemolytic uremic syndrome (HUS), malignant hypertension, and CsA toxicity may lead to an erroneous diagnosis. Lastly, recurrence rates can be complicated by the existence of de novo glomerular disease. These scenarios lead to underdiagnoses and therefore an underreporting of the true recurrence rate. Finally, the duration of follow-up of a particular study is important, since the impact of recurrence on graft survival will increase with longer periods of follow-up.

Using data compiled by the Australian and New Zealand Dialysis and Transplant Registry, Briganti et al. [28] studied incidence, timing, and relative importance of allograft loss due to recurrence of GN in 1,505 renal transplant recipients with biopsy-proven GN as the cause of ESRD. At 10-year post-transplantation, the incidence of allograft loss due to recurrent GN was 8.4 % as compared with 4.1 % for loss due to acute rejection, 15.0 % for loss due to death with a functioning allograft, and 20.3 % for loss due to IF/TA, making recurrent GN the third most common cause of allograft loss in this patient population. Allograft loss due to recurrent GN occurred in patients with focal segmental glomerulosclerosis (FSGS), mesangiocapillary glomerulonephritis type 1 (MCGN-I), MCGN type III, IgA nephropathy, Henoch–Schonlein purpura, membranous nephropathy, and pauci-immune crescentic GN. The greatest incidence of allograft loss occurred among patients with FSGS and MCGN-I, and allograft loss tended to occur earlier in these patients. The 10-year incidence of graft loss from any cause was similar among recipients with biopsy-proven GN and among those with renal failure from other causes. Since the incidence of allograft loss due to GN increased over time, recurrent GN will likely become an increasingly important cause of allograft loss as overall long-term graft rates continue to improve.

Risk Factors for Patient and Graft Survival

Pretransplant Factors

Waiting Time/Preemptive Transplantation

As presented earlier, transplantation has been shown to improve survival when compared with maintenance dialysis for patients with ESRD [10]. Since the incidence of treated ESRD has nearly doubled over the past decade, with no substantial growth in the cadaveric donor kidney pool, the waiting time to receive a renal allograft has been steadily increasing [51]. Earlier, retrospective single-center [9] and small database [8] analyses yielded conflicting results regarding the effect of length of pretransplant dialysis on patient and graft survival. The argument that time on dialysis itself is an independent risk factor for graft loss was strengthened by a subsequent large, retrospective study based on USRDS data showing a clear dose-dependent detrimental effect of dialysis time on transplant outcomes for both patient and graft survival and, somewhat surprising, also for death-censored graft survival [52]. These findings held true for both cadaveric and living transplantation and, importantly, were proportional across different primary disease groups, suggesting that the risk of increased ESRD is not simply related to cumulative disease burden alone (i.e., diabetes mellitus or HTN vs. GN).

These data were further substantiated by Mange et al. [53], who demonstrated in a retrospective cohort study of 8,481 patients that preemptive transplantation in living donor transplant recipients was associated with a 52 % reduction in the risk of allograft failure during the first year after transplantation, an 82 % reduction during the second year, and an 86 % reduction during subsequent years, as compared with transplantation after dialysis. Furthermore, increasing duration of dialysis was associated with increasing odds of acute rejection within 6 months after transplantation, suggesting that dialysis may alter the immune status of patients with chronic kidney disease (CKD) as an explanation for the increased incidence of graft loss. Kasiske et al. [54] studied this issue further by examining outcomes of patients who receive preemptive kidney transplants. Retrospective analysis was performed on 38,836 first kidney transplants carried out between 1995 and 1998. Overall, 13.2 % of the transplants were preemptive, which comprised 7.7 % of the total number of cadaveric transplants and 24 % of the total number of living donor transplants. Preemptive transplant recipients were more likely to be less than 17 years old, white, actively working, privately insured, college graduates, and transplanted with kidneys having fewer HLA mismatches (all patient characteristics shown to favor improved graft survival). However, multivariate analysis demonstrated that the beneficial effect of preemptive transplantation on graft survival was independent of other pretransplant characteristics.

To remove potential donor-related confounding factors present in previous studies, an analysis of 2,405 kidneys pairs harvested from the same donor but transplanted into recipients with different ESRD time was performed [55]. Five- and ten-year unadjusted graft- and death-censored graft survival rates were significantly worse in paired kidney recipients who had undergone more than 24 months of dialysis compared with paired kidney recipients who had undergone less than 6 months of dialysis. Although advanced age, African American race, and higher panel-reactive antibody (PRA) percentage were characteristics of the recipient population, when adjustments in the multivariate analysis for these risk factors were made, the trend was maintained. Important to these findings was the exclusion of six-antigen-matched transplants, since the current national sharing policy results in a higher proportion of such kidneys transplanted preemptively, regardless of recipient waiting time. In a follow-up study using a nontraditional endpoint, death after allograft loss (DAGL), risk factors were analyzed for a total of 78,564 primary renal transplant patients reported to the USRDS from 1988 to 1998 [56]. By Cox model, dialysis for more than 2 years was associated with a more than twofold RR for DAGL, while transplant time was not associated with DAGL. These findings suggest that time with ESRD is a strong, independent, and potentially modifiable risk factor for renal transplant outcomes and emphasize the need for timely referral of all ESRD patients for transplantation.

HLA Matching

Although improvements in immunosuppression have diminished its relative importance, HLA-matching continues to be a major determinant of survival in large retrospective analyses [57]. Held et al. [58] studied a series of Medicare patients receiving a first cadaveric kidney transplant between 1984 and 1990. Both multivariate and univariate estimates indicate that grafts with fewer HLA mismatches tend to survive longer. The survival of grafts with no mismatches is substantially better than that of grafts with one mismatch, whereas the survival of grafts with 1–6 mismatches is more homogeneous. Analysis of the United Network for Organ Sharing (UNOS) registry between 1991 and 1997 demonstrated an 11 % reduction in 3-year graft survival rate ($p<0.001$) between transplants involving 6 compared to 0 HLA mismatches, with the most discernible difference in survival which was observed between recipients with 0–1 HLA mismatch[59].

Through an agreement among US transplant centers, UNOS established a program in 1987 to ship kidneys anywhere in the country to recipients who have the same HLA-A, HLA-B, and HLA-DR antigens as the donor. The HLA-matching policy has been liberalized twice, to include kidneys with the same constellation of HLA antigens as the recipient even though fewer than six antigens were identified and again to include zero-A-, zero-B-, and zero-DR-mismatched kidneys [60]. Takemoto et al. [61] examined the results of the national kidney-sharing program after over 10 years of operation. The survival rate of HLA-matched kidneys was similar regardless of the criteria followed and was significantly higher than those for HLA-mismatched transplants (half-life of 12.5 years vs. 8.6 years, respectively). The benefit of HLA matching was diminished in kidneys from older donors, with the difference in projected 10-year rates of graft survival between HLA-matched and HLA-mismatched recipients greatest (28 %) among those whose donor was 15 years of age or younger and least (10 %) among those whose donor was older than 55 years. There was no significant increase in graft survival associated with HLA matching in black recipients. Finally, no improvement in graft survival was noted when cold ischemia time (CIT) was greater than 36 h. The findings with CIT greater than 36 h were confirmed in a similar study by separate investigators [62].

Several other publications have explored further the clinical contexts in which HLA matching is associated with improved graft survival. Using data from UNOS, Mange et al. [63] compared the outcomes of organs from the same donors for which one kidney was shipped and one was transplanted locally. In their analysis, a significant association between shipment and allograft survival at 1 year was noted for HLA-mismatched but not HLA-matched kidneys. In a single-centered study, Asderakis et al. [64] showed that ignoring HLA match to achieve a shorter CIT for donors greater than 55 years old resulted in a 3.7 % increase in graft survival. Similar results have been reported for other single-centered studies aimed at optimizing HLA-independent risk factors for allograft survival at the expense of HLA matching [65, 66]. In fact, Terasaki et al. [67] showed that survival of grafts from living unrelated donors was comparable to that of parental donor grafts, despite significantly higher major histocompatibility complex (MHC) mismatches in the former group. In this same study, survival rates of zero-antigen-mismatched cadaveric grafts that functioned immediately were similar to those of spousal grafts. However, the survival rate of grafts mismatched for all six antigens that functioned on the first day was higher than that of a perfectly matched graft that did not function immediately. In summary, HLA matching is only one factor in the complex interplay of risk factors important to long-term graft survival, and there is a point of diminished returns for any HLA-matching strategy that increases the overall number of risk factors for graft loss. Even though new technologies of solid-phase assays (e.g., enzyme-linked immunosorbent assay (ELISA) or Luminex) have allowed a more accurate assessment of transplant candidate's immunologic risk pretransplantation, non-HLA antibodies may also be clinically important in the development of allograft rejection, although the extent of their harmful effects is not fully clear.

Donor Source

Live donor (LD) source, even when corrected for ischemic times and delayed graft function (DGF), is one of the strongest factors associated with good graft survival [14, 67]. This advantage occurs despite higher degrees of HLA mismatching in LD kidneys and does not appear to be affected by donor race, donor age, length of cold ischemia, or the use of preoperative donor transfusions [67]. Although better compliance with immunosuppressive medications is a reasonable explanation in the case of spousal donated grafts, survival rates of grafts from other living unrelated donors are similarly high. In all likelihood, the advantages of living donated kidneys are a combination of better-quality kidneys undergoing minimal trauma in a better educated, highly motivated recipient of higher socioeconomic status.

Donor Age

One of the strongest risk factors for poor long-term graft survival is advanced donor age [23, 68, 69]. Kidneys from older donors show an increased frequency of adverse features after transplantation, including DGF and an elevated baseline serum creatinine. Although the reason is not entirely clear, decreased functional reserve due to age and age-related diseases such as HTN and vascular disease probably explains the phenomenon. Alternatively, there may exist accelerated aging after transplantation, which would manifest itself more in an older kidney [70]. Donor age is also a risk factor for recipient death with a functioning allograft [69], which likely reflects the known association of cardiovascular death with CKD [71–73] and, more recently, with elevated serum creatinine at 1-year posttransplantation [74].

Non-heart-Beating Donors

Non-heart-beating donors (NHBD) are those donors who have experienced irreversible cessation of circulatory and respiratory function [75], in contrast to donors with a heat-beat (HBD) in whom death is determined according to neurologic criteria. By definition, a kidney from an NHBD experiences a prolonged phase of insufficient or complete lack of perfusion (i.e., warm ischemia), which is purported to cause irreversible damage and, therefore, poor short-term and long-term graft survival. In fact, the use of NHBD has been restricted almost exclusively to kidney transplantation, given the availability of dialysis for support should the graft not function posttransplantation. The Maastricht protocol is used by the majority of centers performing such transplants and requires a waiting time of 10 min after cessation of cardiac massage and mechanical ventilation before organ retrieval, with the diagnosis of death made by physicians independent of the procurement team [76]. Furthermore, the protocol categorizes donors: category I, death on arrival; category II, unsuccessful resuscitation; category III, cardiac arrest; and category IV, cardiac arrest in a brain-dead donor. The use of NHBD represents an attempt to increase the donor pool in response to the increasing shortage of suitable cadaveric organs. Although there are numerous centers worldwide that have used NHBD since the early 1980s, the inherent ethical issues have prevented the practice from being widely embraced by most US centers.

Several small single-centered studies have addressed the effect of NHBD on graft outcomes, albeit with relatively short follow-up periods [77–81]. An increase in DGF was seen in all cases compared with kidneys from HBD. In two of the studies, in which the majority of NHBD were category II or III, there was no significant difference in patient or graft survival at 1 and 3 years compared with recipients of HBD [79, 80]. In one of the studies, the serum creatinine was marginally higher at 5 years, emphasizing the importance of long-term follow-up in these recipients [79]. Sanchez-Fructuoso et al. [77] excluded donors of greater than 55 years and warm ischemia time greater than 120 min as part of their locally mandated policy whereby subjects who die on the street suddenly are transported immediately to the donation center. In their analysis, there was no significant difference in graft survival at 1 and 5 years for recipients of category I [77]. Weber et al. [76] reported long-term data on 122 NHBD kidney transplants, who received sequential therapy with antithymocyte globulin (ATG) initially, CsA starting at day 10, and triple therapy with CsA thereafter. Case-controlled recipients of HBD received triple therapy immediately post-transplantation. Confirming previous studies, DGF affecting kidneys from HBD was approximately double that affecting kidneys from HBD. Ten-year graft survival was no different for kidneys from NHBD (78.7 %) and HBD (76.7 %). Interestingly, DGF had no effect on graft survival for kidneys from NHBD but was associated with decreased graft survival for those from HBD. More recently, Brook et al. [82] demonstrated higher 6-year graft survival rates in patients with kidneys from NHBD with DGF than in patients with kidneys from HBD with DGF (84 % vs. 62 %, respectively), despite a longer duration of DGF in the NHBD group. Although these results may be influenced by differences in immunosuppression between the two groups, it appears that initial fears held by transplant physicians and patients regarding the use of NHBD are not as great as anticipated and that NHBD represent an untapped source of cadaveric organs.

Marginal Donors

Marginal donors, or expanded criteria donors (ECDs), are defined by UNOS as those donors that, because of certain clinical characteristics, have been demonstrated to increase the risk of late allograft loss (10 years) by 70 % [83]. Some of these donor characteristics are age greater than 50 years, long-standing history of HTN, cerebrovascular accident (CVA) as the cause of death, terminal serum creatinine greater than 1.5 mg/dL, diabetes, or long CIT (e.g., greater than 36 h) [84–86]. Transplantation with organs fulfilling these criteria accounts for nearly one-fifth of cadaveric renal transplants [83]. Although organs from such donors produce results inferior to standard donors, these results remain superior to dialysis in terms of cost [87] and clinical outcome [88].

Using a total of 122,175 patients registered on the UNOS renal transplant waiting list during 1992–1997, Ojo et al. [88] examined the effect of ECD kidneys on survival of recipients relative to those remaining on the waiting list. On the average, recipients of marginal kidney transplants lived 5 years longer than transplant patients who remained on dialysis, whereas ideal cadaveric transplant recipients had a 13-year survival benefit. As expected, the survival benefit of ECD transplantation varied by cause of ESRD, recipient age, and race. Patients with ESRD due to diabetes mellitus had the greatest proportional benefit (RR = 0.62), while those with HTN as the etiology had the longest numerical increase in life expectancy (8.5 years). The survival benefit of younger recipients (aged 18–54) was mitigated by their relatively lower mortality risk on the waiting list, although this group still gained an additional 5–6.5 life years compared with their wait-listed counterparts. The increase in life expectancy was greater for white than black recipients (6 years vs. 3 years). Importantly, receipt of a marginal kidney transplant was not detrimental to patient survival in any subgroup examined.

UNOS has now implemented a policy whereby all consenting ESRD patients awaiting a transplant may be listed for both a marginal and ideal donor kidney [89]. Those patients who decline to be listed for marginal donors will have substantially longer waiting times and therefore higher dialysis-associated mortality. Schnitzler et al. [89] attempted to address the question of how long a patient must wait after refusing an ECD kidney before the poorer outcomes, and increased costs of waiting on dialysis outweigh the benefits gained from receiving a standard donor kidney. Their results showed that the average patient could wait 3.2 years longer for a standard donor over an ECD and expect equivalent quality-adjusted life years. The break-even wait time would be 4.4 years for an average black candidate and 11 months for a 60-year-old candidate. The authors suggested that older recipients may be some of the most appropriate candidates for ECD kidneys. For the time being, any decision to utilize ECD kidneys must take into account the individual patient's perspective as well as society's need to remove patients from dialysis as soon as possible. Moreover, waiting lists for ECD kidneys will need to remain relatively small to allow a substantial shortening of the waiting time for a transplant.

Dual Kidney Transplantation

In effort to expand the cadaveric kidney donor pool further, centers have begun to perform dual kidney transplants [90, 91]. This procedure involves placing two marginal kidneys (usually organs that would otherwise be discarded) into one recipient, with the goal of improving graft survival to an acceptable level not achievable with either kidney alone. In an early prospective, case-control study, Remuzzi et al. [92] reported 6-month patient and graft survival of 100 % and significantly lower serum creatinine levels in dual transplant recipients vs. control recipients. Subsequent studies with longer follow-up periods have confirmed these initial reports [93–96]. Andres et al. [96] used glomerular sclerosis percentage of 15 % or higher to determine whether kidneys from donors greater than 60 years of age would be transplanted as double. Results showed no significant differences in 1-year actuarial patient survival (100, 95, and 98 %) or graft survival (95, 90, and 93 %) between double, single marginal, and single ideal kidney transplants, respectively. Jerius et al. [93] reported superior 2-year graft survival rates for DKT of marginal kidneys (96 %) compared with single marginal kidney transplantation (73 %). It appears from these studies that graft survival after dual transplantation of marginal kidneys is equal or superior to survival after transplantation of single marginal kidneys, although the criteria for

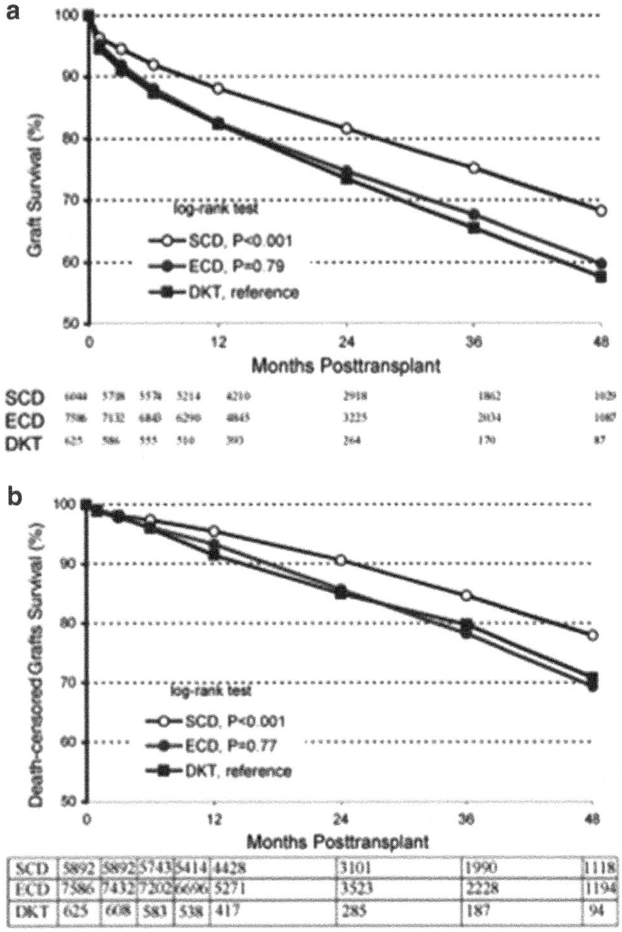

Fig. 1.3 Unadjusted graft survival of DKT, SCD, and ECED transplants (From Gill J, et al. *Transplantation* 2008;85(1)62-68, with permission)

determining which kidneys undergo dual transplantation vary among these centers.

In the United States, a Dual Kidney Registry exists, which, along with the SRTR, allows for comparison of long-term outcome in recipients of dual transplants with that of single kidney transplants. Gill et al. [97] analyzed OPTN/UNOS database from January 2000 to December 2005 and reported that 88 % of 625 patients who underwent DKT had received ECD kidney. The mean donor age was 64.6 ± 7.7 years and the mean terminal creatinine clearance was 70 ± 28 ml/min. Among the 526 who underwent procurement biopsy in the DKT group, 32.5 % had >15 % glomerulosclerosis. In comparison with recipients of single kidney transplants, recipients of dual kidney transplants had similar allograft survival up to 4 years posttransplantation (Fig. 1.3). From the evidence to date, excellent graft survival can be achieved through the dual transplantation of marginal kidneys that otherwise would be discarded. This approach is one of the many being explored to increase the overall cadaveric donor pool.

Recipient Sensitization

Renal transplant candidate sensitization remains a difficult problem for transplant centers, with the three main sources of sensitization being previous transplantation, transfusion, and pregnancy. From the recent UNOS data [21], first transplant recipients who were broadly sensitized (>80 % PRA) had significantly poorer graft survival rates than non-sensitized or more narrowly sensitized patients. The decrease in graft survival was seen with PRA greater than 10 %, and the risk worsened with increasing PRA. The graft loss was more pronounced in living donor compared to cadaveric donor kidney transplants. Approximately one-third of broadly sensitized patients became less sensitized while awaiting transplantation. However, this reduction in PRA percentage transplanted into only modest improvement in graft survival. Despite the introduction of erythropoietin, more than one-third of transplant recipients continue to be transfused, and those patients receiving the greatest number of transfusions had the worst outcomes. This loss of a beneficial "transfusion effect" on graft survival has occurred in the past 5 years. The deleterious effect of transfusions was greatest in parous female recipients, with graft survival worse than that of male and nonparous and non-sensitized parous female patients. It is clear from these data that recipient sensitization has a major impact on graft survival. Recent study by Montgomery et al. [98] showed that desensitization provided a significant survival benefit for patients with HLA sensitization, as compared with waiting for a compatible organ. This survival advantage more than doubled at about 8 years.

Posttransplant Factors

Acute Rejection

AR is the major immunologic risk factor for long-term graft loss [31]. The AR episodes that correlate most strongly with the development of graft loss are those that are one or more late rejection episodes occurring after the first year [99], those that are recurrent [100], those with increased severity of the acute rejection episodes [101, 102], and, probably the most important, those that result in impaired renal function at the time of diagnosis [103] and after therapy [104–109]. This phenomenon may be due to a change in the "y" axis and thus leave patients less reserve to withstand further injury. Hariharan et al. [14] showed that improvement in graft survival was predominantly in those recipients without AR. The progress in immunosuppressive regimens in the last 2 decades has resulted in fewer acute rejection episodes leading to excellent short-term outcomes in renal transplantation [14, 18]. An analysis of the USRDS data from 1988 to 1997 [110] demonstrated that an AR episode in the most recent era confers a higher risk for the subsequent graft loss relative to earlier eras. However, more recent outcome studies [29, 32] may have begun to shed some light on the reasons why we haven't seen improvement in long-term outcomes despite the reduction in AR rates. More recently, antibody-mediated rejection is favored to be more important factor in long-term graft loss as compared to the traditional paradigm of T-cell-mediated rejection.

Delayed Graft Function

Most cadaver and some living donor organ transplants manifest some degree of early dysfunction. In some cases they meet arbitrary criteria for DGF, generally defined as the requirement for dialysis in the first week posttransplantation. DGF is partly an outcome and partly a risk factor, reflecting several influences such as donor tissue quality, donor kidney harvest injury, preservation and implantation details, immune variables, and recipient variables [111]. It is well established that DGF is deleterious to cadaveric renal allograft survival when analyzed as a solitary variable, since DGF increases the incidence of major risk factors for graft survival such as AR [112]. However, some impact of DGF is independent of rejection [113]. Other risk factors for DGF such as CIT do not always impact graft survival; this was recently shown by Kayler et al. [114] who analyzed data of paired deceased-donor kidneys (derived from the same donor transplanted to different recipients) in which one donor resulted in DGF and the other did not, using national Scientific Registry of Transplant Recipients data between 2000 and 2009, and showed that graft survival between paired donor transplants, with and without DGF, was similar. The same group [115] further analyzed paired ECD kidneys from the same registry in the time period 1995–2009 and showed that CIT did not affect graft survival in these patients. These results suggest that DGF, specifically induced by prolonged CIT, has limited bearing on long-term graft outcomes. DGF is associated with powerful factors, such as donor age, recipient race, and sensitization, making dissection of the effects of DGF from the effects of these associated factors extremely difficult.

Several studies have shed light on the complexities associated with DGF and its impact on long-term graft and patient survival. In a single-center retrospective analysis of 405 primary cadaveric kidney transplants, Troppmann et al. [116] found an association of DGF with CIT greater than 24 h and AR. However, graft survival was no worse in those recipients with DGF but no AR. In fact, for recipients with DGF without AR and good clinical graft function at 1-year posttransplantation, death-censored graft survival was 100 % at 6 years. Similar findings were demonstrated by Marcen et al. [117] in a prospective analysis of 461 cadaveric renal transplants. Analyses of large databases have yielded contradictory results, however. Using USRDS data from 37,216 primary cadaveric renal transplants from 1985 to 1992, Ojo et al. [113] found that DGF independently portends a significant reduction in short- and long-term graft survival. Similarly, Shoskes et al. [118], in their analysis of UNOS data from 27,906 primary cadaveric renal transplants between 1994 and 1997, also found DGF to be an important independent predictor of poor graft survival. The discrepancy between large, multicenter registry analyses and single-center reports may lie in the fact that although registry reports have enormous statistical power to avoid sampling errors inherent to single-centered studies, they do not always accurately identify individual factors that contribute to the pathogenesis of DGF because of inconsistent reporting and variation in individual center practices. For instance, Boom et al. [105] used more stringent criteria for DGF than simply the need for dialysis in the first 7 days posttransplantation, which would not be possible using registry data. In their retrospective analysis of 734 cadaveric renal transplants from 1983 to 1987, DGF had an independent effect on graft function at 1 year, but did not seem to influence late graft loss. Long-term graft function was mainly a determinant of creatinine clearance at 1 year, suggesting that the influence of DGF on long-term graft function is through graft function at 1 year.

Other reports have addressed the association of DGF with long-term graft survival in specific transplant subpopulations. Kwon et al. [119] examined the role of DGF in the outcome of 93 consecutive living donor kidney transplants. Consistent with data in cadaveric transplants, DGF was associated with increased risk of AR. However, in the absence of AR, 5-year actuarial graft survival was no different between patients with or without DGF. In their analysis presented in an earlier section, Weber et al. [76] noted nearly double the incidence of DGF among patients who received kidneys from NHBD than among patients who received kidneys from HBD. However, 10-year graft survival was similar in both groups. In the analysis of Dual Kidney Registry data presented earlier [97], DGF was associated with worse graft outcome, presumably due to additive effects on already marginal kidneys. The more recent studies [114, 115] support the concept that DGF may not be a risk factor for long-term graft survival in cases where donated kidneys are not otherwise damaged.

Recipient Age

The elderly are the fastest growing segment of the ESRD population. Renal transplantation in this group of patients not only improves the quality of life [120] but also has a positive impact on patient survival [10]. Elderly renal transplant recipients experience fewer AR episodes than younger recipients [120]. However, despite less immunologic graft loss, death-censored graft loss is not improved [120]. Using USRDS data from 59,509 white patients, an analysis was performed [121]

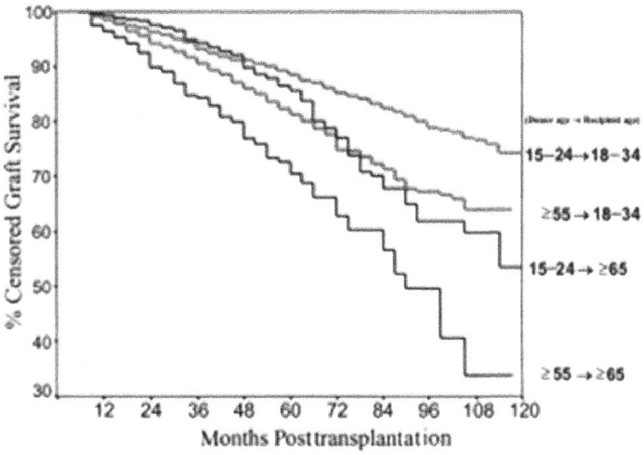

Fig. 1.4 Death-censored graft survival beyond 6 months posttransplantation (From Meier-Kriesche HU, et al. *J Am Geriatr Soc* 2002;50:14, with permission)

to determine whether recipient age itself is an independent risk factor for graft loss. As expected, patient death with a functioning graft was poorer in older age groups. However, results also showed that death-censored graft survival was decreased in this population of patients, with a marked decrease in those patients older than 65 years of age. Compared with ages 18–59, the age group of 50–64 had a 29 % higher RR of graft loss, and ages 65 and above conferred a 67 % RR. This effect was independent of donor age, CIT, DGF, and AR, which are historically strong determinants of long-term allograft survival. Likewise, the worse outcome could not be explained by differences in baseline immunosuppression. In contrast, in black recipients, there was no increased risk for graft loss in the older patients, but rather a 17 % increased risk in the youngest age group. For further confirmation of the independent effect of recipient age on graft loss, an analysis was performed on 11,009 white patients who had received a living donated kidney and had not suffered an AR episode within the first 6 months posttransplantation. In this more homogenous subgroup analysis, older age remained a strong independent risk factor for graft loss.

Earlier studies suggested worse allograft survival in older patients receiving kidneys from older donors [122, 123]. However, these studies were limited by the lack of a control group with younger recipients receiving organs from older donors. In 40,289 primary white renal transplant patients between 1988 and 1997 using the USRDS database [69], both donor and recipient age were significant independent risk factors for chronic allograft loss. As seen in Fig. 1.4, a young kidney (aged 15–25) transplanted into a young recipient (aged 18–35) had the best long-term allograft survival, whereas an older donor kidney (aged 55 and older) transplanted into an older recipient (greater than 65 years) had the worst long-term survival. Thus, donor and recipient age may have an additive detrimental effect on allograft survival that becomes synergistic in grafts surviving beyond 3 years. Similar results were published by Kasiske et al. [124] in an analysis of 74,297 transplant patients during this same time period. As with the previous study, recipients greater than 55 years of age were more likely to die with a functioning graft compared with younger recipients. Both donor and recipient age were found to have important effects on graft survival, although the effects of donor age were much stronger than those of recipient age. However, when intrinsic effects of recipient and donor age were taken into account, giving older kidneys to older recipients had little effect on graft survival in this analysis. Although death-censored graft loss is an important phenomenon, it must be remembered that the major cause of graft loss in the elderly is not rejection but death with a functioning graft.

It was noted in early studies that there was an increased risk for serious infectious complications in the older age group [125]. These findings have been confirmed in other studies [126, 127]. In a single-centered study, intensification of immunosuppressive therapy in elderly recipients increased infectious complications without decreasing the incidence of AR or leading to improvement in graft survival [128]. In contrast, for patients on the waiting list, the risk of infectious death increased only linearly with advancing patient age [129]. As shown in Fig. 1.5, overall mortality and cardiovascular mortality increased with advancing age in both wait-listed patients and transplanted patients, but the degree of increase was not greater for transplant patients. In fact, although the slope for overall mortality was essentially the same for wait-listed and transplanted patients with advancing age, the slope for cardiovascular deaths in transplant patients was nearly half as compared with that in wait-listed patients. These results suggest that with increasing age, patients have an increased benefit in terms of cardiovascular mortality from transplantation. There was no advantage, and in fact a slight increase, in malignancy-related mortality in transplant patients, as evidenced by a steeper age-related slope. This finding suggests that similar to infectious death, the decreased immune function in the older population might make these patients more susceptible to the effects of immunosuppression and therefore the incidence of malignancies.

Recipient Size

In the general population, obesity is defined as a body mass index (BMI) greater than 30 kg/m^2 and is associated with HTN, diabetes, cardiovascular disease, and premature death [130]. Obesity has been shown to be associated with improved survival among patients on dialysis, compared with patients who are nonobese [131–134]. However, in patients with ESRD who undergo renal transplantation, elevated BMI has been associated with a significantly increased

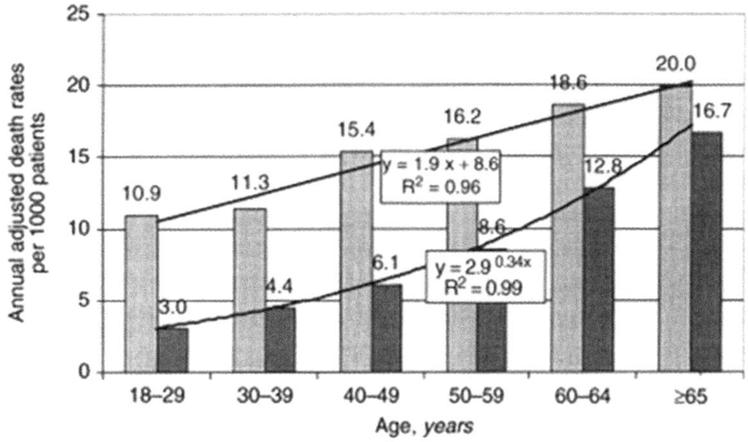

Fig. 1.5 Mortality secondary to infectious disease in wait-listed (*gray bars*) and transplant patients (*black bars*) (From Meier-Kriesche HU, et al. Kidney Int 2001;59:1529, with permission)

risk for patient death [134–136]. Single-centered studies addressing the relationship of BMI to death-censored graft survival have been limited in their conclusions by small sample sizes [137, 138]. In an analysis of 51,927 renal transplant recipients, registered in the USRDS database between 1988 and 1997, BMI was a strong independent risk factor for patient mortality and long-term graft failure independent of patient death after renal transplantation [139]. The relationship between BMI and mortality followed a U-shaped association held true for cardiovascular as well as infectious deaths. Elevated BMI was strongly associated with worse death-censored graft survival. These findings were confirmed in a separate analysis by Kasiske et al. [140], although when donor/recipient body surface area (BSA) was taken into account, the effect of obesity (BMI) on graft failure was no longer statistically significant.

It is clearly important for providers and patients alike to know the relative prognosis for obese transplant recipients compared with nonobese transplant recipients. However, it is perhaps more relevant to individual obese patients to know the prognosis after renal transplantation compared with remaining on dialysis. To address this question, Glanton et al. [141] analyzed USRDS data in a historical cohort study of the association of renal transplantation with patient survival among obese patients enrolled on the waiting list. Results showed that for patients with a BMI greater than 30 kg/m^2 up to 40 kg/m^2, renal transplantation was significantly associated with lower mortality compared with remaining on the renal transplant waiting list. This benefit was seen for obese recipients of cadaveric as well as living donated kidneys, similar to the benefit of renal transplantation previously shown for the entire population of patients on the waiting list [10]. Although other factors that might influence survival after renal transplantation, such as blood pressure and lipid levels, were not assessed in this study, and results for individual patients can never be predicted, it would appear to be in the best interest of obese ESRD patients to undergo renal transplantation.

In the past decade, several investigators have suggested that hyperfiltration injury from "inadequate nephron dosing" may cause progressive injury in transplanted human kidneys, which may explain the association of graft loss with large recipient size. Body size, measured as BSA, correlates with glomerular volume [142, 143], kidney weight [142, 143], and glomerular filtration rate [144]. Therefore, a reasonable test of this hypothesis is to examine the effects on long-term graft survival of placing a kidney from a small donor (low BSA) into a large recipient (high BSA). Several single-centered studies have produced conflicting results [145–149] to lack of statistical power, and large database analyses lacked the necessary patient data until 1994 when UNOS began collecting data on donor size. Using USRDS data from 1994 to 1999, Kasiske et al. [140] investigated whether the effect of size mismatching on patient and graft survival was simply due to an effect of obesity in the recipient per se or whether it could have been due to the effects of size mismatching that were independent of obesity. For those recipients surviving at least 4 months with a functioning graft, the adjusted risk for graft failure was increased 43 % for large recipients (high BSA) of kidneys from small donors (low BSA). Furthermore, this donor/recipient combination carried the highest adjusted RR for death. Donor gender only had an effect on the rate of late allograft failure (decreased rate in females) when donor/recipient BSA were taken into account, lending further support to this hypothesis and perhaps explaining conflicting reports that did not use BSA measurements. The results of this study suggest that a donor kidney can be too small for a large recipient and that donor/recipient size disparity is a likely risk factor for late allograft failure. Kayler et al. analyzed 30,258 living donor transplants [150] and found significantly higher 1- and 5-year graft survival rates in male recipients of male donors compared with other gender pairs. There was no improvement in graft survival demonstrated in male-to-female grafts, however, raising the possibility that other factors such as the effects of sex hormones on immunologic responsiveness, drug metabolism, and hemodynamic responses may be active.

Renal Function

Many renal transplant recipients experience a gradual but steady decline in renal function after transplantation [7]. The rate of decline varies across individuals based on multiple factors including donor quality, recipient comorbidities, immunologic risk, and immunosuppressive regimen [7, 8]. It is now well known that CKD is a risk factor for cardiovascular (CV) death, independent of traditional risk factors such as age, male gender, HTN, diabetes, left ventricular hypertrophy, and hypercholesterolemia. Renal allograft recipients have an increased survival compared with those who remain on the transplant waiting list [10]. However, these patients still have a significant higher mortality compared with the general population, and CV disease accounts for most of this risk [24, 151, 152]. Prior studies have described associations of posttransplant renal function at 12 months with subsequent clinical outcomes. Based on registry data for US transplant recipients in 1988–1998, Hariharan et al. [107] reported a 63 % increase in the relative risk of long-term graft loss (HR 1.63, 95 % CI 1.61–1.65) for each 1.0 mg/dl increment in serum creatinine measured at the first transplant anniversary. In the same year it was demonstrated that loss of graft function with return to dialysis is associated with a significant increase in overall and CV mortality, nearly to the degree seen in ESRD patients [56]. This study raised question of whether increase in CV mortality after graft loss occurs as a continuum of increasing risk with progressive loss of renal function, as suggested by studies in native renal disease.

To address the question of whether decreased renal allograft function is an independent risk factor for patient death, and whether the severity of graft dysfunction is related to CV mortality, an analysis of USRDS data from 1988 to 1998 was performed [74]. Results showed a strong association of renal function at 1 year after renal transplantation with both the incidence and risk of CV death, independent of the many known risk factors. The separation of survival curves began at 2–3 years of follow-up and continued through the 10-year follow-up period, consistent with the expected translation of CV disease to mortality. There was also an increased RR for infection—but not malignancy—related death.

In summary, renal function at 1 year is strongly associated with both long-term graft survival [14] and overall mortality [74] posttransplantation. Improved renal clearance after transplantation may explain the survival benefit conferred by transplantation over patients on the waiting list [10].

Recipient Race

Very early in clinical transplantation, it was noted that both graft and patient survival were lower for black recipients than for white recipients [153, 154]. Since that time, numerous reports have confirmed a higher incidence of AR and worse long-term outcomes in black recipients [155–164]. Potential explanations are varied and but generally include immunologic factors (HLA polymorphisms [165], presensitization [166]), pharmacokinetics of several key immunosuppressive medications [167], prevalence of HTN [158, 159], noncompliance, and socioeconomic status [163]. In a single-centered study [168], significantly shorter renal allograft survival was observed in patients receiving deceased-donor kidneys from African Americans with two APOL1 nephropathy risk variants compared to patients receiving kidneys from African American donors with fewer than two risk variants. Differences in graft survival were seen after approximately 20 months. Accounting for risk variation in APOL1, overall African ancestry did not significantly impact renal allograft survival after transplantation. However, using newer immunosuppressive medications, with dosing tailored by race, the differences in 1-year graft survival are becoming smaller [169, 170]. There is evidence that newer immunosuppressive agents and strategies have improved outcomes in black patients [164, 169], and it is hopeful that newer therapies will further narrow this difference.

Given the need for increased immunosuppression in black recipients to achieve comparable graft survival, an analysis of 68,885 renal transplant recipients using USRDS data was undertaken to examine the risk of death due to infection in this population [171]. Confirming previous reports, results showed significantly worse patient survival (83 % vs. 86 %, respectively, at 5 years) for black recipients compared with white recipients, which was due to the effect of several covariates and not an independent effect of black recipient status. Interestingly, black recipient status conferred a significant, independent, protective effect from dying secondary to infectious causes as compared with white recipients. These results may indicate that more intensive immunosuppressive strategies in black renal transplant recipients might not incur the same infectious mortality risk as in white recipients and could prove successful in further narrowing of the racial gap in long-term graft survival.

Hypertension

The prevalence of hypertension in renal transplant recipients is at least 60–80 % [152, 172]. Usual causes include pretransplant recipient HTN, native kidney disease, allograft dysfunction, steroids, calcineurin inhibitors, weight gain, and transplant renal artery stenosis. HTN has been identified in numerous studies as a risk factor for CV disease and long-term graft failure [152, 172–177], although distinguishing cause and effect in the latter has been difficult. Likewise, there have been no large randomized trials demonstrating that reduction of blood pressure improves long-term graft survival.

Given the high prevalence of CV disease and proteinuria in renal transplant population, beta-blockers and angiotensin-converting enzyme-I are initiated as first-line agents by most centers based on their efficacy in the general population. Although calcium channel blockers are widely used, at least one retrospective analysis [22] identified the dihydropyridine class an independent risk factor for ischemic heart disease.

Immunosuppressive Therapy

In less than a decade, immunosuppressive therapy has advanced from the standard protocol of prednisone, azathioprine, and CsA suspension (Sandimmune) to a choice of several combinations of FDA-approved maintenance medications, including sirolimus, tacrolimus, mycophenolate mofetil (MMF), and CsA microemulsion (Neoral) as well as antilymphocyte preparations for induction therapy. The improvements in short-term kidney graft survival that are now enjoyed are in large part due to these agents. Improvement in long-term graft survival associated with these newer medications, however, has been more difficult to prove, mostly due to lack of statistical power in prospective trials. Several large retrospective analyses have been published that shed some light on the debate whether improvements in allograft and patient survival are indeed the result of advances in immunotherapy.

In a study of transplant registry data from 66,774 patients from 1988 to 1997 [178], MMF was associated with improvement in patient survival and a decreased RR for development of chronic allograft failure (27 %) compared with therapy with azathioprine. Interestingly, this decreased risk was partly caused by an effect independent of decreasing AR. These findings were confirmed in a latter subgroup analysis of black recipients [164], which is important given that black recipient status is an independent risk factor for IF/TA. In a similar analysis of USRDS data [179], both of the newer microemulsion formulations of CsA and tacrolimus were associated with improved 4-year graft survival rates compared with the older Sandimmune formulation of CsA. Despite improvements in short-term outcomes due to introduction of calcineurin inhibitors, there has not been a significant improvement in long-term graft survival. This may be due to toxic effects of medications on patient and graft survival. Newer regimens using reduced exposure to calcineurin inhibitors have been tried. The investigators of the Efficacy Limiting Toxicity Elimination (ELITE)–Symphony study [180, 181] showed that an MMF-based regimen would permit the administration of lower doses of adjunct immunosuppressive agents (e.g., CsA, tacrolimus, and sirolimus), yet still maintain an acceptable rate of acute rejection at 1 and 3 years that was similar to standard immunosuppressive regimen. Studies with newer agents such as belatacept, a selective costimulation blocker, have shown promising results [182–184] with similar patient and graft survival, better renal function, and an improved cardiovascular and metabolic risk profile compared with CsA at 3 years posttransplant even though acute rejection and posttransplant lymphoproliferative disorder (PTLD) was higher in the belatacept group in the first 18 months posttransplant. Studies with newer agents require a longer period of evaluation before conclusions regarding long-term graft and patient survival can be made.

Summary

Dramatic improvements made in the 1-year renal allograft survival over the past 2 decades have shifted attention to long-term graft survival as a more reliable measure of successful transplantation. Despite the recognized limitations of large-scale database retrospective analyses, well-executed studies have identified key risk factors important for long-term patient and graft survival. It is becoming increasingly clear that early transplantation, preservation of optimal renal function, and attempts to decrease CV morbidity and mortality are becoming important goals of new therapeutic strategies. In addition, prevention of recurrent renal disease and BK virus nephropathy are also of greater importance in this era of lowered AR risk. Ultimately, large, prospective, multicentered trial will be necessary to determine whether therapeutic interventions designed to alter these identified risk factors will have the desired effects on long-term graft survival.

References

1. Simmons RG, Abress L. Quality-of-life issues for end-stage renal disease patients. Am J Kidney Dis. 1990;15(3):201–8. PubMed PMID: 2305760. Epub 1990/03/01. eng.
2. Laupacis A, Keown P, Pus N, Krueger H, Ferguson B, Wong C, et al. A study of the quality of life and cost-utility of renal transplantation. Kidney Int. 1996;50(1):235–42. PubMed PMID: 8807593. Epub 1996/07/01. eng.
3. Evans RW, Manninen DL, Garrison Jr LP, Hart LG, Blagg CR, Gutman RA, et al. The quality of life of patients with end-stage renal disease. N Engl J Med. 1985;312(9):553–9. PubMed PMID: 3918267. Epub 1985/02/28. eng.
4. Russell JD, Beecroft ML, Ludwin D, Churchill DN. The quality of life in renal transplantation–a prospective study. Transplantation. 1992;54(4):656–60. PubMed PMID: 1412757. Epub 1992/10/01. eng.
5. Eggers P. Comparison of treatment costs between dialysis and transplantation. Semin Nephrol. 1992;12(3):284–9. PubMed PMID: 1615249. Epub 1992/05/01. eng.
6. Weller JM, Port FK, Swartz RD, Ferguson CW, Williams GW, Jacobs Jr JF. Analysis of survival of end-stage renal disease patients. Kidney Int. 1982;21(1):78–83. PubMed PMID: 7043052. Epub 1982/01/01. eng.
7. Schaubel D, Desmeules M, Mao Y, Jeffery J, Fenton S. Survival experience among elderly end-stage renal disease patients. A controlled comparison of transplantation and dialysis. Transplantation. 1995;60(12):1389–94. PubMed PMID: 8545862. Epub 1995/12/27. eng.

8. Arend SM, Mallat MJ, Westendorp RJ, van der Woude FJ, van Es LA. Patient survival after renal transplantation; more than 25 years follow-up. Nephrol Dial Transplant. 1997;12(8):1672–9. PubMed PMID: 9269647. Epub 1997/08/01. eng.
9. Cosio FG, Alamir A, Yim S, Pesavento TE, Falkenhain ME, Henry ML, et al. Patient survival after renal transplantation: I. The impact of dialysis pre-transplant. Kidney Int. 1998;53(3):767–72. PubMed PMID: 9507225. Epub 1998/03/21. eng.
10. Wolfe RA, Ashby VB, Milford EL, Ojo AO, Ettenger RE, Agodoa LY, et al. Comparison of mortality in all patients on dialysis, patients on dialysis awaiting transplantation, and recipients of a first cadaveric transplant. N Engl J Med. 1999;341(23):1725–30. PubMed PMID: 10580071. Epub 1999/12/02. eng.
11. Cosio FG, Hickson LJ, Griffin MD, Stegall MD, Kudva Y. Patient survival and cardiovascular risk after kidney transplantation: the challenge of diabetes. Am J Transplant. 2008;8(3):593–9. PubMed PMID: 18294155. Epub 2008/02/26. eng.
12. Meier-Kriesche HU, Schold JD, Srinivas TR, Reed A, Kaplan B. Kidney transplantation halts cardiovascular disease progression in patients with end-stage renal disease. Am J Transplant. 2004;4(10):1662–8. PubMed PMID: 15367222. Epub 2004/09/16. eng.
13. Lentine KL, Rocca Rey LA, Kolli S, Bacchi G, Schnitzler MA, Abbott KC, et al. Variations in the risk for cerebrovascular events after kidney transplant compared with experience on the waiting list and after graft failure. Clin J Am Soc Nephrol. 2008;3(4):1090–101. PubMed PMID: 18385393. Pubmed Central PMCID: PMC2440268. Epub 2008/04/04. eng.
14. Hariharan S, Johnson CP, Bresnahan BA, Taranto SE, McIntosh MJ, Stablein D. Improved graft survival after renal transplantation in the United States, 1988 to 1996. N Engl J Med. 2000;342(9):605–12. PubMed PMID: 10699159. Epub 2000/03/04. eng.
15. Denton MD, Magee CC, Sayegh MH. Immunosuppressive strategies in transplantation. Lancet. 1999;353(9158):1083–91. PubMed PMID: 10199367. Epub 1999/04/13. eng.
16. Merion RM, White DJ, Thiru S, Evans DB, Calne RY. Cyclosporine: five years' experience in cadaveric renal transplantation. N Engl J Med. 1984;310(3):148–54. PubMed PMID: 6361559. Epub 1984/01/19. eng.
17. A randomized clinical trial of OKT3 monoclonal antibody for acute rejection of cadaveric renal transplants. Ortho Multicenter Transplant Study Group. N Engl J Med. 1985;313(6):337-42. PubMed PMID: 2861567. Epub 1985/08/08. eng.
18. Meier-Kriesche HU, Schold JD, Srinivas TR, Kaplan B. Lack of improvement in renal allograft survival despite a marked decrease in acute rejection rates over the most recent era. Am J Transplant. 2004;4(3):378–83. PubMed PMID: 14961990. Epub 2004/02/14. eng.
19. Pascual M, Theruvath T, Kawai T, Tolkoff-Rubin N, Cosimi AB. Strategies to improve long-term outcomes after renal transplantation. N Engl J Med. 2002;346(8):580–90. PubMed PMID: 11856798. Epub 2002/02/22. eng.
20. Lamb KE, Lodhi S, Meier-Kriesche HU. Long-term renal allograft survival in the United States: a critical reappraisal. Am J Transplant. 2011;11(3):450–62. PubMed PMID: 20973913. Epub 2010/10/27. eng.
21. Annual Report of the U.S. Organ Procurement and Transplantation Network and the Scientific Registry of Transplant Recipients: Transplant Data 1998-2007. In: Services HaH, editor. Rockville, MD2008.
22. Kasiske BL, Chakkera HA, Roel J. Explained and unexplained ischemic heart disease risk after renal transplantation. J Am Soc Nephrol. 2000;11(9):1735–43. PubMed PMID: 10966499. Epub 2000/08/31. eng.
23. Prommool S, Jhangri GS, Cockfield SM, Halloran PF. Time dependency of factors affecting renal allograft survival. J Am Soc Nephrol. 2000;11(3):565–73. PubMed PMID: 10703681. Epub 2000/03/07. eng.
24. Ojo AO, Hanson JA, Wolfe RA, Leichtman AB, Agodoa LY, Port FK. Long-term survival in renal transplant recipients with graft function. Kidney Int. 2000;57(1):307–13. PubMed PMID: 10620213. Epub 2000/01/05. eng.
25. West M, Sutherland DE, Matas AJ. Kidney transplant recipients who die with functioning grafts: serum creatinine level and cause of death. Transplantation. 1996;62(7):1029–30. PubMed PMID: 8878401. Epub 1996/10/15. eng.
26. Wheeler DC, Steiger J. Evolution and etiology of cardiovascular diseases in renal transplant recipients. Transplantation. 2000;70(11 Suppl):SS41–5. PubMed PMID: 11152230. Epub 2001/01/11. eng.
27. Kahwaji J, Bunnapradist S, Hsu JW, Idroos ML, Dudek R. Cause of death with graft function among renal transplant recipients in an integrated healthcare system. Transplantation. 2011;91(2):225–30. PubMed PMID: 21048529. Epub 2010/11/05. eng.
28. Briganti EM, Russ GR, McNeil JJ, Atkins RC, Chadban SJ. Risk of renal allograft loss from recurrent glomerulonephritis. N Engl J Med. 2002;347(2):103–9. PubMed PMID: 12110738. Epub 2002/07/12. eng.
29. El-Zoghby ZM, Stegall MD, Lager DJ, Kremers WK, Amer H, Gloor JM, et al. Identifying specific causes of kidney allograft loss. Am J Transplant. 2009;9(3):527–35. PubMed PMID: 19191769. Epub 2009/02/05. eng.
30. Solez K, Colvin RB, Racusen LC, Sis B, Halloran PF, Birk PE, et al. Banff '05 Meeting Report: differential diagnosis of chronic allograft injury and elimination of chronic allograft nephropathy ('CAN'). Am J Transplant. 2007;7(3):518–26. PubMed PMID: 17352710. Epub 2007/03/14. eng.
31. Womer KL, Vella JP, Sayegh MH. Chronic allograft dysfunction: mechanisms and new approaches to therapy. Semin Nephrol. 2000;20(2):126–47. PubMed PMID: 10746856. Epub 2000/04/04. eng.
32. Matas AJ, Leduc R, Rush D, Cecka JM, Connett J, Fieberg A, et al. Histopathologic clusters differentiate subgroups within the nonspecific diagnoses of CAN or CR: preliminary data from the DeKAF study. Am J Transplant. 2010;10(2):315–23. PubMed PMID: 20041864. Epub 2010/01/01. eng.
33. Mannon RB, Matas AJ, Grande J, Leduc R, Connett J, Kasiske B, et al. Inflammation in areas of tubular atrophy in kidney allograft biopsies: a potent predictor of allograft failure. Am J Transplant. 2010;10(9):2066–73. PubMed PMID: 20883541. Pubmed Central PMCID: PMC2951299. Epub 2010/10/05. eng.
34. Tullius SG, Tilney NL. Both alloantigen-dependent and -independent factors influence chronic allograft rejection. Transplantation. 1995;59(3):313–8. PubMed PMID: 7871557. Epub 1995/02/15. eng.
35. Cecka JM. The UNOS Scientific Renal Transplant Registry—ten years of kidney transplants. Clinical transplants. 1997:1-14. PubMed PMID: 9919387. Epub 1997/01/01. eng.
36. Legendre C, Thervet E, Skhiri H, Mamzer-Bruneel MF, Cantarovich F, Noel LH, et al. Histologic features of chronic allograft nephropathy revealed by protocol biopsies in kidney transplant recipients. Transplantation. 1998;65(11):1506–9. PubMed PMID: 9645814. Epub 1998/06/30. eng.
37. Womer KL, Stone JR, Murphy B, Chandraker A, Sayegh MH. Indirect allorecognition of donor class I and II major histocompatibility complex peptides promotes the development of transplant vasculopathy. J Am Soc Nephrol. 2001;12(11):2500–6. PubMed PMID: 11675428. Epub 2001/10/25. eng.
38. Lee RS, Womer KL, Yamada K, Maloney ME, Houser SL, Sayegh MH, et al. The role of indirect recognition of donor MHC class II peptides in cardiac transplantation in miniature swine. J Heart Lung Transplant. 2001;20(2):172. PubMed PMID: 11250273. Epub 2001/03/16. Eng.

39. Vella JP, Spadafora-Ferreira M, Murphy B, Alexander SI, Harmon W, Carpenter CB, et al. Indirect allorecognition of major histocompatibility complex allopeptides in human renal transplant recipients with chronic graft dysfunction. Transplantation. 1997;64(6):795–800. PubMed PMID: 9326400. Epub 1997/10/27. eng.
40. Lee RS, Yamada K, Houser SL, Womer KL, Maloney ME, Rose HS, et al. Indirect recognition of allopeptides promotes the development of cardiac allograft vasculopathy. Proc Natl Acad Sci U S A. 2001;98(6):3276–81. PubMed PMID: 11248069. Pubmed Central PMCID: PMC30644. Epub 2001/03/15. eng.
41. Mauiyyedi S, Pelle PD, Saidman S, Collins AB, Pascual M, Tolkoff-Rubin NE, et al. Chronic humoral rejection: identification of antibody-mediated chronic renal allograft rejection by C4d deposits in peritubular capillaries. J Am Soc Nephrol. 2001;12(3):574–82. PubMed PMID: 11181806. Epub 2001/02/22. eng.
42. Russell PS, Chase CM, Winn HJ, Colvin RB. Coronary atherosclerosis in transplanted mouse hearts. II. Importance of humoral immunity. J Immunol. 1994;152(10):5135–41. PubMed PMID: 8176230. Epub 1994/05/15. eng.
43. Dong VM, Womer KL, Sayegh MH. Transplantation tolerance: the concept and its applicability. Pediatr Transplant. 1999;3(3):181–92. PubMed PMID: 10487277. Epub 1999/09/16. eng.
44. Womer KL, Lee RS, Madsen JC, Sayegh MH. Tolerance and chronic rejection. Philos Trans R Soc Lond B Biol Sci. 2001;356(1409):727–38. PubMed PMID: 11375075. Pubmed Central PMCID: PMC1088459. Epub 2001/05/26. eng.
45. Denton MD, Singh AK. Recurrent and de novo glomerulonephritis in the renal allograft. Semin Nephrol. 2000;20(2):164–75. PubMed PMID: 10746858. Epub 2000/04/04. eng.
46. Hariharan S, Adams MB, Brennan DC, Davis CL, First MR, Johnson CP, et al. Recurrent and de novo glomerular disease after renal transplantation: a report from Renal Allograft Disease Registry (RADR). Transplantation. 1999;68(5):635–41. PubMed PMID: 10507481. Epub 1999/10/03. eng.
47. Briggs JD, Jones E. Recurrence of glomerulonephritis following renal transplantation. Scientific Advisory Board of the ERA-EDTA Registry. European Renal Association-European Dialysis and Transplant Association. Nephrol Dial Transplant. 1999;14(3):564–5. PubMed PMID: 10193799. Epub 1999/04/08. eng.
48. Hariharan S, Adams MB, Brennan DC, Davis CL, First MR, Johnson CP, et al. Recurrent and de novo glomerular disease after renal transplantation: a report from renal allograft disease registry. Transplant Proc. 1999;31(1-2):223-4. PubMed PMID: 10083084. Epub 1999/03/20. eng.
49. Odorico JS, Knechtle SJ, Rayhill SC, Pirsch JD, D'Alessandro AM, Belzer FO, et al. The influence of native nephrectomy on the incidence of recurrent disease following renal transplantation for primary glomerulonephritis. Transplantation. 1996;61(2):228–34. PubMed PMID: 8600629. Epub 1996/01/27. eng.
50. Chadban S. Glomerulonephritis recurrence in the renal graft. J Am Soc Nephrol. 2001;12(2):394–402. PubMed PMID: 11158232. Epub 2001/02/07. eng.
51. Cooper L. USRDS. 2001 Annual Data Report. Nephrol News Issues. 2001;15(10):31, 4-5, 8 passim. PubMed PMID: 12098974. Epub 2002/07/09. eng.
52. Meier-Kriesche HU, Port FK, Ojo AO, Rudich SM, Hanson JA, Cibrik DM, et al. Effect of waiting time on renal transplant outcome. Kidney Int. 2000;58(3):1311–7. PubMed PMID: 10972695. Epub 2000/09/06. eng.
53. Mange KC, Joffe MM, Feldman HI. Effect of the use or nonuse of long-term dialysis on the subsequent survival of renal transplants from living donors. N Engl J Med. 2001;344(10):726–31. PubMed PMID: 11236776. Epub 2001/03/10. eng.
54. Kasiske BL, Snyder JJ, Matas AJ, Ellison MD, Gill JS, Kausz AT. Preemptive kidney transplantation: the advantage and the advantaged. J Am Soc Nephrol. 2002;13(5):1358–64. PubMed PMID: 11961024. Epub 2002/04/19. eng.
55. Meier-Kriesche HU, Kaplan B. Waiting time on dialysis as the strongest modifiable risk factor for renal transplant outcomes: a paired donor kidney analysis. Transplantation. 2002;74(10):1377–81. PubMed PMID: 12451234. Epub 2002/11/27. eng.
56. Kaplan B, Meier-Kriesche HU. Death after graft loss: an important late study endpoint in kidney transplantation. Am J Transplant. 2002;2(10):970–4. PubMed PMID: 12482151. Epub 2002/12/17. eng.
57. Meier-Kriesche HU, Ojo AO, Leichtman AB, Magee JC, Rudich SM, Hanson JA, et al. Interaction of mycophenolate mofetil and HLA matching on renal allograft survival. Transplantation. 2001;71(3):398–401. PubMed PMID: 11233900. Epub 2001/03/10. eng.
58. Held PJ, Kahan BD, Hunsicker LG, Liska D, Wolfe RA, Port FK, et al. The impact of HLA mismatches on the survival of first cadaveric kidney transplants. N Engl J Med. 1994;331(12):765–70. PubMed PMID: 8065404. Epub 1994/09/22. eng.
59. Schnitzler MA, Hollenbeak CS, Cohen DS, Woodward RS, Lowell JA, Singer GG, et al. The economic implications of HLA matching in cadaveric renal transplantation. N Engl J Med. 1999;341(19):1440–6. PubMed PMID: 10547408. Epub 1999/11/05. eng.
60. Hata Y, Cecka JM, Takemoto S, Ozawa M, Cho YW, Terasaki PI. Effects of changes in the criteria for nationally shared kidney transplants for HLA-matched patients. Transplantation. 1998;65(2):208–12. PubMed PMID: 9458016. Epub 1998/02/11. eng.
61. Takemoto SK, Terasaki PI, Gjertson DW, Cecka JM. Twelve years' experience with national sharing of HLA-matched cadaveric kidneys for transplantation. N Engl J Med. 2000;343(15):1078–84. PubMed PMID: 11027742. Epub 2000/10/12. eng.
62. Lee CM, Carter JT, Alfrey EJ, Ascher NL, Roberts JP, Freise CE. Prolonged cold ischemia time obviates the benefits of 0 HLA mismatches in renal transplantation. Arch Surg. 2000;135(9):1016–9; discussion 9–20. PubMed PMID: 10982503. Epub 2000/09/12. eng.
63. Mange KC, Cherikh WS, Maghirang J, Bloom RD. A comparison of the survival of shipped and locally transplanted cadaveric renal allografts. N Engl J Med. 2001;345(17):1237–42. PubMed PMID: 11680443. Epub 2001/10/30. eng.
64. Asderakis A, Dyer P, Augustine T, Worthington J, Campbell B, Johnson RW. Effect of cold ischemic time and HLA matching in kidneys coming from "young" and "old" donors: do not leave for tomorrow what you can do tonight. Transplantation. 2001;72(4):674–8. PubMed PMID: 11544430. Epub 2001/09/07. eng.
65. Gillich MS, Heimbach D, Schoeneich G, Muller SC, Klehr HU. Comparison of blood group versus HLA-dependent transplantation and its influence on donor kidney survival. Nephrol Dial Transplant. 2002;17(5):884–6. PubMed PMID: 11981078. Epub 2002/05/01. eng.
66. Voiculescu A, Schlieper G, Hetzel GR, Hollenbeck M, Ivens K, Willers R, et al. Kidney transplantation in the elderly: age-matching as compared to HLA-matching: a single center experience. Transplantation. 2002;73(8):1356–9. PubMed PMID: 11981438. Epub 2002/05/01. eng.
67. Terasaki PI, Cecka JM, Gjertson DW, Takemoto S. High survival rates of kidney transplants from spousal and living unrelated donors. N Engl J Med. 1995;333(6):333–6. PubMed PMID: 7609748. Epub 1995/08/10. eng.
68. Terasaki PI, Gjertson DW, Cecka JM, Takemoto S, Cho YW. Significance of the donor age effect on kidney transplants. Clin Transplant. 1997;11(5 Pt 1):366–72. PubMed PMID: 9361925. Epub 1997/11/15. eng.
69. Meier-Kriesche HU, Cibrik DM, Ojo AO, Hanson JA, Magee JC, Rudich SM, et al. Interaction between donor and recipient age in determining the risk of chronic renal allograft failure. J Am Geriatr Soc. 2002;50(1):14–7. PubMed PMID: 12028241. Epub 2002/05/25. eng.

70. Halloran PF, Melk A, Barth C. Rethinking chronic allograft nephropathy: the concept of accelerated senescence. J Am Soc Nephrol. 1999;10(1):167–81. PubMed PMID: 9890324. Epub 1999/01/16. eng.
71. Sarnak MJ, Levey AS. Cardiovascular disease and chronic renal disease: a new paradigm. Am J Kidney Dis. 2000;35(4 Suppl 1):S117–31. PubMed PMID: 10766010. Epub 2000/04/15. eng.
72. Jungers P, Massy ZA, Nguyen Khoa T, Fumeron C, Labrunie M, Lacour B, et al. Incidence and risk factors of atherosclerotic cardiovascular accidents in predialysis chronic renal failure patients: a prospective study. Nephrol Dial Transplant. 1997;12(12):2597–602. PubMed PMID: 9430858. Epub 1998/02/12. eng.
73. Mann JF, Gerstein HC, Pogue J, Bosch J, Yusuf S. Renal insufficiency as a predictor of cardiovascular outcomes and the impact of ramipril: the HOPE randomized trial. Ann Intern Med. 2001;134(8):629–36. PubMed PMID: 11304102. Epub 2001/04/17. eng.
74. Meier-Kriesche HU, Baliga R, Kaplan B. Decreased renal function is a strong risk factor for cardiovascular death after renal transplantation. Transplantation. 2003;75(8):1291–5. PubMed PMID: 12717218. Epub 2003/04/30. eng.
75. Guidelines for the determination of death. Report of the medical consultants on the diagnosis of death to the President's Commission for the Study of Ethical Problems in Medicine and Biomedical and Behavioral Research. JAMA. 1981;246(19):2184-6. PubMed PMID: 7289009. Epub 1981/11/13. eng.
76. Weber M, Dindo D, Demartines N, Ambuhl PM, Clavien PA. Kidney transplantation from donors without a heartbeat. N Engl J Med. 2002;347(4):248–55. PubMed PMID: 12140300. Epub 2002/07/26. eng.
77. Sanchez-Fructuoso AI, Prats D, Torrente J, Perez-Contin MJ, Fernandez C, Alvarez J, et al. Renal transplantation from non-heart beating donors: a promising alternative to enlarge the donor pool. J Am Soc Nephrol. 2000;11(2):350–8. PubMed PMID: 10665943. Epub 2000/02/09. eng.
78. Mizutani K, Ono Y, Kinukawa T, Hattori R, Nishiyama N, Kamihila O, et al. Use of marginal organs from non-heart-beating cadaveric kidney donors. Transplantation. 2001;72(8):1376–80. PubMed PMID: 11685106. Epub 2001/10/31. eng.
79. Metcalfe MS, Butterworth PC, White SA, Saunders RN, Murphy GJ, Taub N, et al. A case-control comparison of the results of renal transplantation from heart-beating and non-heart-beating donors. Transplantation. 2001;71(11):1556–9. PubMed PMID: 11435964. Epub 2001/07/04. eng.
80. Gok MA, Buckley PE, Shenton BK, Balupuri S, El-Sheikh MA, Robertson H, et al. Long-term renal function in kidneys from non-heart-beating donors: A single-center experience. Transplantation. 2002;74(5):664–9. PubMed PMID: 12352883. Epub 2002/09/28. eng.
81. Cho YW, Terasaki PI, Cecka JM, Gjertson DW. Transplantation of kidneys from donors whose hearts have stopped beating. N Engl J Med. 1998;338(4):221–5. PubMed PMID: 9435327. Epub 1998/01/22. eng.
82. Brook NR, White SA, Waller JR, Veitch PS, Nicholson ML. Non-heart beating donor kidneys with delayed graft function have superior graft survival compared with conventional heart-beating donor kidneys that develop delayed graft function. Am J Transplant. 2003;3(5):614–8. PubMed PMID: 12752318. Epub 2003/05/20. eng.
83. Rosengard BR, Feng S, Alfrey EJ, Zaroff JG, Emond JC, Henry ML, et al. Report of the Crystal City meeting to maximize the use of organs recovered from the cadaver donor. Am J Transplant. 2002;2(8): 701–11. PubMed PMID: 12243491. Epub 2002/09/24. eng.
84. Nyberg SL, Matas AJ, Rogers M, Harmsen WS, Velosa JA, Larson TS, et al. Donor scoring system for cadaveric renal transplantation. Am J Transplant. 2001;1(2):162–70. PubMed PMID: 12099365. Epub 2002/07/09. eng.
85. Berardinelli L, Beretta C, Raiteri M, Carini M. Early and long-term results using older kidneys from cadaver or living donors. Clinical transplants. 2001:157-66. PubMed PMID: 12211778. Epub 2002/09/06. eng.
86. Port FK, Bragg-Gresham JL, Metzger RA, Dykstra DM, Gillespie BW, Young EW, et al. Donor characteristics associated with reduced graft survival: an approach to expanding the pool of kidney donors. Transplantation. 2002;74(9):1281–6. PubMed PMID: 12451266. Epub 2002/11/27. eng.
87. Whiting JF, Woodward RS, Zavala EY, Cohen DS, Martin JE, Singer GG, et al. Economic cost of expanded criteria donors in cadaveric renal transplantation: analysis of Medicare payments. Transplantation. 2000;70(5):755–60. PubMed PMID: 11003352. Epub 2000/09/26. eng.
88. Ojo AO, Hanson JA, Meier-Kriesche H, Okechukwu CN, Wolfe RA, Leichtman AB, et al. Survival in recipients of marginal cadaveric donor kidneys compared with other recipients and wait-listed transplant candidates. J Am Soc Nephrol. 2001;12(3):589–97. PubMed PMID: 11181808. Epub 2001/02/22. eng.
89. Schnitzler MA, Whiting JF, Brennan DC, Lin G, Chapman W, Lowell J, et al. The expanded criteria donor dilemma in cadaveric renal transplantation. Transplantation. 2003;75(12):1940–5. PubMed PMID: 12829891. Epub 2003/06/28. eng.
90. Johnson LB, Kuo PC, Schweitzer EJ, Ratner LE, Klassen DK, Hoehn-Saric EW, et al. Double renal allografts successfully increase utilization of kidneys from older donors within a single organ procurement organization. Transplantation. 1996;62(11):1581–3. PubMed PMID: 8970611. Epub 1996/12/15. eng.
91. Johnson LB, Kuo PC, Dafoe DC, Drachenberg CB, Schweitzer EJ, Alfrey EJ, et al. The use of bilateral adult renal allografts—a method to optimize function from donor kidneys with suboptimal nephron mass. Transplantation. 1996;61(8):1261–3. PubMed PMID: 8610427. Epub 1996/04/27. eng.
92. Remuzzi G, Grinyo J, Ruggenenti P, Beatini M, Cole EH, Milford EL, et al. Early experience with dual kidney transplantation in adults using expanded donor criteria. Double Kidney Transplant Group (DKG). J Am Soc Nephrol. 1999;10(12):2591–8.
93. Jerius JT, Taylor RJ, Murillo D, Leone JP. Double renal transplants from marginal donors: 2-year results. J Urol. 2000;163(2):423–5. PubMed PMID: 10647645. Epub 2000/01/27. eng.
94. Kumar A, Mandhani A, Verma BS, Srivastava A, Gupta A, Sharma RK, et al. Expanding the living related donor pool in renal transplantation: use of marginal donors. J Urol. 2000;163(1):33–6. PubMed PMID: 10604308. Epub 1999/12/22. eng.
95. Dietl KH, Wolters H, Marschall B, Senninger N, Heidenreich S. Cadaveric "two-in-one" kidney transplantation from marginal donors: experience of 26 cases after 3 years. Transplantation. 2000;70(5):790–4. PubMed PMID: 11003359. Epub 2000/09/26. eng.
96. Andres A, Morales JM, Herrero JC, Praga M, Morales E, Hernandez E, et al. Double versus single renal allografts from aged donors. Transplantation. 2000;69(10):2060–6. PubMed PMID: 10852597. Epub 2000/06/14. eng.
97. Gill J, Cho YW, Danovitch GM, Wilkinson A, Lipshutz G, Pham PT, et al. Outcomes of dual adult kidney transplants in the United States: an analysis of the OPTN/UNOS database. Transplantation. 2008;85(1):62–8. PubMed PMID: 18192913. Epub 2008/01/15. eng.
98. Montgomery RA, Lonze BE, King KE, Kraus ES, Kucirka LM, Locke JE, et al. Desensitization in HLA-incompatible kidney recipients and survival. N Engl J Med. 2011;365(4):318–26. PubMed PMID: 21793744. Epub 2011/07/29. eng.
99. Basadonna GP, Matas AJ, Gillingham KJ, Payne WD, Dunn DL, Sutherland DE, et al. Early versus late acute renal allograft rejection: impact on chronic rejection. Transplantation. 1993;55(5):993–5. PubMed PMID: 8497913. Epub 1993/05/01. eng.

100. Matas AJ, Gillingham KJ, Payne WD, Najarian JS. The impact of an acute rejection episode on long-term renal allograft survival (t1/2). Transplantation. 1994;57(6):857–9. PubMed PMID: 8154032. Epub 1994/03/27. eng.
101. van Saase JL, van der Woude FJ, Thorogood J, Hollander AA, van Es LA, Weening JJ, et al. The relation between acute vascular and interstitial renal allograft rejection and subsequent chronic rejection. Transplantation. 1995;59(9):1280–5. PubMed PMID: 7762062. Epub 1995/05/15. eng.
102. Chavers BMM, Gillingham K. Histology of acute rejection (AR) impacts renal allograft survival (GS) in patients (pts) with a single rejection episode (SRE). J Am Soc Nephrol. 1995;6:1076.
103. Heaf JG, Ladefoged J. The effect of acute rejection on long-term renal graft survival is mainly related to initial renal damage. Transpl Int. 1998;11 Suppl 1:S26–31. PubMed PMID: 9664937. Epub 1998/07/17. eng.
104. Cosio FG, Pelletier RP, Falkenhain ME, Henry ML, Elkhammas EA, Davies EA, et al. Impact of acute rejection and early allograft function on renal allograft survival. Transplantation. 1997;63(11): 1611–5. PubMed PMID: 9197355. Epub 1997/06/15. eng.
105. Boom H, Mallat MJ, de Fijter JW, Zwinderman AH, Paul LC. Delayed graft function influences renal function, but not survival. Kidney Int. 2000;58(2):859–66. PubMed PMID: 10916111. Epub 2000/08/01. eng.
106. Giral M, Taddei C, Nguyen JM, Dantal J, Hourmant M, Cantarovich D, et al. Single-center analysis of 468 first cadaveric kidney allografts with a uniform ATG-CsA sequential therapy. Clinical transplants. 1996:257-64. PubMed PMID: 9286575. Epub 1996/01/01. eng.
107. Hariharan S, McBride MA, Cherikh WS, Tolleris CB, Bresnahan BA, Johnson CP. Post-transplant renal function in the first year predicts long-term kidney transplant survival. Kidney Int. 2002;62(1):311–8. PubMed PMID: 12081593. Epub 2002/06/26. eng.
108. Nicol D, MacDonald AS, Lawen J, Belitsky P. Early prediction of renal allograft loss beyond one year. Transpl Int. 1993;6(3):153–7. PubMed PMID: 8499066. Epub 1993/05/01. eng.
109. Humar A, Kerr S, Gillingham KJ, Matas AJ. Features of acute rejection that increase risk for chronic rejection. Transplantation. 1999;68(8):1200–3. PubMed PMID: 10551652. Epub 1999/11/07. eng.
110. Meier-Kriesche HU, Ojo AO, Hanson JA, Cibrik DM, Punch JD, Leichtman AB, et al. Increased impact of acute rejection on chronic allograft failure in recent era. Transplantation. 2000;70(7):1098–100. PubMed PMID: 11045649. Epub 2000/10/25. eng.
111. Halloran PF, Hunsicker LG. Delayed graft function: state of the art, November 10-11, 2000. Summit meeting, Scottsdale, Arizona, USA. Am J Transplant. 2001;1(2):115-20. PubMed PMID: 12099358. Epub 2002/07/09. eng.
112. Shoskes DA, Halloran PF. Delayed graft function in renal transplantation: etiology, management and long-term significance. J Urol. 1996;155(6):1831–40. PubMed PMID: 8618268. Epub 1996/06/01. eng.
113. Ojo AO, Wolfe RA, Held PJ, Port FK, Schmouder RL. Delayed graft function: risk factors and implications for renal allograft survival. Transplantation. 1997;63(7):968–74. PubMed PMID: 9112349. Epub 1997/04/15. eng.
114. Kayler LK, Srinivas TR, Schold JD. Influence of CIT-induced DGF on kidney transplant outcomes. Am J Transplant. 2011;11(12):2657–64. PubMed PMID: 22051325. Epub 2011/11/05. eng.
115. Kayler LK, Magliocca J, Zendejas I, Srinivas TR, Schold JD. Impact of cold ischemia time on graft survival among ECD transplant recipients: a paired kidney analysis. Am J Transplant. 2011;11(12): 2647–56. PubMed PMID: 21906257. Epub 2011/09/13. eng.
116. Troppmann C, Gillingham KJ, Gruessner RW, Dunn DL, Payne WD, Najarian JS, et al. Delayed graft function in the absence of rejection has no long-term impact. A study of cadaver kidney recipients with good graft function at 1 year after transplantation. Transplantation. 1996;61(9):1331–7.
117. Marcen R, Orofino L, Pascual J, de la Cal MA, Teruel JL, Villafruela JJ, et al. Delayed graft function does not reduce the survival of renal transplant allografts. Transplantation. 1998;66(4): 461–6. PubMed PMID: 9734488. Epub 1998/09/12. eng.
118. Shoskes DA, Cecka JM. Deleterious effects of delayed graft function in cadaveric renal transplant recipients independent of acute rejection. Transplantation. 1998;66(12):1697–701. PubMed PMID: 9884262. Epub 1999/01/12. eng.
119. Kwon OJ, Ha MK, Kwak JY, Lee HW. The impact of delayed graft function on graft survival in living donor kidney transplantation. Transplant Proc. 2003;35(1):92–3. PubMed PMID: 12591321. Epub 2003/02/20. eng.
120. Becker BN, Ismail N, Becker YT, MacDonnell RC, Helderman JH. Renal transplantation in the older end stage renal disease patient. Semin Nephrol. 1996;16(4):353–62. PubMed PMID: 8829273. Epub 1996/07/01. eng.
121. Meier-Kriesche HU, Ojo AO, Cibrik DM, Hanson JA, Leichtman AB, Magee JC, et al. Relationship of recipient age and development of chronic allograft failure. Transplantation. 2000;70(2):306–10. PubMed PMID: 10933154. Epub 2000/08/10. eng.
122. Smits JM, De Meester J, Persijn GG, Claas FH, Van Houwelingen HC. The outcome of kidney grafts from multiorgan donors and kidney only donors. Transplantation. 1996;62(6):767–71. PubMed PMID: 8824475. Epub 1996/09/27. eng.
123. Basar H, Soran A, Shapiro R, Vivas C, Scantlebury VP, Jordan ML, et al. Renal transplantation in recipients over the age of 60: the impact of donor age. Transplantation. 1999;67(8):1191–3. PubMed PMID: 10232574. Epub 1999/05/08. eng.
124. Kasiske BL, Snyder J. Matching older kidneys with older patients does not improve allograft survival. J Am Soc Nephrol. 2002;13(4):1067–72. PubMed PMID: 11912268. Epub 2002/03/26. eng.
125. Wedel N, Brynger H, Blohme I. Kidney transplantation in patients 60 years and older. Scand J Urol Nephrol Suppl. 1980;54:106–8. PubMed PMID: 7013026. Epub 1980/01/01. eng.
126. Nyberg G, Nilsson B, Norden G, Karlberg I. Outcome of renal transplantation in patients over the age of 60: a case-control study. Nephrol Dial Transplant. 1995;10(1):91–4. PubMed PMID: 7724038. Epub 1995/01/01. eng.
127. Jassal SV, Opelz G, Cole E. Transplantation in the elderly: a review. Geriatr Nephrol Urol. 1997;7(3):157–65. PubMed PMID: 9493037. Epub 1997/01/01. eng.
128. Meier-Kriesche HU, Friedman G, Jacobs M, Mulgaonkar S, Vaghela M, Kaplan B. Infectious complications in geriatric renal transplant patients: comparison of two immunosuppressive protocols. Transplantation. 1999;68(10):1496–502. PubMed PMID: 10589946. Epub 1999/12/10. eng.
129. Meier-Kriesche HU, Ojo AO, Hanson JA, Kaplan B. Exponentially increased risk of infectious death in older renal transplant recipients. Kidney Int. 2001;59(4):1539–43. PubMed PMID: 11260418. Epub 2001/03/22. eng.
130. Calle EE, Thun MJ, Petrelli JM, Rodriguez C, Heath Jr CW. Body-mass index and mortality in a prospective cohort of U.S. adults. N Engl J Med. 1999;341(15):1097–105.
131. Wolfe RA, Ashby VB, Daugirdas JT, Agodoa LY, Jones CA, Port FK. Body size, dose of hemodialysis, and mortality. Am J Kidney Dis. 2000;35(1):80–8. PubMed PMID: 10620548. Epub 2000/01/06. eng.
132. Leavey SF, McCullough K, Hecking E, Goodkin D, Port FK, Young EW. Body mass index and mortality in 'healthier' as compared with 'sicker' haemodialysis patients: results from the Dialysis Outcomes and Practice Patterns Study (DOPPS). Nephrol

Dial Transplant. 2001;16(12):2386–94. PubMed PMID: 11733631. Epub 2001/12/26. eng.
133. Kutner NG, Zhang R. Body mass index as a predictor of continued survival in older chronic dialysis patients. Int Urol Nephrol. 2001;32(3):441–8. PubMed PMID: 11583369. Epub 2001/10/05. eng.
134. Hakim RM, Lowrie E. Obesity and mortality in ESRD: is it good to be fat? Kidney Int. 1999;55(4):1580–1. PubMed PMID: 10201027. Epub 1999/04/14. eng.
135. Johnson DW, Herzig KA, Purdie DM, Chang W, Brown AM, Rigby RJ, et al. Is obesity a favorable prognostic factor in peritoneal dialysis patients? Perit Dial Int. 2000;20(6):715-21. PubMed PMID: 11216565. Epub 2001/02/24. eng.
136. Fleischmann EH, Bower JD, Salahudeen AK. Risk factor paradox in hemodialysis: better nutrition as a partial explanation. ASAIO J. 2001;47(1):74-81. PubMed PMID: 11199320. Epub 2001/02/24. eng.
137. Howard RJ, Thai VB, Patton PR, Hemming AW, Reed AI, Van der Werf WJ, et al. Obesity does not portend a bad outcome for kidney transplant recipients. Transplantation. 2002;73(1):53–5. PubMed PMID: 11792977. Epub 2002/01/17. eng.
138. Meier-Kriesche HU, Vaghela M, Thambuganipalle R, Friedman G, Jacobs M, Kaplan B. The effect of body mass index on long-term renal allograft survival. Transplantation. 1999;68(9):1294–7. PubMed PMID: 10573066. Epub 1999/11/26. eng.
139. Meier-Kriesche HU, Arndorfer JA, Kaplan B. The impact of body mass index on renal transplant outcomes: a significant independent risk factor for graft failure and patient death. Transplantation. 2002;73(1):70–4. PubMed PMID: 11792981. Epub 2002/01/17. eng.
140. Kasiske BL, Snyder JJ, Gilbertson D. Inadequate donor size in cadaver kidney transplantation. J Am Soc Nephrol. 2002;13(8):2152–9. PubMed PMID: 12138149. Epub 2002/07/26. eng.
141. Glanton CW, Kao TC, Cruess D, Agodoa LY, Abbott KC. Impact of renal transplantation on survival in end-stage renal disease patients with elevated body mass index. Kidney Int. 2003;63(2):647–53. PubMed PMID: 12631130. Epub 2003/03/13. eng.
142. Kasiske BL, Umen AJ. The influence of age, sex, race, and body habitus on kidney weight in humans. Arch Pathol Lab Med. 1986;110(1):55–60. PubMed PMID: 3753571. Epub 1986/01/01. eng.
143. Nyengaard JR, Bendtsen TF. Glomerular number and size in relation to age, kidney weight, and body surface in normal man. Anat Rec. 1992;232(2):194–201. PubMed PMID: 1546799. Epub 1992/02/01. eng.
144. White AJ, Strydom WJ. Normalisation of glomerular filtration rate measurements. Eur J Nucl Med. 1991;18(6):385–90. PubMed PMID: 1879445. Epub 1991/01/01. eng.
145. Nicholson ML, Windmill DC, Horsburgh T, Harris KP. Influence of allograft size to recipient body-weight ratio on the long-term outcome of renal transplantation. Br J Surg. 2000;87(3):314–9. PubMed PMID: 10718800. Epub 2000/03/16. eng.
146. Vianello A, Calconi G, Amici G, Chiara G, Pignata G, Maresca MC. Importance of donor/recipient body weight ratio as a cause of kidney graft loss in the short to medium term. Nephron. 1996;72(2):205–11. PubMed PMID: 8684528. Epub 1996/01/01. eng.
147. Miles AM, Sumrani N, John S, Markell MS, Distant DA, Maursky V, et al. The effect of kidney size on cadaveric renal allograft outcome. Transplantation. 1996;61(6):894–7. PubMed PMID: 8623156. Epub 1996/03/27. eng.
148. Gaston RS, Hudson SL, Julian BA, Laskow DA, Deierhoi MH, Sanders CE, et al. Impact of donor/recipient size matching on outcomes in renal transplantation. Transplantation. 1996;61(3):383–8. PubMed PMID: 8610346. Epub 1996/02/15. eng.
149. Moreso F, Seron D, Anunciada AI, Hueso M, Ramon JM, Fulladosa X, et al. Recipient body surface area as a predictor of posttransplant renal allograft evolution. Transplantation. 1998;65(5):671–6. PubMed PMID: 9521202. Epub 1998/04/01. eng.
150. Kayler LK, Rasmussen CS, Dykstra DM, Ojo AO, Port FK, Wolfe RA, et al. Gender imbalance and outcomes in living donor renal transplantation in the United States. Am J Transplant. 2003;3(4):452–8. PubMed PMID: 12694068. Epub 2003/04/16. eng.
151. Kasiske BL, Guijarro C, Massy ZA, Wiederkehr MR, Ma JZ. Cardiovascular disease after renal transplantation. J Am Soc Nephrol. 1996;7(1):158–65. PubMed PMID: 8808124. Epub 1996/01/01. eng.
152. Kasiske BL. Epidemiology of cardiovascular disease after renal transplantation. Transplantation. 2001;72(6 Suppl):S5–8. PubMed PMID: 11585242. Epub 2001/10/05. eng.
153. Opelz G, Mickey MR, Terasaki PI. Influence of race on kidney transplant survival. Transplant Proc. 1977;9(1):137–42. PubMed PMID: 325754. Epub 1977/03/01. eng.
154. Stuart FP, Hill JL, Reckard CR, Buckingham M, Nakamura S. Race as a risk factor in cadaver kidney transplantation. Arch Surg. 1979;114(4):416–20. PubMed PMID: 373703. Epub 1979/04/01. eng.
155. Butkus DE, Meydrech EF, Raju SS. Racial differences in the survival of cadaveric renal allografts. Overriding effects of HLA matching and socioeconomic factors. N Engl J Med. 1992;327(12):840–5. PubMed PMID: 1508243. Epub 1992/09/17. eng.
156. Gaston RS, Hudson SL, Deierhoi MH, Barber WH, Laskow DA, Julian BA, et al. Improved survival of primary cadaveric renal allografts in blacks with quadruple immunosuppression. Transplantation. 1992;53(1):103–9. PubMed PMID: 1733054. Epub 1992/01/01. eng.
157. Cooper TY, Jordan CL, Willimon CM, Land GA. Comparison of panel-reactive antibody levels in Caucasian and African American renal transplant candidates. Transplantation. 1995;60(4):327–30. PubMed PMID: 7652759. Epub 1995/08/27. eng.
158. Cosio FG, Dillon JJ, Falkenhain ME, Tesi RJ, Henry ML, Elkhammas EA, et al. Racial differences in renal allograft survival: the role of systemic hypertension. Kidney Int. 1995;47(4):1136–41. PubMed PMID: 7783411. Epub 1995/04/01. eng.
159. Cosio FG, Falkenhain ME, Pesavento TE, Henry ML, Elkhammas EA, Davies EA, et al. Relationships between arterial hypertension and renal allograft survival in African-American patients. Am J Kidney Dis. 1997;29(3):419–27. PubMed PMID: 9041219. Epub 1997/03/01. eng.
160. Ojo AO, Port FK, Held PJ, Wolfe RA, Turenne MN, Chung E, et al. Inferior outcome of two-haplotype matched renal transplants in blacks: role of early rejection. Kidney Int. 1995;48(5):1592–9. PubMed PMID: 8544419. Epub 1995/11/01. eng.
161. Kahan BD, Welsh M, Schoenberg L, Rutzky LP, Katz SM, Urbauer DL, et al. Variable oral absorption of cyclosporine. A biopharmaceutical risk factor for chronic renal allograft rejection. Transplantation. 1996;62(5):599–606. PubMed PMID: 8830822. Epub 1996/09/15. eng.
162. Chertow GM, Milford EL. Poorer graft survival in African-American transplant recipients cannot be explained by HLA mismatching. Adv Ren Replace Ther. 1997;4(1):40–5. PubMed PMID: 8996619. Epub 1997/01/01. eng.
163. Young CJ, Gaston RS. Renal transplantation in black Americans. N Engl J Med. 2000;343(21):1545–52. PubMed PMID: 11087885. Epub 2000/11/23. eng.
164. Meier-Kriesche HU, Ojo AO, Leichtman AB, Punch JD, Hanson JA, Cibrik DM, et al. Effect of mycophenolate mofetil on long-term outcomes in African American renal transplant recipients. J Am Soc Nephrol. 2000;11(12):2366–70. PubMed PMID: 11095660. Epub 2000/11/30. eng.

165. Leffell MS, Steinberg AG, Bias WB, Machan CH, Zachary AA. The distribution of HLA antigens and phenotypes among donors and patients in the UNOS registry. Transplantation. 1994;58(10): 1119–30. PubMed PMID: 7974720. Epub 1994/11/27. eng.
166. Katznelson S, Gjertson DW, Cecka JM. The effect of race and ethnicity on kidney allograft outcome. Clinical transplants. 1995:379-94. PubMed PMID: 8794281. Epub 1995/01/01. eng.
167. Pirsch JD, Miller J, Deierhoi MH, Vincenti F, Filo RS. A comparison of tacrolimus (FK506) and cyclosporine for immunosuppression after cadaveric renal transplantation. FK506 Kidney Transplant Study Group. Transplantation. 1997;63(7): 977–83.
168. Reeves-Daniel AM, DePalma JA, Bleyer AJ, Rocco MV, Murea M, Adams PL, et al. The APOL1 gene and allograft survival after kidney transplantation. Am J Transplant. 2011;11(5):1025–30. PubMed PMID: 21486385. Pubmed Central PMCID: PMC3083491. Epub 2011/04/14. eng.
169. Hricik DE, Anton HA, Knauss TC, Rodriguez V, Seaman D, Siegel C, et al. Outcomes of African American kidney transplant recipients treated with sirolimus, tacrolimus, and corticosteroids. Transplantation. 2002;74(2):189–93. PubMed PMID: 12151730. Epub 2002/08/02. eng.
170. Neylan JF. Immunosuppressive therapy in high-risk transplant patients: dose-dependent efficacy of mycophenolate mofetil in African-American renal allograft recipients. U.S. Renal Transplant Mycophenolate Mofetil Study Group. Transplantation. 1997;64(9):1277–82.
171. Meier-Kriesche HU, Ojo A, Magee JC, Cibrik DM, Hanson JA, Leichtman AB, et al. African-American renal transplant recipients experience decreased risk of death due to infection: possible implications for immunosuppressive strategies. Transplantation. 2000;70(2):375–9. PubMed PMID: 10933166. Epub 2000/08/10. eng.
172. Paul LC, Benediktsson H. Post-transplant hypertension and chronic renal allograft failure. Kidney Int Suppl. 1995;52:S34–7. PubMed PMID: 8587280. Epub 1995/12/01. eng.
173. Modena FM, Hostetter TH, Salahudeen AK, Najarian JS, Matas AJ, Rosenberg ME. Progression of kidney disease in chronic renal transplant rejection. Transplantation. 1991;52(2):239–44. PubMed PMID: 1871796. Epub 1991/08/01. eng.
174. Opelz G, Wujciak T, Ritz E. Association of chronic kidney graft failure with recipient blood pressure. Collaborative Transplant Study. Kidney Int. 1998;53(1):217–22. PubMed PMID: 9453022. Epub 1998/02/07. eng.
175. Mange K, Feldman H. Blood pressure and prediction of patient outcome. Kidney Int. 2000;57(6):2655. PubMed PMID: 10844640. Epub 2000/06/09. eng.
176. Perico N, Remuzzi G. Angiotensin II receptor antagonists and treatment of hypertension and renal disease. Curr Opin Nephrol Hypertens. 1998;7(5):571–8. PubMed PMID: 9818206. Epub 1998/11/18. eng.
177. Kasiske BL, Vazquez MA, Harmon WE, Brown RS, Danovitch GM, Gaston RS, et al. Recommendations for the outpatient surveillance of renal transplant recipients. American Society of Transplantation J Am Soc Nephrol. 2000;11 Suppl 15:S1–86. PubMed PMID: 11044969. Epub 2000/10/25. eng.
178. Ojo AO, Meier-Kriesche HU, Hanson JA, Leichtman AB, Cibrik D, Magee JC, et al. Mycophenolate mofetil reduces late renal allograft loss independent of acute rejection. Transplantation. 2000;69(11): 2405–9. PubMed PMID: 10868649. Epub 2000/06/27. eng.
179. Meier-Kriesche HU, Kaplan B. Cyclosporine microemulsion and tacrolimus are associated with decreased chronic allograft failure and improved long-term graft survival as compared with sandimmune. Am J Transplant. 2002;2(1):100–4. PubMed PMID: 12095048. Epub 2002/07/04. eng.
180. Ekberg H, Tedesco-Silva H, Demirbas A, Vitko S, Nashan B, Gurkan A, et al. Reduced exposure to calcineurin inhibitors in renal transplantation. N Engl J Med. 2007;357(25):2562–75. PubMed PMID: 18094377. Epub 2007/12/21. eng.
181. Ekberg H, Bernasconi C, Tedesco-Silva H, Vitko S, Hugo C, Demirbas A, et al. Calcineurin inhibitor minimization in the Symphony study: observational results 3 years after transplantation. Am J Transplant. 2009;9(8):1876–85. PubMed PMID: 19563339. Epub 2009/07/01. eng.
182. Vincenti F, Charpentier B, Vanrenterghem Y, Rostaing L, Bresnahan B, Darji P, et al. A phase III study of belatacept-based immunosuppression regimens versus cyclosporine in renal transplant recipients (BENEFIT study). Am J Transplant. 2010;10(3): 535–46. PubMed PMID: 20415897. Epub 2010/04/27. eng.
183. Durrbach A, Pestana JM, Pearson T, Vincenti F, Garcia VD, Campistol J, et al. A phase III study of belatacept versus cyclosporine in kidney transplants from extended criteria donors (BENEFIT-EXT study). Am J Transplant. 2010;10(3):547–57. PubMed PMID: 20415898. Epub 2010/04/27. eng.
184. Vincenti F, Larsen CP, Alberu J, Bresnahan B, Garcia VD, Kothari J, et al. Three-year outcomes from BENEFIT, a randomized, active-controlled, parallel-group study in adult kidney transplant recipients. Am J Transplant. 2012;12(1):210–7. PubMed PMID: 21992533. Epub 2011/10/14. eng.

Immunological Assessment of the Transplant Patient

2

Rowena Delos Santos, Eric D. Langewisch, and Douglas J. Norman

Introduction

Before a patient can be safely transplanted several aspects of the match between the donor and recipient must be evaluated. These include the ABO blood group match, the major histocompatibility (human leukocyte antigen, HLA) antigen match, and an assessment of the presence, in the serum of a patient, of anti-HLA antibodies that might cause a transplanted kidney to fail. Highly accurate laboratory techniques for determining the suitability of the match are now available in most tissue typing laboratories. Outcomes of kidney transplantation have steadily improved over the years because of improvements in these matching techniques as well as the more commonly cited improvements in immunosuppression and patient care.

The most important immunologic barrier to a successful transplant is the ABO blood group antigen system. Anti-ABO A and B antibodies are naturally made by humans who do not express one or both of those antigens. ABO-incompatible kidneys can be rejected immediately by these antibodies if present in a large amount at the time of transplant. The second important immunologic barrier is the presence of anti-donor HLA antibodies in the serum of a potential recipient. These are not naturally occurring but will be made as a result of exposure to HLA antigens via blood transfusions, pregnancy, and tissue transplants. If present in a high amount at the time of transplant anti-HLA antibodies will cause hyperacute rejection. Mismatched HLA antigens are the next important immunologic barrier to a successful transplant. The fewer HLA antigens on the donor tissue that are mismatched by the recipient, the better the outcome of transplant. Minor histocompatibility antigens are the final immunologic barrier and explain why recipients of HLA-identical sibling kidney transplants still require some, although reduced, immunosuppression. Minor histocompatibility antigens are not well defined but we know that they exist and we strongly suspect that they can be targets of the immune response. The purpose of this chapter is to describe the immunologic barriers to a successful transplant, and the different laboratory methods available to evaluate the compatibility of a donor for a potential recipient.

R. Delos Santos
Washington University in St. Louis,
660 S. Euclid Avenue, St. Louis, MO 63110, USA

E.D. Langewisch • D.J. Norman (✉)
Oregon Health and Science University,
3181 SW Sam Jackson Park Road, Portland, OR 97239, USA
e-mail: normand@ohsu.edu

Barriers to Successful Transplantation

ABO Incompatibility

ABO blood group incompatibility is the initial and most important barrier to a successful transplant. Table 2.1 lists frequencies of ABO blood types within the US population as a whole and their acceptable ABO blood type donors.

ABO blood group B frequencies are higher among individuals of African, Asian, and Central European descent. As an example, approximately 20 % of African Americans type as blood group B. In contrast, native Americans rarely express the blood group B allele. When ABO-incompatible blood is transfused into individuals a severe immune reaction can occur, including acute lung injury and fatal complement-mediated hemolysis. ABO-incompatible organs can be rejected immediately due to the presence of circulating preformed anti-A and/or anti-B antibodies. However in certain circumstances, transplantation across ABO disparate blood groups is possible. Individuals who are ABO blood group B or O may receive a kidney from an ABO A2 donor if their anti-A antibody titer is low (IgG $\leq$ 1:2) [1–4]. The A2 antigen is less reactive with anti-A isoagglutinin and is expressed in lower amounts on the surface of red blood cells and tissue cells [3]. Waiting times and outcomes for A2 kidneys transplanted into O or B recipients between

M.R. Weir and E.V. Lerma (eds.), *Kidney Transplantation: Practical Guide to Management*,
DOI 10.1007/978-1-4939-0342-9_2, © Springer Science+Business Media New York 2014

Table 2.1 Recipient blood groups, their relative frequencies in the population, and compatible blood group donors

Recipient blood group	Percent of population (%)	Donor blood group compatible with recipient
A	42	A, O
B	10	B, O
AB	4	A, B, AB, O
O	44	O

Note: Rh factor status (positive or negative) is not an issue in transplantation

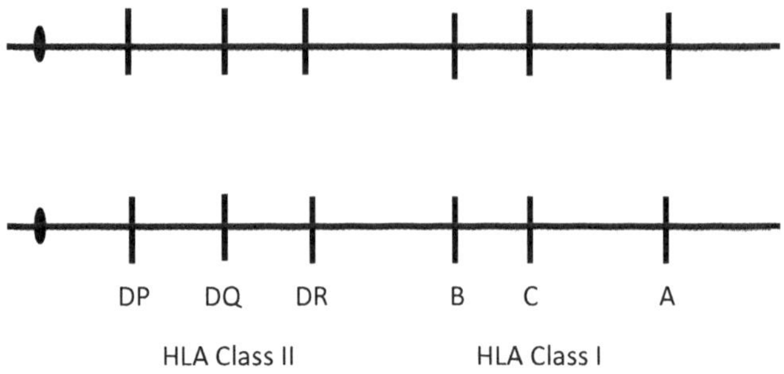

Fig. 2.1 Major histocompatibility complex/human leukocyte antigen on the short arm of chromosome 6 and their relative orientation on the chromosome

1995 and 2006 were examined using the United Network for Organ Sharing (UNOS) database [5]. There were 150,118 first kidney transplant recipients and among these 113 were O recipients of A2 kidneys and 125 were B recipients of A2 kidneys. These recipients had shorter waiting times than their counterparts who received ABO-compatible kidneys (A2 into O median wait time was 0.7 vs. 1.63 years and A2 into B median wait time was 0.74 vs. 1.9 years) [5]. In addition, there was no significant difference in graft or patient survival between the recipients of A2 compared with the ABO-compatible kidneys.

Several groups have developed protocols to transplant kidneys across major ABO barriers [6–11]. These protocols employ methods to reduce naturally occurring anti-A or anti-B antibodies. A variety of techniques and drugs have been used to achieve antibody reduction including plasmapheresis, intravenous immunoglobulin (IVIG), splenectomy, and rituximab [6–11]. These methods of antibody reduction have helped to expand the number of patients who may receive a kidney from a living donor. However, the growing participation of patients in paired donor exchanges may reduce the need for using ABO-incompatible donors.

Major Histocompatibility Complex

Major histocompatibility complex antigens (HLA) pose the next most important barrier to successful transplantation. HLA antigens are encoded by genes located on the short arm of the sixth human chromosome. This region, spanning an area of 3.6 mega base pairs, includes over 100 genes that are involved in the regulation of immunity. These genes are divided into three groups or classes. Class I and II genes encode for HLA molecules that are important in transplantation. Class III genes encode for other proteins related to the immune system, including heat shock proteins, complement factors, and cytokines. Class I HLA molecules consist of a heavy chain with three domains (alpha1, alpha2, alpha3) and an invariable light chain called beta-2 microglobulin (coded on chromosome 15). The alpha3 domain anchors the molecule into the cell, while the alpha1 and alpha2 domains form a peptide binding groove. Class II HLA molecules consist of two chains, an alpha and a beta chain (both coded on the sixth chromosome). Each chain has two domains, with the alpha1 and beta1 domains forming a peptide binding site.

The importance of HLA molecules hinges on their ability to present peptides to T cells. T cells, via their T cell receptor, are only capable of recognizing peptides (self or nonself) when these are presented in the peptide binding regions of HLA molecules [12–14]. T cells are continuously engaging HLA molecules to assess the nature of peptides. T cells will kill cells whose HLA molecules express nonself-peptides, such as viral peptides. This is how a person prevents viruses from spreading from cell to cell. Donor (allo) HLA molecules elicit a very strong immune response. Up to 15 % of all T cells are able to recognize nonself (allo)-HLA and initiate an effector response to a transplanted organ. It is because T cells are constantly surveying HLA molecules that HLA antigens are considered the major histocompatibility antigens.

HLA Class I genes include A, B, and C. HLA Class II genes include DP, DQ, and DR. HLA genes are co-dominantly expressed. Therefore, there are two HLA A molecules, two Bs, and so on. We inherit one number 6 chromosome from each of our parents. One set of HLA genes derived from one number 6 chromosome is called a haplotype. The probability that a sibling has inherited the same two haplotypes as a brother or sister who is in need of a transplant is 25 %, or 1−75 % (the probability that he/she inherited either one, 50 %, or inherited neither, 25 %). The probability that one of the several siblings is HLA identical (a two-haplotype match) is determined by the formula $1-(0.75)^n$, where *n* is the number of siblings. Figure 2.1 illustrates the orientation of the HLA genes on chromosome 6. Figure 2.2 demonstrates the inheritance pattern of the HLA genes.

HLA genes are highly polymorphic, with more than 1,980 unique alleles. These alleles are not randomly distributed, and certain alleles are more frequent than others. In fact, allele

Mother	Father
HLA A2 B7 DR4	HLA A11 B18 DR6
HLA A24 B8 DR51	HLA A36 B40 DR8

Sibling 1	Sibling 2	Sibling 3	Sibling 4
HLA A2 B7 DR4	HLA A2 B7 DR4	HLA A24 B8 DR51	HLA A2 B7 DR4
HLA A11 B18 DR6	HLA A36 B40 DR8	HLA A11 B18 DR6	HLA A11 B18 DR6

Fig. 2.2 The figure demonstrates the inheritance pattern for HLA genes. Each child is a one-haplotype match with its parent. Sibling 1 is a one-haplotype match to siblings 2 and 3, and a two-haplotype match with sibling 4. Sibling 2 is a one-haplotype match with siblings 1 and 4, and a 0 match with sibling 3. Sibling 3 is a one-haplotype match with siblings 1 and 4. Sibling 4 is a one-haplotype match with siblings 2 and 3. The probability that one of the several siblings is HLA identical (a two-haplotype match) is determined by the formula $1-(0.75)^n$, where n is the number of siblings

frequencies differ among different human populations [15]. Each HLA allele is unique in its ability to bind amino acids. The restricted nature of peptide binding favors having several different HLA molecules so many different peptides can be presented. If a person does not possess the ability to present peptides of a virus he/she will die because that virus will escape T cell-mediated elimination. The large number of HLA alleles (capable of presenting peptides) that exist in a population protects the population from extinction due to a specific viral infection. It is overwhelmingly likely that some members of the specific population will express HLA alleles that are capable of presenting peptides of all viruses to T cells. The fact that an individual has 12 distinct genes that code for HLA molecules makes it more likely that at least some peptides from a virus will bind in the peptide grooves of the HLA molecules to be presented to T cells, allowing T cells to kill virally infected cells.

HLA Class I is expressed on the surface of all nucleated cells while HLA Class II is expressed on antigen presenting cells (mononuclear phagocytes, B lymphocytes, dendritic cells) as well as some endothelial cells and thymus epithelium. Of note, HLA Class II is expressed on the endothelial cells of glomeruli and peritubular capillaries [16]. HLA of the transplanted organ can activate the recipient's T cells via the direct and indirect pathways of T cell activation [17]. Recipient T cells residing in lymph nodes can be directly activated by donor passenger cells from the allograft migrating to local draining lymph nodes. The direct pathway is dominant early after transplantation. The indirect pathway is the classic pathway of T and B cell activation used by the immune system to combat microorganisms. Recipient antigen presenting cells process donor antigen first and then present donor peptides to recipient immune cells. This pathway is responsible for rejection episodes that occur later after transplant, after the passenger donor cells are no longer around to directly activate recipient immune cells.

Preformed Anti-HLA Antibodies

The presentation of donor HLA via the direct or indirect pathway can lead to the development of anti-donor HLA antibodies. Anti-HLA antibodies do not occur naturally (as do anti-ABO antibodies). There are three ways that an individual can be exposed to HLA antigens and subsequently develop anti-HLA antibodies. The first is via blood product transfusions. The second is via pregnancy and the third is via tissue transplantation. Preformed anti-HLA antibodies represent another major barrier to a successful transplant either by limiting the number of compatible donors or, worse, by causing early graft failure if transplantation occurs despite the presence of donor-specific anti-HLA antibodies. Donor-specific antibodies (DSAs), if present in high amounts, will cause immediate (hyperacute) graft loss and if present in small amounts will limit the survival of an allograft.

Influence of Mismatched HLA Antigens on Transplant Outcomes

Mismatched donor HLA antigens become a target of the immune response by a recipient. Unfortunately, not all recipients will have the opportunity to receive a 0-antigen-mismatched kidney. The outcomes of this type of transplant are superior as demonstrated by data tracked by the Scientific Registry of Transplant Recipients (SRTR) illustrated by Fig. 2.3 [18].

The best opportunity for finding a minimally mismatched donor is among family members and specifically among siblings. However, for patients who do not have a living donor the national 0-antigen mismatch sharing program provides an opportunity to improve graft survival from a deceased donor. Patients who benefit the most from this program are those who possess anti-HLA antibodies and are therefore limited to a small pool of compatible donors. To qualify for this sharing program a patient must have a calculated panel reactive antibody (cPRA) (see below) of ≥20 % [18]. Not all patients will qualify for this program and even for those who do, if they possess a rare HLA phenotype, it is unlikely that a 0-antigen-mismatched donor will ever be identified. There is good evidence that long-term allograft survival is directly related to the number of HLA mismatches at the time of transplantation. A study of over 30,000 first deceased donor allograft recipients transplanted between 1984 and 1990 showed that 0-antigen mismatch kidneys had 1- and 5-year survivals of 84.3 % and 65.4 %, respectively. The 1- and 5-year survivals for 6-antigen-mismatched kidneys were 76.1 % and 52.3 %, respectively. There was also a stepwise decrease in survival with each mismatched HLA antigen [19]. Another study of nearly 136,000 recipients from 363

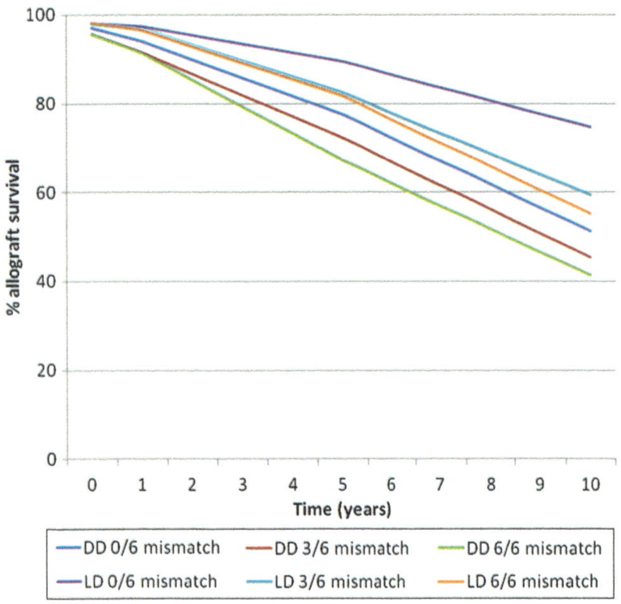

Fig. 2.3 Survival of deceased donor (DD inclusive of non-expanded criteria donor and expanded criteria donor) and living donor (LD) allograft kidneys according to their HLA mismatches with the recipient. Data for this figure was obtained from the OPTN/SRTR 2010 Annual Data Report (ADR) Table 5,10c, d as of October 1, 2010

Table 2.2 Time (years) to transplantation according to percentage of panel reactive antibodies (PRAs)

	Peak PRA			
	Total patients	0–9 %	10–79 %	≥80 %
10th percentile (TT)	0.29	0.31	0.43	0.52
25th percentile (TT)	0.94	0.93	1.32	1.97
50th percentile	3.50	3.18	4.86	Not enough patients to calculate

Data for this table was obtained from the OPTN/SRTR 2010 Annual Data Report (ADR) Table 5.2 as of October 1, 2010. The data is for patients who were registered onto the transplant waiting list in 2005. The panel reactive antibodies (PRAs) of these patients are the peak PRAs. The time to transplantation (TT) is denoted in years. The percentiles represent the time to transplantation for the total population waitlisted, for the time to transplantation for 10 % of the population of waitlisted individuals, time to transplantation for 25 % of the population of waitlisted, and the time to transplantation for 50 % of the waitlisted population

centers, transplanted between 1985 and 1994, reported 5-year allograft survivals of 69.9 % and 54.3 % for a 0- and 6-antigen mismatch, respectively [20]. This study also noted a persistent importance of HLA mismatching for recipients transplanted between 1995 and 2004, well after the introduction of superior immunosuppression, and also a stepwise decrease in 5-year allograft survival with an increasing HLA antigen mismatch [20]. Other studies have shown that greater levels of HLA mismatch are associated with higher rates of rejection [21, 22].

Pretransplant Assessment of Anti-HLA Antibody Status

The pretransplant assessment for anti-HLA antibodies consists of determining the breadth and strength of anti-HLA antibodies that are present and performing a crossmatch prior to transplant to be certain that there are no DSAs.

There are several reasons for determining if anti-HLA antibodies are present in a patient's serum prior to transplant. First, it is known that patients with a high level of anti-HLA antibodies have a higher incidence of rejection [23, 24]. Most transplant programs will give stronger immunosuppression to patients who are sensitized (possess high levels of anti-HLA antibodies). Second, patients who have anti-HLA antibodies receive additional points in the allocation scheme and are prioritized for transplantation with a deceased donor [18]. Third, by determining to which specific HLA antigens a patient has antibodies, it is now possible to list those on the national computer (UNet, the computer program operated by the UNOS, the national organ procurement and transplantation network) as unacceptable antigens [18, 25–28]. Their policies and guidelines regarding the listing of unacceptable antigens can be found on their website. If listed in UNet as an unacceptable antigen for a specific patient, kidneys from donors with that antigen will not be offered to that patient. Moreover, the only way to obtain allocation points for being sensitized is to list unacceptable antigens in UNet (more later). Fourth, and finally, it is very useful for the physicians caring for a patient who is on the waiting list to know if a patient is sensitized. The more sensitized a patient, the longer it will take to find a compatible donor, as illustrated by SRTR data in Table 2.2 [18]. This is important information for both the patient and his/her physician.

The techniques for determining the presence of anti-HLA antibodies have evolved. The commonly used term to describe the breadth of antibodies is PRA. PRA stands for panel reactive antibody and is expressed as a percent. The techniques for the determination of an individual's PRA are illustrated in Fig. 2.4.

The classical method for determining the PRA used a panel of individuals who together possessed as many of the known HLA antigens as possible [29]. Cells from these individuals were put on a tray, each well containing the cells of one individual. Serum from a patient was added to the tray to determine if antibodies were present, the readout being cytotoxicity in the presence of complement. The PRA percent was calculated by simply dividing the number of wells with dead cells by the total number of wells (e.g., 24 wells with dead cells and a total of 48 wells = PRA of 50 %). The cytotoxicity method is less sensitive than techniques that are currently used but the term PRA has endured. Current techniques are bead—instead of cell—based. Polystyrene or latex beads are coated with HLA molecules that are obtained from

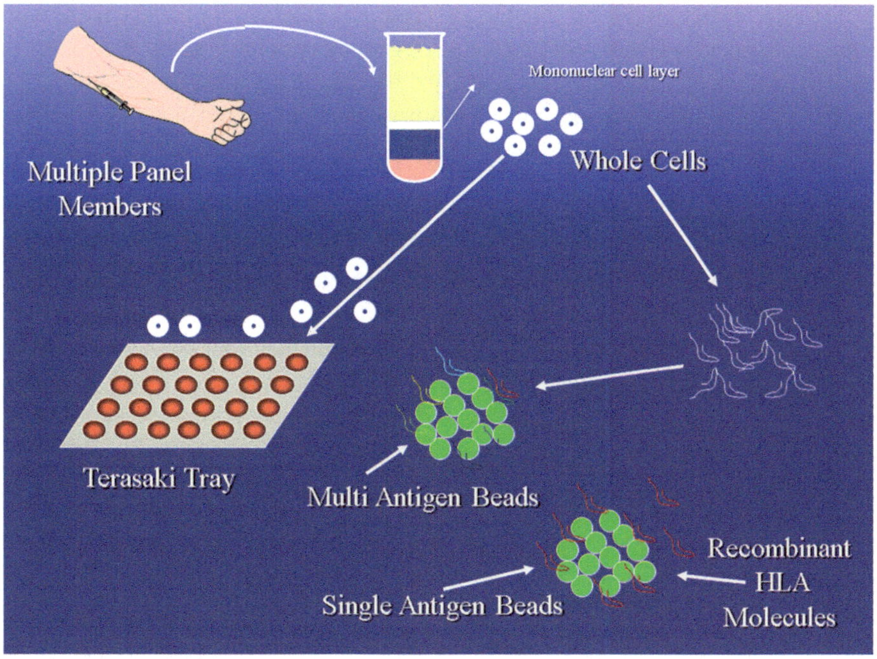

Fig. 2.4 Panel reactive antibodies. Two different techniques: cytotoxicity method and bead-based method. The cytotoxicity method involves the use of whole cells from a panel of donors who together possess as many known HLA antigens as possible. Each donor has his/her cells placed into one well of a tray and mixed with the recipient serum and complement. Cytotoxicity as evidenced by dead donor cells in a tray well represents reactivity of the recipient sera with the donor. The percent PRA is the number of "reactive" wells, or wells with dead cells, divided by the total number of wells. Example: 12 wells with dead cells and a total of 48 wells=PRA of 25 %. The current techniques are bead based. Polystyrene or latex beads are coated with HLA molecules that are obtained from either digested cells from multiple donors (multi-antigen beads) or recombinant techniques (single antigen beads). A mix of either Class I or II beads is chosen to represent as many HLA antigens as possible. The "flow PRA" uses multi-antigen beads, patient serum, fluorochrome-tagged anti-human immunoglobulin antibodies, and a flow cytometer to detect anti-HLA antibodies. In the assay, beads that have antibodies attached indicate that the patient possesses anti-HLA antibody to the HLA bound to the bead. The "reactive beads" emit photons from laser activation of fluorochromes on the antibodies. The PRA percent is calculated by counting the number of beads that have antibodies attached and dividing by the total number of beads present. For instance, if 30 % of the beads have antibodies attached the flow PRA is 30 %

either digested cells (multi-antigen beads) or recombinant techniques (single antigen beads). The "flow PRA" uses multi-antigen beads, patient serum, fluorochrome-tagged anti-human immunoglobulin antibodies, and a flow cytometer to detect anti-HLA antibodies. Multi-antigen beads have either HLA Class I or Class II antigens attached [30, 31]. A mix of either Class I or II beads is chosen to represent as many HLA antigens as possible. The mix does not represent the frequency of HLA antigens in the population because this varies by demographic group. In the assay, beads that have antibodies attached (indicating that a patient has an anti-HLA antibody(ies) that recognizes the HLA antigen(s) that is (are) bound to that bead) emit photons from laser activation of fluorochromes on the antibodies. The PRA percent is calculated by counting the number of beads that have antibodies attached and dividing by the total number of beads present. If 10 % of the beads have antibodies attached the flow PRA is 10 %. Another technique using multi-antigen beads (quick screen) can be used to determine if a patient has anti-HLA antibodies, but the breadth of antibodies (PRA) is not calculated [32]. When either the flow PRA or quick screen is positive a single antigen bead assay is generally run to identify the specific antibodies causing the positive results. Single antigen bead assays use a Luminex platform that in addition to recognizing the presence of antibodies attached to beads can identify intrinsic color of the beads [33, 34]. Polystyrene beads with multiple (up to 1,000) different colors are used in these assays. The advantage of this platform is the ability to attach specific recombinant HLA molecules to beads having a unique color. For example, HLA B7 adherent beads will have a different color from HLA A2 adherent beads. Luminex assays can determine if antibodies are bound to the HLA A2 beads, to the HLA B7 beads, to both, or to multiple other beads with unique colors and unique single HLA antigen specificities.

For patients who are waitlisted on the national computer for a deceased donor a PRA is calculated (cPRA) by entering unacceptable antigens into UNet. The computer is programmed to calculate a cPRA based on the frequency of HLA Class I and Class II antigens expressed by 12,000 US organ donors [18, 35]. The higher the cPRA, the greater the number of points offered to a patient via the allocation scheme. A high cPRA can result from a small number of common HLA antigens (e.g., HLA A2) or from a large number of less common HLA antigens. It is the responsibility of each transplant program to enter unacceptable HLA antigens for each of their waiting patients into UNet. Most patients will have none. Some will have one or more and a few will have many unacceptable antigens. An unacceptable HLA antigen may be defined differently by different programs and currently there is no national standard. HLA antigens will be listed if they exceed a threshold based on the strength or amount of antibody measured. The measure of strength in the Luminex single antigen bead assay is mean fluorescence intensity (MFI). Increasing fluorescence intensity measured by photons emitted by specific beads bound with specific HLA molecules correlates with increasing amounts of antibody to that specific HLA antigen. Each program, in consultation with their tissue typing laboratory director, chooses an MFI threshold above which an HLA antigen will be listed as unacceptable. If the MFI threshold is low, more HLA antigens will be listed and if the threshold is high fewer will be listed. At present MFI thresholds chosen by programs range from as low as 1,000 to as high as 10,000. One distinct advantage of listing unacceptable HLA antigens in UNet is that when a donor kidney is offered to a patient it is highly likely that the final pretransplant crossmatch (see below) will be compatible. However, this is much more likely if the unacceptable MFI threshold is set low and much less likely if the MFI threshold is set high.

When considering a living donor, knowing about antibody specificities can help determine compatibility. A DSA with a high MFI indicates an incompatible match (virtual crossmatch, see below).

The Pretransplant Crossmatch

Before a kidney transplant is performed it is essential that the recipient is found to be devoid of any antibodies that can cause hyperacute rejection or early graft failure. A pretransplant crossmatch is performed using techniques that can detect the presence of DSAs. The tissue typing laboratory generally considers the crossmatch to be the most important test that it performs. Crossmatching techniques have evolved to become substantially more sensitive. Several crossmatching assays are currently available for use and tissue typing laboratories differ regarding which are used. Figure 2.5 provides a list of the different techniques used when performing a crossmatch between a potential donor and a recipient. Each technique is described in the following sections.

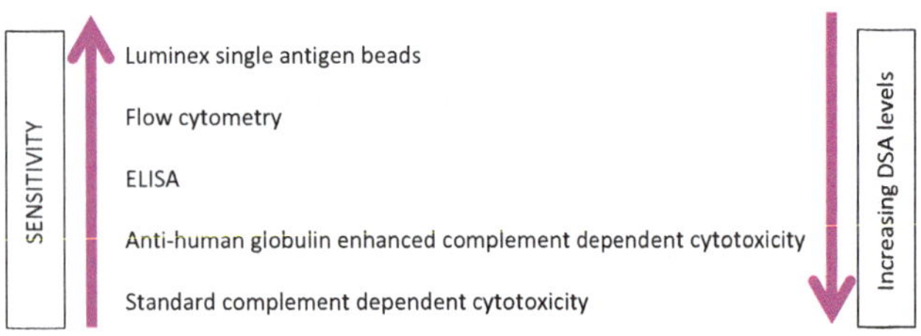

Fig. 2.5 This figure illustrates the increasing sensitivity of immunologic evaluation tests for detecting donor specific antibody (DSA) in the recipient serum. The most sensitive is the single antigen beads, while the least sensitive is the standard complement-dependent cytotoxicity test

Standard Complement-Dependent Cytotoxicity or NIH Crossmatch

The complement-dependent cytotoxicity test (CDC) or standard crossmatch developed in 1964 by Terasaki and McClelland has been used as the standard crossmatch for several decades, shown in Fig. 2.6 [25].

Buffy coat containing lymphocytes from the donor is combined with serum (in several dilutions) from the recipient in a multiwell tray and incubated at room temperature for 30 min followed by the addition of complement and further incubation at room temperature for 60 min. A vital dye (usually eosin) is added along with formalin (permanently fixes cells). Eosin enters cells that have been damaged by complement activation and can be easily identified under an inverted phase microscope. Live cells remain small and refractile and exclude eosin. In their original publication that appeared in the New England Journal of Medicine, Patel and Terasaki conclusively demonstrated the specificity of this technique [36]. Patients were transplanted and a retrospective crossmatch was performed. Patients were divided into two groups based on the presence or absence of anti-HLA antibodies. Among patients with antibodies and with a positive crossmatch immediate graft failure occurred in 80 % and only 10 % of kidneys survived for more than 3 months. This confirmed the need for a crossmatch with the specificity of the standard cytotoxic crossmatch before every transplant. However, among patients with antibodies and a negative crossmatch immediate graft failure occurred in 15 % but among patients without antibodies only 2.4 % failed immediately. These findings indicated that while highly specific (grafts will fail if the test is positive) this test lacked adequate sensitivity. This led to the development of more sensitive crossmatching techniques.

Anti-human Globulin-Enhanced Crossmatch

Adding several washes and increasing incubation times increase the sensitivity of the standard crossmatch [37, 38]. However, the most effective way to increase sensitivity of the cytotoxic crossmatch is with the use of anti-human globulin [39, 40]. The anti-human globulin crossmatch technique is similar to the standard CDC crossmatch, with one additional step. Anti-human globulin is added prior to the addition of complement to augment the cytotoxicity reaction. Complement activation requires cross linking of antibodies.

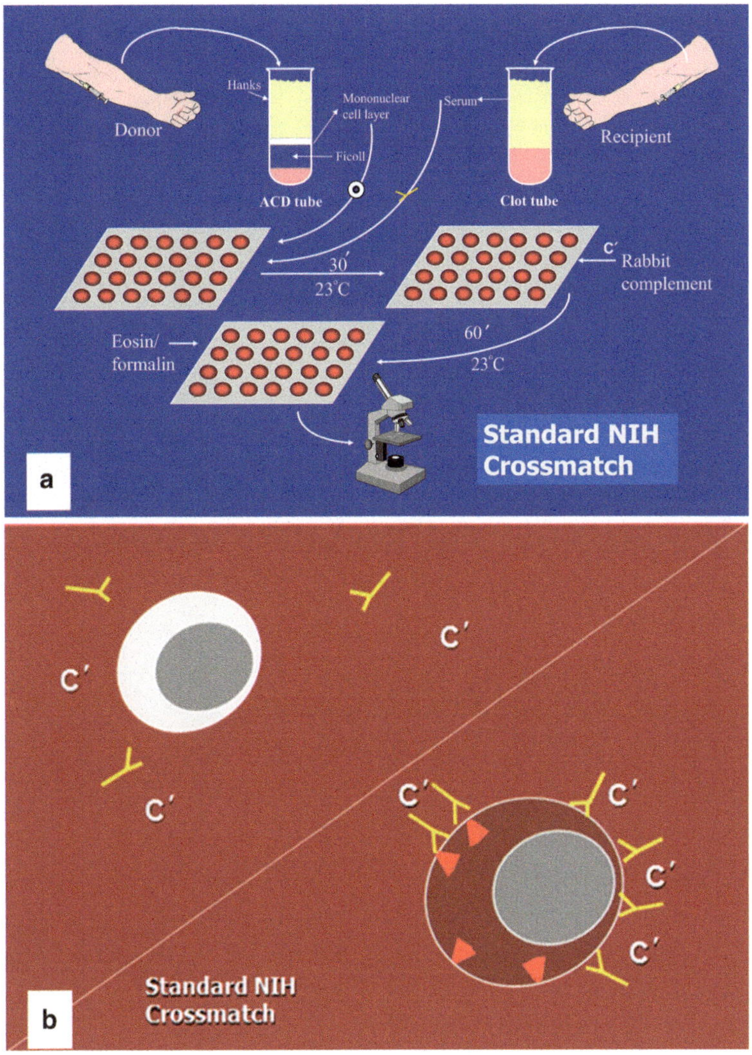

Fig. 2.6 (**a**) Standard NIH Crossmatch. Donor lymphocytes are collected and placed into wells. Recipient serum is then added to the wells and incubated with the lymphocytes. Rabbit complement is then added to this mixture and incubated. After the second incubation, eosin dye and formalin are added to fix the cells and evaluated under the microscope. (**b**) If donor specific antibodies are present, then the combination of donor lymphocytes, recipient sera, and complement leads to a reaction in which the antigen/antibody complex recruits complement that then will form membrane attack complexes that destabilize the cell membrane, allowing eosin dye to enter the cell and lead to cell swelling, which is discernible under phase contrast microscopy

If non-complement binding antibodies (IgG4) or low levels of antibodies are present cytotoxicity might not be seen even if antibodies are donor specific. Anti-human immunoglobulin can create cross linking and complement activation and reveal the presence of a DSA. Figure 2.7 demonstrates the steps in performing the anti-human globulin CDC crossmatch.

In a study that compared the standard complement-dependent microcytoxicity test, the standard test with the addition of antiglobulin, and the standard test with doubled incubation periods 52 of 56 sera tested (93 %) were positive when adding antiglobulin compared with 28/56 (50 %) when the incubation time was extended and 13/56 (23 %) when the standard technique was used [40].

B Cell Cytotoxic Crossmatch

Peripheral blood lymphocytes (PBL) are used for the standard CDC crossmatch and PBL are mostly T lymphocytes (80–85 %). T lymphocytes do not express HLA Class II molecules but B lymphocytes do express Class II. The B cell crossmatch uses PBL that have been enriched for B cells and therefore is able to detect anti-HLA Class II anti-donor antibodies. Moreover, B cells express higher amounts of Class I molecules. Therefore, the B cell crossmatch can also detect low levels of anti-Class I antibodies even when the standard crossmatch might not. The B cell crossmatch is more technically difficult than the standard crossmatch for several reasons. B cells must be enriched using immuno-magnetic beads, incubation is done at 37 °C, fluorescent dyes are used, incubation is longer, and B cells might be damaged by the enrichment technique [41].

Flow Crossmatch Test

The flow crossmatch test is the most sensitive of all of the tests. Donor lymphocytes are mixed with recipient serum followed by the addition of a fluorochrome-tagged anti-human immunoglobulin. After washing, donor cells are run through

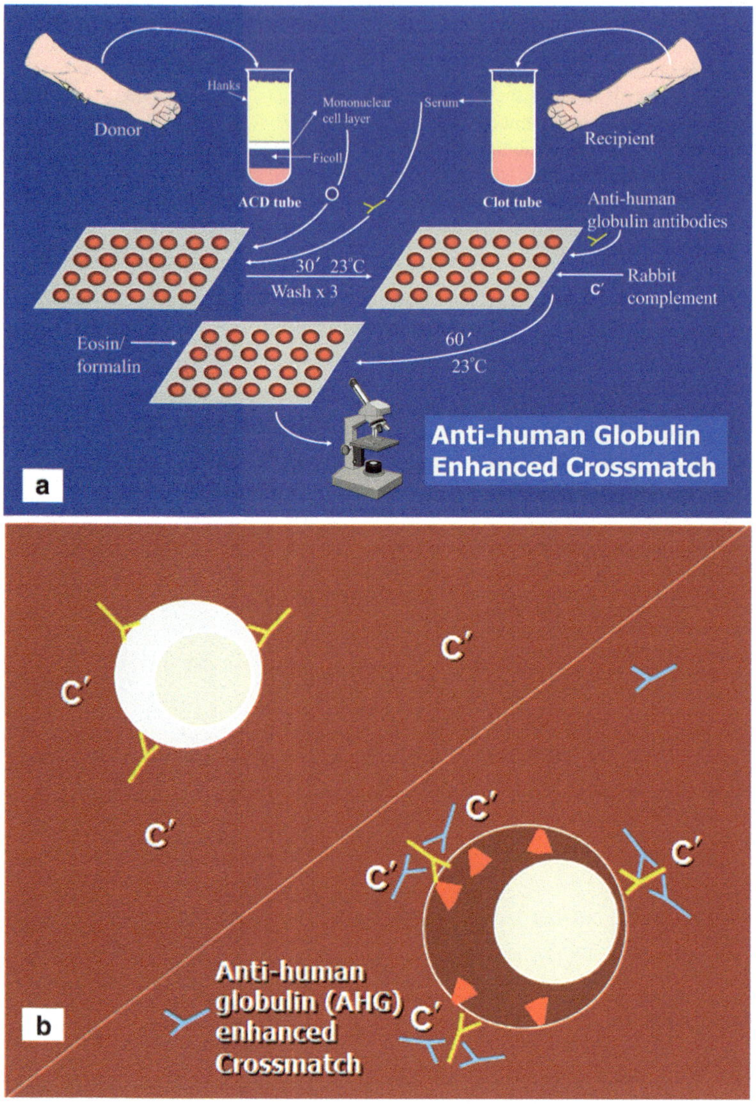

Fig. 2.7 Anti-human globulin-enhanced CDC crossmatch. (**a**) The anti-human globulin-enhanced CDC crossmatch is similar to the CDC crossmatch, except for additional wash steps and the addition of anti-human globulin, which is thought to bind to the recipient HLA-bound antibodies, thereby improving the ability for the immunoglobulins to fix complement. (**b**) The additional anti-human globulin binds to the human immunoglobulin that binds to the recipient HLA. Anti-human globulin increases the sensitivity of the CDC crossmatch

a flow cytometer where cells are counted individually. Cells that are bound by antibodies are identified by laser activation of the fluorochrome. This technique allows detection of very small amounts of DSAs and it can differentiate between T and B cells and between IgM and IgG antibodies [42, 43]. It can also be done with donor cells that have been damaged and could not be used in a cytotoxic crossmatch which requires live cells. Figure 2.8 shows the steps involved in a flow crossmatch.

B cells can nonspecifically bind immunoglobulin via FcγR receptors, which bind to the Fc region on IgG antibodies [44]. Addition of the enzyme pronase, which cleaves FcγR receptors, has led to significant improvement in the sensitivity and specificity of the flow crossmatch [44, 45]. While the general understanding is that a positive standard or antiglobulin crossmatch is a contraindication to transplantation, a positive flow crossmatch may indicate a lower risk of rejection if the standard and antiglobulin crossmatches are both negative. Each transplant center decides which crossmatches to use and how to weigh the importance of each. Table 2.3 lists the different crossmatch test combinations possible and the interpretations of these combinations.

IgM Antibodies and Autoantibodies

IgM antibodies are not considered pathogenic in kidney transplantation [23, 46–48]. However, IgM antibodies can cause a positive cytotoxic crossmatch. Therefore, techniques that remove IgM are necessary. One such technique is the use

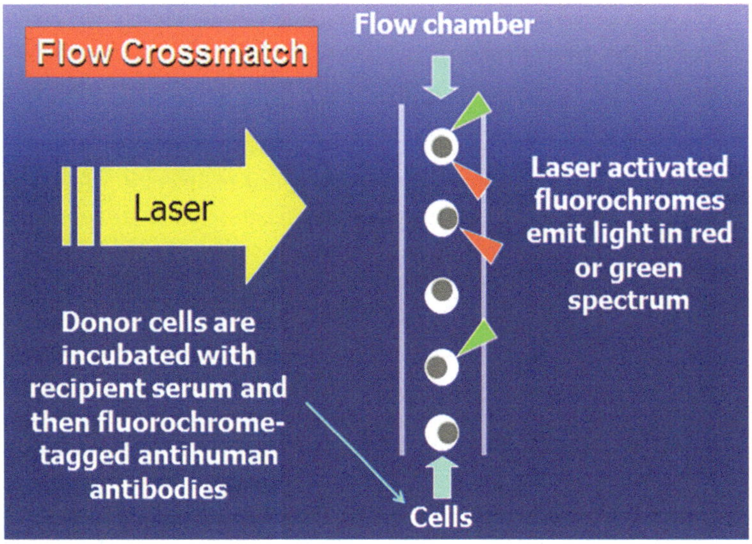

Fig. 2.8 Flow crossmatch illustration. In this test, donor cells are incubated with recipient serum. Fluorochrome-tagged anti-human globulin antibodies are added to the mixture which is then placed into the flow machine. Each cell travels through the machine and undergoes evaluation by two lasers. One laser measures the fluorochrome tag differentiating T cells from B cells. The other laser detects the fluorochromes as they emit their signature within the spectrum that identifies the cells with antibody attached to the HLA

Table 2.3 Various combinations of immunologic tests and possible interpretations

Cytotoxic crossmatch			Flow crossmatch		
Standard	AHG	B cell	T cell	B cell	Interpretation of crossmatch results
+	+	+	+	+	Serum contains significant amount of antibodies to the donor HLA. High risk for hyperacute rejection. Transplantation contraindicated
+	+	0	+	0	Probably not anti-Class I antibodies as B cell crossmatch should also be positive. Perform further antibody testing for antibody specificity
0	0	0	+	+	Probably with a low titer of anti-Class I antibodies and requires further testing. Some risk of hyperacute rejection likely
0	0	+	0	+	Anti-Class II antibody present, or low titer anti-Class I antibody. Check for titer for anti-Class II as this may lead to hyperacute rejection
0	0/+	+	0	0	There is likely an autoantibody, IgM, which is low risk for rejection. Treat with DTT or auto-absorb to remove IgM antibody. May be early sensitizing event prior to class switch from IgM to IgG. If class switch occurs, will be at risk for rejection
0	0	0	0	0	No anti-HLA antibodies present. Low risk for hyperacute rejection

The cytotoxic crossmatch tests include the standard CDC, AHG, and B cell. The flow crossmatch includes the T cell and B cell
AHG anti-human globulin, *0* negative reaction, + positive reaction

of dithiothreitol (DTT) [49]. DTT reduces the disulfide bonds of IgM antibodies, destroying the tertiary structure and reactivity without affecting the IgG reactivity. IgM antibodies, which are reactive at 4 °C (39.2 °F), can also be removed by increasing the incubation temperature to 55 °C (131 °F). It is generally considered important to evaluate the sera of patients who are sensitized to determine if IgM antibodies are present. The flow crossmatch allows the differentiation of IgG from IgM by the reagents used. The fluorochrome-tagged anti-human immunoglobulin used in the assay is specifically directed to IgG only, ignoring IgM.

Occasionally the flow B cell crossmatch is positive but the flow T cell crossmatch is negative. Both T and B lymphocytes express HLA Class I but only B lymphocytes express Class II. The discrepant T and B cell results could be due to the presence of a donor specific anti-HLA Class II antibody (such as an anti-HLA DP, DQ, or DR antibody). However, IgM or IgG autoantibodies might also cause this due to nonspecific binding on B cells. If a donor specific anti-HLA antibody is not found and if treatment with pronase to cleave FcR from the surface of B cells does not reduce the reaction, an autoantibody might be present. Performing an auto-flow crossmatch (recipient lymphocytes and recipient serum) can clarify these findings. An autoantibody will cause a positive flow B and sometimes flow T cell crossmatch. In the absence of a DSA and in the presence of a positive auto-crossmatch it is generally considered safe to disregard the positive crossmatch against a kidney donor. Many kidney transplants have been performed safely under these circumstances.

The Virtual Crossmatch

Because very sensitive techniques are now available to detect (and specifically identify) the presence of anti-HLA antibodies in the serum of a potential kidney transplant recipient it has become reasonable to consider transplant without a physical pretransplant crossmatch. However, several conditions are necessary to allow the safe application of a virtual crossmatch. If no anti-HLA antibodies are present in a patient's serum it would be considered safe to bypass a physical crossmatch if the most sensitive single antigen bead assay was used to detect antibodies. When anti-HLA antibodies have been detected, the donor HLA type is known, and there are no DSAs, a physical crossmatch can also be bypassed. Further, if a high level of a DSA is present it would be permissible to rule out a donor without performing a physical crossmatch. In most other circumstances including if a highly sensitized patient is being considered or if a patient appears to have a low level DSA a physical crossmatch must always be performed. Moreover, whenever a deceased donor is available several potential recipients are considered and among these there are often sensitized patients. So, unless a kidney is being offered for a specific patient who has no anti-HLA antibodies a physical crossmatch must always be performed. It is always prudent to have backup recipients available even in a directed-donor circumstance in case the recipient is ruled out for some reason. Since the backup recipients are not donor directed a physical crossmatch would need to be performed. It may be possible to more fully use the virtual crossmatch in the future but the most sensitive techniques would need to be used to detect anti-HLA antibodies and the donor would need to be fully HLA typed (A, B, C, DP, DQ, and DR). Further cautioning the use of a virtual crossmatch is the possibility that a potential recipient has a non-HLA antibody that might cause rejection [50–54]. These antibodies would not be detected using only HLA beads and there are no bead-based techniques that detect non-HLA antibodies. However, further complicating issues is the fact that non-HLA antigens that might be important in kidney transplantation (e.g., MICA) are not expressed on lymphocytes, possibly rendering the crossmatch useless in their detection anyway.

Donor-Specific Antibodies

Following transplantation patients can make DSA and these can cause acute antibody-mediated rejection and chronic rejection. Noncompliance with immunosuppressive drugs or chronic under-immunosuppression is likely a cause of the development of DSA. Several studies have shown a significant adverse effect of DSA on graft survival [24, 33, 55, 56]. One study evaluated the outcomes over a 30-year period of patients who were previously transplanted and then retransplanted with donor allografts of the same HLA A and B antigens as the first allograft. These patients were at increased risk for rejection and early graft loss [55]. Another study found that patients with preformed DSA even with low anti-donor HLA antibody levels suffered from decreased allograft survival [56]. Another found that recipients who developed de novo anti-HLA antibodies to their allografts were more likely to develop acute rejection than those who did not have DSA (29 % vs. 9.5 %) as well as lower 2-year allograft survival (83 % vs. 98 %) [24]. There is probably a level below which DSAs are not pathogenic but that level has not been exactly identified. Certainly, low levels of DSA will not cause a hyperacute rejection. It is generally assumed that the MFI of a DSA must be greater than 10,000 for it to cause a positive standard cytotoxic crossmatch (the one that is associated with 80 % immediate graft loss). It is for this reason that a living donor might be considered acceptable even if a DSA is present if there are no other donors available and if the MFI is <2,000. Techniques and drugs (plasmapheresis, IVIG, rituximab, bortezomib) are available and have been used successfully to reduce or eliminate anti-HLA antibodies. Since most patients who take their immunosuppressive drugs as prescribed do not make DSA it is likely that standard immunosuppression might also help to decrease low levels of DSA present at transplant.

Conclusions

The practice of transplantation has improved tremendously over the last half century. These improvements have been partly due to the recognition of the importance of HLA and ABO blood group matching. Methods to detect antibodies directed against potential donor HLA have improved, and we now possess the ability to detect very low levels of anti-HLA antibodies. Information gathered from the detection of anti-HLA antibodies have helped in donor allocation and the ability of highly sensitized patients to be offered donor kidneys.

References

1. Alkhunaizi AM, de Mattos AM, Barry JM, Bennett WM, Norman DJ. Renal transplantation across the ABO barrier using A2 kidneys. Transplantation. 1999;67(10):1319–24.
2. Mendez R, Sakhrani L, Chaballout A, Mendez RG. ABO incompatible transplants involving A2 donors. Transplant Proc. 1991;23(2): 1738–41.
3. Nelson PW, Landreneau MD, Luger AM, Pierce GE, Ross G, Shield III CF, et al. Ten-year experience in transplantation of A2 kidneys into B and O recipients. Transplantation. 1998;65(2): 256–60.

4. Slapak M, Digard N, Ahmed M, Shell T, Thompson F. Renal transplantation across the ABO barrier—a 9-year experience. Transplant Proc. 1990;22(4):1425–8.
5. Hurst FP, Sajjad I, Elster EA, Falta EM, Patel P, Abbott KC, et al. Transplantation of A2 kidneys into B and O recipients leads to reduction in waiting time: USRDS experience. Transplantation. 2010;89(11):1396–402.
6. Sonnenday CJ, Warren DS, Cooper M, Samaniego M, Haas M, King KE, et al. Plasmapheresis, CMV hyperimmune globulin, and anti-CD20 allow ABO-incompatible renal transplantation without splenectomy. Am J Transplant. 2004;4(8):1315–22.
7. Tyden G, Kumlien G, Genberg H, Sandberg J, Lundgren T, Fehrman I. ABO incompatible kidney transplantations without splenectomy, using antigen-specific immunoadsorption and rituximab. Am J Transplant. 2005;5(1):145–8.
8. Uchida J, Machida Y, Iwai T, Naganuma T, Kitamoto K, Iguchi T, et al. Desensitization protocol in highly HLA-sensitized and ABO-incompatible high titer kidney transplantation. Transplant Proc. 2010;42(10):3998–4002.
9. Flint SM, Walker RG, Hogan C, Haeusler MN, Robertson A, Francis DM, et al. Successful ABO-incompatible kidney transplantation with antibody removal and standard immunosuppression. Am J Transplant. 2011;11(5):1016–24.
10. Fuchinoue S, Ishii Y, Sawada T, Murakami T, Iwadoh K, Sannomiya A, et al. The 5-year outcome of ABO-incompatible kidney transplantation with rituximab induction. Transplantation. 2011;91(8):853–7.
11. Montgomery JR, Berger JC, Warren DS, James NT, Montgomery RA, Segev DL. Outcomes of ABO-incompatible kidney transplantation in the United States. Transplantation. 2012;93(6):603–9.
12. Marrack P, Kappler J. The antigen-specific, major histocompatibility complex-restricted receptor on T cells. Adv Immunol. 1986;38:1–30.
13. Hedrick SM. Specificity of the T cell receptor for antigen. Adv Immunol. 1988;43:193–234.
14. Davis MM, Bjorkman PJ. A model for T cell receptor and MHC/peptide interaction. Adv Exp Med Biol. 1989;254:13–6.
15. Cao K, Hollenbach J, Shi X, Shi W, Chopek M, Fernández-Viña MA. Analysis of the frequencies of HLA-A, B, and C alleles and haplotypes in the five major ethnic groups of the United States reveals high levels of diversity in these loci and contrasting distribution patterns in these populations. Hum Immunol. 2001;62(9):1009–30.
16. Muczynski KA, Cotner T, Anderson SK. Unusual expression of human lymphocyte antigen class II in normal renal microvascular endothelium. Kidney Int. 2001;59(2):488–97.
17. Auchincloss Jr H, Sultan H. Antigen processing and presentation in transplantation. Curr Opin Immunol. 1996;8(5):681–7.
18. Organ Procurement and Transplantation Network (OPTN) and Scientific Registry of Transplant Recipients (SRTR). OPTN/SRTR 2010 annual data report. Department of Health and Human Services, Health Resources and Services Administration, Healthcare Systems Bureau, Division of Transplantation; 2012. [cited 2012 November 16]. Available from: http://www.srtr.org/annual_Reports/default.aspx.
19. Held PJ, Kahan BD, Hunsicker LG, Liska D, Wolfe RA, Port FK, et al. The impact of HLA mismatches on the survival of first cadaveric kidney transplants. N Engl J Med. 1994;331(12):765–70.
20. Opelz G, Dohler B. Effect of human leukocyte antigen compatibility on kidney graft survival: comparative analysis of two decades. Transplantation. 2007;84(2):137–43.
21. Paramesh AS, Zhang R, Baber J, Yau CL, Slakey DP, Killackey MT, et al. The effect of HLA mismatch on highly sensitized renal allograft recipients. Clin Transplant. 2010;24(6):E247–52.
22. Wissing KM, Fomegne G, Broeders N, Ghisdal L, Hoang AD, Mikhalski D, et al. HLA mismatches remain risk factors for acute kidney allograft rejection in patients receiving quadruple immunosuppression with anti-interleukin-2 receptor antibodies. Transplantation. 2008;85(3):411–6.
23. Scornik JC, Salomon DR, Lim PB, Howard RJ, Pfaff WW. Posttransplant antidonor antibodies and graft rejection. Evaluation by two-color flow cytometry. Transplantation. 1989;47(2):287–90.
24. Cooper JE, Gralla J, Cagle L, Goldberg R, Chan L, Wiseman AC. Inferior kidney allograft outcomes in patients with de novo donor-specific antibodies are due to acute rejection episodes. Transplantation. 2011;91(10):1103–9.
25. Cecka JM, Kucheryavaya AY, Reinsmoen NL, Leffell MS. Calculated PRA: initial results show benefits for sensitized patients and a reduction in positive crossmatches. Am J Transplant. 2011;11(4):719–24.
26. Cecka JM. Calculated PRA, (CPRA): the new measure of sensitization for transplant candidates. Am J Transplant. 2010;10(1):26–9. PubMed PMID: 46824236.
27. Gebel HM, Bray RA. The evolution and clinical impact of human leukocyte antigen technology. Curr Opin Nephrol Hypertens. 2010;19(6):598–602 [English].
28. U.S. Organ Procurement and Transplantation Network and the Scientific Registry of Transplant Recipient. Rockville, MD: Department of Health and Human Services, Health Resources and Services Administration, Healthcare Systems Bureau, Division of Transplantation; Richmond, VA: United Network for Organ Sharing; Ann Arbor, MI: University Renal Research and Education Association; 2012 [cited 2012 November 16].
29. Terasaki PI, McClelland JD. Microdroplet assay of human serum cytotoxins. Nature. 1964;204:998–1000.
30. Pei R, Wang G, Tarsitani C, Rojo S, Chen T, Takemura S, et al. Simultaneous HLA class I and class II antibodies screening with flow cytometry. Hum Immunol. 1998;59(5):313–22.
31. Pei R, Lee J, Chen T, Rojo S, Terasaki PI. Flow cytometric detection of HLA antibodies using a spectrum of microbeads. Hum Immunol. 1999;60(12):1293–302.
32. Colombo MB, Haworth SE, Poli F, Nocco A, Puglisi G, Innocente A, et al. Luminex technology for anti-HLA antibody screening: evaluation of performance and of impact on laboratory routine. Cytometry B Clin Cytom. 2007;72(6):465–71. PubMed PMID: 17397064. Epub 2007/04/03. eng.
33. Caro-Oleas JL, Gonzalez-Escribano MF, Gentil-Govantes MA, Acevedo MJ, Gonzalez-Roncero FM, Blanco GB, et al. Clinical relevance of anti-HLA donor-specific antibodies detected by Luminex assay in the development of rejection after renal transplantation. Transplantation. 2012;94(4):338–44. PubMed PMID: 22814330. Epub 2012/07/21. eng.
34. Caro-Oleas JL, Gonzalez-Escribano MF, Toro-Llamas S, Acevedo MJ, Martinez-Bravo MJ, Aguilera I, et al. Donor-specific antibody detection: comparison of single antigen assay and Luminex crossmatches. Tissue Antigens. 2010;76(5):398–403. PubMed PMID: 20630037. Epub 2010/07/16. eng.
35. Lefaucheur C, Antoine C, Suberbielle C, Glotz D. Mastering the risk of HLA antibodies in kidney transplantation: an algorithm based on pretransplant single-antigen flow bead techniques. Am J Transplant. 2011;11(8):1592–8. PubMed PMID: 21668626. Epub 2011/06/15. eng.
36. Patel R, Terasaki PI. Significance of the positive crossmatch test in kidney transplantation. N Engl J Med. 1969;280(14):735–9. PubMed PMID: 4886455. Epub 1969/04/03. eng.
37. Amos DB, Bashir H, Boyle W, MacQueen M, Tiilikainen A. A simple micro cytotoxicity test. Transplantation. 1969;7(3):220–3.
38. Ting A, Hasegawa T, Ferrone S, Reisfeld RA. Presensitization detected by sensitive crossmatch tests. Transplant Proc. 1973;5(1):813–7.
39. Fuller TC, Phelan D, Gebel HM, Rodey GE. Antigenic specificity of antibody reactive in the antiglobulin-augmented lymphocytotoxicity test. Transplantation. 1982;34(1):24–9.

40. Johnson AH, Rossen RD, Butler WT. Detection of alloantibodies using a sensitive antiglobulin microcytotoxicity test: identification of low levels of pre-formed antibodies in accelerated allograft rejection. Tissue Antigens. 1972;2(3):215–26.
41. Pellegrino MA, Belvedere M, Pellegrino AG, Ferrone S. B peripheral lymphocytes express more HLA antigens than T peripheral lymphocytes. Transplantation. 1978;25(2):93–5.
42. Garovoy MR, Rheinschmidt MA, Bigos M, Perkins H, Colombe B, Feduska N, et al. Flow cytometry analysis: high technology crossmatch technique facilitating transplantation. Transplant Proc. 1983;15:1939–44.
43. Iwaki Y, Cook DJ, Terasaki PI, Lau M, Terashita GY, Danovitch G, et al. Flow cytometry crossmatching in human cadaver kidney transplantation. Transplant Proc. 1987;19(1 Pt 1):764–6.
44. Lobo PI, Spencer CE, Stevenson WC, McCullough C, Pruett TL. The use of pronase-digested human leukocytes to improve specificity of the flow cytometric crossmatch. Transpl Int. 1995;8(6):472–80.
45. Vaidya S, Cooper TY, Avandsalehi J, Barnes T, Brooks K, Hymel P, et al. Improved flow cytometric detection of HLA alloantibodies using pronase: potential implications in renal transplantation. Transplantation. 2001;71(3):422–8.
46. Groth J, Schonemann C, Kaden J, May G. Dynamics of donor-reactive IgG, IgA and IgM antibodies against T and B lymphocytes early after clinical kidney transplantation using flow cytometry. Transplant Immunol. 1996;4(3):215–9.
47. Roelen DL, van Bree J, Witvliet MD, Habraken I, van Beelen E, van't Sant PH, et al. IgG antibodies against an HLA antigen are associated with activated cytotoxic T cells against this antigen IgM are not. Transplantation. 1994;57(9):1388–92.
48. Reddy KS, Clark KR, Cavanagh G, Forsythe JL, Proud G, Taylor RM. Successful renal transplantation with a positive T-cell cross match caused by IgM antibodies. Transplant Proc. 1995;27(1):1042–3.
49. Kosmoliaptsis V, O'Rourke C, Bradley JA, Taylor CJ. Improved Luminex-based human leukocyte antigen-specific antibody screening using dithiothreitol-treated sera. Hum Immunol. 2010;71(1):45–9. PubMed PMID: 19808074. Epub 2009/10/08. eng.
50. Mizutani K, Shih RNJ, Pei R, Lee J, Ozawa M, Terasaki P. MICA and MICB antibodies in patients who rejected kidney transplants. Hum Immunol. 2003;64(10 Suppl):S79.
51. Zou Y, Heinemann FM, Grosse-Wilde H, Sireci G, Wang Z, Lavingia B, et al. Detection of anti-MICA antibodies in patients awaiting kidney transplantation, during the post-transplant course, and in eluates from rejected kidney allografts by Luminex flow cytometry. Hum Immunol. 2006;67(3):230–7. PubMed PMID: 16698447. Epub 2006/05/16. eng.
52. Alheim M, Johansson SM, Hauzenberger D, Grufman P, Holgersson J. A flow cytometric crossmatch test for simultaneous detection of antibodies against donor lymphocytes and endothelial precursor cells. Tissue Antigens. 2010;75:269–77.
53. Zou Y, Stastny P. Screening for antibodies against MICA by Luminex flow cytometry. Methods Mol Biol. 2012;882:279–88.
54. Zou Y, Stastny P, Susal C, Dohler B, Opelz G. Antibodies against MICA antigens and kidney-transplant rejection. N Engl J Med. 2007;357(13):1293–300. PubMed PMID: 17898098. Epub 2007/09/28. eng.
55. House AA, Chang PC, Luke PP, Leckie SH, Howson WT, Ball EJ, et al. Re-exposure to mismatched HLA class I is a significant risk factor for graft loss: multivariable analysis of 259 kidney retransplants. Transplantation. 2007;84(6):722–8.
56. Singh N, Djamali A, Lorentzen D, Pirsch JD, Leverson G, Neidlinger N, et al. Pretransplant donor-specific antibodies detected by single-antigen bead flow cytometry are associated with inferior kidney transplant outcomes. Transplantation. 2010;90(10):1079–84.

3 Recipient Evaluation

Eliyahu V. Khankin and Didier A. Mandelbrot

Abbreviations

CKD	Chronic kidney disease
CMV	Cytomegalovirus
EBV	Epstein–Barr virus
ECD	Expanded criteria donor
EKG	Electrocardiogram
ESRD	End-stage renal disease
FSGS	Focal segmental glomeruloscelrosis
HIV	Human immunodeficiency virus
PKD	Polycystic kidney disease
PSA	Prostate-specific antigen
SCD	Standard criteria donor
SPEP	Serum protein electrophoresis
UPEP	Urine protein electrophoresis

The Decision Between Transplantation and Dialysis: Risks and Benefits

Kidney transplantation is the treatment of choice for patients with ESRD [1]. Compared to dialysis, transplantation improves quality of life and reduces mortality [2] for most patients. However, some patients would not be expected to benefit from transplantation, so risks and benefits of transplantation versus dialysis should be carefully assessed before deciding on which modality of renal replacement therapy is best for an individual. Since mortality from kidney transplantation is increased compared to dialysis for the first few months after surgery [2], the decision to proceed with transplantation sometimes involves a trade-off between short-term risks and long-term benefits.

The success of transplantation has led to increased demand from patients, but the supply of organs has not increased nearly as quickly, producing a greater shortage of organs every year (OPTN/SRTR Annual report Tables 1.3, 1.6, 1.7 [3]). Given this limited resource, potential recipients must also be carefully evaluated to detect and treat coexisting illnesses, which may affect survival after transplantation.

Several published guidelines have addressed the process of evaluating a potential transplant recipient [4, 5]. Issues to address before transplant include surgical, medical, and psychosocial contraindications. Each category includes absolute as well as relative contraindications, and often further evaluation and treatment can resolve temporary contraindications before proceeding with transplant. In addition, individual patients and transplant programs may approach relative contraindications differently and not have the same tolerance for risk. This chapter focuses on medical issues, since other are addressed elsewhere in this book.

The initial evaluation should also consider a recipient's options for the source of an organ and the expected waiting times for each source, since the timing of transplantation may have a substantial impact on its benefits, especially in the elderly.

The Medical Evaluation

All patients undergoing evaluation for kidney transplantation should undergo a thorough history, physical, and laboratory examination. Particular attention should be devoted to areas related to decision making about transplantation, including cardiovascular disease, infections, malignancies, and recurrent renal disease. The laboratory evaluation (Table 3.1) includes a complete blood count, full chemistry panel, PT/PTT, and testing for infectious diseases. In addition, tissue typing is performed, including evaluation of blood group, HLA type, as well as anti- HLA antibody levels. Patients should undergo chest X-ray and EKG, further cardiac testing

E.V. Khankin • D.A. Mandelbrot (✉)
Department of Medicine, The Transplant Center, Beth Israel Deaconess Medical Center, 110 Francis Street, Boston, MA 02215, USA
e-mail: dmandelb@bidmc.harvard.edu

M.R. Weir and E.V. Lerma (eds.), *Kidney Transplantation: Practical Guide to Management*, DOI 10.1007/978-1-4939-0342-9_3, © Springer Science+Business Media New York 2014

Table 3.1 Diagnostic testing

Required
Tissue typing
Comprehensive metabolic panel
Complete blood count, PT/PTT/INR
Serologies: hepatitis B and C, HIV, RPR, CMV, EBV
Electrocardiogram
Chest X-ray
Recommended screening for colorectal, breast, cervical, and prostate cancer
In selected patients
Dental evaluation if poor dentition
Dermatology evaluation if suspicious lesions
Testing for TB (PPD or interferon release assay) if prior exposure
Renal imaging if high risk for malignancy
Testing for parasitic and fungal disease if prior exposure

is often needed, as detailed elsewhere. Particular attention should be paid to testing for infections and malignancies, as detailed below.

Cardiovascular Disease

Cardiovascular disease is the leading cause of death for both dialysis and renal transplant patients [6, 7]. Much of the survival benefit of transplantation is likely due to the long-term reduction in cardiac stress resulting from dialysis [2]. However, many patients with chronic kidney disease (CKD) have such severe cardiovascular disease that perioperative mortality precludes transplantation. As a result, cardiovascular disease is the most common reason for disqualifying a patient for transplantation [8]. While assessing the risk, it is important to remember that the presence of renal failure makes the perioperative evaluation and risk stratification of these patients different from general population [9]. The details of cardiovascular testing and therapy are discussed in Chap. 10.

Before proceeding with transplantation on a patient at elevated risk for cardiovascular disease, such as diabetics, smokers, the elderly, and those on dialysis for a long time, noninvasive cardiac testing should be performed. Patients with positive findings usually require coronary angiography to determine the extent of coronary disease and perform therapeutic interventions. While the trend in general cardiology is for decreased invasive testing and percutaneous coronary interventions [10], especially for asymptomatic patients, the approach to pre-transplant cardiac evaluation is often more aggressive. In part, this is due to the high rate of CKD patients who are diabetics and might have silent ischemia, and patients who have minimal physical activity, so may not report symptoms. In patients at particularly high cardiovascular risk, some advocate proceeding with cardiac catheterization as "first-line" screening test [7]. Once treatable causes of cardiac disease have been addressed, patients should be advised about their perioperative risk of heart attack and death. This risk assessment often requires the input of a cardiology consultant [11].

Many CKD patients are also at increased risk for cerebrovascular disease, but no data demonstrates a benefit of routine screening for cerebrovascular disease in asymptomatic transplant candidates. However, patients with a history of stroke or transient ischemic attack (TIA) should have imaging of their carotid arteries and be counseled about the risk of peri-transplant stroke. Peripheral vascular disease (PVD) is also an important part of the pre-transplant evaluation. PVD increases the risk of infections and can cause technical difficulties in the creation of the arterial anastomosis and hypoperfusion of the graft. In addition, a steal syndrome has been described, in which perfusion of the graft reduces distal flow sufficiently to cause or worsen limb ischemia [12]. In those with known PVD, CT scans can demonstrate the location of vascular calcifications, but angiography may be required to accurately delineate the arterial anatomy and flow. Groups at high risk for PVD, including diabetics, smokers, and the elderly, as well as those with symptoms of claudication, should be considered for noninvasive peripheral artery testing and vascular surgery consultation.

Cigarette smoking has been shown to contribute to graft loss and death, so cessation of smoking should be advised and facilitated with available resources [13]. Some programs will deny transplantation to patients who refuse to quit smoking, while others only deny transplantation to smokers with known cardiovascular or lung disease. Smoking cessation is an undeniable benefit to patients, but those who are unable to quit are potentially denied a life-prolonging organ if smoking cessation is required; many programs will strongly encourage cessation, but do not make it an absolute requirement.

Infections

Infections are the second most common cause of death for ESRD patients [14] and may worsen with immunosuppression at the time of the transplantation. Pre-transplant evaluation should therefore include the diagnosis and treatment of any ongoing infections. Transplantation may have to be delayed until an acute infection, such as a wound infection, can be fully resolved. Infections that cannot be resolved, such as chronic osteomyelitis, are usually a contraindication to transplantation. In some cases, such an HIV, the infection was previously considered an absolute contraindication to transplantation, but more recent studies [15] demonstrate that with good control of the infection, even without a cure, transplantation can be safely performed.

The pre-transplant evaluation is an important time to ensure completeness of immunizations. Vaccine response rates are significantly reduced by immunosuppression after transplant, and live vaccines are not safe to administer to immunosuppressed patients. Vaccines, which must be administered regularly, such as tetanus and pneumococcus, should be updated. For other vaccinations, immune status can be evaluated so that vaccination can be performed as needed. Required serological screening includes hepatitis B, hepatitis C, HIV, RPR, CMV, and EBV. This testing can detect lack of immune status, which requires vaccination, for example, for hepatitis B. It can also detect infections that may be treatable, such as hepatitis B or C. CMV and EBV screening are mostly relevant for posttransplant management. Consideration should also be given to screening for hepatitis A, measles, mumps, rubella and varicella and vaccinating those who are not immune.

A number of latent infections such as TB are usually asymptomatic in a patient with CKD, but can become severe infections after immunosuppression for transplantation. Although low-risk patients may not need screening, a careful exposure history and CXR should be reviewed, and a low threshold should exist for performing further testing, such as a PPD or interferon release assay (such as Quantiferon Gold). Potential exposure history should also prompt testing and appropriate treatment for parasitic infections such as strongyloides and endemic mycoses such as histoplasmosis and coccidiomycosis [16]. Many insurance companies require a formal dental evaluation in all pre-transplant patients to rule out occult abscess, and certainly patients with possible mouth lesions or no recent dental care should see a dentist before transplantation.

Malignancies

Malignancy is more common in patients with ESRD than the general population, so detection of malignancies and reduction of risk factors for cancer are an important part of the pre-transplant evaluation. In addition, immunosuppression increases the risk of cancers [17] and existing malignancies can follow a more aggressive course. For example, squamous cell carcinoma is 20 times more common in transplant recipients than the general population and is more likely to metastasize [18]. There are two main mechanisms by which immunosuppressive medications increase the risk for and severity of malignancies. The first is that immune surveillance for newly arising tumor antigens is impaired. The second is that infections are more common in immunosuppressed patients, and a number of infections are the direct cause of malignancies, such as Kaposi's sarcoma and EBV-driven posttransplant lymphomas.

Because of the increased cancer risk from immunosuppression, ongoing malignancy is usually a contraindication to proceeding with transplantation. However, many patients that have been successfully treated for cancer are suitable

Table 3.2 Minimum waiting time for transplantation after malignancy

Malignancy	Minimum waiting time
Renal cell carcinoma	Symptomatic <5 cm—2 years
	Symptomatic >5 cm—5 years
	Incidental, no capsule penetration—none
Bladder cancer	Invasive bladder cancer—2 years
	In situ/noninvasive—none
Cervical cancer	5 years (may be 2 years for low grade)
Uterine body	2 years
Testicular cancer	2 years
Thyroid cancer	2 years
Sarcomas	5 years (may be 2 years for low grade)
Breast cancer	5 years (may be 2 years for low grade)
Colorectal cancer	5 years (may be 2 years for low grade)
Prostate cancer	2 years
	Focal cancer—may not require waiting time
Multiple myeloma	Usually a contraindication to transplant
Lymphomas	5 years (may be 2 years)
Skin cancer	Basal cell—none
	Localized squamous cell—2 years
	Malignant melanoma—5 years
Lung cancer	2 years

candidates. Published guidelines [4] provide suggestions as to appropriate time to wait between cancer cure and transplantation. In addition, detailed information about a specific patient can be obtained by querying the Israel Penn International Transplant Tumor Registry (IPITTR) formerly known as Cincinnati Transplant Tumor Registry (CTTR). In making a decision regarding the waiting time, the risk of recurrence must be balanced with overall benefits from the transplant. The goal of this waiting period is to ensure that early recurrence is detected before proceeding with transplantation, but later recurrence is always a possibility. In general, a minimal time of 2 years is recommended for most malignancies, with exception of localized and in situ malignancies, which do not require waiting time. A 5-year wait is often recommended for malignancies with higher later recurrence risk, such as metastatic or large tumors.

Recommendations regarding waiting time after selected malignancies are summarized in Table 3.2.

The evaluation should focus on malignancies relevant to the patient's gender, age, environmental exposures, and family history. This might include a pelvic exam and Pap smear, breast exam and mammography for women, digital rectal exam and PSA for men, and colorectal screening. Guidelines for cancer screening change over time, and thorough review of evidence-based workup is available elsewhere [19]. In addition, given the dramatically increased incidence of skin cancer after transplantation, we recommend dermatologist evaluation in anyone with questionable skin lesions. The dialysis population has a particularly high risk for cancer of the kidney and urinary tract, especially when ESRD is a result of toxic, infectious, or cystic process [20]. Screening individual patients for renal and urinary tract malignancies with a CT scan should be considered, especially if appropriate history or symptoms are present. Serum protein electrophoresis (SPEP) and urine protein electrophoresis (UPEP) should also be considered, particularly in older patients in whom the cause of kidney disease is unclear, such as those labeled as hypertension. While MGUS is usually not a contraindication to transplantation, multiple myeloma usually is.

Recurrent Disease in the Graft

While knowing the cause of kidney failure is not always essential for providing optimal ESRD care, establishing this cause can be critical in pre-transplant counseling. Some kidney diseases, such as PKD, never recur in transplants, so such patients can be reassured. In contrast, diabetes, which is the most common cause of ESRD in the United States, has a high likelihood of recurrence, although rarely causes early graft failure. Diabetics should be informed of this and the fact that pancreas transplantation of type I diabetics can prevent recurrent diabetic nephropathy. Despite this risk of recurrence, diabetics represent the group of patients that derives the greatest survival benefit from transplantation compared to dialysis [2]. Glomerular diseases have different rates of recurrence, and episodes of recurrence have different rates of graft failure. For example, primary FSGS recurs in approximately 40 % of patients, leading to graft failure in close to 50 % of these recurrences. Patients with recurrent FSGS in a first kidney transplant have an approximately 70 % risk of recurrence in a second graft [21–23]. Recurrent IgA nephropathy, if defined as IgA predominant staining on biopsy, occurs in about 50 % of cases, but is much less likely to cause graft failure than is FSGS. With rare exceptions such as primary oxalosis, which inevitably recur and cause graft failure, the risk of recurrent disease does not preclude transplantation. However, repeat transplantation of a patient who lost a first graft to recurrent FSGS should only be performed with careful informed consent.

Additional Medical Considerations

Patients with a life expectancy of less than 2 years should generally not undergo transplantation. This category includes untreatable malignancy, uncontrolled infection, and severe and irreversible extrarenal conditions. End-stage diseases of the heart, lung, or liver are all absolute contraindications to renal transplant alone. However, in these patients, combined transplantation of the effect organ and a kidney may be considered. Cardiovascular disease is unique in this context, as cardiac function can be shown to improve with kidney transplantation [24]. With moderate heart disease, in which heart transplantation is not a consideration, the short-term risk of perioperative death or heart attack must be balanced against long-term survival benefits. Similarly, the presence of moderate lung or liver disease, in which transplantation of those organs is not considered, may increase the patient's mortality, but this must be balanced against the mortality reduction benefit as a result of receiving a transplant rather than being on dialysis.

Given the continued increase in obesity rates in the United States, overweight transplant candidates are common. Obesity in renal transplant recipients increases the risk of wound complications [25] and probably slightly reduces graft survival [26]. Obesity also increases the risk of cardiovascular disease. BMI is commonly used to assess obesity, and weight loss should be encouraged and facilitated in those with a BMI over 30, which defines obesity. Different cutoffs, such as 35 or 40, are used by different programs as absolute contraindications to transplantation [27]. However, some flexibility in interpreting BMI is required, since some patients may be extremely broad boned and muscular, while others may have disproportionate volume of abdominal fat. Abdominal circumference may be helpful in distinguishing these types, but this measurement is poorly standardized, so a subjective assessment is usually relied upon. Bariatric surgery is sometimes recommended for those who are particularly heavy and unable to lose weight.

Psychosocial Evaluation

The psychosocial evaluation is an important part of the pretransplant evaluation, since these nonmedical factors can have an important impact on graft survival. Patients with unstable psychiatric disease or home situations are at increased risk of graft loss, which can leave them worse off than if they had never been transplanted. In addition to wasting a precious organ, the patients may have to undergo a second surgery to remove the kidney and will be exposed to the side effects of immunosuppression and risks being sensitized, making future transplant more difficult.

Patients with a history of psychiatric disease, such as depression or schizophrenia, should be evaluated by a specialist, to ensure that the disease is well controlled before proceeding with transplantation and that follow-up care is adequate. Active drug abuse, especially of nephrotoxins such as cocaine and heroin, is an absolute contraindication to transplantation; however, successful treatment of drug abuse may permit future transplantation. Homelessness, a volatile home environment, and other significant social stressors should also be addressed before transplantation, since the postoperative period requires frequent and high-quality communication between the patient and transplant center.

Future adherence of candidates after transplantation is often difficult to predict, but previous poor adherence, especially with a prior transplant, should be carefully assessed. Risk factors such as missed physician and dialysis appointments and medication nonadherence should be corrected or explained before proceeding with transplant.

Kidney Sources

A discussion about different possible sources of organs, and the expected waiting times for each, is an essential part of the pre-transplant evaluation. This discussion can effect decisions as to whether or not to list someone at all, since an elderly candidate with no potential living donors, in a region with long waiting times, may not want to bother going through the steps of the transplant evaluation. In addition, the discussion can affect decisions about dialysis access, since a patient with no potential donors will likely need early creation of an arteriovenous fistula, while someone with many eligible living donors may never need any dialysis access because they undergo preemptive transplantation.

The benefits of receiving a live donor versus deceased donor kidney, including shorter wait times and longer graft survival, should be emphasized to all candidates for transplantation. Promoting living donation benefits both the individual recipient and the wait-listed population, since one less person needs to receive a deceased donor kidney. Candidates often require support and advice in looking for a live donor and should understand that live donors do not need to be genetically related. Potential transplant recipients should also understand that ABO or HLA incompatibilities do not necessarily preclude transplantation, since paired live donor exchange and desensitization programs are available [28, 29].

If living donation is not an option, candidates also need to decide whether they wish to be listed only for a standard criteria donor (SCD) kidney, or also be placed on the list for an extended criteria donor (ECD) kidney. The details of these types of kidneys are discussed in Chap. 9, but recipients must understand that ECD kidneys will provide shorter graft survival, but substantially reduce waiting times for transplantation. Young, healthy patients are generally not considered for ECD transplantation, unless dialysis is very poorly tolerated. Listing for ECD kidneys is usually recommended for those who are expected to decline more rapidly during upcoming years on dialysis, such as diabetics and older candidates. In these patients, ECD transplantation can be shown to improve patient survival [30].

Candidates waiting for deceased donor transplantation may eventually be asked to consider accepting a CDC high-risk kidney, so discussing this possibility ahead of time is also useful. Patients must understand that careful testing of deceased donors reduces the risk of infection to extremely low levels, but that risk can never be completely eliminated. They should understand that a CDC high-risk donor may have a higher risk of transmitting infection, but that accepting such a kidney can also significantly shorten waiting times.

Transplantation of organs from a donor who has hepatitis C is relatively rare. However, potential recipients who have hepatitis C and are not candidates for successful treatment of hepatitis C may be able to dramatically reduce their waiting time for deceased donor transplantation by accepting a hepatitis C-positive donor.

Timing of Transplant

Several studies have shown that graft and patient outcomes are better if kidney transplantation is performed earlier, before patients spend a prolonged time on dialysis [31]. Preemptive transplantation allows patients to avoid dialysis altogether and has the additional benefit of avoiding placement of dialysis access. Given the long waiting times that are typical for deceased donor transplantation, preemptive transplantation usually requires the availability of a live donor. The benefits of early transplantation sometimes have to be balanced against the risk of transplanting too soon and prematurely exposing the recipient to the risks of surgery and immunosuppression. In the fortunate situation where both donor and recipient are ready for transplant, we usually follow the recipient closely for the development of uremic symptoms or electrolyte abnormalities and then proceed expeditiously with transplant.

Conclusions

Much of the evaluation of a potential kidney transplant recipient can be described as an art rather than a science. Many candidates could be described as borderline, based on factors such as age and comorbidities, as there is limited data to guide the decision as to whether transplantation or dialysis would best serve a specific candidate. Nevertheless, we believe that the first principle to consider in evaluating a candidate is whether transplantation or dialysis is the best choice for that individual. The optimal allocation of organs that are a scarce resource is important and is the focus of the OPTN and other public health authorities. However, we believe that the scarcity of organs should only be a secondary consideration in the recipient evaluation, relevant only for those at highest risk. Restricting kidney transplants to young healthy individuals would shorten wait lists, but disadvantage large segments of the ESRD population.

The balance between risks and benefits is a cornerstone of the discussion with potential transplant recipients and should be addressed during the first session since some patients may decide not to proceed with the evaluation due to the risks.

References

1. Suthanthiran M, Strom TB. Renal transplantation. N Engl J Med. 1994;331(6):365–76. PubMed PMID: 7832839.
2. Wolfe RA, Ashby VB, Milford EL, Ojo AO, Ettenger RE, Agodoa LY, et al. Comparison of mortality in all patients on dialysis, patients on dialysis awaiting transplantation, and recipients of a first cadaveric transplant. N Engl J Med. 1999;341(23):1725–30. PubMed PMID: 10580071.
3. SRTR 2009 annual report (available at http://www.ustransplant.org/annual_reports/current/default.htm). 2009.
4. Kasiske BL, Cangro CB, Hariharan S, Hricik DE, Kerman RH, Roth D, et al. The evaluation of renal transplantation candidates: clinical practice guidelines. Am J Transplant. 2001;1 Suppl 2:3–95. PubMed PMID: 12108435.
5. EBPG (European Expert Group on Renal Transplantation), European Renal Association (ERA-EDTA), European Society for Organ Transplantation (ESOT). European Best Practice Guidelines for Renal Transplantation (part 1). Nephrol Dial Transplant. 2000;15 Suppl 7:1–85.
6. Hildreth CM. Prognostic indicators of cardiovascular risk in renal disease. Front Physiol. 2011;2:121. PubMed PMID: 22294981. Pubmed Central PMCID: 3257971.
7. Karthikeyan V, Ananthasubramaniam K. Coronary risk assessment and management options in chronic kidney disease patients prior to kidney transplantation. Curr Cardiol Rev. 2009;5(3):177–86. PubMed PMID: 20676276. Pubmed Central PMCID: 2822140.
8. Holley JL, Monaghan J, Byer B, Bronsther O. An examination of the renal transplant evaluation process focusing on cost and the reasons for patient exclusion. Am J Kidney Dis. 1998;32(4):567–74. PubMed PMID: 9774116.
9. Kasiske BL, Ramos EL, Gaston RS, Bia MJ, Danovitch GM, Bowen PA, et al. The evaluation of renal transplant candidates: clinical practice guidelines.. Patient Care and Education Committee of the American Society of Transplant Physicians. J Am Soc Nephrol. 1995;6(1):1–34. PubMed PMID: 7579061.
10. Fleisher LA, Beckman JA, Brown KA, Calkins H, Chaikof E, Fleischmann KE, et al. ACC/AHA 2007 guidelines on perioperative cardiovascular evaluation and care for noncardiac surgery: Executive summary: A report of the American College of Cardiology/American Heart Association Task Force on Practice Guidelines (Writing Committee to Revise the 2002 Guidelines on Perioperative Cardiovascular Evaluation for Noncardiac Surgery): Developed in Collaboration With the American Society of Echocardiography, American Society of Nuclear Cardiology, Heart Rhythm Society, Society of Cardiovascular Anesthesiologists, Society for Cardiovascular Angiography and Interventions, Society for Vascular Medicine and Biology, and Society for Vascular Surgery. Circulation. 2007;116(17):1971–96. PubMed PMID: 17901356.
11. Lentine KL, Costa SP, Weir MR, Robb JF, Fleisher LA, Kasiske BL, et al. Cardiac disease evaluation and management among kidney and liver transplantation candidates: a scientific statement from the American Heart Association and the American College of Cardiology Foundation. J Am Coll Cardiol. 2012;60(5):434–80. PubMed PMID: 22763103. Epub 2012/07/06. eng.
12. Goldsmith PJ, Fraser SM, Fitzpatrick M, Scott DJ, Ahmad N. Acute lower limb ischemia following pediatric renal transplantation. Pediatr Transplant. 2010;14(7):E93–5. PubMed PMID: 19496979. Epub 2009/06/06. eng.
13. Sung RS, Althoen M, Howell TA, Ojo AO, Merion RM. Excess risk of renal allograft loss associated with cigarette smoking. Transplantation. 2001;71(12):1752–7. PubMed PMID: 11455254.
14. Dalrymple LS, Go AS. Epidemiology of acute infections among patients with chronic kidney disease. Clin J Am Soc Nephrol. 2008;3(5):1487–93. PubMed PMID: 18650409.
15. Stock PG, Barin B, Murphy B, Hanto D, Diego JM, Light J, et al. Outcomes of kidney transplantation in HIV-infected recipients. New Engl J Med. 2010;363(21):2004–14. PubMed PMID: 21083386. Pubmed Central PMCID: 3028983.
16. Avery RK. Prophylactic strategies before solid-organ transplantation. Curr Opin Infect Dis. 2004;17(4):353–6. PubMed PMID: 15241081.
17. Martinez OM, de Gruijl FR. Molecular and immunologic mechanisms of cancer pathogenesis in solid organ transplant recipients. Am J Transplant. 2008;8(11):2205–11. PubMed PMID: 18801025.
18. Vajdic CM, van Leeuwen MT, McDonald SP, McCredie MR, Law M, Chapman JR, et al. Increased incidence of squamous cell carcinoma of eye after kidney transplantation. J Natl Cancer Inst. 2007;99(17):1340–2. PubMed PMID: 17698951. Epub 2007/08/19. eng.
19. Wong G, Chapman JR, Craig JC. Cancer screening in renal transplant recipients: what is the evidence? Clin J Am Soc Nephrol. 2008;3 Suppl 2:S87–S100. PubMed PMID: 18309007. Pubmed Central PMCID: 3152279.
20. Stewart JH, Buccianti G, Agodoa L, Gellert R, McCredie MR, Lowenfels AB, et al. Cancers of the kidney and urinary tract in patients on dialysis for end-stage renal disease: analysis of data from the United States, Europe, and Australia and New Zealand. J Am Soc Nephrol. 2003;14(1):197–207. PubMed PMID: 12506152.
21. Striegel JE, Sibley RK, Fryd DS, Mauer SM. Recurrence of focal segmental sclerosis in children following renal transplantation. Kidney Int Suppl. 1986;19:S44–50. PubMed PMID: 3528625.
22. Lewis EJ. Recurrent focal sclerosis after renal transplantation. Kidney Int. 1982;22(3):315–23. PubMed PMID: 6757526.
23. Newstead CG. Recurrent disease in renal transplants. Nephrol Dial Transplant. 2003;18 Suppl 6:vi68–74. PubMed PMID: 12953046.
24. Wali RK, Wang GS, Gottlieb SS, Bellumkonda L, Hansalia R, Ramos E, et al. Effect of kidney transplantation on left ventricular systolic dysfunction and congestive heart failure in patients with end-stage renal disease. J Am Coll Cardiol. 2005;45(7):1051–60. PubMed PMID: 15808763. Epub 2005/04/06. eng.
25. Bunnapradist S, Danovitch GM. Evaluation of adult kidney transplant candidates. Am J Kidney Dis. 2007;50(5):890–8. PubMed PMID: 17954303.
26. Halme L, Eklund B, Kyllonen L, Salmela K. Is obesity still a risk factor in renal transplantation? Transpl Int. 1997;10(4):284–8. PubMed PMID: 9249938.
27. Scandling JD. Kidney transplant candidate evaluation. Semin Dial. 2005;18(6):487–94. PubMed PMID: 16398711.
28. Bohmig GA, Wahrmann M, Bartel G. Transplantation of the broadly sensitized patient: what are the options? Curr Opin Org Transplant. 2011;16(6):588–93. PubMed PMID: 21971512.
29. Montgomery RA, Lonze BE, Jackson AM. Using donor exchange paradigms with desensitization to enhance transplant rates among highly sensitized patients. Curr Opin Org Transplant. 2011;16(4):439–43. PubMed PMID: 21666478.
30. Merion RM, Ashby VB, Wolfe RA, Distant DA, Hulbert-Shearon TE, Metzger RA, et al. Deceased-donor characteristics and the survival benefit of kidney transplantation. JAMA. 2005;294(21):2726–33. PubMed PMID: 16333008.
31. Meier-Kriesche HU, Kaplan B. Waiting time on dialysis as the strongest modifiable risk factor for renal transplant outcomes: a paired donor kidney analysis. Transplantation. 2002;74(10):1377–81. PubMed PMID: 12451234.

4 Wait List Management

John J. Friedewald, Darshika Chhabra, and Baris Ata

Abbreviations

CDC	Centers for Disease Control and Prevention
CPRAs	Calculated panel reactive antibodies
DCD	Donation after cardiac death
DSA	Donor service area
ECD	Expanded criteria donors
eGFR	Estimated glomerular filtration rate
EPTS	Estimated posttransplant survival
HLA	Human leukocyte antigen
KDPI	Kidney donor profile index
MPSC	Membership and Professional Standards Committee
NOTA	National Organ Transplant Act
OPO	Organ procurement organization
OPTN	Organ Procurement and Transplantation Network
PRA	Panel reactive antibodies
PSR	Program-specific reports
SCD	Standard criteria donor
SRTR	Scientific Registry of Transplant Recipients
UNOS	United Network for Organ Sharing
WIP	Work-in-progress

J.J. Friedewald, M.D. (✉)
Northwestern University Feinberg School of Medicine,
676 N. St. Clair, Arkes Pavilion 1900, Chicago, IL 60611, USA
e-mail: jfriedew@nmh.org

D. Chhabra, M.D., M.P.H.
Kidney Transplant Program, Advocate Christ Medical Center,
Department of Medicine, Section of Nephrology,
University of Illinois at Chicago, 4400 W 95th Street, Suite 112,
Oak Lawn, IL 60453, USA
e-mail: darshika.chhabra@advocatehealth.com

B. Ata
Booth School of Business, The University of Chicago,
5807 South Woodlawn Ave, Chicago, IL 60637, USA
e-mail: Baris.Ata@chicagobooth.edu

Background

The US Transplant System

The transplant system consists of a large network of transplant centers, organ procurement organizations (OPO), and donor hospitals. The Organ Procurement and Transplantation Network (OPTN) is the unified transplant network established by the US Congress under the National Organ Transplant Act (NOTA) of 1984. The OPTN links all professionals involved in organ donation and transplantation. United Network for Organ Sharing (UNOS), a private nonprofit organization, administers the OPTN under contract with the Health Resources and Services Administration of the US Department of Health and Human Services. Every transplant center and OPO is a member of UNOS. For ease of administration, UNOS has established 11 geographic regions that are further subdivided into local donor service areas (DSAs).

National Wait List

Transplant candidates waiting for a kidney transplant from a deceased donor are registered on a national transplant waiting list. UNOS maintains this list in the United States and matches donors to recipients. Each transplant center's waiting list is part of this national list. In 2011, 35,013 new registrations were added to the list (based on OPTN data as of September 11, 2012). This list encompasses patients who are both active and inactive (Status 7). Inactive patients consist of candidates who are temporarily unable to receive a transplant due to medical, social, or other conditions. During this period, patients do accrue waiting time; however, only the active patients are allocated organs. Most of the explosive growth in the waiting list has been among candidates listed as inactive, as shown in Fig. 4.1.

M.R. Weir and E.V. Lerma (eds.), *Kidney Transplantation: Practical Guide to Management*,
DOI 10.1007/978-1-4939-0342-9_4,

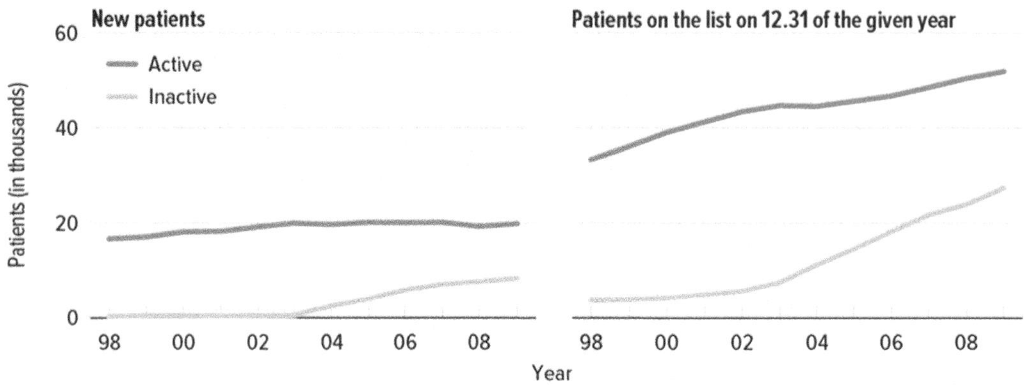

Fig. 4.1 United Network for Organ Sharing national kidney wait list additions and composition by active status

Facts and Figures

Since UNOS began keeping records in 1987, over 500,000 organ transplants have been performed in the United States. More than 28,000 recipients receive lifesaving organ transplants each year. As of early June 2012, over 92,000 patients were registered with UNOS on the kidney transplant wait list. In 2011, 16,814 kidney transplants were performed, which included 11,043 from deceased donors (based on OPTN data as of May 25, 2012).

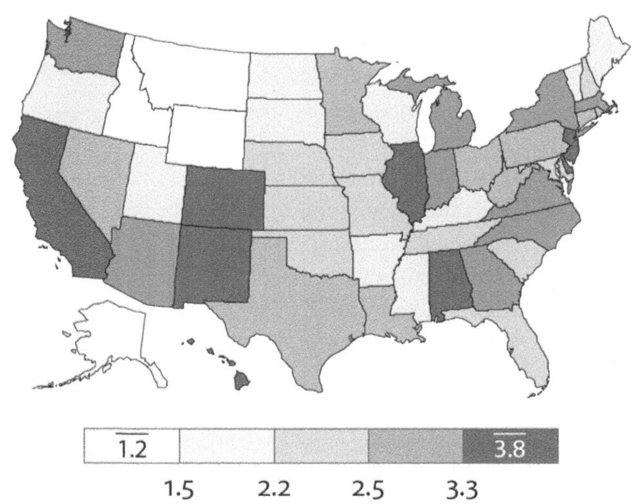

Fig. 4.2 Unadjusted median wait times in years for adults transplanted in 2009, by state of transplant center [1]

Wait Times

Because deceased donor kidney allocation is prioritized locally, the median wait time for kidney transplant varies across the country (Fig. 4.2) [1]. Efforts to equalize wait time across geographic regions have been met with both logistical and political resistance. The median wait time in 2009 was 2.3 years [1]. This varies by blood type, with blood groups O and B patients waiting the longest (5 and 6 years, respectively) compared to 1 and 3 years for blood types AB and A, respectively [2]. Wait time for Caucasians is about 40 % less than other races. Sensitized patients (i.e., patients who have anti-HLA antibodies as a result of blood transfusions, pregnancy, or prior transplants) may wait longer than patients who have low level of antibodies (PRA or panel reactive antibodies).

Kidney Allocation

Kidneys are allocated on a local, regional, and national level. When possible, kidneys are offered locally first to minimize organ preservation time, which is associated with better graft survival. The exception is sensitized recipients of zero human leukocyte antigen (HLA)-mismatched kidneys who are given priority to these close biological matches. Blood type, HLA matching, degree of sensitization, pediatric recipients, and time waiting on the list are factors taken into account in UNOS' computer-based network for allocating donated organs. Every organ sharing institution is electronically linked via this secure, real-time environment over the internet so that donated organs can be placed as efficiently and as quickly as possible.

Point System for Kidney Allocation

The 1984 NOTA mandates that organ allocation take into account both efficiency (graft and patient survival) and equity (fair distribution) [3]. The allocation system was designed to balance fairness with medical utility and improved organ survival. Potential recipients receive one point for each year they wait on the list. A few regions that have an approved variance in allocation define wait time as the time since initiating dialysis. Extra points are awarded to patients who are broadly sensitized (more than 80 % panel reactive antibody level and a negative crossmatch) and to pediatric patients. The system also includes points for better HLA-DR-matched recipients to promote longer graft survival, thereby promoting improved organ utility.

Listing Practices

Potential recipients undergo an evaluation to determine their candidacy for kidney transplantation and once listed, they may be required to undergo periodic testing. The evaluation process strives to identify patients who may benefit the most from transplantation, separating them from patients who may be placed at risk. Policies may vary between transplant centers within a region and across the country. Listing practices take into account median wait times and allocation variances within the region, as well as list size, while optimizing resource utilization. Some centers perform an intensive evaluation up front, which may delay time to listing. Others prefer to list with minimal or no workup and complete the evaluation later. For example, cardiac workup for low- or moderate-risk candidates at initial listing may not be required in an OPO with lengthy median wait times. However, this depends on predictability within the OPO and does not take into account zero antigen mismatch offers.

Acceptance Criteria

Acceptance criteria at a given transplant center will vary based on a number of factors and are often subjective. The risk tolerance of the transplant center and clinicians is an important factor here. This is also one of the major system points where patient preference comes into play. Of particular relevance are ECD and CDC increased-risk organs. Because the transplant center must convey a relative risk to a potential recipient when making the offer, acceptance often depends on how the information is conveyed and in what context. As an example, for a very highly sensitized candidate, a CDC increased-risk donor organ with which they are compatible often represents their best chance at improving their overall survival compared to staying on maintenance dialysis. Informed consent is critical in these instances and quite challenging when taking into account levels of literacy and numeracy in candidates trying to grasp concepts that often challenge transplant professionals. Developing and periodically updating protocols for guidance can help keep acceptance patterns in line with the overall goals of the transplant center.

Acceptance criteria can also be affected by external factors. Transplant centers are monitored on their performance, specifically short-term patient and graft survival. Program-specific reports (PSRs) are generated by the Scientific Registry of Transplant Recipients (SRTR) and reviewed by the Membership and Professional Standards Committee (MPSC) of UNOS. The PSRs are publically available and have been used by insurance providers, the lay press, and the general public to evaluate transplant center performance. There is ongoing debate about the accuracy of the formulae used to generate a center's expected outcomes, and there are initiatives at UNOS and the SRTR to improve on the methods of patient risk stratification that inform the PSRs. But currently, there is a very real disincentive for transplant centers to use high-risk organs. Poor short-term outcomes are not just harmful to patients but also can jeopardize the viability of a transplant center. The deceased donor transplant system in the United States is plagued by a high rate of discarded organs, and beyond inefficiencies in the distribution system, many blame this institutional risk aversion for high discard rates. With so many candidates dying on the wait list, improving organ acceptance and utilization rates remains a vital task.

Lists Within the List

Centers may manage subgroups of patients within their list differently, e.g., patients consenting to expanded criteria donors (ECD), donation after cardiac death (DCD), and Centers for Disease Control and Prevention (CDC) increased-risk donors (donors exhibiting a behavior placing them at increased risk for HIV, hepatitis B and C). Patients with a lower life expectancy can anticipate a lesser absolute gain in life-years from transplantation. Mortality on the wait list has been reported to be around 6 % per year, as much as 10 % per year for diabetic patients, increasing with older age [4]. More effort and cost may be required to maintain older candidates with multiple comorbidities on the list. All these are factored into the complex algorithm of a center's listing, wait list maintenance, and acceptance criteria.

ECD Listing Variability

An extended criteria donor (ECD) kidney is a kidney from a deceased donor older than 60 years or between 50 and 59 years with any two of the following risk factors: history of hypertension, death from a cerebrovascular accident, or a terminal serum creatinine more than 1.5 mg/dL. Only patients who have previously consented to ECD kidneys are offered them. These kidneys are allocated based on wait time alone to increase predictability of which candidates will be at the top of

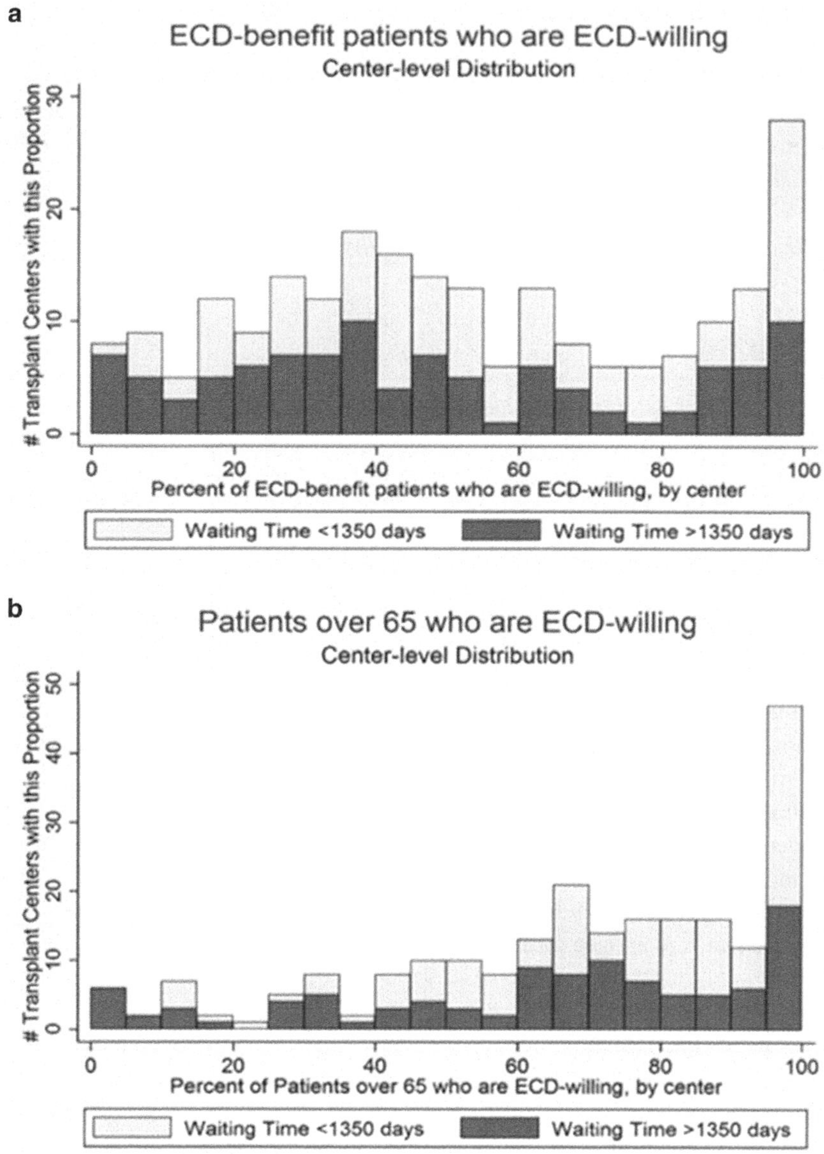

Fig. 4.3 Variability in extended criteria donor (ECD) listing by center [9]

the list. Compared to standard criteria donor (SCD) kidneys, ECD kidneys carry the benefit of a shorter wait time. Although these organs have a 1.7-fold or higher risk of graft loss compared with SCD organs [5], they still provide a survival advantage over maintenance dialysis [6]. It is critical to allocate these organs to patients who would most benefit from them, i.e., older adults, diabetics, and patients at centers with long waiting times [7]. Generally, younger patients stand to benefit more by waiting for an SCD kidney compared to older patients [8]. An exception to this may be an elderly patient who is in a region with relatively short wait times where it may be in their interest to wait longer for a higher quality organ. ECD listing practices vary significantly across the United States due to variation in risk tolerance, adherence to evidence-based practice, and the complexity involved (Fig. 4.3) [9].

Sensitized Patients

Sensitized patients (i.e., patients who have anti-HLA antibodies as a result of blood transfusions, pregnancy, or prior transplants) may wait twice as long as patients who have low level of PRA, as they are more likely to have positive crossmatch results. The virtual crossmatch or calculated PRA (CPRA) test identifies specific donor HLA antigens in the wait-listed recipient, and these are reported to UNOS if it is determined that they are likely to engender a positive crossmatch. To avoid unnecessary testing, expense, and loss of time, highly sensitized patients are not included in a match run if the donor possesses antigens against which the recipient has preformed antibody (virtual crossmatch), thereby increasing the probability of a negative final crossmatch.

Timing of Transplantation

Preemptive Transplants (Just-in-Time Theory)

There are numerous advantages to preemptive kidney transplantation (transplantation before dialysis) including a survival advantage [10]. However, there are concerns that preemptive transplantation performed too soon (at higher levels of estimated glomerular filtration rates, eGFR) may not translate into an added benefit to the recipients. Achieving "just-in-time" kidney transplantation with living donors is a challenge and more so with deceased donors. A candidate may be placed on the wait list and accrue points for waiting time once the eGFR is below 20 mL/min/1.73 m^2. The ability to receive a preemptive kidney transplant often hinges on early listing for transplant and local waiting times.

Reevaluation

As wait time for deceased donor organs continues to increase, the complexity of managing candidates for long periods of time on the wait list increases. This is coupled with an ever-aging pool of candidates that have more medical comorbidities. As an example, an elderly, diabetic candidate may need cardiac clearance prior to a transplant surgery event. However, with several years to wait, when does a transplant center perform this testing? And how often should it be repeated? These answers have implications for cost, transplant center staffing, patient convenience, and even patient safety when considering invasive testing. Different strategies evolve at individual transplant centers based on their milieu, including median wait time and candidate characteristics. One effective strategy at our center has been to generate a list of candidates nearing the top of each blood group on the wait list. Those patients are brought into a clinic for an examination and to order updated tests. Then, when an offer is made, the transplant team has recent knowledge of the health and readiness of that candidate.

Communication with the referring nephrologist or other provider is also more important than ever. With so many candidates inactive on the list, keeping their status accurate and managing intercurrent medical events can consume a large amount of time and resources for transplant center staff.

Multiple Listing

Without the prospect of a living donor, many candidates list in multiple DSAs to decrease their waiting time for transplant. Multiple listing requires the ability to travel and navigate the health care system, and so is not a reality for many patients. However, given the difficult and wide geographic disparities, multiple listing is still a good option for patients that are able to do so.

New Allocation System

UNOS has been involved in a long and comprehensive review of the kidney allocation process. Substantial resources have been applied to improving the current system. Unfortunately, over the last three decades, a disproportionate emphasis has been placed on wait time in the allocation of kidneys based simply on the massive growth of the list (Fig. 4.4). The proposed new system (still not approved at the time of writing this chapter) would strive to maintain access for all candidates, while trying to maximize outcomes from each kidney. To do this, a continuous scale, the kidney donor profile index (KDPI), will be used to replace the older, binary SCD/ECD classification of kidneys. The KPDI takes into account ten donor variables that better predict the relative risk of graft failure. The top 20 % of kidneys based on KDPI will be allocated first (but not exclusively) to candidates with the longest estimated posttransplant survival (EPTS). The EPTS is calculated based on four factors: age, time on dialysis, presence of diabetes, and previous transplant status. By allocating long lasting kidneys to the longest living candidates, we can realize many more graft years of life that are lost when recipients die with a functioning graft. This in turn will also decrease candidates returning to the wait list after graft failure, thus increasing transplant opportunities for others on the list. Candidates will continue to be rank ordered as they are currently based on waiting time, CPRA points (with a sliding scale of points for increasing CPRA), and HLA-DR matching.

Principles of Inventory Management and Applications to the Wait List

The workings of the transplant waiting list exhibits important similarities to that of the work-in-progress (WIP) inventory at a manufacturing plant. Therefore, the same core principles can guide the management of both. Managing the WIP inventory at a manufacturing plant aims at matching supply and demand, trying to eliminate any mismatch between the two. In the transplant system, the supply of organs is significantly lower than the demand for them. The objective is to reduce this imbalance and match the supply and demand, as in the case of manufacturing.

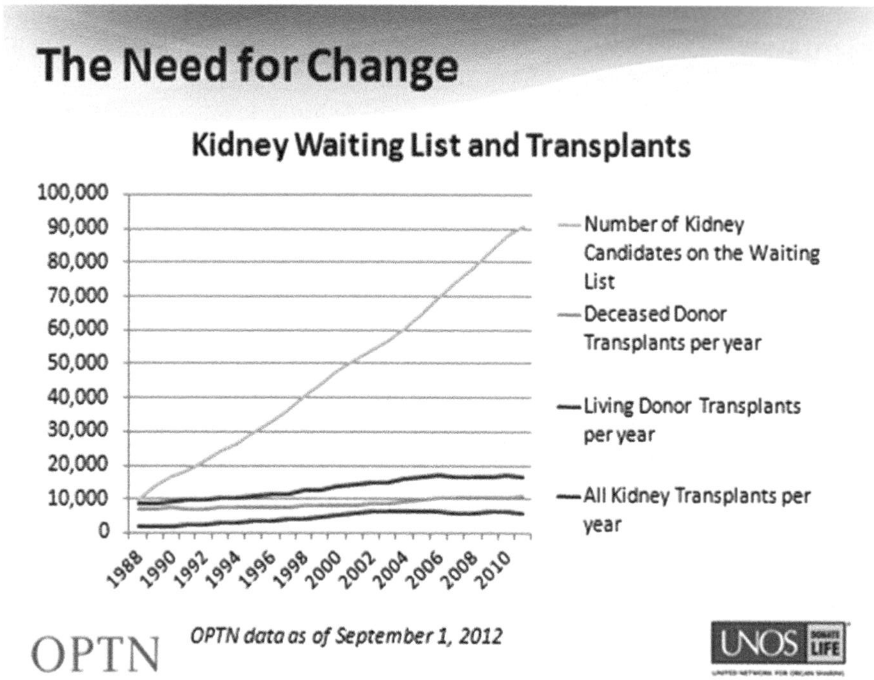

Fig. 4.4 Number of kidney transplant candidates on the waiting list and number of transplants performed per year

A key metric widely used in the inventory management literature is the inventory turns (11). Following that literature, an analogous metric for managing the transplant wait list is the patient-inventory turns defined as

Patient-inventory turns = Effective transplant rate/Number of patients on the list.

The higher the turns are, the more efficient the management of the wait list becomes.

A crucial aspect of the transplant wait list is that the candidates (and the organs available for transplant) are heterogeneous. Moreover, the allocation policy (i.e., UNOS' point system) determines the composition of the list. Different allocation policies lead to different compositions of patient demographics on the wait list. Therefore, for a more effective wait list (or patient inventory) management, we propose a more refined metric that calculates the patient-inventory turns for each demographic (e.g., different blood types, CPRAs, age groups) separately. In that calculation, the numerator and the denominator are the number of transplants received in a year by and the average candidate inventory for that demographic, respectively.

The turn numbers for the various patient groups not only identify the patient demographics suffering most on the wait list and help track the performance of various patient groups over time, but it helps assess the disparity among various demographics. Different turn numbers for different patient demographics facilitate a tailored approach, whereby patients with different demographics can benefit from different wait list management strategies. As an aside, other important performance metrics such as waiting time, wait list mortality, and percentage of patients receiving a transplant are strongly correlated with the patient-inventory turns, i.e., high turns imply low waiting times and wait list mortality and a higher percentage of patients receiving a transplant.

The most effective way of increasing turns, and hence, improving performance, is to increase the effective transplant rate, which will reduce the patient inventory in the long term too. An increase in living donors certainly increases the transplant rate, but this can be achieved in several other ways, e.g., increasing the usage of ECD or DCD organs. This requires educating the candidates about such options and encouraging them to list for ECD organs, particularly given the wide disparity in ECD listing practices previously mentioned. Furthermore, such an effort can be focused more toward the candidate demographics for whom the patient-inventory turns are low, because those candidates are the ones with long expected waits and high wait list mortality rates. Such a focused approach will likely reduce the implementation cost of this effort while simultaneously increasing its effectiveness. Increasing the transplant rate can also be achieved by increasing the utilization of the organs offered to the wait list (i.e., by minimizing organ wastage).

This, in turn, relates to the transplantability (or readiness for transplant) of patients. For example, making sure that the patients' up-to-date information, fresh blood samples for crossmatching, etc. are available increases their chances of receiving a transplant. However, making sure that patients are ready for transplant at all times may be costly. Once again, the patient-inventory turns metric for the various demographics can be used to facilitate a tailored approach for different candidates. Those candidates who belong to demographic groups with high turns should be kept active at all times. In contrast, for those patients with low turns, it may be cost-effective to delay the work necessary to activate them. In the latter case, when to activate a patient can be decided by a careful comparison of the lead time of getting the candidate ready for transplant and his expected remaining time on the waiting list (if he were ready for transplant). A related consideration is that the patients' information should be updated periodically, and those ineligible for transplant should be removed from the wait list. This increases the turns metric because it reduces the denominator. More importantly, it leads to a more accurate measure of performance.

Summary

The number of kidney transplant candidates on the UNOS waiting list far exceeds the number of transplants performed each year. Organ allocation is a complex system, aiming at balancing efficiency and equity. The transplant community is scrutinizing the system, working toward maximizing outcomes from each organ, while maintaining access for all. Improved management of the wait list can increase opportunities for transplant for candidates while simultaneously streamlining resource utilization at transplant centers.

References

1. U S Renal Data System, USRDS 2011 annual data report: atlas of chronic kidney disease and end-stage renal disease in the United States. Bethesda, MD: National Institutes of Health, National Institute of Diabetes and Digestive and Kidney Diseases, 2011
2. Leichtman AB, Cohen D, Keith D, O'Connor K, Goldstein M, McBride V, et al. Kidney and pancreas transplantation in the United States, 1997-2006: the HRSA breakthrough collaboratives and the 58 DSA Challenge. Am J Transplant. 2008;8(4 Pt 2):946–57. PubMed PMID: 18336698.
3. National Organ Transplant Act (NOTA). 1984.
4. Danovitch GM, Cohen DJ, Weir MR, Stock PG, Bennett WM, Christensen LL, et al. Current status of kidney and pancreas transplantation in the United States, 1994-2003. Am J Transplant. 2005;5(4 Pt 2):904–15. PubMed PMID: 15760417.
5. Port FK, Bragg-Gresham JL, Metzger RA, Dykstra DM, Gillespie BW, Young EW, et al. Donor characteristics associated with reduced graft survival: an approach to expanding the pool of kidney donors. Transplantation. 2002;74(9):1281–6. PubMed PMID: 12451266.
6. Ojo AO, Hanson JA, Meier-Kriesche H, Okechukwu CN, Wolfe RA, Leichtman AB, et al. Survival in recipients of marginal cadaveric donor kidneys compared with other recipients and wait-listed transplant candidates. J Am Soc Nephrol. 2001;12(3):589–97. PubMed PMID: 11181808.
7. Merion RM, Ashby VB, Wolfe RA, Distant DA, Hulbert-Shearon TE, Metzger RA, et al. Deceased-donor characteristics and the survival benefit of kidney transplantation. JAMA. 2005;294(21):2726–33. PubMed PMID: 16333008.
8. Schold JD, Meier-Kriesche HU. Which renal transplant candidates should accept marginal kidneys in exchange for a shorter waiting time on dialysis? Clin J Am Soc Nephrol. 2006;1(3):532–8. PubMed PMID: 17699256.
9. Grams ME, Womer KL, Ugarte RM, Desai NM, Montgomery RA, Segev DL. Listing for expanded criteria donor kidneys in older adults and those with predicted benefit. Am J Transplant. 2010;10(4):802–9. PubMed PMID: 20148808. Pubmed Central PMCID: PMC3146063.
10. Friedewald JJ, Reese PP. The kidney-first initiative: what is the current status of preemptive transplantation? Adv Chronic Kidney Dis. 2012;19(4):252–6. PubMed PMID: 22732045. Pubmed Central PMCID: PMC3384698.

Approach to the Highly Sensitized Patient

5

Nadia Chaudhri and Joseph M. Nogueira

Introduction

All recipients of non-genetically identical solid organ transplants are at risk for rejection *initiated by alloantigens* and must be pharmacologically immunosuppressed to prevent rejection mediated by T cell recognition of these non-self HLA molecules or peptides as foreign. However, a potential transplant recipient may also be at risk for rejection *initiated by alloantibodies* if they were exposed pretransplant to foreign antigens that are also present on the allograft. When these preexisting alloantibodies are directed against ABO group antigens, HLA class I antigens, endothelial-monocyte antigens and perhaps HLA class II antigens that are also present on the allograft, they can initiate immediate (hyperacute) or delayed humoral immune responses against the graft [1, 2]. Patients who possess such alloantibodies prior to transplantation are considered to be "sensitized". Highly sensitized patients, especially those who have high levels of circulating anti-HLA class I antibodies, face significant difficulties in finding a compatible donor and encounter a worse prognosis for the organ after transplantation [3, 4]. According to the Organ Procurement and Transplant Network (UNOS data), graft survival rates for patients transplanted between 1997-2004 in the United States were 72.2 % at five years for those with a PRA of 0–9 % versus 65.7 % for those with a PRA of 10–80 % [5]. As such, these patients present difficult challenges to transplant physicians and to organ allocation systems. Until recent years, these patients faced hopelessly long waits for a crossmatch-negative kidney. However, in the past several years much progress has been made in managing highly sensitized patients by more optimally pairing the recipient with a compatible organ and, more recently, by suppressing the powerful humoral immune response elicited by the alloantibodies.

N. Chaudhri, M.D. • J.M. Nogueira, M.D. (✉)
Division of Nephrology, Department of Medicine,
University of Maryland, 22 South Greene Street, Room N3W143,
Baltimore, MD, USA
e-mail: jnogueir@medicine.umaryland.edu

Definition, Quantitation, and Monitoring of Sensitization

Sensitization is defined as the presence of preformed alloantibodies in the serum of a prospective transplant recipient [3]. In other words, it is pretransplant humoral alloimmunization. These alloantibodies are usually anti-HLA class I antibodies but may also include anti-HLA class II or non-HLA antibodies [3]. They are formed in response to prior exposure to foreign antigens encountered during events such as blood transfusions, prior transplants, and pregnancies [6]. (Of note, in addition to this humoral sensitization, there also appears to be donor-reactive T cell sensitization ("cellular sensitization"), which is measured with a delayed type hypersensitivity assay [7]. To what degree this phenomenon may be present pretransplant and manifest posttransplant is not clear.)

Anti-HLA antibodies are conventionally known as panel-reactive antibodies, or PRA, and they are quantified as the percentage of PRA that are reactive. Historically, this has been determined by testing the potential recipient's serum against a panel of lymphocytes harvested from 40 to 60 HLA-typed individuals who were chosen to represent the widest variety of HLA antigens, and an antibody-activated, complement-dependent cytotoxic (CDC) assay is used to detect antibodies against donor lymphocyte surface antigens in the recipient serum. The breadth of variety of antibodies present in the potential recipient's serum is determined by calculating the percent of donors in the panel whose cells are killed. Currently there are a variety of assays used to measure the PRA [8]. A discussion of the intricacies of the various methods is beyond the scope of this chapter and is addressed in an earlier chapter. However, in order to clarify what each test can reveal about a given recipient's level of sensitization, a discussion of some salient aspects of the methods that may be used in this setting will follow.

M.R. Weir and E.V. Lerma (eds.), *Kidney Transplantation: Practical Guide to Management*,
DOI 10.1007/978-1-4939-0342-9_5, © Springer Science+Business Media New York 2014

The *NIH standard technique*, which has been used in much of its present form since the 1960s, essentially involves isolating each donor's peripheral T cells, placing them in individual wells of a plate, adding recipient serum, incubating, adding rabbit complement to induce killing of cells if complement-fixing antibodies directed against the donor lymphocytes are present in the recipient serum, and then distinguishing live from dead cells using a vital dye. A technologist then identifies which individual donor wells demonstrated cytotoxicity and scores the PRA as the fraction (expressed as percentage) of donors whose cells elicit a positive reaction. The sensitivity of this technique in identifying anti-donor antibodies suffers if the antibodies are not efficient enough or are not present in sufficient numbers to activate complement. The *antihuman globulin (AHG)-enhanced technique* includes the addition of antihuman immunoglobulin antibody to augment the ability of the recipient antibodies to activate complement by providing cross-linking molecules, and thereby, it increases the sensitivity of detecting these alloantibodies. Both of these cytotoxic assays (especially the more sensitive AHG-enhanced technique) will generally detect not only antibodies directed against HLA but also those directed against other non-HLA antigens that reside on lymphocytes. The latter antigens should not be present on the allograft cells and may therefore be clinically irrelevant. Also, the assays may not differentiate between immunoglobulin G (IgG) and IgM antibodies, and this distinction can be important because IgM antibodies are generally considered to be benign in this context as they are generally not directed at HLA antigens and are often drug induced. Dithiothreitol (DTT) destroys IgM and therefore is added to eliminate the effect of IgM in these PRA assays. However, it may also cause a weak IgG antibody response to disappear, thereby diminishing the sensitivity of the assay.

The *flow cytometry technique* uses soluble HLA molecules that are bound to beads, which are used in place of live donor T cells. The HLA molecules are either class I or class II and are, as with the cytotoxic assays, chosen from typed individuals with a wide spectrum of HLA antigens. Recipient serum and then antihuman antibodies labeled with a fluorochrome are then incubated with beads, and finally the antibody-labeled beads are passed through a flow cytometer that measures the intensity of light emitted from the fluorochromes and mathematically converts it into a percent PRA. Still another method uses *enzyme-linked immunoabsorption* (ELISA) methodology rather than flow cytometry to detect antibodies. The main advantage of these two molecular HLA (as opposed to live cellular) assays in the field of pretransplant PRA testing is that they specifically detect anti-HLA antibodies and not other molecules on the lymphocyte that have no significance in alloreactivity. Other advantages are that (1) the flow cytometry and ELISA techniques are considered to be more sensitive than the complement-dependent cytotoxicity assays, (2) they can distinguish between IgG and IgM antibodies, and (3) they can determine if the antibodies are directed against HLA class I or class II or both. Moreover, because ELISA reactions can be examined in a multiwell plate, determination of the specificity of HLA antibodies is possible with this technique.

Although various regulatory bodies (UNOS, HCFA, etc.) may dictate which tests to use and how often they should be done, a PRA should generally be measured at least every 3 months on all patients on the cadaveric waiting list. Because kidney transplant candidates with high PRAs statistically face longer wait list times for compatible organs, they are given priority in the cadaveric renal allograft allocation system for potentially compatible organs. As discussed later, PRA levels are instrumental in guiding cost- and (cold ischemia) time-efficient crossmatching immediately prior to deceased donor renal transplantation, and they impact greatly on posttransplant allograft outcome.

Various terms and definitions have been used to grade the degree of sensitization. Although there appears to be a graded or stepwise effect on outcomes [9], the term "highly sensitized" or "broadly sensitized" is applied to those who have a PRA of at least 30–50 %. A designation of "unsensitized" has been applied to patients with a PRA of 0 % up to 10 %. Some authors hold that the peak pretransplant PRA is more predictive of graft outcome than the PRA level at the time of surgery [8, 10] and that therefore the sensitization status a given patient may best be determined by the highest pretransplant PRA. Other investigators have argued that only those antibodies present in the serum at the time of transplantation (current crossmatch) are relevant to outcome [11]. The peak PRA may be less pertinent if histocompatibility laboratories have a conscientious sampling and screening program that excludes recipients from receiving allografts that harbor mismatched antigens against which the recipient has ever developed specific antibodies [12].

Importance of Sensitization

UNOS data indicate that approximately 20 % of patients on the transplant wait list have a PRA of greater than 20 % and in France more than 50 % of patients have reactive PRAs [48]. Although hyperacute rejection (HAR) with immediate and universal graft loss historically was a common occurrence in these patients, this problem has been largely eliminated using sensitive crossmatch techniques. Still, sensitized patients wait longer for compatible allograft [3] and are at increased risk for early acute humoral rejection [13–17] and have worse short-term and long-term outcomes [4].

The presence of anti-HLA antibodies present posttransplant is associated with acute and chronic rejection as well as decreased graft survival in various organs transplanted, including kidneys [18]. Renal transplant patients with post-transplant HLA alloantibodies were 5–6 times more likely to develop chronic rejection [19, 20]. Animal and in vitro human models suggest that a repair response to donor-specific antibodies may result in arterial thickening associated with chronic rejection [21]. To what extent patients with pretransplant sensitization may be at risk for this phenomenon of posttransplant alloantibody-induced graft pathology and to what extent posttransplant humorally mediated rejection involves a de novo versus an amnestic response is not yet clear. Highly sensitized patients are clearly at increased risk for antibody-mediated (humoral) rejection, and a thorough discussion of this is beyond the scope of this chapter.

Causes of Sensitization

There are three primary sources of sensitization of kidney transplant patients: pregnancy, blood transfusions, and prior transplants [8, 22]. All three of these situations may present the potential recipient's immune system with "a look at" foreign antigens, including HLA molecules. If the potential recipient is not immunosuppressed, he or she will appropriately produce antibodies against these alloantigens. These sensitizing events appear to have a cumulative and interacting impact on the PRA.

Blood transfusions: Early in the history of solid organ transplantation, the "transfusion effect" was observed by Opelz et al. [23] and others [24] when they demonstrated a benefit on graft outcome if preoperative blood transfusions were given in combination with immunosuppressive drugs or X-radiation [25, 26]. The mechanism of this beneficial effect has still to this day not been elucidated. It has been theorized that (a) it may allow for preselection of a population with a high response (that later will presumably fail crossmatch when reexposed to antigens), (b) it may induce clonal deletion or activate suppressor mechanisms of alloreactive T cells, or (c) it may block allo- or anti-idiotypic antibodies [27]. Whatever the case, over the years, it has also become clear that blood transfusions may also induce sensitization, and by the late 1990s, the previously noted beneficial "transfusion effect" had given way to a deleterious effect, with worsening graft survival associated with the greater numbers of transfusions in sensitized and nonsensitized patients [28].

Prior transplants and pregnancies: The rate of sensitization seems greater in regraft as compared to initial graft recipients. The sensitizing effect of pregnancy appears to be more important in initial transplants than in retransplants. Increasing numbers of transfusions are associated with increasing PRAs, and the effect seems to be modulated by sex and pregnancies [28]. It has been hypothesized that pregnant women may be sensitized at the time of delivery with exposure to parental HLA antigens expressed by fetal cells [29].

Other as yet unidentified factors: Among patients receiving their first kidney transplant with no known history of blood transfusions, approximately 20 % of nulliparous women and 13 % of men were sensitized (PRA > 10 %) [27]. It is not clear how such a large proportion of patients lacking risk factors became sensitized. As this observation was noted in patients who actually received a kidney and as the prevalence of sensitization is overall higher in wait-listed patients, it is likely that a higher percent of such patients on the transplant wait list may be sensitized. Certainly, underreporting of these sensitizing events may have occurred. Additional factors in women may have included unrecognized pregnancies, alloantigenic stimulation from sperm, or an augmenting estrogen effect [30].

Pathogenesis of Sensitization

Essentially, sensitization develops when a non-immunosuppressed patient is exposed to foreign human cells that have HLA molecules and other surface antigens that are recognized as nonself. A humoral response ensues, and it appears to be initiated via the T cell-dependent, Th2 cytokine-driven humoral response (as opposed to T cell-independent B cell activation). Recent studies have demonstrated that a Bcl-6-expressing T cell subset found with B cell follicles (i.e., T follicular helper cells (Tfh)) is important in the development of germinal center B cells. However, because B cells and plasma cells have short life spans, it is not clear how a patient may sustain an anti-HLA antibody response and thus a high PRA without ongoing antigenic stimulation. Possible explanations include (a) the persistence of residual donor protein antigens in long-lived follicular dendritic cells, (b) the presence of cross-reactive environmental antigens, or (c) the development of chimerism (the presence of donor stem cells in the host) or microchimerism (small numbers of such cells) [31]. In support of theory of a chimeric mechanism, one group has identified non-genomic DNA in sensitized patients (Y chromosome material in sensitized females) [30], and another group demonstrated more than two HLA-DR antigens in a higher percentage of sensitized as compared to nonsensitized individuals [32]. In addition, it has been described that a small proportion of plasma cells become established as long-term antibody factories, producing IgG, in the bone marrow, or within a number of limited niches (i.e., allografts, inflamed tissues), and antibodies are the critical mediators of humoral immunity [33]. Tertiary lymphoid organs have also been observed in human renal allografts suggesting possible direct B cell activation in the graft [34]. B cells produce VEGF-A and lymphotoxin-β, which drive lymphoid organ formation and lymphangiogenesis, pointing to a role in how they develop within allografts [33].

Immunobiology of Rejection in Sensitized Recipients

In 1966, it was reported that sensitized recipients of renal allografts may undergo fulminant rejection within minutes or hours of implantation [35], and it became clear that the process, known as HAR, was the result of the preexisting antibodies that bind to donor allograft endothelium and activate complement cascade with subsequent rapid immune and ischemic destruction of the graft. With the implementation and refinement of pretransplant crossmatching techniques, this disaster has become exceedingly rare. Still, a highly sensitized patient who does eventually receive a kidney transplant faces a more hostile posttransplant immunologic environment with a higher risk of rejection, including the accelerated humoral form (ACCR). Although HAR and ACCR are probably on the same continuum in terms of pathophysiology (both induced by preformed alloantibodies), the onset and tempo differ. It may be that the level of preexisting antibodies at the time of engraftment may determine whether HAR (if levels are high) or ACCR develop. If anti-donor alloantibody levels are low (perhaps too low to be identified with a cytotoxic crossmatch), then ACCR may develop as titers rise to a level sufficient to activate complement following reexposure to the antigen on the allograft [3]. Some investigators define HAR as rejection within 24 h and ACCR as rejection within the first few days. In both forms of early rejection, microthrombi with aggregates of fibrin, red blood cells, and platelets occlude small arteries and glomeruli; polymorphonuclear neutrophils (PMNs) accumulate within glomeruli, juxtaglomerular arterioles, and intertubular capillaries. Meanwhile, medium and large vessels are spared. Typically, complement C4d is observed with immunofluorescence staining in the peritubular capillaries (PTCs) and circulating anti-donor antibodies can be detected on crossmatching [26]. (Of note, important diagnostic criteria of acute humoral rejection include PTC C4d deposition, granulocytes in PTC, and severe renal allograft dysfunction [36].) If the process is not reversed, intense vasospasm and intravascular microthrombi causes ischemic necrosis of the parenchyma and permanent loss of graft function.

The time course of events during early allograft rejection in heart allografts transplanted into highly sensitized patients has been elucidated, and it probably parallels that which occurs in renal allografts in this setting. Early in the course of the process, the graft endothelial cells are coated with dense deposits of IgM, IgG, and complement C3, with only trace amounts of fibrin. Then, fibrin deposition on capillary and small vessel endothelium increases progressively such that by 18–24 h, dense fibrin deposits occlude essentially all capillaries and venules. Graft cellularity rapidly increases, with the appearance of polymorphonuclear leukocytes (PMNs) within the first hour after engraftment. By 3–6 h, cell adhesion molecules such as E-selectin and ICAM-1 appear, and this is followed by deposition of the extracellular matrix proteins laminin and fibronectin and then the massive influx of PMNs and mononuclear cells (>75 % macrophages, 10–20 % T cells/natural killer cells, <1 % B cells). Cytokines clearly are involved in this rejection process as well, with expression of tumor necrosis factor (TNF)-α, interleukin (IL)-12, IL-1β, IL-6, IL-2, and interferon (INF)-γ [26].

Although the humoral arm of the immune system has received most of the attention in discussions of the mechanism of early rejection in these highly sensitized patients, it has become clear that cellular immunity is also involved. Although preformed antibodies initiate the process, current theories posit an interdependence of the two pathways with key roles for CD4 T cells and macrophages along with their cytokine mediators in the initiation and control of B cell differentiation and immunoglobulin production. In fact, both Th1 and Th2 cytokine elaboration profiles are observed. Contrary to what would be expected in a largely humorally mediated rejection, the Th1 subsets (which include IL-2 and INF-γ and which promote cell-mediated immunity and tend to suppress the humoral response) seem to dominate the Th2 subsets (which typically promote antibody production by B cells). These Th1 cytokines as well as IL-12 seem to effect an isotype switch of IgG to the IgG2b subclass, which appears to deposit at intragraft epithelial cells and seems to be very effective in inducing complement activation [26].

Strategies to Optimize Outcomes in Sensitized Patients

Limit alloimmunizing events: Avoiding transfusions and pregnancies in patients who may eventually need kidney transplantations may lessen exposure to alloantigens. Two studies [37, 38] have suggested cyclosporine administration with pretransplant transfusions ("under cyclosporine cover") may prevent the development of alloimmunization and furthermore may improve posttransplant graft survival and increase anti-idiotypic antibody activity. In the second study cited above [35], cyclosporine was started 4 days prior to transfusion and continued until 1 month after. The feasibility and safety of this strategy in patients with advanced chronic kidney disease or hyperkalemia who are not yet on dialysis obviously may be problematic, and it does not appear to have achieved widespread use. Although to our knowledge no studies have shown convincing benefits of leukoreduction (to remove HLA-bearing leukocytes) of transfused products on sensitization rates in this population, leukocyte filtering of blood products is routinely done [39].

Pretransplantation Crossmatching

The pretransplant crossmatch tests for the presence of donor-directed antibodies in the sera of a potential transplant recipient may doom the allograft to early humoral rejection and more rapid graft failure. It is used primarily to prevent hyperacute rejection, an immediate and irreversible HLA class I antibody-mediated rejection of the allograft. While universal use of basic crossmatching techniques has relegated hyperacute rejection to the history books, more sophisticated techniques of crossmatching have extended their use to also identifying the presence of less potent alloantibodies that do not produce hyperacute rejection but may predict less fulminant adverse immunologic outcomes [7].

While nonsensitized patients are extremely unlikely to have positive crossmatches, the highly sensitized patient is much more likely to be eliminated from consideration for transplantation from a given deceased donor or living donor by a positive pretransplant crossmatch. So as not to deprive a highly sensitized patient any realistic hope of ever receiving an allograft, organ allocation systems and individual clinicians may have to accept less than optimal highly sensitive crossmatch results and the attendant increased immunologic risk. An understanding of the implications of the results of the various crossmatching techniques is critical in optimizing the matching of these highly sensitized recipients with an organ.

The basic procedure of the CDC crossmatch techniques is essentially the same as the PRA tests that were discussed above, with the important difference being that the recipient's serum is tested against the specific donor candidate's lymphocytes rather than against a panel of anonymous individuals' lymphocytes. The NIH standard technique is the least sensitive but the most specific crossmatch assay. If recipient's serum produces a complement-mediated cytotoxic reaction with this test, then it strongly suggests the presence of anti-HLA antibodies and is highly predictive of hyperacute rejection. A positive result has been considered an absolute contraindication to transplant of renal, pancreas, and heart transplants (although aggressive treatments may be capable of converting a positive to a negative result in certain settings). However, the test may fail to detect small amounts of HLA class I or II antibodies such that a negative test cannot exclude the possibility of poor immunologic outcome. In the late 1960s, when this test was first used clinically, sensitized patients demonstrated an 80 % immediate graft failure rate if the pretransplant NIH standard crossmatch was positive. However, a negative test in a sensitized patient was still associated with a 15 % immediate graft failure rate (i.e., many grafts would still be squandered if allocated to sensitized patients with a negative assay) [1].

The AHG-enhanced technique (as discussed previously) increases the sensitivity of the NIH assay by adding AHG to crosslink antibodies that may not have been numerous or efficient enough to activate complement by themselves. When the AHG-enhanced assay is positive after the standard NIH test was negative, the antibodies that were insufficient to cause lysis of cells in the unenhanced test are likewise probably not capable of causing hyperacute rejection. Nevertheless, the presence of these antibodies in the recipient seems to adversely impact graft survival to the extent that it is widely considered prudent to forgo transplantation of the recipient–donor pair.

The above crossmatch assays generally use live donor T cells as targets for recipient alloantibodies, but in certain circumstances, B cells may be substituted for T cells. The latter is known as the *B cell crossmatch*, and it is used to detect anti-HLA II antibodies. Resting T cells express only HLA class I and not class II antigens on their surface. Class I HLA molecules are present on the endothelial and interstitial cells of the transplanted organ, and these are felt to be the primary targets of the alloimmune response. Class II molecules have a much more restricted tissue distribution than class I molecules, but can be induced to be expressed on injured endothelium and interstitial cells of renal allografts. Although class I antigens appear to be responsible for most episodes of HAR, anti-HLA class II antibodies appear to also adversely impact graft survival, with a more delayed rather than immediate effect (although there have been rare reports of HLA class II antibody-induced hyperacute rejection). Substituting B cells, which express class II antigens, for T cells in the CDC assay allows for the detection of anti-donor class II antibodies. Among recipients with a negative standard T cell crossmatch, those with a negative B cell crossmatch demonstrated improved 2-year survival as compared to those with a positive result. The test seems to be most discriminating in retransplant patients [40–42].

Flow cytometry technology may be used in place of the CDC assay to identify the presence of donor-directed antibodies in recipient serum. When using the flow cytometry crossmatch (FCXM), recipient serum is mixed with lymphocytes from the potential donor, and then this mixture is incubated with fluorochrome-labeled, xeno (mouse, goat, or other species) antihuman immunoglobulin antibodies. When recipient antibodies bind to antigens on the donor lymphocytes, fluorochrome-labeled AHG antibodies will conjugate with the recipient antibodies. The lymphocytes (rather than the HLA-coated beads used to determine the PRA, as discussed above) are then passed through the flow cytometer. If the lymphocytes have alloantibody-AHG complexes attached, the fluorochrome will be activated by the flow cytometer laser beam and emit photons that will be measured as a quantitation of the amount of anti-donor antibody present in the serum. Donor lymphocytes may include T cells, B cells, or both, depending on whether the clinician hopes to identify HLA class I or HLA class I and II antibodies. As opposed to the CDC crossmatch techniques, live donor lymphocytes are not needed for the flow cytometry crossmatching and previously frozen donor cells may be used. This may be a critical advantage in certain situations when live donor lymphocytes are not available or if posttransplant testing for donor-specific alloreactivity is needed (e.g., to assist in the diagnosis of humoral rejection). This technique is able to detect very low levels of circulating antibodies and is therefore very sensitive and may be positive when CDC crossmatches are negative. The FCXM, however, lacks specificity, and a positive result does not necessarily doom the graft to immediate rejection. A review of UNOS Scientific Transplant Registry data in the late 1990s [43] indicated that a positive FCXM (T cell or B cell) was associated with suboptimal allograft function as evidenced by an increased need for posttransplant dialysis, higher incidence of primary nonfunction, longer hospital stays, and a higher incidence of rejection. The impact of graft survival was greatest among retransplanted patients (60 % 3-year graft survival with a positive FCXM versus 79 % with a negative FCXM, $p=0.003$) although significant differences were also noted in primary transplants (76 % 3-year graft survival with positive FCXM versus 81 % with negative FCXM, $p<0.001$). Although a subsequent single-center retrospective study suggested that a positive FCXM (of course with a negative AHG-enhanced CDC crossmatch) did not have a negative impact on graft survival or rejection frequency [44], a more recent prospective single-center study indicated that low-level preformed alloantibodies detected by FCXM represents a risk for rejection even in those patients with no additional immunologic risk factors and that the risk seemed to be due to donor-specific memory rather than to a direct effect of the antibodies [45].

Properly using these tests is critical. It is important not to waste precious organs by failing to identify an incompatible match, and it is likewise important to not deny the highly sensitized patient a rare opportunity to get an acceptable allograft because of a false positive crossmatch. The University of Maryland has adopted a policy of selective application of the FCXM to optimize allograft selection, cost, and cold ischemia time. Because of the higher pretest probability of HLA alloimmunization in highly sensitized patients and thus the lower risk for false positives (i.e., a higher positive predictive value), the FCXM is performed in potential recipients with a PRA over 40 %. Additionally, all potential recipients who had a prior transplant receive the FCXM because a positive test seems to be a more strongly negative prognostic factor in this population. The FCXM is performed simultaneously with the AHG crossmatch if sequential AHG-then-flow testing would increase cold ischemic time. The combination of negative AHG crossmatch and positive flow crossmatch is not considered an absolute contraindication as the anti-donor antibody level is relatively low (below the detection level for the less sensitive AHG assay) in this situation such that hyperacute rejection is unlikely. Depending on the situation, the transplant surgeon decides whether to bypass the potential recipient or to proceed with the transplant under cover of antilymphocyte antibody ± rituximab induction and plasmapheresis (to prevent accelerated humoral rejection).

Immunosuppression: Aspects of immunosuppression of highly sensitized kidney transplant patients include desensitization therapy prior to transplantation, induction therapy with transplantation, maintenance therapy after transplantation, and rescue therapy in the event of acute humoral rejection. In addition to the standard immunosuppressive agents used, the following modalities have been found to be useful in controlling the antibody-mediated response in certain highly sensitized patients in the desensitization, induction, and rescue phases of therapy.

Intravenous immunoglobulins (IVIg): IVIgs are commercially prepared mixtures of IgG derived from pooled human plasma from at least 50,000 to 100,000 screened donors, and they probably contain the entire complement of antibodies that are found in normal human serum. While the composition is >90 % intact IgG, some dimers or aggregates, a few F(ab')2 fragments, and traces of IgM and IgA are also present. Multiple theories have been proposed to explain the immunomodulatory effects of IVIg, and the mechanism may vary depending on the setting and the indication of use. Its mechanism of action in the setting of the sensitized transplant patient may involve reduction or neutralization of alloantibodies via anti-idiotypic binding, inhibition of inflammatory cytokine generation, inhibitory binding of complement components with inhibition of complement-mediated injury, and inhibition of antibody production. It is now recognized that IVIg can also modify antigen-presenting cell and B cell activity. It causes a number of inhibitory effects on B cells through upregulation of the inhibitory receptor FcγIIB, leading to crosslinking and then apoptosis of plasma cells. IVIg can also inhibit growth factors for B cell development and maturation [46]. There are data demonstrating inhibitor effects of IVIg on T cell proliferation in culture, which was associated with significant reduction in co-stimulatory and adhesion molecules. It has also recently been shown in vitro and in vivo (in humans with autoimmune disease) to enhance the expansion and effector function of Tregs [46]. IVIg has shown success in treating steroid and antilymphocyte–antibody-resistant rejection episodes, suggesting that IVIg exerts its antirejection effects via different mechanisms than that of standard anti-T cell therapies [47]. Whatever the exact mechanism, the beneficial effects of IVIg on the alloimmune response appear to persist long after the half-life of the IgG, suggesting that it has the ability to produce long-term suppression of antibody production.

At least five trials have used IVIg in the treatment of highly sensitized patients as part of a desensitizing protocol:

1. Leffell et al. at Johns Hopkins [48] provided plasmapheresis and IVIg until crossmatch was negative and they gave methylprednisolone 500 mg per day for three doses to four patients before or during this course. Maintenance immunosuppression consisted of triple therapy with tacrolimus, mycophenolate mofetil (MMF), and prednisone. All four patients were transplanted and subsequently developed antibody-mediated rejection that was treated successfully with IVIg/plasmapheresis with no graft loss and serum creatinines ranging from 0.8 to 1.2 mg/dL at follow-up periods ranging from 4.4 to 17 months.
2. Schweitzer et al. at the University of Maryland [49] utilized a protocol in 15 AHG-crossmatch positive live donor kidney transplant recipients that included preconditioning with plasmapheresis three times weekly for a maximum of six treatments along with IVIg, tacrolimus, MMF, and prednisone. The 11 patients who were successfully desensitized were given 10 days of OKT3 following living donor transplantation. Three patients developed antibody-mediated rejection, and each case was successfully rescued with additional plasmapheresis, OKT3, or antithymocyte globulin (ATG), and IVIg. A fourth patient developed mild acute cellular rejection that was treated successfully with pulse steroids. All 11 patients were dialysis free and the group had a mean serum creatinine of 1.6±0.2 (range 1.1–2.4) mg/dL at mean follow-up period of 13.3±2.4 months. The protocol was well tolerated without excessive infectious complications. Of note, two patients received cadaveric pancreas transplants simultaneously with the kidney transplantation. One was lost to accelerated chronic rejection, and the other to early thrombosis which may have been caused by antibody-mediated rejection.
3. Glotz et al. from Hospital Europeén Georges Pompidou [50] utilized a regimen of IVIg given as three monthly courses of 2 g/kg body weight. Thirteen of 15 patients with a PRA of at least 50 % were successfully desensitized (defined as at least 50 % decrease in PRA) and underwent immediate transplantation, 11 of whom received the first available ABO-matched, IgG T cell crossmatch-negative cadaveric kidney and two of whom received a living donor kidney against which pretreatment crossmatch was positive. Posttransplant immunosuppression consisted of Thymoglobulin®, tacrolimus, MMF, and steroids. One graft was lost from thrombosis and one from rejection. All other patients had uneventful courses, without any episodes of rejection at a mean follow-up of more than 1 year.
4. The NIH sponsored a randomized, double-blind, placebo-controlled clinical trial (the IGO2 study) to compare IVIg versus placebo in highly sensitized patients awaiting kidney transplantation. Between 1997 and 2000, 101 patients with ESRD who were highly sensitized to HLA antigens (PRA ≥ 50 %) received either 2 g/kg body weight of IVIg monthly for 4 months or placebo infusions. If transplanted, patients were given additional monthly infusions for 4 months. IVIg significantly reduced PRA levels in study subjects compared with placebo. Sixteen IVIG patients (35 %) and eight placebo patients (17 %) were transplanted. Seven graft failures occurred (four IVIG, three placebo) among adherent patients, with similar 2-year graft survival rates (80 % IVIG, 75 % placebo). Viable transplants functioned normally with a mean ± SEM serum creatinine of 1.68 ± 0.28 for IVIG versus 1.28 ± 0.13 mg/dl for placebo after a median follow-up of 2 years posttransplant. They concluded that IVIg was effective in reducing anti-HLA antibody levels and improving transplantation rates in highly sensitized patients with ESRD. In addition, IVIg desensitizes highly sensitized patients and offers them significant transplantation opportunities without excessive graft loss [51].
5. Montogmery et al. from Johns Hopkins Hospital enrolled 211 HLA-sensitized patients who underwent living donor kidney transplantation (215 patients were desensitized, 4 did not undergo transplantation). They compared rates of death between the group undergoing desensitization and two matched control groups from the UNOS kidney transplant waiting list who either continued with dialysis or who underwent transplantation. Patients received plasmapheresis and then IVIg at a dose of 100 mg/kg after each pheresis session. Numbers of treatments varied depending on the level of donor-specific anti-HLA antibody at baseline, with the goal of conversion to a negative crossmatch before transplantation. MMF and tacrolimus were given with PP before transplantation and induction therapy consisted of daclizumab or Thymoglobulin with intraop and post-op steroids. The average calculated PRA was 82 and 32 % of patients had PRA of 98 % or more. During the overall study periods, desensitization was associated with a significant increase in the rate of patient survival, as compared with the rates in the dialysis-only group and the dialysis organ transplantation group. The survival rates in the treatment group were similar up to 12 months with the dialysis-only group and up to 18 months with the dialysis-or-transplant group, but were higher in the treatment group compared to both control groups, thereafter. The survival benefit was preserved in all three subgroups based on the level of donor specific anti-HLA antibiody [52].

As can be seen, various regimens that employ IVIg in combination with other modalities such as plasmapheresis and immunosuppressive drugs resulted in the successful transplantation of patients who would otherwise have been considered non-transplantable.

The main side effects associated with IVIg therapy have been infusion-related reactions that can usually be controlled with slowing the rate of infusion or treating with anti-inflammatory drugs, very rare anaphylactic transfusion reactions, acute renal failure which appears to be secondary to tubular toxicity related to osmolarity of sucrose-containing preparations and which can be prevented by avoiding such preparations, and acute thrombotic events such as myocardial infarction, deep vein thrombosis, central retinal vein occlusion, stroke, and pulmonary embolism. Various IVIg preparations are available, and these vary in terms of diluent, sodium content, sugar moiety, and content and osmolarity. The side effect profiles differ significantly among the preparations, with higher concentration sucrose mixtures having a higher incidence of acute tubular necrosis and lower concentration products causing more problems with volume overload. Difficulties obtaining Medicare and private insurance coverage for this expensive drug have limited its usefulness in the highly sensitized potential renal transplant [43].

Protein A immunoabsorption and plasma exchange have been used in combinations with other modalities and are very effective in rapidly removing alloantibodies from serum. These modalities have shown success in the desensitization regimens as well as rescue/treatment regimens in patients with humoral rejection.

Rituximab is a chimeric murine human monoclonal antibody directed against the B cell surface molecule CD20. CD20 is not found on pro-B cells or mature plasma cells, so rituximab attacks peripheral B cells and does not prevent the regeneration of B cells from precursors or directly affect immunoglobulin levels. Several groups have reported reduction in DSA titers, and there is a fair amount of published data on its use in combination with IVIg and/or plasma exchange for desensitization and treatment of ABMR. For example, Vo et al. showed that high-dose IVIg in conjunction with anti-CD20 antibody, rituximab, improved transplantation rates of highly allosensitized living and deceased donor kidney transplant candidates. Twenty patients received 2 g/kg body weight IVIg and two infusions of rituximab. PRA levels decreased significantly following treatment, and 16 patients were transplanted within 4 months of treatment, though 13 of 16 recipients had persistent positive crossmatches at the time of transplantation. The AMR rate after transplantation was 31 % but the 1-year allograft survival was 94 % [53]. Addition of rituximab to the IVIg (NIH protocol) improved transplant rates for deceased donors to 73% [54]. Thielke et al. reported that a negative crossmatch was successfully achieved in 51 of 57 positive crossmatch patients treated with antithymocyte and anti-CD20 antibody induction therapy in addition to plasma exchange and low-dose IVIg. The rate of allograft survival was 93 % at 1 year and 81 % at 2 years [55]. Stanley Jordan's group from Cedars-Sinai Medical Center is currently conducting a placebo-controlled, multicenter, randomized clinical trial of high-dose IVIg ± rituximab for desensitization to help determine if rituximab is superior to IVIg alone in improving rates of transplantation for highly sensitized deceased donor candidates on the UNOS waiting list (NCT01178216). A preconditioning regimen consisting of rituximab infusions and a splenectomy was also found to be effective in allowing transplantation and preventing early rejection (which would be expected to be humorally mediated) in a recipient of an ABO-incompatible kidney transplantation after conventional preconditioning regimen with plasmapheresis had failed [56].

In addition to these novel treatments, antilymphocyte–antibody induction is probably necessary to prevent reformation of removed antibodies and to suppress cell-mediated rejection in these high-risk patients. In a randomized, controlled clinical trial, ATG showed benefit when added to cyclosporine, steroids, and azathioprine in sensitized kidney recipients: the ATG group demonstrated lower incidence of biopsy-proven rejection (38 % in ATG versus 64 % in controls), 1-year graft survival (89 % in ATG versus 76 % in controls), and 1-year inulin clearances (49 ± 18 in ATG versus 37 ± 15 in controls) at the expense of higher incidence of leukopenia and thrombocytopenia with ATG administration [57]. Nevertheless, OKT3 is favored by other experts because of its documented superiority in the setting of vascular rejection (which may be humorally mediated) and its success as part of the University of Maryland regimen that successfully allowed successful transplantation in high PRA patients with a positive crossmatch. Potent triple-drug maintenance immunosuppression therapy with a calcineurin inhibitor, MMF, and steroids is probably indicated to prevent later rejection in this immunologically high-risk population.

University of Maryland experience with sensitized patient: In a retrospective comparative cohort study, we examined the long-term results of living donor kidney transplant recipients who had undergone desensitization therapy for positive FC crossmatch. We compared results to transplant outcomes in a group of matched recipients with negative crossmatch who were chosen in a blind fashion by 1:1 matching for age, gender, race, year of transplantation, and retransplantation status from a pool of 946 LDKT patients transplanted at our center. A total of 41 live donor kidney recipients with preoperative desensitization regimen for removal of donor-specific alloantibody, as detailed in

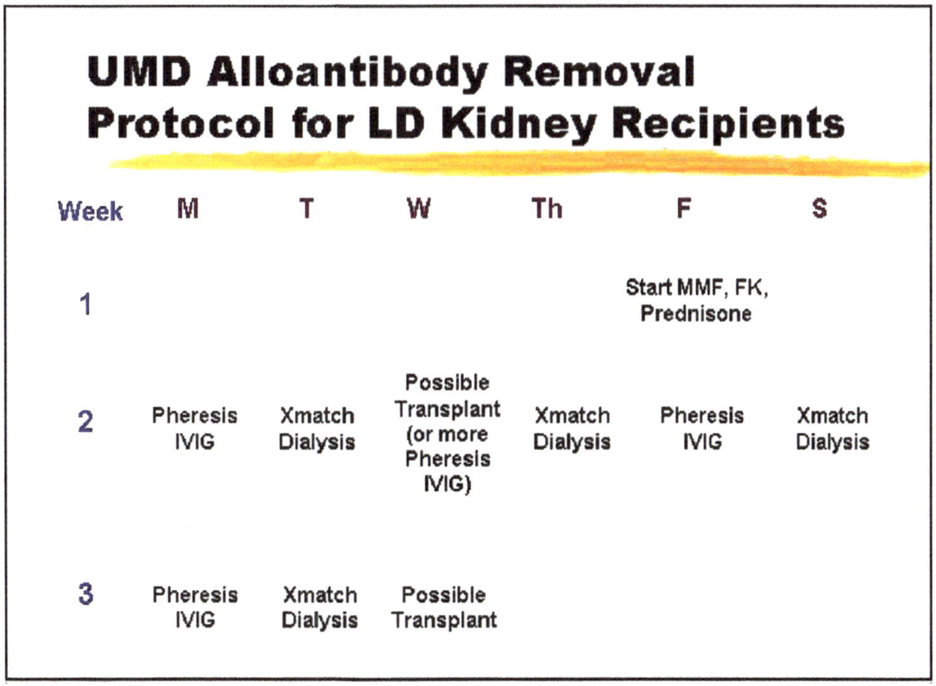

Fig. 5.1 University of Maryland alloantibody removal protocol for live donor kidney recipients who have a positive crossmatch with their donor

Fig. 5.2 Graft survival in positive crossmatch cases compared with controls

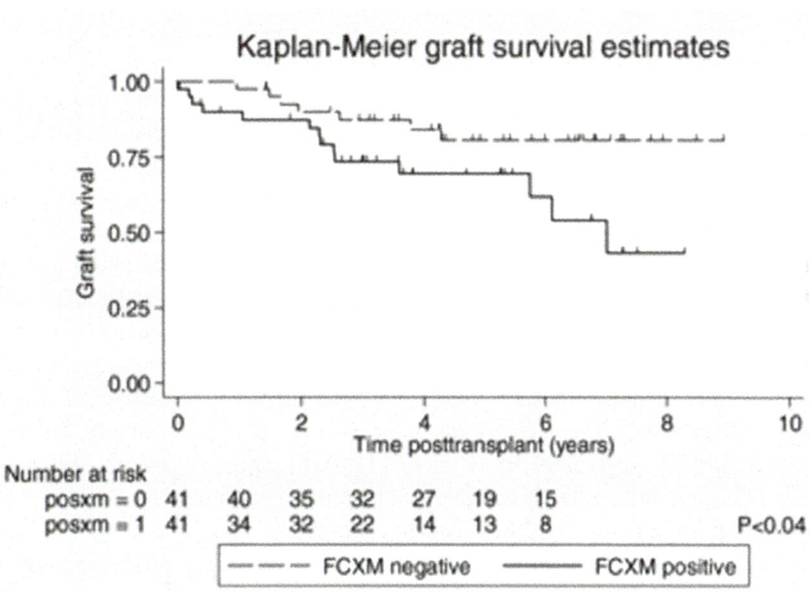

Fig. 5.1. Prior to desensitization, 33 patients were positive for T-flow crossmatch, 35 patients were positive for B cell crossmatch, and 27 patients were both T and B cell FC crossmatch positive. After desensitization and prior to operation, 18 patients remained T-FCXM positive and 17 patients remained B-FCXM positive and 15 had both tests positive, though with reduced median channel value (MCV).

Patients were followed for up to 9 years. Serum creatinine at 1, 3, and 5 years posttransplant was not statistically different between the positive crossmatch group and controls. As shown in Fig. 5.2, positive crossmatch recipients had significantly worse graft survival than matched controls ($p = 0.04$). Graft survival at 1 year was 89.9 % for the presensitized patient and 97.6 % for the controls. At 5 years, it

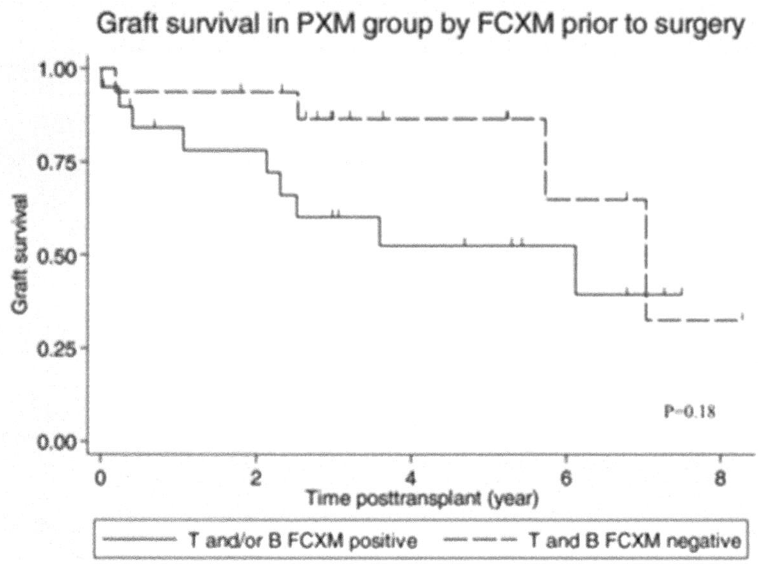

Fig. 5.3 Graft survival in positive crossmatch group in those who achieved negative crossmatch versus those with persistently positive flow crossmatch at the time of transplant following course of desensitization

was 69.4 % and 80.6 %, respectively. After adjusting for acute cellular rejection, presensitization was associated with inferior graft survival during the observation period (HR for graft loss: 2.6, $p=0.04$, 95 % CI 1.03–6.4). Acute antibody-mediated rejection was a strong predictor for worse graft survival in the positive crossmatch group (HR: 9.1, $p<0.001$, 95 % CI 2.9–28.8). One- and 5-year graft survival rates for positive T cell FC crossmatch patients were 90.6 % and 69.2 % and 87.5 % and 72.9 %, respectively, for patients with positive B cell FC crossmatch. Of the factors examined as possible predictors of poor outcome within the positive crossmatch group (i.e., age, sex, race, BMI, pretransplant diabetes), negative crossmatch and PP/IVIg prior to transplant surgery were associated with improved graft survival when compared with positivity in either both T and B cell crossmatch, though it was not statistically significant (HR: 0.45, $p=0.2$, 95 % CI 0.13–1.6). Previous transplantation was significantly associated with graft loss (HR 3.4, $p<0.05$, 95 % CI 1.0–11.8). In patients with DSA and those without identifiable DSA, there was no difference in graft survival rates. Patients who had a negative T and B cell crossmatch before surgery had a nonstatistically significant trend toward better graft survival rates than those with low-grade positivity, as shown in Fig. 5.3. We noted shortcomings of this study included limited power to detect true differences (given the small number of cases) and the lack of protocol biopsies and posttransplant DSA monitoring which could adversely affect outcomes. Overall, the study suggests that desensitization of positive FC crossmatch can provide fair short-term results but suboptimal medium to long-term outcomes that are inferior to LDKT. The 5-year survival rates seem comparable to non-ECD and perhaps better than ECD DDKT [58].

Future Directions

If regimen of administering IVIG to patients on the transplant wait list (such as those protocols of monthly infusions with dialysis described above) is found to be effective, logistically feasible, cost-effective in clinical practice, then perhaps this could be an option for highly sensitized kidney transplant candidates who are unable to find a living donor. Also, given the evidence that chimerism or microchimerism may be involved in the genesis of sustained sensitization and given the inability to produce long-term suppression of sensitization with our current regimens, some authors have suggested that actively eliminating chimerism in sensitized patients may provide an alternative strategy to control alloimmunization [31]. Immunopotentiating agents such as interferon or administration of antibodies with specificity of chimeric HLA are two strategies that could be employed in the near future.

References

1. Patel R, Terasaki PI. Significance of the positive crossmatch test in kidney transplantation. N Engl J Med. 1969;280:735–9.
2. Iwaki Y, Igurio T, Terasaki PI. Effect of sensitization on kidney allografts. In: Terasaki PI, editor. Clinical Transplants 1985. Los Angeles: UCLA Tissue Typing Laboratory; 1986. p. 139.
3. Sayegh MH, Colvin RB. Case 8–2003: A35-year-old man with early dysfunction of a second renal transplant. N Engl J Med. 2003;348:1033–44.
4. Cecka JM. The UNOS Scientific Renal Transplant Registry—2000. Clin Transpl 2000;1–18
5. UNOS data: Scientific Registry of Transplant Recipients: Transplant Data 1988–2012. Department of Health and Human Services,

Health Resources and Services Administration, 15 June 2012. Web. 25 June 2012. http://optn.transplant.hrsa.gov
6. Iwaki Y, Terasaki PI. Sensitization effect. In: Terasaki PI, editor. Clinical kidney transplants 1986. Los Angeles: UCLA Tissue Typing Laboratory; 1987. p. 257 ("Organ Procurement and Transplantation Network." United States Department of Health and Human Services).
7. Pelletier RP, Hennessy PK, Adams PW, et al. High incidence of donor-reactive delayed-type hypersensitivity in transplant patients. Am J Transplant. 2002;2(10):926–33.
8. Norman DJ. Clinical immunogenetics. In: Norman DJ, Turka LA, editors. Primer on transplantation. 2nd ed. Mt. Laurel: American Society of Transplantation; 2001. p. 51–9.
9. Katznelson S, Bhaduri S, Cecka JM. Clinical aspects of sensitization. In: Cecka JM, Terasaki PI, editors. Clinical transplants 1997. Los Angeles: UCLA Tissue Typing Laboratory; 1998. p. 285–96.
10. Ogura K. Sensitization. In: Terasaki PI, Cecka JM, editors. Clinical transplants 1992. Los Angeles: UCLA Tissue Typing Laboratory; 1993. p. 357.
11. Cardella CJ, Falk JA, et al. Successful renal transplantation in patients with T-cell reactivity to donor. Lancet. 1982;2:240.
12. Chapman JR. A different view of sensitization after transplant rejection? (editorial). Transplantation. 2001;71(7):825–6.
13. Crespo M, Pascual M, Tolkoff-Rubin N, et al. Acute humoral rejection in renal allograft recipients. I. Incidence, serology and clinical characteristics. Transplantation. 2001;71:652–8.
14. Mauiyyedi S, Crespo M, Collins AB, et al. Acute humoral rejection in kidney transplantation. II. Morphology, immunopathology, and pathologic classification. J Am Soc Nephrol. 2002;13:779–87.
15. Halloran PF, Wadgymar A, Ritchie S, Falk J, Solez K, Srinivasa NS. The significance of the anti-class I antibody response. I. Clinical and pathologic features of anti-class I-mediated rejection. Transplantation. 1990;49:85–91.
16. Halloran PF, Schlaut J, Solez K, Srinivasa NS. The significance of the anti-class I response. II. Clinical and pathologic features of renal transplants with anti-class I-like antibody. Transplantation. 1992;53:550–5.
17. Bohmig GA, Exner M, Watschinger B, Regele H. Acute humoral renal allograft rejection. Curr Opin Urol. 2002;12:95–9.
18. McKenna RM, Takemoto SK, Terasaki PI. Anti-HLA antibodies after solid organ transplantation. Transplantation. 2000;69(3):319–26.
19. Abe M, Kawai T, Futatsuyama K, et al. Postoperative production of anti-donor antibody and chronic rejection in renal transplantation. Transplantation. 1997;63(11):1616.
20. Kerman RH, Susskind B, Kerman DH, et al. Anti-HLA antibodies detected in posttransplant renal allograft recipient sera correlate with chronic rejection. Transplant Proc. 1997;29(1–2):1515.
21. Harris PE, Bian H, Reed EF. Induction of high affinity fibroblast growth factor receptor expression and proliferation in human endothelial cells by anti-HLA antibodies: a possible mechanism for transplant atherosclerosis. J Immunol. 1997;159(11):5697.
22. Iwaki Y, Terasaki PI. Sensitization effect. In: Treasaki PI, editor. Clinical kidney transplants 1986. Los Angeles: UCLA Tissue Typing Laboratory; 1987. p. 257.
23. Opelz G, Sengar DPS, Mickey MR, Terasaki P. Effect of blood transfusion on subsequent kidney transplantations. Transplant Proc. 1973;5:253–9.
24. Scornik JC, Salomon DR, Howard RJ, et al. Prevention of transfusion-induced broad sensitization in renal transplant candidates. Transplantation. 1989;47:617–20.
25. Olewole SF, Lau HT, Reemtsma K, et al. Effect of ultraviolet-B-irradiated donor-specific blood transfusions and peritransplant immunosuppression with cyclosporine on rat cardiac allograft survival. Transplantation. 1988;45:293–7.
26. Lasek W, Jakobisiak M, Grochowska M, et al. The influence of pretransplant and posttransplant immunosuppression on cardiac graft survival in the donor-specific transfusion model in mice. Comparison of the effects of cyclophosphamide, procarbazine, cyclosporine and cortisone. Transplantation. 1989;47:913–5.
27. Stadlbauer TH, Kupiec-Weglinski JW. Immunobiology of sensitization in transplant recipients. Am J Med Sci. 1997;313(5):268–74.
28. HardyS LSH, Terasaki PI. Sensitization 2001. In: Cecka JM, Terasaki PI, editors. Clinical transplants 2001. Los Angeles: UCLA Tissue Typing Laboratory; 2001. p. 247.
29. Sanfilippo F, Vaughn WK, Bollinger RR, et al. Comparative effects of pregnancy, transfusion and prior graft rejection on sensitization and renal transplant results. Transplantation. 1982;34:360–6.
30. Nakayama M, Otsuka K, Sato K, et al. Activation by estrogen of the number and function of forbidden T cell clones in intermediate receptor cells. Cell Immunol. 1996;172:163.
31. Inman B, Halloran B, Melk A, et al. Microchimerism in sensitized renal patients. Transplantation. 1999;67(10):1381–3.
32. SivaSai KS, Jendrisak M, Duffy BF, et al. Chimerism in peripheral blood of sensitized patients waiting for renal transplantation: clinical implications. Transplantation. 2000;69(4):538–44.
33. Clatworthy MR. Targeting B, cells and antibody in transplantation. Am J Transplant. 2011;11(7):1359–67.
34. Thaunat O, Field AC, Dai J, Louedec L, Patey N, Bloch MF, et al. Lymphoid neogenesis in chronic rejection: Evidence for a local humoral alloimmune response. Proc Natl Acad Sci U S A. 2005;102:14723–8.
35. Kissmeyer-Nielsen F, Olsen S, Petersen VP, et al. Hyperacute rejection of kidney allografts associated with pre-existing humoral antibodies against donor cells. Lancet. 1966;2:662–5.
36. Bohmig GA, Regele H, Exner M, et al. C4d-positive acute humoral renal allograft rejection: effective treatment by immunoadsorption. J Am Soc Nephrol. 2001;12:2482–9.
37. Niaudet P, Dudley J, Charbit M, et al. Pretransplant blood transfusions with cyclosporine in pediatric renal transplantation. Pediatr Nephrol. 2000;14:451–6.
38. Al Murzairiai IA, Innes A, Hillis A, et al. Renal transplantation: cyclosporin A and antibody development after donor-specific transfusion. Kidney Int. 1989;35:1057–63.
39. Smith R. Filtering white cells from blood for transfusion. [Editorial]. BMJ. 1993;360(6881):810.
40. Braun WE, Dejelo CL, Williams TC. B cell crossmatch in renal transplantation. Lancet. 1977;2:241.
41. Buckingham JM, Geiss WP, Giacchino JL, et al. B-cell directed antibodies and delayed hyperacute rejection: A case report. J Surg Res. 1979;27:268.
42. Russ GR, Nicholls C, Sheldon A, et al. Positive B lymphocyte crossmatch and glomerular rejection in renal transplant recipients. Transplant Proc. 1987;19:785.
43. Cook DJ, Fettouh HI, Gjertson DW, et al. (1998) Flow cytometry crossmatching in the UNOS Kidney Transplant Registry. Clin Transpl. 413–9.
44. Kerman RH, Susskind B, Buyse I, et al. Flow cytometry-detected IgG is not a contraindication to renal transplantation. Transplantation. 1999;68(12):1855–8.
45. Scornik JC, Clapp W, Patton PR, et al. Outcome of kidney transplants in patients known to be flow cytometry crossmatch positive. Transplantation. 2001;71(8):1098–102.
46. Jordan SC. Novel immunotherapeutic approaches to improve rates and outcomes of transplantation in sensitized renal allograft recipients. Discov Med. 2012;70(13):235–45.
47. Jordan S, Cunningham-Rundles C, Mc ER. Utility of intravenous immune globulin in kidney transplantation: efficacy, safety and cost implications. Am J Transplant. 2003;3:653–64.
48. Leffell MS, King KE, Burdick J, et al. Plasmapheresis and intravenous immune globulin provides effective rescue therapy for refractory humoral rejection and allows kidneys to be successfully transplanted into cross-match-positive recipients. Transplantation. 2000;70:887–95.

49. Schweitzer EJ, Wilson JS, Fernandez-Vina M, et al. A high panel-reactive antibody rescue protocol for cross-match-positive live donor kidney transplants. Transplantation. 2000;70:1531–6.
50. Glotz D, Antoine C, Julia P, et al. Desensitization and subsequent kidney transplantation of patients using intravenous immunoglobulins. Am J Transplant. 2002;2:758–60.
51. Jordan SC, et al. Evaluation of intravenous immunoglobulin as an agent to lower allosensitization and improve transplantation in highly sensitized adult patients with end-stage renal disease: report of the NIH IG02 trial. J Am Soc Nephrol. 2004;15: 3256–62.
52. Jordan SC, et al. Desensitization in HLA-incompatible kidney recipients and survival. N Engl J Med. 2011;365:318–26.
53. Vo AA, et al. Rituximab and intravenous immune globulin for desensitization during renal transplantation. N Engl J Med. 2008;359:242–51.
54. Reinsmoen N, et al. Acceptable donor-specific antibody levels allowing for successful deceased and living donor kidney transplantation after desensitization therapy. Transplantation. 2008;86: 820–5.
55. Thielke J, et al. Living donor kidney transplantation across positive crossmatch: The University of Illinois at Chicago experience. Transplantation. 2009;87:268–73.
56. Sawada T, Fuchinoue S, Teraoka S. Successful A1-to-O ABO-incompatible kidney transplantation after a preconditioning regimen consisting of anti-CD20 monoclonal antibody infusions, splenectomy, and double-filtration plasmapheresis. Transplantation. 2002;74(9):1207–10.
57. Thibaudin D, Alamartine E, de Filippis JP, et al. Advantage of antithymocyte globulin induction in sensitized kidney recipients: a randomized prospective study comparing induction with and without antithymocyte globulin. Nephrol Dial Transplant. 1998;13(3): 711–5.
58. Haririan A, et al. Positive cross-match living donor kidney transplantation: longer term outcomes. Am J Transplant. 2009;9: 536–42.

Part II

Simultaneous Paired Kidney Exchange

6

Jennifer E. Verbesey and Matthew Cooper

Paired kidney exchange (PKE) has been developed to help increase the utilization of the possible kidney donor pool in a given population. Its goal is to allow recipients who have incompatible living donors to successfully come to transplantation by matching with a donor from another incompatible pair. It has been estimated that approximately 1/3 of recipients who come forward with a living donor will be unable to move forward with their intended donor due to either blood type incompatibility or a positive crossmatch [4,16,17]. The main tenet of an exchange is that a donor who is not suitable for their intended recipient will give their kidney to another recipient and that person's intended donor will give back to the first donor. Multiple incompatible pairs may participate in a similar fashion with all donors and recipients being matched for transplantation. When multiple transplants result, a "chain" is formed. Chains have the advantage of allowing every recipient to be screened against multiple donors and allowing each person to find the "best match" [10,15].

It has been estimated that over 50 % of participants in a large pool (>1,000 pairs) could be expected to match if included in an exchange. Groups that have traditionally low match rates despite participation in large exchanges tend to include highly sensitized patients and blood type O recipients with type A donors [5,11,18]. Highly sensitized patients within a match may compete for any donors that have an unusual HLA genotype for that population [11]. Gentry et al. found that most pools will have an excess of type O recipients (61 % vs. 44 % in the general population) and fewer O donors (30 % vs. 66 %) translating into low success rates for O recipients that enter the match with a type A donor [4,11].

J.E. Verbesey, M.D. • M. Cooper, M.D. (✉)
MedStar Georgetown Transplant Institute, Georgetown University School of Medicine, 3800 Reservoir Road, NW—2 Main, Washington, DC 20007, USA
e-mail: Jennifer.E.Verbesey@gunet.georgetown.edu; Matthew.Cooper@gunet.georgetown.edu

Potential Benefactors of PKE

There are several groups of patients who could possibly benefit from an exchange and include the following:

1. Recipients who are of different blood type than their intended donor.
2. Recipients who have a positive crossmatch with their intended donor.
3. Nondirected or Good Samaritan donors, i.e., donors who come forward without a designated recipient.
4. Compatible donor/recipient pairs that agree to join an exchange only so other incompatible pairs might benefit from a swap. The original recipient may benefit, however, in the identification of a "better" match even though he or she is compatible with their original donor. For example, the exchange kidney may be from a younger donor, have more amenable anatomy, or be a better size match [3]. It is also possible that, after a full explanation, some compatible pairs may opt to participate in an exchange simply with the knowledge that their exchange will benefit others. A donor may, therefore, represent a highly sensitized patient's "needle in the haystack" and can lead to two transplants instead of one. Some are motivated to participate in an exchange by these altruistic reasons. With this in mind, it is the policy at many centers to explain and ask all pairs to consider being part of an exchange regardless of compatibility. It has been estimated by Gentry et al. that approximately 50 % of compatible pairs could medically benefit by participating in a swap or exchange and another 10 % would be able to help other pairs if they came forward altruistically [6].

Creating a database of all potential pairs for exchange is crucial for the success of the program. Many centers utilize complex computer matching programs that help organize and identify potential pairs. Another key component for success is maintenance of a collegial and cooperative relationship with the HLA laboratory. Optimally, HLA personnel are directly involved with the screening of pairs while the clinical

M.R. Weir and E.V. Lerma (eds.), *Kidney Transplantation: Practical Guide to Management*,
DOI 10.1007/978-1-4939-0342-9_6,

team continuously updates pairs for donation and transplantation. As staff is continuously informed of added pairs, the lab can routinely perform virtual crossmatches in an effort to identify a potential donor for a sensitized recipient. This is particularly important for highly sensitized individuals as this group may be screened against all possible donors who have indicated a willingness to participate in a match, regardless if they are deemed compatible with their original intended recipient. Collaboration with the HLA lab is paramount for the success of any exchange program.

Strategies for the Incompatible Pair

Multiple strategies have been employed in an effort to convert an incompatible pair into one suitable for direct donor transplantation. Historically, either the recipient was paired with another donor through an exchange or completed a desensitization process so that the original donor could be utilized. Increasingly, a combination of these two methods has been employed to identify another incompatible donor for the intended recipient for whom the potential of successful desensitization was more likely than the original intended donor. Highly sensitized patients, most commonly those who have had a previous transplant, multiple transfusions, or previous pregnancies, may still need to be desensitized to receive a kidney even in an exchange; however multiple possible donors allow for choosing a donor that has the best chance of success with this process.

Desensitizing a patient can be approached via several popular and publicized methods. Procedures include plasmapheresis (PP), intravenous immunoglobulin (IVIg), rituximab, bortezomib, and/or splenectomy in a variety of combinations, schedules, and reported success. Almost all protocols include the use of IVIg and PP. Complements to this therapy vary by center. Many utilize rituximab, a drug originally approved for the treatment of leukemias and lymphomas. Rituximab is an anti-CD20 agent which acts as a depleting agent via the destruction of B-cells. CD-20 is expressed on all mature B-cells, and these cells are the target of treatment. Rituximab is used in combination with other treatments since it has no effect on plasma cells or circulating antibody [22]. Bortezomib is a proteasome inhibitor currently FDA approved for the treatment of multiple myeloma. When utilized in desensitization protocols, Bortezomib induces plasma cell apoptosis. Limited experience has been reported, but several centers have published on the success of desensitization with the use of bortezomib [14]. Many of these were attempts with combination therapy, whereby bortezomib was used to deplete plasma cells, PP to eliminate circulating antibody, and rituximab to deplete mature B-cells and inhibit further antibody production. A summary of generally accepted desensitization methods is found in Fig. 6.1.

In order for a patient to undergo PP, central venous catheter placement similar to dialysis access is necessary. PP temporarily quells HLA formation and decreases antibody strength [24]. As the effect of PP is transient, sessions are often completed every other day for a predetermined quantity based on the strength of the antibody once a proposed surgical date has been chosen. ABO titers and/or HLA antibody "strength" (often reported in mean fluorescence intensity (MFI)) is measured prior to the initiation of PP, and the number of treatments is planned based upon the published experience but oftentimes, based upon the past experience of the center. The endpoint is usually when a negative crossmatch is achieved although many authors have reported successful transplantation following a low-level positive crossmatch. Following each plasmapheresis session, IVIg is administered [11]. IVIg is thought to neutralize complement-fixing antibodies, modulate expression and function of Fc receptors, interfere with the complement and cytokine cascade, and generally inhibit normal function of both T- and B-cells [8]. For many centers, there exists a maximum initial titer for which a desensitization attempt is thought permissible and safe. As Montgomery et al. noted, "In general, the success of the transplant has been shown to be inversely proportional to the original strength of the donor-specific antibody" [12].

While HLA strength generally predicts success of desensitization in crossmatch positive patients, ABO incompatibility tends to be an easier problem to solve. Many O recipients who have blood type-incompatible donors can be successfully desensitized and either receive an allograft from their original donor or identify a donor with which they are more likely to successfully be desensitized through the exchange process [11]. With the exception of individual case reports, ABO incompatibility was thought to be an absolute contraindication to transplant prior to the late 1980s. In 1987, Alexandre et al. first described the use of PP to reduce anti-A or anti-B antibody titers and allow successful transplantation [20]. It was already known that not all blood type incompatibility conferred equal risk. For example, blood group A_2 donors could at times donate directly to O recipients since antigen expression tended to be much weaker than the A_1 phenotype [19]. When necessary, the same desensitization techniques will be employed to facilitate a direct donation to the intended recipient (PP, IVIg, rituximab, bortezomib, splenectomy) [1]. With newer desensitization treatment modalities, many studies have shown equivalent patient and graft survival for ABO-incompatible transplants when compared to ABO compatible [7,21]. In contrast to HLA antibody, accommodation to donor blood type occurs, whereby rejection episodes due to ABO antibodies become much less likely. Due to this success, ABO-incompatible transplants with or without desensitization are increasingly common.

Fig. 6.1 Summary of the potential interventions in desensitization protocols [13]

Intervention	Category	Mechanism	Dosing	Side Effects
Plasmapheresis (PP)	Antibody removal	Reduces antibody load by plasma exchange	Alternate days based on DSA	Well tolerated. Complications due to vascular access and volume removal.
IVIG	Antibody inhibition and Anti B-cell therapy	Neutralizes complement, inhibits both T and B cells	High dose (2gm/kg) or low dose (100mg/kg). Low dose usually used with PP.	Well tolerated. Volume overload.
Rituximab	Anti B-Cell therapy	Anti-CD20 monoclonal antibody that depletes mature B cells	375 mg/m^2/wk for 2-4 weeks	Reactivation of latent viruses. Acute infusion reactions. Anaphylaxis.
Bortezomib	Anti-plasma cell therapy	Proteosome inhibitor that causes plasma cell apoptosis.	1.3 mg/m2/wk, 4 doses given over 2 weeks (standard myeloma dosing)	Gastrointestinal upset. Neuropathy. Hematological toxicity.
Splenectomy	Antibody removal and Anti B-cell therapy	Reduction in antibody levels	N/A	Sepsis from encapsulated organisms. Surgical complications.

Desensitization is not a process to be undertaken lightly. There are many potential side effects and complications associated with the overall immunosuppressive burden that is inherent in all desensitization procedures. A large bore catheter is necessary for PP if a native fistula/graft is not in place. This procedure is associated with potential morbidity. As recipient serum may thrombose as it passes through the plasmapheresis machine, citrate is infused. The citrate binds calcium in the blood, rendering it unavailable to the body's natural clotting factors and therefore resulting in a relative thrombophilic state. As the procedure is being completed with a concomitant surgery, there is a greater risk of postoperative bleeding and/or poor wound healing. Bortezomib, for example, can cause a severe peripheral neuropathy, with some requiring physical/occupational therapy several weeks or months. Although generally reversible, it may cause a severe disability for an extended period of time, coinciding with efforts to recover from a surgery when complications associated with inactivity are most probable. Therefore, it is important that when patients are being selected to undergo desensitization, a decision is made not only based upon the potential for therapeutic success but also a critical review of the general health status of the individual.

Organizing a PKE

The simplest PKE is an exchange between two incompatible pairs. This situation arises when Donor A cannot donate to Recipient A and Donor B cannot donate to Recipient B. An exchange may occur if it is determined that Donor A and Recipient B are a blood type match with a negative cross-match and the same is true with Donor B and Recipient A, as seen in Fig. 6.2.

Occasionally, a nondirected or "Good Samaritan" donor can help to initiate what has been termed a "chain." A chain can be "open" which includes the need for one or multiple "bridge donors" or a chain can be "closed" which often results in a living donor ultimately donating to a recipient on the deceased donor waiting list. A nondirected donor is an individual who presents for donation without an intended recipient. Without expectation of financial or material reward, a nondirected donor chooses to put themselves "in harm's way" for the good of another. It is expected, as well, that the nondirected donor plays no role in the choice of the recipient to begin the proposed chain. Based upon the number of incompatible pairs available in the pool for PKE and the successful matches that are

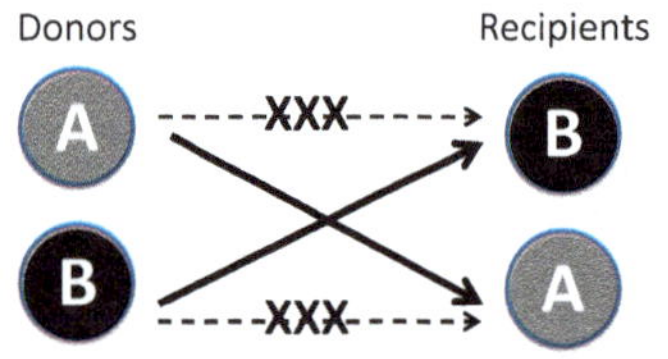

Fig. 6.2 A simple swap—Donor blood type A (*grey*) was incompatible for Recipient blood type B (*black*). Similarly, Donor blood type B (*black*) was incompatible for Recipient blood type A (*grey*). Intended donors are exchanged permitting two successful ABO-compatible living donor transplants

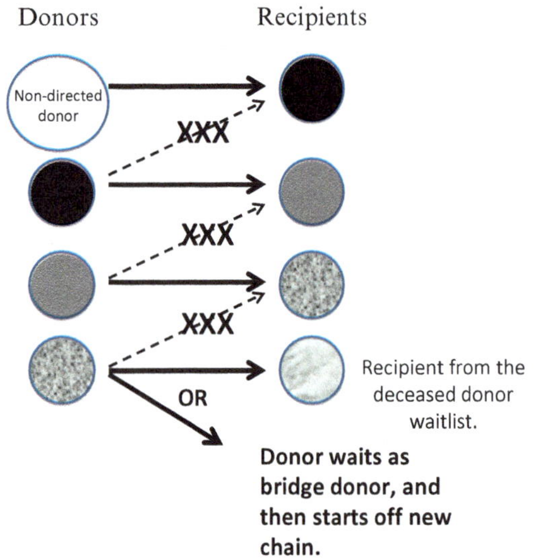

Fig. 6.3 Donor chain initiated with a nondirected or altruistic donor. Following multiple exchanges for incompatible pairs, the final donor may donate to a recipient on the deceased donor waitlist and "close" the chain or remain as a bridge donor and leave the chain "open" to continue with additional pairs at a later date

achieved, a nondirected donor may initiate a chain that leads to multiple transplants. The final recipient's unmatched donor remains at the end of this chain. This donor can then either donate their kidney to someone chosen from the center's waitlist, thereby "closing" the chain, or the donor can remain as a "bridge donor." A bridge donor is defined by Woodle et al. as a donor "who agrees not to donate his/her kidney at the same time as their loved one receives a kidney, but rather at a later date" [23]. A bridge donor is someone who then may start or reinitiate a chain in the future, in the same fashion as the nondirected donor who began the chain (Fig. 6.3). The advantage of an open chain includes the ability to add new pairs as they become available without an expectation that all transplants involved will be done simultaneously as is usually practiced for smaller swaps to avoid the potential scenario in which a donor whose recipient has already received a living donor kidney through PKE rescinds their offer for donation thereby resulting in a non-transplanted recipient whose donor is "lost" having donated previously. Chains as described above can occur across multiple centers, multiple time zones, and multiple dates sometimes taking months to complete and/or maintaining donors in a "bridge" state for weeks or months until more pairs can be added to continue the chain.

With success in the matching of incompatible pairs via PKE, clinicians have recently begun to incorporate the use of compatible living donor pairs to facilitate more transplants particularly the difficult to match highly sensitized, blood type O recipient. Compatible pairs that have consented to participate in an exchange can be continually reviewed to determine if they allow for further matches to be made. The advantage of involving these pairs, beyond simply increasing the size of the pool, is that they tend to normalize the blood type proportions within the pool. In addition, compatible pairs may participate in PKE to improve the "age matching" of intended donors and recipients and to increase the HLA match between non-related donors. Recipients have nearly a 40 % chance of decreasing the age of their donor significantly or identifying a zero-mismatch donor which has demonstrated a survival advantage following living donor transplantation [11].

How Is the Exchange Performed?

Exchanges may be performed within one center or extend locally, regionally, or nationally. For countries that are geographically close, there are certainly international opportunities as well. The size of the registry, or number of pairs listed, is directly correlated to the number of compatible pairs that can be transplanted which has prompted the efforts to create a national PKE program to gain access to a greater number of pairs. As mentioned, for swaps or small exchanges, an effort is often made to complete the transplants simultaneously or, within hours of each other, to minimize the potential of donor dropout following the transplantation of their intended recipient although data has demonstrated that this is an extremely rare occurrence. With larger chains, it is logically not feasible to complete the surgeries at the same time or even the same date, and a single chain may be spread out among several hospitals over several days, weeks, or even months. This then allows hospitals greater flexibility in scheduling and relieves a great deal of pressure in the operating room. Even in the case of bridge donors, very low rates of "reneging" have been demonstrated, even when donors are asked to wait long periods of time.

Currently, multiple national organizations have been formed to facilitate national chains. Melcher et al. recently reported on 54 chains that led to 272 kidney transplants from 57 centers over the course of 3 years organized through the National Kidney Registry [10]. A computer-based algorithm was utilized to match recipients with incompatible donors, altruistic donors, and compatible pairs willing to be screened for inclusion. There are several other national organizations (countries other than the United States have run similar successful national programs [2]). UNOS runs its own Kidney Paired Donation (KPD) program. In this program, recipients are given prioritization points based upon factors including HLA match, degree of sensitization, pediatric status, length of wait time, and geographic proximity to the matched donor.

Logistically, large exchanges can be very challenging. Donors may decide to travel to the site of their intended recipient or the donated organ will travel to the recipient center similar to that of deceased donor allografts. Although one of the recognized advantages of living donation is short ischemic times, most donors prefer to remain local in proximity of their personal support systems following surgery [11]. Segev et al. reported that shipped living donor kidneys as part of an exchange did not demonstrate an increased rate of delayed graft function, resulting in a more liberal policy regarding transportation of living donor kidneys rather than encouraging donors to travel a distance [16–18].

Challenges Associated with Paired Kidney Exchanges

There are several inherent problems with exchanges as the success depends on the coordinated efforts of multiple individuals (donors, recipients, and hospital staff) to come to fruition. Recipients must maintain candidacy throughout the waiting period either prior to or during and exchange that may cause a "break" in the chain and either a dissolution of the original plan or efforts made to "fix the break" with alternative pairs. Donors, too, must not only remain medically able to donate but also remain willing, as there may be a waiting time of several months to years before the surgical procedure. Both doctors and institutions must remain committed to the process financially in the assignment of personnel specifically tasked to PKE. In addition, financially, exchanges can become quite complex as cost reporting for donor charges may be transferred from the initial donor center to the center in which the organ was ultimately transplanted [9]. Many exchanges will involve the transportation of living donor organs to other programs which requires a plan for safety, reliability, and efficiency.

Conclusions

PKE is an exciting new frontier being explored in an effort to increase the number of patients that can successfully receive a kidney transplant and the benefits associated with a living donor organ. By matching recipients with donors through simple swaps or longer chains, we allow patients, who would have otherwise been turned away due to a positive crossmatch or ABO incompatibility with their potential donor, an opportunity for compatibility. Exchanges performed in combination with desensitization protocols or across ABO-incompatible barriers have further increased the success rate. Great debate ensues surrounding the issue of center, local, regional, or national control of PKE programs although all have met with various levels of success. Currently, all are being utilized, and with further development, it may become clear which is the most advantageous to the greatest number of potential recipients. Notwithstanding the inherent problems expected with a proposed endeavor such as a large PKE, the rewards are priceless for those recipients that may have otherwise never been fortunate to have been given the "gift of life."

References

1. Crew RJ, Ratner LE. ABO-incompatible kidney transplantation: current practice and the decade ahead. Curr Opin Organ Transplant. 2010;15:526–30.
2. de Klerk M, Witvliet MD, Haase-Kromwijk BJ, Claas FH, Weimar W. A highly efficient living donor kidney exchange program for both blood type and crossmatch incompatible donor-recipient combinations. Transplantation. 2006;82(12):1616–20.
3. Gentry SE, Montgomery RA, Segev DL. Kidney paired donation: fundamentals, limitations, and expansions. Am J Kidney Dis. 2011;57(1):144–51.
4. Gentry SE, Montgomery RA, Swihart BJ, Segev DL. The roles of dominos and nonsimultaneous chains in kidney paired donation. Am J Transplant. 2009;9:1330–6.
5. Gentry SE, Segev DL, Montgomery RA. A comparison of populations served by kidney paired donation and list paired donation. Am J Transplant. 2005;5:1914–21.
6. Gentry SE, Segev DL, Simmerling M, Montgomery RA. Expanding kidney paired donation through participation by compatible pairs. Am J Transplant. 2007;7:2361–70.
7. Gloor JM, Stegall MD. ABO incompatible kidney transplantation. Curr Opin Nephrol Hypertens. 2007;16(6):529–34.
8. Kazatchkine MD, Kaveri SV. Immunomodulation of autoimmune and inflammatory diseases with intravenous immune globulin. N Engl J Med. 2001;345(10):747–55.
9. Mast DA, Vaughan W, Busque S, et al. Managing finances of shipping living donor kidneys for donor exchanges. Am J Transplant. 2011;11:1810–4.
10. Melcher ML, Leeser DB, Gritsch HA. Chain transplantation: initial experience of a large multicenter program. Am J Transplant. 2012;12:2429–36.
11. Montgomery RA. Living donor exchange programs: theory and practice. Br Med Bull. 2011;98:21–30.
12. Montgomery RA, Lonze BE, Jackson AM. Using donor exchange paradigms with desensitization to enhance transplant rates among highly sensitized patients. Curr Opin Organ Transplant. 2011;16:439–43.
13. Puttarajappa C, Shapiro R, Tan HP. Antibody-mediated rejection in kidney transplantation: a review. J Transplant. 2012;2012:193724.
14. Raghavan R, Jeroudi A, Achkar K, Gaber AO, Patel SJ, Abdellatif A. Bortezomib in kidney transplantation. J Transplant 2010;2010. pii: 698594.
15. Roth AE, Sonmez T, Unver MU, Delmonico FL, Saidman SL. Utilizing list exchange and nondirected donation through 'chain' paired kidney donations. Am J Transplant. 2006;6(11):2694–705.

16. Segev DL, Gentry SE, Melancon JK, Montgomery RA. Characterization of waiting times in a simulation of kidney paired donation. Am J Transplant. 2005;5(10):2448–55.
17. Segev DL, Gentry SE, Warren DS, Reeb B, Montgomery RA. Kidney paired donation and optimizing the use of live donor organs. JAMA. 2005;293:1883–90.
18. Segev DL, Veale JL, Berger JC, et al. Transporting live donor kidneys for kidney paired donation: initial national results. Am J Transplant. 2011;11:356–60.
19. Shin M, Kim SJ. ABO incompatible kidney transplantation—current status and uncertainties. J Transplant. 2011;2011:970421.
20. Thielke J, Kaplan B, Benedetti E. The role of ABO-incompatible living donors in kidney transplantation: state of the art. Semin Nephrol. 2007;27(4):408–13.
21. Tyden G, Donauer J, Wadstrom J, et al. Implementation of a protocol for ABO-incompatible kidney transplantation—a three center experience with 60 consecutive transplantations. Transplantation. 2007;83(9):1153–5.
22. Vo AA, Lukovsky M, Toyoda M, et al. Rituximab and intravenous immune globulin for desensitization during renal transplantation. N Engl J Med. 2008;359:242–51.
23. Woodle ES, Daller JA, Aeder M, et al. Ethical considerations for participation of nondirected living donors in kidney exchange programs. Am J Transplant. 2010;10:1460–7.
24. Zachary AA, Montgomery RA, Ratner LE, et al. Specific and durable elimination of antibody to donor HLA antigens in renal-transplant patients. Transplant. 2003;76:1519–25.

Ethical Issues and Transplant Tourism

7

Dominique E. Martin and Francis L. Delmonico

Traveling to a Foreign Destination for Organ Transplantation

For some patients awaiting organ transplantation, traveling to a foreign country may either be perceived or become an expedient solution to a life-threatening problem. Although organ transplantation services may be available in a domestic healthcare jurisdiction, the shortage of organs compels patients to consider transplantation in a foreign destination. Some may have a relative living abroad who is willing to donate a kidney and yet cannot travel to the home country of the potential recipient. Others may have been judged medically unfit to receive, for example, a liver transplant in their own healthcare system because of systemic malignancy. Patients who travel to a foreign destination to undergo transplantation and fit the following description are referred to as "transplant tourists": they purchase a transplantation package that includes an organ obtained through a commercial system of (living or deceased) procurement and/or distribution, with access to those organs made possible by a monetary transaction. The vendor or "donor" of the organ is paid usually through a broker.

The precise number of such transplant tourists is unknown annually. The commercial systems of such transplantation are clandestine without any demographic data transparently reported. Some years ago, the WHO speculated that the proportion of customers in the global market for human organs comprised up to 10 % of organ transplants worldwide [1]. The well-established evidence concerning the perceived benefits and realistic hazards of transplant tourism for recipients and organ vendors is discussed in this chapter, including a review of the efforts to prevent harmful travel abroad. In conclusion, an outline of the ethical strategies required to address the problem of cross-border trade in organs is provided.

Myths About the Organ Market

The mythical market for organs is conceived as a mutually beneficial exchange—an economic win–win scenario between relatively wealthy patients in need of an organ transplant (residing in a country suffering from a shortage of organs) and relatively poor but healthy individuals in other countries in need of money. This conception is founded on the following assumptions that are refuted by a now well-established experience.

Markets Do Not Make Use of Surplus Organs

Although shortages of organs are the main factor driving patients to seek transplantation abroad, the relative ease of obtaining a transplant overseas is not due to a corresponding surplus of organs in destination countries. Data from the Global Observatory on Donation and Transplantation [2] show that destination countries for transplant tourists, like the Philippines, India, China, and Egypt, rank among the lowest in the world with respect to rates of donation and transplantation activities per million population. Transplant tourists usually travel from countries with a high economic development index to locations that do not have a surplus of organs but rather a surplus of the poor.

Foreign patients who purchase access to deceased donor organs directly impact domestic patients in need of transplantation. In the absence of formal waiting lists and equitable organ allocation systems, wealthy foreign patients may "outprice" poorer locals. Locals may also be reluctant to donate organs that are likely to be purchased by foreigners rather than allocated to members of their own community,

D.E. Martin (✉)
Centre for Health and Society, School of Population and Global Health, The University of Melbourne, Parkville, VIC, Australia
e-mail: Dominique.martin@unimelb.edu.au

F.L. Delmonico
Department of Surgery, Harvard Medical School, Massachusetts General Hospital, Boston, MA, USA

M.R. Weir and E.V. Lerma (eds.), *Kidney Transplantation: Practical Guide to Management*,
DOI 10.1007/978-1-4939-0342-9_7, © Springer Science+Business Media New York 2014

resulting in lower supplies. Commercial activities may discourage deceased donation by impairing trust in the integrity of organ procurement ([3], p. 961). Markets in organs obtained from living "donors" also impair public access to transplantation for domestic patients, as individuals who sell organs such as a kidney or part of a liver to a foreign patient are then unable to donate to a relative or member of their own community. Immediate financial pressures in poor societies are likely to encourage selling rather than related donation. Furthermore, markets for foreign transplant patients may divert limited healthcare resources away from the priority healthcare needs of local communities and may impair access through higher prices for health care.

Although providing payment for organs in some poor communities has increased supplies of kidneys from living vendors, for example, in Iran, the assumption that markets are therefore necessary to increase supplies is mistaken. For example, in Spain, and more recently Croatia, systematic changes in policy and procurement practices have resulted in dramatic increases in the supply of organs from deceased donors such that these two countries have the highest donation rates in the world [4]. Rates of living donation of kidneys in countries such as Turkey and the Netherlands are greater than those of paid kidney vendors in Iran [2]. Nor is there evidence that payment is a requirement for motivating donation in particular cultures, as the successful program of living-related unpaid kidney donation at the Sindh Institute of Urology and Transplantation in Pakistan demonstrates [5]. Pakistan's history as a major destination for "transplant tourists" is indicative of the socioeconomic vulnerability of its population rather than a cultural reluctance to donate organs in the absence of payment.

Transplant Tourism Is Not Indicative of Moral Pluralism

Where international travel for health care involves ethically contentious activities, cultural diversity and respect for moral pluralism have been invoked as justifications for allowing or even facilitating trade [6]. The existence of illicit organ markets in some countries is not, however, evidence of moral pluralism. Thus, transplant tourism is not a matter of seeking out a foreign society that shares an individual's personal moral preferences regarding organ markets. Organ trading is legally prohibited in the countries to which foreign patients travel, and selling organs is associated with religious condemnation and social stigma in the communities in which organs are sold. The ability to buy an organ abroad is indicative of economically mediated power to circumvent ethically underpinned prohibitions in one's own country and to undermine such prohibitions abroad. These prohibitions are aimed at protecting vulnerable individuals and communities who may be harmed by organ markets, rather than restricting individual liberty.

Cross-Border Trade in Organs Is Not a Mutually Beneficial Exchange

The majority of living kidney vendors are ultimately harmed by their participation in organ markets. The decision to sell an organ may be nominally voluntary; however, it frequently occurs in the setting of impaired or constrained autonomy. Inadequate consenting procedures and coercive economic factors such as the treatment of organs as debt collateral ([7], p. 676) exacerbate vulnerabilities such as illiteracy and social disenfranchisement in vendor communities. Living organ vendors are inadequately screened and lack appropriate follow-up care. They are often cheated of promised payments and suffer long-term impairments to health, economic and social status, employment opportunities, and psychological well-being. These consequences are revealed in studies of kidney vendors from Pakistan [8, 9], India [10], Colombia [11], the Philippines [12], Iran [13], and Turkey and Eastern Europe [14]. In the case of commercial transplant travel to China, the execution of prisoners to provide organs for foreign patients offers only financial benefits to the other parties involved. The use of organs from executed prisoners has provoked such widespread condemnation [15] that transplant travel there has decreased markedly in recent years and the Chinese government has expressed plans to eradicate the practice altogether [16].

Furthermore, the purchase of an organ abroad is not necessarily beneficial to recipients. Although problematic continuity of care in the setting of illicit cross-border healthcare provision and poor selection of transplant recipients [17] may play a part in poorer outcomes for transplant "tourists," the higher rates of infection and graft failure associated with purchased organs seem largely due to the qualities of organs deemed suitable for sale. Naqvi et al. [9] found high rates of hepatitis infection and ill health among kidney vendors in Pakistan and concluded that as many as 25 % of vendors would have been excluded using appropriate standards of donor screening. In the market, financial incentives encourage both vendors and brokers of organs to withhold relevant health information, to avoid screening, and to accept organs for sale that expose recipients to life-threatening infections and complications.

In 2012, Dr. Mitwalli from Riyadh personally reported the case of a 15-year-old Saudi Arabian girl who traveled to China and received a kidney transplant obtained from an unrelated living "donor." She returned with urinary sepsis and biopsy of the transplanted kidney revealed cytomegalovirus infection and interstitial fibrosis. She subsequently died. Numerous studies from countries including Canada, Saudi Arabia, the United States, Taiwan, Malaysia, Turkey, and the United Kingdom confirm that transplant "tourists" suffer higher rates of infection, graft failure, and other complications [18].

The negative impact of "transplant tourism" extends beyond the immediate participants. Reliance on outsourcing discourages investment in the technical infrastructure, societal education, and cultural evolution required to build effective and sustainable systems of deceased and living organ donation. Increasing transplant tourism from Israel at the beginning of the last decade resulted in falling rates of living-related kidney donation and stagnant rates of deceased donation domestically [19]. After removing insurance coverage for foreign transplants and financial disincentives to living donation and rewarding registered donors with priority in organ waiting lists through new legislation in 2008, Israel has witnessed significant growth in living and deceased donation within the country, with 68 % more transplants performed in 2011 than the previous year [20].

Not All Travel for Transplantation Is Unethical

In condemning harmful "transplant tourism," it is important to note that some patients may travel abroad for transplantation and organs may be exchanged across international borders in ethically responsible circumstances. Examples include situations where living-related donor and recipient pairs are separated by nationality or country of residence, but where there is evidence of close emotional ties and the absence of financial motivations or coercive elements; international paired kidney donation chains [21]; and regional organ sharing programs such as EuroTransplant ([22], pp. 361–362), which are designed to minimize discard of organs and to help address urgent needs through equitable and cooperative mechanisms. In some cases, patients may seek transplantation abroad, bringing with them their own living-related donors, due to a lack of transplantation services in their own country (e.g., [23]). Efforts to ensure transparency in these circumstances are critical to avoid corruption. In the cross-border setting, it can be especially difficult for transplantation programs to identify coercive or commercial relationships between prospective foreign donors and recipients. Effective screening of such pairs is best performed by responsible medical authorities in their country of origin, who should also take responsibility for maintaining follow-up care of recipients and donors.

Finally, some countries offer limited compassionate access to transplantation programs for foreign patients. With the possible exception of patients who unexpectedly suffer life-threatening organ failure while traveling or living abroad (e.g., [24], p. 3), patients who are granted access to a foreign transplant program are likely to be selected at least in part as a result of their capacity to pay for transplantation services. That is, the organs offered to foreign patients are not allocated according to equitable criteria, and more medically urgent cases or better candidates for transplantation from foreign countries will miss out as a result of poverty.

Although the number of organs allocated to foreign patients in the United States, for example, is sometimes balanced by the number donated by foreigners within the country, programs that offer even limited access to organs for foreign patients risk impairing access for local patients who form part of the potential donor community. In 2008, for example, analysis of UNOS data revealed that 44 nonresident alien donors provided 134 organs for transplantation in the United States, whereas 198 nonresident aliens received deceased donor organs. Transparency in such programs is critical to sustain public trust that organs will primarily be shared among members of the potential donor community and to ensure that allocation to foreign patients occurs equitably and is not influenced by the potential profits inherent in selling health care to foreign patients. Systems should be carefully implemented and monitored to prevent efforts to circumvent the equitable allocation of organs and the integrity of the donation and transplantation program through the purchase of medical visas and/or the effective purchase of citizenship rights by foreign patients. With this aim in mind, UNOS has recently revised their policy to better promote transparency and equity in the treatment of nonresidents [25].

A Note on Citizenship and "Foreign" Patients

Each country is responsible for determining the rights of citizens and governing access to healthcare and transplantation services. However, it is important to recognize that citizenship is not always indicative of foreignness in social communities. Those who reside in a country and make their lives there through social interactions, employment, education, and other practices may rightly be considered members of a potential deceased donor population and, in the spirit of reciprocity and justice, may well be deserving of equitable access to the deceased donor organ pool if in need of transplantation. Conversely, ownership of a passport may confer citizenship rights to individuals who have long resided abroad and who make no social, economic, or other contributions to a country in which they may be legally eligible for transplantation.

Prevention of Harmful Travel for Transplantation

The Role of Prohibitory Legislation

Legislation to prohibit organ sales, to prioritize access to transplantation for domestic patients, and to establish deceased donation programs has played a key role in preventing the growth of cross-border organ trading. For example, legislation in Brazil, Pakistan, China, and the Philippines has resulted in significant decreases in transplant travel to these countries (e.g., [26, 27], p. 125, [28], p. 927, [29]). Effective prohibition relies on a number of factors including willingness to investigate and prosecute violations of the law by domestic authorities as well as evidence that illegal activities are taken seriously, for example, through the imprisonment of organ brokers and transplant surgeons and the closure of transplantation programs in hospitals where illegal activities occur.

As yet, only Spain and Israel have extended extraterritorial jurisdiction to the crime of organ trading, but this option may one day be explored by other countries [30, 31]. When citizens from a country where organ trade is prohibited travel abroad to purchase an organ in a country in which trade is also illegal, efforts to facilitate prosecution of the crime by both countries should in theory be unproblematic. Instead, illegal organ trading has long been a neglected transnational crime. Targeting of organ brokers and transplant professionals engaged in the trade is likely to be most cost-effective and rightly takes priority in law enforcement. Reluctance to condemn patients who purchase an organ stems naturally from recognition that their actions are driven by the promise of lifesaving treatment. However, those who violate laws against organ trading should be held accountable. This is especially the case as participation in illegal organ markets is not a "victimless" crime, with organ vendors frequently subject to coercion, exploitation, and other harmful consequences.

Increasingly, efforts to prevent cross-border organ trade have focused on the criminalization of organ trafficking. In Australia, for example, a bill prohibiting organ trafficking was recently introduced to parliament [32]. Existing international treaties (e.g., [33]) and domestic laws against human trafficking help to provide the infrastructure required to investigate and prosecute transnational crimes that involve trafficking in persons for their organs. Francis and Francis [34] argue that the International Criminal Court could be helpful in strengthening domestic efforts to combat trafficking. Anti-trafficking laws will serve to supplement existing prohibitive legislation on organ trading by facilitating international efforts to prevent trade. Nevertheless, like domestic legislation, anti-trafficking laws will only prove effective with sufficient investment in their implementation within national borders.

Enhancing Access to Organ Transplantation

Prohibitions are rendered more effective when countries strive to discourage travel for transplantation abroad by removing any economic incentives to travel and by enhancing access to transplantation domestically. Israel, for example, complemented its removal of funding for transplantation abroad by introducing policy designed to encourage participation in deceased donation [35, 36]. As noted above, this has had a demonstrably positive impact on access to transplantation within Israel.

Prohibition and discouragement of harmful practices also relies on the influence of professional organizations that may sanction medical practitioners through exclusion from academic journals and meetings and through the reporting of cases that violate law to the relevant authorities [37]. Removing disincentives to donation through reimbursement of direct expenses incurred by living donors, investing in the infrastructure required to enhance deceased donation, and striving to prevent organ failure through the treatment and prevention of chronic and infectious diseases such as hypertension and diabetes are critical if countries are to progress towards self-sufficiency in organ donation and transplantation [38]. Self-sufficiency, or being able to meet the needs of one's own community for transplantation without relying on foreign populations, represents the most reliable and sustainable system of donation and transplantation. When transplantation and donation activities occur within national or regional borders, a sense of community solidarity may effectively be fostered which encourages donation and facilitates the promotion of equity in access to transplantation. Activities can more effectively be monitored to ensure transparency, promote quality of care, ensure follow-up of patients, and engage in regular evaluation to enhance efficiency and efficacy.

Inspiration, Not Resignation

Every society engaged in transplantation, through its government, has a responsibility to oversee and assure a just distribution of deceased organs and the proper care of the live donor. This responsibility is grossly neglected in the global market for organs; however, despite the persistence of transplant tourism, enormous progress has been made worldwide with respect to enhanced access to organ transplantation and prevention of unethical practices. A fine example of successful new strategies to improve organ availability includes the new approach to transplantation and donation in Croatia (see Box 7.1), which has increased the national donation rate there from 2.7pmp in 2000 to 28.6 in 2010 ([39], p. 48).

Box 7.1 Some key strategies adopted by Croatia ([39], p. 51)

- Presumed consent legislation
- National public donation awareness program
- National donor registry, waiting list, and allocation program
- National transplant coordinator appointed in the Ministry of Health
- Training programs for donor coordinators
- Coordinators nominated in each intensive care unit
- Reimbursement of living donor expenses

The effect of Croatia's multifaceted strategic plan demonstrates that inspiration rather than resignation is key to achieving progress towards self-sufficiency. The pursuit of self-sufficiency in organ transplantation within any country relies upon a communal appreciation of the value of organ donation after death and societal promotion of principles and values such as reciprocity and solidarity. Organ-specific registries of transplants should be mandatorily assembled for annual review of collected data. Such data should be used to assess performance of the appropriate stakeholders, develop donation and transplantation policy, and improve patient care. This national framework should be established by legislation with the oversight authority vested in the Ministry of Health or its designated representative organization. The prohibition of transplant tourism becomes a vital component of such national legislation.

International guidelines such as the WHO Guiding Principles [40]; national legislation and policy such as that of Israel, Pakistan, and the Philippines; and international professional collaborations such as the development of the Declaration of Istanbul [37] have all made a substantial impact on the global organ trade. Although the nature of illicit markets is such that evidence is only sporadically and incompletely gathered, we know that fewer foreign patients now undergo organ transplantation in China, the Philippines, and Pakistan. Simply restraining the growth of markets is an achievement, but further diminishing them while enhancing legitimate transplant activities worldwide remains a challenging and long-term endeavor.

References

1. World Health Organization (WHO). WHO proposes global agenda on transplantation. 2007. Mar 30. http://www.who.int/mediacentre/news/releases/2007/pr12/en/index.html. Accessed Nov 6, 2012.
2. Global observatory on organ donation and transplantation. Organ donation and transplantation activities. 2010. http://www.transplant-observatory.org/Pages/home.aspx. Accessed Nov 6, 2012.
3. Epstein M, Martin D, Danovitch G. Caution: deceased donor organ commercialism. Transpl Int. 2011;24:958–64. doi:10.1111/j.1432-2277.2011.01294.x.
4. Matesanz R, Domínguez-Gil B, Coll E, de la Rosa G, Marazuela R. Spanish experience as a leading country: what kind of measures were taken? Transpl Int. 2011;24:333–43. doi:10.1111/j.1432-2277.2010.01204.x.
5. Rizvi SAH, Anwar Naqvi SA, Zafar MN, Hussain Z, Hashmi A, Akhtar F, Hussain M, Ahmed E. Pakistan abolishes kidney market and ushers in new era of ethical transplantation. Int J Organ Transplant Med. 2010;1:193–7.
6. Pennings G. Reproductive tourism as moral pluralism in motion. J Med Ethics. 2002;28:337–41. doi:10.1136/jme.28.6.337.
7. Cohen L. Where it hurts: Indian material for an ethics of organ transplantation. Zygon. 2003;38:663–88. doi:10.1111/1467-9744.00527.
8. Naqvi SAA, Ali B, Mazhar F, Zafar MN, Rizvi SAH. A socioeconomic survey of kidney vendors in Pakistan. Transpl Int. 2007;20:934–9. doi:10.1111/j.1432-2277.2007.00529.x.
9. Naqvi SAA, Rizvi SAH, Zafar MN, Ahmed E, Ali B, Mehmood K, Awan MJ, Mubarak B, Mazhar F. Health status and renal function evaluation of kidney vendors: a report from Pakistan. Am J Transplant.2008;8:1444–50.doi:10.1111/j.1600-6143.2008.02265.x.
10. Goyal M, Mehta RL, Schneiderman LJ, Sehgal AR. Economic and health consequences of selling a kidney in India. JAMA. 2002;288:1589–93. doi:10.1001/jama.288.13.1589.
11. Mendoza RL. Colombia's organ trade: evidence from Bogota and Medellìn. J Public Health. 2010;18:375–84. doi:10.1007/s10389-010-0320-3.
12. Padilla BS. Regulated compensation for kidney donors in the Philippines. Curr Opin Organ Transplant. 2009;14:120–3. doi:10.1097/MOT.0b013e328329256f.
13. Zargooshi J. Quality of life of Iranian kidney "donors". J Urol. 2001;166:1790–9.
14. Scheper-Hughes N. Rotten trade: millennial capitalism, human values and global justice in organs trafficking. J Hum Rights. 2003;2:197–226. doi:10.1080/1475483032000078189.
15. Danovitch GM, Shapiro M, Lavee J. The use of executed prisoners as a source of organ transplants in China must stop. Am J Transplant. 2011;11:426–8. doi:10.1111/j.1600-6143.2010.03417.x.
16. Bradsher K. China moves to stop transplants of organs after executions. The New York Times [Internet]. 2012 Mar 23. http://www.nytimes.com/2012/03/24/world/asia/china-moves-to-stop-transplants-of-organs-after-executions.html?pagewanted=all&_moc.semityn. Accessed Nov 6, 2012.
17. Rizvi SA, Naqvi SA, Zafar MN, Mazhar F, Muzaffar R, Naqvi R, Akhtar F, Ahmed E. Commercial transplants in local Pakistanis from vended kidneys: a socioeconomic and outcome study. Transpl Int. 2009;22:615–21. doi:10.1111/j.1432-2277.2009.00836.x.
18. Anker AE, Feeley TH. Estimating the risks of acquiring a kidney abroad: a meta-analysis of complications following participation in transplant tourism. Clin Transplant. 2012;26:E232–41. doi:10.1111/j.1399-0012.2012.01629.x.
19. Mor E. Transplant tourism: effect on transplant practice and organ donation in Israel. www.esot.org/files/elpat/Content_Files/BOXA9presentation_Mor_slides.pdf. Accessed July 31, 2012.
20. Even D. Dramatic increase in organ transplants recorded in Israel in 2011. Haaretz [Internet] 2012. Jan 12. http://www.haaretz.com/print-edition/news/dramatic-increase-in-organ-transplants-recorded-in-israel-in-2011-1.406824. Accessed July 31, 2012.
21. Sisson P. Pair are part of first international kidney transplant chain. North County Times. [Internet]. 2012. June 1. http://www.nctimes.com/news/local/rancho-bernardo/health-pair-are-part-of-first-international-kidney-transplant-chain/article_05ea95c4-2b7a-5208-b082-f19e950c0297.html. Accessed July 31, 2012.
22. Roels L, Rahmel A. The European experience. Transplant Int. 2011;24:350–67. doi:10.1111/j.1432-2277.2011.01225.x.
23. Vyas H. 8 year old from Mauritius gets liver donation from his mother. Times of India. [Internet] 2012. Jul 2. http://articles.timesofindia.indiatimes.com/2012-07-02/bangalore/32507575_1_donor-liver-liver-transplantation-liver-donation. Accessed July 31, 2012.
24. Transplantation Society of Australia and New Zealand. Organ transplantation from deceased donors: consensus statement on eligibility criteria and allocation protocols. Version 1.2—May 16. 2012. www.tsanz.com.au/downloads/16thMayTSANZConsensusStatementVs1.2_000.pdf. Accessed July 31, 2012.
25. Organ Procurement and Transplantation Network. OPTN/UNOS Board approves new requirements for liver allocation, transplantation of non-resident candidates. 2012. Jun 27. http://optn.transplant.hrsa.gov/news/newsDetail.asp?id=1572. Accessed July 31, 2012.
26. Abbud-Filho M, Campos HH, Garcia VD, Pestana JO. Payment for donor kidneys: only cons. Kidney Int. 2006;70:603. doi:10.1038/sj.ki.5001635.
27. Rizvi AHS, Naqvi ASA, Zafar NM, Ahmed E. Regulated compensated donation in Pakistan and Iran. Curr Opin Organ Transplant. 2009;14:124–8. doi:10.1097/MOT.0b013e328326f6ef.

28. Budiani-Saberi D, Delmonico FL. Organ trafficking and transplant tourism: a commentary on the global realities. Am J Transplant. 2008;8:925–9. doi:10.1111/j.1600-6143.2008.02200.x.
29. Chua A. Re: the Filipino Connection. BMJ 2010. Sept 3. http://www.bmj.com/rapid-response/2011/11/02/rethe-filipino-connection. Accessed Nov 6, 2012.
30. Cohen IG. Can the Government ban organ sale? Recent court challenges and the future of US law on selling human organs and other tissue. Am J Transplant. 2012;12:1983–7. doi:10.1111/j.1600-6143.2012.04092.x.
31. McHale JV. Organ transplantation, the criminal law, and the health tourist. Cambridge Quarterly of Healthcare Ethics, 2013;22(01), 64–76.
32. Willingham R. New laws criminalise slave practices. The Sydney Morning Herald.[Internet]. 2012. May 30. http://www.smh.com.au/opinion/political-news/new-laws-criminalise-slave-practices-20120529-1zhge.html. Accessed Nov 6, 2012.
33. United Nations. Protocol to prevent, suppress and punish trafficking in persons, especially women and children, supplementing the United Nations Convention against transnational organized crime. 2000. www.uncjin.org/documents/conventions/dcatoc/final_documents_2/convention_ traff_eng.pdf. Accessed Jul 31, 2012.
34. Francis LP, Francis JG. Stateless crimes, legitimacy, and international criminal law: the case of organ trafficking. Crim Law Philos. 2010;4:283–95. doi:10.1007/s11572-010-9100-y.
35. Jotkowitz A. Notes on the new Israeli organ donation law-2008. Transplant Proc. 2008;40:3297–8. doi:10.1016/j.transproceed.2008.08.128.
36. Lavee J, Ashkenazi T, Gurman G, Steinberg D. A new law for allocation of donor organs in Israel. Lancet. 2010;375:1131–3. doi:10.1016/S0140-6736(09)61795-5.
37. Danovitch GM, Al-Mousaw M. The declaration of Istanbul—early impact and future potential. Nat Rev Nephrol. 2012;8:358–61. doi:10.1038/nrneph.2012.59.
38. FL, Dominguez-Gil B, Matesanz R, Noel L. A call for government accountability to achieve national self-sufficiency in organ donation. Lancet. 2011; 378:1414–18. doi: 10.1016/S0140-6736(11)61486-4.
39. Busic M, Lovrencic-Huzjan A. Action taken to boost donor rate in Croatia. In: Randhawa G, editor. Organ donation and transplantation—public policy and clinical perspectives. Intech. 2012. http://www.intechopen.com/books/organ-donation-and-transplantation-public-policy-and-clinical-perspectives/action-taken-to-boost-donor-rate-in-croatia. Accessed Nov 6, 2012, p. 47–68.
40. World Health Organization. WHO guiding principles on human cell, tissue and organ transplantation. 2010. http://www.who.int/entity/transplantation/Guiding_PrinciplesTransplantation_WHA63.22en.pdf. Accessed Nov 6, 2012.

8 Live Donor Transplantation

Scott Reule, Arthur Matas, and Hassan N. Ibrahim

Trends in Donation

Given the limited supply of deceased donor allografts, efforts to increase organ supply to match the demands of those recipients in need have focused on increasing the live donor pool. Internationally, the number of live kidney donation has risen, with a 50 % increase in 62 % of 69 countries [2]. In the United States, Taler et al. reviewed kidney donation trends over the past 5 decades among three large transplant centers [3]. This group examined approximately 8,951 donors from 1963 through 2007. A review of quartiles for year of transplant revealed a number of findings, including a significant increase in the total number of donors over time with an approximate threefold increase from 1963–1974 to 1975–1985 and a twofold increase from 1986–1996 to 1997–2007. Eighty-six percent of donors were Caucasian and the majority of donors were female. Approximately 80 % of the donors were biologically related to the recipient. However there was an increase in non-related donors in the most recent era. There was increasing trend for age from 1975–1985 to 1997–2007 (increasing from 35.9 to 41.5 years of age), likely reflecting the larger pool of donors in the group of 41–60 years old. The percentage of donors 60 years and older was stable at 3–4 %. In addition, mean BMI, fasting blood glucose, and SBP increased over time. When reviewing data in two donor age groups (≤60 years of age or >60 years of age), a similar proportion of obesity, with less hypertension and glucose intolerance was seen in those donors ≤60 years old [3]. National trends are very similar. Using Organ Procurement and Transplant Network (OPTN) and United Network for Organ Sharing (UNOS) national registries, Segev et al. reviewed 80,347 live kidney donors between April 1, 1994, and March 31, 2009 [4]. Similar to the results above, they found a general increase in donor age over time, with 13.9 % of donors older than 50 in 1994 compared to 22.8 % in 2008.

Screening

Efforts to standardize the screening process of living donors began in 2006, with the Health Resources and Services Administration (HRSA) issuing recommendations to the Secretary of Health and Human Services and the OPTN. The primary goal was to establish a set of equitable guidelines that would meet the needs of recipients. In 2007, in accordance with the recommendations issued, UNOS and OPTN began working on a uniform set of guidelines for the evaluation of potential living donors. This includes evaluation of current transplant centers' informed-consent process and medical and psychosocial evaluation, with planned follow-up of living donors.

The initial screening of prospective kidney donors includes a thorough medical history with a particular focus on a kidney-specific disease history including but not limited to existing kidney disease, hypertension, diabetes, family history of kidney disease, autoimmune disease, cardiac or pulmonary disease, bleeding and clotting disorders, and history of malignancy. Education regarding the organ donation and transplantation process begins at this level as well. In addition, a thorough psychosocial evaluation by a social worker and occasionally a psychologist with experience in organ transplantation to evaluate if there are any possible coercion to donate. This includes assessment of various possible barriers to successful organ donation including history of substance abuse, high-risk behaviors, or poor psychosocial support system. A basic physical exam, with assessment of blood pressure and BMI, is performed. General laboratory testing includes a metabolic panel, complete blood count, and coagulation assessment is performed. A urinalysis with

S. Reule, M.D. • H.N. Ibrahim, M.D., M.S. (✉)
Division of Renal Diseases and Hypertension,
University of Minnesota, 717 Delaware Street, S.E., Suite 353,
Mail Delivery Code 1932, Minneapolis, MN 55414, USA
e-mail: ibrah007@umn.edu

A. Matas, M.D.
Department of Surgery, University of Minnesota,
Minneapolis, MN, USA

M.R. Weir and E.V. Lerma (eds.), *Kidney Transplantation: Practical Guide to Management*,
DOI 10.1007/978-1-4939-0342-9_8, © Springer Science+Business Media New York 2014

microscopic evaluation and assessment of urinary protein excretion is a must. Blood typing to ensure compatibility with the recipient is obtained. A chest X-ray and electrocardiogram are performed, as well. A formal cardiac evaluation may be required in donors greater than 55 years. This cardiac evaluation may include echocardiography or stress testing. Anatomic assessment of the kidneys is performed to assess for any structural abnormalities or stones. Renal imaging, generally through the use of computerized tomography or magnetic resonance, is performed to clearly delineate vascular anatomy. A final crossmatch with the recipient is also performed.

Glomerular filtration assessment is generally performed using creatinine-based glomerular filtration equations, isotopic methods, or 24 h creatinine clearance. Candidate donors with normal or near-normal estimated GFR for the accepted criterion will need a repeat assessment as estimation equations are inadequate. Most transplant centers accept a GFR of 80 mL/min; however, some centers may accept a lower threshold GFR [5]. There is evidence of a 2.28 relative risk of graft loss if donor GFR <80 mL/min [6]. In addition, the method to assess kidney function has important considerations as well. There is a shift towards utilizing creatinine-based formulas and movement away from 24 urinary creatinine clearance due to its known limitations. The Cockcroft–Gault and the Modification of Diet in Renal Disease (MDRD) GFR estimating formulas are most widely used for estimation of kidney function. Lin et al. assessed the utility of these equations in 117 potential kidney donors. The donors underwent iothalamate or DTPA GFR studies as part of the routine kidney donor evaluation [7]. The MDRD equations were more accurate, being within 30 and 50 % of measured GFR in comparison to the Cockcroft–Gault. The MDRD equations consistently underestimated GFR while the Cockcroft–Gault equation overestimated it. The limitations of the creatinine-based formulas are apparent, as the MDRD formula was developed for use in patient with a GFR <60 mL/min. Formal GFR measurements should be performed, especially if the Cockcroft–Gault estimation predicts a GFR <80 mL/min. The newer Chronic Kidney Disease Epidemiologic Collaboration (CKD-EPI) has generated interest as an attractive alternative to the existing creatinine-based formulas. Lujan et al. performed a cross-sectional analysis of 85 potential kidney donors and compared iothalamate measure GFR to both the CKD-EPI and MDRD equations. Their results indicate that the CKD-EPI equation had a lower bias (3.3 vs. 10.2 mL/min/1.73 m^2), higher precision, and higher accuracy (100 % vs. 89 %) than MDRD [8]. In addition, the correlation coefficients between measured GFR and estimates based on the CKD-EPI and MDRD equations were $r=0.89$ and $r=0.68$, respectively. An important observation was the finding that the ability of the estimating equation to appropriately discriminate values of GFR <90 mL/min as a cutoff for kidney donation led to 5.9 % misclassification using the CKD-EPI equation versus 21.2 % through the use of the MDRD equation [8]. While the number of donor evaluations in this study is small and the threshold cutoff GFR for rejection of kidney donation is slightly higher than what most centers will accept, the findings in this study are important as the CKD-EPI equation may lead to less misclassification and the inclusion of more candidates for donation.

Surgical Risk

Most transplant centers perform donor nephrectomies laparoscopically as this technique has been associated with decreased postsurgical pain, discomfort, and possibly earlier return to work [9, 10]. Early literature regarding outcomes related to surgical techniques was reviewed by Matas et al. [11]. In their survey of 2,828 living donors' nephrectomies, 52.3 % were performed open, 20.7 % were hand-assisted, and 27 % were non-hand-assisted. Of the donors undergoing laparoscopic nephrectomy, two died due to surgical complications and one was in a persistent vegetative state. Reoperation was needed in 0.4 % of the cases, 1 % of the hand-assisted and 0.9 % of the non hand-assisted nephrectomies. Readmission rates were higher in the laparoscopic nephrectomy group (1.6 % vs. 6 %) as a result of an increase in gastrointestinal complications [11]. Segev et al. reported on the mortality associated with live kidney donation in 80,347 live donors over a 15-year time period [4]. In the first 90 days following donor nephrectomy, risk of death was 3.1 per 10,000 donors (95 % CI, 2.0–4.6). This result significantly exceeded the matched NHANES III cohort of 0.4 per 10,000 donors (95 % CI, 0.1–1.1; $p<0.001$). However, at 1-year follow-up, the risk of death was similar in both the matched and live donor cohort (4.6 vs. 6.5 per 10,000 donors; $p=0.11$). Additional observations included a statistically significantly higher surgical mortality observed in men versus women. No significant differences were observed by age, smoking status, BMI, or systolic blood pressure. In summary, as the majority of transplant centers perform laparoscopic nephrectomy, it is reasonable to quote these numbers for all potential donors.

Consequences of Living with One Kidney

Given the selfless nature as well as unnecessary surgical risk imparted on the donor, potential long-term implications of live kidney donation such as development of chronic kidney disease and survival need to be discussed with potential donors. It is unclear if unilateral nephrectomy performed for organ donation and its associated loss of glomerular mass is similar to loss of functional glomerular mass due to chronic kidney disease. Whether donors experience adverse events such as incident chronic kidney disease or decreased survival as a result of donation is highly doubted. A number of studies with carefully matched controls have suggested that donors may outlive both general population as well as carefully selected controls [4, 12–16].

Early studies of both short- and long-term consequences of unilateral nephrectomy used animal models or evaluated outcomes in patients undergoing nephrectomy under non-donor circumstances. In one large Danish study of 232 patients undergoing nephrectomy benign disease, those with preserved kidney function in the remaining kidney experienced no significant decrease in survival [17]. In addition, other studies of unilateral nephrectomy for benign disease have not shown deterioration in kidney function [18, 19]. More pertinent to donors, Fehrman-Ekholm et al. analyzed 459 live kidney donors between 1964 and 1994 [12]. Forty-one donors died over this time period. The 20-year survival was 85 % versus 66 % in comparison to their Swedish general population controls. A Japanese study by Okamoto et al. of 601 live kidney donors between 1970 and 2006 reported similar findings with a 20-year survival of 86.4 % [13]. Ibrahim et al. reported on the vital status of 3,700 kidney donors over 4 decades [14]. In this large single-center study from the University of Minnesota, the 20-year survival was 93.5 % for donors versus 89.5 % controls matched for age, gender, and race. The 30-year survival of donors and controls was 82.5 % versus 76.2 %. At 40 years, survival proportions for donors and controls were 50.1 % versus 55.8 %. It should be noted that the donor population was 98.8 % white. This study also selected donors from its cohort and measured numerous health and quality of life measures. Compared with age-, gender-, race-, and BMI-matched controls, donor outcomes were similar.

These studies face not only the limitations of being a single-center experience but also the significant racial homogeneity of the population. Segev et al. reported on 80,000 kidney donors from national registries with comparison to age and comorbidity-matched controls [4]. These were further stratified by age, sex, and race. No differences were found in overall long-term survival in donors and controls after a median follow-up of 6.3 years. The survival probabilities demonstrated by six major long-term follow-up studies of kidney donors are represented in Fig. 8.1.

Significant limitations regarding the selection of controls for comparison to carefully screened kidney donors have been a major concern regarding the long-term survival of kidney donors. It is possible that validity of studies addressing improved survival in kidney donors may reflect the overall excellent health of kidney donors, the meticulous medical screening and the use of general population controls as opposed to better matched controls.

Risk of Progression and Proteinuria

Garg et al. reported on 5,048 donors with a mean follow-up of 7 years post donation [20]. They demonstrated a pooled incidence of proteinuria of 12 % (95 % CI 8–16 %) and an average 24 h urine protein of 154 mg/dL. The pooled risk of albuminuria in 67 donors was 3.9 % (95 % CI 1.2–12.6 %) in comparison to controls. In regard to GFR, the level reported depended heavily on the proportion of missing data; studies with more data missing reported a larger decrement in GFR. The average GFR reported was 86 mL/min and 78.8 % of donors had a GFR >60 ml/min. Okamoto et al. showed that 3.1 % of their donors developed proteinuria and 0.7 % had a serum creatinine above 2 mg/dL [13]. Ibrahim et al. measured urinary albumin excretion rate and iohexol GFR (iGFR) in 255 randomly selected kidney donors [14]. Mean donor age was 41.1 ± 11.0 years at the time of donation and 53.2 ± 10.0 years at the time of GFR measurement. Women comprised 61.6 % of the donors and 98.8 % were white. Time since donation was 12.1 ± 9.2 years. Those donors <10 years from donation comprised 56.9 %; 21.6 % of the donors were 11–20 years from donation and 15.3 % were 21–30 years from donation. Only 6.2 % were 31–45 years from donation. Serum creatinine at the time of donation was 0.90 ± 0.2 mg/dL and eGFR was 84.0 ± 13.8 mL/min/1.73 m^2. iGFR measurement revealed serum creatinine of 1.10 ± 0.20 mg/dL and eGFR was 63.7 ± 11.9 mL/min/1.73 m^2 at the time of donation. Donors with the greatest compensatory increase in eGFR were more likely to be younger at the time of donation. The majority of donors (85.5 %) had an iGFR >60 mL/min/1.73 m^2 with only 0.8 % having an iGFR of 30–45 mL/min/1.73 m^2 and 14.5 %, 46–60 mL/min/1.73 m^2, and none had a measured iGFR <30 mL/min/1.73 m^2. A total of 87.3 % were normoalbuminuric, 11.5 % were microalbuminuric, and only 1.2 % were macroalbuminuric. None of the donors had both a measured GFR <45 mL/min/1.73 m^2 and albuminuria. The results of this study are reassuring in that previously published studies may have demonstrated changes in proteinuria due to the method of assessment and of adjustment for BMI. The risk of having a GFR <60 mL/min/1.73 m^2 was associated with older age, OR = 1.15 (95 % CI, 1.08–1.21), $p < 0.0001$; higher BMI, OR = 1.12 (95 % CI, 1.02–1.23); and female gender ($p = 0.03$). Time from donation was associated with the development of albuminuria with an OR = 1.12 (95 % CI, 1.05–1.20), $p = 0.0004$, and women were less likely to develop albuminuria [14].

These findings may not be representative of other ethnic groups, however. Parasuraman et al. demonstrated a greater loss of eGFR in 54 African American donors compared to Caucasian donors 2–3 years after donation (39.8 vs. 30.4 mL/min, $p = 0.001$) [21]. Predonation eGFR <100 mL/min and

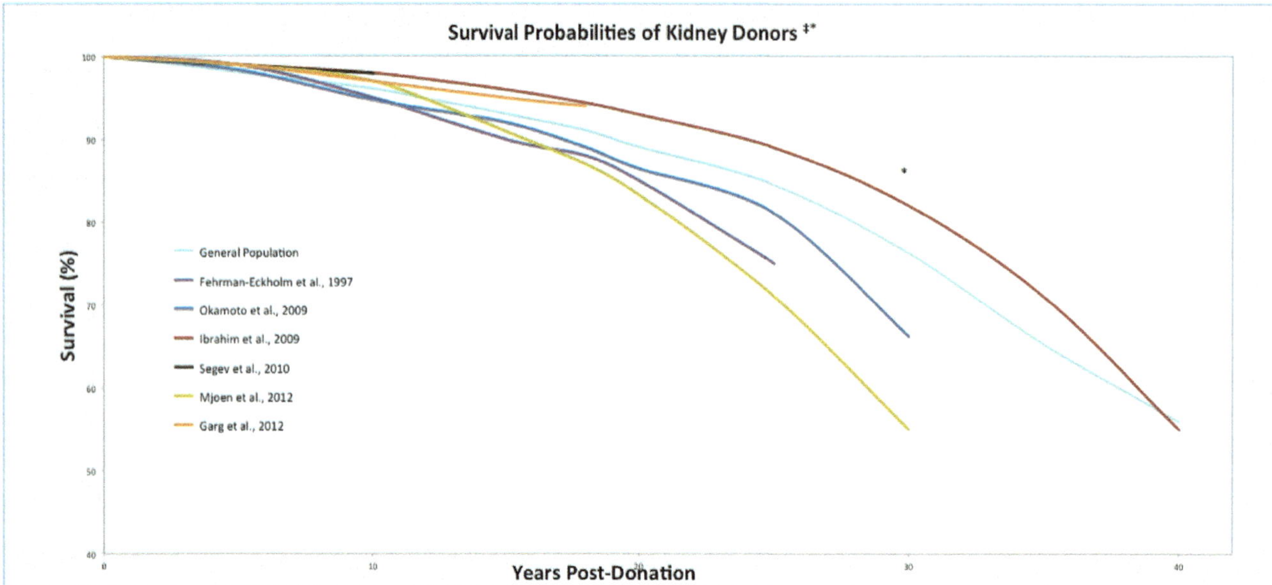

Study	Mean/Median Follow Up (y)	Controls	Mean/Median Age (y) at Donation	Donor Survival (%)
Fehrman-Eckholm *et al.* 1964-2005, n=459	12	Swedish Population[a]	78% <59 years	20 years = 85
Okamoto *et al.* 1970-2006, n=601	13.7	Japanese Population[a]	52 ± 10	20 years = 86.4
Ibrahim *et al.* 1963-2007, n=3698	12.2	Human Mortality Database[b]	41.1 ± 11	20 years = 93.5
Segev *et al.* 1994-2009, n=80347	6.3	NHANES III/DMF[c]	79.5% <50 years	12 years = 97.9
Mjoen *et al.* 1963-2007, n=2269	14.7	Norwegian Population[d]	47.6 ± 12.6	20 years = 83.3
Garg *et al.* 1992-2009, n=2028	6.5	Canadian Population[e]	43	15 years = 95

‡ = direct comparisons cannot be made given differences in baseline characteristics
§ = estimates based on Kaplan Meier curves published
* = younger age at time of donation
[a]Age, sex, and calendar year-bsed expected survival.
[b]Age, sex, race, and BMI using National Center for Health Statistics
[c]United Network for Organ Sharing
[d]Age, gender, and year of birth
[e]Age, sex, index date, population density of residence, income, and conditions precluding kidney donation

Fig. 8.1 Survival probabilites of kidney donors from six large studies

age at time of donation were associated with eGFR <60 mL/min in African American donors. With over 50 years of experience in kidney donation, the question regarding whether an increased risk of ESRD after donation lingers. This has stemmed mainly from the lack of routine follow up of kidney donors, analogous to what we do for recipients, and perhaps due to the commonly held belief that donors do indeed do well and are not at increased risk for ESRD or excess mortality. Three large single center studies, two large US registry-based studies and a more recent study from Canada have affirmed the belief regarding any adverse outcomes for kidney donors [1–6]. In addition, kidney donors do not appear to be at high risk for the complications seen in those with CKD such as fractures, kidney stones or acute kidney injury requiring dialysis [7, 8].

The study of Mjoen et al. challenges our convictions regarding donor outcomes in the domains of ESRD, overall mortality and also cardiovascular mortality [9]. Before commenting specifically about this study, it is worth pointing out two other recent observations that have also suggested increased risk of ESRD in donors. Muzaale et al. matched a cohort of 96,217 US donors who underwent nephrectomy between 1994–2011 with NHANES controls matched on age, gender, race, education, BMI, systolic blood pressure and also smoking history [10]. ESRD incidence at 15 years was 0.31 % vs. 0.04 % in controls; a 15 fold higher risk. This excess risk was consistent across different racial groups. More recently, Reese et al. matched 3,368 donors who were above 50 years of age at the time of donation to healthy controls drawn from the National Institutes of Health sponsored Health and Retirement Study. After a mean follow up of 7.8 years, 20 donors developed ESRD; a 7.4 fold increase in risk compared to controls. Both groups, however, enjoyed a similar survival.

The study of Mjoen et al. is at great odds with all other previous studies as it is the first study to ever demonstrate both excess risk of ESRD and mortality in kidney donors [9]. In this study 1901 donors were matched with 32,621 healthy controls and follow up duration was 15.1 years in donors and 24.9 years in controls. Donors incurred a 30 % increase in risk of death, a 40 % increase risk of death from cardiovascular disease and an over an 11 fold increase in the risk of ESRD. In total, 9 donors developed ESRD. These data should be considered seriously as an ideal study to really answer the question of ESRD and mortality risk is yet to be done as single center data has longer follow up but less events and registry based data has more events but are certainly plagued by their short follow up.

Does Donation Place the Kidney Donor at Higher Cardiovascular Risk?

The association of reduced renal function as a consequence of donor nephrectomy and cardiovascular disease without the clustering of known risk factors that are common in CKD is unknown. Go et al. and many others reported an inverse relationship in GFR and hazard ratio of death and cardiovascular disease [22]. Donor nephrectomy and loss of glomerular mass as a result of surgery may not impart similar risk on kidney donors, however. Mjøen et al. followed 2,269 Norwegian donors for a median of 14.3 years and found that overall mortality, as well as cardiovascular mortality, was lower in donors than the general population matched for age and gender [15]. Garg et al. reported on long-term outcomes with healthy matched controls. Using registry data beginning in 1991 and applying extensive exclusion criteria, the authors attempted to select for the "healthiest" segment of the population in Ontario, Canada. A total of 2,028 kidney donors were matched to population controls with exhaustive exclusion criteria applied. Prior conditions that would have otherwise eliminated kidney donation were excluded as controls. Through diagnostic and procedural codes for visits related to hypertension, cancer, cardiovascular disease, pulmonary disease, liver disease, and rheumatologic and genitourinary disease, the authors were able to include patients as controls representing a potentially healthier control group. They also were able to obtain data on the number of physician visits as a method of establishing access to care. This criterion resulted in exclusion of approximately 85 % of the population in question. The remaining controls were matched to living donors in a 10:1 ratio. Median follow-up was 6.5 years with a maximum of 17.7 years of follow-up time. Using outcomes of both first cardiovascular event and mortality, the observed event rates were lower in donors. In addition, there appeared to be no difference in major cardiovascular event in both donors and controls when censored for death. Together, these studies provide compelling data to show that survival in donors is excellent, when compared to carefully selected controls.

Special Donor Situations

Older Kidney Donors

While it is known that there is some, though not universal, loss of kidney function with aging, the consequences of donor nephrectomy in the elderly are unknown. Efforts to expand the live donor kidney pool have included use of "non-ideal" donors including those with hypertension, increased body mass, and older age. Studies reviewing the use of donors aged greater than 70 years old have yielded mixed results. Some studies have suggested that these particular allografts perform as well as ones from younger donors but others have shown increased rates of chronic allograft dysfunction. Berger et al. analyzed a large cohort of data from the Scientific Registry of Transplant Recipients (SRTR), that included older donors, predominantly women, with increased prevalence of hypertension, and more often white. The authors compared graft loss and death in a competing risk model. The 1-, 5-, and 10-year risks of graft failure among recipients of kidneys from live donors greater than 70 years of age were 7.4, 14.9, and 33.3 %, whereas the 1-, 5-, and 10-year graft failure rates from live donors between the ages 50 and 59 years old were 5.0, 12.0, and 21.6 %. Importantly, graft failure rates of those recipients of older donors were similar to non-ECD donors. These results were significant in that there were higher rates of allograft failure from donors ≥70 years of age in comparison to matched controls ages 50–59 years old. Interestingly there was no difference in graft failure rates for donors ≥65 years old [23].

Obesity

As the prevalence of obesity increases, the number of obese candidate donors is likely to increase as well. The association between obesity and end-stage kidney disease in non-donors has been demonstrated. Screening over 175,000 subjects in California over a period of 1964–1973, Hsu et al. demonstrated that there is an increasing association with obesity and end-stage kidney disease beginning at a BMI >25 kg/m^2, with those subjects whose BMIs ≥35 kg/m^2 having the highest relative risk of ESKD at 4.39 (95 % CI; 3.38–5.70) [24]. In addition to the association of obesity with various health consequences, there are also significant structural and functional consequences to the kidney [25]. Data from Kambham et al. reveal a possible increase in glomerular volume and findings of focal segmental glomerulosclerosis [26].

There are surgical considerations as well. Heimbach et al. demonstrated that laparoscopic donor nephrectomy to be generally safe; however donors with BMI >35 kg/m^2 may experience both slightly longer operative times and higher percentage of procedure related surgical outcomes. In addition, obese donors demonstrated no difference in renal function or the prevalence of albuminuria at 6–12 months [27]. In a small, single-center study, O'Brien et al. reviewed the outcomes of seven donor nephrectomies in morbidly obese patients (BMI >40 kg/m^2). There did not appear to be any significant differences in mean operation time, blood loss, or hospital stay. There was also no significant changes in kidney function during follow-up (mean 20 months) [28]. Young et al. performed a systematic review of kidney donors with isolated medical abnormalities (IMA). Their analysis included information from ten studies on outcomes in obese kidney donors. Only two of the ten studies reviewed included long-term follow-up and the information reported regarding GFR decline was conflicting [29].

Hypertension

Hypertension is a risk factor for end-stage kidney disease. In addition, inadequately controlled blood pressure is associated with adverse cardiovascular events. Current recommendations require clinic blood pressure evaluation of potential donors on two separate occasions. Textor et al. evaluated patients undergoing donor nephrectomy between January 2001 and December 2002 [3]. Only 24 of the 148 living donors reviewed were found to be hypertensive after approximately 10 months of follow-up. There was no change in ambulatory blood pressure monitoring while awake, and blood pressure in hypertensive donors actually improved by 10 mmHg systolic and 5 mmHg diastolic blood pressure with both non-pharmocologic and drug therapy. Although starting at a lower estimated GFR, there was no effect of blood pressure for predicting GFR before and after nephrectomy in hypertensive donors, adjusted for age [3]. In addition there was no difference in protein excretion on hypertensive donors. There is a paucity of data regarding long-term follow-up of hypertensive kidney donors likely related to the exclusion of candidates with hypertension, and while these results are encouraging, it is important to remember that this is a highly selected population of patients with no evidence of proteinuria, generally preserved GFR, and only have modest hypertension. Young and colleagues reported on the significant heterogeneity including the definitions of hypertension used as well as length of follow-up in hypertensive kidney donors [29]. Of the long-term follow-up studies, one demonstrated an increase in serum creatinine of 14 μmol/L in hypertensive patients versus normotensive patients. One study reported on blood pressure assessment 1 year post donation revealing that there was a decrease in systolic and diastolic blood pressure of 5 and 6 mmHg in hypertensive donors [29].

These findings have significant implications in the evaluation of possible kidney donors. In most transplant centers, donors with hypertension are generally excluded donation however donors with well-controlled hypertension may be considered for kidney donation. Importantly, there appear to be a large number of patients who may have elevated clinic blood pressure alone. In a recent study of 178 potential kidney donors utilizing ambulatory blood pressure monitoring, 62 % of those patients characterized as having hypertension by clinical assessment were found to have "white-coat hypertension" [30]. In addition, approximately 17 % of donors with normal clinic blood pressure were found to have "masked" hypertension [30].

Recommendations from the Amsterdam Forum on the Care of the Live Kidney Donor regarding hypertension include [31]:

1. Patients with a blood pressure >140/90 by ambulatory blood pressure should generally not be accepted as donors; the preferred method of measurement is ambulatory blood pressure monitoring particularly in those aged >50 years and/or with high office blood pressure readings.
2. Those candidate donors with controlled hypertension may be considered if age >50 years, GFR ≥80 mL/min, and no evidence of proteinuria defined as urinary albumin of <30 mg/day.
3. Donors with hypertension should be regularly followed up by a physician.

Nephrolithiasis

Potential donors with evidence of bilateral nephrocalcinosis on imaging of the abdomen and those with a known history of kidney stones that have high recurrence potential such as cystine stones, hyperoxaluria-related stones, renal tubular acidosis, or infectious stones are generally excluded from donation. Subjects with a history of a single kidney stone in the absence of the previously mentioned conditions may be considered for donation. Those donors with asymptomatic nephrolithiasis during evaluation may be allowed to donate in the presence of a favorable urinary stone profile, as well as favorable stone size profile, namely, <15 mm. Recently,

Rule et al. reviewed the association between symptomatic stone formers and CKD using a population-based historical cohort and matched controls. Using both diagnostic codes and increased creatinine values for a period of ≥3 months as criteria, they demonstrated a 51–68 % increased risk for CKD by diagnosis codes and a 25–44 % increased risk for CKD using creatinine-based criteria [32]. Furthermore, this increased risk of development of CKD was not explained by comorbidities including diabetes, hypertension, and obesity [32]. An association between nephrolithiasis and ESKD was recently demonstrated as well. El-Zoghby et al. demonstrated that an increased risk of ESKD in stone formers was observed over a 9-year period after adjustment for diabetes, hypertension, hyperlipidemia, gout, and CKD with an HR of 2.09; (95 % CI 1.45–3.01) [33]. Therefore, accepting those with stones as kidney donors should be considered when other options are exhausted.

Malignancy

As part of the screening process for kidney donation, screening for a history of malignancy in the donor as well as a family history of malignancy is performed. Candidate donors should undergo age- and gender-appropriate malignancy screening tests. This includes a chest X-ray, flexible sigmoidoscopy, or colonoscopy for those above 50. Mammography and a pelvic exam for females above the age of 20 should also be done. If the donor has a history of malignancy, oncologic evaluation may be considered. Importantly, a prior history of malignancy may exclude kidney donation in certain circumstances. Those donors with a history of melanoma, testicular cancer, hematologic malignancy, renal cell carcinoma, choriocarcinoma, bronchial cancer, breast cancer, or monoclonal gammopathy should generally be excluded from donation unless 2–5 years of remission has elapsed. Prior history of treated or cured malignancy, thereby decreasing potential transmission to the recipient including early-stage colon cancer, nonmelanoma skin cancer, or carcinoma in situ of the cervix, may be considered for donation.

Hematuria

Workup for microscopic hematuria in donors is similar to the general population. Urine dipstick testing should be performed on two occasions to confirm the presence of microscopic hematuria. Positive results should be confirmed with analysis of the urinary sediment. Evidence of dysmorphic red cells, as well as proteinuria, casts, or decreased kidney function may be an indication of a glomerular pathology warranting further workup and potential kidney biopsy.

While current recommendations for workup of hematuria include a full urologic workup and screening for malignancy, Loo et al. used risk factors for the development of urothelial malignancy to develop a risk index as a means to stratify patients as high or low risk for malignancy detection [34]. Using a prospective cohort of 2,630 patients evaluated for hematuria, 2.1 % had a neoplasm detected and 1.9 % had histopathologic confirmation of a urothelial tract malignancy. Predictive factors including age >50 years, recent gross hematuria, and male gender were used to develop a Hematuria Risk Index. The risk index was then validated in 1,784 patients. Of the patients identified as low risk (32 %), 0.2 % had a detected neoplasm. Fourteen percent were identified as high risk, with 11.1 % found to have a malignancy [34]. The results indicate that extensive testing and additional cost may be avoided through use of the proposed risk index. Persistent microscopic hematuria (>3 months duration) may be present in up to 3 % of the general population and may have important implications in the development of ESKD. In over one million Israeli adults screened for entry into military service, Vivante et al. demonstrated an increased risk of ESKD. Adjusting for age, sex, paternal country of origin, year of enrollment, BMI, and BP at baseline revealed a hazard ratio of 18.5 (95 % CI, 12.4–27.6) [35]. ESKD attributed to glomerular disease for individuals with isolated microscopic hematuria occurred with incidence rates of 19.6 versus 0.55 per 100,000 person-years (HR: 32.4, 95 % CI, 18.9–55.7).

Koushik et al. noted in 512 potential donors that 14 (2.7 %) continued to have microscopic hematuria for >1 month [36]. Urinary tract imaging and full urologic workup was performed, and if the potential donor still wanted to donate, and the results of the urologic testing were unremarkable, a kidney biopsy was performed. Two of the donors experienced resolution of hematuria after treatment for urinary tract infections and two candidates declined donation. Kidney biopsy was performed in the remaining with normal finding observed in two donors, four had thin basement membrane nephropathy; one nonhomogeneous basement membrane abnormalities; IgA nephropathy was found in one, 5 of 16 glomeruli with global sclerosis; one in a patient with a family history of Schimke's Syndrome, 7 of 30 glomeruli with global sclerosis; and one thin basement membrane nephropathy. Only four of the ten who underwent kidney biopsy donated.

Pregnancy After Kidney Donation

It is important to counsel donors regarding a possible increased risk of adverse pregnancy-related issues after kidney donation. Early studies that were small in number indicated no significant increased risk of pregnancy after kidney donation; however, recently, Ibrahim et al. surveyed donors from 1963 to 2007 and included information on predonation pregnancy as well as post donation pregnancies regarding pregnancy. The authors compared pregnancy outcomes of 1,785 donors and 3,213 reported pregnancies. Fetal, and maternal outcomes were similar to the general population; however in those pregnancies post kidney donation, there was an association with lower likelihood of full-term delivery (73.7 % vs. 84.6 %, $p = 0.0004$) and a higher likelihood of fetal loss, including death, miscarriage, and abortion (19.2 % vs. 11.3 %, $p < 0.0001$). Those pregnancies post donation were also associated with a higher risk of gestational diabetes (2.7 % vs. 0.7 %, $p = 0.0001$), gestational hypertension (5.7 % vs. 0.6 %, $p < 0.0001$), proteinuria (4.3 % vs. 1.1 %, $p < 0.0001$), and preeclampsia (5.5 % vs. 0.8 %, $p < 0.0001$) [37]. Similar results have been reported from Norway (ref). Although this study is retrospective and single center in nature, it provides important information when counseling female subjects on the risks of kidney donation.

Smoking

The association between smoking and various health conditions is well established. Given the known perioperative consequences of long-term tobacco use such as ventilator dependence and pneumonia, donors with a history of shortness of breath or chronic cough should be evaluated with a chest X-ray and possible pulmonary function testing prior to surgery. Importantly, smoking is also strongly associated with renal cell carcinoma [38, 39]. The relative risk of incident renal cell carcinoma in those with a history of tobacco use compared to those with no history is 1.38 (95 % CI, 1.09–1.36). Smoking is also associated with development of chronic kidney disease [40, 41]. Haroun et al. demonstrated a relative risk for the development of ESRD in men and women of 2.4 and 2.9, respectively [41]. Mechanistically, tobacco use may contribute to increased endothelial dysfunction, oxidative stress, and hemodynamic-mediated injury in the glomeruli [42, 43]. Smoking has been associated with increased surgical complications as well. However, in the setting of kidney donation, tobacco use in patients undergoing laparoscopic donor nephrectomy did not seem to lead to adverse postsurgical outcomes. In a review of 221 laparoscopic donor nephrectomies with a known tobacco use history, Taber et al. did not demonstrate a significant increased risk in operative time, mean length of hospital stay, blood loss, or use of narcotics [44]. Regardless, candidate donors should be counseled on the adverse effects of tobacco abuse and encourage smoking cessation prior to planned nephrectomy.

Financial Considerations

Part of the screening of potential donors includes evaluation of potential donor's financial circumstances, including healthcare insurance coverage as well as discussions regarding the financial implications of organ donation. Additional efforts to increase the donor pool have also included policy-driven changes such as tax incentives for potential kidney donors. The significant expense and lost wage associated with kidney donation is poorly characterized and the ability of donors to bear such burden financially is unclear. The National Organ Transplant Act (NOTA) excludes the use of monetary compensation or other "valuable consideration" for organ donation. This act excludes compensation related to travel, housing, or lost wages. Although it is currently illegal to offer payment for organ donation, many states currently have tax policies in place that propose to allow for tax breaks for expenses related to living donation. Currently there are 16 states that offer tax incentives (currently up to $10,000 in tax deductions with the exception of Iowa which offers a tax credit) for expenses incurred during the donation process. The impact of policies such as these on donation rates is not well known.

To further characterize the financial status of donors and their recipients, Gill et al. described the income of 54,483 living donor transplants in the United States from 2000 to 2009 [45]. Median household income data was linked to the 2000 United States census by ZIP code and divided into quintiles. Donor–recipient location and income level were described as "concordant" if the donor–recipients resided in the same ZIP code or the same median household income level. Those with "discordant" location or income level were those donor–recipient groups residing in different ZIP codes or of different household income level. They showed a similar proportion of transplants in which the recipient had a higher income than their donor compared to transplants in which the donor income was higher than that of the recipient, suggesting a limited ability of recipients to compensate potential donors based on lost wages, travel expenses or other expenses related to donation. Furthermore of those in which the recipient have a higher income than the donor, these differences were not substantial, and only 10 % of transplants had a median household difference in income of greater than $40,000. Factors associated with a large "income discordant" pairing of donor–recipient (>$40,000) included older age, male gender, education, preemptive kidney transplantation and Asian race.

The impact of nephrectomy on the ability to secure both life insurance policies and health care insurance has been an increasingly important issue. In Canadian study of the insurance status of donors, Yang et al. found no difference in the numbers of life insurance policies between 40 donors and controls in major Canadian cities. In reviewing the health care insurance status of donors, Gibney et al. reviewed the insurance status of 10,021 live kidney donations between July 2004 and September 2006. A total of 17.6 % of donors over this time period lacked health care insurance, although the sample likely underrepresented those without health care insurance and may also have not reflected those acquiring healthcare insurance after nephrectomy. In their study, they found a clear graded association for age, with the youngest donors more likely to have insurance. Males were also more likely to lack healthcare insurance [46]. In comparison with white living kidney donors, they also found that donors of African American, Hispanic and Asian ethnicity had a higher frequency of lack of coverage. In addition, those donors with a BMI >30, preexistent hypertension, and those with a eGFR <60 mL/min had similar rates of insurance as other LKD. In comparison with general US population insurance rates, the authors further characterized insurance patterns based on regional variation. They were able to show that donors, in general, were insured at a slightly higher frequency than the general population with the exception of highly populous areas such as the Great Lakes region (37 % vs. 14.8 %), California and the desert Southwest (27 % vs. 23.9 %), and the northeast region including New York (19.5 % vs. 18.1 %) [46]. The implementation of the Affordable Care Act will make this issue a thing of the past.

Conclusion

Increasing the numbers of available live donors as well as improving safety to those willing to donate must go hand and hand. Efforts may include but are not limited to a protocol-based evaluation that includes uniform guidelines for evaluation, continued medical follow-up after donation, and establishing donor registries.

References

1. Taler SJ, Messersmith EE, Leichtman AB, Gillespie BW, Kew CE, Stegall MD, et al. Demographic, metabolic, and blood pressure characteristics of living kidney donors spanning five decades. Am J Transplant.2013;13(2):390–8.doi:10.1111/j.1600-6143.2012.04321.x.
2. Horvat LD, Shariff SZ, Garg AX. Global trends in the rates of living kidney donation. Kidney Int. 2009;75(10):1088–98. doi:10.1038/ki.2009.20.
3. Textor SC, Taler SJ, Driscoll N, Larson TS, Gloor J, Griffin M, et al. Blood pressure and renal function after kidney donation from hypertensive living donors. Transplantation. 2004;78(2):276–82.
4. Segev DL, Muzaale AD, Caffo BS, Mehta SH, Singer AL, Taranto SE, et al. Perioperative mortality and long-term survival following live kidney donation. JAMA. 2010;303(10):959–66. doi:10.1001/jama.2010.237.
5. Knoll G, Cockfield S, Blydt-Hansen T, Baran D, Kiberd B, Landsberg D, et al. Canadian Society of Transplantation: consensus guidelines on eligibility for kidney transplantation. CMAJ. 2005;173(10):S1–25. doi:10.1503/cmaj.1041588.
6. Norden G, Lennerling A, Nyberg G. Low absolute glomerular filtration rate in the living kidney donor: a risk factor for graft loss. Transplantation. 2000;70(9):1360–2.
7. Lin J, Knight EL, Hogan ML, Singh AK. A comparison of prediction equations for estimating glomerular filtration rate in adults without kidney disease. J Am Soc Nephrol. 2003;14(10):2573–80.
8. Lujan PR, Chiurchiu C, Douthat W, de Arteaga J, de la Fuente J, Capra RH, et al. CKD-EPI instead of MDRD for candidates to kidney donation. Transplantation. 2012;94(6):637–41. doi:10.1097/TP.0b013e3182603260.
9. Chung E, Grant AB, Hibberd AD, Sprott P. Why potential live renal donors prefer laparoscopic nephrectomy: a survey of live donor attitudes. BJU Int. 2007;100(6):1344–6. doi:10.1111/j.1464-410X.2007.07126.x.
10. Wilson CH, Sanni A, Rix DA, Soomro NA. Laparoscopic versus open nephrectomy for live kidney donors. Cochrane Database Syst Rev. 2011;(11):CD006124. doi:10.1002/14651858.CD006124.pub2.
11. Matas AJ, Bartlett ST, Leichtman AB, Delmonico FL. Morbidity and mortality after living kidney donation, 1999–2001: survey of United States transplant centers. Am J Transplant. 2003;3(7):830–4.
12. Fehrman-Ekholm I, Elinder CG, Stenbeck M, Tyden G, Groth CG. Kidney donors live longer. Transplantation. 1997;64(7):976–8.
13. Okamoto M, Akioka K, Nobori S, Ushigome H, Kozaki K, Kaihara S, et al. Short- and long-term donor outcomes after kidney donation: analysis of 601 cases over a 35-year period at Japanese single center. Transplantation. 2009;87(3):419–23. doi:10.1097/TP.0b013e318192dc95.
14. Ibrahim HN, Foley R, Tan L, Rogers T, Bailey RF, Guo H, et al. Long-term consequences of kidney donation. N Engl J Med. 2009;360(5):459–69. doi:10.1056/NEJMoa0804883.
15. Mjoen G, Reisaeter A, Hallan S, Line PD, Hartmann A, Midtvedt K, et al. Overall and cardiovascular mortality in Norwegian kidney donors compared to the background population. Nephrol Dial Transplant. 2012;27(1):443–7. doi:10.1093/ndt/gfr303.
16. Garg AX, Meirambayeva A, Huang A, Kim J, Prasad GV, Knoll G, et al. Cardiovascular disease in kidney donors: matched cohort study. BMJ. 2012;344:e1203.
17. Andersen B, Hansen JB, Jorgensen SJ. Survival after nephrectomy. Scand J Urol Nephrol. 1968;2(2):91–4.
18. Narkun-Burgess DM, Nolan CR, Norman JE, Page WF, Miller PL, Meyer TW. Forty-five year follow-up after uninephrectomy. Kidney Int. 1993;43(5):1110–5.
19. Baudoin P, Provoost AP, Molenaar JC. Renal function up to 50 years after unilateral nephrectomy in childhood. Am J Kidney Dis. 1993;21(6):603–11.
20. Garg AX, Muirhead N, Knoll G, Yang RC, Prasad GV, Thiessen-Philbrook H, et al. Proteinuria and reduced kidney function in living kidney donors: a systematic review, meta-analysis, and meta-regression. Kidney Int. 2006;70(10):1801–10. doi:10.1038/sj.ki.5001819.
21. Parasuraman R, Venkat KK. Utility of estimated glomerular filtration rate in live kidney donation. Clin J Am Soc Nephrol. 2008;3(6):1608–9. doi:10.2215/cjn.04840908.
22. Go AS, Chertow GM, Fan D, McCulloch CE, Hsu CY. Chronic kidney disease and the risks of death, cardiovascular events, and hospitalization. N Engl J Med. 2004;351(13):1296–305. doi:10.1056/NEJMoa041031.
23. Berger JC, Muzaale AD, James N, Hoque M, Wang JM, Montgomery RA, et al. Living kidney donors ages 70 and older: recipient and donor outcomes. Clin J Am Soc Nephrol. 2011;6(12):2887–93. doi:10.2215/cjn.04160511.

24. Hsu CY, Iribarren C, McCulloch CE, Darbinian J, Go AS. Risk factors for end-stage renal disease: 25-year follow-up. Arch Intern Med. 2009;169(4):342–50. doi:10.1001/archinternmed.2008.605.
25. Chagnac A, Weinstein T, Korzets A, Ramadan E, Hirsch J, Gafter U. Glomerular hemodynamics in severe obesity. Am J Physiol Renal Physiol. 2000;278(5):F817–22.
26. Kambham N, Markowitz GS, Valeri AM, Lin J, D'Agati VD. Obesity-related glomerulopathy: an emerging epidemic. Kidney Int. 2001;59(4):1498–509.doi:10.1046/j.1523-1755.2001.0590041498.x.
27. Heimbach JK, Taler SJ, Prieto M, Cosio FG, Textor SC, Kudva YC, et al. Obesity in living kidney donors: clinical characteristics and outcomes in the era of laparoscopic donor nephrectomy. Am J Transplant. 2005;5(5):1057–64. doi:10.1111/j.1600-6143.2005.00791.x.
28. O'Brien B, Mastoridis S, Crane J, Hakim N, Papalois V. Safety of nephrectomy in morbidly obese donors. Exp Clin Transplant. 2012;10(6):579–85.
29. Young A, Storsley L, Garg AX, Treleaven D, Nguan CY, Cuerden MS, et al. Health outcomes for living kidney donors with isolated medical abnormalities: a systematic review. Am J Transplant. 2008;8(9):1878–90. doi:10.1111/j.1600-6143.2008.02339.x.
30. Ommen ES, Schroppel B, Kim JY, Gaspard G, Akalin E, de Boccardo G, et al. Routine use of ambulatory blood pressure monitoring in potential living kidney donors. Clin J Am Soc Nephrol. 2007;2(5):1030–6. doi:10.2215/cjn.01240307.
31. Delmonico F. A report of the Amsterdam forum on the care of the live kidney donor: data and medical guidelines. Transplantation. 2005;79(6 Suppl):S53–66.
32. Rule AD, Krambeck AE, Lieske JC. Chronic kidney disease in kidney stone formers. Clin J Am Soc Nephrol. 2011;6(8):2069–75. doi:10.2215/cjn.10651110.
33. El-Zoghby ZM, Lieske JC, Foley RN, Bergstralh EJ, Li X, Melton III LJ, et al. Urolithiasis and the risk of ESRD. Clin J Am Soc Nephrol. 2012;7(9):1409–15. doi:10.2215/cjn.03210312.
34. Loo RK, Lieberman SF, Slezak JM, Landa HM, Mariani AJ, Nicolaisen G, et al. Stratifying risk of urinary tract malignant tumors in patients with asymptomatic microscopic hematuria. Mayo Clin Proc. 2013;88(2):129–38. doi:10.1016/j.mayocp.2012.10.004.
35. Vivante A, Afek A, Frenkel-Nir Y, Tzur D, Farfel A, Golan E, et al. Persistent asymptomatic isolated microscopic hematuria in Israeli adolescents and young adults and risk for end-stage renal disease. JAMA. 2011;306(7):729–36. doi:10.1001/jama.2011.1141.
36. Koushik R, Garvey C, Manivel JC, Matas AJ, Kasiske BL. Persistent, asymptomatic, microscopic hematuria in prospective kidney donors. Transplantation. 2005;80(10):1425–9.
37. Ibrahim HN, Akkina SK, Leister E, Gillingham K, Cordner G, Guo H, et al. Pregnancy outcomes after kidney donation. Am J Transplant. 2009;9(4):825–34.
38. Flaherty KT, Fuchs CS, Colditz GA, Stampfer MJ, Speizer FE, Willett WC, et al. A prospective study of body mass index, hypertension, and smoking and the risk of renal cell carcinoma (United States). Cancer Causes Control. 2005;16(9):1099–106. doi:10.1007/s10552-005-0349-8.
39. Hunt JD, van der Hel OL, McMillan GP, Boffetta P, Brennan P. Renal cell carcinoma in relation to cigarette smoking: meta-analysis of 24 studies. Int J Cancer. 2005;114(1):101–8. doi:10.1002/ijc.20618.
40. Ejerblad E, Fored CM, Lindblad P, Fryzek J, Dickman PW, Elinder CG, et al. Association between smoking and chronic renal failure in a nationwide population-based case–control study. J Am Soc Nephrol. 2004;15(8):2178–85. doi:10.1097/01.asn.0000135048.35659.10.
41. Haroun MK, Jaar BG, Hoffman SC, Comstock GW, Klag MJ, Coresh J. Risk factors for chronic kidney disease: a prospective study of 23,534 men and women in Washington County, Maryland. J Am Soc Nephrol. 2003;14(11):2934–41.
42. Nagasawa Y, Yamamoto R, Rakugi H, Isaka Y. Cigarette smoking and chronic kidney diseases. Hypertens Res. 2012;35(3):261–5. doi:10.1038/hr.2011.205.
43. Orth SR. Effects of smoking on systemic and intrarenal hemodynamics: influence on renal function. J Am Soc Nephrol. 2004;15 Suppl 1:S58–63.
44. Taber DJ, Ashcraft E, Cattanach LA, Baillie GM, Weimert NA, Lin A, et al. No difference between smokers, former smokers, or nonsmokers in the operative outcomes of laparoscopic donor nephrectomies. Surg Laparosc Endosc Percutan Tech. 2009;19(2):153–6. doi:10.1097/SLE.0b013e31819f42f4.
45. Gill JS, Gill J, Barnieh L, Dong J, Rose C, Johnston O, et al. Income of living kidney donors and the income difference between living kidney donors and their recipients in the United States. Am J Transplant. 2012;12(11):3111–8. doi:10.1111/j.1600-6143.2012.04211.x.
46. Gibney EM, Doshi MD, Hartmann EL, Parikh CR, Garg AX. Health insurance status of US living kidney donors. Clin J Am Soc Nephrol. 2010;5(5):912–6. doi:10.2215/cjn.07121009.

Extended Criteria Donors in Renal Transplantation

9

Todd E. Pesavento

It has long been an accepted reality that the demand for kidney transplantation exceeds the supply of organs available. Equally disturbing is the acceptance of the reliance on kidneys from "marginal" kidney donors. While these kidneys are important in helping to meet the ever growing demand for renal transplantation, it is essential for the transplant professional to understand the risks and benefits of extended criteria donor kidneys (typically referred to as "ECD kidneys"), the groups of patients that may be the best recipients of these organs, and medical management strategies that will allow for long-lasting function of these kidneys.

At the beginning of the twenty-first century, there was a growing awareness of the value of utilizing nontraditional living donors, e.g., spousal donors [1], nondirected donors [2], utilizing techniques to allow donation to highly sensitized recipients [3], and the use of donor exchange programs [4, 5]. With these individuals being more readily accepted as realistic donor candidates, the number of living kidney donors actually exceeded the number of deceased donors [5, 6]. However, as concern over long-term living donor safety has grown, the number of living donors has declined. In 2010, the number of deceased donors accounted for 65 % of the total number of kidneys transplanted with about 18 % of these donors being expanded criteria donor (ECD) which has not substantially changed in the last decade [7–9].

History and Classification

In an attempt to allow more patients to be transplanted and reduce organ discard rates, in 2002 the Organ Procurement and Transplantation Network/United Network for Organ Sharing (OPTN/UNOS) implemented an ECD program. This new ECD policy was based on donor factors previously shown to have significant prognostic importance for graft survival, namely, donor age, cause of death, renal function, and history of hypertension. As a result of these analyses, ECDs were defined as any kidney donor 60 years of age or older, or a donor equal to or greater than 50 years old and at least two of the following characteristics: (1) terminal creatinine >1.5 mg/dL, (2) cerebrovascular accident as the cause of death, and (3) history of arterial hypertension. Each of these criteria had been shown to portend a relative risk of graft loss exceeding 1.7 compared to "ideal donors" [10–12] (Table 9.1). Donation after cardiac death (DCD) is distinct from the ECD category and will not be extensively discussed in this chapter.

While the ECD/SCD classification is simple and convenient for practitioners and patients, the dichotomous categorization fails to account for fact that organs may be misclassified by the rigid diagnostic criteria. It is now clear that some SCD kidneys may have functional characteristics of ECD organs (Fig. 9.1) and some ECD kidneys could be inadvertently discarded for fear of poor function and outcome. Baskin-Bay et al. noted nearly 11 % of deceased donor kidneys had worse posttransplant survival rates but were not classified as ECD [13].

To more accurately characterize donor kidneys, Rao et al. [14] have proposed a more granular index of risk, a continuous kidney donor risk index (KDRI). This index, based on data from the Scientific Registry of Transplant Recipients (SRTR), incorporates ten donor and four transplant characteristics that have been demonstrated to be independently and significantly associated with graft failure or death compared to a healthy 40-year-old donor. These factors include donor age, race, history of hypertension, history of diabetes, serum creatinine, cerebrovascular cause of death, height, weight, donation after cardiac death, hepatitis C virus status, human leukocyte antigen B and DR mismatch, cold ischemia time, and double or en bloc transplant. Analyzing nearly 70,000 deceased donors over a 10-year period, the authors noted the minimum KDRI was 0.5 and the maximal value was 4.2, although smaller and larger values were possible.

T.E. Pesavento, M.D. (✉)
Comprehensive Transplant Center, Ohio State University, 395 West 12th Avenue, Columbus, OH 43210, USA
e-mail: todd.pesavento@osumc.edu

M.R. Weir and E.V. Lerma (eds.), *Kidney Transplantation: Practical Guide to Management*,
DOI 10.1007/978-1-4939-0342-9_9, © Springer Science+Business Media New York 2014

Table 9.1 Definition of extended criteria kidney donor

	A	B
Age	60 or older	50–59 and two of the following characteristics
Creatinine		>1.5 mg/dL
Hypertension		History of hypertension
Cause of donor death		Cerebrovascular death

ECD donors are considered present if the donor has characteristics from either column A or B
The risk of graft failure is 70 % higher than a standard criteria donor

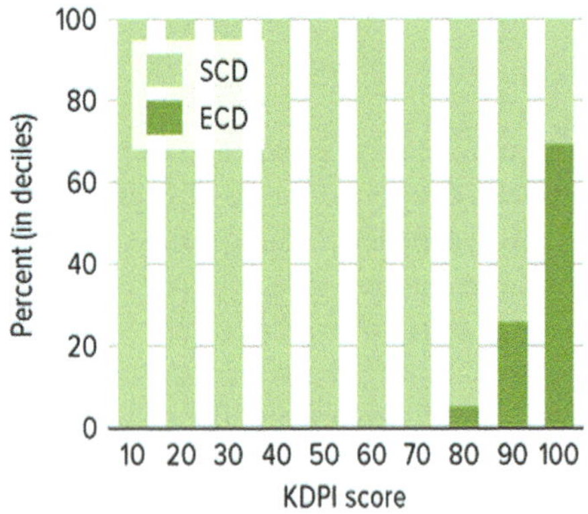

Fig. 9.1 Kidney donor profile index (KDPI) scores for ECD and SCD kidneys. KDPI scores mapped from kidney donor profile risk for 2011. The lower KDPI score represents kidneys with better functional and demographic characteristics. Higher scores are more likely to represent kidneys with less favorable characteristics. Reference Matas et al. [7]

It was noted the median KDRI was 1.05, which compares closely to the graft failure rate of the reference donor with a KDRI of 1.00. The KDRI is now remapped into a cumulative percentage scale from 0 to 100 using a kidney donor profile index (KDPI). This KDPI is easier to explain to patients as a donor with a KDPI of 80 % would have a higher expected graft failure rate than 80 % of kidneys recovered during the last year. See Fig. 9.1 for graphic representation.

Currently, UNOS has proposed a new kidney allocation policy which incorporates the KDRI classification. The public comment period closed in December of 2012 and a UNOS Board decision is expected in June of 2013 [15].

Benefits of ECD Organs

While understanding the variables used to classify ECD kidneys and the implications on graft outcome is important, applying this information for transplanting the appropriate organ in the best recipient is the ultimate goal. Ojo et al. provided the first evidence that transplanting "marginal" kidneys resulted in a tangible benefit. In his seminal study, waitlisted patients who received a kidney from older donors with either hypertension, diabetes, or prolonged cold ischemia had an average 5-year survival benefit compared to those patients who remained on the waiting list [16]. In 2005 Merion et al. further defined the benefits of transplantation using extended criteria donors [17].

Notable findings from the Merion study included a 17 % reduction in adjusted long-term mortality for recipients of ECD transplants compared to those who were waitlisted and may have eventually received a non-ECD organ. While there was a long-term improvement in mortality, the perioperative morality risk was 5.2-fold higher during the first 2 weeks posttransplant compared to the waitlisted group. This excess mortality risk eventually declined, and by 33 weeks the mortality risk equaled that in the waitlisted group. However, the substantial early risk resulted in a cumulative mortality that did not become equal in the two groups until 3.5 years posttransplant.

Management of ECD Organs

Understanding which organs are classified as ECD and the allocation system that distributes these organs is important but, ultimately, what is paramount is the appropriate management of these kidneys and choosing immunosuppression that will allow for both excellent short- and long-term graft survival.

Although it is convenient to address management of the recipient's kidney transplant at the time of implantation, it is more appropriate to consider how the organ is preserved as this factor can have a crucial impact in the cascade of events during the first few days and weeks following transplantation. At the present time, there still remains no clear consensus as to whether static cold storage versus hypothermic machine perfusion (so-called pulsatile perfusion) is superior for organ preservation. While there are advantages to each method, improving short- and long-term outcomes remains the overall goal. Moers et al. helped to answer this important question in a well-done, large-scale, prospective randomized trial of 336 kidney donors in which each of the paired kidneys were randomized to either cold storage or machine perfusion [18]. After 1 year of follow-up, there was a significant reduction in delayed graft function, improved graft survival, and reduction of serum creatinine in the first 2 weeks following transplantation. In a follow-up to their initial study, the authors analyzed graft survival at 3 years [19]. Importantly, overall graft survival continued to be significantly better in the machine preservation group. Even more impressive was the improvement in graft survival from expanded donor kidneys in the machine preservation group compared to cold storage (86 % vs. 76 % with an adjusted hazard ratio of 0.38, $P=0.01$). The authors then followed-up this study with an economic analysis that determined a net cost savings of over $8,000 for ECD using machine preservation [20].

A potential advantage of machine preservation is ex vivo perfusion of substrate to reduce ischemia-reperfusion injury and assessment of dynamic flow characteristics that can help make more informed decisions regarding acceptance of organ offers. However, neither histological assessment of donor kidneys nor machine perfusion characteristics have been reproducibly validated or have sufficient positive predictive value [21–23].

Irrespective of how the organ is preserved, cold ischemia time remains an important determinant of delayed graft function. Several studies have quantified the impact of duration of cold ischemia time in ECD transplants, and while there is a graded effect for increasing periods of ischemia, times greater than 10 h appear to have a significant effect [24, 25].

Impact of Donor Age

Kidneys from older donors are physiologically and immunologically different than kidneys from younger donors, and these changes make these kidneys more susceptible to damage and reduce the likelihood of meaningful recovery. Older kidneys have glomerular, interstitial, and vascular senescence [26, 27], reduced glomerular filtration rates, and overall worse renal function compared to younger recipients [27, 28]. A large study of older donors in Spain examined 3,365 transplants from donors older than 60 years, and at 1 year, their creatinine was significantly higher compared to younger donors, 2.1 versus 1.6 mg/dL ($P<0.0001$) [29]. In addition to preexisting damage, older kidneys are at an increased risk for acute rejection [26, 27]. Fijter et al. demonstrated kidneys from donors >age 50 had a 1.53 times higher rate of rejection compared to younger donors [27].

One option available to allow a successful outcome with ECD organs is the transplantation of dual kidneys when one alone may not allow for satisfactory outcomes. This approach reduces organ discard rates while still achieving the goal of successful transplants in appropriate candidates. Tan et al. reported on their sizeable experience using dual kidney ECD transplants compared to standard donors. The 8-year actuarial graft survival was not different between the two groups, but waiting time was significantly reduced by 224 days ($P<0.01$) [30].

Potential Implications of Using ECD Organs

A significant concern of transplant centers is that the utilization of extended criteria donor kidneys may result in poor outcomes that are publicly reported and used by the Center for Medicaid and Medicare Services (CMS) to determine if sanctioning and removal of public funding should occur. Schold et al. analyzed data from the SRTR from January 2007 to July 2009 and determined that 23 % of all adult kidney programs were considered to be low-performing centers as defined by lower than expected 1-year patient or graft survival [31]. These so-called low-performing centers had a reduction of over 22 transplants during the study period compared to an increase of nearly eight additional transplants at other centers. These low-performing centers had a decrease of all donor types, but ECD transplants declined by nearly five during this study period, suggesting that centers may view these kidneys as having unnecessary risk. This compared to an increase of nearly four additional ECD transplants at other centers. Therefore, understanding appropriate donor and recipient management strategies may help to reduce the risk associated with these kidneys.

Defining which patient group benefits (and just as importantly, who is harmed) from ECD kidney transplants is essential if transplant centers properly educate the patients and advise them to be listed for ECD transplants. Merion et al. analyzed over 109,000 waitlisted patients from 1995 to 2002 to determine which patients would benefit from ECD transplants [17]. After reviewing the results of nearly 8,000 transplants, they were able to demonstrate that the cumulative survival benefit of ECD compared to SCD transplants did not occur until 3.5 years, but the overall mortality risk was reduced by 17 % for patients who received an ECD transplant versus remaining on the waiting list. Significant benefit was specifically shown in the subgroup of patients under the following conditions: (1) median waiting times greater than 1,350 days: patients greater than age 40 and older, non-Hispanic, all races, and both sexes, and (2) median waiting times less than 1,350: only recipients with diabetes as the cause of ESRD demonstrated significant benefit. Figure 9.2 summarizes the proposed algorithm for ECD kidneys. Diabetics as a group experienced a 23 % reduction in long-term mortality when receiving an ECD kidney, likely due to the shorter waiting time and avoidance of dialysis complications. Patients less than age 40 did not benefit from ECD transplantation despite a shorter waiting time.

Traditionally, ECDs have referred to deceased donors, but with the ever expanding recipient waiting list, centers are now utilizing living donors that are older, obese, more often hypertensive, and with reduced renal function than previously. These living donors are now referred to as "medically complex" rather than extended criteria living donors. Regardless of the label, these living donor kidneys are at risk for delayed graft function, reduced long-term function, and less able to withstand challenges due to reduced nephron mass [32–34].

Although the data delineating which patients are the best candidates for ECD transplants has been available for over 7 years, there is still wide variability on how this is applied to candidates at the time of listing which has consequences for the patients' overall waiting time and long-term survival.

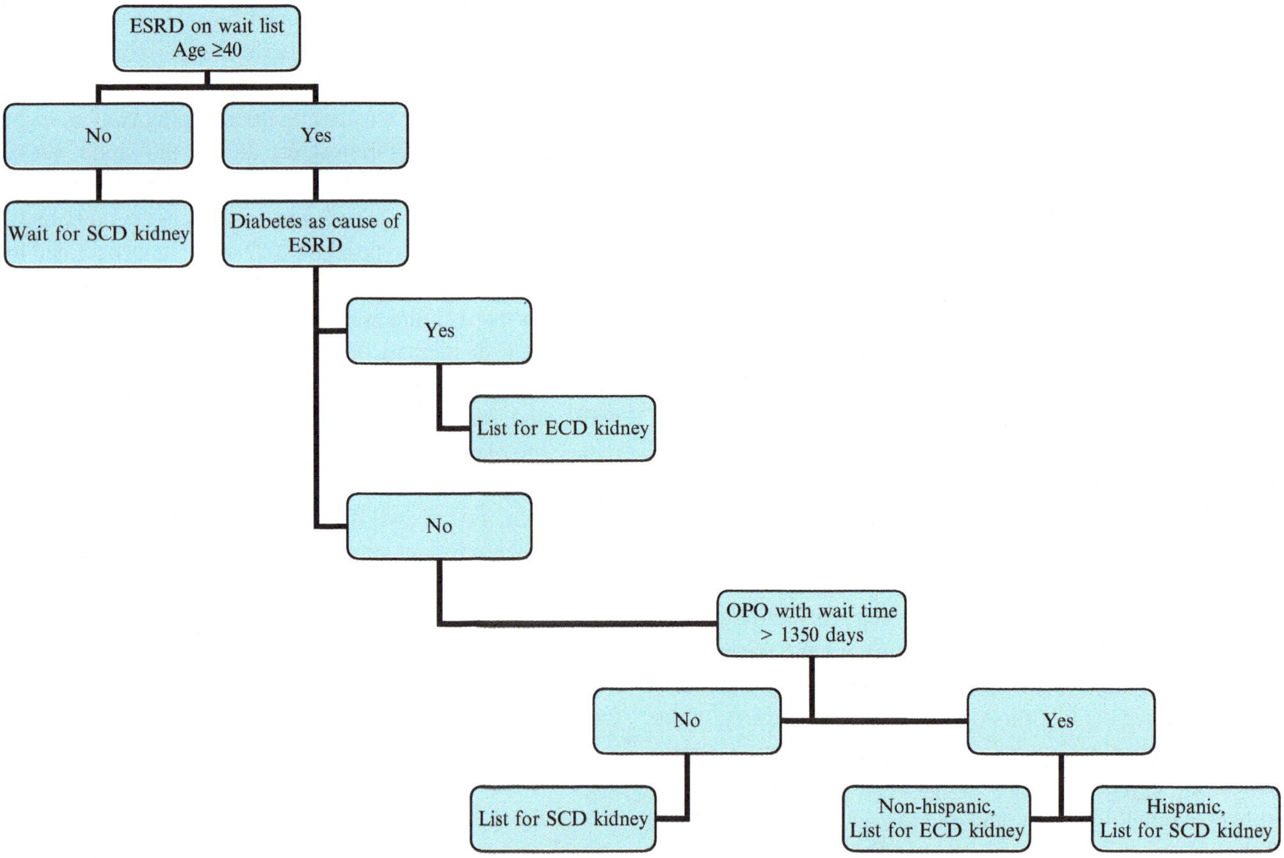

Fig. 9.2 Algorithm for listing patient for extended criteria donor kidney. Adapted from Merion et al. [17]

One large study demonstrated that only 50 % of patients that by Merion's criteria [17] would benefit from an ECD kidney were listed for such an organ. Neither diabetic status nor length of the waitlist had any significant association with being listed for an ECD kidney [35]. Therefore, education of transplant professionals and patients is important to realize benefit from these organs.

Immunosuppressive Management

Immunosuppressive management that reduces acute rejection episodes and minimizes ischemic damage is the cornerstone of successful management of these fragile organs. The cardiovascular impact of renal dysfunction is not widely appreciated. A retrospective study of nearly 59,000 renal transplant recipients in the United States Renal Data System registry noted that a serum creatinine greater than 1.5 mg/dL at 1 year was strongly associated with cardiovascular death [36]. Therefore, minimizing renal dysfunction is important not only for graft survival but reducing patient mortality.

While there are multiple strategies to achieve these goals, the general concepts that most agree are useful include induction therapy to allow the delayed introduction of calcineurin inhibitors (CNI) and ultimately calcineurin elimination or minimization.

Delayed CNI introduction is possible with depleting antibody agents. A relatively large prospective trial using either rabbit anti-thymocyte globulin or alemtuzumab as the induction agent with delayed introduction of tacrolimus resulted in comparable rates of delayed graft function, acute rejections, and graft survival rates with a mean follow-up of 24 months in ECD kidneys compared to SCDs [37].

Recently, a novel immunosuppressive agent, belatacept has been used in renal transplantation as a costimulatory blocker that binds to CD80 and CD86 and has been demonstrated to allow for calcineurin inhibitor minimization. In the BENEFIT-EXT study, patients receiving an ECD kidney transplant were randomized to either belatacept or cyclosporine. At 3 years acute rejection rates were similar in each group, graft survival was not different at 82–80 %, but calculated GFR was 11 mL/min/1.73 m^2 higher in the belatacept versus cyclosporine group. Moreover, this difference in GFR persisted and widened over time, from 8 ml/min at 1 year to 11 mL/min at 3 years [38].

In an open-label phase II trial, patients between 6 and 36 months posttransplant were randomized to either continue their calcineurin inhibitor or to change to belatacept.

There was a significant improvement in overall renal function in the belatacept group. Although the trial did not exclusively enroll patient with ECD transplants, the subgroup of patients converted to belatacept with a GFR less than 45 did experience an improvement in GFR compared to the CNI group (3.7 vs. 2.8 mL/min). The group with the greatest gain in GFR has renal function at baseline between 45 and 60 with a gain of 10.0 versus 1.9 mL/min. Of note, 7 % of patients in the belatacept conversion group experienced an acute rejection episode (vs. none in the CNI group), although there were no graft losses overall [39].

Conversion from a calcineurin inhibitor to other non-nephrotoxic agents is appealing, but the clinically available options are limited at this point [40]. The mammalian target of rapamycin (mTOR) agents, sirolimus/everolimus would appear to be reasonable agents. However, if conversion from CNIs is to be accomplished, data from the CONVERT trial gives some guidance in which type of patient is not appropriate [41]. In this trial, patients between 6 and 120 months posttransplant were randomized to remaining on a CNI or to sirolimus. Overall, at 2 years, patients randomized to sirolimus had a significantly higher GFR (62.6 vs. 59.9 mL/min) compared to the CNI group; this benefit was even more pronounced in the subgroup of patients with a baseline GFR >40 mL/min and U prot/creat ≤0.11 (63.8 vs. 59.0 mL/min). However, in patients with a GFR between 20 and 40 mL/min, the study was halted as 16.7 % of the sirolimus group reached the primary endpoint of acute rejection, graft loss, or death compared to 0 % in the CNI group. Also, in the overall study, proteinuria rose significantly in the sirolimus group.

Lessons from Other Countries

Given a relatively fixed supply of deceased donor kidneys, one strategy to raise the total number of "graft years" from these transplants is to age match the donor and recipient. The rationale for this approach is to better match the nephron supply with the metabolic and physiologic demand of the recipient. It also acknowledges that older recipients receiving kidneys from younger donors may not fully utilize the organ due to death with a functioning graft. In 1999 the Eurotransplant Senior Program (ESP) was initiated in which deceased donor kidneys from donors over 65 years of age were allocated to nonimmunized recipients older than 65 in their local area to minimize cold ischemia time [42]. The results of this so-called old to old strategy reduced cold ischemia time by 7 h, waiting time in elderly patients was shortened by 250 days, and prompt initial function and delayed graft function was improved in the "old to old" group.

Using this strategy, older patients receiving kidneys from older donors have comparable 8-year actual graft survival compared to patients who receive kidneys from younger donors [43]. However, younger patients have significantly worse graft survival when they receive kidneys from older donors (RR 1.97, $P<0.001$) [44]. This kidney matching program, in part, is responsible for a significantly lower risk rate of death with a functioning graft. At 10 years posttransplant, patients in the USA compared to Spain have a significantly higher risk of death with a functioning graft, with a hazard ratio of 2.31 ($P<0.001$). However, when graft survival is death censored, 10-year survival is the same at 76 % [45].

A retrospective analysis of the Australia and New Zealand Dialysis and Transplant Registry from 1991 to 2005 reviewed the outcomes of 4,466 recipients of deceased donor kidney transplants, including 781 ECD organs. Acute rejections were significantly more common with donor age and ECD status ($P<0.001$) [26]. Although graft survival and estimated GFR was lower at 1 year, by 5 years there were no significant differences in either of these measures. This is in contrast to donors aged 60 or older where death-censored graft survival was significantly greater compared to non-ECD counterparts (HR 3.43, $P<0.001$) and eGFR was significantly less than ECD age 50–59 (31.1 vs. 36.9 mL/min, $P<0.05$).

Conclusion

Due to the ever expanding kidney transplant waiting list and the likely changes to the kidney allocation schema, it is vital that transplant professional become more aware of the value and limitations of extended criteria kidney donors. In appropriate patients, these organs can shorten waiting times, increase patient survival, and achieve acceptable short- and long-term outcomes. Aggressive donor management with pulsatile perfusion, reduced cold ischemia times, and use of non-nephrotoxic immunosuppressive agents are all important factors in attaining successful results. While the patients who receive these kidneys are more medically challenging, the rewards are well worth the effort needed to realize success.

Acknowledgment The data and analyses reported in the 2011 Annual Data Report of the Organ Procurement and Transplantation Network and the US Scientific Registry of Transplant Recipients have been supplied by the Minnesota Medical Research Foundation and UNOS under contract with HHS/HRSA. The authors alone are responsible for reporting and interpreting these data; the views expressed herein are those of the authors and not necessarily those of the US Government.

References

1. Terasaki PI, Cecka JM, Gjertson DW, Takemoto S. High survival rates of kidney transplants from spousal and living unrelated donors. N Engl J Med. 1995;333:333–6.
2. Dams PL, Cohen DJ, Danovitch GM, Deington MD, Gaston RS, Jacobs CL, Luskin RS, Metzger RA, Peters TG, Siminoff LA, Veatch RM, Tothberg-Wegman L, Bartlett ST, Brigham L, Burdick J,

Gunderson S, Harmon W, Matas AJ, Thistlehwaite JR, Delmonico FL. The nondirected live-kidney donor: ethical considerations and practice guidelines. Transplantation. 2002;74:582–90.
3. Marfo K, Lu A, Ling M, Akalin E. Desensitization protocols and their outcome. Clin J Am Soc Nephrol. 2011;6:922–36.
4. Massie AB, Gentry SE, Montgomery RA, Bingaman AA, Segev DL. Center-level utilization of kidney paired donation. Am J Transplant. 2013. doi:10.1111/ajt.12189.
5. Wallis CB, Samy KP, Roth AE, Rees MA. Kidney paired donation. Nephrol Dial Transplant. 2011;26:2091–9.
6. Davis CL, Delmonico FL. Living-donor kidney transplantation: a review of the current practices for the live donor. J Am Soc Nephrol. 2005;16:2098–110.
7. Matas AJ, Smith JM, Skeans MA, Lamb KE, Gustafson SK, Samana CJ, Stewart DE, Snyder JJ, Israni AK, Kasiske BL. OPTN/SRTR 2011 annual data report: kidney. Am J Transplant. 2013;13 Suppl 1:11–46.
8. Kasiske BL, Skeans MA, Leighton TR, Ghimire V, Leppke SN, Israni AK. OPTN/SRTR 2011 annual data report: international data. Am J Transplant. 2013;13 Suppl 1:199–225.
9. Israni AK, Zaun DA, Rosendale JD, Snyder JJ, Ksaiske BL. OPTN/SRTR 2011 annual data report: deceased organ donation. Am J Transplant. 2013;13 Suppl 1:179–98.
10. Port FK, Bragg-Gresham JL, Metzger RA, Dykstra DM, Gillespie BW, Young EW, Delmonico FL, Wynn JJ, Merion RM, Wolfe RA, Held PJ. Donor characteristics associated with reduced graft survival: an approach to expanding the pool of kidney donors. Transplantation. 2002;74:1281–6.
11. Metzger RA, Delmonico FL, Feng S, Port FK, Wynn JJ, Merion RM. Expanded criteria donors for kidney transplantation. Am J Transplant. 2003;3 Suppl 4:S114–25.
12. Pascual J, Zamora J, Pirsch JD. A systematic review of kidney transplantation from expanded criteria donors. Am J Kidney Dis. 2008;52:553–86.
13. Baskin-Bay ES, Kremers W, Stegall MD, Nyberg SL. United network for organ sharing's expanded criteria donors: is stratification useful. Clin Transplant. 2005;19:406–12.
14. Rao PS, Schaubel DE, Guidinger MK, Andreoni KA, Wolfe RA, Merion RM, Port FK, Sung RS. A comprehensive risk quantification score for deceased donor kidneys: the kidney donor risk index. Transplantation. 2009;88:231–6.
15. Heaphy ELG, Goldfarb DA, Poggio ED, Buccini LD, Flechner SM, Schold JD. The impact of deceased donor kidney risk significantly varies by recipient characteristics. Am J Transplant. 2013;13(4):1001–11. doi:10.1111/ajt. 12154.
16. Ojo AK, Hanson JA, Meier-Kriesche HU, Okechukwu CN, Wolfe RA, Leichtman AB, Agodoa LY, Kaplan B, Port FK. Survival in recipients of marginal cadaveric donor kidneys compared with other recipients and wait-listed candidates. J Am Soc Nephrol. 2001;12:589–97.
17. Merion RM, Ashby VB, Wolfe RA, Distant DA, Hulbert-Shearon TE, Metzger RA, Ojo AO, Port FK. Deceased-donor characteristics and the survival benefit of kidney transplantation. JAMA. 2005;294:2726–33.
18. Moers C, Smits JM, Maathuis MHJ, Treckmann J, van Gelder F, Napieralski BP, van Kasterop-Kutz M, van der Heide JJH, Squifflet JP, van Heurn E, Kirste GR, Rahmel A, Leuvenink HGD, Paul A, Pirenne J, Ploeg RJ. Machine perfusion or cold storage in deceased-donor kidney transplantation. N Engl J Med. 2009;360:7–19.
19. Moers C, Pirenne J, Paul A, Ploeg RJ. Machine perfusion or cold storage in deceased-donor kidney transplantation. N Engl J Med. 2012;366:770–1.
20. Groen H, Moers C, Smits JM, Treckmann J, Monbaliu D, Rahmel A, Paul A, Pirenne J, Ploeg RJ, Buskens E. Cost-effectiveness of hypothermic machine preservation versus static cold storage in renal transplantation. Am J Transplant. 2012;12:1824–30.
21. Strattta RJ, Moore PS, Farney AC, Rogers J, Hartman EL, Reeves-Daniel A, Gautreaux MD, Iskandar SS, Adams PL. Influence of pulsatile perfusion preservation on outcomes in kidney transplantation from expanded criteria donors. J Am Coll Surg. 2007;204:873–84.
22. Shapiro R, Halloran PF, Delmonico FL, Bromber JS. The "two, one, zero" decision: what to do with suboptimal deceased donor kidneys. Am J Transplant. 2010;10:1959–60.
23. Tso PL, Dar WA, Henry ML. With respect to elderly patients: finding kidneys in the context of new allocation concepts. Am J Transplant. 2012;12:1091–8.
24. Kim SM, Ahn S, Min SI, Park D, Park T, Min SK, Kim SJ, Ha J. Cold ischemic time is critical in outcomes of expanded criteria donor renal transplantation. Clin Transplant. 2013;27:132–9.
25. Kayler LK, Magliocca J, Zendejas I, Srinivas TR, Schold JD. Impact of cold ischemia time on graft survival among ECD transplant recipients: a paired kidney analysis. Am J Transplant. 2011;11:2647–56.
26. Collins MG, Chang SH, Russ GR, McDonald SP. Outcomes of transplantation using kidneys from donors meeting expanded criteria in Australia and New Zealand, 1991 to 2005. Transplantation. 2009;87:1201–9.
27. De Fijter JW, Mallaat MJK, Noxiadis IIN, Ringers J, Rosendaal FR, Claas FHJ, Paul LC. Increased immunogenicity and cause of graft loss of old donor kidneys. J Am Soc Nephrol. 2001;12:1538–46.
28. Woo YM, Gill JS, Johnson N, Pereira BJG, Hariharan S. The advanced age deceased kidney donor: current outcomes and future opportunities. Kidney Int. 2005;67:2407–14.
29. Oppenheimer F, Alijam P, Peinado CA, Bustamante JB, Albiach JFC, Perich LG. The impact of donor age on the results of renal transplantation. Nephrol Dial Transplant. 2004;19 Suppl 3:11–5.
30. Tan JC, Alfrey EJ, Dafoe DC, Millan MT, Scandling JD. Dual-kidney transplantation with organs from expanded criteria donors: a long-term follow-up. Transplantation. 2004;78:692–6.
31. Schold JD, Buccini LD, Srinivas TR, Srinivas RT, Poggio ED, Flechner SM, Soria C, Segev DL, Fung J, Goldfarb DA. The association of center performance evaluations and kidney transplant volume in the United States. Am J Transplant. 2013;13:67–75.
32. Textor S, Taler S. Expanding criteria for living kidney donors: what are the limits? Transplant Rev. 2008;22:187–91.
33. O'Brien B, Mastoridis S, Sabharwal A, Hakim N, Taube D, Papalois V. Expanding the donor pool: living donor nephrectomy in the elderly and the overweight. Transplantation. 2012;93:1158–65.
34. Berger JC, Muzaale AD, James N, Hoque M, Garonzik Wang JM, Montgomery RA, Massie AB, Hall EC, Segev DL. Living kidney donors ages 70 and older: recipient and donor outcomes. Clin J Am Soc Nephrol. 2011;6:2887–93.
35. Grams ME, Massie AB, Schold JD, Chen BP, Segev DL. Trends in the inactive kidney transplant waitlist and implications for candidate survival. Am J Transplant. 2013;13(4):1012–8. doi:10.1111/ajt 12143.
36. Meier-Kriesche HU, Baliga R, Kaplan B. Decreased renal function is a strong risk factor for cardiovascular death after renal transplantation. Transplantation. 2003;75(8):1291–5.
37. Stratta RJ, Rohr MS, Sundberg AK, Farney AC, Hartmann EL, Moore PS, Rogers J, Iskandar SS, Gautreaux MD, Kiger DF, Doares W, Anderson TK, Hairston G, Adams PL. Intermediate-term outcomes with expanded criteria deceased donors in kidney transplantation. A spectrum or specter of quality? Ann Surg. 2006;243:594–603.
38. Pestana JOM, Grinyo JM, Vanrenterghem Y, Becker T, Campistol MJ, Florman S, Garcia VD, Kamar N, Lang P, Manfro RC, Massari P, Rial MDC, Schnitzler MA, Vitko S, Duan T, Block A, Harler MB, Durrbach A. Three-year outcomes from BENEFIT-EXT: a phase III study of belatacept versus cyclosporine in recipients of extended criteria donor kidneys. Am J Transplant. 2012;12:630–9.

39. Rostaing L, Massari P, Garcia VD, Mancilla-Urrea E, Nainan G, del Carmen RM, Steinberg S, Vincenti F, Shi R, Di Russo G, Thomas D, Grinyo J. Switching from calcineurin inhibitor-based regimens to a belatacept-based regimen in renal transplant recipients: a randomized phase II study. Clin J Am Soc Nephrol. 2011;6:430–9.
40. Heemann U, Viklicky O. The role of belataceptin transplantation: results and implications of clinical trials in the context of other new biological immunosuppressant agents. Clin Transplant. 2013;27:E3–11.
41. Schena FP, Pascoe MD, Alberu J, del Carmen RM, Oberbauer R, Brennan DC, Campistol JM, Racusen L, Polinsky MS, Goldberg-Alberts R, Li H, Scarola J, Neylan JF. Conversion from calcineurin inhibitors to sirolimus maintenance therapy in renal allograft recipients: 24-month efficacy and safety results from the CONVERT trial. Transplantation. 2009;87:233–42.
42. Smits JMA, Persijn, GG, van Houwelingen JC, Claas FHJ, Frei U on behalf of all the Eurotransplant Senior Program Centers. Evaluation of the Eurotransplant Senior Program. The results of the first year. Am J Transplant. 2002;2:664–70.
43. Lim W, Chang S, Chadban S, Campbell S, Dent H, Russ GR, McDonald SP. Donor-recipient age matching improves year of graft function in deceased-donor kidney transplantation. Nephrol Dial Transplant. 2010;8:50–7.
44. Waiser J, Schreiber M, Budde K, Fritsche L, Bohler T, Hauser I, Neumayer H-H. Age-matching in renal transplantation. Nephrol Dial Transplant. 2000;15:696–700.
45. Ojo AO, Morale JM, Gonzalez-Molina M, Steffick DE, Luan FL, Merion RM, Ojo T, Moreso F, Arias M, Campistol JM, Hernandez D, Seron D. Comparison of the long-term outcomes of kidney transplantation: USA versus Spain. Nephrol Dial Transplant. 2013;28:213–20.

Preoperative Cardiovascular Evaluation and Management

10

Krista L. Lentine, Todd C. Villines, Kevin C. Abbott, and Salvatore P. Costa

Introduction

Cardiovascular disease is a leading cause of morbidity and mortality among patients with end-stage renal disease (ESRD) including transplant candidates and recipients. Although transplantation improves cardiovascular risk in the long term compared with dialysis [1–5], cardiovascular diseases in aggregate comprise the most common cause of death in patients with functioning allografts at all times after kidney transplant, accounting for 30 % of mortality overall, with highest rates in the peritransplant period [6]. Among kidney transplant recipients, the highest risk of cardiovascular events occurs in the first months after transplant, but risk persists in the longer term [2, 3, 7]. Based on Medicare billing claims, the 3-year cumulative incidence of myocardial infarction has been estimated at 8.7–16.7 % after kidney transplant listing and 4.7–11.1 % after kidney transplantation [2, 8].

Achieving clinically and cost-effective management of cardiovascular disease in kidney transplant candidates is a challenging endeavor due to the large size of the target population, prevalent disease burden, and the often extended waiting periods between initial candidate evaluation and transplantation surgery. The number of total listings for kidney transplantation increased more than fivefold since 1991, such that per Organ Procurement and Transplant Network (OPTN) records, more than 99,000 persons are awaiting these organs in the U.S. in January 2014 [9]. Kidney transplant candidates are also waiting longer for organ offers, such that the time between evaluation and surgery is also growing longer [9]. Further, there is a paucity of randomized clinical trials addressing the efficacy of cardiac screening, surveillance, coronary revascularization, and medical management among patients with ESRD, and extrapolation from trials performed in other populations or observational studies is often necessary to formulate practice recommendations. In this context, substantial heterogeneity in pretransplant cardiac evaluations has been shown by surveys and retrospective study of Medicare claims [10–13].

Recently, the American Heart Association (AHA) and American College of Cardiology Foundation (ACCF) convened a working group of cardiologists, nephrologists, hepatologists, and intensivists to compose a Scientific Statement on "Cardiac Disease Evaluation and Management Among Kidney and Liver Transplantation Candidates" [14]. The current chapter provides a practical summary of some of the key recommendations in this Scientific Statement relevant to kidney transplant candidates, focused as a practical guide for the clinician.

Evaluation for Active Cardiac Conditions

The primary goal of the preoperative cardiac evaluation is to establish whether an active cardiac condition is present. Clinical assessment should occur during the initial evaluation and should also be repeated before anticipated transplantation to assess for interval changes in cardiovascular conditions. "Active" conditions include unstable coronary syndromes (e.g., unstable or severe angina (Canadian

K.L. Lentine, M.D., Ph.D. (✉)
Center for Outcomes Research, Abdominal Transplant Program, Saint Louis University School of Medicine, Salus Center, 3545 Lafayette Avenue, St. Louis, MO 63104, USA

Abdominal Transplant Program, Saint Louis University School of Medicine, St. Louis, MO, USA
e-mail: lentinek@slu.edu

T.C. Villines, M.D.
Cardiology Service, Department of Medicine, Walter Reed National Military Medical Center, Bethesda, MD, USA

K.C. Abbott, M.D., M.P.H.
Nephrology Service, Department of Medicine, Walter Reed National Military Medical Center, Bethesda, MD, USA

S.P. Costa, M.D.
Cardiology Section, Department of Medicine, Dartmouth Hitchcock Medical Center, Hanover, NH, USA

M.R. Weir and E.V. Lerma (eds.), *Kidney Transplantation: Practical Guide to Management*, DOI 10.1007/978-1-4939-0342-9_10, © Springer Science+Business Media New York 2014

Cardiovascular Society Class III/IV) or recent myocardial infarction (MI), decompensated heart failure, significant arrhythmias, and severe valvular heart disease). The presence of one or more of these conditions is associated with high rates of perioperative cardiovascular morbidity and mortality and may require delay or cancelation of surgery. As described in the 2012 AHA/ACCF Scientific Statement, a thorough history and physical examination are recommended to evaluate for the presence of active cardiac conditions in potential transplant candidates (Table 10.1) [14].

Table 10.1 Recommendations for preoperative and perioperative cardiovascular evaluation and management in kidney transplant candidates summarized from the 2012 AHA/ACCF Scientific Statement "Cardiac Disease Evaluation and Management Among Kidney and Liver Transplantation Candidates" [14]

Topic	Recommendation	Evidence grading
Clinical assessment for active cardiac conditions	• A thorough history and physical examination are recommended to identify active cardiac conditions before kidney transplantation • Clinical assessment should occur during the initial evaluation and be repeated immediately before anticipated transplantation	Class I, Level of Evidence C
Preoperative noninvasive stress testing in the evaluation of kidney transplantation candidates without active cardiac conditions	• Noninvasive imaging stress testing may be considered in kidney transplant candidates with no active cardiac conditions based on the presence of multiple CAD risk factors regardless of functional status • Relevant risk factors among transplant candidates include diabetes, prior cardiovascular disease, >1 year on dialysis, left ventricular hypertrophy, age >60 years, smoking, hypertension, and dyslipidemia • The specific number of risk factors that should be used to prompt testing remains to be determined, but ≥3 is considered reasonable	Class IIb, Level of Evidence C
Noninvasive stress testing for cardiac surveillance after listing for kidney transplantation	• Currently the usefulness of periodically screening asymptomatic kidney transplant candidates for myocardial ischemia while on the transplant waiting list to improve the risk of major adverse cardiac events is uncertain	Class IIb, Level of Evidence C
Preoperative 12-lead ECG at evaluation	• Preoperative resting 12-lead ECG is recommended for potential kidney transplant candidates with known coronary heart disease, known peripheral arterial disease, or any cardiovascular symptoms	Class I, Level of Evidence C
Preoperative 12-lead ECG at evaluation	• Preoperative resting 12-lead ECG is reasonable in potential kidney transplant candidates without known cardiovascular disease	Class IIa, Level of Evidence C
12-lead ECG for cardiac surveillance after listing	• Annual performance of 12-lead ECG after listing for kidney transplantation may be reasonable	Class IIb, Level of Evidence C
Preoperative echocardiography at evaluation	• It is reasonable to perform preoperative assessment of left ventricular function by echocardiography in potential kidney transplantation candidates	Class IIa, Level of Evidence B
Echocardiography for cardiac surveillance after listing	• There is no evidence for or against surveillance by repeated left ventricular function tests after listing for kidney transplantation	
Preoperative cardiac CT at evaluation	• The usefulness of noncontrast CT coronary artery calcium scoring and cardiac CT angiography is uncertain for the assessment of pretransplant cardiovascular risk	Class IIb, Level of Evidence B
Preoperative measurement of cardiac biomarkers at evaluation	• Measurement of a cTnT level at the time of evaluation for kidney transplant may be considered as an additional prognostic marker	Class IIb, Level of Evidence B
Recommendations for referral to a cardiologist	• Kidney transplantation candidates who have an LVEF less than 50 %, evidence of ischemic left ventricular dilation, exercise-induced hypotension, angina, or demonstrable ischemia in the distribution of multiple coronary arteries should be referred to a cardiologist for evaluation and long-term management according to ACC/AHA guidelines for the general population	Class I, Level of Evidence B
Recommendations for referral to a cardiologist	• Coordination of care: It may be reasonable for each program to identify a primary cardiology consultant for questions related to potential kidney transplantation candidates	Class IIb, Level of Evidence C
Revascularization before transplantation surgery	• Coronary revascularization before transplantation surgery should be considered in patients who meet the criteria outlined in the "2011 ACCF/AHA Guidelines for Coronary Artery Bypass Graft Surgery"	Class I, Level of Evidence B

(continued)

Table 10.1 (continued)

Topic	Recommendation	Evidence grading
Revascularization before transplantation surgery	• It is recognized that in some asymptomatic transplantation candidates, the risk of coronary revascularization may outweigh the risk of transplantation and these risks must be weighed by the multidisciplinary transplantation team on a case-by-case basis until further studies are performed in this population	
Revascularization before transplantation surgery	• CABG is probably recommended in preference to PCI to improve survival in patients with multivessel CAD and diabetes mellitus	Class IIa, Level of Evidence B
Revascularization before transplantation surgery	• CABG to improve survival and/or to relieve angina despite optimal medical therapy may be reasonable for patients with ESRD with significant (>50 %) left main stenosis or significant (>70 %) stenoses in 3 major vessels or in the proximal left anterior descending artery plus 1 other major vessel, regardless of left ventricular systolic function	Class IIb, Level of Evidence B
Timing of transplant surgery in relation to PCI	• In patients in whom coronary revascularization with PCI is appropriate for mitigation of cardiac symptoms and who need transplantation surgery in the subsequent 12 months, a strategy of balloon angioplasty or BMS placement followed by 4–12 weeks of dual antiplatelet therapy is probably indicated	Class IIa, Level of Evidence B
Timing of transplant surgery in relation to PCI	• Transplantation surgery is not recommended within 4 weeks of coronary revascularization with balloon angioplasty	Class III, Level of Evidence B
Timing of transplant surgery in relation to PCI	• Transplantation surgery within 3 months of BMS placement and within 12 months of DES placement is not recommended, particularly if the anticipated time of post-stent dual antiplatelet therapy will be shortened	Class III, Level of Evidence B
Antiplatelet therapy in relation to recent PCI	• In patients who have received DES and who must undergo urgent surgical procedures that mandate the discontinuation of thienopyridine therapy, it is reasonable to continue aspirin if at all possible and to restart the thienopyridine as soon as possible	Class IIa, Level of Evidence C
Antiplatelet therapy in relation to recent PCI	• In cases when urgent surgery must be performed in patients taking aspirin and thienopyridines after coronary stent placement and who are at high risk for bleeding complications, a strategy of stopping the thienopyridine 5 days before surgery and continuing aspirin perioperatively may be reasonable. The thienopyridine should be restarted as soon as possible postoperatively	Class IIb, Level of Evidence B
Antiplatelet therapy in relation to recent PCI	• It may be reasonable to perform kidney transplantation surgery without interruption of clopidogrel therapy if the risk of bleeding is low	Class IIb, Level of Evidence C

BMS, bare-metal stent; *CABG*, coronary artery bypass grafting; *CAD*, coronary artery disease; *CT*, computed tomography; *cTnT*, cardiac troponin T; *DES*, drug-eluting stent; *ECG*, electrocardiogram; *ESRD*, end-stage renal disease; *LVEF*, left ventricular ejection fraction; *PCI*, percutaneous coronary intervention

Noninvasive Testing for Coronary Artery Disease in Asymptomatic Kidney Transplant Candidates: Modalities and Testing Accuracy

Several consensus-based recommendations for cardiac risk assessment among kidney transplant candidates have been offered in the past decade (Table 10.2). The 2001 American Society of Transplantation "Guidelines for the Evaluation of Renal Transplant Candidates" advanced recommendations that (1) "high-risk patients," defined as those with diabetes, prior ischemic heart disease, or ≥2 traditional cardiovascular risk factors, should have a cardiac stress test; (2) patients with positive stress tests should be studied by invasive coronary angiography; and (3) patients with critical coronary lesions should undergo revascularization prior to transplantation [15]. In 2005, the National Kidney Foundation/Kidney Disease Outcomes Quality Initiative (NKF/KDOQI) "Clinical Practice Guidelines for Cardiovascular Disease in Dialysis Patients" recommended that patients on the kidney transplant waitlist with a history of diabetes mellitus or known coronary artery disease (CAD) undergo noninvasive cardiac stress testing at baseline and then subsequently every 12 months until transplantation [16]. NKF/DOQI also recommended a similar evaluation strategy for transplantation candidates deemed at high risk per Framingham criteria (≥2 traditional risk factors, left ventricular ejection fraction (LVEF) ≤40 %, or peripheral arterial disease) [16].

In contrast, the 2007 American College of Cardiology (ACC)/AHA "Guidelines on Perioperative Cardiovascular Evaluation and Care for Noncardiac Surgery" promote an algorithm that considers the presence of active cardiac conditions, the type of noncardiac surgery, patient functional

Table 10.2 Published recommendations for noninvasive testing in asymptomatic kidney transplant candidates

Reference	Recommendations
2012 AHA/ACCF Scientific Statement [14]	• Noninvasive stress testing may be considered in kidney transplantation candidates with no active cardiac conditions on the basis of the presence of multiple CAD risk factors regardless of functional status (Class IIb, Level of Evidence C)
	• Relevant risk factors among transplantation candidates include diabetes mellitus, prior cardiovascular disease, >1 year on dialysis, LV hypertrophy, age >60 years, smoking, hypertension, and dyslipidemia; the specific number of risk factors that should be used to prompt testing remains to be determined, but the committee considers ≥3 to be reasonable
2007 ACC/AHA Perioperative Guidelines for Noncardiac Surgery [17]	• No testing recommended if functional status ≥4 METS
	• If functional status <4 METS or unknown, then consideration of noninvasive stress testing is recommended based on the following clinical risk factors:
	– Ischemic heart disease
	– Compensated or prior heart failure
	– Diabetes
	– Renal insufficiency
	– Cerebrovascular disease
	• Recommendations for testing are stronger if ≥3 clinical risk factors are present but may be considered in those with 1–2 risk factors
2007 Lisbon Conference [59]	Acknowledges that there are no data establishing that screening of asymptomatic patients in itself prevents cardiac events. Testing should be considered in highest-risk patients with the following conditions:
	• Diabetes
	• Prior cardiovascular disease
	• Multiple cardiac risk factors, such as diabetes, >1 year on dialysis, LV hypertrophy, age >60 years, smoking, hypertension, and dyslipidemia
	Does not specify number of risk factors to justify testing
2005 NKF/KDOQI Guidelines [16]	Noninvasive stress testing recommended for:
	• All patients with diabetes. Repeat every 12 months
	• All patients with known CAD:
	– If not revascularized, repeat every 12 months
	– If prior PCI, repeat every 12 months
	– If prior CABG, repeat after first 3 years, then every 12 months
	• Repeat every 24 months in "high-risk" nondiabetic patients, defined as:
	– ≥2 traditional risk factors
	– Known history of CAD
	– LVEF ≤40 %
	– Peripheral vascular disease
2001 AST Guidelines [122]	• Noninvasive stress testing recommended for patients at "high risk," defined as renal disease from diabetes, prior history of ischemic heart disease, or ≥2 risk factors
	• Coronary angiography for possible revascularization before transplantation recommended for patients with a positive stress test
	• Revascularization before transplantation recommended for patients with critical coronary lesions
2000 European Best Practice Guidelines [123]	• Thallium scanning recommended for patients with history of myocardial infarction or "high-risk" clinical features
	• Coronary angiography recommended if thallium scanning positive
	• Revascularization advised if lesions are suitable

Reproduced with permission from [14]

CABG, coronary artery bypass grafting; *CAD*, coronary artery disease; *LV*, left ventricular; *PCI*, percutaneous coronary intervention

capacity, and clinical risk profile [17]. These ACC/AHA guidelines identify four "active" cardiac conditions warranting specific evaluation and treatment before noncardiac surgery, including unstable coronary syndromes (unstable or severe angina or MI within the past 30 days), decompensated heart failure, significant arrhythmia, and severe valvular heart disease. If none of the active cardiac conditions are present, the ACC/AHA algorithm then risk stratifies patients on the basis of functional capacity. If functional status is estimated as at least four metabolic equivalents (METS, where four is equivalent to the ability to climb a flight of stairs) in a patient without an active cardiac condition, then no further testing is recommended. Patients with lower or unknown functional capacity who are scheduled for intermediate-risk surgery (reported cardiac perioperative morbidity rates generally 1–5 %) are also generally recommended to proceed with surgery, regardless of the number of risk markers. However, consideration of noninvasive testing is given a Class IIb/ Level of Evidence (LOE) recommendation "if it will change management." Kidney transplantation is typically considered an intermediate-risk surgery.

A recent single-center study quantified the frequency of recommended testing and the observed results of cardiac testing (primarily dobutamine stress echocardiography (DSE) or myocardial perfusion scintigraphy (MPS)) that would result from application of different clinical practice guidelines among 204 consecutive patients who were determined to be free of active cardiac conditions by a cardiologist at the time of transplant evaluation [18]. Active cardiac conditions were defined according to the ACC/AHA criteria [17]. If followed precisely, 20 % of patients met criteria for cardiac testing by ACC/AHA guidelines for noncardiac surgery, whereas use of the NKF/KDOQI guidelines would have resulted in testing 100 % of the sample. Among the 178 (87 %) patients who underwent stress tests, the prevalence of ischemia was similar among those for whom testing was and was not recommended per the ACC/AHA guidelines, 10.3 % vs. 9.4 %, respectively. The relatively low use of coronary revascularization after pretransplant cardiac evaluation also raises concern for the clinical and cost-effectiveness of pretransplant cardiac evaluation as currently applied. Several registry-based and single-center observational studies have found that only 2.9–9.5 % of patients who receive pretransplant cardiac stress testing or angiography proceeded to percutaneous coronary intervention (PCI) or surgical bypass [13, 19–22].

In formulating current recommendations regarding noninvasive testing for CAD in kidney transplant candidates, the 2012 AHA/ACCF Scientific Statement on "Cardiac Disease Evaluation and Management Among Kidney and Liver Transplantation Candidates" [14] weighed the following considerations:

1. Noninvasive cardiac stress testing by DSE or MPS has prognostic value for cardiac events and mortality but imperfect sensitivity and specificity for detecting angiographically defined CAD in patients with ESRD.
2. Associations of coronary stenoses by invasive coronary angiography with subsequent survival in ESRD patients are also inconsistent, likely because plaque instability is more important for major adverse cardiac event (MACE) risk than angiographic stenosis and most plaque disruption events (erosion or rupture) producing acute coronary syndromes are not localized to sites of angiographic stenosis.
3. Coronary revascularization in asymptomatic patients has failed to show benefit before surgery or among nonsurgical patients, except in a small subset of patients with high-risk anatomic lesions.

Accuracy of Noninvasive Testing for CAD in Kidney Transplantation Candidates

Among studies evaluating associations between cardiac stress testing results and angiographically defined obstructive CAD in cohorts with chronic kidney disease (CKD) stage 5 (glomerular filtration rate (GFR) <15 mL/min/1.73 m^2 or dialysis dependence), DSE and MPS have sensitivities varying from 0.44 to 0.89 and 0.29 to 0.92 and specificities ranging from 0.71 to 0.94 and 0.67 to 0.89, respectively, for identifying one or more coronary stenoses ≥70 % [23–31]. In a recent meta-analysis assessing the pooled sensitivity and specificity of DSE and MPS in kidney transplant candidates, both DSE and MPS had moderate sensitivity and specificity in detecting significant coronary artery stenosis on invasive coronary angiography in patients who are kidney transplant candidates (DSE (13 studies), pooled sensitivity 0.79 (95 % CI 0.67 to 0.88) and pooled specificity 0.89 (95 % CI 0.81 to 0.94); MPS (9 studies), pooled sensitivity 0.74 (95 % CI 0.54 to 0.87) and pooled specificity 0.70 (95 % CI 0.51 to 0.84)) [32]. When limited to studies that defined CAD as ≥70 % stenosis on coronary angiography, there was little change in these pooled estimates of accuracy (DSE (nine studies), pooled sensitivity 0.76 (95 % CI 0.60 to 0.87) and specificity 0.88 (95 % CI 0.78 to 0.94); MPS (seven studies), pooled sensitivity 0.67 (95 % CI 0.48 to 0.82) and pooled specificity 0.77 (95 % CI 0.61 to 0.88)) [32]. There was evidence that DSE had improved accuracy over MPS ($p=0.02$) when all studies were included in the analysis, but this was not significant when the authors excluded studies which did not verify all results with coronary angiography or use a reference standard threshold of ≥70 % stenosis ($p=0.09$) [32].

The operational characteristics of the type of stress imaging may differ in ESRD compared with non-ESRD patients. In one study of coronary flow reserve in 64 patients with normal epicardial arteries, 57 % (12/21) of those with diabetic nephropathy had high resting coronary basal flow with no incremental response to adenosine compared with 18 % (2/11) of diabetic patients without renal failure and 9 % (3/32) of nondiabetic patients [33], suggesting impaired vasodilator reserve in diabetic ESRD patients. Overall, the accuracy of inotropic stress echocardiography for the purpose of screening to identify high-risk coronary anatomy may be somewhat superior to that of vasodilator stress nuclear perfusion imaging; however, patient-specific variables, such as echocardiography imaging quality or prior testing results, may guide providers in the selection of stress imaging modality. Comparative studies using contemporary imaging technology (e.g., attenuation correction in MPS) are needed.

Despite the imperfect accuracy of stress testing for the detection of coronary stenoses, abnormal MPS and DSE test results have shown prognostic value for cardiac events and mortality in the ESRD population [21, 27, 30, 31, 34–39].

In a meta-analysis of 12 studies employing either thallium-201 MPS or DSE, ESRD patients with inducible ischemia had approximately six times the risk of myocardial infarction and four times the risk of cardiac death as patients without inducible defects, and patients with fixed defects had nearly five times the risk of cardiac death [40]. The percentage of ischemic segments by DSE was an independent predictor of mortality among 485 patients with advanced renal failure and offered prognostic information beyond clinical characteristics alone [41]. In a study of 126 ESRD patients who underwent 99 m-technetium MPS as part of their pretransplant assessment, the presence of a reversible defect was associated with three times the risk of posttransplant cardiac events and nearly twice the risk of death compared with normal test results [42].

Imperfect Correlations of Coronary Stenosis with Subsequent MACEs in ESRD Patients

Angiographic studies from the 1970s have documented a high prevalence of coronary stenoses among patients on long-term dialysis [43–47]. More recently, angiographically significant CAD was found in 53 % of a sample of 30 incident ESRD patients without known cardiac history who consented to screening angiography, including 10 (83 %) of the 12 participants with diabetes, although notably angiographic significance was liberally defined as lesions >50 % [48]. Recent reports of angiography in patients undergoing transplant evaluation identified angiographically significant CAD in 42–81 % of samples, with a higher prevalence in subgroups defined as "high risk" by clinical criteria and with use of more liberal angiographic definitions of CAD [22, 29, 30, 49–53].

Despite the high prevalence of CAD in ESRD patients, reported associations of angiographic coronary stenoses with subsequent clinical events in ESRD patients have varied. In one prospective study of 126 renal transplant candidates clinically classified as moderate (age ≥50 years) or high (diabetes, extracardiac vascular disease, or known CAD) coronary risk, MPS, DSE, and coronary angiography were performed in all participants [29]. Clinical risk stratification and coronary angiography predicted MACE after median follow-up of 46 months, but results of MPS and DSE were not significantly correlated with MACE. Several observational studies reported increased unadjusted risk of all-cause mortality and MACE in patients with angiographic CAD [30, 50], while other studies found correlations of angiography and outcomes only in certain patient subgroups, such as those with proximal CAD [49] or with nondiabetic renal failure [51]. Several recent studies have found no associations of CAD with survival of ESRD patients and kidney transplant candidates [22, 52, 53].

Lack of Evidence that Coronary Revascularization Benefits *Asymptomatic* Patients Before Surgery or in General, Except for a Small Subset of Patients with High-Risk Anatomic Lesions

There are significant gaps in the literature regarding the outcomes of prophylactic coronary revascularization before kidney transplantation. Only one small randomized trial of revascularization has been performed in this patient population. In 1992, Manske et al. randomly assigned 31 insulin-dependent diabetic transplant candidates with CAD (>75 % stenosis) to revascularization or medical therapy with a calcium channel blocker and aspirin [54]. Ultimately, 10 of 13 medically managed and 2 of 13 revascularized patients reached the primary MACE endpoint including unstable angina, myocardial infarction, or cardiac death. The contemporary relevance of these findings is limited by the small sample size, high event rate among the medically managed group, and subsequent advances that have occurred in medical management of CAD.

While there are no contemporary randomized trials of prophylactic coronary revascularization in kidney transplant candidates, several observational studies have described outcomes after coronary revascularization in selected cohorts of potential kidney transplant candidates. In an observational study of 300 patients who underwent multimodality testing as part of the candidate evaluation at one center, crude survival was not different in patients who underwent revascularization compared with those who underwent angiography without revascularization or no angiography [22]. Among 3,698 patients evaluated for kidney transplant at a single center in 2001–2004, MPS was performed in 60 %, and 7 % of the sample subsequently underwent coronary angiography. The presence and severity of CAD on angiography were not predictive of survival, and coronary revascularization was associated with survival only in patients with 3-vessel CAD [52].

A recent study described one center's experience (2006–2009) under a protocol in which potential kidney transplant candidates were evaluated by angiography based on the presence of any of the following criteria: age >50 years, diabetes mellitus, any cardiac symptoms, or electrocardiogram (ECG) evidence of ischemia or prior infarction [55]. Among the 657 patients who underwent angiography, significant CAD (defined as >75 % stenosis of one or more coronary arteries, >50 % left main stem stenosis, or an equivocal lesion with flow limitation) was found in 28 %, of whom 55 % were asymptomatic and without prior CAD history. Patients with significant CAD who underwent revascularization followed by transplant ($n=51$, 1-year survival 100 %, 3-year survival 97 %) or by continued waiting ($n=177$, 1-year survival 95 %, 3-year survival 81 %) had superior survival to the 16 patients who declined revascularization (1-year survival 75 %, 3-year survival 37 %). While this study demonstrates excellent survival in transplant recipients who received preemptive revascularization, the lack of a comparator group of similar patients who did not undergo angiography before transplant prevents inferences regarding the impact of the management approach on outcomes.

In stable general population samples, recent randomized trials have failed to support benefit of revascularization over contemporary medical management, including the CARP and DECREASE-V trials performed among patients awaiting major vascular surgery [56, 57]. Randomized comparison of PCI plus optimal medical therapy among 2,238 patients with stable CAD (≥70 % stenosis in at least one proximal epicardial coronary artery and objective evidence of myocardial ischemia) also found no benefit on the risk of MACE over 4.6 years compared with optimal medical therapy alone [57]. Secondary analysis of 320 participants with CKD defined as estimated glomerular filtration rate (eGFR) <60 mL/min/1.73 m^2 found that, while CKD was associated with increased risk of death or nonfatal MI, the incidence of death or MI in CKD patients did not differ by treatment arm [58].

Weighing these data, the 2012 AHA/ACCF writing group acknowledged that there are "no definitive data at this time for or against screening for myocardial ischemia among kidney transplant candidates who are free of active cardiac conditions" [14]. However, until more data are available, the authors recommended consideration of CAD risk factors to target screening of patients with the highest pretest likelihood of prognostically significant CAD. Risk factors for CAD deemed relevant to transplant candidates in a 2007 report from an international collaboration of the NKF and the Transplantation Society called the Lisbon Report include diabetes, prior cardiovascular disease, >1 year on dialysis, left ventricular hypertrophy, age >60, smoking, hypertension, and dyslipidemia [59]. When compared with the ACC/AHA "Guidelines on Perioperative Cardiovascular Evaluation and Care for Noncardiac Surgery," screening transplant candidates with multiple risk factors defined by the Lisbon report appeared to improve sensitivity and specificity for the identification of CAD (sensitivity 94 % vs. 77 %; specificity 33 % vs. 24 %) and reduce the overall frequency of testing in a retrospective analysis of data from one center [18]. The Class IIb/LOE C recommendation of the 2012 AHA/ACCF Scientific Statement on consideration of noninvasive stress testing in kidney transplant candidates with no active cardiac conditions based on the presence of multiple CAD risk factors regardless of functional status is shown in Table 10.1. The Scientific Statement also recommends a randomized trial of the impact of screening for CAD on pre- and posttransplant MACE among potential transplant candidates, such as a randomized comparison of four approaches to the preoperative cardiovascular evaluation: (1) cardiac catheterization for all candidates, including fractional flow reserve measurement in indeterminate lesions, (2) noninvasive imaging stress testing (DSE or MPS) for all patients, (3) noninvasive stress testing based on presence of ≥3 cardiac risk factors, and (4) ACC/AHA cardiac evaluation and care algorithm for noncardiac surgery [14].

Cardiac Surveillance After Listing for Kidney Transplantation

Along with the uncertainty regarding which asymptomatic patients to screen for CAD the optimal frequency for repeat noninvasive testing among kidney transplant candidates on the waiting list is not known. The NKF/KDOQI guidelines recommended repeat stress testing with imaging once a year among subgroups on the transplant list including diabetic patients regardless of symptoms [16]. These guidelines parallel recommendations from the American Society of Transplantation's 2002 conference on waitlist management [60].

Notably, among patients without organ failure, the cardiac event rate (cardiac death or nonfatal MI) was only 0.6 % over 2–3 years in 7,376 patients after a normal MPS, suggesting that the "warranty" on a normal imaging stress test is at least 2 years in the general population [61] however, only 10 % of participants in this study were diabetic. A large cohort study found low and similar cardiac event rates among diabetic and nondiabetic persons up to 2 years after normal stress MPS, although the diabetic cohort experienced a greater event rate after 2 years [61]. Outcomes after a normal MPS also vary with renal function. In an observational cohort study of the Veterans Affairs database with an average of 2 years of follow-up, annualized cardiac mortality after a normal MPS (defined as no scar or ischemia) rose in a graded manner with declining renal function: eGFR ≥90 mL/min/1.73 m^2, 0.4 %; eGFR 60–89 mL/min/1.73 m^2, 0.9 %; eGFR 30–59 mL/min/1.73 m^2, 2.2 %; and eGFR <30 mL/min/1.73 m^2, 4.7 % [62].

In a cohort study from Brisbane, Australia, including 107 CKD patients with baseline and repeat DSE tests after mean follow-up time of 1.8 years, 19 % of the 73 CKD patients with normal baseline DSE results developed inducible ischemia or new scar on repeat testing [63]. Despite the potential for conversion of normal noninvasive tests to abnormal at a rate of approximately 10 % per year, an argument that "periodic cardiac surveillance testing after waitlist may be unnecessary" is supported by a prospective, observational study of patients on the kidney transplant waitlist in British Columbia in 1998–2001 [64]. Among kidney transplant candidates with normal cardiac stress testing at listing, the reference cardiac surveillance guideline recommended annual testing in those with diabetes, testing every 2 years in those with ischemic heart disease or peripheral vascular disease, and testing every 3 years in others. Surveillance based on ongoing clinical assessment resulted in fewer investigations than suggested by guidelines over a mean follow-up period of 3.7 years. Total cardiovascular event rates after listing did not differ in subsets who received the recommended frequency of cardiac tests compared with those in whom testing was guided by symptoms. Weighing these data, the 2012 AHA/ACCF Scientific Advisory Committee on pretransplant cardiac evaluation concluded that the usefulness of periodically screening asymptomatic kidney transplant candidates for myocardial ischemia while on the transplant waiting list to improve the risk of MACE is currently uncertain (Table 10.1) [14].

Use Other Testing in the Pretransplant Cardiac Evaluation

Resting Electrocardiogram

While there are limited data on the association of preoperative ECG with posttransplant outcomes, data are available on the natural history and prognostic value of baseline ECG abnormalities in dialysis patients. In one study of 12-lead ECG findings among 221 chronic hemodialysis patients compared with patients non-dialysis requiring CKD and patients without kidney disease, the prevalence of ECG abnormalities was 65 %, 41 %, and 5 %, respectively [65]. Significant differences between dialysis patients and normal controls included left ventricular hypertrophy (19 % vs. 0.7 %), evidence of ischemia (7.2 % vs. 0.6 %), premature ventricular contractions (6.8 % vs. 0.3 %), nonspecific ST-T changes (6 % vs. 0.3 %), atrial fibrillation (5.4 % vs. 0 %), left atrial enlargement (2.7 % vs. 0 %), and old MI (1.4 % vs. 0 %). Eighty-seven hemodialysis patients were followed by serial ECG for an average of 7.5 years, during which 39 % maintained normal ECGs, 31 % had abnormal but stable ECGs, 25 % had worsening of their ECG findings, and 5 % had apparent improvement. In another study of 1,738 asymptomatic diabetic patients who were free of known CAD, the presence of pathologic Q waves on ECG was the strongest independent correlate of abnormal "high-risk" MPS results (OR 3.92) [66]. Sixty-one percent of patients with high-risk MPS results were found to have angiographic evidence of left main CAD, 3-vessel CAD, or 1- or 2-vessel with proximal left anterior descending CAD.

Given the low cost and the prognostic implications of ECG abnormalities, the 2012 AHA/ACCF Scientific Statement on pretransplant cardiac evaluation recommends a preoperative resting ECG among all potential transplant candidates but with a stronger evidence class among those with symptoms or known atherosclerotic vascular disease (Table 10.1) [14]. Serial ECG changes in dialysis patients can be expected and thus periodic monitoring of ECGs (e.g., annually) while on the waitlist may be appropriate, although there are no data to support an optimal time interval between repeated ECG tests.

Exercise Treadmill Testing and Exercise Stress Echocardiography

Exercise as the form of cardiovascular stress including exercise treadmill stress testing (ETT) alone or in combination with stress echocardiography or MPS, is the most commonly used method for the performance of stress testing, in ambulatory general population patients in whom there is no evidence of left bundle branch block or significant resting ST segment deviation. Exercise duration and the occurrence and severity of exercise-induced chest discomfort and ECG changes provide important diagnostic and prognostic information. However, there is limited data regarding the diagnostic and prognostic value of regular ETT in pretransplant populations. Based on documented improvements in test accuracy using stress imaging modalities as compared to ETT and the high rate of baseline ST segment abnormalities and left ventricular hypertrophy in pretransplant patients that may limit accuracy of ETT, the use of ETT has not been widely studied in this population [30]. In addition, the majority of studies evaluating stress echocardiography and MPS have used inotropic or vasodilator stress imaging likely as a way to standardize stress imaging protocols among the study populations [32]. Given the increased cost (and risks in the case of dobutamine administration) associated with pharmacologic stress imaging, studies evaluating the accuracy and prognostic value of exercise stress imaging protocols among appropriately selected patients requiring kidney transplantation are needed.

Resting Echocardiography

Multiple studies have consistently demonstrated the diagnostic and prognostic value of resting echocardiography among dialysis patients [30, 67, 68]. The "NKF/KDOQI Clinical Practice Guidelines for Cardiovascular Disease in Dialysis Patients" recommend that a resting echocardiogram be performed in all patients at the initiation of dialysis, once the patient has achieved dry weight (ideally within 1–3 months of dialysis initiation) [16]. Two reports from one large center using stress MPS in potential candidates meeting AST criteria for pretransplant ischemia evaluation found left ventricular systolic dysfunction, defined as LVEF less than 40–45 %, in 16–18 % of patients [69, 70]. The majority (61–63 %) of these patients did not have evidence of ischemia by perfusion imaging. Median survival in patients with LVEF <40 % was 49 months compared with 72 months in patients with higher LVEF; after adjustment for ischemia and other risk factors, the relative risk of mortality increased by 2.5 % for each percent decline in LVEF [70]. Further, the 2007 ACC/AHA guidelines on preoperative evaluation in patients undergoing noncardiac surgery recommend the performance of testing to assess left ventricular function among patients with unexplained dyspnea or with known heart failure and a change in functional status [17]. As described in the 2012 AHA/ACCF Scientific Statement, it is reasonable to perform preoperative echocardiography in potential kidney transplantation candidates (Table 10.1) [14].

Other Imaging: Cardiac CT

In addition to MPS and DSE, noninvasive image-based testing for CAD is available using cardiac computed tomography (CT) (Table 10.3). Noncontrast CT for detection and quantification of coronary artery calcification (CAC scoring) has been shown to significantly improve cardiovascular risk prediction as compared to the Framingham score and highly sensitive C-reactive protein in asymptomatic patients without kidney disease [71–73]. Elevated CAC scores (median Agatston score 595, interquartile range 76–1,600) were

Table 10.3 Advantages and disadvantages of available methods for detecting coronary artery disease

Method	Advantages	Disadvantages
Myocardial perfusion scintigraphy (MPS)	• Noninvasive	• Confers exposure to ionizing radiation
• Exercise (E) *OR*	• Assesses ischemic burden and left ventricular function	• Attenuation artifacts (breast, bowel, motion) may limit accuracy
• Pharmacologic (P) stress (adenosine, persantine, or dobutamine)	• Has prognostic value • Adenosine/persantine MPS preferred in patients with left bundle branch block • Assesses functional status (E)	• Requires delayed imaging to assess for myocardial viability • (P) form does not assess functional capacity • Expensive
Stress echocardiography	• Noninvasive	• Poor image quality with some comorbidities (e.g., obesity, chronic obstructive pulmonary disease)
• Exercise (E) *OR*	• Higher specificity compared to MPS	• Peak exercise images may be technically challenging to obtain
• Dobutamine (D) stress	• No exposure to ionizing radiation • Assesses ischemic burden, left ventricular function, and valvular function • Prognostic value demonstrated in some studies among patients with advanced kidney failure • Assessment of myocardial viability may be obtained with low-dose dobutamine at time of scan • Assesses functional status (E)	• (D) side effects may be intolerable (e.g., arrhythmias, hypotension, hypertension, stress cardiomyopathy)
Cardiac computed tomography (CT)	• Rapid, noninvasive means of defining cardiac and extracardiac anatomy	• Confers exposure to ionizing radiation
• Noncontrast CT for coronary artery calcium (CAC) scoring *OR*	• Highly sensitive for coronary atherosclerosis detection and quantification	• Confers exposure to iodinated contrast for angiography
• Coronary CT angiography (CTA)	• Retrospectively ECG-gated protocols allow assessment of left ventricular function • Prospective ECG-triggered protocols and other dose-sparing techniques markedly reduce radiation exposure	• Prognostic value of CAC scoring is controversial, and coronary CTA is untested in patients with advanced kidney failure • Image quality may be limited in patients with cardiac arrhythmias, poor heart rate control, advanced coronary calcification, and obesity
Invasive coronary angiography	• Gold standard for identifying obstructive coronary artery disease • Percutaneous coronary intervention may be performed at the time of angiography if needed • Measures of cardiac and valvular hemodynamics (e.g., left ventricular filling pressures) may be obtained • Allows for ad hoc assessment of lesion functional significance using fractional flow reserve-guided revascularization (FFR)	• Invasive and confers risks of major complications (e.g., vascular damage with major bleeding, arterial dissection, stroke, arrhythmia, myocardial infarction, death) • Confers exposure to radiation and iodinated contrast • Does not assess myocardial viability • Expensive

Reproduced with permission from [124]

identified in a sample of 205 adult maintenance hemodialysis patients [74], and similar studies have reported markedly greater coronary calcification in ESRD compared with non-ESRD patients, with greatest disparities according to ESRD status in young cohorts [75–77]. Although one study reported Agatston CAC scores to be an independent predictor of death in chronic hemodialysis patients [78], the role of calcium scoring as a prognostic marker in the ESRD population is uncertain [79]. Other studies report poor correlation between CAC scores and the likelihood of angiographic CAD in patients with advanced kidney disease [80–82], a finding that may reflect the high burden of medial vascular calcification in ESRD compared to the intimal atherosclerotic plaque calcification seen in the non-ESRD population [83]. Modern (64–320-slice and dual-source) coronary computed tomography angiography (CTA) is a highly accurate and prognostically informative noninvasive tool for the diagnosis of CAD when used to evaluate symptomatic patients with low-to-intermediate pretest probability of obstructive coronary stenosis [84–86]. However, coronary CTA has not been adequately studied in patients with significant kidney disease, and its accuracy may be limited in this population due to a high burden of calcified coronary atherosclerosis. Further, the safety of CTA in patients with advanced kidney disease is a concern related to the attendant exposure to iodinated contrast. The "ACCF/SCCT/ACR/AHA/ASE/ASNC/NASCI/SCAI/SCMR 2010 Appropriate Use Criteria for Cardiac Computed Tomography" consider coronary CTA as an option among patients undergoing cardiac surgery for noncoronary indications (e.g., valve replacement) when the pretest CAD risk is either intermediate (appropriate) or low (uncertain) but deem that there are currently no appropriate indications for coronary CTA as part of the preoperative evaluation for noncardiac surgery [87]. Currently, the usefulness of noncontrast CT for CAC scoring and coronary CT angiography is uncertain for the assessment of pretransplant cardiovascular risk (Table 10.1) [14].

Cardiac Biomarkers

Several biomarkers, namely, the cardiac troponins (cTn), have been proposed as tools in the cardiac evaluation of kidney transplant candidates for specific applications including risk stratification within protocols for initial disease screening, surveillance after listing, and as a reference against which to compare levels if symptoms of an acute coronary syndrome arise. Risk stratification of asymptomatic patients with biomarkers is distinct from the diagnosis of acute coronary syndromes. While cTns are excreted by the kidney, the source of elevations in the bloodstream even in ESRD patients appears to be the myocardium. A dynamic rise and fall in cTn with appropriate clinical signs or symptoms suggests an acute coronary syndrome, but persistent elevations in cTn may result from other sources of prognostically important cardiac stress such as volume overload, uncontrolled hypertension, or left ventricular hypertrophy [88]. Persistent elevations of cTnT isoform levels correlate with all-cause and cardiac mortality in asymptomatic dialysis patients. A meta-analysis of 28 studies found that cTnT >0.10 ng/mL in ESRD patients predicts more than twice the mortality risk of ESRD patients with lower cTnT levels [89]. The prognostic value of cTnI has been less consistent, perhaps due to lack of assay standardization and/or use of a broader range of threshold values in studies to date. Based on such data, the Food and Drug Administration approved use of cTnT levels for mortality prognostication in persons with chronic renal failure in 2004.

Several studies have examined associations of cTnT with mortality before and after kidney transplantation. In a retrospective study of 644 patients on the transplant waitlist at one center, each increment in cTnT level (<0.01, 0.01–0.03, 0.04–0.09, and ≥0.10 ng/mL) was associated with 64 % higher adjusted relative risk of transplant-censored mortality [53]. Each increment in cTnT measured before transplantation was associated with 58 % higher relative risk of MACE during an average for 28 months of posttransplant follow-up [90]. Another study of 379 prevalent transplant recipients found that mortality at 3.8-year follow-up was nearly 3 times higher in patients with cTnT ≥0.03 at study enrollment vs. <0.01 ng/mL [91]. The clinical and prognostic implications of novel ultrasensitive troponin assays in patients with advanced kidney disease and patients awaiting kidney transplantation have not yet been well studied [92]. While cTn levels may have prognostic importance, it remains uncertain how biomarker assessment should be used to direct therapies or the use of more expensive or invasive diagnostic testing before or after kidney transplantation (Table 10.1) [14].

Coronary Angiography: Use and Considerations

Coronary angiography is the gold standard modality for detecting coronary stenosis, but despite the imperfect performance of noninvasive testing described above, commonly suggested algorithms for cardiac evaluation of asymptomatic kidney transplant candidates reserve coronary angiography for patients with abnormal noninvasive testing [19, 93, 94]. The rationale for noninvasive testing prior to angiography relates to concerns for procedure-related risks and costs. Contrast-induced nephropathy has been reported to complicate angiography in 2–50 % of samples depending on case definition and patient mix [95–98]. The risk of contrast-induced acute kidney injury is inversely related to a patient's eGFR [99] and is of particular concern in patients with stages

4 and 5 CKD because of the potential for accelerating the need for dialysis. Other clinical and periprocedural risk factors for contrast-induced nephropathy include diabetes mellitus, intravascular volume depletion, hemodynamic instability, concomitant use of nephrotoxic drugs, and high contrast loads [99, 100]. Recent small, retrospective studies have suggested that minimization of the risk of contrast-induced acute kidney injury from coronary angiography among kidney transplant candidates may be possible with careful patient selection and careful management before, during, and after the procedure [101, 102]. However, the risk of contrast-induced acute kidney injury after pretransplant coronary angiography has not been evaluated in prospective studies with large numbers of patients and control groups.

Rather than offer explicit recommendations on the use of coronary angiography for pretransplant evaluation, the 2012 AHA/ACCF Scientific Statement Committee on pretransplant cardiac evaluation [14] recommended that kidney transplantation candidates with LVEF <50 %, evidence of ischemic left ventricular dilation, exercise-induced hypotension, angina, or demonstrable ischemia in the distribution of multiple coronary arteries should be referred to a cardiologist for evaluation and long-term management according to ACC/AHA guidelines for the general population [103–105] (Table 10.1). To facilitate consistency in care, the 2012 AHA/ACCF Scientific Statement also recommended that transplant programs attempt to identify a primary cardiology consultant for questions related to potential kidney transplantation candidates (Table 10.1) [14].

Pretransplant Coronary Revascularization

In addition to the uncertainty regarding benefits of pretransplant coronary revascularization on clinical outcomes, as discussed above, there are technical and procedural complexities related to revascularization among ESRD patients being considered for transplantation.

PCI vs. CABG in Patients with ESRD

The optimal coronary revascularization strategy remains controversial in kidney transplant candidates for a number of reasons: Patients with ESRD are often excluded from large cardiology trials [106], the one randomized trial in this patient population included only 31 patients and was performed in the early 1990s prior to modern medical therapy and current revascularization techniques [54], randomized trials on prophylactic revascularization prior to surgery in other high-risk populations have not demonstrated a clear benefit beyond optimal medical therapy [56, 107], and lastly, the majority of transplant candidates with CAD are asymptomatic and only identified through preoperative "screening" initiatives [55]. Although there is some support in the literature for coronary revascularization in patients with a large area of "silent" ischemia identified on noninvasive testing in the general population, some of these patients are referred directly for angiography without a functional assessment.

Accepting the current limitations in the literature as noted above, some themes have emerged from observational studies and registry data. One theme is that kidney transplant patients appear similar to patients with diabetes in general such that those with high-risk coronary anatomy (left main disease, 3-vessel disease, or 2-vessel disease including proximal LAD) have demonstrated a significant survival benefit with coronary artery bypass grafting (CABG) over PCI [52, 108–110]. This observation may be due to the high prevalence of diabetes in the kidney transplant candidate population, but detailed subgroup analyses have not been published to suggest that nondiabetic ESRD patients should be treated differently, and multiple studies have demonstrated CKD to be an independent predictor of CAD regardless of diabetic status [111]. A new study of USRDS data for 23,033 dialysis patients who underwent coronary revascularization from 2004 to 2009 (6178 CABG, 5011 bare-metal stents (BMS), 11 844 drug-eluting stents (DES)) found that in-hospital mortality was higher after CABG compared with PCI, but long-term survival was superior if CABG included use of an internal mammary graft [112]. Thus the long-term outcome data involving CABG and PCI in the ESRD population may be evolving. However, given that multiple randomized controlled trials in patients with diabetes support a long-term survival advantage with CABG [113], the AHA/ACCF Scientific Advisory Committee on pretransplant cardiac evaluation recommended that CABG is the preferred method of revascularization in patients with diabetes mellitus with left main, 3-vessel CAD and 2-vessel CAD involving the proximal left anterior descending artery, and should be strongly considered in terms of durability and the reduced incidence of recurrent revascularization procedures in all transplantation candidates needing coronary revascularization [14]. In addition, left ventricular dysfunction attributed to high-risk coronary stenosis is usually further support for CABG as the preferred revascularization approach.

A second theme is that regardless of whether CABG or PCI is selected for coronary revascularization, patients with ESRD (especially those on dialysis) have long-term outcomes that are significantly worse than the general population. For example, a study of coronary revascularization using USRDS data reported unadjusted 5-year survival of 28 % for ESRD patients who underwent CABG [112], which is markedly lower than the 5-year survival of 85–90 % after CABG in the general population [114]. Other investigators have demonstrated that dialysis patients have roughly three times the mortality after CABG compared with post-CABG mortality in the general population, even after controlling for other variables [115]. Similar observations have been made for PCI. A recent study of a large subset of long-term dialysis patients ($N=5{,}182$) reported 30-month death rates of 49 % with DES and 56 % with BMS ($p<0.001$), significantly higher than the post-PCI mortality in the general population (12 % with DES and 15 % with BMS, $p<0.01$) [116]. These data suggest that when PCI is appropriate, there may be an advantage to DES among ESRD patients (possibly due to the high prevalence of cormorbid diabetes, a factor associated with benefit from DES over BMS), but the risks and benefits of long-term thienopyridines (at least 1 year with DES vs. shorter durations with BMS) and technical considerations regarding size of coronary vessels and complexity of disease (i.e., bifurcation lesions) must be taken into consideration. Overall, significant work remains to be done to improve survival rates with CABG or PCI in all ESRD patients.

A third theme in the literature is that in the absence of high-risk coronary anatomy, there does not appear to be a survival advantage to revascularization as compared to optimal medical therapy. The COURAGE trial was a pivotal trial supporting this concept, studying patients with chronic stable angina with ischemia on noninvasive stress testing [57]. The main benefit of revascularization in this patient group was short-term relief of angina symptoms. Secondary analysis of patients with 320 participants with CKD, defined as eGFR <60 mL/min/1.73 m^2 demonstrated similar results [58]. Therefore, kidney transplant candidates with no cardiac symptoms who demonstrate ischemia on noninvasive testing and do not have high-risk anatomy may equally benefit from optimal medical therapy as from PCI.

In the general population, patients with asymptomatic ischemia or stable angina do not appear to benefit from prophylactic preoperative coronary revascularization unless cardiac catheterization reveals high-risk anatomy. The anatomic subsets and revascularization strategies that confers survival advantages are discussed in detail in the "2011 ACCF/AHA Guideline for Coronary Artery Bypass Graft Surgery" and "2011 ACCF/AHA/SCAI Guideline for Percutaneous Coronary Intervention", weighing the risks and benefits of CABG vs. PCI based on the coronary anatomy, complexity of PCI (SYNTAX score), and surgical risk (STS risk calculator) [103, 104]. Pending more direct data from the ESRD population, the 2012 AHA/ACCF Scientific Statement on pretransplant cardiac evaluation recommended that the indications for CABG and PCI in the pretransplant setting should be identical to those developed by the harmonized ACCF/AHA CABG and ACCF/AHA/SCAI PCI revascularization guidelines (Table 10.1). It is recognized that in some asymptomatic transplantation candidates, the risk of coronary revascularization may outweigh the risk of transplantation and these risks must be weighed by the multidisciplinary transplantation team on a case-by-case basis until further studies are performed in this population.

Interval Between PCI and Subsequent Surgery

The need for noncardiac surgery in patients who have recently undergone PCI is commonly encountered and requires careful consideration of the type of coronary intervention performed when contemplating optimal surgical timing. In patients who have undergone balloon angioplasty without stent implantation, it is recommended that surgical procedures be delayed for 4–6 weeks to allow for vessel healing. Daily antiplatelet therapy, which is indicated indefinitely for patients who undergo any form of PCI, should be continued perioperatively unless the risk of bleeding complications is felt to be prohibitive. Dual antiplatelet therapy (DAPT), which is mandated after intracoronary stent implantation, is not required following angioplasty without stenting when performed in patients without an acute coronary syndrome.

In an attempt to reduce the rate of restenosis seen with balloon angioplasty, most patients who undergo PCI will receive either a BMS or DES, a distinction that carries important considerations regarding the duration of DAPT and surgical timing. Stent thrombosis, which typically presents in an emergent fashion as an ST elevation myocardial infarction or as sudden death, typically occurs within the first 2 weeks following BMS and is exceedingly rare (<0.1 % in most case series) >4 weeks after BMS when most stents have full endothelial coverage. Therefore, in order to ensure adequate stent endothelialization and reduce perioperative coronary risk, it is be reasonable to delay surgery for 3 months, but not >6 months, the time period when BMS restenosis typically occurs.

The timing of surgery following DES implantation is more challenging. Due to delayed stent endothelialization inherent to this stent platform resulting in an increased risk of stent thrombosis for at least 12 months following DES implantation, DAPT (aspirin plus either clopidogrel 75 mg daily, prasugrel 10 mg daily, or ticagrelor 90 mg twice/day) is mandated for at least 12 months following DES implantation.

Studies assessing the risk of perioperative complications following BMS and DES have consistently demonstrated an inverse relationship between the time from PCI to noncardiac surgery and perioperative MACE rates, with important distinctions in risk duration and timing between patients receiving BMS vs. DES PCI [117–120]. Two retrospective studies from the Mayo Clinic analyzed the risk of cardiac complications after noncardiac surgery in the 2 years following BMS and DES implantation. Among BMS recipients, the frequency of perioperative MACE (death, MI, stent thrombosis, repeat revascularization) was temporally related to the time following BMS implantation and subsequent noncardiac surgery (<30 days, 10.5 %; 30–90 days, 3.8 %; and >90 days, 2.8 %) [118]. The authors concluded that noncardiac surgery should be delayed for 90 days following PCI using BMS, findings consistent with current recommendations. Among patients who received a DES, MACE was lowest when noncardiac surgery was performed >1 year following DES implantation [117]. Similarly, in a single-center observational study from the Netherlands ($n=550$; 376 DES, 174 BMS), MACE rates for intervals between BMS PCI and noncardiac surgery <30 days, 30 days to 3 months, and >3 months were 50 %, 14 %, and 4 %, respectively. In the DES PCI group, MACE risk decreased at a slower rate: 35 %, 13 %, 15 %, 6 %, and 9 % for patients undergoing surgery within <30 days, 30 days to 3 months, 3–6 months, 6–12 months, and >12 months, respectively.

Based on the current literature, the 2012 AHA/ACCF Scientific Statement on pretransplant cardiac evaluation recommends against the performance of kidney transplantation within 4 weeks of balloon angioplasty, within 3 months of BMS, and within 12 months of DES implantation (Class III; LOE B), particularly if the anticipated time of post-stent DAPT will be reduced (Table 10.1) [14].

Antiplatelet Therapy in the Context of Recent PCI

As mentioned above, treatment with DAPT is recommended for a minimum of 1 month after BMS implantation and ≥12 months following DES implantation, with premature discontinuation of antiplatelet agents consistently identified as one of the strongest predictors of stent thrombosis. The optimal duration of DAPT beyond 12 months following DES has not been determined. Continuation of DAPT beyond 1 year may be considered in patients deemed at relatively higher risk for stent thrombosis in whom the risk-to-benefit ratio of DAPT is felt to be acceptable by the patient and physician. It is important to note that current guidelines advocate that all patients who undergo any type of PCI (BMS or DES) for acute coronary syndrome should ideally receive 12 months of DAPT to prevent recurrent acute coronary events [104].

In light of the above considerations, the 2007 AHA/ACC/SCAI/ACS/ADA Science Advisory on the "Prevention of Premature Discontinuation of Dual Antiplatelet Therapy in Patients With Coronary Artery Stents" [121] outlined several recommendations regarding DAPT that were also similarly recommended by the 2012 AHA/ACCF Scientific Statement on pretransplant cardiac evaluation (Table 10.1) [14]. First, when the need for kidney transplantation falls within the time frame of recommended DAPT (particularly for those who have received DES) or the patient is beyond the mandated DAPT time frame but is felt to be at high risk for stent thrombosis (e.g., left main stent; stent in the only remaining conduit for myocardial perfusion), consideration should be given to performing kidney transplantation without interruption of clopidogrel-based DAPT if the risk of bleeding is low. In cases when urgent surgery must be performed in patients taking DAPT and the patient is deemed to be at high risk for surgical bleeding complications, stopping the thienopyridine 5 days prior to surgery and continuing aspirin may be reasonable. If the thienopyridine is stopped, it should be restarted as soon as possible postoperatively. There is no evidence that warfarin or other anticoagulants, antithrombotics, or glycoprotein IIb/IIIa agents are effective to mitigate the risk of stent thrombosis after discontinuation of oral antiplatelet medications.

Summary

Cardiovascular disease is the most common cause of death after kidney transplantation. The presence of symptoms of cardiovascular disease is an important prognostic marker that warrants cardiac evaluation. Current noninvasive methods for screening for CAD have prognostic value for mortality among asymptomatic patients with kidney failure but imperfect sensitivity and specificity for detecting angiographically verified coronary stenoses. Associations of angiographically defined CAD with subsequent survival in this population are also inconsistent, likely because many plaque ruptures that produce myocardial infarction are not localized to sites of angiographic stenoses. The efficacy and best methods of myocardial revascularization have not been examined in large, contemporary clinical trials among patients with CKD. Biomarkers, such as cardiac troponins, have prognostic value in ESRD, but require further study to determine clinical applications in directing more expensive and invasive cardiac evaluation. At this time, it is reasonable to consider noninvasive stress testing in asymptomatic kidney transplantation candidates based on the presence of three or more CAD risk factors to target screening of the subgroups with highest pretest probability of prognostically significant CAD. Coronary revascularization before transplantation surgery should be considered in patients who meet the criteria outlined in the "2011 ACCF/AHA Guidelines for Coronary Artery Bypass Graft Surgery." A suggested approach to cardiac evaluation before kidney transplantation based on currently available evidence is summarized in Fig. 10.1. Pursuit of more evidence, ideally from randomized clinical trials, is an urgent priority to strengthen the evidence base for pretransplant cardiac evaluation and the management of cardiovascular disease before, during, and after transplant.

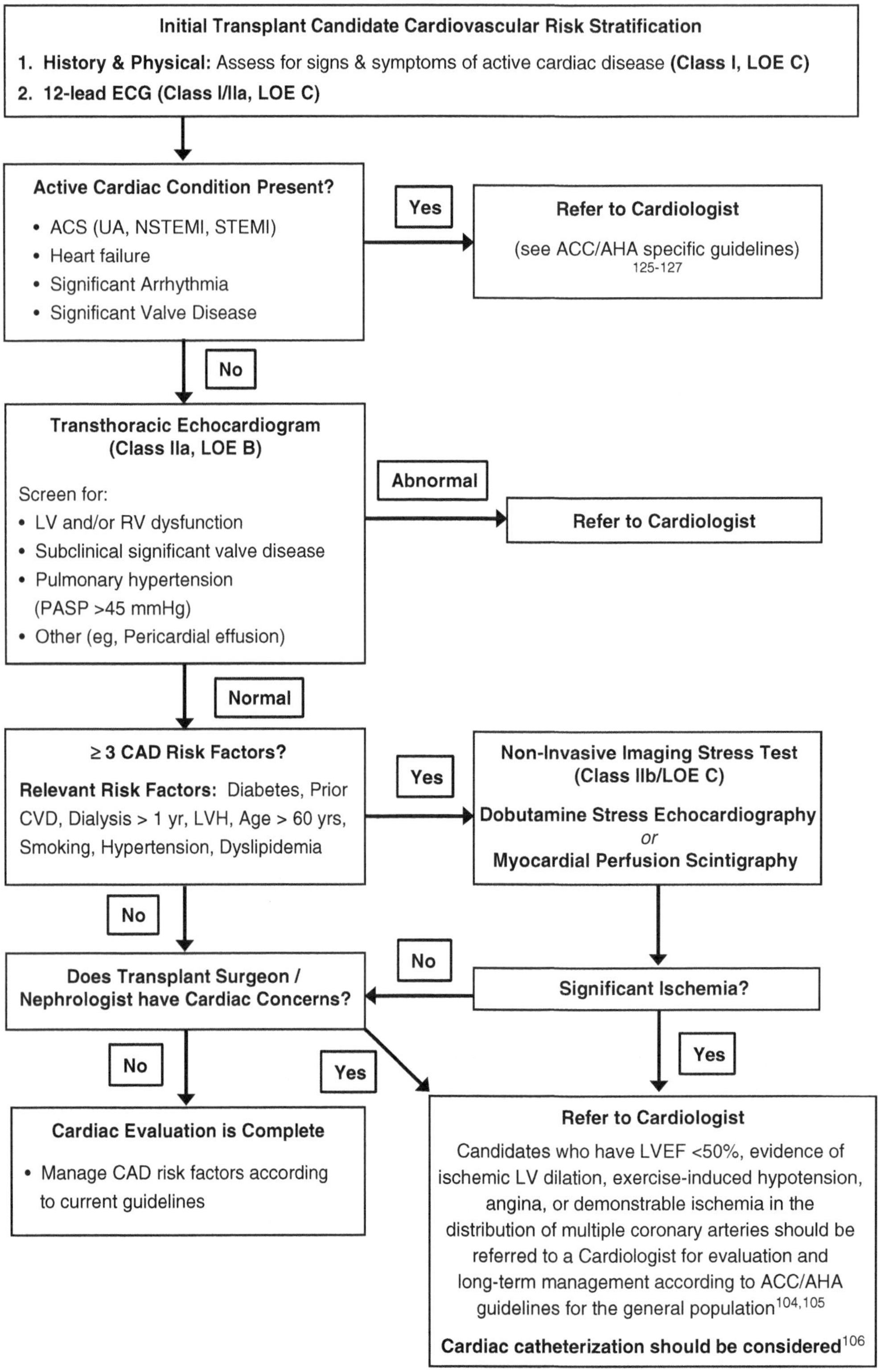

Fig. 10.1 Suggested approach to cardiac evaluation before kidney transplantation. *ACC/AHA*, American College of Cardiology/American Heart Association; *ACS*, acute coronary syndrome; *CAD*, coronary artery disease; *CVD*, cardiovascular disease; *ECG*, electrocardiogram; *LV*, left ventricular; *LVEF*, left ventricular ejection fraction; *LVH*, left ventricular hypertrophy; *LOE*, level of evidence; *NSTEMI*, non-ST elevation myocardial infarction; *PASP*, pulmonary artery systolic pressure; *RV*, right ventricular; *STEMI*, ST elevation myocardial infarction; *UA*, unstable angina

References

1. Meier-Kriesche HU, Schold JD, Srinivas TR, Reed A, Kaplan B. Kidney transplantation halts cardiovascular disease progression in patients with end-stage renal disease. Am J Transplant. 2004;4:1662–8.
2. Lentine KL, Brennan DC, Schnitzler MA. Incidence and predictors of myocardial infarction after kidney transplantation. J Am Soc Nephrol. 2005;16:496–506.
3. Lentine KL, Schnitzler MA, Abbott KC, et al. De novo congestive heart failure after kidney transplantation: a common condition with poor prognostic implications. Am J Kidney Dis. 2005;46:720–33.
4. Lentine KL, Rocca Rey LA, Kolli S, et al. Variations in the risk for cerebrovascular events after kidney transplant compared with experience on the waiting list and after graft failure. Clin J Am Soc Nephrol. 2008;3:1090–101.
5. Lentine KL, Xiao H, Brennan DC, et al. The impact of kidney transplantation on heart failure risk varies with candidate body mass index. Am Heart J. 2009;158:972–82.
6. Ramanathan V, Goral S, Tanriover B, et al. Screening asymptomatic diabetic patients for coronary artery disease prior to renal transplantation. Transplantation. 2005;79:1453–8.
7. Lentine KL, Schnitzler MA, Abbott KC, et al. Incidence, predictors, and associated outcomes of atrial fibrillation after kidney transplantation. Clin J Am Soc Nephrol. 2006;1:288–96.
8. Kasiske BL, Maclean JR, Snyder JJ. Acute myocardial infarction and kidney transplantation. J Am Soc Nephrol. 2006;17:900–7.
9. (OPTN) OPaTN. Organ Procurement and Transplant Network Database, Current US waiting list, kidney transplants. http://optn.transplant.hrsa.gov/latestData/rptData.asp. Accessed 20 Jan 2014.
10. Ramos EL, Kasiske BL, Alexander SR, et al. The evaluation of candidates for renal transplantation. The current practice of U.S. transplant centers. Transplantation. 1994;57:490–7.
11. Danovitch GM, Hariharan S, Pirsch JD, et al. Management of the waiting list for cadaveric kidney transplants: report of a survey and recommendations by the Clinical Practice Guidelines Committee of the American Society of Transplantation. J Am Soc Nephrol. 2002;13:528–35.
12. Zarifian A, O'Rourke M. Managing the kidney waiting list. Prog Transplant. 2006;16:242–6.
13. Lentine KL, Schnitzler MA, Brennan DC, et al. Cardiac evaluation before kidney transplantation: a practice patterns analysis in Medicare-insured dialysis patients. Clin J Am Soc Nephrol. 2008;3:1115–24.
14. Lentine KL, Costa SP, Weir MR, et al. Cardiac disease evaluation and management among kidney and liver transplantation candidates: a scientific statement from the American Heart Association and the American College of Cardiology Foundation. Circulation. 2012;126:617–63.
15. Kasiske BL, Cangro CB, Hariharan S, et al. The evaluation of renal transplantation candidates: clinical practice guidelines. Am J Transplant. 2001;1 Suppl 2:3–95.
16. K/DOQI Workgroup. K/DOQI clinical practice guidelines for cardiovascular disease in dialysis patients. Am J Kidney Dis. 2005;45:S1–153.
17. Fleisher LA, Beckman JA, Brown KA, et al. ACC/AHA 2007 guidelines on perioperative cardiovascular evaluation and care for noncardiac surgery: executive summary: a report of the American College of Cardiology/American Heart Association Task Force on Practice Guidelines (writing committee to revise the 2002 guidelines on perioperative cardiovascular evaluation for noncardiac surgery) developed in collaboration with the American Society of Echocardiography, American Society of Nuclear Cardiology, Heart Rhythm Society, Society of Cardiovascular Anesthesiologists, Society for Cardiovascular Angiography and Interventions, Society for Vascular Medicine and Biology, and Society for Vascular Surgery. J Am Coll Cardiol. 2007;50:1707–32.
18. Friedman A, ZLotnick D, Palac R, Costa S. A study in contradictions: rates of noninvasive stress testing in renal transplant candidates are dependent on which set of national guidelines are applied. Clin J Am Soc Nephrol. 2011;6:1185–91.
19. Kasiske BL, Malik MA, Herzog CA. Risk-stratified screening for ischemic heart disease in kidney transplant candidates. Transplantation. 2005;80:815–20.
20. Lewis MS, Wilson RA, Walker K, et al. Factors in cardiac risk stratification of candidates for renal transplant. J Cardiovasc Risk. 1999;6:251–5.
21. Patel AD, Abo-Auda WS, Davis JM, et al. Prognostic value of myocardial perfusion imaging in predicting outcome after renal transplantation. Am J Cardiol. 2003;92:146–51.
22. Patel RK, Mark PB, Johnston N, et al. Prognostic value of cardiovascular screening in potential renal transplant recipients: a single-center prospective observational study. Am J Transplant. 2008;8:1673–83.
23. Marwick TH, Steinmuller DR, Underwood DA, et al. Ineffectiveness of dipyridamole SPECT thallium imaging as a screening technique for coronary artery disease in patients with end-stage renal failure. Transplantation. 1990;49:100–3.
24. Boudreau RJ, Strony JT, duCret RP, et al. Perfusion thallium imaging of type I diabetes patients with end stage renal disease: comparison of oral and intravenous dipyridamole administration. Radiology. 1990;175:103–5.
25. Vandenberg BF, Rossen JD, Grover-McKay M, Shammas NW, Burns TL, Rezai K. Evaluation of diabetic patients for renal and pancreas transplantation: noninvasive screening for coronary artery disease using radionuclide methods. Transplantation. 1996;62:1230–5.
26. Dahan M, Viron BM, Faraggi M, et al. Diagnostic accuracy and prognostic value of combined dipyridamole-exercise thallium imaging in hemodialysis patients. Kidney Int. 1998;54: 255–62.
27. Herzog CA, Marwick TH, Pheley AM, White CW, Rao VK, Dick CD. Dobutamine stress echocardiography for the detection of significant coronary artery disease in renal transplant candidates. Am J Kidney Dis. 1999;33:1080–90.
28. Worthley MI, Unger SA, Mathew TH, Russ GR, Horowitz JD. Usefulness of tachycardic-stress perfusion imaging to predict coronary artery disease in high-risk patients with chronic renal failure. Am J Cardiol. 2003;92:1318–20.
29. De Lima JJ, Sabbaga E, Vieira ML, et al. Coronary angiography is the best predictor of events in renal transplant candidates compared with noninvasive testing. Hypertension. 2003;42:263–8.
30. Sharma R, Pellerin D, Gaze DC, et al. Dobutamine stress echocardiography and the resting but not exercise electrocardiograph predict severe coronary artery disease in renal transplant candidates. Nephrol Dial Transplant. 2005;20:2207–14.
31. Ferreira PA, de Lima VC, Campos Filho O, et al. Feasibility, safety and accuracy of dobutamine/atropine stress echocardiography for the detection of coronary artery disease in renal transplant candidates. Arq Bras Cardiol. 2007;88:45–51.
32. Wang LW, Fahim MA, Hayen A, et al. Cardiac testing for coronary artery disease in potential kidney transplant recipients. Cochrane Database Syst Rev. 2011;(12):CD008691.
33. Ragosta M, Samady H, Isaacs RB, Gimple LW, Sarembock IJ, Powers ER. Coronary flow reserve abnormalities in patients with diabetes mellitus who have end-stage renal disease and normal epicardial coronary arteries. Am Heart J. 2004;147(6):1017–23.
34. Morrow CE, Schwartz JS, Sutherland DE, et al. Predictive value of thallium stress testing for coronary and cardiovascular events in uremic diabetic patients before renal transplantation. Am J Surg. 1983;146:331–5.

35. Reis G, Marcovitz PA, Leichtman AB, et al. Usefulness of dobutamine stress echocardiography in detecting coronary artery disease in end-stage renal disease. Am J Cardiol. 1995;75:707–10.
36. Bates JR, Sawada SG, Segar DS, et al. Evaluation using dobutamine stress echocardiography in patients with insulin-dependent diabetes mellitus before kidney and/or pancreas transplantation. Am J Cardiol. 1996;77:175–9.
37. Tita C, Karthikeyan V, Stroe A, Jacobsen G, Ananthasubramaniam K. Stress echocardiography for risk stratification in patients with end-stage renal disease undergoing renal transplantation. J Am Soc Echocardiogr. 2008;21:321–6.
38. Marwick TH, Lauer MS, Lobo A, Nally J, Braun W. Use of dobutamine echocardiography for cardiac risk stratification of patients with chronic renal failure. J Intern Med. 1998;244:155–61.
39. Rakhit DJ, Armstrong KA, Beller E, Isbel NM, Marwick TH. Risk stratification of patients with chronic kidney disease: results of screening strategies incorporating clinical risk scoring and dobutamine stress echocardiography. Am Heart J. 2006;152:363–70.
40. Rabbat CG, Treleaven DJ, Russell JD, Ludwin D, Cook DJ. Prognostic value of myocardial perfusion studies in patients with end-stage renal disease assessed for kidney or kidney-pancreas transplantation: a meta-analysis. J Am Soc Nephrol. 2003;14:431–9.
41. Bergeron S, Hillis GS, Haugen EN, Oh JK, Bailey KR, Pellikka PA. Prognostic value of dobutamine stress echocardiography in patients with chronic kidney disease. Am Heart J. 2007;153:385–91.
42. Wong CF, Little MA, Vinjamuri S, Hammad A, Harper JM. Technetium myocardial perfusion scanning in prerenal transplant evaluation in the United Kingdom. Transplant Proc. 2008;40: 1324–8.
43. Bennett WM, Kloster F, Rosch J, Barry J, Porter GA. Natural history of asymptomatic coronary arteriographic lesions in diabetic patients with end-stage renal disease. Am J Med. 1978;65:779–84.
44. Weinrauch L, D'Elia JA, Healy RW, Gleason RE, Christleib AR, Leland Jr OS. Asymptomatic coronary artery disease: angiographic assessment of diabetics evaluated for renal transplantation. Circulation. 1978;58:1184–90.
45. Braun WE, Phillips DF, Vidt DG, et al. Coronary artery disease in 100 diabetics with end-stage renal failure. Transplant Proc. 1984;16:603–7.
46. Lorber MI, Van Buren CT, Flechner SM, et al. Pretransplant coronary arteriography for diabetic renal transplant recipients. Transplant Proc. 1987;19:1539–41.
47. Manske CL, Wilson RF, Wang Y, Thomas W. Prevalence of, and risk factors for, angiographically determined coronary artery disease in type I-diabetic patients with nephropathy. Arch Intern Med. 1992;152:2450–5.
48. Ohtake T, Kobayashi S, Moriya H, et al. High prevalence of occult coronary artery stenosis in patients with chronic kidney disease at the initiation of renal replacement therapy: an angiographic examination. J Am Soc Nephrol. 2005;16:1141–8.
49. Charytan D, Kuntz RE, Mauri L, DeFilippi C. Distribution of coronary artery disease and relation to mortality in asymptomatic hemodialysis patients. Am J Kidney Dis. 2007;49:409–16.
50. Gowdak LH, de Paula FJ, Cesar LA, et al. Screening for significant coronary artery disease in high-risk renal transplant candidates. Coron Artery Dis. 2007;18:553–8.
51. Gowdak LH, de Paula FJ, Cesar LA, et al. Diabetes and coronary artery disease impose similar cardiovascular morbidity and mortality on renal transplant candidates. Nephrol Dial Transplant. 2007;22:1456–61.
52. Hage FG, Smalheiser S, Zoghbi GJ, et al. Predictors of survival in patients with end-stage renal disease evaluated for kidney transplantation. Am J Cardiol. 2007;100:1020–5.
53. Hickson LJ, Cosio FG, El-Zoghby ZM, et al. Survival of patients on the kidney transplant wait list: relationship to cardiac troponin T. Am J Transplant. 2008;8:2352–9.
54. Manske CL, Wang Y, Rector T, Wilson RF, White CW. Coronary revascularisation in insulin-dependent diabetic patients with chronic renal failure. Lancet. 1992;340:998–1002.
55. Kumar N, Baker CS, Chan K, et al. Cardiac survival after preemptive coronary angiography in transplant patients and those awaiting transplantation. Clin J Am Soc Nephrol. 2011;6: 1912–9.
56. McFalls EO, Ward HB, Moritz TE, et al. Coronary-artery revascularization before elective major vascular surgery. N Engl J Med. 2004;351:2795–804.
57. Boden WE, O'Rourke RA, Teo KK, et al. Optimal medical therapy with or without PCI for stable coronary disease. N Engl J Med. 2007;356:1503–16.
58. Sedlis SP, Jurkovitz CT, Hartigan PM, et al. Optimal medical therapy with or without percutaneous coronary intervention for patients with stable coronary artery disease and chronic kidney disease. Am J Cardiol. 2009;104:1647–53.
59. Abbud-Filho M, Adams PL, Alberu J, et al. A report of the Lisbon Conference on the care of the kidney transplant recipient. Transplantation. 2007;83:S1–22.
60. Gaston RS, Danovitch GM, Adams PL, et al. The report of a national conference on the wait list for kidney transplantation. Am J Transplant. 2003;3:775–85.
61. Hachamovitch R, Hayes S, Friedman JD, et al. Determinants of risk and its temporal variation in patients with normal stress myocardial perfusion scans: what is the warranty period of a normal scan? J Am Coll Cardiol. 2003;41:1329–40.
62. Hakeem A, Bhatti S, Dillie KS, et al. Predictive value of myocardial perfusion single-photon emission computed tomography and the impact of renal function on cardiac death. Circulation. 2008;118:2540–9.
63. Rakhit DJ, Marwick TH, Armstrong KA, Johnson DW, Leano R, Isbel NM. Effect of aggressive risk factor modification on cardiac events and myocardial ischaemia in patients with chronic kidney disease. Heart. 2006;92:1402–8.
64. Gill JS, Ma I, Landsberg D, Johnson N, Levin A. Cardiovascular events and investigation in patients who are awaiting cadaveric kidney transplantation. J Am Soc Nephrol. 2005;16:808–16.
65. Abe S, Yoshizawa M, Nakanishi N, et al. Electrocardiographic abnormalities in patients receiving hemodialysis. Am Heart J. 1996;131:1137–44.
66. Rajagopalan N, Miller TD, Hodge DO, Frye RL, Gibbons RJ. Identifying high-risk asymptomatic diabetic patients who are candidates for screening stress single-photon emission computed tomography imaging. J Am Coll Cardiol. 2005;45:43–9.
67. Foley RN, Parfrey PS, Harnett JD, et al. Clinical and echocardiographic disease in patients starting end-stage renal disease therapy. Kidney Int. 1995;47:186–92.
68. Yamada S, Ishii H, Takahashi H, et al. Prognostic value of reduced left ventricular ejection fraction at start of hemodialysis therapy on cardiovascular and all-cause mortality in end-stage renal disease patients. Clin J Am Soc Nephrol. 2010;5:1793–8.
69. Siedlecki A, Foushee M, Curtis JJ, et al. The impact of left ventricular systolic dysfunction on survival after renal transplantation. Transplantation. 2007;84:1610–7.
70. de Mattos AM, Siedlecki A, Gaston RS, et al. Systolic dysfunction portends increased mortality among those waiting for renal transplant. J Am Soc Nephrol. 2008;19:1191–6.
71. Budoff MJ, Shaw LJ, Liu ST, et al. Long-term prognosis associated with coronary calcification: observations from a registry of 25,253 patients. J Am Coll Cardiol. 2007;49:1860–70.
72. Polonsky TS, McClelland RL, Jorgensen NW, et al. Coronary artery calcium score and risk classification for coronary heart disease prediction. JAMA. 2010;303:1610–6.
73. Blaha MJ, Budoff MJ, DeFilippis AP, et al. Associations between C-reactive protein, coronary artery calcium, and cardiovascular

events: implications for the JUPITER population from MESA, a population-based cohort study. Lancet. 2011;378:684–92.
74. Raggi P, Boulay A, Chasan-Taber S, et al. Cardiac calcification in adult hemodialysis patients. A link between end-stage renal disease and cardiovascular disease? J Am Coll Cardiol. 2002;39: 695–701.
75. Braun J, Oldendorf M, Moshage W, Heidler R, Zeitler E, Luft FC. Electron beam computed tomography in the evaluation of cardiac calcification in chronic dialysis patients. Am J Kidney Dis. 1996;27:394–401.
76. Goodman WG, Goldin J, Kuizon BD, et al. Coronary-artery calcification in young adults with end-stage renal disease who are undergoing dialysis. N Engl J Med. 2000;342:1478–83.
77. Oh J, Wunsch R, Turzer M, et al. Advanced coronary and carotid arteriopathy in young adults with childhood-onset chronic renal failure. Circulation. 2002;106:100–5.
78. Matsuoka M, Iseki K, Tamashiro M, et al. Impact of high coronary artery calcification score (CACS) on survival in patients on chronic hemodialysis. Clin Exp Nephrol. 2004;8:54–8.
79. Greenland P, Bonow RO, Brundage BH, et al. ACCF/AHA 2007 clinical expert consensus document on coronary artery calcium scoring by computed tomography in global cardiovascular risk assessment and in evaluation of patients with chest pain: a report of the American College of Cardiology Foundation Clinical Expert Consensus Task Force (ACCF/AHA Writing Committee to Update the 2000 Expert Consensus Document on Electron Beam Computed Tomography) developed in collaboration with the Society of Atherosclerosis Imaging and Prevention and the Society of Cardiovascular Computed Tomography. J Am Coll Cardiol. 2007;49:378–402.
80. Haydar AA, Hujairi NM, Covic AA, Pereira D, Rubens M, Goldsmith DJ. Coronary artery calcification is related to coronary atherosclerosis in chronic renal disease patients: a study comparing EBCT-generated coronary artery calcium scores and coronary angiography. Nephrol Dial Transplant. 2004;19:2307–12.
81. Sharples EJ, Pereira D, Summers S, et al. Coronary artery calcification measured with electron-beam computerized tomography correlates poorly with coronary artery angiography in dialysis patients. Am J Kidney Dis. 2004;43:313–9.
82. Tong LL, Mehrotra R, Shavelle DM, Budoff M, Adler S. Poor correlation between coronary artery calcification and obstructive coronary artery disease in an end-stage renal disease patient. Hemodial Int. 2008;12:16–22.
83. Shroff RC, McNair R, Figg N, et al. Dialysis accelerates medial vascular calcification in part by triggering smooth muscle cell apoptosis. Circulation. 2008;118:1748–57.
84. Vanhoenacker PK, Heijenbrok-Kal MH, Van Heste R, et al. Diagnostic performance of multidetector CT angiography for assessment of coronary artery disease: meta-analysis. Radiology. 2007;244:419–28.
85. Meijboom WB, Weustink AC, Pugliese F, et al. Comparison of diagnostic accuracy of 64-slice computed tomography coronary angiography in women versus men with angina pectoris. Am J Cardiol. 2007;100:1532–7.
86. Hulten EA, Carbonaro S, Petrillo SP, Mitchell JD, Villines TC. Prognostic value of cardiac computed tomography angiography: a systematic review and meta-analysis. J Am Coll Cardiol. 2011;57:1237–47.
87. Taylor AJ, Cerqueira M, Hodgson JM, et al. ACCF/SCCT/ACR/AHA/ASE/ASNC/NASCI/SCAI/SCMR 2010 appropriate use criteria for cardiac computed tomography. A report of the American College of Cardiology Foundation Appropriate Use Criteria Task Force, the Society of Cardiovascular Computed Tomography, the American College of Radiology, the American Heart Association, the American Society of Echocardiography, the American Society of Nuclear Cardiology, the North American Society for Cardiovascular Imaging, the Society for Cardiovascular Angiography and Interventions, and the Society for Cardiovascular Magnetic Resonance. J Am Coll Cardiol. 2011;56:1864–94.
88. Jaffe AS, Babuin L, Apple FS. Biomarkers in acute cardiac disease: the present and the future. J Am Coll Cardiol. 2006;48:1–11.
89. Khan NA, Hemmelgarn BR, Tonelli M, Thompson CR, Levin A. Prognostic value of troponin T and I among asymptomatic patients with end-stage renal disease: a meta-analysis. Circulation. 2005;112:3088–96.
90. Hickson LT, El-Zoghby ZM, Lorenz EC, Stegall MD, Jaffe AS, Cosio FG. Patient survival after kidney transplantation: relationship to pretransplant cardiac troponin T levels. Am J Transplant. 2009;9:1354–61.
91. Connolly GM, Cunningham R, McNamee PT, Young IS, Maxwell AP. Troponin T is an independent predictor of mortality in renal transplant recipients. Nephrol Dial Transplant. 2008;23:1019–25.
92. Bonaca M, Scirica B, Sabatine M, et al. Prospective evaluation of the prognostic implications of improved assay performance with a sensitive assay for cardiac troponin I. J Am Coll Cardiol. 2010;55:2118–24.
93. Lewis MS, Wilson RA, Walker KW, et al. Validation of an algorithm for predicting cardiac events in renal transplant candidates. Am J Cardiol. 2002;89:847–50.
94. Le A, Wilson R, Douek K, et al. Prospective risk stratification in renal transplant candidates for cardiac death. Am J Kidney Dis. 1994;24:65–71.
95. Parfrey PS, Griffiths SM, Barrett BJ, et al. Contrast material-induced renal failure in patients with diabetes mellitus, renal insufficiency, or both. A prospective controlled study. N Engl J Med. 1989;320:143–9.
96. Nikolsky E, Aymong ED, Dangas G, Mehran R. Radiocontrast nephropathy: identifying the high-risk patient and the implications of exacerbating renal function. Rev Cardiovasc Med. 2003;4 Suppl 1:S7–14.
97. Mehran R, Aymong ED, Nikolsky E, et al. A simple risk score for prediction of contrast-induced nephropathy after percutaneous coronary intervention: development and initial validation. J Am Coll Cardiol. 2004;44:1393–9.
98. Dangas G, Iakovou I, Nikolsky E, et al. Contrast-induced nephropathy after percutaneous coronary interventions in relation to chronic kidney disease and hemodynamic variables. Am J Cardiol. 2005;95:13–9.
99. McCullough PA, Adam A, Becker CR, et al. Risk prediction of contrast-induced nephropathy. Am J Cardiol. 2006;98:27K–36.
100. Tan N, Liu Y, Zhou YL, et al. Contrast medium volume to creatinine clearance ratio: a predictor of contrast-induced nephropathy in the first 72 hours following percutaneous coronary intervention. Catheter Cardiovasc Interv. 2012;79(1):70–5.
101. Kumar N, Dahri L, Brown W, et al. Effect of elective coronary angiography on glomerular filtration rate in patients with advanced chronic kidney disease. Clin J Am Soc Nephrol. 2009;4: 1907–13.
102. Lorenz EC, Stegall MD, Cosio FG, Gloor JM, Larson TS, Taler SJ. The effect of coronary angiography on renal function in preemptive renal transplant candidates. Clin Transplant. 2011;25: 594–9.
103. Hillis LD, Smith PK, Anderson JL, et al. 2011 ACCF/AHA guideline for coronary artery bypass graft surgery. A report of the American College of Cardiology Foundation/American Heart Association Task Force on Practice Guidelines. Developed in collaboration with the American Association for Thoracic Surgery, Society of Cardiovascular Anesthesiologists, and Society of Thoracic Surgeons. J Am Coll Cardiol. 2011;58:e123–210.
104. Levine GN, Bates ER, Blankenship JC, et al. 2011 ACCF/AHA/SCAI guideline for percutaneous coronary intervention. A report of the American College of Cardiology Foundation/American

Heart Association Task Force on Practice Guidelines and the Society for Cardiovascular Angiography and Interventions. J Am Coll Cardiol. 2011;58:e44–122.
105. Patel MR, Bailey SR, Bonow RO, et al. ACCF/SCAI/AATS/AHA/ASE/ASNC/HFSA/HRS/SCCM/SCCT/SCMR/STS 2012 appropriate use criteria for diagnostic catheterization: a report of the American College of Cardiology Foundation Appropriate Use Criteria Task Force, Society for Cardiovascular Angiography and Interventions, American Association for Thoracic Surgery, American Heart Association, American Society of Echocardiography, American Society of Nuclear Cardiology, Heart Failure Society of America, Heart Rhythm Society, Society of Critical Care Medicine, Society of Cardiovascular Computed Tomography, Society for Cardiovascular Magnetic Resonance, and Society of Thoracic Surgeons. J Am Coll Cardiol. 2012;59:1995–2027.
106. Charytan D, Kuntz RE. The exclusion of patients with chronic kidney disease from clinical trials in coronary artery disease. Kidney Int. 2006;70:2021–30.
107. Poldermans D, Schouten O, Vidakovic R, et al. A clinical randomized trial to evaluate the safety of a noninvasive approach in high-risk patients undergoing major vascular surgery: the DECREASE-V Pilot Study. J Am Coll Cardiol. 2007;49:1763–9.
108. Szczech LA, Reddan DN, Owen WF, et al. Differential survival after coronary revascularization procedures among patients with renal insufficiency. Kidney Int. 2001;60:292–9.
109. Reddan DN, Szczech LA, Tuttle RH, et al. Chronic kidney disease, mortality, and treatment strategies among patients with clinically significant coronary artery disease. J Am Soc Nephrol. 2003;14:2373–80.
110. Herzog CA, Ma JZ, Collins AJ. Long-term outcome of renal transplant recipients in the United States after coronary revascularization procedures. Circulation. 2004;109:2866–71.
111. Debella YT, Giduma HD, Light RP, Agarwal R. Chronic kidney disease as a coronary disease equivalent—a comparison with diabetes over a decade. Clin J Am Soc Nephrol. 2011;6:1385–92.
112. Shroff GR, Solid CA, Herzog CA. Long-term survival and repeat coronary revascularization in dialysis patients after surgical and percutaneous coronary revascularization with drug-eluting and bare metal stents in the United States. Circulation. 2013;127: 1861–9.
113. Flaherty JD, Davidson CJ. Diabetes and coronary revascularization. JAMA. 2005;293:1501–8.
114. Eagle KA, Guyton RA, Davidoff R, et al. ACC/AHA 2004 guideline update for coronary artery bypass graft surgery: a report of the American College of Cardiology/American Heart Association Task Force on Practice Guidelines (committee to update the 1999 guidelines for coronary artery bypass graft surgery). Circulation. 2004;110:e340–437.
115. Liu JY, Birkmeyer NJ, Sanders JH, et al. Risks of morbidity and mortality in dialysis patients undergoing coronary artery bypass surgery. Northern New England Cardiovascular Disease Study Group. Circulation. 2000;102:2973–7.
116. Tsai TT, Messenger JC, Brennan JM, et al. Safety and efficacy of drug-eluting stents in older patients with chronic kidney disease: a report from the linked CathPCI Registry-CMS claims database. J Am Coll Cardiol. 2011;58:1859–69.
117. Rabbitts JA, Nuttall GA, Brown MJ, et al. Cardiac risk of noncardiac surgery after percutaneous coronary intervention with drug-eluting stents. Anesthesiology. 2008;109:596–604.
118. Nuttall GA, Brown MJ, Stombaugh JW, et al. Time and cardiac risk of surgery after bare-metal stent percutaneous coronary intervention. Anesthesiology. 2008;109:588–95.
119. van Kuijk JP, Flu WJ, Schouten O, et al. Timing of noncardiac surgery after coronary artery stenting with bare metal or drug-eluting stents. Am J Cardiol. 2009;104:1229–34.
120. Anwaruddin S, Askari AT, Saudye H, et al. Characterization of post-operative risk associated with prior drug-eluting stent use. JACC Cardiovasc Interv. 2009;2:542–9.
121. Grines CL, Bonow RO, Casey Jr DE, et al. Prevention of premature discontinuation of dual antiplatelet therapy in patients with coronary artery stents: a science advisory from the American Heart Association, American College of Cardiology, Society for Cardiovascular Angiography and Interventions, American College of Surgeons, and American Dental Association, with representation from the American College of Physicians. J Am Coll Cardiol. 2007;49:734–9.
122. Kendrick E. Cardiovascular disease and the renal transplant recipient. Am J Kidney Dis. 2001;38:S36–43.
123. EBPG Expert Group on Renal Transplantation. European best practice guidelines for renal transplantation. Section I: evaluation, selection and preparation of the potential transplant recipient. I.5. Risk factors/relative contra-indications. Nephrol Dial Transplant. 2000;15 Suppl 7:3–38.
124. Lentine KL, Hurst FP, Jindal RM, et al. Cardiovascular risk assessment among potential kidney transplant candidates: approaches and controversies. Am J Kidney Dis. 2010;55: 152–67.
125. Anderson JL, Adams CD, Antman EM, et al. 2011 ACCF/AHA focused update incorporated into the ACC/AHA 2007 guidelines for the management of patients with unstable angina/non-ST-elevation myocardial infarction: a report of the American College of Cardiology Foundation/American Heart Association Task Force on Practice Guidelines. Circulation. 2011;123:e426–579.
126. Jessup M, Abraham WT, Casey DE, et al. 2009 focused update: ACCF/AHA guidelines for the diagnosis and management of heart failure in adults: a report of the American College of Cardiology Foundation/American Heart Association Task Force on Practice Guidelines: developed in collaboration with the International Society for Heart and Lung Transplantation. Circulation. 2009;119:1977–2016.
127. Bonow RO, Carabello BA, Chatterjee K, et al. 2008 focused update incorporated into the ACC/AHA 2006 guidelines for the management of patients with valvular heart disease: a report of the American College of Cardiology/American Heart Association Task Force on Practice Guidelines (writing committee to revise the 1998 guidelines for the management of patients with valvular heart disease): endorsed by the Society of Cardiovascular Anesthesiologists, Society for Cardiovascular Angiography and Interventions, and Society of Thoracic Surgeons. Circulation. 2008;118:e523–661.

Part III

Surgical Issues in the Transplant Recipient

11

Sunil S. Karhadkar and David B. Leeser

Pretransplant Care

The treatment of the kidney transplant recipient by the transplant surgeon begins with the pretransplant evaluation. At this time, the surgeon along with nephrologists, social workers, dietitians, transplant coordinators, and cardiologists performs a thorough workup to determine a patient's suitability for cadaveric or living donor renal transplantation. The evaluation process is used to select appropriate patients for placement on the waiting list or further preparation toward living donor transplantation and is covered in detail elsewhere in this text. Issues of specific importance to the surgeon include the patient's previous surgical history, vascular examination, overall risk for anesthetic complications, and the presence of any pathologic process that might require pretransplant surgical treatment (i.e., inguinal hernia, biliary disease, peripheral vascular disease, symptomatic polycystic kidney disease).

Surgical Disease in the Pretransplant Period

Abdominal Wall Hernia

Patients found to have any type of abdominal wall hernia during evaluation for organ transplant should be referred for evaluation and repair by a qualified surgeon. The incidence of incarceration, obstruction, and strangulation in abdominal wall hernias is significant enough to mandate a surgical repair even in the absence of symptoms. Additionally, the risks are magnified in the posttransplant patient due to the impact of steroids and immunosuppressants [1]. Therefore, all hernias should be repaired prior to transplantation. Factors that should be specifically considered are (a) presence of coexisting liver disease and ascites and (b) peritoneal dialysis and presence of peritoneal fluid. In both of these situations, medical management should be exhausted before consideration of a hernia repair.

Biliary Disease

The treatment of biliary disease in the patient with renal failure being evaluated for possible kidney transplantation is still controversial. General agreement exists that symptomatic cholelithiasis should be treated by laparoscopic cholecystectomy. Patient history should include questions that elicit a history of right upper quadrant pain, intolerance of fatty foods, jaundice, or pancreatitis. The presence of any of these in the history should prompt evaluation with a right upper quadrant ultrasound and cholescintigraphy. Cholescintigraphy has a sensitivity and specificity of approximately 97 % and 90 %, respectively, in the diagnosis of acute cholecystitis and biliary dyskinesia.

The difficulties lie in the treatment of asymptomatic cholelithiasis in the pretransplant period. Many institutions perform screening abdominal ultrasonography as part of the pretransplant evaluation. Gallstones have been estimated to be present in anywhere from 7 to 40 % of transplant candidates [2–4]. The potential for serious complications from symptomatic gallstone disease in the transplant recipient has been well described in the literature and includes gangrenous cholecystitis, choledocholithiasis and cholangitis, pancreatitis, loss of the allograft, and death [5–9]. The potential for serious adverse events and the relatively low morbidity and mortality have led to the suggestion that prophylactic laparoscopic cholecystectomy should be performed in all candidates for solid organ transplant prior to transplantation [5, 10]. Others have concluded that the morbidity and mortality of asymptomatic gallstones are overstated and that the percentage of patients prevented from developing complications does not justify the risk of prophylactic surgery, since up to

S.S. Karhadkar • D.B. Leeser, M.D., F.A.C.S. (✉)
University of Maryland Medical Center,
29 South Greene Street, Suite 200, Baltimore, MD 21201, USA
e-mail: dleeser@smail.umaryland.edu

M.R. Weir and E.V. Lerma (eds.), *Kidney Transplantation: Practical Guide to Management*,
DOI 10.1007/978-1-4939-0342-9_11, © Springer Science+Business Media New York 2014

82 % will never develop symptoms [2]. Therefore, the treatment of pretransplant cholelithiasis is center specific. At our center, we do not currently perform prophylactic laparoscopic cholecystectomy prior to renal transplantation. During the era of muromonab-CD3 (OKT3) induction, posttransplant cholecystitis was relatively more frequent, whereas now with widespread use of induction agents that do not lead to cytokine release (i.e., interleukin-2 receptor antibody), we have dropped prophylactic cholecystectomy for asymptomatic cholelithiasis.

Peripheral Vascular Disease

PVD is common in patients with end-stage renal disease (ESRD) and is associated with significant morbidity and mortality. In the United States, the overall prevalence of PVD among patients initiating dialysis is approximately 14–15 % and 25 % in patients on chronic hemodialysis. The pretransplant history should include questions regarding nonhealing ulcers on the lower extremities, claudication, rest pain, and any current or past tobacco use. Physical examination should include upper and lower extremity pulse examination. A positive history should prompt noninvasive vascular studies, which include ankle-brachial indices (ABI) with Doppler-derived segmental pressures of both lower extremities.

The diagnosis of PVD in patients with ESRD is not simple because ABI to diagnose PVD may be less useful due to the high prevalence of medial arterial calcification. This abnormality can result in falsely elevated lower extremity blood pressure readings due to arterial incompressibility. If femoral pulses are diminished, then the patient should also have a computed tomography (CT) angiogram or a magnetic resonance angiography (MRA) of the abdominal aorta. If peripheral vascular disease is confirmed, the treatment plan is an area of debate.

The survival of the patients with ESRD following lower extremity bypass for limb salvage has been reported to be 69 %, 18 %, and 5 % at 1, 3, and 5 years, respectively [11]. Most prior studies of revascularization in patients with renal failure have been small, retrospective, and conducted at single medical centers. The results of revascularization have been mixed. A systematic review of 16 retrospective surgical case series of infrainguinal bypass in ESRD patients reported pooled estimates of 79 %, 77 %, and 42 % for 1-year graft patency, 1-year limb salvage, and 2-year patient survival, respectively [12].

The poor outcome may be contributed to by the increased mortality from ESRD, but has led some to suggest consideration of early amputation in this patient population [12, 13]. Others have acknowledged the higher mortality rates in patients with ESRD and peripheral vascular disease, but continue to advocate attempts at limb salvage in this patient group. Limb salvage rates are reported to be between 71 and 80 % at 2 years [11, 14]. Since kidney transplantation is known to improve survival substantially over hemodialysis, we recommend aggressive treatment of PVD in renal transplant candidates.

Candidates for renal transplantation should also be evaluated for aortic aneurysm. Important risk factors for aneurysm formation are the presence of hypertension and a history of smoking in the patient. In the perioperative workup, in patients found to have infrarenal aortic aneurysmal disease, the repair can be done as part of a simultaneous aneurysm repair and living donor transplant or as a staged procedure while a patient waits for a cadaver kidney. We have performed simultaneous aortic bypass and living donor transplantation in nine patients and aortic repair followed by cadaveric renal transplant in six patients. Five-year survival was 90 % in this group of patients. Two grafts were lost secondary to polyomavirus and noncompliance. Repair of aortic aneurysm is also possible in patients that have previously received a renal allograft. In these cases, the procedure must be planned to minimize the ischemic period experienced by the kidney that receives blood from the iliac artery below the aneurysm repair site. If the iliac arteries are involved with the aneurysm, the kidney may need to be re-transplanted during the aneurysm repair. These procedures should involve the combined efforts of a vascular and transplant surgeon [15, 16]. Infrarenal AAA amenable to endovascular stent graft placement (EVAR) based on anatomy, angulation, and landing zone can also undergo simultaneous or staged renal transplantation. Protection for the grafted kidney from ischemic or reperfusion injury may be achieved by permanent or temporary axillofemoral, femorofemoral, aortoiliac bypass, cold perfusion, local cold preservation, or autotransplantation [16].

Vascular pathology that can also be found in the population with ESRD is cerebrovascular occlusive disease. Patients with ESRD have a relative risk of stroke that is 6.1 times greater than the general population [17]. Forty-four percent to 61 % of patients with renal failure have measurable plaque in the carotid artery [18]. Patients should be queried about any history of stroke or symptoms of transient ischemic attack. The patient should be examined for carotid bruits or if a significant history of peripheral vascular or cardiovascular occlusive disease exists, a carotid duplex ultrasound should be performed to rule out carotid artery stenosis. If significant stenosis is found, the patient should be referred to a vascular surgeon for evaluation for carotid endarterectomy. For symptomatic patients, a stenosis of 50 % or greater should be considered for treatment by endarterectomy [19]. In patients without symptoms, a stenosis of 70 % or greater should be considered for treatment by endarterectomy as long as the treating surgeon has a stroke rate of less than 3 %. These recommendations are consistent with the Asymptomatic Carotid Artery Stenosis Trial and the North

American Symptomatic Carotid Endarterectomy Trial [20]. Patients over the age of 80, recurrent stenosis, neck irradiation, and on dialysis should be offered carotid artery stenting. The SAPPHIRE and CREST trials found that CAS was not inferior to CEA in patients with symptomatic or asymptomatic carotid stenosis considered to be at high risk for carotid surgery [21].

Polycystic Kidney Disease

Patients with renal failure secondary to polycystic kidney disease should be asked about symptoms related to their disease process, which may warrant native nephrectomy. In some cases, patients complain of early satiety, respiratory compromise, hematuria, urinary tract infections, and abdominal pain as a result of the native kidneys. The patient should be examined for palpable masses on either side of the midline and to ascertain whether there will be adequate room for the graft. In cases where the kidneys have enlarged to extent as to cause symptoms or are causing hematuria or infection, the patient should be evaluated by a computed tomography (CT) scan and native nephrectomy considered. The native nephrectomy can be planned as a staged procedure, can be done at the time of kidney transplantation, or performed after transplant when the physiologic condition of the patient has improved. Treatment of patients with polycystic kidney needing native nephrectomy should involve discussion between a urologist and transplant surgeon [22].

Renal Artery Stenosis

Finally, patients with severe hypertension on three drugs or more, with diastolic pressures greater than 100 with onset before age 30 or after age 55, with rapid decline in renal function, with episodes of flash pulmonary edema, or with cardiovascular or PVD should prompt consideration of renovascular hypertension. Renovascular hypertension occurs when uni- or bilateral stenosis or occlusion of the renal arteries results in a diminution of the pressure experience by the juxtaglomerular complex. The resultant secretion of renin activates angiotensinogen to angiotensin I. Angiotensin I is then converted to angiotensin II which causes direct arteriolar vasoconstriction and also stimulates the release of aldosterone which causes sodium and water retention. Renal artery stenosis (RAS) is caused most commonly by atherosclerotic disease in 75–95 % of cases and fibromuscular dysplasia in 5–20 %. The 2006 American College of Cardiology/American Heart Association (ACC/AHA) guidelines state that testing for RAS is *only* indicated if a corrective procedure would be performed if clinically significant renovascular disease were detected. The gold standard for diagnosing RAS is renal arteriography. However, a variety of less invasive tests have been evaluated for testing purposes including duplex Doppler ultrasonography, computed tomographic angiography (CTA), or magnetic resonance angiography (MRA) [23, 24].

In patients with established renal failure, the diagnosis is confirmed by angiography alone, and the renal scan can be omitted. In the presence of renal failure and confirmed renovascular hypertension, strong consideration should be given to nephrectomy prior to or concurrently with renal transplantation. Surgical revascularization (or removal of a completely occluded atrophic kidney) appears to have similar efficacy to percutaneous transluminal angioplasty [25].

The 2005 ACC/AHA guidelines recommended surgery in patients with atherosclerotic RAS who have multiple small renal arteries, early primary branching of the main renal artery, or require aortic reconstruction near the renal arteries for other indications. In some cases, renal function can be restored by performing renal artery angioplasty and stenting to the affected kidney. The preservation of native renal function should be attempted whenever possible. Occasionally, patients with ESRD can come off hemodialysis after correction of RAS [25, 26].

Peritransplant Care

Aside from brief visits to update a patient's workup while on the waiting list, the surgeon's interaction with the transplant candidate is minimal until a call from an organ procurement organization (OPO) identifies the candidate as a possible recipient for a kidney. When a kidney becomes available, the surgeon and a transplant coordinator contact potential recipients and their nephrologists to determine their immediate medical readiness for transplant. The patient should also be asked about their desire to proceed with the organ being offered if the donor fits expanded criteria. The patient is then brought to the hospital while crossmatching is performed to ensure that no barrier exists to a successful transplant. Crossmatching is performed in order to prevent the occurrence of hyperacute antibody-mediated rejection and accelerated forms of acute rejection in the transplanted organs due to the presence of preformed anti-human leukocyte antigen (HLA) antibodies in the recipient to donor lymphocytes. Three types of crossmatching procedures currently exist. The first is the direct complement-dependent lymphocytotoxicity (CDC) test in which recipient sera is placed with donor lymphocytes and the cells are monitored for the occurrence of complement-mediated cell lysis. The second crossmatch procedure is the anti-human globulin (AHG)-enhanced CDC in which rabbit complement is used to increase the sensitivity of the test. Finally, the most sensitive test is the flow cytometric crossmatch in which recipient sera are placed with donor lymphocytes and then fluorescent antibodies are used to detect recipient antibodies adherent to the donor lymphocytes. Most centers use the AHG test for patients without a history of prior sensitization from previous transplants, blood transfusions, or pregnancies. However, if patients are found to have anti-HLA antibodies on a panel of reactive antibodies (PRA), which measures the presence of antibodies to common HLA types, then the type of crossmatch used is center dependent. The specificity of anti-HLA antibodies can also be identified so that donors with these HLA types can be excluded from consideration. Our practice is to perform a flow cytometric crossmatch on all patients with a history of prior transplantation or a PRA greater than 40 %, while other centers feel that the flow crossmatch is too time-consuming and too sensitive. Once the patient arrives at the hospital, a thorough history is taken and a physical performed. The history should include attention to any interim cardiac events, recent illnesses, active PVD, and the date and time of the patient's last hemodialysis treatment. These questions should elicit any recent changes in the recipient's medical condition that would preclude transplantation due to an acute illness or recent event that would make risk of anesthesia too high. The patient should also be queried for the amount of urine produced on a daily basis to aid in post-operative management. Physical exam should be comprehensive with particular attention to signs of congestive heart failure and include a lower extremity vascular examination and the presence and type of dialysis access. Laboratory tests should include a complete blood count (CBC); basic metabolic panel; calcium, magnesium, and phosphorous levels; coagulation tests; and type and crossmatch. If there is any indication of fluid overload or a potassium level greater than 5.4, nephrology should be contacted immediately and hemodialysis should be considered prior to the transplant procedure [27]. Once the above is done, our practice is to complete and review a pretransplant checklist (Fig. 11.1). The patient's name, medical record number, and social security number are checked and recorded from the hospital admission data. Blood type is checked on the admission type and screen. The patient's serologies are then recorded from original laboratory reports. The donor United Network for Organ Sharing (UNOS) number is recorded from the data available in the UNOS database, and the match of the patient's name and social security number with the organ is confirmed with the OPO. The serologies and blood type of the donor are recorded from primary source documents of the donor hospital to ensure a proper match between donor and recipient. The crossmatch data is reviewed and recorded. Once these aspects of the checklist are recorded, the information is reviewed with the patient, while maintaining appropriate donor confidentiality; as part of the informed consent process and consent for transplantation, consent for expanded criteria (hepatitis B- or hepatitis C-positive donors) is obtained. The checklist process ensures the transplantation of appropriate organs into appropriate patients. Once the evaluation by the transplant surgeon is complete, orders are written for the patient to receive prophylactic perioperative antibiotics, steroids, and an immunosuppressive induction agent like basiliximab or antithymocyte immunoglobulin or alemtuzumab intraoperatively.

Operative Procedures

Prior to bringing the patient to the operating room, the organ is removed from storage on iced preservative solution and placed in a basin with slush for back table preparation. The perinephric fat is removed and the hilar fat is dissected away from the artery and vein to free an adequate length to perform vascular anastomoses. Arterial and venous branches to the adrenal gland are ligated and divided and the gland removed. The gonadal vein is identified and ligated. The gonadal vein can be saved should an extension graft be needed for arterial reconstruction. Excessive periureteral tissue is also removed, taking care to preserve the immediate periureteral tissue, which carries the blood supply. The kidney is also inspected for any pathology not seen by the procuring surgeon that would preclude transplantation prior to the patient's arrival in the operating room. The patient is brought to the operating room and general anesthesia is induced. A central venous or Swan-Ganz catheter is placed. An arterial line is optional. A Foley catheter is placed and approximately 200 cm^3 of antibiotic solution is placed in the bladder. Alternatively, a three-way Foley can be used and attached to a bag of GU irrigant solution. Compression stockings and sequential compression devices are placed on the patient's lower extremities. The abdomen is prepped and draped. Perioperative antibiotics, steroids, and, if desired, thymocyte-depleting induction agents are given to the patient. Routinely, a right lower quadrant hockey stick incision is made. The right side is preferred since the iliac vessels tend to be more superficial allowing the construction of the vascular anastomoses to be carried out more easily. Using cautery, the incision is carried down through the aponeurosis of the external oblique. The abdominal oblique musculature is then divided to expose the peritoneum. The peritoneum is swept medially, so that the abdominal cavity is never entered and the iliac vessels can be exposed in the iliac fossa. In females, the round ligament is divided, and in males, the spermatic cord is preserved and mobilized medially. The inferior epigastric vessels can be ligated or preserved. If the patient has had a previous subcostal incision, which implies previous ligation of the superior epigastric artery and vein, the inferior epigastric vessels should be preserved to prevent ischemic necrosis of the anterior abdominal wall. The perivascular lymphatics are ligated to prevent postoperative lymphocele.

University of Maryland Medical Center

Deceased Donor Transplant – Final Checklist

This form must be completed by the transplant surgeon prior to the time of surgery and must be included in the patient's medical record.

RECIPIENT

NAME:_______________

MRN:_______________

D.O.B.:_______________

SS #:_______________

#1 ABO Date: ________ #2 ABO Date: ________

SEROLOGY:

HCV Ab:	☐ POSITIVE	☐ NEGATIVE
HCV PCR*	☐ POSITIVE	☐ NEGATIVE
CMV:	☐ POSITIVE	☐ NEGATIVE
EBV:	☐ POSITIVE	☐ NEGATIVE
HIV Ab:	☐ POSITIVE	☐ NEGATIVE
HIV PCR:	☐ POSITIVE	☐ NEGATIVE
HBsAb:	☐ POSITIVE Titer:	☐ NEGATIVE
HBcAb:	☐ POSITIVE	☐ NEGATIVE
HBsAg:	☐ POSITIVE	☐ NEGATIVE
RPR:	☐ POSITIVE	☐ NEGATIVE
FTA:	☐ POSITIVE	☐ NEGATIVE

DECEASED DONOR

ORGAN:_______________

UNOS #:_______________

IF KIDNEY: ☐ RIGHT ☐ LEFT

ABO:_______________

SEROLOGY:

HCV Ab:	☐ POSITIVE	☐ NEGATIVE	
HCV PCR	☐ POSITIVE	☐ NEGATIVE	☐ NOT TESTED
CMV:	☐ POSITIVE	☐ NEGATIVE	
EBV:	☐ POSITIVE	☐ NEGATIVE	☐ NOT TESTED
HIV:	☐ POSITIVE	☐ NEGATIVE	
HIV PCR:	☐ POSITIVE	☐ NEGATIVE	☐ NOT TESTED
HBsAb:	☐ POSITIVE	☐ NEGATIVE	☐ NOT TESTED
HBV PCR:	☐ POSITIVE	☐ NEGATIVE	☐ NOT TESTED
HBcAb:	☐ POSITIVE	☐ NEGATIVE	
HBsAg:	☐ POSITIVE	☐ NEGATIVE	
RPR:	☐ POSITIVE	☐ NEGATIVE	

*** BOTH HCV Ab AND HCV PCR MUST BE POSITIVE FOR HCV POSITIVE DONOR**

CROSSMATCH:

☐ AHG ☐ POSITIVE ☐ NEGATIVE
☐ FLOW (PRA ≥ 40 or Re-Transplant): ☐ POSITIVE ☐ NEGATIVE
☐ PREVIOUS TRANSPLANTS: ☐ NO ☐ YES

☐ **EXPANDED CRITERIA:** ☐ YES (Informed Consent) ☐ NO
☐ **CDC HIGH RISK:** ☐ YES (Informed Consent) ☐ NO
☐ **HBcAb:** ☐ YES (Informed Consent) ☐ NO
☐ **HCV:** ☐ YES (Informed Consent) ☐ NO

I certify that the above information has been verified from primary source documents.

_______________ Attending Surgeon Signature   _______ Date   _______ Time

_______________ Attending Surgeon Printed Name

EP3A (rev. 02/12) Page 1 of 1

Fig. 11.1 University of Maryland pretransplant checklist

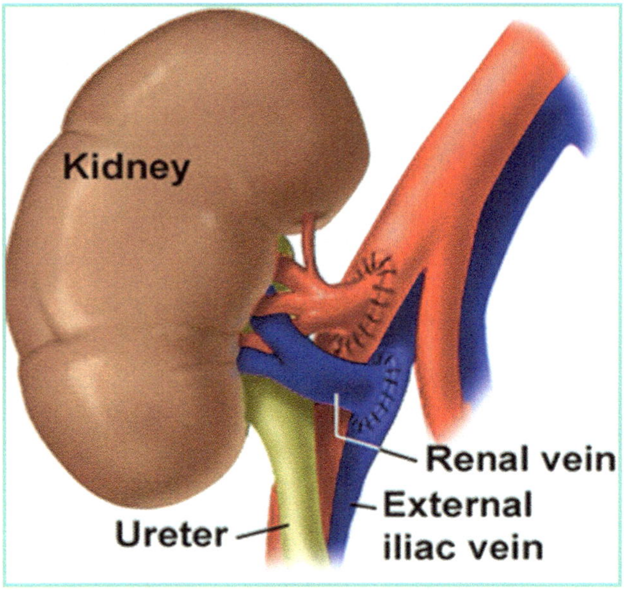

Fig. 11.2 Kidney allograft in situ

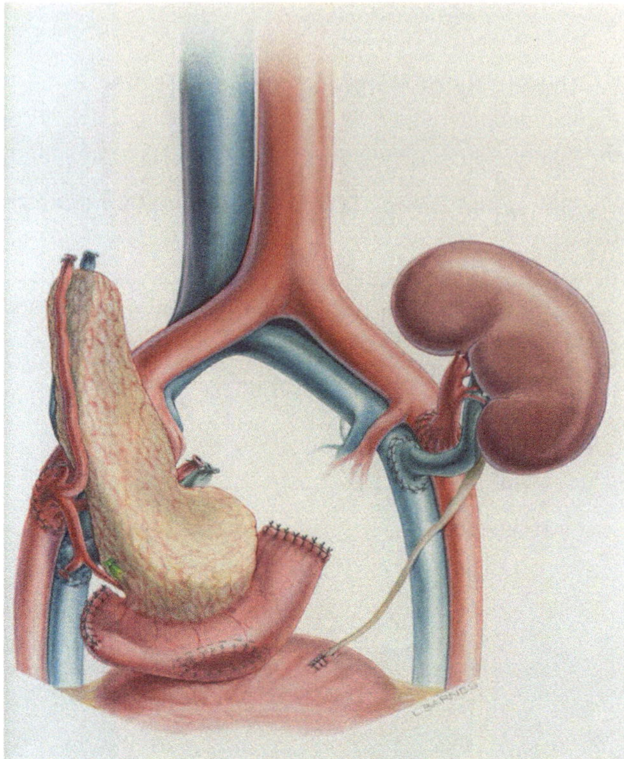

Fig. 11.3 Simultaneous pancreas and kidney transplant with systemic venous drainage and bladder drainage of the exocrine pancreas

Standard vascular techniques are used to create anastomoses between the renal vessels and the external iliac vessels using fine monofilament nonabsorbable suture (Fig. 11.2). The kidney is reperfused and hemostasis achieved using sutures, electrocautery, and prothrombotic agents. At the time of reperfusion of the kidney, the patient is given mannitol as a free radical scavenger and furosemide (Lasix) to promote postreperfusion diuresis. Once the kidney is reperfused and hemostasis achieved, the bladder is exposed at the inferomedial aspect of the wound for creation of a neoureterocystostomy to drain urine into the bladder. The ureterocystic anastomosis is created by incising the posterior aspect of the ureter longitudinally for approximately 1.0–1.5 cm. This spatulation allows for the creation of a large ureterocystic anastomosis with absorbable monofilament suture. The bladder wall musculature is then brought together over the top of the anastomosis to create a tunnel, which will minimize reflux of urine into the distal ureter from the bladder. The kidney can be placed on the left side if there is a contraindication to placing the kidney on the right. This is done if previous incisions have been made in the right lower quadrant, if the patient may receive a pancreas transplant in the future, or if the patient has had a previous kidney placed on the right side. The fascia and skin are then closed, and the patient is taken to the recovery room. When a simultaneous kidney and pancreas transplant is being performed, the pancreas is prepared along with the kidney. During back table preparation of the pancreas, one of the donor's iliac arterial bifurcations is used to create a vascular conduit to the donor superior mesenteric and splenic arteries in order to provide arterial flow to the pancreas. The portal vein, which will drain the pancreas, is also freed from the surrounding structures in order to allow for the construction of an anastomosis. Once the pancreas is prepared, a midline incision is made in the abdomen. The right iliac artery and vein are exposed through the abdominal cavity. The donor common iliac artery is anastomosed to the recipient's common iliac artery (Y-graft). If the pancreas will be drained into the systemic venous circulation, then anastomosis is created between the portal vein and the recipient's common iliac vein (systemic drainage) (Fig. 11.3). When the pancreas is drained systemically, the head lies in the right lower quadrant of the abdomen, and the tail is directed cephalad in the right pericolic gutter. Alternatively, the superior mesenteric vein can be exposed at the base of the transverse mesocolon and the portal vein drained into the recipient's portal vein via the superior mesenteric vein (portal drainage) (Fig. 11.4). In the case of portal drainage, the head of the pancreas lies at the base of the transverse mesocolon and the tail lies caudad toward the right lower quadrant. The organ is then reperfused and hemostasis achieved. Portal venous drainage is advocated because the insulin is delivered directly to the liver in a physiologic manner and drainage into the liver is reported to have an immunologic advantage [28–30]. The past two decades of pancreas transplantation has seen a gradual increase in enteric drainage of the pancreas allograft. The use of the bladder to drain the pancreas can be performed when

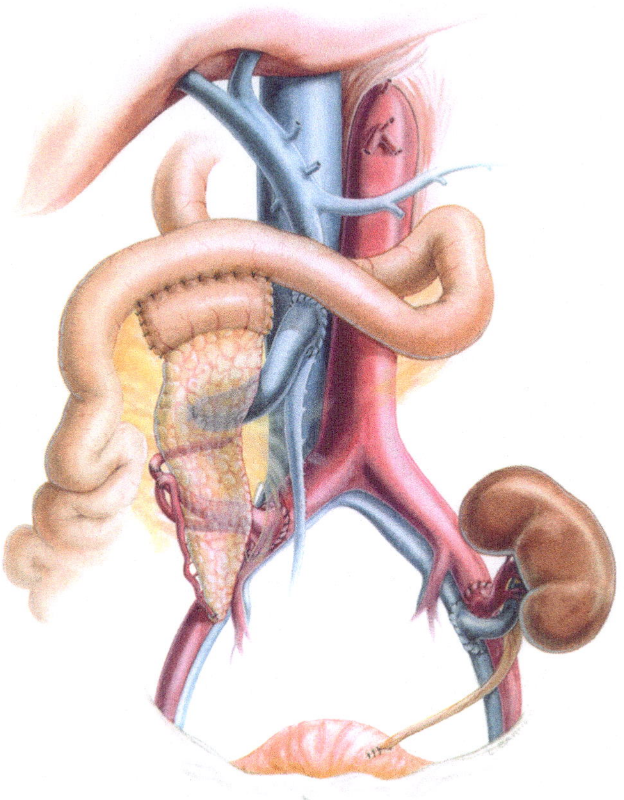

Fig. 11.4 Simultaneous pancreas and kidney transplant with portal venous drainage and enteric drainage of the exocrine pancreas

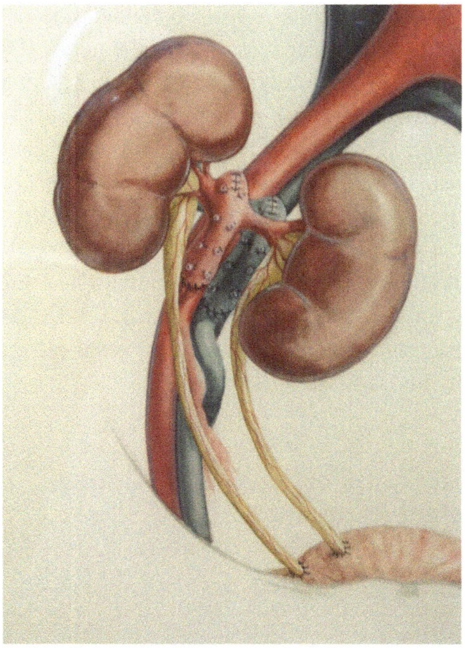

Fig. 11.5 Pediatric en bloc kidney transplant

the donor duodenum is compromised. In these situations, the surgeon may feel that the patient would be at increased risk for an enteric leak. However, enteric drainage of the pancreas has been shown to be safe and effective in many centers, and the need to convert 24 % of patients from bladder to enteric drainage in a subsequent operation is avoided [29–31]. Once the pancreas is implanted, the kidney is placed in the left lower quadrant within the peritoneum or retroperitoneally by dissecting the peritoneum off the anterior abdominal wall in the left lower quadrant to expose the iliac vessels on the left. We prefer to put the kidney in the retroperitoneum for two reasons: (a) the kidney is held in place by the peritoneum and cannot undergo torsion on its vascular pedicle, and (b) the pancreas and the kidney are in separate compartments should there be a peripancreatic infection or fluid collection.

The most common renal transplants are done with a single renal artery being implanted on the common external or common iliac artery. However, the occurrence of two or more renal arteries is common. When using a cadaver kidney, the two arteries can be anastomosed to the iliac artery using a common patch of aorta. When a living donor has multiple renal arteries, the arteries may be implanted using two separate arteriotomy sites. At times, one or both of the arteries may be too short for the anastomosis to be constructed or the caliber of the vessel too small to create an anastomosis. In these cases, a piece of donor gonadal vein or recipient saphenous vein can be used to lengthen the artery or create a larger caliber conduit for construction of an anastomosis. We advocate using a vein conduit routinely when an artery is less than 3 mm in diameter. Alternatively, an end-to-side anastomosis can be created between the smaller artery and the main renal artery, or two arteries can be opened longitudinally and sutured together to make a common orifice for anastomosis with the iliac artery [32]. The presence of multiple renal arteries and the method used to implant them are important to know when ordering postoperative sonograms to evaluate the kidney. The sonographer must know not to end the exam after seeing only one artery. The exam can also confirm flow within the cortex supplied by the different arteries in order to help confirm flow in all implanted vessels. The presence of a small inferior polar renal artery is particularly important since in many cases this vessel provides arterial flow to the ureter. Another special case is a pediatric donor. In the majority of cases, the kidneys can be split to provide single grafts to two separate recipients. However, below the age of 2 or 3 years or a weight of 12–15 kg, the kidneys can be transplanted en bloc or separately [33–38]. The decision to split pediatric donor kidneys is center and surgeon specific [39]. En bloc kidneys are transplanted as a pair and the aorta and vena cava are used as the vascular conduits. Technically, en bloc transplants require strict attention to detail when preparing the kidneys on the back table. The anastomoses of the donor aorta and vena cava to the iliac vessel result in the kidneys lying on either side of the iliac vessels within the retroperitoneum of the pelvis (Fig. 11.5). Care must be taken to ensure that the kidneys do not twist on their respective vascular pedicle, which would result in thrombosis to prevent torsion, and sutures are placed between perinephric tissue and tissues in the retroperitoneum to accomplish nephropex. Attention to the position of the kidneys as the peritoneum is released and allowed to come back laterally over the kidneys is essential. The presence of a pediatric en bloc graft is another important detail to know when ordering and viewing transplant renal ultrasounds in these patients.

Surgical Complications in the Kidney Transplant Recipient

Hemorrhage

Aside from a problem with the patient's airway, the presence of occult bleeding is the most pressing development in the immediate postoperative period following renal transplantation and requires prompt attention by the surgical team caring for the patient. Since the renal allograft may be unable to make urine or unable to concentrate urine, the patient's urine output may not be a good indicator of volume status. Decreasing trends in central venous pressure, hypotension, and tachycardia should prompt an aggressive workup to rule out bleeding as a cause. Hemoglobin levels should be checked, physical exam performed to rule out a palpable hematoma in the area of the graft, and an ultrasound performed to look for perinephric fluid and blood. The patient's EKG should be repeated and cardiac enzymes sent in order to rule out myocardial infarction as a cause of hypotension. If hypovolemia, hypotension, and tachycardia coexist, the patient should be aggressively resuscitated with crystalloid and packed red cells and returned emergently to the operating room. Bleeding that results in hypovolemic shock can result from the rupture of the arterial anastomosis, the loosening of a tie placed on the end of a divided vessel, or the rupture of the kidney from severe acute tubular necrosis. All of these situations require surgical reexploration. The majority of bleeding episodes following renal transplantation does not result in development of hemorrhagic shock, but presents with a modest decrease in hemoglobin accompanied by patient discomfort and a palpable fullness over the graft consistent with a hematoma. Postoperative transplant hematoma should be evacuated and the wound irrigated in the operating room. The hematoma can become secondarily infected and impair function of the allograft by compressing the renal vein, resulting in outflow resistance and increasing vascular congestion. Delay should be avoided because venous congestion can ultimately result in thrombosis of the transplanted kidney.

Wound complications can become a significant problem in the transplant patient. Careful handling of tissues to prevent necrotic debris in the wound along with irrigation of the wound to remove all blood and clots and to dilute any microorganisms from the skin is essential. Our preference is for closure of the fascia with interrupted monofilament suture. The subcutaneous tissue is re-approximated to close the dead space and the skin is closed with a running monofilament subcuticular suture. This helps prevent serous drainage from the wound and in our center has helped reduce wound separation and superficial wound infection rates.

When wound complications develop, the length of time required for wound closure is prolonged because of steroids and immunosuppressants. Multiple studies have shown that obesity is the most significant risk factor for wound complications [1, 40]. The effects of various immunosuppressants on wound healing have also been studied and the results are mixed. Some studies show increased complications with the use of rapamycin and mycophenolate mofetil, while others show no difference [1, 40, 41]. If a wound discharge is discovered, the fluid is sent for measurement of creatinine, culture, and Gram stain. Elevated creatinine is indicative of a urine leak, which is covered below. An ultrasound or CT scan can also be performed to ascertain whether the fluid is coming from a subcutaneous collection or a subfascial location. If the amount of fluid is substantial, soaking multiple dressings per day, then the patient is taken to the operating room for exploration of the wound and reclosure. The fascia is left intact unless the fluid is coming through a defect in the fascia itself. All attempts are made to close the wound unless a significant purulent infection is found in the subcutaneous or subfascial space in which case the skin is left open and the wound packed with moist gauze. Subfascial closed suction drainage should also be considered.

Ureteral Complications

The measurement of an elevated creatinine in the fluid from a transplant wound is diagnostic of a urine leak. If the diagnosis is in question, a radionuclide scan can be performed to confirm the diagnosis. Historically, the incidence of ureteral complications following renal transplantation ranges from 0.9 to 30 %. The current rate of ureteral complications is approximately 10 % [42–44]. These complications include urinary leak and urinary obstruction. In the immediate transplant period, urinary leak is the most common urologic complication, and the patient should be returned to the operating room for revision of the neoureterocystostomy. If a urine leak presents several weeks after a transplant, the patient should be evaluated with cystoscopy and or percutaneous nephrostomy. These procedures will define the problem by demonstrating any stenoses that can accompany a urine leak. A ureteral stent can also be placed, which will help locate the ureter intraoperatively. Urine leak following renal transplantation is usually secondary to ischemic necrosis of the ureter. Drainage of the kidney once the ureter has necrosed can be accomplished by mobilizing the bladder so that it can reach the healthy ureter (psoas hitch), using the native ureter as a conduit to the bladder and, though rare, creating a tube from a flap of bladder to create a conduit to the bladder (Boari flap). Biopsy of the renal allograft can be required at any time following renal transplantation and should be performed as part of any subsequent operative procedures. The most common reason for renal biopsy in the immediate transplant period is delayed graft function as defined by the need for hemodialysis. Delayed graft function can be secondary to a technical problem with the graft, acute tubular necrosis, or acute cellular or humoral rejection. Patients with poor urine output and the need for continued hemodialysis should be evaluated with sonography as stated before and should also undergo biopsy of the renal allograft between 7 and 10 days postoperatively to rule out rejection as a cause of poor graft function. If rejection is found on biopsy, the patient should be treated with steroids or thymocyte-depleting medications. In the majority of cases, percutaneous renal allograft biopsy under ultrasound guidance with a small caliber spring-loaded biopsy needle is a benign procedure. However, in a minority of patients, the procedure can be complicated by the development of a perinephric hematoma, arteriovenous fistula, or bleeding into the peritoneal cavity if the biopsy needle violates the peritoneum during the biopsy procedure. Any of these occurrences can require immediate attention. Patients who develop symptoms of hypovolemia, abdominal pain, or graft bruit or mass following renal transplant biopsy need to be evaluated with transplant ultrasound and admitted to the hospital. Serial measurement of hemoglobin and hematocrit should also be carried out. The majority of bleeding following renal transplant biopsy stops spontaneously. Some patients do require transfusion to maintain adequate hemoglobin concentrations. In limited instances, the patient with a post-biopsy bleed requires exploration for suture closure of the biopsy site in the renal capsule. The presence of intraperitoneal blood should heighten the concern of the clinician. When intraperitoneal bleeding occurs, the peritoneum has been violated and the peritransplant capsule is not intact to tamponade the bleeding. However, these cases can be handled by laparoscopic exploration and suture closure of the peritoneal defect in many instances. The presence of an arterial venous fistula on renal ultrasound should prompt evaluation of the renal graft by arteriography. These fistulas are best treated by embolization by an experienced interventional radiologist [45].

Lymphocele can develop in up to 20 % of patients in the first several weeks to months following transplantation [46]. Many of these fluid collections are small, do not cause any physical symptoms to the patient or compromise renal function, and do not require treatment. Lymphoceles develop from failure of the peri-iliac lymphatics to close following exposure of the iliac vessels during the transplant procedure. The development of lymphoceles is contributed to by the retardation of wound healing caused by immunosuppressive drugs. The use of sirolimus in the peritransplant immunosuppressive regimen has been found to increase the incidence of lymphocele to 38 % [47]. Lymphoceles causing pain and swelling over the graft or compromising renal function must be treated. Rarely, lymphocele can present as an acute abdomen [48]. The diagnosis is made with ultrasound and analysis of fluid aspirate. Attempts at percutaneous aspiration will eliminate some lymph collections permanently and can be combined with sclerotherapy [46]. Lymphoceles that do not respond to percutaneous drainage or percutaneous catheter drainage require open or laparoscopic transabdominal fenestration [46, 49]. Fenestration of the lymphocele requires widely opening a window between the peritoneum and the lymphocele cavity. In this way, any fluid produced in the cavity is absorbed by the peritoneal surface. With time, the entire cavity becomes lined by the peritoneum. Open fenestration should be employed over the laparoscopic technique when the lymphocele is accompanied by a significant wound infection or if the lymphocele is small and close to hilar structures which could be injured during a laparoscopic approach [49]. The recurrence of lymphocele following fenestration is less than 10 % [46, 49].

Acute Illness in the Transplant Patient

A common problem facing the physician treating patients with solid organ transplants is when they present to the emergency department with an acute illness. Complaints can include fever, abdominal pain, nausea, vomiting, diarrhea, upper respiratory tract infection, urinary tract infection, and gastrointestinal (GI) bleeding. This section will discuss the surgical problems associated with these complaints and when surgical consultation and intervention are required.

Febrile Illness

Patients with delayed graft function requiring several weeks of hemodialysis while the graft recovers are often discharged from the hospital with a tunneled hemodialysis catheter in place. These patients can present to the emergency department or the dialysis center with low-grade fever. Fever in a patient several weeks post-op from a renal transplant should prompt a complete workup to include CBC, blood culture and fungal culture both peripherally and through the catheter, cytomegalovirus (CMV) antigen, urinalysis, and urine culture. The patient should be queried about his or her daily urine output and predialysis. Creatinine should be measured to see if the graft has recovered function. When a tunneled hemodialysis catheter is present in a patient with fever, the catheter should be removed immediately unless another clear source of infection is present. Although some reports advocate antibiotic treatment in order to sterilize an infected line, the immunosuppressed patient should not be treated in this fashion [50]. The immunosuppressed patient can harbor occult line sepsis that can quickly progress to septic shock, systemic inflammatory response syndrome, and multiple organ dysfunction. If the patient reports improving graft function, then hemodialysis may no longer be required. If hemodialysis is needed, a temporary hemodialysis catheter can be placed contralateral to the kidney or in the neck.

Abdominal Pain

Transplant patients also present in the emergency department with complaints of abdominal pain and symptoms of gastroenteritis. The patient who presents in this manner is concerning because even when the patient appears to be doing fairly well clinically, the immunosuppressants can mask a significant pathologic process. The differential diagnosis can include toxicity from mycophenolate mofetil, viral gastroenteritis, CMV infection, diverticulitis, appendicitis, cholecystitis, peptic ulcer disease, posttransplant lymphoproliferative disease (PTLD), and rejection [6, 51–72]. In addition to a complete history and physical examination, the patient should be evaluated with routine laboratory studies, CMV antigen, blood and urine culture, stool culture (check for ova and parasites), and a computed tomography of the abdomen with oral contrast should be performed. The patient should be admitted to the hospital, and empiric broad-spectrum antibiotic and antiviral treatment considered. Patients with findings of free air should be taken to the operating room for repair of a ruptured viscus. Causes of free air in the transplant patient include infectious colitis, perforated peptic ulcer, infectious enteritis, and lymphoproliferative disease [51–54]. Perforated ulcer should be treated with resection or repair using omental patch. Proton pump inhibitors and anti *H. pylori* treatment have significantly reduced the need for performing vagotomy. Gastric ulcers should be biopsied, and culture for *Helicobacter pylori* should be taken in all cases of peptic ulcer disease. The patient should be treated with intravenous proton pump inhibitors and antibiotic therapy for *Helicobacter pylori* begun [57–59]. Perforated areas of bowel should be resected with primary anastomosis in the small bowel and ascending colon performed. Perforation of the descending colon should be treated with resection and diverting colostomy. If PTLD is suspected, frozen section should be performed. Postoperatively, immunosuppression should be reduced to allow the immune system to clear infection and sepsis. In most cases of PTLD, immunosuppression should be eliminated. Stress dose steroids should be given if the patient had been taking steroids as part of the immunosuppressive regimen. Colorectal carcinoma should be treated according to standard protocols [60]. Specimens should be routinely sent for bacterial, mycobacterial, and fungal culture in addition to standard pathologic evaluation. Histology should include staining for CMV infection.

Transplant patients can develop symptomatic diverticulitis, as can their nonimmunosuppressed counterparts, since 30–50 % of patients over age 50 have diverticula [61]. Patients with acute diverticulitis classically present with left lower quadrant pain and tenderness along with fever. This constellation of symptoms has earned diverticulitis the nickname of left-sided appendicitis. Although standard of care for acute uncomplicated diverticulitis is for sigmoid resection only in patients with complications, we advocate elective resection following the initial episode in the immunosuppressed patient as patients who have received organ transplants are at higher risk for perforation and abscess formation. The clinical presentation of these patients is further complicated by the often indolent, smoldering nature of acute episodes of diverticulitis and the lack of usual signs of the disease such as fever and elevated white blood cell count [62, 63]. These patients can have more fulminant courses than normal patients, and their second episode could be life threatening or result in loss of the allograft.

GI Hemorrhage

GI bleeding presents in the transplant recipient as well [56, 64–68]. In general, the treatment of the transplant patient with GI bleeding is no different from that of a nonimmunosuppressed patient. The patient should first be evaluated for hemodynamic stability and the need for immediate resuscitation with crystalloid or packed red blood cells. The patient's upper GI tract should be ruled out as a source by placing a nasogastric tube and lavage with a liter of water. Confirmed upper GI bleeds should be evaluated by upper endoscopy, which can also provide treatment. A negative nasogastric lavage can safely rule out a bleeding source proximal to the ligament of Treitz in most instances. Lower GI bleeding can be secondary to diverticula, mesenteric ischemia, arterial venous malformations, colorectal carcinoma, Kaposi's sarcoma, or infectious colitis, which is more common in the transplant population [64, 66, 68–71]. The pancreas transplant population is also subject to bleeding from the duodenal cuff of the allograft [72, 73]. Bleeding from this site can be extremely vexing to the clinician who does not consider the enterically drained pancreas as a possible source of lower GI bleeding. Patients with lower GI bleeding should be resuscitated with crystalloid and blood until stable. The majority of lower GI bleeds resolve spontaneously. Lower GI bleeds should be evaluated with a radionuclide scan [74]. If this test is positive, an arteriogram should be performed. In the patient with an enterically drained pancreas, the arteriogram should include injection of the arterial supply, to the pancreas, which arises in most cases from the right common or external iliac artery. Profuse bleeding from the allograft duodenal segment can be treated with coil embolization in the unstable patient or the patient with a blood transfusion requirement high enough to mandate surgical resection. When the inferior pancreaticoduodenal artery of the allograft is embolized, the patient will require exploration and resection of the transplant pancreatic head and duodenum and possibly the entire gland. A transplant surgeon should be included in this decision process if possible.

The transplant patient with abdominal pain both acute and chronic can be manifesting symptoms of mesenteric ischemia. In some instances, these patients present with lower GI bleeding [75, 76]. If GI bleeding is massive, then the patient should be treated as above. The patient who has mild to moderate GI bleeding should undergo colonoscopy, which can be diagnostic and therapeutic depending on the source of the bleeding. Patients found to have ischemia or colitis on colonoscopy would have immediate surgical evaluation. In some instances, aggressive surgical therapy is lifesaving. The watch and wait approach can be lethal in the immunosuppressed patient that may not manifest significant findings on physical exam.

Parathyroid Disease in the Kidney Transplant Recipient

Patients with ESRD develop secondary hyperparathyroidism due to chronic overstimulation of normal parathyroid glands. The pathophysiology does not involve an intrinsic defect in the parathyroid glands themselves. Patients with long standing secondary hyperparathyroidism can subsequently develop tertiary hyperparathyroidism due to autonomous hypersecretion by the parathyroid glands despite correction of the underlying etiology. Patients who undergo renal transplantation after several years of hemodialysis will have tertiary hyperparathyroidism in up to 2.5 % of cases [77]. Secondary hyperparathyroidism develops as the levels of 1,25-vitamin D3 produced in the kidney fall, and gut absorption of calcium is impaired. As renal failure progresses, hyperphosphatemia develops, stimulating increased parathyroid hormone (PTH) secretion by decreasing ionized calcium levels and by a phosphorous-dependent direct stimulation of PTH secretion in the parathyroid gland. Secondary hyperparathyroidism is treated with oral calcium supplementation, phosphate binders, and vitamin D supplementation. In renal transplant recipients, 30 % will have persistent hypercalcemia following transplantation. Less than 5 % of these recipients of renal transplants will develop tertiary hyperparathyroidism requiring surgical intervention [78]. A study of 4,344 transplant recipients found that 38 patients had persistent hypercalcemia defined as a serum calcium level greater than 12.0 mg/dL persisting for more than 1 year posttransplant, acute hypercalcemia (greater than 125 mg/dL) in the immediate transplant period, or symptomatic hypercalcemia [79]. Symptoms of hypercalcemia include bone and joint pain, pathologic fractures, generalized weakness, severe pruritus, neuropsychiatric problems, and GI complaints. Patients fitting the above criteria should undergo subtotal parathyroidectomy or total parathyroidectomy, with intraoperative serum PTH determination to ensure removal of all glands, followed by autografting of parathyroid tissue in the forearm or neck [80, 81]. The recurrence of hyperparathyroidism following autografting is 5–10 % [82].

References

1. Flechner SM, Zhou L, Derweesh I, et al. The impact of sirolimus, mycophenolate mofetil, cyclosporine, azathioprine, and steroids on wound healing in 513 kidney-transplant recipients. Transplantation. 2003;76:1729–34.
2. Greenstein SM, Katz S, Sun S, et al. Prevalence of asymptomatic cholelithiasis and risk of acute cholecystitis after kidney transplantation. Transplantation. 1997;63:1030–2.
3. Girardet RE, Rosenbloom P, DeWeese BM, et al. Significance of asymptomatic biliary tract disease in heart transplant recipients. J Heart Transplant. 1989;8:391–9.
4. Steck TB, Constanzo-Nordin MR, Keshavarzian A. Prevalence and management of cholelithiasis in heart transplant patients. J Heart Lung Transplant. 1991;10:1029–32.
5. Graham SM, Flowers JL, Schweitzer E, Bartlett ST. The utility of prophylactic laparoscopic cholecystectomy in transplant candidates. Am J Surg. 1995;169:44–9.
6. Colon R, Frazier OH, Kahan BD, et al. Complications in cardiac transplant patients requiring general surgery. Surgery. 1988;103:32–8.
7. Merrell SW, Ames SA, Nelson EW, et al. Major abdominal complications following cardiac transplantation. Arch Surg. 1989;124:889–94.
8. Villar HV, Neal DD, Levinson M, et al. Gastrointestinal complications after human transplantation and mechanical heart replacement. Am J Surg. 1989;157:168–74.
9. Sekela ME, Hutchins DA, Young JB, Noon GP. Biliary surgery after cardiac transplantation. Arch Surg. 1991;126:571–3.
10. Lowell JA, Stratta RJ, Taylor RJ, et al. Cholelithiasis in the pancreas and kidney recipients with diabetes. Surgery. 1993;114:858–63.
11. Ramdev P, Rayan SS, Sheahan M, et al. A decade experience with infrainguinal revascularization in dialysis-dependent patient population. J Vasc Surg. 2002;36:969–74.
12. Albers M, Romiti M, Bragança Pereira CA, et al. A meta-analysis of infrainguinal reconstruction in patients with end-stage renal disease. Eur J Vasc Endovasc Surg. 2001;22(4):294–300.

13. Johnson BL, Glickman MH, Bandyk DF. Failure of foot salvage in patients with end-stage renal disease after surgical revascularization. J Vasc Surg. 1995;22:280–6.
14. Sanchez LA, Goldsmith J, Rivers SP, et al. Limb salvage in end-stage renal disease: is it worthwhile? J Cardiovasc Surg. 1992;33:344–8.
15. Sidhu RS, Lindsay TF, Rubin B, et al. Aortic and iliac reconstruction after kidney transplantation: experience with an algorithm for renal protection. Ann Vasc Surg. 2003;17:165–70.
16. Gallagher KA, Ravin RA, Schweitzer E, et al. Outcomes and timing of aortic surgery in renal transplant patients. Ann Vasc Surg. 2011;25(4):448–53.
17. Seliger SL, Gillen DL, Laongstreth WT, et al. Elevated risk of stroke among patients with end-stage renal disease. Kidney Int. 2003;64:603–9.
18. Hojs R, Hojs-Fabjan T, Balon BP. Atherosclerosis in patients with end-stage renal failure prior to initiation of hemodialysis. Ren Fail. 2003;25:247–54.
19. Barnett HJM, Taylor W, Eliasziw M, et al. Benefit of carotid endarterectomy in patients with symptomatic moderate or severe stenosis. N Engl J Med. 1998;339:1415–25.
20. Executive Committee for the Asymptomatic Carotid Atherosclerosis Study. Endarterectomy for asymptomatic carotid artery stenosis. JAMA. 1995;273:1421–8.
21. Brott TG, Hobson II RW, Howard G, et al. Stenting versus endarterectomy for treatment of carotid artery stenosis. N Engl J Med. 2010;363:11–23.
22. Glassman DT, Nipkow L, Bartlett ST, Jacobs SC. Bilateral nephrectomy with concomitant renal graft transplantation for autosomal dominant polycystic kidney disease. J Urol. 2000;164:661–4.
23. Weir MR, Salzberg DJ. Management of hypertension in the transplant patient. J Am Soc Hypertens. 2011;5:425–32.
24. Herrmann SM, Textor SC. Diagnostic criteria for renovascular disease: where are we now? Nephrol Dial Transplant. 2012;27(7): 2657–73.
25. Cherr GS, Hansen KJ, Craven TE, et al. Surgical management of atherosclerotic renovascular disease. J Vasc Surg. 2002;35: 236–45.
26. Ritchie J, Green D, Kalra PA. Current views on the management of atherosclerotic renovascular disease. Ann Med. 2012;44(1): 98–110.
27. Shapiro R. The transplant procedure. In: Shapiro R, Simmons RL, Starzl TE, editors. Renal transplantation. Stamford, CT: Appleton & Lange; 1997. p. 103–40.
28. Philosophe B, Farney AC, Schweitzer EJ, et al. Superiority of portal venous drainage over systemic venous drainage in pancreas transplantation. Ann Surg. 2001;234:689–96.
29. Kuo PC, Johnson LB, Schweitzer EJ, et al. Simultaneous pancreas/kidney transplantation-a comparison of enteric and bladder drainage of exocrine pancreatic secretions. Transplantation. 1997;63: 238–43.
30. Gaber AO, Shokouh-Amiri MH, Hathaway DK, et al. Results of pancreas transplantation with portal venous and enteric drainage. Ann Surg. 1995;221:613–24.
31. Sollinger HW, Odorico JS, Knechtle SJ, et al. Experience with 500 simultaneous pancreas-kidney transplants. Ann Surg. 1998;228:284–96.
32. Kuo PC, Cho ES, Flowers JL, et al. Laparoscopic living donor nephrectomy and multiple renal arteries. Am J Surg. 1998;176: 559–63.
33. Jordan ML, Shapiro R, Sundberg R, et al. Transplantation of pediatric en bloc kidneys under FK506 immunosuppression. Transplant Proc. 1991;23:3089–90.
34. Ngheim D. En bloc transplantation of kidneys from donors weighing less than 15 kg into adult recipients. J Urol. 1991;145:14–6.
35. Kinne DW, Spanos PK, DeShazo MM, et al. Double renal transplant from pediatric donors to adult recipients. Am J Surg. 1974;127:292–5.
36. Lindstrom BL, Ahonen J. The use of both kidneys obtained from pediatric donors as en bloc transplant to adult recipients. Scand J Urol Nephrol. 1975;29:71.
37. Dreikhorn J, Rohl L, Horsch R. The use of double renal transplant from pediatric cadaver donor. Br J Urol. 1977;49:361.
38. Schneider JR, Sutherland DE, Simmons RL, Fryd DS, Najarian JS. Long-term success with double pediatric cadaver donor renal transplant. Ann Surg. 1983;197:439–42.
39. Balachandran VP, Aull MJ, Goris M. Successful transplantation of single kidneys from pediatric donors weighing less than or equal to 10 kg into standard weight adult recipients. Transplantation. 2010;90(5):518–22.
40. Johnson DW, Isbel NM, Brown AM, et al. The effect of obesity on renal transplant outcomes. Transplantation. 2002;74:675–81.
41. Troppmann C, Pierce JL, Gandhi MM, et al. Higher wound complication rates with sirolimus immunosuppression after kidney transplantation: a matched-pair pilot study. Transplantation. 2003; 76:426–9.
42. Thomolla JV, Lingeman IE, Leapman SB, Filo RS. The manifestation and management of urological complications in renal transplant recipients. Use of the urological armamentarium. J Urol. 1985;134:944.
43. Kayler L, Kang D, Molmeti E, et al. Kidney transplant ureteroneocystostomy techniques and complications: review of the literature. Transplant Proc. 2010;42(5):1413–20.
44. Streeter EH, Little DM, Cranston DW, Morris PJ. The urologic complications of renal transplantation: a series of 1535 patients. BJU Int. 2002;90:627–34.
45. Ettore GC, Francioso G, Francavilla I, et al. Renal arteriovenous fistulas after renal biopsy. Percutaneous embolization. Radiol Med. 2000;100:357–62.
46. Doehn C, Fornara P, Fricke L, Jocham D. Laparoscopic fenestration of post transplant lymphoceles. Surg Endosc. 2002;16:690–5.
47. Langer RM, Kahan BD. Incidence, therapy, and consequences of lymphocele after sirolimus-cyclosporine-prednisone immunosuppression in renal transplant recipients. Transplantation. 2002; 74:804–8.
48. Indudhara R, Menon M, Khauli RB. Posttransplant lymphocele presenting as "acute abdomen". Am J Nephrol. 1994;14:154–6.
49. Fuller TF, Kang SM, Hirose R, et al. Management of lymphoceles after renal transplantation: laparoscopic versus open drainage. J Urol. 2003;169:2022–5.
50. Mermal LA, Farr BM, Sherertz RJ, et al. Guidelines for the management of intravascular catheter-related infections. J Intraven Nurs. 2001;24:180–205.
51. Fan CW, Chen JS, Wang JY, Fan HA. Perforated rectal lymphoma in a renal transplant recipient: report of a case. Dis Colon Rectum. 1997;40:1258–60.
52. Scott-Conner CE, Fabrega AJ. Gastrointestinal problems in the immunocompromised host—a review for surgeons. Surg Endosc. 1996;1:959–64.
53. Ahsan N, Blanchard RL, Mai ML. Gastrointestinal tuberculosis in renal transplantation: a case report and review. Clin Transplant. 1995;9:349–52.
54. Soravia C, Baldi A, Kartheuser A, et al. Acute colonic complications after kidney transplantation. Acta Chir Belg. 1995;95: 157–61.
55. Feduska NJ, Amend WJ, Vincenti F, et al. Peptic ulcer disease in kidney and transplant recipients. Am J Surg. 1984;148:51–7.
56. Stuart FP, Reckerd CR, Schulak JA, Ketel BL. Gastroduodenal complications in kidney transplant recipients. Ann Surg. 1981;194:339–44.
57. Logan RPH, Hirschi AM. Epidemiology of *Helicobacter pylori* infection. Curr Opin Gastroenterol. 1996;12:1–5.
58. *Helicobacter pylori* in peptic ulcer disease. NIH Consensus Development panel on Helicobacter pylori in peptic ulcer disease. JAMA. 1994;272:65–9.

59. Peek RM, Blaser MJ. Pathophysiology of *Helicobacter pylori* induced gastritis and peptic ulcer disease. Am J Med. 1997;102: 200–7.
60. Saidi RF, Dudrick PS, Goldman MH. Colorectal cancer after renal transplantation. Transplant Proc. 2003;35:1410–2.
61. Huges LE. Postmortem survey of diverticular disease of the colon. Gut. 1969;10:336.
62. Seth AA, Longo W, Floch MH. Diverticular disease and diverticulitis. Am J Gastroenterol. 2008;103(6):1550–6.
63. Ferzoco LB, Raptopoulos V, Silen W. Acute diverticulitis. N Engl J Med. 1998;338:1521.
64. Stylianos S, Forde KA, Benvenisty AI, Hardy MA. Lower gastrointestinal hemorrhage in the renal transplant recipient. Arch Surg. 1988;123:739–44.
65. McClellan SL, Komorowski RA, Farmer SG, et al. Severe bleeding diathesis associated with invasive aspergillosis in transplant patients. Transplantation. 1985;39:406–10.
66. Sutherland DE, Chan FY, Fourcar E, et al. The bleeding cecal ulcer in transplant patients. Surgery. 1979;86:386–98.
67. Matsumoto C, Swanson SJ, Agodoa LY, et al. Hospitalized gastrointestinal bleeding and procedures after renal transplantation in the United States. J Nephrol. 2003;16:49–56.
68. Carlton PK, Whelchel JD. Massive colonic diverticular hemorrhage in a transplant patient. Am Surg. 1978;44:159–61.
69. Escudero-Fabre A, Cummings O, Kirklin JK, et al. Cytomegalovirus colitis presenting a hematochezia and requiring resection. Arch Surg. 1992;127:102–4.
70. Calzona A, Naso P, Puliatti C, et al. Massive gastrointestinal hemorrhage in a renal transplant recipient due to visceral Kaposi's sarcoma. Endoscopy. 2002;34:179.
71. Stock KJ, Scott MA, Davis SF, et al. Hemorrhagic colitis due to a novel *Escherichia coli* serotype (0121:H19) in a transplant patient. Transpl Int. 2001;14:44–7.
72. McBeth BD, Stem SA. Lower gastrointestinal hemorrhage from an arterioenteric fistula in a pancreatorenal transplant recipient. Ann Emerg Med. 2003;42:587–91.
73. Barone GW, Webb JW, Hudec WA. The enteric drained pancreas transplant: another potential source of gastrointestinal bleeding. Am J Gastraenterol. 1998;93:1369–71.
74. Bingener-Casey J, Esterl RM, Kenneth Washburn W, et al. Tc-99m-labeled red blood cell scanning localizes hemorrhage between the distal ileum and duodenal stump of an enteric-drained pancreas transplant. Clin Nucl Med. 2002;27:205–6.
75. Hellstrom PM, Rubio C, Odar-Cederlof I, Slezak P. Ischemic colitis of the cecum after renal transplantation masquerading as malignant disease. Dig Dis Sci. 1991;36:1644–8.
76. Margolis DM, Etheredge EE, Garza-Garza R, et al. Ischemic bowel disease following nephrectomy or renal transplant. Surgery. 1977; 82:667–73.
77. Decker PA, Cohen EP, Dffek KM, et al. Subtotal parathyroidectomy in renal failure: still needed after all these years. World J Surg. 2001;25:708–12.
78. Gioviale MC, Bellavia M, Damiano G, et al. Post-transplantation tertiary hyperparathyroidism. Ann Transplant. 2012;17(3):111–9.
79. Kerby JD, Rue LW, Blair H, et al. Operative treatment of tertiary hyperparathyroidism: a single center experience. Ann Surg. 1998;227:878–86.
80. Diethelm AG, Adams PL, Murad TM, et al. Treatment of secondary hyperparathyroidism in patients with chronic renal failure by total parathyroidectomy and parathyroid autograft. Ann Surg. 1981;193: 777–93.
81. Clary BM, Garner SC, Leight GS. Intraoperative parathyroid hormone monitoring during parathyroidectomy for secondary hyperparathyroidism. Surgery. 1997;122:1034.
82. Moffett JM, Suliburk J. Parathyroid autotransplantation. Endocr Pract. 2011;17(1):83–9.

Mechanisms of Immunosuppressive Drugs

12

Adam Weltz, Joseph Scalea, Mihaela Popescu, Jiangnan Xu, and Jonathan S. Bromberg

Glucocorticoids

Corticosteroids (CS) are the products of the adrenal cortex which have broad immunosuppressive and anti-inflammatory effects and were one of the first classes of immunosuppressive drugs developed [1]. Glucocorticoids (GC) represent both natural and synthetic steroids that activate gluconeogenesis including prednisone and methylprednisolone, and they have widely been used as part of the immunosuppressive regimen to suppress transplant organ rejection. However, GC also have various adverse effects on cardiovascular diseases, bone metabolism, and increased risk of infection [2, 3]; thus, despite their effectiveness in preventing acute rejection, starting in the late 1990s, GC doses have often been reduced, withdrawn, or discontinued in many induction and maintenance transplant immunosuppression protocols [4].

Structure and Immunosuppressive Mechanisms: Unbound GC enter cells through passive diffusion, and corticosteroid-binding globulin (CBG)-bound GC can also enter cells via receptor-mediated transport or endocytosis [1, 5–7]. In the cytosol, GC bind to glucocorticoid receptors (GR); the activated receptor dimer then translocates into the nucleus, binds to glucocorticoid response elements (GRE) of various genes, and transactivates their expression [1, 6]. The activated receptor also interacts with specific transcription factors (such as AP-1 and NF-κB) and prevents the transcription of proinflammatory genes including cytokines, chemokines, cell adhesion molecules, and complement factors [6, 8]. GC anti-inflammatory properties also include suppression of prostaglandin synthesis, stabilization of lysosomal membranes, reduction of histamine and bradykinin release, suppression of dendritic cell (DC) antigen presentation, and suppression of CD4 T cell proliferation, trafficking, and activation [9–12].

Metabolism and Side Effects: Prednisone is the most widely used GC and is metabolized in the liver, primarily to its major active metabolite, prednisolone, and they are associated with many adverse effects. Due to their abilities to suppress both adaptive and innate immunity, GC are associated with an increased risk of infections including hepatitis C virus (HCV) infection [13], cytomegalovirus (CMV) infection, and HCV recurrence [14–18]. GC also diminish wound healing by inhibiting circulating monocytes, the influx of macrophages, growth factor and cytokine production, phagocytosis, fibroblast responses, capillary proliferation, and collagen synthesis [19–23].

GC have many other adverse effects related to their primary activity of inducing multiple processes related to gluconeogenesis (Table 12.1), particularly in patients receiving these drugs in high doses or over a long period of time. Systemic (oral and parenteral) GC treatment may lead to adrenal insufficiency, avascular necrosis, cushingoid changes, cataracts, decrease in bone density, dermal thinning, ecchymosis, fluid retention, glaucoma, hyperglycemia, hypertension, skin fragility, violaceous dermal striae, and secondary cardiovascular complications including myocardial infarction and cerebrovascular disease [12]. There remains uncertainty regarding the relative safety of low-dose GC use (<10 mg/day of prednisone or equivalent). Several studies have shown that long-term GC use, even in low doses, remains a significant risk for serious adverse effects [24, 25], while other analyses show little documented toxicity from very low-dose GC use [26].

Use for Immunosuppressive Therapy in Kidney Transplantation: Large doses of GC are used in many transplant

A. Weltz • J. Scalea • M. Popescu • J. Xu
Department of Surgery, University of Maryland School of Medicine, Baltimore, MD, USA

J.S. Bromberg, M.D., Ph.D. (✉)
Division of Transplantation, Department of Surgery, University of Maryland School of Medicine, 29 South Greene Street, Suite 200, Baltimore, MD 21201, USA
e-mail: jbromberg@smail.umaryland.edu

M.R. Weir and E.V. Lerma (eds.), *Kidney Transplantation: Practical Guide to Management*, DOI 10.1007/978-1-4939-0342-9_12, © Springer Science+Business Media New York 2014

Table 12.1 Characteristics of available biological immunosuppressive drugs used in kidney transplantation

Drug	Description	Mechanism of action	Use in induction	Use in rejection	Use in maintenance	Adverse effects
Polyclonal antithymocyte globulin [rabbit] (Thymoglobulin®)	Polyclonal IgG from rabbits immunized with human thymocytes	Blocks various T cell, non-T cell, and MHC membrane proteins leading to prolonged depletion	X	X		Cytokine release syndrome, thrombocytopenia, leukopenia, reactivation and development of viral disease
Alemtuzumab (Campath®)	Humanized monoclonal antibody against CD52	Binds to CD52 on B cells, T cells, macrophages, natural killer cells, and granulocytes and triggers antibody-dependent lysis	X			Neutropenia, thrombocytopenia, anemia, nausea, vomiting, diarrhea, headache, and dizziness
Basiliximab (Simulect®)	Chimeric monoclonal antibody against CD25	Binds to the alpha subunit of the IL-2 receptor on the surface of activated T cells and acts as a receptor antagonist	X			Headache, hypertension, peripheral edema
Belatacept (Nulojix®)	Fusion protein which binds to CD80 and CD86 receptors on APCs	Binds to CD80 and CD86, blocking CD28 interaction between APCs and T cells needed to activate T lymphocytes			X	Infusion reactions, peripheral edema, hyper- or hypotension, headache, electrolyte abnormalities, diarrhea, and abdominal pain

centers perioperatively and immediately postoperatively, consisting one intraoperative dose of 5–10 mg/kg of intravenous methylprednisolone, followed with a transition to 1 mg/kg/day of oral prednisone. This is subsequently reduced to physiological doses or approximately 5 mg/day of prednisone by 1 year or less.

To minimize toxicity and reduce overall immunosuppression, strategies aimed at minimizing or avoiding GC in kidney transplantation have been increasingly applied in the past decade [27–32]. More selective immunosuppressive agents and antibody induction therapy enabled the use of GC to be further minimized via several different strategies: very low-dose maintenance (reducing the prednisone dose to 20 mg/day on postoperative days 3–5 with tapering to 5 mg/day by 1 month or 2), complete withdrawal early after transplantation (several weeks to months) or at a later time (after 1 year), and complete avoidance. However, GC withdrawal following kidney transplantation still remains a controversial issue, and the general policy is to individualize therapy based on a careful assessment of the risk–benefit ratio, such as immunological risk of rejection (prior transplants, high PRA) and risk of side effects (recipients with obesity, diabetes, cardiovascular disease).

When acute cellular rejection (ACR) occurs, pulse methylprednisolone (3–5 mg/kg intravenously daily for 3–5 days) is the first-line therapy for management of active episodes, either alone or in combination with other immunosuppressive agents. After a steroid pulse, oral steroids are tapered rapidly to the same dosage the patient had been taking prior to the episode. The expected reversal rate for the first episode of ACR is approximately 60 % with steroid therapy [33]. If rejection resists steroid treatment, administration of antilymphocyte antibodies could be used as second-line therapy [34–36].

Antimetabolites

Antimetabolites function by inhibition of purine metabolism. Purine (adenine and guanine) synthesis may occur by de novo or salvage pathways. Whereas some cells have the ability to synthesize purines via both pathways, lymphocytes lack the salvage pathway. Thus, by blocking de novo purine synthesis, lymphocyte proliferation, expansion, and activation are inhibited or decreased.

Antimetabolites are used routinely in the management of organ transplant recipients. The rationale, discovery, and development of azathioprine in the 1950s led to the 1988 Nobel Prize in medicine for Gertrude Elion and George Hitchings.

Azathioprine

Mechanism of Action and Structure: Azathioprine was originally described as a therapy for childhood acute leukemia [37]. However, with the advent of kidney transplantation, early observations demonstrated the drug's ability to prolong renal allograft survival [38].

Azathioprine blocks de novo purine synthesis in addition to blocking co-stimulation of T cells. A structural analog of mercaptopurine, azathioprine is metabolized through multiple steps yielding biologically active metabolites. One of these metabolites, 6-thio-GTP inserts into T cell DNA and prevents DNA replication [39]. Metabolites of azathioprine have also been shown to inhibit Rac-1 activity by binding GTPases [37, 39, 40]. Rac1 inhibition then sets in motion a cascade culminating with mitochondrial-driven T cell apoptosis [39].

More recently, data have suggested that 6-thio-GTP may also inhibit CD28, an important co-stimulation signaling mediator required for T cell activation [37].

Dosage: Azathioprine is typically given orally at 3–5 mg/kg/day immediately following transplantation. With time dosing may be decreased to 1–3 mg/kg/day. The agent is given as a once- or twice-per-day oral pill. In some cases, azathioprine may be given prior to transplantation.

Mycophenolate Mofetil

Mechanism of Action and Structure: Like azathioprine, mycophenolate mofetil also acts as a purine metabolism inhibitor. The agent is a prodrug which is rapidly broken down to mycophenolic acid which subsequently inhibits inosine monophosphate dehydrogenase (IMPDH). IMPDH is the first of two enzymes required for metabolism of inosine monophosphate to guanine monophosphate in the pathway of de novo purine synthesis. Thus, the result of adding mycophenolic acid to lymphocyte populations is inhibition of DNA replication via decreased availability of nucleotides [41, 42].

Dosage: CellCept is available in oral and IV forms. The oral forms are typically given twice daily and are available as 250 and 500 mg pills. Additionally, an oral suspension is also available. The maximum adult dose is 3 g/24 h. Mycophenolate is also available IV and should be reconstituted with D5W. Myfortic is given twice daily at a dose of 720 mg, for a total daily dose of 1,440 mg. The drug is available in either 180 or 360 mg dosages. Myfortic is an enteric-coated formulation which decreases gastrointestinal symptoms (see caveats in "Side Effects" below).

Administration: While both drugs (CellCept and Myfortic) may be used for rejection prevention, CellCept is FDA approved for heart, kidney, and liver rejection prophylaxis, whereas Myfortic is only FDA approved for kidney rejection prophylaxis. Neither drug has been approved for the treatment of rejection [43].

Antimetabolites are primarily used as a maintenance immunosuppressive administered starting at the time of transplantation and are not considered induction therapies. These agents are typically given in conjunction with calcineurin inhibitors and corticosteroids in what is classically referred to as "triple therapy." Medication adherence is critically important. In a quantitative analysis of drug adherence patterns, missed doses of azathioprine were clearly linked to development of rejection, graft failure, and death [44].

A 1997 pooled analysis of three multinational phase III studies demonstrated that rejection rates for patients taking mycophenolate mofetil were approximately one-half that of patients taking azathioprine [45]. Based on these data, many centers switched patients from azathioprine to mycophenolate mofetil. Although there was a small improvement in graft survival in the mycophenolate mofetil arm, the difference was not statistically significant. In the analysis of the follow-up study to the Mycophenolate Steroids Sparing (MYSS) study, authors demonstrated similar long-term outcomes for patients receiving either azathioprine or mycophenolate, if the patient was also receiving a cyclosporine microemulsion, a newer form of this calcineurin inhibitor [46, 47]. It should be noted that most centers use tacrolimus instead of cyclosporine and most registry data over the last decade support the widespread practice that tacrolimus plus mycophenolate derivatives is the most efficacious regimen for maintenance immunosuppression.

Side Effects: Antimetabolite therapies for transplantation are generally well tolerated clinically. They are known to cause GI upset, bone marrow suppression, and hepatotoxicity. As for other classes of immunosuppressives, antimetabolite therapies are also associated with the development of infection and malignancy. GI upset (diarrhea in particular) is well documented in some patients that receive antimetabolites and may lead to decreased dosing in a large percentage of cases [48]. Some data have shown that higher doses may be achieved with fewer GI symptoms, and avoidance of missed doses, if patients switch to enteric-coated mycophenolate [49]. The antimetabolites may also lead to bone marrow suppression, so monitoring of cell counts is always required.

Calcineurin Inhibitors

Tacrolimus and cyclosporine are the two drugs in this class utilized in renal transplantation management.

Mechanism of Action: Tacrolimus and cyclosporine exert their immunosuppressive action through inhibition of calcineurin–calmodulin activation. Tacrolimus and cyclosporine bind to intracellular targets called immunophilins. Cyclosporine binds to cyclophilin, and tacrolimus binds to FK-binding protein (FKBP). The calcium-sensitive phosphatase calcineurin, also called protein phosphatase 2B, is implicated in eukaryotic activation, including lymphocyte activation, heart–valve morphogenesis, angiogenesis, and neural and muscle development. Calcineurin is dependent on calcium and calmodulin for activation. When the cell surface receptors of T cells are stimulated, there is an influx of calcium into the cell cytoplasm that binds to calmodulin (calcium-modulating protein). Calmodulin is a messenger protein expressed in all cells. The calcium–calmodulin complex activates the phosphatase activity of calcineurin, which then cleaves a phosphate group from the regulatory domain of NFAT (nuclear factor of activated T cells) in the cytoplasm. The dephosphorylated NFAT is then translocated into the nucleus where it acts as a transcription factor for various immunologically important genes. By inhibiting calcineurin, the transcription of genes, such as IL-2, needed for T cell proliferation and differentiation is suppressed.

Tacrolimus

Also known as FK-506 or fujimycin, tacrolimus was isolated in 1984 from a Japanese soil sample that contained the bacteria *Streptomyces tsukubaensis*. Common trade names in the USA are Prograf and Protopic with several other generic versions now available.

Pharmacokinetics: Tacrolimus is rapidly absorbed from the small intestine [50] and has a bioavailability ranging from 7 to 27 % in adult kidney transplant patients. Tacrolimus is metabolized solely in the liver and the metabolites are primarily excreted in the bile. The elimination half-life of tacrolimus is approximately 8.5 h and is prolonged in hepatic dysfunction [51]. Tacrolimus has its greatest bioavailability in a fasting state and presence of food decreases absorption [52]. Absorption also seems to vary with ethnicity. The mean tacrolimus exposure after a single oral dose in healthy Latin American and African American subjects was 18 and 39 % less than in Caucasians [53]. This may arise from differences in intestinal CYP3A or P-glycoprotein activities. Tacrolimus is lipophilic and after absorption in the intestine undergoes extensive distribution in the body including placenta and breast milk [54]. In the blood, most of it is bound to RBCs and to plasma proteins, namely, α-acid glycoprotein and albumin [55]. Presystemic metabolism by cytochrome P450 (CYP) 3A4 isoenzymes and P-glycoprotein occurs in the intestinal mucosa [5]. P-glycoprotein lowers the intracellular levels of tacrolimus by pumping drug back into the intestinal lumen for further metabolism by CYP3A4. Thereafter, CYP3A4 (and to a lesser extent CYP3A5) isoenzymes in the liver provide extensive metabolism [55]. There are at least 15 metabolites, the major metabolite being 13-*O*-demethyl-tacrolimus. The terminal half-life of tacrolimus in kidney transplant recipients is approximately 8.7 h. Biliary excretion and fecal elimination are responsible for the major clearance of metabolites, whereas renal excretion plays only a small role (feces 92.4 %, urine 2.3 %, <1 % unchanged) [56].

Use for Induction and Maintenance: Two popular regimens currently exist. The older standard regimen uses high doses of calcineurin inhibitors, steroids, and antimetabolites; and the other uses low doses of the aforementioned immunosuppressive agents with antilymphocyte antibodies. The latter is found to be superior to the regimen using high-dose conventional immunosuppressives [57–59] to prevent allograft rejection and is generally used by most centers. Tacrolimus is generally ineffective to treat acute rejection, although some uncontrolled series and case reports suggest that very high doses may sometimes be effective.

Tacrolimus is available in oral form as capsules and 5 mg/mL IV solution in the USA. Oral formulations are preferred over intravenous. When switching from IV to PO, the first dose of oral therapy should be given 8–12 h after discontinuing the IV infusion. African American patients may require larger doses to maintain trough concentration. Due to its potential for nephrotoxicity, consideration should be given to dosing tacrolimus at the lower end of the therapeutic dosing range in patients having preexisting renal impairment.

In liver dysfunction, there are reduced clearance and prolonged half-life so patients with severe hepatic impairment may require lower doses of tacrolimus. Close monitoring of blood concentrations is warranted.

Monitoring of whole blood trough concentrations is required to assist in the clinical evaluation of toxicity, efficacy, and failure. In conjunction with mycophenolate, goal tacrolimus trough levels for the first year are typically in the 4–11 ng/mL range, with individual programs adopting slightly different goals and protocols according to the assay used to measure serum levels, the type of induction immunosuppression used, and the immunological risk of the recipient.

Side Effects: The most common adverse reactions (≥30 %) are infection, tremor, hypertension, abnormal renal function, constipation, diarrhea, headache, abdominal pain, insomnia, nausea, hypomagnesemia, hypophosphatemia, peripheral edema, asthenia, pain, hyperlipidemia, hyperkalemia, myocardial hypertrophy, and pure red cell aplasia.

Other side effects are anaphylaxis with intravenous formulations, posttransplant insulin-dependent diabetes mellitus, alopecia, and risk of malignancy. Nephrotoxicity was reported in approximately 52 % of kidney transplantation patients on tacrolimus in the USA. Due to the potential for additive or synergistic impairment of renal function, care should be taken when administering tacrolimus with drugs that may be associated with renal dysfunction.

Concurrent use with strong CYP3A4 inhibitors (e.g., grapefruit juice, ritonavir, ketoconazole, itraconazole, voriconazole, clarithromycin) or inducers (e.g., rifampin, rifabutin) is not recommended without close monitoring of tacrolimus trough concentrations. Exposure to mycophenolic acid may be higher with concurrent tacrolimus or in patients changing therapy from cyclosporine to tacrolimus.

Cyclosporine

Cyclosporine (CyA) is a cyclic polypeptide immunosuppressant produced by the fungus *Beauveria nivea.*

Pharmacokinetics: The absorption of cyclosporine from the gut is incomplete and variable. Due to its lipophilic nature, cyclosporine is largely distributed extravascularly. Compared to an intravenous infusion, the absolute bioavailability of the oral solution is approximately 30 %. In plasma, approximately 90 % is bound to proteins, primarily lipoproteins. Approximately 33–47 % is in plasma, 4–9 % in lymphocytes, 5–12 % in granulocytes, and 41–58 % in erythrocytes. At high concentrations, the uptake by leucocytes and erythrocytes becomes saturated. The disposition of cyclosporine from blood is biphasic with a terminal half-life of approximately 19 h (range: 10–27 h). Elimination is primarily biliary with only 6 % of the dose excreted in the urine. Peak concentrations (C_{max}) in blood and plasma are achieved at about 3.5 h. C_{max} and area under the plasma or blood concentration/time curve (AUC) increase with the administered dose; for blood, the relationship is curvilinear (parabolic) between 0 and 1,400 mg. As determined by a specific assay, C_{max} is approximately 1.0 ng/mL/mg of dose for plasma and 1.4–2.7 ng/mL/mg of dose for blood (for low to high doses).

Cyclosporine is extensively metabolized but there is no major metabolic pathway. Only 0.1 % of the dose is excreted in the urine as unchanged drug. About 15 metabolites are characterized in human urine.

Use for Induction and Maintenance: Cyclosporine has modified (Neoral®) and non-modified formulations (Sandimmune®) which are not bioequivalent. The modified preparation has better bioavailability and, in general, has completely supplanted the non-modified form. Both oral and intravenous formulations are available. Dosing is between 10 and 14 mg/kg/day.

Plasma concentrations should be monitored closely and adjusted as necessary, until desired trough level is obtained. The blood levels are very assay specific. Whole blood 24-h trough levels of 100–200 ng/mL as determined by high-pressure liquid chromatography (HPLC) are often targeted, but therapeutic trough level depends on the type of assay used and is best if referred to the specific institutional protocol. Cyclosporine is not used for the treatment of acute rejection.

Side Effects: Apart from risk of infections and malignancies for all immunosuppressants, common side effects are hirsutism, gingival hyperplasia, hypertension, posttransplant diabetes mellitus, and renal dysfunction. Less common are GI distress, tremors, paresthesias, muscle cramps, hypomagnesemia, seizures, leucopenia, headache, and acne.

mTOR Inhibitors

Rapamycin

Structure and Function: The 23-member macrolide rapamycin (also called sirolimus) is the prototypic example of the mTOR inhibitor (mTORi) family of drugs. Initial tests with rapamycin showed it inhibited proliferation in multiple cell types and led to the discovery of the mammalian target of rapamycin (mTOR). Examinations of mTOR revealed it to be a serine/threonine kinase vital to many aspects of cellular growth and metabolism and marked mTOR as a new target for immunosuppression. Like the CNI family member tacrolimus, sirolimus, and other mTORi, such as everolimus, function requires binding to the protein chaperone FKBP12. The sirolimus/FKBP12 protein complex then interrupts the binding of mTOR to the regulatory-associated protein of TOR (raptor) preventing formation of the mTOR complex-1 (mTORC1), one of the two signaling complexes that require mTOR incorporation. Overall, currently available pharmacologic mTORi (sirolimus and everolimus) demonstrate general suppression of cell proliferation induced by exposure to growth factors [60–64].

Mechanisms of Action: mTORC1 is a component of the phosphoinositide 3-kinase (PI3K) signaling pathway activated by receptor recognition of growth factors, cytokines, and Toll-like receptor ligands. By blocking mTORC1 activity, mTORi drugs prevent activation of multiple proteins involved in regulating the cell cycle, including the P70 ribosomal protein S6 protein kinase 1 (S6K1), eukaryotic initiation factor 4E binding protein 1 (eIF1A), and multiple cyclin-dependent kinases (CDK). Inhibition of these proteins is associated with a severe reduction in protein synthesis and cell cycle arrest in the G1 phase. While mTOR acts a ubiquitous cellular signaling component, increased cellular metabolic demands associated with immune cell activation result in a preferential reliance on mTOR activation for immune cell survival and function. As a consequence mTORi have been shown to effectively inhibit clonal expansion of T cells and modulate T cell trafficking resulting in sequestration of T cells within lymphoid tissue [65]. Further, exposure to mTORi during antigenic stimulation of T cells results in hyporesponsiveness to subsequent stimulation [66, 67]. The mTORi-mediated induction of hyporesponsiveness has also been linked to increased induction and/or survival of FOXP3+ regulatory T cells [68–75]. These findings suggest that mTORi lower the ratio of effector to suppressive T cells.

In addition to T cells, studies have demonstrated that inhibition of mTOR signaling can negatively impact B cell activity [76]. Inhibition of mTOR also decreases the number of circulating neutrophils and inhibits neutrophil GM-CSF-associated tissue migration [77]. For antigen-presenting cells (APC) such as DC and monocytes/macrophages, the effects of mTOR inhibitors are more complex. Studies suggest that mTOR inhibition can block GM-CSF, IL-1, and IL-4 induced DC maturation and subsequent activation of T cells. However, treatment with mTORi has also been shown to increase DC and monocyte production of inflammatory cytokines, including TNF-α, IL-6, IL-12, and IL-23, while blocking production of the anti-inflammatory cytokine IL-10 [78]. Indeed, mTORi treatment has been reported to inhibit the immunosuppressive effects of corticosteroids on these cell types [79]. As such, mTORi can have both anti- and proinflammatory effects on DCs and monocytes [80, 81].

Finally, parenchymal cell involvement in inflammation is modulated by treatment with mTORi [82–84]. Specifically, mTORi treatment decreases the responsiveness of fibroblasts to wound-associated growth factors, preventing cell replacement and wound closure during tissue remodeling [85, 86]. This inhibition reduces VEGF production at the wound site and subsequent vascular tissue recovery [87] and is associated with delayed wound healing.

Overall, mTORi has significant immunosuppressive effects on lymphocyte-mediated acute graft rejection [75, 88] but may increase the chances of long-term graft loss [89–91].

Use for Induction, Maintenance, and Rejection Therapy: While mTOR inhibitors exhibit significant immunosuppressive capabilities, they are typically not utilized as induction therapeutics because of their interference with wound healing. mTORi are used in immunosuppression maintenance, often in combination with drugs targeted to alternate pathways of immunosuppression, such as mycophenolate mofetil [92, 93]. While multiple combinations of immunosuppressive drugs have been examined [94–99], as yet a combination with clearly superior safety and/or efficacy remains undefined. Several studies have examined the use of mTORi as a total or eventual replacement for CNI during maintenance immunosuppression in order to limit CNI-associated nephrotoxicity [99–102]; however, success has been limited by increased rejection and undesirable drug interactions.

Dosing and Levels: The current manufacturer of sirolimus suggests administration of sirolimus in conjunction with cyclosporine and corticosteroids. Dosing depends on the relative risk of immunological complications within an individual patient. For high-risk patients, initial suggested dosing includes a loading dose of 15 mg followed by daily maintenance doses of 5 mg. For lower-risk patients, suggested dosing includes a 6 mg loading dose followed by daily 2 mg doses. For both groups, blood trough levels of sirolimus should be determined 5–7 days after the initial administration and adjusted to give 3–7 ng/mL concentrations for the first year of treatment.

For everolimus, which has a much shorter half-life, the manufacturer suggests administration of 0.75 mg twice daily as maintenance therapy. Blood trough levels of everolimus should be determined 4–5 days after the initial administration and adjusted to give 3–8 ng/mL concentrations.

Side Effects: The effects of mTORi on parenchymal cells result in delayed wound healing and increased incidence of lymphoceles [103]. Additionally, the use of mTORi is also associated with anemia [104], leukopenia, and thrombocytopenia [94]. Further, sirolimus is associated with proteinuria [105, 106], increased incidence of posttransplant pneumonitis [107], and gastrointestinal tract ulcer and inflammation. In addition, sirolimus treatment is associated with enhanced nephrotoxicity of cyclosporine [108, 109]. In contrast, there is also evidence that sirolimus decreases the incidence and growth of tumors.

Treatment with sirolimus also results in dose-dependent hyperlipidemia, possibly contributing to cardiovascular morbidity [96]. Additionally, mTORi treatment increases incidence of reduced insulin sensitivity and disruption of beta cell function resulting in an increased incidence of posttransplant diabetes [110, 111].

The use of mTORi has been associated with increased incidence of bacterial, viral, protozoal, and fungal infections. However, there have also been suggestions that mTORi can ameliorate transplant immunosuppression-associated development of posttransplant lymphoproliferative disease (PTLD) [112, 113] and CMV infections [114].

Depleting Antibodies

Antithymocyte Globulins

Polyclonal antibodies are derived by immunizing animals with human thymocytes and then collecting the resultant IgG from the serum. Two preparations are available commercially: rabbit-derived antithymocyte globulin (ATG-R, Thymoglobulin®) and horse-derived thymoglobulin (Atgam®).

Mechanism of Action: Polyclonal preparations include a wide variety of antibodies and specificities including T cell molecules (i.e., CD2, CD3, CD4, CD8, TCR, CD28, CD40, CD80, CD86, CD154), non-T cell molecules (i.e., CD16, CD20), and class I and class II major histocompatibility complex (MHC) molecules [115–117]. It is uncertain which of these specificities leads to the therapeutic effect of lymphocyte depletion. Potential mechanisms include Fc-receptor-mediated complement-dependent lysis and opsonization and phagocytosis by macrophages. The extensive T cell depletion can persist for months after administration. These agents also likely have other mechanisms of immunosuppressive action such as receptor blockade or activation-induced anergy or cell death.

Use: Antithymocyte preparations are used for both induction and rejection therapy. The rabbit-derived preparation is favored over the horse-derived product because of improved tolerance and efficacy when used for either indication [34, 118, 119].

Dosage: Though rabbit-derived antithymocyte globulin is not labeled for induction therapy, it is commonly used for this purpose in clinical practice. The course of therapy is usually 1.5–2.5 mg/kg/day for 3–10 days for a total dose of 6–15 mg/kg [119]. When treating an acute rejection episode, the duration of treatment can vary from 7 to 14 days [117]. Polyclonal preparation administration is generally through a large-caliber central vein to prevent thrombophlebitis but can also be administered peripherally when diluted and formulated with heparin, hydrocortisone, or bicarbonate solutions [120].

Adverse Effects: Most common antithymocyte acute side effects are due to transient cytokine release as a result of cell surface receptor cross-linking [117]. Chills, fevers, urticaria, rash, and headache are common but can be ameliorated by premedication with corticosteroids, antihistamines, and antipyretics. Pulmonary edema and severe hypertension or hypotension can also occur and range from mild to life-threatening. However, this risk is minimized with repeated dosing as the number of target cells decreases. Additionally, because of their long-lasting immunosuppressive effects, polyclonal antibodies are associated with an increased risk of reactivation and development of viral disease caused by herpes simplex virus, CMV, Epstein–Barr virus (EBV), and varicella. Hematologic complications are also common and may warrant dose reductions to counter leukopenia and thrombocytopenia.

Alemtuzumab

Mechanism of Action: Alemtuzumab (Campath®) is a humanized monoclonal antibody directed against the surface glycoprotein CD52 [121]. Alemtuzumab binds to CD52 present on various cells (i.e., B cells, T cells, macrophages, natural killer cells, granulocytes) and triggers an antibody-dependent lysis. Alemtuzumab's depletional effect can last for up to 1 year.

Use: Although labeled for use in the treatment of B cell chronic lymphocytic leukemia, alemtuzumab is commonly used for induction immunosuppression therapy but not acute rejection in renal transplant recipients [122, 123].

Dosage: Despite a lack of consensus on the dosing of alemtuzumab, common regimens include doses of 20–30 mg on the day of transplantation and then again on postoperative day 1 or 4 [124–126]. A single 30 mg intraoperative dose is a common regimen in clinical practice.

Adverse Effects: Alemtuzumab causes marked lymphocyte depletion leading to neutropenia, thrombocytopenia, and anemia [121–123]. Acute side effects include nausea, vomiting, diarrhea, headache, and dizziness.

Muromonab-CD3

Muromonab-CD3 (Orthoclone®) was the first biological agent marketed for use in clinical medicine and thus has significant historical significance and figures prominently in older literature from the 1980s through the end of the 1990s. It was primarily utilized for the treatment of ACR in renal transplantation. Muromonab is a murine monoclonal antibody that binds to the CD3 cell surface antigen of T cells [127, 128]. Once the drugs bind, the antibody mediates both activation-induced cell death and complement-dependent cell lysis and leads to T cell depletion from the peripheral circulation. This agent was particularly noted for inducing an intense cytokine syndrome. Muromonab is entirely mouse derived and can lead to significant adverse effects including the development of an antibody response directed against the drug upon administration. This agent has been discontinued from the market secondary to its severe side effect profile and declining use in clinical practice.

Nondepleting Antibodies

Basiliximab

Mechanism of Action: Basiliximab (Simulect®) is a chimeric monoclonal antibody (70 % human and 30 % murine components) that binds to the alpha subunit of the IL-2 receptor on the surface of activated T lymphocytes (i.e., CD25) and acts as a receptor antagonist [129].

Use: Basiliximab is labeled for induction therapy in renal transplant recipients [129]. Since CD25 primarily has a role in naïve T cell early activation, basiliximab does not have a role in the treatment of rejection [130].

Dosage: Basiliximab is given as a 20 mg IV dose intraoperatively (2 h before renal transplantation) followed by a second 20 mg dose on posttransplantation day 4 [131]. Administration of both doses of basiliximab leads to complete saturation of the CD25 receptor for 5–8 weeks [129, 131].

Adverse Effects: Basiliximab is well tolerated and no cytokine release occurs since it does not mediate T cell activation [129]. There is no increase in infectious complications or delayed wound healing, while the risk of PTLD is similar as when no induction is employed [132]. There is a theoretical concern that this agent may inhibit or deplete suppressive regulatory T cells since they express very high levels of CD25; however, this has not been observed in clinical practice.

Daclizumab

Daclizumab (Zenapax®) is a monoclonal antibody (90 % human and 10 % murine components) that was used for induction therapy in renal transplant recipients [133]. Its mechanism of action and side effect profile are similar to basiliximab. However, daclizumab has a longer and more cumbersome dosing regimen in comparison to basiliximab. Daclizumab was withdrawn for the market secondary to high production costs and low demand.

Belatacept

Belatacept (Nulojix®) is the newest addition to the available options for maintenance immunosuppression therapy. Its unique mechanism of action, route of administration, and limited adverse effect profile make it a viable option in preventing kidney transplant rejection.

Mechanism of Action: Belatacept is not an antibody, but rather a fusion protein of the extracellular domain of CTLA4 with the Fc portion of IgG. This agent binds to CD80 and CD86 receptors on APC, therefore blocking the required CD28-mediated interaction between APCs and T cells needed to activate T lymphocytes [134, 135]. Overall, belatacept acts as a T cell co-stimulation blocker. The saturation of CD80 and CD86 receptors is concentration dependent.

Use: Belatacept is approved for prevention of kidney transplant rejection in combination with basiliximab induction, mycophenolate, and corticosteroids [134].

Dosage: Belatacept is the only intermittent intravenous maintenance therapy for solid organ transplantation [134]. Belatacept infusions are required more frequently during the immediate posttransplant period (i.e., initial phase) but then taper to monthly infusions after 4 months (i.e., maintenance phase). The initial phase consists of 10 mg/kg/dose on the day of transplant and then followed with a dose on day 5 (~96 h after first dose), at the end of week 2, week 4, week 8, and week 12. The maintenance phase consists of 5 mg/kg/dose every 4 weeks (±3 days) beginning at week 16 posttransplant. Belatacept is dosed based on actual body weight with the dose rounded to the nearest 12.5 mg to match the marketed disposable syringe sizes.

Adverse Effects: An increased incidence of PTLD has been associated with the use of belatacept in clinical trials [134, 136–139]. Belatacept is contraindicated in EBV seronegative patients since this population was found to have particularly high PTLD risk. Infusion-related reactions are rare and usually present as mild to moderate. Other potential side effects include peripheral edema, hyper- or hypotension, headache, electrolyte abnormalities (e.g., hypokalemia, hyperkalemia, hypophosphatemia, hypocalcemia), diarrhea, and abdominal pain. Based on clinical trial data, it does not appear that belatacept poses a higher risk of infection (e.g., urinary tract infections, CMV, upper respiratory infections) in comparison to cyclosporine maintenance immunosuppression.

Though long-term data is needed to establish belatacept's role in maintenance immunosuppression therapy, its use may help avoid some of the side effects seen with calcineurin inhibitors (i.e., nephrotoxicity, neurotoxicity, metabolic disorders) as well as drug–drug interactions. Belatacept's dosing may improve patient compliance while the absence of drug monitoring may reduce the burden on both patients and clinicians.

Biological agents are valuable in induction, maintenance, and rescue therapies in renal transplant patients. In clinical practice, it is always crucial to evaluate the potential risk versus benefits of these agents and tailor immunosuppressive therapy to each patient.

Eculizumab

Mechanism of Action and Structure: Complement is required for antibody-mediated tissue damage during rejection. This antibody-initiated process is mediated by the classical pathway of complement activation. The development of the membrane attack complex (MAC) is a crucial step of the classical pathway of complement activation. The MAC consists of C5, 6, 7, 8, and 9. Eculizumab is a humanized monoclonal antibody which contains human constant regions and murine variable regions and is FDA approved for the treatment of paroxysmal nocturnal hemoglobinuria. This agent binds to and prevents cleavage of C5 subsequently inhibiting MAC formation [140, 141].

Dosages: Eculizumab is only available as an IV infusion and dosing likely varies between programs. In one trial of eculizumab for renal transplantation in patients with a history of catastrophic antiphospholipid syndrome, the drug was given preoperatively at a dose of 1,200 mg, followed by a single 900 mg dose on postoperative day 1. Thereafter, patients receive 900 mg weekly with transition to 1,200 mg biweekly dosing in the maintenance phase [142].

Administration: Like bortezomib, administration of eculizumab is currently considered experimental therapy for prevention of antibody-mediated rejection (AMR) in the sensitized patient. In small case series, the drug has been shown to prevent AMR when compared with highly sensitized patients that received plasma exchange in addition to conventional immunosuppression [140, 143].

Side Effects: Eculizumab has been associated with headache, fever, infection, and sensitization. In a recent phase III study of eculizumab for the treatment of paroxysmal nocturnal hemoglobinuria, investigators observed that 49 % of patients experienced headache within the first week of drug administration. This figure dropped to 15 %, however, during the second week. Nasopharyngitis (32 %) and fever (19 %) were also reported during the first week. In the same study, authors found that 89 patients (92 %) experienced an infection after starting eculizumab; however, nearly 75 % of these were mild in nature and only 23 % were thought to be related to the drug. Only 1 % of patients experienced a severe infection [144]. The development of serious meningococcal infection has been reported following eculizumab therapy [145]. Based on these concerns, the FDA recommends vaccination against meningococcus at least 2 weeks prior to initiation of eculizumab. The development of anti-eculizumab antibodies has been reported in approximately 2 % of drug recipients [144].

Intravenous Immunoglobulin

Mechanism of Action: Intravenous immunoglobulin (IVIG) formulations are derived from human plasma from thousands of donors and have numerous clinical applications [146, 147]. When given as replacement, IVIG confers passive immunity by providing antibodies from the donor pool. However, the mechanisms of the anti-inflammatory and immunomodulatory effects of IVIG are not fully defined. Theories include inhibition of complement activation and complement-mediated inflammation, modification of cell-mediated immune responses, inhibition of deleterious antibody production, and induction of regulatory T cells.

Use: IVIG is approved for immunoglobulin replacement therapy, yet this indication accounts for less than half of its current use [146, 147]. IVIG is used in various treatment regimens including immunodeficiency, autoimmunity, and inflammatory disorders. In solid organ transplantation, IVIG has several applications. Patients who are sensitized to human leukocyte antibodies resulting from pregnancy, previous transplants, or blood transfusions have longer wait times on the transplantation list. IVIG has been used for its immunomodulatory properties in combination with plasmapheresis and rituximab as part of desensitization protocols for this patient population [148]. Additionally, high-dose IVIG is commonly used in AMR treatment in combination with plasmapheresis and rituximab with data supporting the modification of donor-specific antibody levels and improvement of long-term allograft survival [149, 150]. Hypogammaglobulinemia has been linked to increased risk for infection in solid organ transplant patients and may be related with long-term immunosuppression [151–154]. IVIG therapy can provide passive immunity in patients with CMV, parvovirus B19, and BKV.

Dosage: Dosing of IVIG is based on clinical indication and varies greatly across medical centers. Dosing for hypogammaglobulinemia is usually 500 mg/kg monthly while doses ranging from 100–300 mg/kg to as high as 1–2 g/kg may be necessary for anti-inflammatory effects in AMR [146, 150].

Adverse Effects: Since higher doses of IVIG are needed to obtain anti-inflammatory effects, these doses can lead to infusion-related complications including thrombotic events, bronchospasm, and hemolytic anemia [155, 156]. Adverse events can be related to the IVIG formulation used and varies depending on excipients and osmolality. In current clinical practice, most products are isosmolar and have good tolerability. It is particularly important to use IVIG preparations that have low concentrations of mannitol or other carbohydrates as these may cause acute tubular necrosis (ATN). Additionally, hemolytic anemia can occur due to anti-blood group antibodies that are part of the IVIG products and the risk is increased in formulations with higher titers.

Rituximab

Mechanism of Action: Rituximab (Rituxan®) is a chimeric monoclonal antibody that targets CD20, a surface glycoprotein expressed on circulating pre-B and mature B cells [157–159]. Though their role is not completely elucidated, CD20+ B cells serve as precursors to antibody-producing plasma cells and have antigen-presenting cell abilities. These properties can potentially play a role in AMR and ACR. Administration of rituximab leads to a depletion of CD20+ B cells from the circulation. This effect is hypothesized to involve complement-dependent cytotoxicity, drug-induced apoptotic death of B cells, and antibody-dependent cellular cytotoxicity.

Use: Initially approved for the treatment of non-Hodgkin's lymphoma, rituximab has also been proven effective in the treatment of rheumatoid arthritis, autoimmune hemolytic anemia, and idiopathic thrombocytopenic purpura. Furthermore, its off-label use is widely applied in transplant. Rituximab has been used in conjunction with plasmapheresis in AMR treatment and in desensitization protocols for ABO-incompatible donor recipient pairs or transplants across a positive crossmatch [160–163]. Rituximab has also been used as a primary treatment for PTLD in addition to immunosuppression reduction [163, 164].

Dosage: Rituximab is administered peripherally and dosed typically at 375 mg/m^2 [162, 163]. The duration of therapy varies greatly depending on indication.

Adverse Effects: Rituximab can lead to cytokine release syndrome due to tumor burden in patients with lymphoma or PTLD. However, side effects in non-oncology patients are less severe and usually occur with the first dose. Most common adverse effects are infusion reactions, transient hypotension, low-grade fever, mild tachycardia, and arthralgias [165, 166].

Proteasome Inhibitors

Bortezomib

Mechanism of Action and Structure: Bortezomib is a proteasome inhibitor that induces G2-M cell cycle arrest and apoptosis. Bortezomib is approved for the treatment of non-Hodgkin's lymphoma and multiple myeloma and has been used in clinical and experimental transplantation models as an immunosuppressant, specifically for the prevention of AMR. Bortezomib inhibits the 20S subunit of the proteasome which leads to bcl-2 phosphorylation and cleavage, and subsequent apoptosis [167]. This drug is effective against highly metabolically active cells involved in high levels of protein production, such as antibody-producing plasma cells. The goal of treatment with bortezomib is to target plasma cells. The drug has promise for patients that are highly sensitized. In a study of recipients with refractory AMR and ACR, investigators saw improvement in following treatment with bortezomib. This drug is not widely used and is generally considered experimental.

Dosage: Bortezomib is typically at 1.3 mg/m^2 for four doses.

Administration: Bortezomib is only available as an IV infusion and is not currently FDA approved for transplantation.

Side Effects: Bortezomib may cause thrombocytopenia, neutropenia, gastrointestinal symptoms, and neurological symptoms such as neuropathy and reversible posterior leukoencephalopathy. In a phase I/II trial of bortezomib-based lung cancer treatment, thrombocytopenia was the most commonly reported toxicity (58 % of patients) followed by lymphopenia and neutropenia [168]. Gastrointestinal symptoms are generally mild to moderate, such as progressive constipation, but may be as severe as paralytic ileus [169]. Bortezomib has also been associated with the development of bortezomib-induced peripheral neuropathy (BIPN). Generally, neuropathic pain is relieved with narcotics (specifically controlled-release oxycodone) during therapy but nearly always resolves with cessation of the agent [170, 171].

References

1. Baxter JD. The effects of glucocorticoid therapy. Hosp Pract (Off Ed). 1992;27(9):111–4, 115–8, 123 passim.
2. Opelz G, Dohler B, Laux G. Long-term prospective study of steroid withdrawal in kidney and heart transplant recipients. Am J Transplant. 2005;5(4 Pt 1):720–8.
3. Matas AJ, Kandaswamy R, Gillingham KJ, McHugh L, Ibrahim H, Kasiske B, et al. Prednisone-free maintenance immunosuppression-a 5-year experience. Am J Transplant. 2005;5(10): 2473–8.
4. Augustine JJ, Hricik DE. Steroid sparing in kidney transplantation: changing paradigms, improving outcomes, and remaining questions. Clin J Am Soc Nephrol. 2006;1(5):1080–9.
5. Breuner CW, Orchinik M. Plasma binding proteins as mediators of corticosteroid action in vertebrates. J Endocrinol. 2002; 175(1):99–112.
6. Rhen T, Cidlowski JA. Antiinflammatory action of glucocorticoids—new mechanisms for old drugs. N Engl J Med. 2005; 353(16):1711–23.
7. Henley DE, Lightman SL. New insights into corticosteroid-binding globulin and glucocorticoid delivery. Neuroscience. 2011;180:1–8.
8. Almawi WY, Melemedjian OK, Rieder MJ. An alternate mechanism of glucocorticoid anti-proliferative effect: promotion of a Th2 cytokine-secreting profile. Clin Transplant. 1999;13(5): 365–74.
9. Geissler EK, Schlitt HJ. Immunosuppression for liver transplantation. Gut. 2009;58(3):452–63.
10. Taylor AL, Watson CJ, Bradley JA. Immunosuppressive agents in solid organ transplantation: mechanisms of action and therapeutic efficacy. Crit Rev Oncol Hematol. 2005;56(1):23–46.
11. Segal BH, Sneller MC. Infectious complications of immunosuppressive therapy in patients with rheumatic diseases. Rheum Dis Clin North Am. 1997;23(2):219–37.
12. Poetker DM, Reh DD. A comprehensive review of the adverse effects of systemic corticosteroids. Otolaryngol Clin North Am. 2010;43(4):753–68.
13. Henry SD, Metselaar HJ, Van Dijck J, Tilanus HW, Van Der Laan LJ. Impact of steroids on hepatitis C virus replication in vivo and in vitro. Ann N Y Acad Sci. 2007;1110:439–47.
14. Vivarelli M, Burra P, La Barba G, Canova D, Senzolo M, Cucchetti A, et al. Influence of steroids on HCV recurrence after liver transplantation: a prospective study. J Hepatol. 2007;47(6):793–8.
15. Segev DL, Sozio SM, Shin EJ, Nazarian SM, Nathan H, Thuluvath PJ, et al. Steroid avoidance in liver transplantation: meta-analysis and meta-regression of randomized trials. Liver Transpl. 2008;14(4):512–25.
16. Klintmalm GB, Washburn WK, Rudich SM, Heffron TG, Teperman LW, Fasola C, et al. Corticosteroid-free immunosup-

pression with daclizumab in HCV(+) liver transplant recipients: 1-year interim results of the HCV-3 study. Liver Transpl. 2007;13(11):1521–31.
17. Llado L, Fabregat J, Castellote J, Ramos E, Xiol X, Torras J, et al. Impact of immunosuppression without steroids on rejection and hepatitis C virus evolution after liver transplantation: results of a prospective randomized study. Liver Transpl. 2008;14(12): 1752–60.
18. Sgourakis G, Radtke A, Fouzas I, Mylona S, Goumas K, Gockel I, et al. Corticosteroid-free immunosuppression in liver transplantation: a meta-analysis and meta-regression of outcomes. Transpl Int. 2009;22(9):892–905.
19. Atkinson JB, Kosi M, Srikanth MS, Takano K, Costin G. Growth hormone reverses impaired wound healing in protein-malnourished rats treated with corticosteroids. J Pediatr Surg. 1992;27(8): 1026–8.
20. Nguyen H, Lim J, Dresner ML, Nixon B. Effect of local corticosteroids on early inflammatory function in surgical wound of rats. J Foot Ankle Surg. 1998;37(4):313–8.
21. Goforth P, Gudas CJ. Effects of steroids on wound healing: a review of the literature. J Foot Surg. 1980;19(1):22–8.
22. Suh DY, Hunt TK, Spencer EM. Insulin-like growth factor-I reverses the impairment of wound healing induced by corticosteroids in rats. Endocrinology. 1992;131(5):2399–403.
23. Lenco W, McKnight M, Macdonald AS. Effects of cortisone acetate, methylprednisolone and medroxyprogesterone on wound contracture and epithelization in rabbits. Ann Surg. 1975;181(1):67–73.
24. Saag KG, Koehnke R, Caldwell JR, Brasington R, Burmeister LF, Zimmerman B, et al. Low dose long-term corticosteroid therapy in rheumatoid arthritis: an analysis of serious adverse events. Am J Med. 1994;96(2):115–23.
25. McDougall R, Sibley J, Haga M, Russell A. Outcome in patients with rheumatoid arthritis receiving prednisone compared to matched controls. J Rheumatol. 1994;21(7):1207–13.
26. Da Silva JA, Jacobs JW, Kirwan JR, Boers M, Saag KG, Ines LB, et al. Safety of low dose glucocorticoid treatment in rheumatoid arthritis: published evidence and prospective trial data. Ann Rheum Dis. 2006;65(3):285–93.
27. Vincenti F. Immunosuppression minimization: current and future trends in transplant immunosuppression. J Am Soc Nephrol. 2003;14(7):1940–8.
28. Pascual J, Quereda C, Zamora J, Hernandez D. Steroid withdrawal in renal transplant patients on triple therapy with a calcineurin inhibitor and mycophenolate mofetil: a meta-analysis of randomized, controlled trials. Transplantation. 2004;78(10):1548–56.
29. Meier-Kriesche HU, Li S, Gruessner RW, Fung JJ, Bustami RT, Barr ML, et al. Immunosuppression: evolution in practice and trends, 1994-2004. Am J Transplant. 2006;6(5 Pt 2):1111–31.
30. Schold JD, Santos A, Rehman S, Magliocca J, Meier-Kriesche HU. The success of continued steroid avoidance after kidney transplantation in the US. Am J Transplant. 2009;9(12): 2768–76.
31. Knight SR, Morris PJ. Steroid avoidance or withdrawal after renal transplantation increases the risk of acute rejection but decreases cardiovascular risk. A meta-analysis. Transplantation. 2010; 89(1):1–14.
32. Pascual J, Royuela A, Galeano C, Crespo M, Zamora J. Very early steroid withdrawal or complete avoidance for kidney transplant recipients: a systematic review. Nephrol Dial Transplant. 2012;27(2):825–32.
33. Gray D, Shepherd H, Daar A, Oliver DO, Morris PJ. Oral versus intravenous high-dose steroid treatment of renal allograft rejection. The big shot or not? Lancet. 1978;1(8056):117–8.
34. Gaber AO, First MR, Tesi RJ, Gaston RS, Mendez R, Mulloy LL, et al. Results of the double-blind, randomized, multicenter, phase III clinical trial of Thymoglobulin versus Atgam in the treatment of acute graft rejection episodes after renal transplantation. Transplantation. 1998;66(1):29–37.
35. Norman DJ, Barry JM, Bennett WM, Leone M, Henell K, Funnell B, et al. The use of OKT3 in cadaveric renal transplantation for rejection that is unresponsive to conventional anti-rejection therapy. Am J Kidney Dis. 1988;11(2):90–3.
36. Basu S, Golovina T, Mikheeva T, June CH, Riley JL. Cutting edge: Foxp3-mediated induction of pim 2 allows human T regulatory cells to preferentially expand in rapamycin. J Immunol. 2008;180(9):5794–8.
37. Maltzman JS, Koretzky GA. Azathioprine: old drug, new actions. J Clin Invest. 2003;111(8):1122–4.
38. Murray JE, Merrill JP, Harrison JH, Wilson RE, Dammin GJ. Prolonged survival of human-kidney homografts by immunosuppressive drug therapy. N Engl J Med. 1963;268:1315–23.
39. Poppe D, Tiede I, Fritz G, Becker C, Bartsch B, Wirtz S, et al. Azathioprine suppresses ezrin-radixin-moesin-dependent T cell-APC conjugation through inhibition of Vav guanosine exchange activity on Rac proteins. J Immunol. 2006;176(1):640–51.
40. Aarbakke J, Janka-Schaub G, Elion GB. Thiopurine biology and pharmacology. Trends Pharmacol Sci. 1997;18(1):3–7.
41. Ransom JT. Mechanism of action of mycophenolate mofetil. Ther Drug Monit. 1995;17(6):681–4.
42. Ji Y, Gu J, Makhov AM, Griffith JD, Mitchell BS. Regulation of the interaction of inosine monophosphate dehydrogenase with mycophenolic acid by GTP. J Biol Chem. 2006;281(1):206–12.
43. Panel PBMSHGatMA. Mycophenolate sodium (Myfortic). National PBM Drug Monograph, VHA; 2007.
44. Nevins TE, Thomas W. Quantitative patterns of azathioprine adherence after renal transplantation. Transplantation. 2009;87(5):711–8.
45. Halloran P, Mathew T, Tomlanovich S, Groth C, Hooftman L, Barker C. Mycophenolate mofetil in renal allograft recipients: a pooled efficacy analysis of three randomized, double-blind, clinical studies in prevention of rejection. The International Mycophenolate Mofetil Renal Transplant Study Groups. Transplantation. 1997;63(1):39–47.
46. Brennan DC, Koch MJ. Is mycophenolate mofetil really necessary in renal transplantation? A review of the MYSS follow-up study. Nat Clin Pract Nephrol. 2007;3(11):602–3.
47. Remuzzi G, Cravedi P, Costantini M, Lesti M, Ganeva M, Gherardi G, et al. Mycophenolate mofetil versus azathioprine for prevention of chronic allograft dysfunction in renal transplantation: the MYSS follow-up randomized, controlled clinical trial. J Am Soc Nephrol. 2007;18(6):1973–85.
48. Bunnapradist S, Ambuhl PM. Impact of gastrointestinal-related side effects on mycophenolate mofetil dosing and potential therapeutic strategies. Clin Transplant. 2008;22(6):815–21.
49. Ortega F, Sanchez-Fructuoso A, Cruzado JM, Gomez-Alamillo JC, Alarcon A, Pallardo L, et al. Gastrointestinal quality of life improvement of renal transplant recipients converted from mycophenolate mofetil to enteric-coated mycophenolate sodium drugs or agents: mycophenolate mofetil and enteric-coated mycophenolate sodium. Transplantation. 2011;92(4):426–32.
50. Kolars JC, Awni WM, Merion RM, Watkins PB. First-pass metabolism of cyclosporin by the gut. Lancet. 1991;338(8781):1488–90.
51. Hooks MA. Tacrolimus, a new immunosuppressant—a review of the literature. Ann Pharmacother. 1994;28(4):501–11.
52. Bekersky I, Dressler D, Mekki Q. Effect of time of meal consumption on bioavailability of a single oral 5 mg tacrolimus dose. J Clin Pharmacol. 2001;41(3):289–97.
53. Mancinelli LM, Frassetto L, Floren LC, Dressler D, Carrier S, Bekersky I, et al. The pharmacokinetics and metabolic disposition of tacrolimus: a comparison across ethnic groups. Clin Pharmacol Ther. 2001;69(1):24–31.
54. Scott LJ, McKeage K, Keam SJ, Plosker GL. Tacrolimus: a further update of its use in the management of organ transplantation. Drugs. 2003;63(12):1247–97.

55. Vicari-Christensen M, Repper S, Basile S, Young D. Tacrolimus: review of pharmacokinetics, pharmacodynamics, and pharmacogenetics to facilitate practitioners' understanding and offer strategies for educating patients and promoting adherence. Prog Transplant. 2009;19(3):277–84.
56. Staatz CE, Tett SE. Clinical pharmacokinetics and pharmacodynamics of tacrolimus in solid organ transplantation. Clin Pharmacokinet. 2004;43(10):623–53.
57. Webster AC, Playford EG, Higgins G, Chapman JR, Craig JC. Interleukin 2 receptor antagonists for renal transplant recipients: a meta-analysis of randomized trials. Transplantation. 2004;77(2):166–76.
58. Webster AC, Ruster LP, McGee R, Matheson SL, Higgins GY, Willis NS et al. Interleukin 2 receptor antagonists for kidney transplant recipients. Cochrane Database Syst Rev. 2010;(1):CD003897.
59. Szczech LA, Berlin JA, Aradhye S, Grossman RA, Feldman HI. Effect of anti-lymphocyte induction therapy on renal allograft survival: a meta-analysis. J Am Soc Nephrol. 1997;8(11):1771–7.
60. Powell JD, Delgoffe GM. The mammalian target of rapamycin: linking T cell differentiation, function, and metabolism. Immunity. 2010;33(3):301–11.
61. Weichhart T, Saemann MD. The multiple facets of mTOR in immunity. Trends Immunol. 2009;30(5):218–26.
62. Saemann MD, Haidinger M, Hecking M, Horl WH, Weichhart T. The multifunctional role of mTOR in innate immunity: implications for transplant immunity. Am J Transplant. 2009;9(12): 2655–61.
63. Thomson AW, Turnquist HR, Raimondi G. Immunoregulatory functions of mTOR inhibition. Nat Rev Immunol. 2009;9(5): 324–37.
64. Schmelzle T, Hall MN. TOR, a central controller of cell growth. Cell. 2000;103(2):253–62.
65. Sinclair LV, Finlay D, Feijoo C, Cornish GH, Gray A, Ager A, et al. Phosphatidylinositol-3-OH kinase and nutrient-sensing mTOR pathways control T lymphocyte trafficking. Nat Immunol. 2008;9(5):513–21.
66. Zheng Y, Collins SL, Lutz MA, Allen AN, Kole TP, Zarek PE, et al. A role for mammalian target of rapamycin in regulating T cell activation versus anergy. J Immunol. 2007;178(4):2163–70.
67. Zheng Y, Delgoffe GM, Meyer CF, Chan W, Powell JD. Anergic T cells are metabolically anergic. J Immunol. 2009;183(10): 6095–101.
68. Valmori D, Tosello V, Souleimanian NE, Godefroy E, Scotto L, Wang Y, et al. Rapamycin-mediated enrichment of T cells with regulatory activity in stimulated CD4+ T cell cultures is not due to the selective expansion of naturally occurring regulatory T cells but to the induction of regulatory functions in conventional CD4+ T cells. J Immunol. 2006;177(2):944–9.
69. Tresoldi E, Dell'Albani I, Stabilini A, Jofra T, Valle A, Gagliani N, et al. Stability of human rapamycin-expanded CD4+CD25+ T regulatory cells. Haematologica. 2011;96(9):1357–65.
70. Battaglia M, Stabilini A, Migliavacca B, Horejs-Hoeck J, Kaupper T, Roncarolo MG. Rapamycin promotes expansion of functional CD4+CD25+FOXP3+ regulatory T cells of both healthy subjects and type 1 diabetic patients. J Immunol. 2006;177(12):8338–47.
71. Battaglia M, Stabilini A, Draghici E, Gregori S, Mocchetti C, Bonifacio E, et al. Rapamycin and interleukin-10 treatment induces T regulatory type 1 cells that mediate antigen-specific transplantation tolerance. Diabetes. 2006;55(1):40–9.
72. Battaglia M, Stabilini A, Roncarolo MG. Rapamycin selectively expands CD4+CD25+FoxP3+ regulatory T cells. Blood. 2005;105(12):4743–8.
73. Kang J, Huddleston SJ, Fraser JM, Khoruts A. De novo induction of antigen-specific CD4+CD25+Foxp3+ regulatory T cells in vivo following systemic antigen administration accompanied by blockade of mTOR. J Leukoc Biol. 2008;83(5):1230–9.
74. Delgoffe GM, Kole TP, Zheng Y, Zarek PE, Matthews KL, Xiao B, et al. The mTOR kinase differentially regulates effector and regulatory T cell lineage commitment. Immunity. 2009;30(6):832–44.
75. Morelon E, Lefrancois N, Besson C, Prevautel J, Brunet M, Touraine JL, et al. Preferential increase in memory and regulatory subsets during T-lymphocyte immune reconstitution after Thymoglobulin induction therapy with maintenance sirolimus vs cyclosporine. Transpl Immunol. 2010;23(1–2):53–8.
76. Zhang S, Readinger JA, DuBois W, Janka-Junttila M, Robinson R, Pruitt M, et al. Constitutive reductions in mTOR alter cell size, immune cell development, and antibody production. Blood. 2011;117(4):1228–38.
77. Gomez-Cambronero J. Rapamycin inhibits GM-CSF-induced neutrophil migration. FEBS Lett. 2003;550(1–3):94–100.
78. Weichhart T, Haidinger M, Katholnig K, Kopecky C, Poglitsch M, Lassnig C, et al. Inhibition of mTOR blocks the anti-inflammatory effects of glucocorticoids in myeloid immune cells. Blood. 2011;117(16):4273–83.
79. Weichhart T, Costantino G, Poglitsch M, Rosner M, Zeyda M, Stuhlmeier KM, et al. The TSC-mTOR signaling pathway regulates the innate inflammatory response. Immunity. 2008;29(4): 565–77.
80. Fischer R, Turnquist HR, Taner T, Thomson AW. Use of rapamycin in the induction of tolerogenic dendritic cells. Handb Exp Pharmacol. 2009;188:215–32.
81. Haidinger M, Poglitsch M, Geyeregger R, Kasturi S, Zeyda M, Zlabinger GJ, et al. A versatile role of mammalian target of rapamycin in human dendritic cell function and differentiation. J Immunol. 2010;185(7):3919–31.
82. Mohacsi PJ, Tuller D, Hulliger B, Wijngaard PL. Different inhibitory effects of immunosuppressive drugs on human and rat aortic smooth muscle and endothelial cell proliferation stimulated by platelet-derived growth factor or endothelial cell growth factor. J Heart Lung Transplant. 1997;16(5):484–92.
83. Schuler W, Sedrani R, Cottens S, Haberlin B, Schulz M, Schuurman HJ, et al. SDZ RAD, a new rapamycin derivative: pharmacological properties in vitro and in vivo. Transplantation. 1997;64(1):36–42.
84. Vogelbacher R, Wittmann S, Braun A, Daniel C, Hugo C. The mTOR inhibitor everolimus induces proteinuria and renal deterioration in the remnant kidney model in the rat. Transplantation. 2007;84(11):1492–9.
85. Azzola A, Havryk A, Chhajed P, Hostettler K, Black J, Johnson P, et al. Everolimus and mycophenolate mofetil are potent inhibitors of fibroblast proliferation after lung transplantation. Transplantation. 2004;77(2):275–80.
86. Salas-Prato M, Assalian A, Mehdi AZ, Duperre J, Thompson P, Brazeau P. Inhibition by rapamycin of PDGF- and bFGF-induced human tenon fibroblast proliferation in vitro. J Glaucoma. 1996;5(1):54–9.
87. Goren I, Muller E, Schiefelbein D, Gutwein P, Seitz O, Pfeilschifter J, et al. Akt1 controls insulin-driven VEGF biosynthesis from keratinocytes: implications for normal and diabetes-impaired skin repair in mice. J Invest Dermatol. 2009;129(3):752–64.
88. Vogelbacher R, Meister S, Guckel E, Starke C, Wittmann S, Stief A, et al. Bortezomib and sirolimus inhibit the chronic active antibody-mediated rejection in experimental renal transplantation in the rat. Nephrol Dial Transplant. 2010;25(11):3764–73.
89. Meier-Kriesche HU, Steffen BJ, Chu AH, Loveland JJ, Gordon RD, Morris JA, et al. Sirolimus with neoral versus mycophenolate mofetil with neoral is associated with decreased renal allograft survival. Am J Transplant. 2004;4(12):2058–66.
90. Meier-Kriesche HU, Schold JD, Srinivas TR, Howard RJ, Fujita S, Kaplan B. Sirolimus in combination with tacrolimus is associated with worse renal allograft survival compared to mycopheno-

late mofetil combined with tacrolimus. Am J Transplant. 2005;5(9):2273–80.

91. Srinivas TR, Schold JD, Guerra G, Eagan A, Bucci CM, Meier-Kriesche HU. Mycophenolate mofetil/sirolimus compared to other common immunosuppressive regimens in kidney transplantation. Am J Transplant. 2007;7(3):586–94.
92. Weir MR, Diekmann F, Flechner SM, Lebranchu Y, Mandelbrot DA, Oberbauer R, et al. mTOR inhibition: the learning curve in kidney transplantation. Transpl Int. 2010;23(5):447–60.
93. Grinyo JM, Cruzado JM. Mycophenolate mofetil and sirolimus combination in renal transplantation. Am J Transplant. 2006;6(9):1991–9.
94. Kahan BD. Efficacy of sirolimus compared with azathioprine for reduction of acute renal allograft rejection: a randomised multicentre study. The Rapamune US Study Group. Lancet. 2000;356(9225):194–202.
95. MacDonald AS. A worldwide, phase III, randomized, controlled, safety and efficacy study of a sirolimus/cyclosporine regimen for prevention of acute rejection in recipients of primary mismatched renal allografts. Transplantation. 2001;71(2):271–80.
96. Groth CG, Backman L, Morales JM, Calne R, Kreis H, Lang P, et al. Sirolimus (rapamycin)-based therapy in human renal transplantation: similar efficacy and different toxicity compared with cyclosporine. Sirolimus European Renal Transplant Study Group. Transplantation. 1999;67(7):1036–42.
97. Kreis H, Cisterne JM, Land W, Wramner L, Squifflet JP, Abramowicz D, et al. Sirolimus in association with mycophenolate mofetil induction for the prevention of acute graft rejection in renal allograft recipients. Transplantation. 2000;69(7): 1252–60.
98. Ciancio G, Burke GW, Gaynor JJ, Ruiz P, Roth D, Kupin W, et al. A randomized long-term trial of tacrolimus/sirolimus versus tacrolimus/mycophenolate versus cyclosporine/sirolimus in renal transplantation: three-year analysis. Transplantation. 2006;81(6): 845–52.
99. Larson TS, Dean PG, Stegall MD, Griffin MD, Textor SC, Schwab TR, et al. Complete avoidance of calcineurin inhibitors in renal transplantation: a randomized trial comparing sirolimus and tacrolimus. Am J Transplant. 2006;6(3):514–22.
100. Budde K, Becker T, Arns W, Sommerer C, Reinke P, Eisenberger U, et al. Everolimus-based, calcineurin-inhibitor-free regimen in recipients of de-novo kidney transplants: an open-label, randomised, controlled trial. Lancet. 2011;377(9768):837–47.
101. Weir MR. Mycophenolate mofetil-based immunosuppression with sirolimus in renal transplantation: a randomized, controlled Spare-the-Nephron trial. Kidney Int. 2011;79(8): 897–907.
102. Flechner SM, Glyda M, Cockfield S, Grinyo J, Legendre C, Russ G, et al. The ORION study: comparison of two sirolimus-based regimens versus tacrolimus and mycophenolate mofetil in renal allograft recipients. Am J Transplant. 2011;11(8):1633–44.
103. Dean PG, Lund WJ, Larson TS, Prieto M, Nyberg SL, Ishitani MB, et al. Wound-healing complications after kidney transplantation: a prospective, randomized comparison of sirolimus and tacrolimus. Transplantation. 2004;77(10):1555–61.
104. Augustine JJ, Knauss TC, Schulak JA, Bodziak KA, Siegel C, Hricik DE. Comparative effects of sirolimus and mycophenolate mofetil on erythropoiesis in kidney transplant patients. Am J Transplant. 2004;4(12):2001–6.
105. Letavernier E, Pe'raldi MN, Pariente A, Morelon E, Legendre C. Proteinuria following a switch from calcineurin inhibitors to sirolimus. Transplantation. 2005;80(9):1198–203.
106. Izzedine H, Brocheriou I, Frances C. Post-transplantation proteinuria and sirolimus. N Engl J Med. 2005;353(19):2088–9.
107. Weiner SM, Sellin L, Vonend O, Schenker P, Buchner NJ, Flecken M, et al. Pneumonitis associated with sirolimus: clinical characteristics, risk factors and outcome—a single-centre experience and review of the literature. Nephrol Dial Transplant. 2007; 22(12):3631–7.
108. Andoh TF, Burdmann EA, Fransechini N, Houghton DC, Bennett WM. Comparison of acute rapamycin nephrotoxicity with cyclosporine and FK506. Kidney Int. 1996;50(4):1110–7.
109. Andoh TF, Lindsley J, Franceschini N, Bennett WM. Synergistic effects of cyclosporine and rapamycin in a chronic nephrotoxicity model. Transplantation. 1996;62(3):311–6.
110. Johnston O, Rose CL, Webster AC, Gill JS. Sirolimus is associated with new-onset diabetes in kidney transplant recipients. J Am Soc Nephrol. 2008;19(7):1411–8.
111. Fraenkel M, Ketzinel-Gilad M, Ariav Y, Pappo O, Karaca M, Castel J, et al. MTOR inhibition by rapamycin prevents beta-cell adaptation to hyperglycemia and exacerbates the metabolic state in type 2 diabetes. Diabetes. 2008;57(4):945–57.
112. Majewski M, Korecka M, Joergensen J, Fields L, Kossev P, Schuler W, et al. Immunosuppressive TOR kinase inhibitor everolimus (RAD) suppresses growth of cells derived from posttransplant lymphoproliferative disorder at allograft-protecting doses. Transplantation. 2003;75(10):1710–7.
113. Krams SM, Martinez OM. Epstein-Barr virus, rapamycin, and host immune responses. Curr Opin Organ Transplant. 2008; 13(6):563–8.
114. Webster AC, Lee VW, Chapman JR, Craig JC. Target of rapamycin inhibitors (sirolimus and everolimus) for primary immunosuppression of kidney transplant recipients: a systematic review and meta-analysis of randomized trials. Transplantation. 2006;81(9): 1234–48.
115. Kirk AD. Induction immunosuppression. Transplantation. 2006;82(5):593–602.
116. Hardinger KL. Rabbit antithymocyte globulin induction therapy in adult renal transplantation. Pharmacotherapy. 2006;26(12): 1771–83.
117. Genzyme. Thymoglobulin® (anti-thymocyte globulin [rabbit]) [package insert]; 2008.
118. Brennan DC, Flavin K, Lowell JA, Howard TK, Shenoy S, Burgess S, et al. A randomized, double-blinded comparison of Thymoglobulin versus Atgam for induction immunosuppressive therapy in adult renal transplant recipients. Transplantation. 1999;67(7):1011–8.
119. Hardinger KL, Rhee S, Buchanan P, Koch M, Miller B, Enkvetchakul D, et al. A prospective, randomized, double-blinded comparison of thymoglobulin versus Atgam for induction immunosuppressive therapy: 10-year results. Transplantation. 2008;86(7):947–52.
120. Wiland AM, Fink JC, Philosophe B, Farney AC, Schweitzer EJ, Colonna JO, et al. Peripheral administration of thymoglobulin for induction therapy in pancreas transplantation. Transplant Proc. 2001;33(1–2):1910.
121. Millennium and ILEX Partners L. Campath® (alemtuzumab) [package insert]; 2001.
122. Morris PJ, Russell NK. Alemtuzumab (Campath-1H): a systematic review in organ transplantation. Transplantation. 2006;81(10): 1361–7.
123. Ciancio G, Burke III GW. Alemtuzumab (Campath-1H) in kidney transplantation. Am J Transplant. 2008;8(1):15–20.
124. Watson CJ, Bradley JA, Friend PJ, Firth J, Taylor CJ, Bradley JR, et al. Alemtuzumab (CAMPATH 1H) induction therapy in cadaveric kidney transplantation—efficacy and safety at five years. Am J Transplant. 2005;5(6):1347–53.
125. Margreiter R, Klempnauer J, Neuhaus P, Muehlbacher F, Boesmueller C, Calne RY. Alemtuzumab (Campath-1H) and tacrolimus monotherapy after renal transplantation: results of a prospective randomized trial. Am J Transplant. 2008;8(7): 1480–5.

126. Tan HP, Donaldson J, Basu A, Unruh M, Randhawa P, Sharma V, et al. Two hundred living donor kidney transplantations under alemtuzumab induction and tacrolimus monotherapy: 3-year follow-up. Am J Transplant. 2009;9(2):355–66.
127. Vallhonrat H, Williams WW, Cosimi AB, Tolkoff-Rubin N, Ginns LC, Wain JC, et al. In vivo generation of C4d, Bb, iC3b, and SC5b-9 after OKT3 administration in kidney and lung transplant recipients. Transplantation. 1999;67(2):253–8.
128. Webster AC, Pankhurst T, Rinaldi F, Chapman JR, Craig JC. Monoclonal and polyclonal antibody therapy for treating acute rejection in kidney transplant recipients: a systematic review of randomized trial data. Transplantation. 2006;81(7):953–65.
129. Novartis. Simulect® (basiliximab) [package insert]; 2005.
130. Suri-Payer E, Amar AZ, Thornton AM, Shevach EM. CD4+CD25+ T cells inhibit both the induction and effector function of autoreactive T cells and represent a unique lineage of immunoregulatory cells. J Immunol. 1998;160(3):1212–8.
131. Ramirez CB, Marino IR. The role of basiliximab induction therapy in organ transplantation. Expert Opin Biol Ther. 2007; 7(1):137–48.
132. Cherikh WS, Kauffman HM, McBride MA, Maghirang J, Swinnen LJ, Hanto DW. Association of the type of induction immunosuppression with posttransplant lymphoproliferative disorder, graft survival, and patient survival after primary kidney transplantation. Transplantation. 2003;76(9):1289–93.
133. Wiseman LR, Faulds D. Daclizumab: a review of its use in the prevention of acute rejection in renal transplant recipients. Drugs. 1999;58(6):1029–42.
134. Co B-MS. Nulojix® (belatacept) [package insert]. 2011.
135. Latek R, Fleener C, Lamian V, Kulbokas III E, Davis PM, Suchard SJ, et al. Assessment of belatacept-mediated costimulation blockade through evaluation of CD80/86-receptor saturation. Transplantation. 2009;87(6):926–33.
136. Ferguson R, Grinyo J, Vincenti F, Kaufman DB, Woodle ES, Marder BA, et al. Immunosuppression with belatacept-based, corticosteroid-avoiding regimens in de novo kidney transplant recipients. Am J Transplant. 2011;11(1):66–76.
137. Vincenti F, Charpentier B, Vanrenterghem Y, Rostaing L, Bresnahan B, Darji P, et al. A phase III study of belatacept-based immunosuppression regimens versus cyclosporine in renal transplant recipients (BENEFIT study). Am J Transplant. 2010;10(3):535–46.
138. Vincenti F, Larsen C, Durrbach A, Wekerle T, Nashan B, Blancho G, et al. Costimulation blockade with belatacept in renal transplantation. N Engl J Med. 2005;353(8):770–81.
139. Durrbach A, Pestana JM, Pearson T, Vincenti F, Garcia VD, Campistol J, et al. A phase III study of belatacept versus cyclosporine in kidney transplants from extended criteria donors (BENEFIT-EXT study). Am J Transplant. 2010;10(3):547–57.
140. Asgari E, Zhou W, Sacks S. Complement in organ transplantation. Curr Opin Organ Transplant. 2010;15(4):486–91.
141. Kelly R, Richards S, Hillmen P, Hill A. The pathophysiology of paroxysmal nocturnal hemoglobinuria and treatment with eculizumab. Ther Clin Risk Manag. 2009;5:911–21.
142. Montgomery RA. Eculizumab to enable renal transplantation in patients with history of catastrophic antiphospholipid antibody syndrome. http://www.clinicaltrials.gov (NCT01029587).
143. Stegall MD, Diwan TS, Burns JM. Prevention of acute humoral rejection with C5 inhibition. Am J Transplant. 2009;9:241–2 (Abstract presented at American Transplant Congress).
144. Brodsky RA, Young NS, Antonioli E, Risitano AM, Schrezenmeier H, Schubert J, et al. Multicenter phase 3 study of the complement inhibitor eculizumab for the treatment of patients with paroxysmal nocturnal hemoglobinuria. Blood. 2008;111(4):1840–7.
145. Dmytrijuk A, Robie-Suh K, Cohen MH, Rieves D, Weiss K, Pazdur R. FDA report: eculizumab (Soliris) for the treatment of patients with paroxysmal nocturnal hemoglobinuria. Oncologist. 2008;13(9):993–1000.
146. Shehata N, Palda VA, Meyer RM, Blydt-Hansen TD, Campbell P, Cardella C, et al. The use of immunoglobulin therapy for patients undergoing solid organ transplantation: an evidence-based practice guideline. Transfus Med Rev. 2010;24 Suppl 1:S7–27.
147. Jordan SC, Toyoda M, Vo AA. Intravenous immunoglobulin a natural regulator of immunity and inflammation. Transplantation. 2009;88(1):1–6.
148. Jordan SC, Tyan D, Stablein D, McIntosh M, Rose S, Vo A, et al. Evaluation of intravenous immunoglobulin as an agent to lower allosensitization and improve transplantation in highly sensitized adult patients with end-stage renal disease: report of the NIH IG02 trial. J Am Soc Nephrol. 2004;15(12):3256–62.
149. Durandy A, Kaveri SV, Kuijpers TW, Basta M, Miescher S, Ravetch JV, et al. Intravenous immunoglobulins—understanding properties and mechanisms. Clin Exp Immunol. 2009;158 Suppl 1:2–13.
150. Jordan SC, Reinsmoen N, Peng A, Lai CH, Cao K, Villicana R, et al. Advances in diagnosing and managing antibody-mediated rejection. Pediatr Nephrol. 2010;25(10):2035–45. quiz 2045–48.
151. Mawhorter S, Yamani MH. Hypogammaglobulinemia and infection risk in solid organ transplant recipients. Curr Opin Organ Transplant. 2008;13(6):581–5.
152. Smith JM, Jordan SC. Intravenous immunoglobulin as treatment for BK virus: nephropathy. Pediatr Transplant. 2009;13(1):11–3.
153. Radha R, Jordan S, Puliyanda D, Bunnapradist S, Petrosyan A, Amet N, et al. Cellular immune responses to cytomegalovirus in renal transplant recipients. Am J Transplant. 2005;5(1):110–7.
154. Barsoum NR, Bunnapradist S, Mougdil A, Toyoda M, Vo A, Jordan SC. Treatment of parvovirus B-19 (PV B-19) infection allows for successful kidney transplantation without disease recurrence. Am J Transplant. 2002;2(5):425–8.
155. Vo AA, Cam V, Toyoda M, Puliyanda DP, Lukovsky M, Bunnapradist S, et al. Safety and adverse events profiles of intravenous gammaglobulin products used for immunomodulation: a single-center experience. Clin J Am Soc Nephrol. 2006;1(4):844–52.
156. Kahwaji J, Barker E, Pepkowitz S, Klapper E, Villicana R, Peng A, et al. Acute hemolysis after high-dose intravenous immunoglobulin therapy in highly HLA sensitized patients. Clin J Am Soc Nephrol. 2009;4(12):1993–7.
157. Grillo-Lopez AJ, White CA, Varns C, Shen D, Wei A, McClure A, et al. Overview of the clinical development of rituximab: first monoclonal antibody approved for the treatment of lymphoma. Semin Oncol. 1999;26(5 Suppl 14):66–73.
158. Deans JP, Li H, Polyak MJ. CD20-mediated apoptosis: signalling through lipid rafts. Immunology. 2002;107(2):176–82.
159. Maloney DG, Smith B, Rose A. Rituximab: mechanism of action and resistance. Semin Oncol. 2002;29(1 Suppl 2):2–9.
160. Sonnenday CJ, Warren DS, Cooper M, Samaniego M, Haas M, King KE, et al. Plasmapheresis, CMV hyperimmune globulin, and anti-CD20 allow ABO-incompatible renal transplantation without splenectomy. Am J Transplant. 2004;4(8):1315–22.
161. Tyden G, Kumlien G, Genberg H, Sandberg J, Lundgren T, Fehrman I. ABO incompatible kidney transplantations without splenectomy, using antigen-specific immunoadsorption and rituximab. Am J Transplant. 2005;5(1):145–8.
162. Becker YT, Becker BN, Pirsch JD, Sollinger HW. Rituximab as treatment for refractory kidney transplant rejection. Am J Transplant. 2004;4(6):996–1001.
163. Becker YT, Samaniego-Picota M, Sollinger HW. The emerging role of rituximab in organ transplantation. Transpl Int. 2006;19(8):621–8.
164. Svoboda J, Kotloff R, Tsai DE. Management of patients with post-transplant lymphoproliferative disorder: the role of rituximab. Transpl Int. 2006;19(4):259–69.

165. Vieira CA, Agarwal A, Book BK, Sidner RA, Bearden CM, Gebel HM, et al. Rituximab for reduction of anti-HLA antibodies in patients awaiting renal transplantation: 1. Safety, pharmacodynamics, and pharmacokinetics. Transplantation. 2004;77(4):542–8.
166. Agarwal A, Vieira CA, Book BK, Sidner RA, Fineberg NS, Pescovitz MD. Rituximab, anti-CD20, induces in vivo cytokine release but does not impair ex vivo T-cell responses. Am J Transplant. 2004;4(8):1357–60.
167. Piperdi B, Ling YH, Liebes L, Muggia F, Perez-Soler R. Bortezomib: understanding the mechanism of action. Mol Cancer Ther. 2011;10(11):2029–30.
168. Piperdi B, Walsh WV, Bradley K, Zhou Z, Bathini V, Hanrahan-Boshes M, et al. Phase-I/II study of Bortezomib in combination with carboplatin and bevacizumab as first-line therapy in patients with advanced non-small-cell lung cancer. J Thorac Oncol. 2012;7(6):1032–40.
169. Perfetti V, Palladini G, Brunetti L, Sgarella A, Brugnatelli S, Gobbi PG, et al. Bortezomib-induced paralytic ileus is a potential gastrointestinal side effect of this first-in-class anticancer proteasome inhibitor. Eur J Gastroenterol Hepatol. 2007;19(7):599–601.
170. Cavaletti G, Jakubowiak AJ. Peripheral neuropathy during bortezomib treatment of multiple myeloma: a review of recent studies. Leuk Lymphoma. 2010;51(7):1178–87.
171. Cartoni C, Brunetti GA, Federico V, Efficace F, Grammatico S, Tendas A, et al. Controlled-release oxycodone for the treatment of bortezomib-induced neuropathic pain in patients with multiple myeloma. Support Care Cancer. 2012;20:2621–6.

Delayed Graft Function and Kidney Transplantation

13

Sunita K. Singh, Edward H. Cole, and S. Joseph Kim

Introduction

Delayed graft function (DGF) generally refers to dysfunction of the allograft with or without oliguria in the early postoperative period. This is typically due to ischemia–reperfusion injury in the donor kidney resulting from the organ recovery process but also may be secondary to other factors (e.g., obstruction by hematoma). Despite the advances in immunosuppression and superior graft survival over time, DGF has significant short- and long-term consequences and continues to be an important challenge for the clinician in the modern era of kidney transplantation. The purpose of this chapter is to provide a clinically oriented overview of DGF. We will review the definitions of DGF and their limitations, pathophysiology, risk factors, and clinical evaluation, as well as outline prevention/management approaches. Finally, we will discuss the impact of DGF on patient and allograft outcomes.

Defining DGF

DGF is most commonly defined as the need for dialysis in the first 7 days post-transplantation [1]. However, this definition is one of many that exist in the literature. In a systematic review by Yarlagadda et al. [2], over 18 unique definitions for DGF were identified which included dialysis-based definitions, creatinine-based definitions, or a combination of the two. At present, there is no uniformly accepted definition and the ambiguity in defining DGF is a significant challenge when comparing and interpreting results of observational studies and clinical trials.

The existing definitions of DGF used in the literature, whether dialysis or creatinine based, have significant limitations that are noteworthy. Firstly, the current definitions do not allow the clinician to differentiate DGF from other causes of graft dysfunction. This is of particular concern since early postoperative graft dysfunction carries an extensive differential diagnosis (Table 13.1). Secondly, the existing dialysis-based definitions may result in misclassification of patients. Patients with good graft function needing dialysis for indications such as hyperkalemia or volume overload may be falsely identified as having DGF. Conversely, those patients with residual renal function prior to transplantation may not necessarily require dialysis in the first 7 days post-transplant despite having poor graft function. This misclassification bias is well highlighted in a study that identified patients with DGF using medical records as the gold standard and comparing with UNOS registry data. Although the false-positive rate of the 7-day DGF definition was low (5 %), the false-negative rate was high (44 %), suggesting that a significant proportion of patients were misclassified as not having DGF [3].

Thirdly, the need for dialysis is somewhat subjective, which may impact documented rates of DGF. Akkina et al. [4] found the incidence of DGF to be two- to threefold higher when comparing two transplant programs in the same US city, despite similar donor and recipient parameters, laboratory data, and graft survival. The specific indications for dialysis could not be elicited from the dataset; however, these findings suggest that physician thresholds in prescribing dialysis post-transplantation may significantly impact DGF rates. Although novel biomarker techniques for the diagnosis of DGF have been studied in order to overcome the limitations noted above, none are yet clinically available. Thus, dialysis-based definitions continue to be most commonly used. Nevertheless, it seems clear that, in the absence of an ideal biomarker, a broader definition, incorporating both

S.K. Singh • E.H. Cole • S.J. Kim (✉)
Division of Nephrology, Department of Medicine, University of Toronto, Toronto, ON, Canada
e-mail: joseph.kim@uhn.ca

M.R. Weir and E.V. Lerma (eds.), *Kidney Transplantation: Practical Guide to Management*, DOI 10.1007/978-1-4939-0342-9_13, © Springer Science+Business Media New York 2014

Table 13.1 Differential diagnosis for graft dysfunction in the early post-transplant period

Acute tubular necrosis
Urological/surgical complications • Urinary leak • Lymphocele • Ureteral obstruction • Catheter obstruction • Bleeding/hematoma
Vascular causes • Hypovolemia/hypoperfusion • CNI toxicity (vasoconstriction) • Thrombosis of the renal artery or vein • Thrombotic microangiopathy/hemolytic-uremic syndrome (CNI use)
Recurrent disease
Acute rejection
Acute interstitial nephritis

function and the need/reason for dialysis, would be more accurate and useful.

Pathophysiology of DGF

The coupled effect of warm and cold ischemia, as well as reperfusion of the kidney allograft after transplantation, results in a complex cascade of biochemical and structural changes at the cellular level. These changes predispose recipients to DGF, which is typically associated with histological findings of acute tubular necrosis (ATN) and intertubular neutrophilic infiltration [5, 6]. A wide spectrum of histopathologic changes, from mild to severe, has been associated with the clinical syndrome of DGF. These changes are more likely to be present after prolonged periods of cold ischemia [5, 7].

Ischemia results in intracellular hypoxia, which triggers multiple downstream effects including activation of anaerobic glucose metabolism and cellular depletion of ATP. Due to anaerobic metabolism, lactic acid is produced and intracellular acidosis ensues. Lytic enzymes are then activated which promote the generation of reactive oxygen species and result in tissue damage. Furthermore, cellular depletion of ATP results in inhibition of the Na/K ATPase which is essential in maintaining membrane potential. This allows sodium and water to enter the cell causing significant cellular edema. The intracellular osmolality of the cell also rises due to accumulation of adenosine, inorganic phosphate, and other intermediate compounds thus exacerbating the edema. The consequences of these processes include disruption of the cytoskeleton and cellular/mitochondrial membranes.

Reperfusion also plays an important role in renal injury. As oxidative metabolism is restored, a substantial and rapid release of reactive oxygen species including hydrogen peroxide and superoxide anions occurs, resulting in apoptosis. Furthermore, the generation of reactive oxygen species triggers a profound release of inflammatory cytokines recruiting neutrophils, monocytes, NK cells, and T cells to the allograft. Recruited leukocytes bind to adhesion molecules on endothelial cells plugging capillaries and increasing permeability of the endothelium. Ultimately, as a result of this complex pro-inflammatory cascade, damage to tubular cells and the vascular endothelium occurs. Furthermore, increases in endothelin and thromboxane, coupled with a decrease in prostacyclin, result in vasoconstriction, further aggravating tissue injury [1, 6, 8, 9].

The mechanisms of injury in DGF are complex and depicted schematically in Fig. 13.1. Although an in-depth description of the cellular and molecular mechanisms of injury in DGF is beyond the scope of this chapter, comprehensive reviews by Siedlecki et al. and Perico et al. highlight these mechanisms in greater detail [1, 6].

Epidemiology of DGF

There is significant variability in the rates of DGF in the literature, ranging from 2 to 50 % depending on the transplant center or database [1]. This is in part due to the heterogeneity in the definitions of DGF in the literature as well as differences across donor subtype. Given the ongoing shortage of organs available for transplantation, the use of expanded criteria donor (ECD) and donation after cardiac death (DCD) kidneys has increased over time, which heavily influences rates of DGF [7, 10, 11]. Thus, despite improvements in overall graft survival, DGF rates continue to increase, in part, due to the composition of the deceased donor pool.

In 2009, the USRDS reported DGF rates of 22 % in recipients of deceased donor kidneys [10]. DCD kidneys are associated with the highest rates of DGF, occurring in 37 % of recipients [10]. The obligate warm ischemia time with DCD kidneys, defined as the time between circulatory arrest and the commencement of cold storage, enhances the ischemia–reperfusion injury resulting in the highest rates of DGF across any subgroup of donor kidneys [12]. Brain death results in a variety of hemodynamic and hormonal derangements, including a systemic inflammatory response and a surge in catecholamine levels, resulting in severe vasoconstriction and hypoperfusion of the allograft [13, 14]. Therefore, DGF also occurs in kidneys from brain dead donors, with rates of 20 and 31 % in standard criteria donor (SCD) and ECD kidneys, respectively [10].

Although DGF occurs most commonly in recipients of deceased donor kidney transplants, it also occurs in living donor kidney transplants, albeit to a much lesser degree. The USRDS reported a DGF rate in living donor kidney transplants of 3.4 % [10]. The risk factors for DGF in living

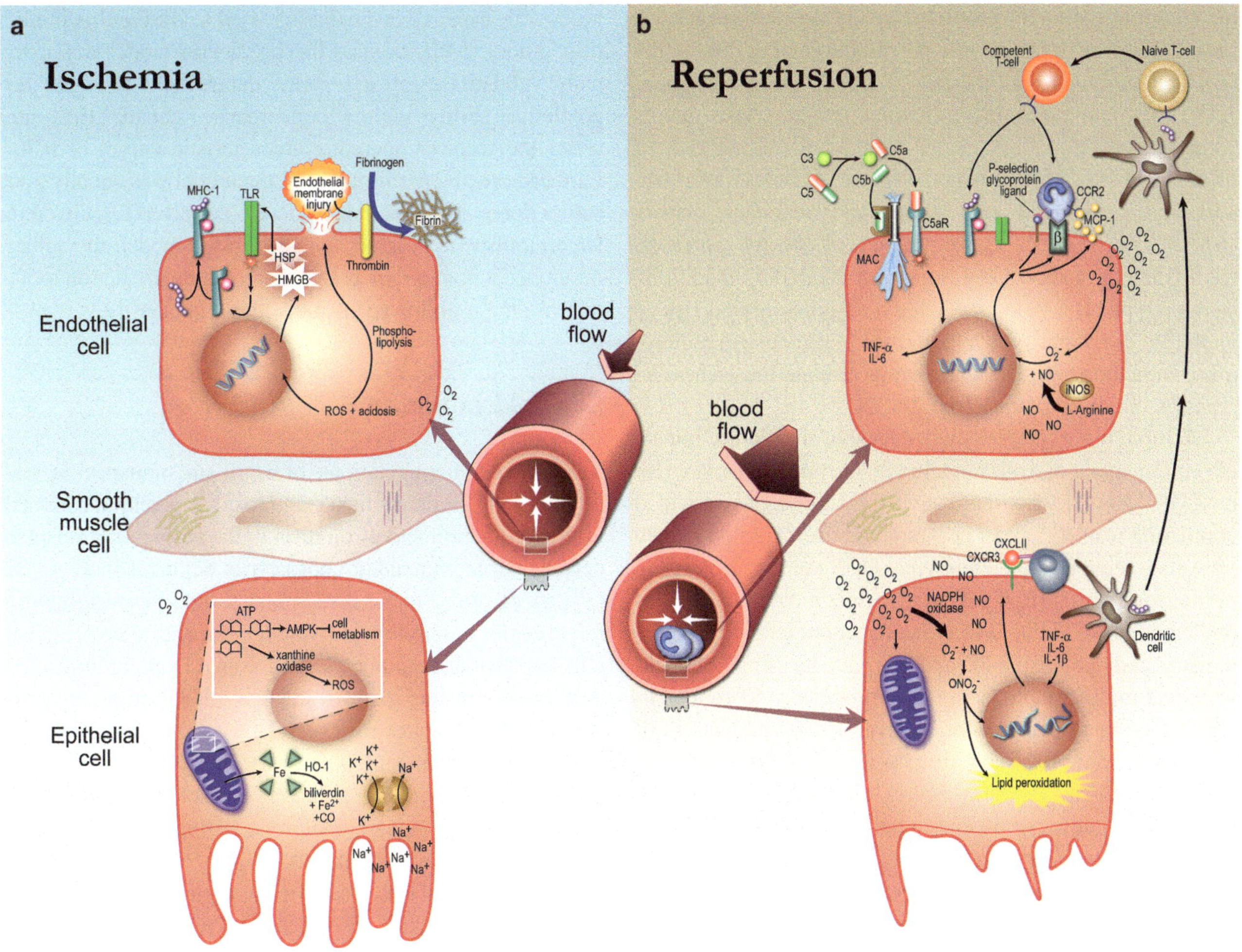

Fig. 13.1 Ischemia–reperfusion injury in delayed graft function. Cellular hypoxia triggers anaerobic metabolism resulting in cellular depletion of ATP, impairment of the Na/K ATPase, and generation of reactive oxygen species, which results in cellular edema and tissue injury. During reperfusion, reactive oxygen species trigger a profound release of inflammatory cytokines that recruit inflammatory cells causing damage to tubular cells and the vascular endothelium. Reproduced with permission from Siedlecki et al. Delayed Graft Function in the Kidney Transplant. American Journal of Transplantation, 2011. 11:p.2279–2296

donor kidney transplants are likely distinct from those in deceased donor kidney transplants [10, 15–17]. However, the implications of DGF on kidney transplant outcomes may be just as significant [16, 18, 19].

Causes and Risk Factors: Transplant, Donor, and Recipient Factors

In addition to donor subtype, various recipient, donor, and transplant factors have been associated with an increased risk of DGF. Cold ischemia time (CIT) is one of the strongest risk factors for the development of DGF [20, 21]. In a large USRDS retrospective cohort study of 37,216 patients, CIT was found to be an independent risk factor for DGF with adjusted odds ratios of 1.38–3.48. Furthermore, the longer duration of CIT resulted in worse outcomes, with an increased risk of DGF of 23 % for every 6-h increase in CIT [21]. In the same study, donor age of >50 years was also a significant risk factor for DGF with an odds ratio of 2.07 (95 % CI: 1.89, 2.27; *P* value <0.001) [21]. This finding has been subsequently demonstrated in several more recent observational studies. [22, 23] There is also evidence that HLA-mismatched kidneys are associated with a higher risk of DGF than zero-mismatched kidneys [23–25].

In order to elucidate the role of recipient factors as determinants of DGF, Doshi et al. conducted a retrospective cohort study of pairs of kidney transplant recipients who shared the same donor, but only one recipient developed DGF [20]. Although there are limitations to this study, including potential confounding due to unmeasured variables, significant amounts of missing data, and lack of information on potential technical problems at the time of surgery, it provides new insights into the potential role of recipient factors as determinants for the risk of DGF. In this analysis of 5,382 recipient pairs, the following recipient risk factors were independently associated with an increased risk of DGF: male sex, African American race, diabetes, prior sensitization, prolonged wait time, and recipient obesity (BMI > 30 kg/m^2). As the prevalence of obesity increases, recent data have shown that obesity in the donor, in addition to the recipient, is also associated with an increased risk of DGF [26–28]. It has been hypothesized that obesity results in a pro-inflammatory state that may potentiate the ischemia–reperfusion injury in the allograft [29].

Multiple observational studies have evaluated the impact of pre-transplant dialysis modality on the post-transplant risk of DGF [30–35]. Two large registry studies have yielded conflicting results. Snyder et al. studied over 252,000 kidney transplant recipients and found that DGF rates were lower in peritoneal dialysis (PD) patients when compared to patients on hemodialysis (HD) [34]. However, more recently, a large registry study compared PD and HD patients using both conventional multivariable models and propensity score matching in a contemporary cohort of over 14,000 patients [33]. This study did not show any association between pre-transplant dialysis modality and risk of DGF. It is possible that residual confounding due to the observational nature of these studies may explain the variability in the results. The impact of pre-dialysis modality remains a largely unresolved issue at this time. It has been hypothesized that higher rates of DGF in HD patients may be attributable to the resulting state of volume depletion and predisposition to ischemic injury. Van Loo et al. demonstrated that in HD patients, ultrafiltration in the 24-h period prior to transplantation was associated with an increased incidence of DGF in comparison to HD patients without ultrafiltration [36]. Conversely, maintaining adequate intravascular volume via CVP monitoring (>8 mmHg) appears to reduce the risk of DGF [37]. Thus, avoidance of aggressive ultrafiltration prior to transplant, and the maintenance of adequate intravascular volume post-transplant, is a reasonable approach to decrease the risk of DGF.

Given the multitude of recipient, donor, and transplant risk factors identified in various reports, Irish et al. [23] derived a risk prediction model in recipients of deceased donor kidneys to quantify the risk of DGF. Using data from a cohort of 24,653 adult recipients of deceased donor kidneys captured in the UNOS database, 18 variables were included in the final predictive model. The five most significant predictor variables included CIT, terminal serum creatinine, recipient BMI, DCD kidney, and donor age. However, it is important to note that certain variables, which may be predictive of DGF, are not necessarily captured in the registry used to derive this prediction model. Nonetheless, the prediction model was externally validated using a separate dataset and showed good predictive ability with a concordance statistic (i.e., area under the receiver operating characteristic curve) of 0.704. Furthermore, the performance of the model was equally good across donor subtypes (i.e., ECD, DCD, and SCD). Given the large number of variables included in the model, the authors developed a nomogram as well as an online prediction tool to improve the usability of the model for clinicians [23].

Clinical Evaluation

The clinical manifestations of DGF are nonspecific, and therefore the clinician must exclude other potential causes of graft dysfunction and/or oliguria in the early post-transplant period. A recommended approach is depicted in Fig. 13.2 [38]. A careful volume assessment should be performed to rule out the possibility of hypovolemia and if present, volume expansion should be pursued. Renal Doppler ultrasound is an important step in the evaluation of DGF in order to rule out vascular complications such as arterial or venous thrombosis or urological complications such as urinary leak, lymphocele, hematoma, or ureteric obstruction. If urological complications are found, additional testing (e.g., cystoscopy with retrograde pyelogram) should be considered to delineate the urological abnormality prior to further surgical intervention. Additionally, if the patient is on a calcineurin inhibitor (CNI), drug levels can be measured to aid in the assessment of CNI toxicity. In the absence of an identifiable cause, a kidney transplant biopsy should be performed to rule out certain etiologies such as acute rejection or thrombotic angiopathy (see section "Management of DGF") [38]. The timing of renal biopsy is variable depending on the clinical scenario and the transplant center. In our center, we favor a biopsy at approximately 7 days post-transplant in patients with persistent graft dysfunction. Given the low incidence of DGF in living donor kidney transplant recipients, a comprehensive search for alternate explanations in this population is of utmost importance.

Prevention of DGF

When kidneys are recovered, they are generally flushed and cooled with a preservation solution, a process referred to as static cold storage. Cooling of the organ is protective by decreasing the metabolic rate at the cellular level during the ischemic period [6]. A number of preservation solutions have been developed to offset the biochemical changes that occur as

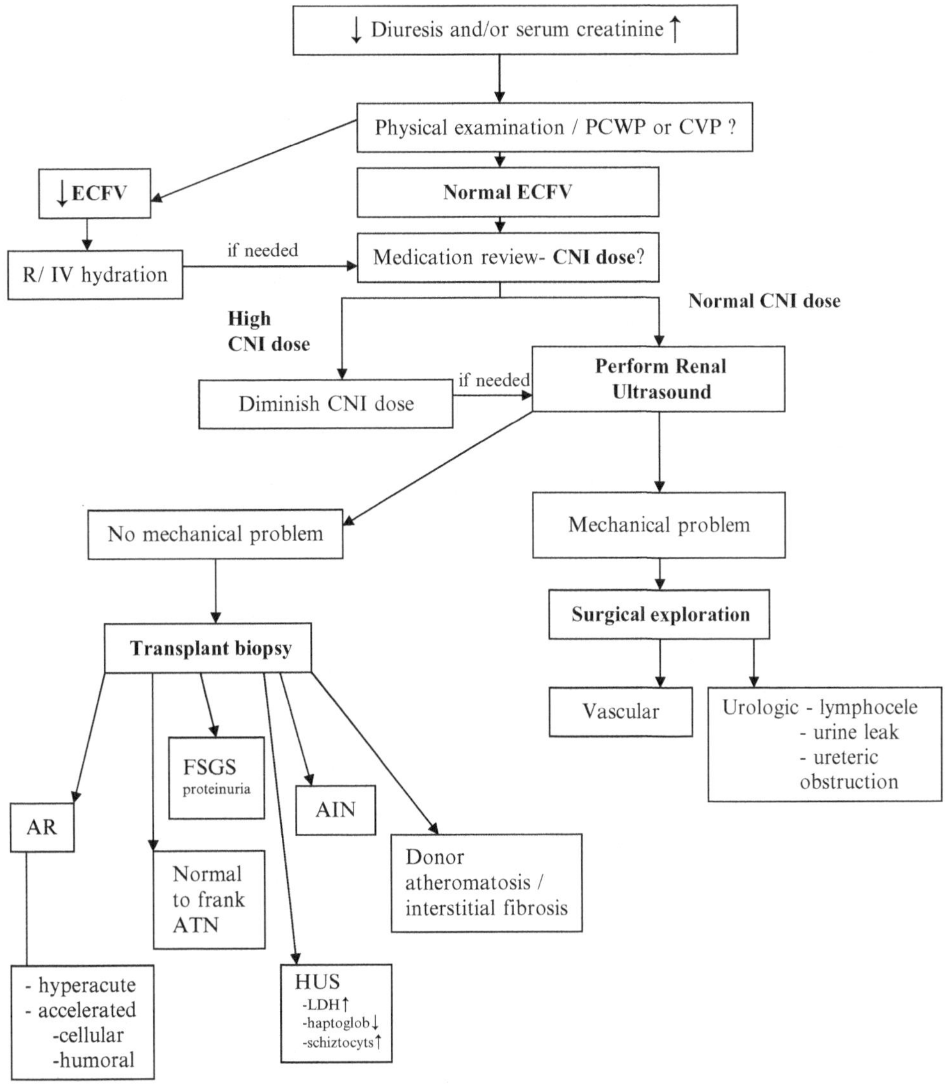

Fig. 13.2 Management of delayed graft function. *AIN* acute interstitial nephritis, *AR* acute rejection, *ATN* acute tubular necrosis, *CNI* calcineurin inhibitor, *CVP* central venous pressure, *ECFV* extracellular fluid volume, *FSGS* focal segmental glomerulosclerosis, *HUS* hemolytic-uremic syndrome, *PCWP* pulmonary capillary wedge pressure, *Screat* serum creatinine. Reproduced with permission from Peeters, P., et al., Delayed graft function in renal transplantation. Current Opinion in Critical Care, 2004. 10(6): p. 489–98

a result of ischemia, with the intent to decrease DGF rates. Commonly used preservation solutions include the Eurocollins (EC) solution, University of Wisconsin (UW) solution, Celsior solution, and histidine-tryptophan-ketoglutarate (HTK) solution. Although the differences among these solutions at a biochemical level are beyond the scope of this chapter, multiple studies have attempted to determine the most effective solution for decreasing the rates of DGF with variable results [39–41]. A recent meta-analysis of 15 studies showed an increased risk of DGF with the EC solution when compared to UW and HTK. However, no significant difference in DGF risk was found between UW, HTK, and Celsior solutions [42]. The randomized controlled trials (RCTs) included in the meta-analysis were generally of poor quality with variable reporting of blinding, the use of intention-to-treat analysis, and allocation concealment. Although multiple RCTs of acceptable size were included in this meta-analysis, the pooling of data cannot overcome the poor quality of the individual studies; thus, the results cannot be considered definitive.

The use of pulsatile machine perfusion (PMP) rather than cold storage has been explored in a number of large, well-designed, international, multicenter RCTs. Among SCD and ECD kidneys, two RCTs have demonstrated benefit in reducing DGF rates by using PMP rather than cold storage [43, 44]. Furthermore, a cost analysis of PMP utilization in ECD kidneys was associated with a decrease in hospitalization expenditures [45]. For DCD kidneys, however, similar high quality RCTs have yielded conflicting results. Watson et al. showed no benefit in PMP in comparison to cold storage in preventing DGF in recipients of DCD kidneys [46]. However, Moers et al. [43] and Jochmans et al. [47] showed significant improvements in DGF rates with PMP. The reasons for these conflicting data are not entirely clear but may at least partially relate to differences in study design and the populations studied. Nevertheless, the weight of the evidence suggests that PMP may reduce the risk of DGF and its associated costs in select kidney transplants.

The use of vasodilatory drugs has been extensively studied in the prevention of DGF. In particular, multiple, small, randomized trials have demonstrated that calcium channel blockers are potentially effective in the prevention of DGF. However, a significant limitation in the interpretation of the results is the small number of patients included in these studies. Furthermore, many of these studies were conducted prior to the increased use of ECD and DCD kidneys, thus limiting their generalizability. In order to overcome this issue, a systematic review was conducted, which included 13 RCTs comparing calcium channel blockers to placebo or no treatment [48]. Overall, the use of calcium channel blockers was associated with a decrease in DGF (risk ratio 0.55, 95 % CI: 0.42–0.73). However, there was significant heterogeneity among the studies included for analysis and the overall quality of the studies was poor. In particular, there were substantial differences in the definition of DGF used, the type of calcium channel blocker administered, the route of drug delivery (PO, IV, or in the preservation solution), and timing of delivery (i.e., pretreatment of recipient vs. treatment of donors). In addition, whether blinding had occurred was unclear in several studies. Given the potential adverse effects of using calcium channel blockers in the post-transplant period (e.g., increase in CNI levels), as well as the lack of large, high quality, and contemporary RCTs demonstrating benefit, these agents have generally not been used for the prevention of DGF [48].

Other vasodilatory agents, such as endothelin agonists, adenosine receptor antagonists, and atrial natriuretic peptide, have also been studied but their efficacy has not been well established. Additionally, given the importance of reactive oxygen species and the inflammatory response in the pathogenesis of DGF, multiple anti-inflammatory and antioxidant therapies are also being actively studied for potential future therapeutic use [6].

Use of dopamine in the donor has also been explored as a strategy to decrease the incidence of DGF. Dopamine optimizes renal perfusion, protects endothelial cells from oxidative stress, down-regulates endothelial adhesion molecules, and alters chemokine release, which are plausible mechanisms to explain the effect of dopamine to reduce the risk of DGF. In addition to small observational studies, a multicenter RCT of 264 patients evaluated the impact of a continuous infusion of dopamine in the donor until cross clamping had occurred [49, 50]. The results of this study showed that low dose dopamine was associated with a decrease in DGF rates. A subgroup analysis demonstrated that the effect of dopamine was more pronounced in kidney transplants with mean CIT of >21.2 h. However, the small sample size and open-label design were significant limitations of this study. Thus, this observation requires further substantiation before implementing it into routine clinical practice.

Management of DGF

The management of DGF is largely supportive. When clinically indicated, hemodialysis should be performed, although peritoneal dialysis is also appropriate if the peritoneal membrane has not been disturbed. Furthermore, in order to minimize any further ischemic injury, hemodynamic instability and use of nephrotoxic drugs should be avoided [1, 6]. Crystalloid solution should be used for volume expansion if needed rather than colloid solutions. At present, although there are some observational studies suggesting the benefits of albumin infusion to decrease DGF rates, there are no large controlled clinical trials to support its use. Furthermore, there are no data to suggest that colloids in general are beneficial in this setting. Loop diuretics are commonly used in the post-transplant period to stimulate diuresis; however, similar to ATN in native kidneys, studies have not suggested a beneficial impact in reducing DGF rates [51]. Although delaying the introduction of CNIs until renal function begins to improve is a common practice, the immediate initiation of CNIs likely does not prolong the recovery phase of DGF and in fact may decrease the risk of early acute rejection episodes when basiliximab induction is used [52, 53].

Generally, immunosuppression in the early post-transplant period is modified in patients at risk for or experiencing DGF. Given the known increased immunogenicity of the allograft as a result of DGF [24], the use of induction therapy has been extensively studied, most commonly with interleukin-2 receptor blockers (IL2RB) and rabbit antithymocyte globulin (rATG) [54]. A meta-analysis of eight RCTs found no difference in DGF rates between the two induction agents (two doses of basiliximab 20 mg vs. 6–9 mg/kg of rATG) with a pooled relative risk of 1.15 (95 % CI: 0.88–1.52; $P=0.31$) [55].

Table 13.2 Common preventive and therapeutic interventions in DGF

Intervention	Best evidence to date	Quality of evidence[a]	Summary of findings	Comments
Preservation solutions	Systematic review and meta-analysis of ten RCTs and five non-RCTs [42]	Moderate	UW and HTK superior to EC in preventing DGF; no difference in UW, HTK, and Celsior solutions	Quality of the majority of studies was poor; no information on blinding or intention-to-treat
Calcium channel blockers	Cochrane Systematic Review of 13 RCTs [48]	Low	Decrease in DGF with CCB use	Significant heterogeneity and small sample size of included studies, lack of studies in modern era of transplantation
Pulsatile machine perfusion (PMP): SCD and ECD kidneys	RCTs [43, 44]	High	PMP (vs. cold storage) reduced risk of DGF	Large, multicenter, high quality RCTs
Pulsatile machine perfusion: DCD kidneys	RCTs [43, 46, 47]	High; conflicting	PMP beneficial vs. cold storage in decreasing risk of DGF in two large RCTs, but one large negative RCT	Conflicting results of large, well-designed, multicenter RCTs
Dopamine	RCT [50]	Low	Low dose dopamine in the donor reduced DGF rates	Small, open-label, unblinded study; further data needed to support use
Basiliximab vs. rATG	Meta-analysis of eight RCTs [55]	Moderate	No difference in DGF between basiliximab and rATG	Further data needed to determine best induction therapy in the setting of DGF
Daclizumab vs. rATG	RCT [56]	Moderate	Decrease in DGF rates in rATG arm	DGF was secondary endpoint

[a]Quality of evidence as per GRADE criteria [66]

A more recent randomized controlled study comparing rATG vs. daclizumab demonstrated lower rates of DGF in the rATG arm (rATG 8.75 mg/kg vs. daclizumab 5 mg/kg) [56]. More research is needed to clarify the role of IL2RB in the setting of DGF.

The timing of induction therapy with rATG may influence the risk of DGF. Goggins et al. conducted a small RCT to evaluate this issue in a cohort of kidney transplant recipients. It showed that rATG decreases the incidence of DGF when administered intraoperatively (prior to reperfusion) vs. postoperatively (6 h after reperfusion) [57]. However, the trial was small in size and did not relate its short-term findings to long-term outcomes.

These preventive and therapeutic interventions, as well as the quality of evidence supporting their use, are summarized in Table 13.2.

Outcomes of DGF

In the short-term, DGF is clearly associated with higher transplant costs, prolonged hospitalization, and increase in patient morbidity [58, 59]. However, the impact of DGF on long-term outcomes in recipients of deceased donor kidneys has been controversial. Although some studies have found that patients without DGF enjoy better graft survival than those with DGF, other studies have shown no impact on long-term outcomes [60–62]. Furthermore, DGF potentially results in increased immunogenicity of the allograft due to the upregulation of HLAs on the vascular endothelium and release of inflammatory cytokines, which may increase the risk of acute rejection. However, the latter has not been a consistent finding in the literature [1].

In order to shed light on this controversial issue, a systematic review and meta-analysis of 33 studies evaluated the impact of DGF on graft survival, patient survival, renal function, and acute rejection episodes [63]. The impact of DGF on graft survival was significant with a pooled relative risk of 1.41 (95 % CI: 1.27–1.56; $P=0.002$). Multiple sensitivity analyses that accounted for acute rejection episodes, year of publication, follow-up time, and donor subtype resulted in similar findings. The impact of DGF on serum creatinine was also significant. Over an average follow-up time of 3.5 years, serum creatinine was higher in the DGF group than the non-DGF group. In this analysis, DGF was not associated with patient survival; however, it should be noted that follow-up time was 5 years, which may limit the ability to detect a difference in patient survival. DGF was also associated with a 38 % increase in acute rejection rates [46].

DGF is also strongly associated with death with graft function (DWGF) in both deceased and living donor kidney transplant recipients. In a retrospective cohort study of 50,246 deceased donor kidney transplant recipients, the hazard ratio for DWGF was 1.56 (95 % CI: 1.45–1.63) in patients with DGF vs. no DGF [47]. The risk for DWGF remained significantly elevated even among patients who achieved reasonable kidney function (eGFR 30–60 mL/min) at 6 and 12 months post-transplant. Similarly, DGF was strongly associated with an increased risk of DWGF among 44,630 living donor kidney transplant recipients. Although the highest risk of DWGF was in the early post-transplant period, the increased risk persisted over the long term [18, 64]. The causes of death were most commonly infection/sepsis and CVD/stroke in both studies. The reasons for this observed association are not entirely clear. It has been hypothesized that DGF may cause extrarenal organ dysfunction akin to patients with other forms of acute kidney injury and predispose patients to adverse long-term outcomes [65].

Conclusion

DGF continues to be a common problem in kidney transplantation. It has been shown that the central pathophysiological process of ischemia–reperfusion injury results in inferior patient and allograft survival. However, over time a better understanding of the complex mechanisms of DGF has allowed for the development of potential novel therapies. Ongoing research exploring gene expression and biomarkers of acute kidney injury will allow for a better understanding of the underlying risk for DGF in a donor–recipient pair. As well, current animal and human studies of antioxidant, anti-inflammatory, vasodilatory, and antiapoptotic agents show promise as therapeutic agents to reduce the burden of DGF in the kidney transplant population.

References

1. Perico N, et al. Delayed graft function in kidney transplantation. Lancet. 2004;364(9447):1814–27.
2. Yarlagadda SG, et al. Marked variation in the definition and diagnosis of delayed graft function: a systematic review. Nephrol Dial Transplant. 2008;23(9):2995–3003.
3. Israni AK, et al. Association of donor inflammation- and apoptosis-related genotypes and delayed allograft function after kidney transplantation. Am J Kidney Dis. 2008; 52(2):331–9.
4. Akkina SK, et al. Similar outcomes with different rates of delayed graft function may reflect center practice, not center performance. Am J Transplant. 2009;9(6):1460–6.
5. Koo DD, et al. Ischemia/reperfusion injury in human kidney transplantation: an immunohistochemical analysis of changes after reperfusion. Am J Pathol. 1998;153(2):557–66.
6. Siedlecki A, Irish W, Brennan DC. Delayed graft function in the kidney transplant. Am J Transplant. 2011;11(11):2279–96.
7. Ounissi M, Gargah T, Barbouch S, Boubaker K, Cherif M, Bacha MM, Abderrahim E, Ben Hamida F, Lakhoua R, Ben Abdallah T, Kheder A. Acute tubular necrosis in kidney transplantation. Tunis Med. 2012;90(6):463–7.
8. Shoskes DA, Halloran PF. Delayed graft function in renal transplantation: etiology, management and long-term significance. J Urol. 1996;155(6):1831–40.
9. Kosieradzki M, Rowinski W. Ischemia/reperfusion injury in kidney transplantation: mechanisms and prevention. Transplant Proc. 2008;40(10):3279–88.
10. Kwon OJ, et al. The impact of delayed graft function on graft survival in living donor kidney transplantation. Transplant Proc. 2003;35(1):92–3.
11. Snoeijs MGJ, et al. Kidney transplantation from donors after cardiac death: a 25-year experience. Transplantation. 2010;90(10): 1106–12.
12. Rojas-Pena A, et al. Extracorporeal support: improves donor renal graft function after cardiac death. Am J Transplant. 2010;10(6): 1365–74.
13. Pratschke J, Tullius SG, Neuhaus P. Brain death associated ischemia/reperfusion injury. Ann Transplant. 2004;9(1):78–80.
14. Nijboer WN, et al. Effect of brain death on gene expression and tissue activation in human donor kidneys. Transplantation. 2004;78(7):978–86.
15. Park HS, et al. Delayed graft function in living-donor renal transplantation: 10-year experience. Transplant Proc. 2012;44(1):43–6.
16. Senel FM, et al. Delayed graft function: predictive factors and impact on outcome in living-related kidney transplantations. Ren Fail. 1998;20(4):589–95.
17. Sharma AK, et al. Evaluation of factors causing delayed graft function in live related donor renal transplantation. Saudi J Kidney Dis Transpl. 2010;21(2):242–5.
18. Narayanan R, et al. Delayed graft function and the risk of death with graft function in living donor kidney transplant recipients. Am J Kidney Dis. 2010;56(5):961–70.
19. Brennan TV, et al. Early graft function after living donor kidney transplantation predicts rejection but not outcomes. Am J Transplant. 2004;4(6):971–9.
20. Doshi MD, et al. Recipient risk factors associated with delayed graft function: a paired kidney analysis. Transplantation. 2011;91(6):666–71.
21. Ojo AO, et al. Delayed graft function: risk factors and implications for renal allograft survival. Transplantation. 1997;63(7):968–74.
22. Robert R, et al. A pair analysis of the delayed graft function in kidney recipient: the critical role of the donor. J Crit Care. 2010;25(4):582–90.
23. Irish WD, et al. A risk prediction model for delayed graft function in the current era of deceased donor renal transplantation. Am J Transplant. 2010;10(10):2279–86.
24. Shoskes DA, Cecka JM. Deleterious effects of delayed graft function in cadaveric renal transplant recipients independent of acute rejection. Transplantation. 1998;66(12):1697–701.
25. Shoskes DA, et al. HLA matching determines susceptibility to harmful effects of delayed graft function in renal transplant recipients. Transplant Proc. 1995;27(1):1068–9.
26. Weissenbacher A, et al. Recipient and donor body mass index as important risk factors for delayed kidney graft function. Transplantation. 2012;93(5):524–9.
27. Gore JL, et al. Obesity and outcome following renal transplantation. Am J Transplant. 2006;6(2):357–63.
28. Chang SH, Coates PTH, McDonald SP. Effects of body mass index at transplant on outcomes of kidney transplantation. Transplantation. 2007;84(8):981–7.
29. Vgontzas AN, et al. Chronic systemic inflammation in overweight and obese adults. JAMA. 2000;283(17):2235. author reply 2236.
30. Binaut R, et al. Comparative study of chronic ambulatory peritoneal dialysis versus hemodialysis patients after kidney transplantation: clinical and financial assessment. Transplant Proc. 1997;29(5): 2428.
31. Bleyer AJ, et al. Dialysis modality and delayed graft function after cadaveric renal transplantation. J Am Soc Nephrol. 1999;10(1): 154–9.
32. Van Biesen W, et al. Peritoneal dialysis favorably influences early graft function after renal transplantation compared to hemodialysis. Transplantation. 2000;69(4):508–14.
33. Molnar MZ, et al. Dialysis modality and outcomes in kidney transplant recipients. Clin J Am Soc Nephrol. 2012;7(2):332–41.

34. Snyder JJ, et al. A comparison of transplant outcomes in peritoneal and hemodialysis patients. Kidney Int. 2002;62(4):1423–30.
35. Resende L, et al. Influence of dialysis duration and modality on kidney transplant outcomes. Transplant Proc. 2009;41(3):837–9.
36. Van Loo AA, et al. Pretransplantation hemodialysis strategy influences early renal graft function. J Am Soc Nephrol. 1998;9(3): 473–81.
37. Bacchi G, et al. The influence of intraoperative central venous pressure on delayed graft function in renal transplantation: a single-center experience. Transplant Proc. 2010;42(9):3387–91.
38. Peeters P, et al. Delayed graft function in renal transplantation. Curr Opin Crit Care. 2004;10(6):489–98.
39. Ploeg RJ, et al. Effect of preservation solution on results of cadaveric kidney transplantation. The European Multicentre Study Group. Lancet. 1992;340(8812):129–37.
40. de Boer J, et al. Eurotransplant randomized multicenter kidney graft preservation study comparing HTK with UW and Euro-Collins. Transpl Int. 1999;12(6):447–53.
41. Faenza A, et al. Kidney preservation with University of Wisconsin and Celsior solution: a prospective multicenter randomized study. Transplantation. 2001;72(7):1274–7.
42. O'Callaghan JM, Knight SR, Morgan RD, Morris PJ. Preservation solutions for static cold storage of kidney allografts: a systematic review and meta-analysis. Am J Transplant. 2012;12:896–906.
43. Moers C, et al. Machine perfusion or cold storage in deceased-donor kidney transplantation. N Engl J Med. 2009;360(1):7–19.
44. Treckmann J, et al. Machine perfusion versus cold storage for preservation of kidneys from expanded criteria donors after brain death. Transpl Int. 2011;24(6):548–54.
45. Buchanan PM, et al. Association of lower costs of pulsatile machine perfusion in renal transplantation from expanded criteria donors. Am J Transplant. 2008;8(11):2391–401.
46. Watson CJE, et al. Cold machine perfusion versus static cold storage of kidneys donated after cardiac death: a UK multicenter randomized controlled trial. Am J Transplant. 2010;10(9):1991–9.
47. Jochmans I, et al. Machine perfusion versus cold storage for the preservation of kidneys donated after cardiac death: a multicenter, randomized, controlled trial. Ann Surg. 2010;252(5):756–64.
48. Shilliday IR, Sherif M. Calcium channel blockers for preventing acute tubular necrosis in kidney transplant recipients. Cochrane Database Syst Rev. 2007;4, CD003421.
49. Schnuelle P, et al. Impact of donor dopamine on immediate graft function after kidney transplantation. Am J Transplant. 2004; 4(3):419–26.
50. Schnuelle P, et al. Effects of donor pretreatment with dopamine on graft function after kidney transplantation: a randomized controlled trial. JAMA. 2009;302(10):1067–75.
51. Schnuelle P, Johannes van der Woude F. Perioperative fluid management in renal transplantation: a narrative review of the literature. Transpl Int. 2006;19(12):947–59.
52. Andres A, et al. A randomized trial comparing renal function in older kidney transplant patients following delayed versus immediate tacrolimus administration. Transplantation. 2009;88(9):1101–8.
53. Borobia AM, et al. Trough tacrolimus concentrations in the first week after kidney transplantation are related to acute rejection. Ther Drug Monit. 2009;31(4):436–42.
54. Brennan DC, et al. Rabbit antithymocyte globulin versus basiliximab in renal transplantation. N Engl J Med. 2006;355(19):1967–77.
55. Liu Y, et al. Basiliximab or antithymocyte globulin for induction therapy in kidney transplantation: a meta-analysis. Transplant Proc. 2010;42(5):1667–70.
56. Noel C, et al. Daclizumab versus antithymocyte globulin in high-immunological-risk renal transplant recipients. J Am Soc Nephrol. 2009;20(6):1385–92.
57. Goggins WC, et al. A prospective, randomized, clinical trial of intra-operative versus postoperative Thymoglobulin in adult cadaveric renal transplant recipients. Transplantation. 2003;76(5):798–802.
58. Rosenthal JT, et al. The high cost of delayed graft function in cadaveric renal transplantation. Transplantation. 1991;51(5):1115–8.
59. Almond PS, et al. Economic impact of delayed graft function. Transplant Proc. 1991;23(1 Pt 2):1304.
60. Boom H, et al. Delayed graft function influences renal function, but not survival. Kidney Int. 2000;58(2):859–66.
61. Howard RJ, et al. Delayed graft function is associated with an increased incidence of occult rejection and results in poorer graft survival. Transplant Proc. 1993;25(1 Pt 2):884.
62. Giral-Classe M, et al. Delayed graft function of more than six days strongly decreases long-term survival of transplanted kidneys. Kidney Int. 1998;54(3):972–8.
63. Yarlagadda SG, et al. Association between delayed graft function and allograft and patient survival: a systematic review and meta-analysis. Nephrol Dial Transplant. 2009;24(3):1039–47.
64. Tapiawala SN, et al. Delayed graft function and the risk for death with a functioning graft. J Am Soc Nephrol. 2010;21(1):153–61.
65. Grams ME, Rabb H. The distant organ effects of acute kidney injury. Kidney Int. 2012;81(10):942–8.
66. Guyatt GH, et al. GRADE: an emerging consensus on rating quality of evidence and strength of recommendations. BMJ. 2008; 336(7650):924–6.

Evaluation and Initial Management of Graft Dysfunction

14

Alexander C. Wiseman and James E. Cooper

How to Understand It: Defining Graft Dysfunction

In a busy clinic, inpatient setting, transplant center, or urgent/emergent care setting, nephrologists often treat kidney transplant recipients in whom a concern is raised regarding graft dysfunction. In contrast to the general nephrology patient presenting with acute kidney injury (AKI), for which there have been active workgroups and guidelines that ultimately have led to a definition of AKI reflected in the RIFLE criteria (risk, injury, functional decline, loss, end-stage) [1], and guidelines for management of glomerular diseases such as diabetes, membranous nephropathy, and minimal change disease based upon quantification of proteinuria [2], there is not a universal definition for graft dysfunction in the kidney transplant setting. Recognizing a few differences in these presentations can help us to understand why there is not a similar definition in the transplant setting:

1. While the causes of allograft AKI can be due to the same etiologies as native AKI, allograft AKI also has unique causes that are specific to the transplant (examples include acute rejection, viral infection, and surgical complications) (Table 14.1), while native AKI is often due to systemic diseases or indirect renal insults (such as hemodyamic or nephrotoxic factors).
2. The differential diagnosis of allograft AKI changes with time following transplant, whereas the differential diagnosis of native AKI (prerenal, renal, and postrenal) can often be considered without regard to the chronology of a specific event.
3. The level of proteinuria that is associated with future graft dysfunction has been incompletely defined, unlike specific causes of native kidney diseases.
4. AKI in the allograft recipient often is an asymptomatic outpatient presentation, unlike native AKI which is typically an inpatient or emergency room presentation.

With these differences in mind and in the absence of a workgroup-defined definition, one must rely upon general consensus regarding the degree to which transplant graft dysfunction is clinically significant and requires further investigation. A reasonable working definition of transplant graft dysfunction is:

1. A rise in serum creatinine of 20 % over an established baseline, or
2. A failure of the serum creatinine to fall following transplant surgery, or
3. Proteinuria >300 mg per day (with caveats regarding the timing of measurement of proteinuria post-transplant, discussed below)

The Differential Diagnosis of Transplant Graft Dysfunction

A logical approach to the patients with allograft dysfunction can begin by considering transplant-related causes of prerenal, renal, and postrenal injury (Table 14.1).

Prerenal: The most common cause of prerenal azotemia in kidney transplantation is due to calcineurin inhibitor (CNI) use. This includes the medications cyclosporine (Neoral, Gengraf) and tacrolimus (Prograf). While the chronic effect of CNIs upon graft function is a subject of research and debate, it is well accepted that CNIs can cause AKI by vasoconstrictive effects on the afferent arteriole. These changes can occur within what is considered therapeutic trough ranges of these agents (e.g., a change in tacrolimus trough from 5 to 9 ng/ml). Other transplant-specific causes of AKI include complications of the surgical procedure such as arterial or venous thrombosis and anastamotic stricture (e.g., transplant renal artery stenosis). General causes of prerenal azotemia are quite common, including hypoperfusion related to

A.C. Wiseman (✉) • J.E. Cooper
Division of Renal Diseases and Hypertension, Transplant Center, University of Colorado, Denver, CO, USA
e-mail: Alexander.wiseman@ucdenver.edu

M.R. Weir and E.V. Lerma (eds.), *Kidney Transplantation: Practical Guide to Management*,
DOI 10.1007/978-1-4939-0342-9_14,

Table 14.1 Differential diagnosis of kidney transplant acute kidney injury

	Diagnosis	Immediate 0-1 week	Early 1-12 weeks	Late >12 weeks
Pre-Renal	Volume depletion, hypotension	xx	x	x
	Renal artery thrombosis	xx	x	
	CNI effects	xx	x	x
Renal	Delayed Graft Function (DGF)	xx		
	Acute Rejection •Cellular •Antibody-mediated	 x xx	 xx x	 x x
	Recurrent Primary Kidney Disease	(x)*	x	xx
	Infection •Urinary Tract Infection (UTI) •Polyoma Virus (BK)	 xx 	 xx x	 x xx
Post-Renal	Obstruction (lymphocele, ureteral stricture, urine leak, hematoma)	xx	x	

*focal segmental glomerulosclerosis

Table 14.2 Timeline of immunosuppression regimens and allograft outcomes

Era	Immunosuppression Developments	1 Year Acute Rejection	1 Year Graft Survival
1960's 1970's	Azathiaprine/Prednisone/ATG (horse)	75-100%	30-50%
1980's	Cyclosporine and OKT3 introduced	50%	80%
1990's	Mycophenolate, Tacrolimus, ATG (rabbit) introduced	25%	90%
2000's	IL-2 receptor Antibodies, Sirolimus introduced	10-15%	95%

hypovolemia and/or hypotension. Often small changes in volume status, renal blood flow, or blood pressure can result in AKI while patients are exposed to CNIs.

Intrarenal: Consideration of the potential location of renal injury can be helpful in formulating a differential diagnosis of graft dysfunction.

Tubulointerstitial: AKI related to ischemia reperfusion injury leading to acute tubular necrosis is related to donor factors such as age, cold ischemia time, and degree of warm ischemia time in the setting of donors who undergo organ procurement following circulatory arrest (see Chaps. 9 and 13, "Delayed Graft Function"). Acute cellular rejection remains a critical consideration in the assessment of transplant AKI. Tubulointerstitial inflammation in this setting is a predominantly T-lymphocyte-mediated process that has become less common over previous decades with the introduction of more potent immunosuppressive agents [3] (Table 14.2). However, depending upon risk factors of the donor and recipient and the immunosuppressive agents used, acute rejection rates may range from 10 % for the lowest risk patients to 40 % for the highest risk patients within the first year. With potent immunosuppression comes an increased risk of infection, another common intrarenal cause of graft AKI. The allograft is sensitive to ascending bacterial infections due to the lack of a natural ureterovesicular valve to prevent reflux, and transplant pyelonephritis can present rapidly after the early signs of cystitis, causing tubulointerstitial injury. Viral infections (commonly BKV, less commonly cytomegalovirus or adenovirus) also can cause AKI due to tubulointerstitial injury. Rarely, post-transplant lymphoproliferative disorder may present with graft dysfunction due to extensive lymphocyte infiltration of the allograft (see Chap. 25).

Vascular: More severe forms of acute rejection that are reflected by monocyte infiltration to the intimal layers of the arterioles (Banff grade II) or neutrophil infiltration of the peritubular capillaries (suggestive of antibody-mediated rejection, see Chap. 29) can occur and often are associated with under-immunosuppression. Severe forms can present as a thrombotic microangiopathy (TMA). Drug-associated TMA must also be considered, as there appears to be an association of TMA with CNI, with some reports of a higher propensity of TMA when CNIs are used in conjunction with MTOR inhibitors (sirolimus, everolimus) [4].

Glomerular: The finding of proteinuria with or without a change in GFR requires consideration of the patient's primary disease that led to renal failure, as a number of glomerulopathies may recur following transplant (see Chap. 15). The possibility of the development of a de novo glomerulonephritis must also be considered. Additionally, the potential development of transplant glomerulopathy, often associated with indolent antibody-mediated injury causing glomerular basement membrane duplication, is common following transplant and associated with a particularly poor graft prognosis [5].

Postrenal: Specific transplant-related causes of postrenal graft dysfunction include ureteral stricture, which may be due to anastamotic complications or to ureteral ischemia. While not definitive, an association of BKV infection/reactivation and ureteral stricture has been reported [6]. The ureter may become obstructed by compression of a fluid collection in the weeks following surgery, including hematoma, seroma, or lymphocoele. Finally, injury to the ureter can lead to urinary leak and urinoma formation, which may also compress the ureter leading to allograft dysfunction. This latter complication often presents clinically with pain at the site of urine leak, as urine can cause severe irritation of the peritoneal membrane.

Beyond these transplant-related causes of graft dysfunction, the differential diagnosis of AKI for native kidney disease should also be considered, including drug toxicities, IV contrast exposure, bladder dysfunction or prostatic hypertrophy, and systemic diseases that may influence renal blood flow.

The Influence of Time Post-transplant in the Differential Diagnosis of Allograft Dysfunction

A comprehensive assessment of the possible causes of allograft dysfunction is important since many of these etiologies can present at any time following transplant. However, the frequency of most of these causes follows a pattern that can aid the clinician in focusing upon likely causes depending on whether the assessment is immediately (within 1 week) following transplant, early (1–12 weeks) following transplant, or late (after 3 months) from transplant (Table 14.1).

Immediate Causes of Graft Dysfunction (Within 1 Week Following Surgery)

During the first week following transplant, prerenal causes predominate, due to ischemia–reperfusion injury-related acute tubular necrosis, hemodynamic effects, and rare circumstances of vascular complications. Hematoma formation may cause ureteral compression as early as 1 week following surgery. Heavy proteinuria due to recurrent focal glomerulosclerosis can lead to hemodynamic effects at this time. Of note, it may be difficult to distinguish proteinuria from native kidney versus transplant source in the setting of the patient transplanted prior to the need for dialysis or with residual renal function. In general, proteinuria from native kidneys tends to dissipate over 4–12 weeks after surgery presumed due to alterations in renal perfusion [7]. However, severe nephrotic range proteinuria even early following transplant requires consideration of transplant graft etiology.

Early Causes of Graft Dysfunction (1–12 Weeks Following Surgery)

After the immediate post-transplant window, other causes of graft dysfunction begin to predominate. Most importantly, the incidence of acute rejection is highest in the period 1–12 weeks following surgery. In otherwise low-risk recipients, acute cellular rejection occurs due to inadequate immunosuppression and the prevalence decreases precipitously from 3 to 12 months and in the years that follow. While acute rejection may occur in 10–15 % of low-risk patients within the first year, 80 % of those with rejection will present during the first 3 months following transplant [8]. Antibody-mediated rejection may occur during this window particularly in patients who have undergone pre-transplant desensitization protocols to permit transplant in the setting of preexisting HLA antibodies to the donor. CNI-related effects commonly cause fluctuations in renal function as doses are optimized and titrated during. Finally, postrenal effects related to ureteral complications due to lymphocoele formation and/or ureteral leak often present during this time window.

Late Causes of Graft Dysfunction (After 12 Weeks from Surgery)

After the early post-transplant period, surgical and anatomic causes of graft dysfunction diminish, the risk of acute rejection dissipates, and CNI levels generally become more stable. At this point, the causes of graft dysfunction more closely approach those noted in native kidney injury. However, infectious etiologies become more problematic as the immunosuppressive burden accumulates. Viral infections, in particular BKV, often present 3–12 months following surgery. BKV reactivation can lead to tubulointerstitial nephritis in susceptible individuals whose immunosuppression is kept at moderate to high levels, with a

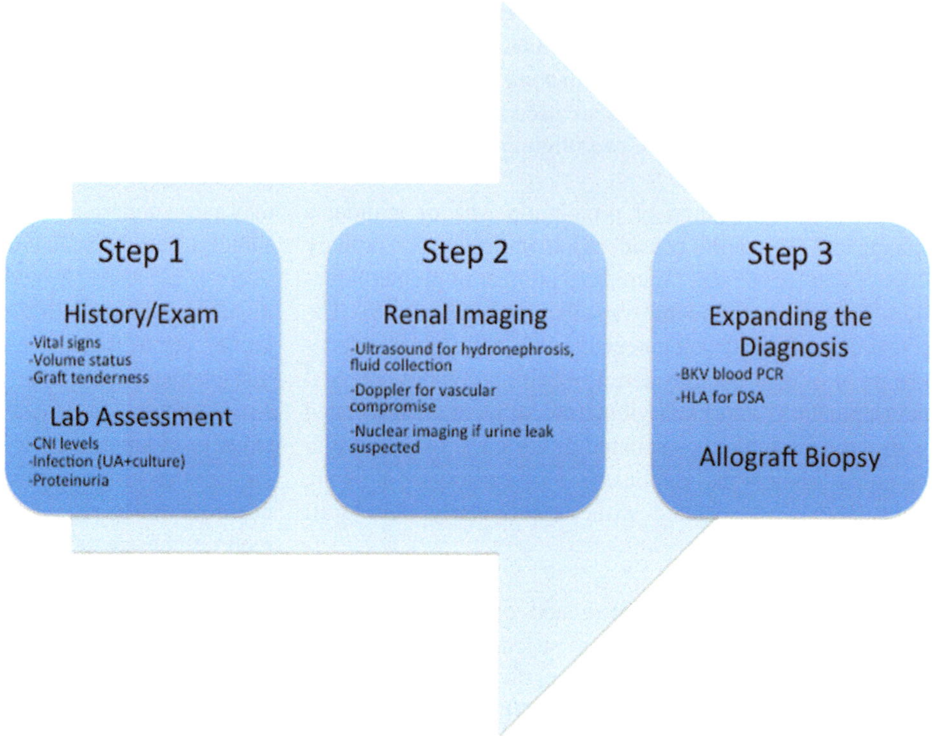

Fig. 14.1 Stepwise approach to the patient with kidney allograft dysfunction

peak in overt graft dysfunction from 6 to 12 months following transplant [9]. Bacterial urinary tract infections remain a persistent problem beyond 3 months from transplant; recurrent infections may require long-term suppressive antibiotic therapy. Recurrent glomerular diseases such as ANCA-related glomerulonephritis, membranoproliferative glomerulonephritis, and atypical hemolytic uremic syndrome are sporadic and can recur at any time post-transplant. Finally, while transplant glomerulopathy may rarely present within the first year following transplant, the incidence and severity increase in the years following transplant.

While the consideration of the temporal relationship of causes of graft dysfunction is helpful in predicting the most *likely* etiology, a high level of awareness of all these processes is necessary as many of the causes of graft dysfunction can appear at atypical periods. Clearly, acute rejection can occur at any time following transplant when there have been alterations in medication dosing, adherence, or absorption/metabolism, and BKV nephritis has been reported as late as 9 years following transplant [10]. Extending throughout these eras include the common causes of hemodynamic insults, including fluctuations in CNI exposure.

Management

Based on the differential diagnosis outlined above, a stepwise approach to the patient with graft dysfunction can be applied based on the frequency of these events post-transplant (Fig. 14.1).

Step 1: History, physical examination, and screening laboratory testing

Assessment of vital signs and clinical findings should focus upon potential hemodynamic, infectious, or structural causes of graft dysfunction. Important questions to address in the history include new medications or change in medication dosing that may have occurred (with specific questions regarding nonsteroidal anti-inflammatory agents and ACE/ARB use due to effects on renal blood flow/perfusion pressure, as well as nondihydropyridine calcium channel blocker and antifungal agents due to effects on CNI metabolism), recent potential hemodynamic insults such as vomiting or diarrhea (which can alter CNI metabolism and effect exposure), and any recent history of medication nonadherence. Key physical examination measures include blood pressure and pulse, assessment for graft tenderness (Table 14.3), examination for abdominal bruit, and assessment of skin turgor and edema. Initial laboratory assessment should consist of CNI trough level measurement, urinalysis dipstick followed by microscopy and culture if pyuria, nitrite, or leukocyte esterase is present, and assessment for proteinuria with spot urine/protein creatinine ratio if urine dipstick demonstrates proteinuria at 2+ or greater.

Step 1 will define prerenal effects, CNI effects, and infectious causes, and initially begin to assess for a potential glomerular cause of graft dysfunction.

Step 2: Renal imaging

If the diagnosis of graft dysfunction cannot be made with confidence in step 1, one should proceed with imaging of the kidney with ultrasound to assess for structural causes of graft dysfunction. If hydronephrosis is identified, assessment for fluid collections (simple fluid collections, such as lymphocoele or urinoma, or complex collections, either hematoma or abscess) versus ureteral strictures versus lower tract pathology (atonic bladder, prostatic hypertrophy) should be pursued as potential causes.

Step 3: Expanding the differential diagnosis

If the results from steps 1 and 2 are unrevealing, consideration of less common causes of graft dysfunction must be pursued. These include BKV nephropathy and other unusual viral infections (such as adenovirus or even less commonly CMV), post-transplant lymphoproliferative disease, or TMA. While noninvasive testing is available for BKV via polymerase chain reaction (PCR), in the setting of graft dysfunction if the diagnosis has not been clarified with step 1 and step 2 then a renal transplant biopsy should be pursued.

Table 14.3 Differential diagnosis of allograft pain

Early	Late
Ruptured Graft	Rejection of failed graft (after weaning immunosuppression)
Acute (large) arterial or venous bleed	Large stone
Acute arterial (iliac) thrombosis	**Anytime**
Urinoma	Pyelonephritis
Graft necrosis	Fluid collection (blood, urine)
Severe hyper-acute rejection	Pathologic events adjacent to graft (appendix, hernia, SBO)

Maintaining a High Degree of Suspicion for Acute Rejection

While the incidence of acute rejection is falling as mentioned above, missing this diagnosis has long-term consequences for allograft longevity and therefore should be considered throughout the stepwise process outlined above. Depending on the degree and rate of rise in serum creatinine, particularly if there are day-by-day changes in creatinine without other etiology identified, acute rejection must be ruled out by biopsy and steps 1–3 may be performed within a 12–24 h period.

In the future, noninvasive diagnosis of allograft pathology may have important implications for the transplant community as kidney transplant biopsy can be costly, time-consuming, and associated with patient morbidity, discomfort, and inconvenience. Numerous reports have described biomarkers detected in either peripheral blood or urine and are associated with varying levels of sensitivity and specificity (Table 14.4). Larger trials, however, are required to validate biomarker use in clinical practice. Until such time, allograft biopsy remains the gold standard for diagnosis of allograft rejection and dysfunction.

When to Consider Empiric Treatment for Acute Rejection

Occasionally a biopsy may not be immediately feasible due to anticoagulation or a poor window for performing a biopsy safely (bowel or fluid collections overlying the kidney). In these circumstances, it is reasonable to give a trial of antirejection therapy provided other causes of graft dysfunction (hypovolemia, obstruction, infection, CNI nephrotoxicity, glomerulonephritis) have been ruled out. Blood for BKV and HLA testing donor-specific antibody should be performed

Table 14.4 Biomarker studies in acute kidney allograft rejection

Biomarker	Method	Sensitivity	Specificity	n
Perforin[1]	Urine mRNA by PCR	83	83	22
Granzyme B[1]	Urine mRNA by PCR	79	77	22
Any 2 of either perforin, FasL, or granzyme B[2]	Peripheral blood mRNA by PCR	100	95	31
FOXP3[3]	Urine mRNA by PCR	90	73	83
IL-6[4]	Peripheral blood Luminex	92	63	64
DUSP1, MAPK9, NKTR, PBEF1, and PSEN1[5]	Peripheral blood microarray gene transcript profiling	91	94	367

[1]N Engl J Med. 2001;344(13):947
[2]Transplantation. 1998;66(5):562
[3]N Engl J Med. 2005;353(22):2342
[4]Clin J Am Soc Nephrol. 2012;7(6):1018
[5]*Am J Transplant 2012; 12: 2710–2718*

since either of these findings would potentially alter management and lead one to either reduce (in the case of BKV) or expand (in the case of donor-specific antibody) immunosuppressive therapy.

Initial Management of Immunosuppression

Often the evaluation of graft dysfunction is an evolving process that occurs over days, and clinical decision-making regarding immunosuppression must be made empirically in the interim. For cases in which bacterial infections or hemodynamic causes are clearly contributory, one reasonable strategy is to reduce or hold the CNI for a brief period (1–3 days) while definitive treatment (antibiotics and/or fluid resuscitation) proceeds, in order to prevent additional potentiation of injury via CNI-induced vasoconstriction. When a postrenal cause of renal dysfunction is identified, alterations in immunosuppression are less likely to be necessary, and urgent management of hydronephrosis should be the priority rather than manipulation of immunosuppression. In setting of an undefined etiology of renal dysfunction, it is most appropriate to maintain immunosuppression and proceed with biopsy rather than empirically adjust based upon suspicion of over-immunosuppression (viral-induced injury) or under-immunosuppression (acute rejection).

Why Is It Important? The Consequences of a Missed Diagnosis

Allograft dysfunction requires urgent evaluation and a heightened sense of awareness of a patient's baseline renal function and proteinuria status. Too often, a subacute rise in serum creatinine is considered "near baseline" while in reality the "baseline" continues to deteriorate, often referred to as "creeping creatinine." Often, changes in serum creatinine reflect injury patterns that have been ongoing for prolonged periods and are difficult to resolve once dysfunction is present. Classic examples include BKV nephropathy, antibody-mediated rejection, and chronic obstruction. Additionally, acute rejection that evolves to include severe tubulointerstitial and vascular injury has long-term consequences upon the longevity of the allograft [8, 11]. By approaching each kidney transplant patient in an organized fashion, ideally one can avoid the pitfall of under-recognition of evolving injury patterns.

References

1. Bellomo R, Ronco C, Kellum JA, Mehta RL, Palevsky P. Acute renal failure - definition, outcome measures, animal models, fluid therapy and information technology needs: the Second International Consensus Conference of the Acute Dialysis Quality Initiative (ADQI) Group. Crit Care. 2004;8:R204–12.
2. KDOQI clinical practice guidelines for chronic kidney disease: evaluation, classification, and stratification http://www.kidney.org/professionals/kdoqi/guidelines_commentaries.cfm
3. The Scientific Registry of Transplant Recipients 2010 Annual Report http://www.srtr.org/annual_reports/2010/
4. Fortin MC, Raymond MA, Madore F, et al. Increased risk of thrombotic microangiopathy in patients receiving a cyclosporin-sirolimus combination. Am J Transplant. 2004;4:946–52.
5. Cosio FG, Gloor JM, Sethi S, Stegall MD. Transplant glomerulopathy. Am J Transplant. 2008;8:492–6.
6. Pahari A, Rees L. BK virus-associated renal problems–clinical implications. Pediatr Nephrol. 2003;18:743–8.
7. Shamseddin MK, Knoll GA. Posttransplantation proteinuria: an approach to diagnosis and management. Clin J Am Soc Nephrol. 2011;6:1786–93.
8. Meier-Kriesche HU, Schold JD, Srinivas TR, Kaplan B. Lack of improvement in renal allograft survival despite a marked decrease in acute rejection rates over the most recent era. Am J Transplant. 2004;4:378–83.
9. Wiseman AC. Polyomavirus nephropathy: a current perspective and clinical considerations. Am J Kidney Dis. 2009;54:131–42.
10. Bansal S, Lucia MS, Wiseman A. A case of polyomavirus-associated nephropathy presenting late after transplantation. Nat Clin Pract Nephrol. 2008;4:283–7.
11. McDonald S, Russ G, Campbell S, Chadban S. Kidney transplant rejection in Australia and New Zealand: relationships between rejection and graft outcome. Am J Transplant. 2007;7:1201–8.

15 Recurrent and De Novo Diseases After Renal Transplantation

Geoffrey K. Dube and David J. Cohen

Recurrent/De Novo Glomerulonephritis

Prevalence

The true prevalence of recurrent and de novo diseases, especially glomerulonephritis (GN), and the impact of these diseases on allograft survival may be underestimated for several reasons. First, many patients present late in the course of their native kidney disease and do not undergo native kidney biopsy; thus, the original disease is unknown, making it impossible to distinguish recurrent disease from de novo disease. Second, many patients do not undergo biopsy of a failing allograft, so the precise causes leading to allograft failure are never identified. Similarly, biopsies may not be performed in patients with asymptomatic urinary abnormalities and a well-functioning allograft. Third, when allograft biopsies are performed, multiple disease processes may be recognized, and the presence of recurrent disease may be overlooked or unrecognized. If recurrent disease is identified, it may be difficult to determine to what extent it is contributing to allograft dysfunction. Fourth, centers differ in how frequently they perform immunofluorescence (IF) and electron microscopy (EM) on allograft biopsies, so many cases of recurrent disease may go unrecognized. Finally, clinicians may differ as to whether histologic evidence of disease recurrence, in the absence of any clinical manifestations, constitutes recurrent disease. Table 15.1 shows a classification scheme for recurrent and de novo diseases.

Single-center and multicenter series have reported recurrent GN rates ranging from 1.8 to 20 %, depending on the criteria used to diagnose recurrence, and the duration of post-transplant follow-up. In the Renal Allograft Disease Registry (RADR), a consortium of six American transplant centers, the rate of recurrent and de novo GN was 3.4 % at a mean follow-up of 65 months [1]. Briganti et al., in analyzing registry data from Australia and New Zealand, found that 8.4 % of allografts were lost due to recurrent GN at 10 years post-transplant [2]. The analysis did not include patients with recurrent disease who did not lose their grafts, but the fact that the incidence of graft loss from recurrent GN continued to increase over time suggests that the overall incidence of recurrent GN in this population was higher than 8.4 %. The risk for recurrence (either clinical or histological) for various diseases is shown in Table 15.2. There have been no registry reports on de novo disease, and in the RADR recurrent and de novo diseases were analyzed together, making it difficult to determine the overall prevalence of de novo disease.

Clinical Presentation

Recurrent and de novo glomerular diseases have similar clinical findings as native kidney disease, with a combination of proteinuria, microscopic or gross hematuria, and/or graft dysfunction. The time to histologic or clinical recurrence of glomerular disease can range from immediately postoperative (focal segmental glomerulosclerosis (FSGS)) to more than a decade after transplant (IgA nephropathy (IgAN) or diabetic nephropathy). True de novo disease, as opposed to recurrence of native kidney disease, tends to occur later after transplant, although cases of de novo anti-glomerular basement membrane (GBM) disease in patients with Alport's disease have been described in the first month after transplant. The development of drug-induced de novo thrombotic microangiopathy (TMA), due to calcineurin-inhibitors or mTOR inhibitors, usually occurs within the first few months post-transplant.

G.K. Dube, M.D. • D.J. Cohen, M.D. (✉)
Division of Nephrology, Columbia University Medical Center, 622 West 168th Street, PH4-124, New York, NY 10032, USA
e-mail: Djc5@columbia.edu

M.R. Weir and E.V. Lerma (eds.), *Kidney Transplantation: Practical Guide to Management*,
DOI 10.1007/978-1-4939-0342-9_15, © Springer Science+Business Media New York 2014

Table 15.1 Classification of recurrent and de novo diseases after transplant

Primary glomerular disease	Systemic disease	Metabolic disease	De novo disease
Focal segmental glomerulosclerosis	Systemic lupus erythematosus	Diabetic nephropathy	Membranous nephropathy
IgA nephropathy	Henoch–Schonlein purpura	Oxalosis	Anti-GBM disease
MPGN type I	Atypical HUS	Fabry's disease	HUS
Dense deposit disease	Amyloidosis/LCDD		Diabetic nephropathy
Membranous nephropathy	Anti-GBM disease		
Fibrillary GN	ANCA vasculitis		
	Scleroderma		

IgA immunoglobulin A, *GBM* glomerular basement membrane, *MPGN* membranoproliferative glomerulonephritis, *HUS* hemolytic-uremic syndrome, *LCDD* light chain deposition disease, *ANCA* antineutrophil cytoplasmic antibody

Table 15.2 Risk of disease recurrence

Disease	Risk in percentage
FSGS	30–50
IgA nephropathy	30–50
MPGN type I	20–50
Membranous nephropathy	10–40
Dense deposit disease	80–100
Atypical HUS	50
ANCA-associated vasculitis	10–20
SLE	10–30
HSP	20–80
Diabetes mellitus	40
Oxalosis	80–100
Fabry's disease	<5

FSGS focal segmental glomerulosclerosis, *IgA* immunoglobulin A, *MPGN* membranoproliferative glomerulonephritis, *HUS* hemolytic-uremic syndrome, *ANCA* antineutrophil cytoplasmic antibody, *SLE* systemic lupus erythematosus, *HSP* Henoch–Schonlein purpura
Percentages include both clinical and histologic recurrences

Impact on Graft Outcomes

Despite advances in understanding the pathogenesis of many renal diseases, treatment options for many recurrent diseases remain limited and disease recurrence frequently leads to allograft dysfunction and ultimately failure. In RADR, the 5-year graft survival in patients with recurrent disease was 39.8 % compared with 67.6 % in patients without recurrent disease. The relative risk for graft failure was 1.9, and the relative risk for graft failure for individual diseases was significantly higher for membranoproliferative GN (MPGN) (2.37), FSGS (2.25), and hemolytic-uremic syndrome (HUS) (5.36) [1]. Analysis of registry data from Australia found an 8.4 % rate of graft failure from recurrent disease over 10 years. In that analysis, the relative risk of graft failure was significantly higher for FSGS (2.03) and MPGN type I (2.91) [2]. For certain diseases, recurrence may be more common with live donors (especially living-related donors) as compared with deceased donors. Indeed, some authors have found that recurrent disease is the most common cause of graft failure in recipients of HLA-identical living-related transplants [3]. However, despite the higher risk of graft failure from recurrent disease, overall graft survival for all primary diseases tends to be higher with living donors as compared with deceased donors. Figure 15.1a shows the relative risk of allograft failure from recurrent disease, as compared with other common causes of graft failure. Figure 15.2 shows the relative risk of allograft failure from recurrent glomerulonephritis for different subtypes of glomerular disease.

There are fewer data on the impact of de novo disease on graft survival. Early reports of de novo TMA likely included many patients with antibody-mediated rejection, making it difficult to determine the relative contribution of each to graft failure. De novo TMA, when caused by medications, has an excellent prognosis when the drug is able to be withdrawn completely [4]. Graft loss is rare in patients with de novo TMA localized to the kidney, although it may occur in some patients with systemic manifestations of TMA [5]. De novo diabetic nephropathy progresses more rapidly than native kidney disease and has a poorer prognosis [6]. De novo membranous nephropathy, which may represent a form of chronic rejection (discussed below), has a poor prognosis, with up to 40 % progressing to graft failure [7].

Impact of Immunosuppression on Disease Recurrence

While improvements in induction and maintenance immunosuppression have greatly improved renal allograft outcomes, these advances do not appear to have translated into any decrease in recurrent disease. Analysis of USRDS data from 1990 to 2003 found a 10-year incidence of allograft failure from recurrent GN of 2.6 %. The use of prednisone, cyclosporine, tacrolimus, sirolimus, azathioprine, or mycophenolate was not associated with any difference in graft failure from recurrent disease. Additionally, there was no difference in the risk of graft failure between cyclosporine and tacrolimus or between azathioprine and mycophenolate [8].

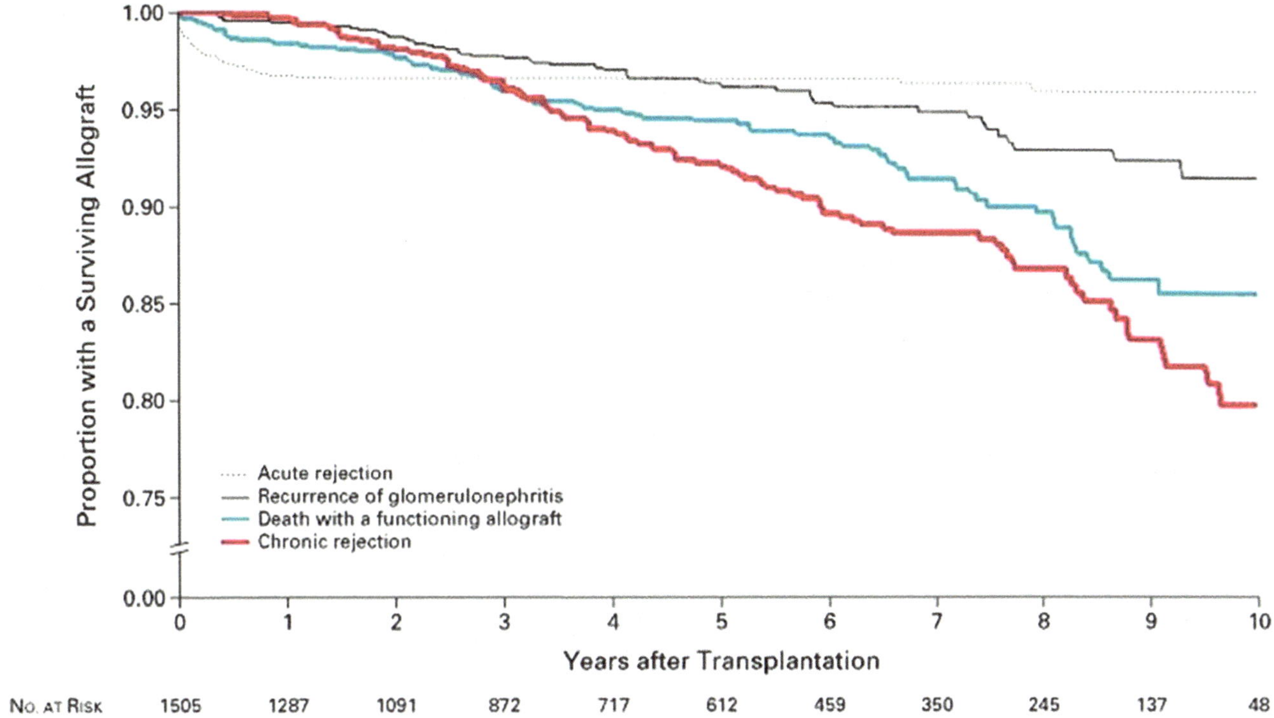

Fig. 15.1 Allograft failure due to recurrent disease, as compared with allograft failure due to other causes. Briganti EM et al. N Engl J Med 2002;347:103-109

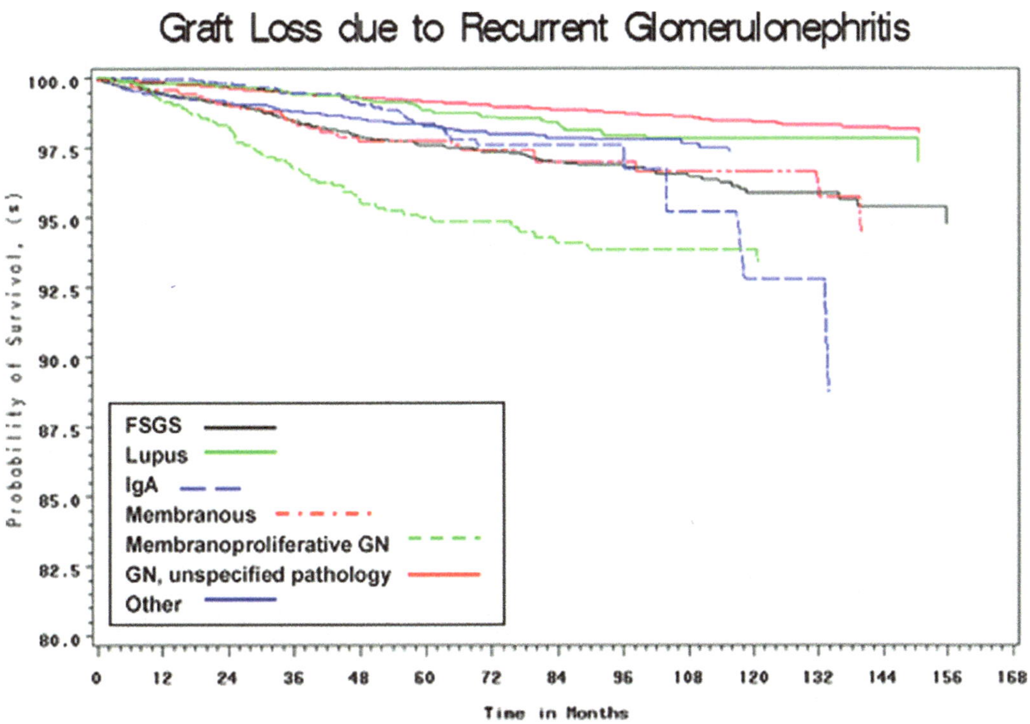

Fig. 15.2 Allograft failure from recurrent disease, by subtype of glomerular disease. American Journal of Transplantation. Volume 9, Issue 4, pages 804-811, 6 Mar 2009 DOI: 10.1111/j.1600-6143.2009.02554.x. http://onlinelibrary.wiley.com/doi/10.1111/j.1600-6143.2009.02554.x/full#f1

Table 15.3 Possible pathogenetic factors and potential therapeutic interventions used for various recurrent and de novo diseases

Disease	Pathogenesis	Potential therapies
FSGS	Circulating serum factor	Plasmapheresis, rituximab, galactose
Membranous nephropathy	Anti-PLA2R antibodies	Rituximab
IgA nephropathy	Aberrantly glycosylated IgA1	
MPGN type I	Circulating immune complexes, dysregulation of alternative complement pathway	Eculizumab
Dense deposit disease	Dysregulation of alternative complement pathway	Eculizumab, rituximab
Atypical HUS	Dysregulation of alternative complement pathway	Eculizumab
Lupus	Autoantibodies	
Anti-GBM disease	Antibody to alpha5 chain of type IV collagen	Plasmapheresis, cyclophosphamide
ANCA vasculitis	P-ANCA, C-ANCA	Plasmapheresis, cyclophosphamide, rituximab
Diabetes mellitus	Hyperglycemia	Pancreas transplantation, with or after kidney transplantation

FSGS focal segmental glomerulosclerosis, *PLA2R* M-type phospholipase A2 receptor, *IgA* immunoglobulin A, *MPGN* membranoproliferative glomerulonephritis, *HUS* hemolytic-uremic syndrome, *GBM* glomerular basement membrane, *ANCA* antineutrophil cytoplasmic antibody

Although the choice of immunosuppression medication did not impact the risk of graft failure from recurrent disease, the risk of graft failure from recurrent disease was lower in transplants performed in more recent years.

Although registry data have not shown an increased risk of graft loss from recurrent disease in patients not maintained on prednisone, Kukla et al. reported higher rates of recurrent glomerular disease in patients on a steroid-free regimen: 1-, 5-, and 7-year recurrence rates were 6.7, 13.7, and 19.2%, compared with 2.4, 3.8, and 5.3 % in historic controls maintained on prednisone. Rates of histologic recurrence were significantly higher at all time points for FSGS, membranous, and IgAN, and were numerically, though not statistically, higher at all time points for MPGN. Despite the higher rate of disease recurrence, there was no difference in allograft survival at 7 years [9].

Pascual et al. reported on the effect of induction therapy on the risk of recurrent disease in 443 recipients with ESRD secondary to biopsy-proven glomerular disease. Clinical recurrence of glomerular disease was numerically higher with use of alemtuzumab (8.7 %) or basiliximab (10.1 %) compared with use of thymoglobulin (1.5 %). Mean follow-up was significantly shorter with alemtuzumab, raising concern that larger differences in recurrence rates could develop over time [10].

Pathogenesis and Treatment

The pathogenesis and treatment differ for each recurrent disease. Table 15.3 summarizes current understanding of the pathogenesis of the individual diseases discussed below, as well as potential treatment options based on our current understanding of each disease.

Primary Glomerular Diseases

Focal Segmental Glomerulosclerosis

FSGS recurs in 20–50 % of patient after transplant. The wide range of reported recurrence rates is likely explained by the fact that some patients had secondary forms of FSGS in the native kidney, which would not be expected to recur. Recurrent FSGS is characterized by the early onset of heavy proteinuria in association with graft dysfunction. Disease recurrence typically occurs within the first year post-transplant. FSGS may recur within the first 24 h of transplant, and foot process effacement may be found on intraoperative biopsies [11]. Biopsies taken early in the course of disease recurrence may appear normal by light microscopy, with histologic evidence of the disease being limited to extensive foot process effacement by EM. However, as the disease progresses, classic lesions of FSGS will become apparent on light microscopy.

The finding that FSGS can recur immediately post-transplant suggested the presence of a circulating factor causing the initial podocyte injury [12]. Savin et al. reported finding a circulating permeability factor in the serum of some patients with recurrent FSGS that increased glomerular permeability to albumin [13]. Recently, Wei et al. found that levels of serum-soluble urokinase receptor (suPAR) are elevated in many patients with primary FSGS and that higher levels pre-transplant increased the risk of post-transplant recurrence. Animal models confirmed the ability of circulating suPAR to activate podocyte β3 integrin, leading to foot process effacement, proteinuria, and FSGS [14].

While these findings suggest that suPAR may be the permeability factor responsible for some cases of recurrent

FSGS, recurrent disease can also develop in patients whose FSGS is due to an underlying genetic defect. Congenital nephrotic syndrome of the Finnish type, due to mutations in nephrin, recurs in 25 % of patients. Disease recurrence appears to be limited to patients with the Fin-major/Fin-major genotype, who have complete absence of nephrin in their native kidneys and develop circulating anti-nephrin antibodies directed against the transplant [15]. Jungraithmayr et al. screened 53 patients for mutations in NPHS2. Recurrence rates were 0 % in patients with homozygous, heterozygous, or compound heterozygous mutations in NPHS2 and 45 % in patients without any NPHS2 mutations; graft failure was also significantly higher in patients without NPHS2 mutations [16]. While recent research has identified mutations in the TRPC6, CD2AP, ACTN4, and IFN2 genes leading to FSGS, there are currently no data on whether mutations in these genes affect the risk of disease recurrence after transplant.

The clinical risk factors for recurrent FSGS include younger age, rapid progression of original disease, Caucasian race, and a history of prior graft loss due to recurrent disease. Early reports suggested that graft loss from recurrent FSGS may be higher with living-related donors, especially HLA-identical donors. However, a large registry analysis found that, after correction for other risk factors, a living donor had no association with graft loss from recurrent disease [17]. Further analysis revealed that long-term graft survival was significantly better with 0-mismatch live donors as compared with nonidentical live donors or any type of deceased donor. While long-term graft survival is excellent, at 10 years 12.7 % of grafts may be lost due to recurrent disease, and the risk of allograft failure from recurrent disease is significantly greater with FSGS compared with most other forms of primary glomerular disease [18].

The most commonly used treatment for recurrent FSGS is plasmapheresis, which leads to partial or complete remission in 60–70 % of patients. Plasmapheresis is usually administered three times a week until the patient is in clinical remission, followed by a gradual reduction in the frequency of treatments. While many patients are able to discontinue plasmapheresis without triggering a relapse, some patients require chronic plasmapheresis in order to maintain a clinical remission. The efficacy of plasmapheresis is in theory due to decreasing the concentration of the circulating factor causing podocyte injury. Wei et al. reported that two patients with recurrent FSGS had remissions with plasmapheresis associated with a reduction in suPAR to near physiologic levels, while two patients in whom suPAR remained elevated despite plasmapheresis did not experience remission [14]. While these findings are intriguing, it remains to be determined whether monitoring suPAR levels will be useful in guiding clinical management of recurrent FSGS.

Other treatment options for recurrent FSGS include high-dose steroids and intravenous cyclosporine for 14 days [19]. Rituximab has been tried as either initial or salvage therapy for patients with recurrent FSGS, either at the time of initial recurrence or in the setting of a relapse. In a review of the published literature to-date, complete remission of proteinuria was seen in 43.5 % of patients, with partial remission seen in an additional 20.5 %. However, plasmapheresis was given concurrently in 38/39 patients. On multivariate analysis, younger age and normal serum albumin at the time of recurrence were the only two factors predictive of a response to rituximab [20]. There is a single case report of oral galactose being used successfully to treat recurrent FSGS, possibly by binding to the circulating permeability factor [21].

It is uncertain whether pre-transplant plasmapheresis has any beneficial effect on the likelihood of recurrence. Gohh et al. reported that 7/10 patients considered at high risk for recurrence, including 3/6 patients who had lost a prior graft to recurrent disease, were free of recurrent FSGS and had excellent graft function after receiving eight perioperative plasmapheresis treatments [22]. By contrast, Hickson et al. found that FSGS recurred in 6/7 high-risk patients treated with preemptive plasmapheresis therapy [23]. As these studies did not report suPAR levels, it remains unclear whether pre-transplant plasmapheresis to reduce suPAR levels will impact the risk or timing of recurrent disease.

Immunoglobulin A Nephropathy

IgAN is the most frequent primary glomerulonephritis. IgAN is now understood to be a systemic disease in which patients develop elevated serum levels of galactose-deficient IgA1. Antibodies directed against galactose-deficient IgA1 then form, leading to the development of pathogenic immune complexes, which deposit in the mesangium, and induce cellular activation and glomerular injury [24].

Recurrence rates of IgAN vary considerably depending on the time from transplantation to allograft biopsy, whether recurrence is defined clinically or histologically, and whether histologic recurrence requires evidence of IgAN by light microscopy or requires only evidence of IgA deposits by IF or EM. Ortiz et al. examined 65 protocol biopsies performed a median of 6.9 months after transplant. Defining IgAN as the presence of 1+ mesangial deposits for IgA by IF, they found recurrent IgAN in 32.3 % of patients, with 52 % lacking clinical findings, and 65 % having normal histology by light microscopy [25]. Coppo et al., when including microscopic hematuria plus proteinuria >0.5 g/day in the diagnosis of recurrent disease, found a 50 % recurrence rate by IF in protocol biopsies performed a mean of 2.9

years after transplant [26]. The recurrence rate in biopsies performed for clinical indications ranges from 13 to 50 %, although in some cases recurrent disease was not the predominant explanation for graft dysfunction.

The prevalence of clinical recurrence increases over time, and may be diagnosed more than 10 years after transplant. Recurrence occurs more frequently in younger patients and patients with a more rapid progression of their native kidney disease, including those with underlying crescentic GN [27]. Biopsy-proven recurrent disease is more common in patients who receive a zero HLA-mismatch live donor transplant [28]. The presence of latent IgA deposits in the allograft at the time of transplant (i.e., donor transmitted) may be associated with a higher risk of recurrent disease [29]. Only one study has examined the relationship of aberrantly glycosylated IgA1 to recurrent disease. In a study of 61 patients with histologic recurrence of IgAN, there was no significant increase in the risk of recurrent disease associated with higher levels of aberrantly glycosylated IgA1. However, certain genetic polymorphisms of IL-10 and TNF-α were associated with protection from early recurrence of IgAN [26]. The risk of recurrent disease is higher in patients who lost a prior allograft due to recurrent IgAN. Other pre-transplant characteristics, including gender, ethnicity, and source of allograft, are not consistently predictive of recurrence.

Angiotensin-converting enzyme inhibitors or angiotensin-receptor blockers are often prescribed in an effort to reduce blood pressure and proteinuria in recurrent IgAN. In one Japanese study of recurrent IgAN, 16 patients underwent tonsillectomy. Proteinuria decreased in all 16 patients, compared with no change in proteinuria in 12 patients who did not undergo tonsillectomy [30]. If disease recurrence is associated with a rapid course and the presence of crescents on biopsy, high-dose steroids and cyclophosphamide have been tried, similar to their use in native kidney disease. However, there is no data to confirm their efficacy in recurrent disease.

Due to the categorization of patients with mesangial IgA deposits and no clinical disease as having recurrent disease, overall, recurrence of IgAN has not been shown to increase the risk of allograft failure in the first decade after transplant. Indeed, 5-year graft survival may be better in patients with IgAN compared with other primary diseases. However, with longer follow-up graft survival becomes comparable to and may be worse than other diseases. Ponticelli et al. found slightly lower 10-year graft survival with IgAN when compared with recipients with ESRD from all other causes (75 % vs. 82 %) [27]. Choy et al. reported 17-year graft survival of 61 % compared with 70 % in non-IgAN patients, with the graft survival curves crossing at 12 years [31]. These data suggest that the detrimental impact of recurrent IgAN on graft survival may become more apparent with longer-term follow-up.

Berthoux et al. found a significantly lower rate of clinically recurrent IgAN at 5 years with thymoglobulin (9 %) compared with either IL2-receptor antagonists (41 %) or no induction agent (14 %) [32]. By contrast, Ortiz et al., using protocol biopsies, found histologic recurrence in 28.6 % of patients induced with thymoglobulin at a mean of 6.9 months after transplant [25]. Kukla et al. found that histologic recurrence of IgAN was significantly more common in patients who underwent early steroid withdrawal, with recurrent disease seen in 8.8 % of patients at 5 years compared with 3.3 % of patients maintained on steroids. However, there was no impact on graft survival [9]. By contrast, registry data have showed an increased risk of allograft failure in patients who underwent steroid withdrawal at any time after transplant. However, the absolute risk of graft failure from recurrent disease was low [33]. Taken together, the current data suggest that choice of induction or maintenance immunosuppressive agents plays at most a small role in the risk of graft failure from recurrent IgAN.

Membranous Nephropathy

Membranous nephropathy is characterized histologically by subepithelial immune-deposits in the GBM. Beck et al. have identified circulating autoantibodies directed against the M-type phospholipase A2 receptor in 70 % of patients with idiopathic native kidney membranous nephropathy [34]. Levels of anti-PLA2R antibodies correlate with disease activity, and several recent findings suggest that these autoantibodies are pathogenic [35, 36].

Following transplantation, the histologic recurrence rate of membranous nephropathy may be as high as 42 % at a mean of 13 months post-transplant when patients are evaluated by protocol biopsy. Disease recurrence was identified as early as 2 months post-transplant, and six of eight recurrences occurred in the first year. However, disease recurrence was also identified more than 5 years after transplant [37]. Moroni et al. found a recurrence rate of 34 % in patients who underwent biopsy for proteinuria or graft dysfunction at mean of 26.2 months after transplant [38]. While the rate of clinical recurrence is less than the rate of histologic recurrence, this study suggests that the reported rate of recurrent membranous will continue to rise with longer periods of follow-up.

No identifiable risk factors have consistently been associated with an increased risk of recurrent membranous. Some authors have found an association of recurrent membranous with anti-PLA2R antibodies. Debiec et al. found that five of ten cases of recurrent membranous were associated with anti-PLA2R antibodies. However, they also found that three patients with anti-PLA2R antibodies did not recur. In patients with antibodies present prior to transplant, the titer did not predict time to recurrence [39]. Kukla et al. found a higher rate of clinical recurrence in patients who underwent rapid steroid withdrawal (31 % vs. 10 % at 7 years), although there was no impact on graft survival [9].

Briganti et al. found that overall 12.5 % of patients with membranous nephropathy experienced allograft failure due to recurrent disease over 10 years of follow-up [2]. Moroni et al. found that 50 % of patients who experienced recurrent disease lost their grafts due to disease recurrence [38]. Patients with graft failure from recurrent disease had earlier recurrences and higher levels of proteinuria at the time of diagnosis. However, membranous nephropathy as a cause of ESRD is not associated with an increased risk of graft failure compared with other primary glomerular diseases, and 10-year graft survival is approximately 60% for patients with membranous nephropathy. There are no prospective studies of treatment of recurrent membranous. Several case reports have suggested that rituximab may be beneficial in some patients with recurrent membranous [40, 41]. Other authors have reported success with the use of angiotensin-converting enzyme inhibitors, high-dose steroids, and cyclophosphamide.

Recurrent membranous nephropathy must be distinguished from de novo disease. It is difficult to determine precisely the frequency of de novo membranous, as some cases undoubtedly represent recurrent disease in patients who did not undergo native kidney biopsy. Case series have estimated that de novo membranous occurs in 0.7–9.3 % of recipients [7]. Honda et al. found that de novo membranous occurs late after transplant, at a mean of 102 months, and presents with varying degrees of proteinuria and graft dysfunction. De novo membranous most likely represents a form of alloimmune response, as histologic findings of acute or chronic antibody-mediated rejection were seen in the majority of patients with de novo membranous, and 30 % had evidence of donor-specific antibodies. The outcome of de novo membranous, especially in those who also had donor-specific antibodies, is generally poor [42].

Membranoproliferative Glomerulonephritis

MPGN is a histologically defined disease that is diagnosed based on a characteristic pattern of injury seen on biopsy. Traditionally, MPGN was classified as type I, type II (also known as dense deposit disease (DDD), discussed below), or type III based on EM findings. Recent studies have pointed to the role of the alternative complement pathway in MPGN. Given these findings, a more practical clinical approach may be to view MPGN as either immune-complex-mediated or complement-mediated [43]. While this classification system may better reflect the underlying pathophysiology of MPGN, there are no data on the risk of recurrent disease based on this schema.

The prevalence and course of recurrent MPGN type I were described in several single-center analyses. Moroni et al. reported a recurrence rate of 23.5 %, occurring at a mean of 40 months (range 3.5–105) after transplant [44]. Using protocol biopsies, Lorenz et al. found a recurrence rate of 41.4 %, with only half of the recurrences having clinical findings at the time of diagnosis. All recurrences were diagnosed within the first 14 months after transplant, with the earliest recurrence documented at 1 week post-transplant [45]. Little et al. found a recurrence rate of 49 %, occurring at a median of 4.7 years post-transplant [46]. While MPGN type I may recur early after renal transplant, these data suggest that histologic recurrence may precede clinical recurrence by several years. Reported risk factors for disease recurrence include younger age at initial diagnosis, use of living-related donors, and the degree of mesangial proliferation and crescent formation on native kidney biopsy [44, 46]. In patients who lost a prior allograft to recurrent MPGN type I, the risk of disease recurrence in a second allograft is over 80 %, and nearly all these grafts will fail due to recurrent disease. Developing recurrent MPGN portends a poor prognosis, with graft failure rates ranging from 50 to 67 % [44, 46]. Overall, approximately 15 % of recipients with MPGN will lose their graft to recurrent disease in the first 10 years after transplant, with two-thirds of these failures occurring in the first 2 years after transplant. In registry studies, the hazard ratio for graft loss was 2.91 for patients with MPGN type I compared with other forms of primary GN [2].

High-dose steroids, cyclophosphamide, plasmapheresis, and rituximab have all been used to treat recurrent MPGN, though no treatment has been shown consistently to slow disease progression. Given recent findings linking MPGN to alternative complement pathway dysregulation, it is possible that there may be a role for complement inhibition in the treatment of recurrent MPGN [47].

Dense Deposit Disease

DDD, also known as MPGN type II, is characterized by the presence of electron-dense material in the GBM. DDD is characterized by hyperactivation of the alternative complement pathway. In DDD, the activity of C3 convertase is increased, either by the presence of C3 nephritic factor or by genetic or acquired defects in complement factor H activity [48].

Histologic recurrence of DDD is common, with the reported recurrence rate varying from 18 to 100 %. Although complement C3 levels are low in most patients with DDD, in the largest study to-date neither pre-transplant nor post-transplant C3 levels were significantly correlated with disease recurrence. Similarly, age, gender, donor source, time from presentation to ESRD, or the presence of crescents on native kidney biopsy was not predictive of clinical recurrence [49]. There is no reported association between different induction or maintenance immunosuppressive medications and the risk of recurrence.

Historically, treatment of recurrent DDD, such as with pulse-dose steroids or switching from cyclosporine to tacrolimus, has had limited success. Recent advances in understanding the pathogenesis of DDD have led to more targeted treatment approaches. Plasma infusion has been used in patients with defects in factor H activity to replace the missing or mutant protein. Plasma exchange may be used in patients with elevated levels of C3 nephritic factor. Given the link between DDD and hyperactivity of the alternative complement pathway, eculizumab, a monoclonal antibody directed against C5, has been used successfully in some patients as treatment for recurrent DDD [50]. While it is not yet known whether any specific underlying defect in the complement regulation will be predictive of a clinical response to eculizumab, early data suggest that elevated levels of serum membrane attack complex prior to treatment are associated with a greater likelihood of response [51].

Secondary Glomerular Diseases

Systemic Lupus Erythematosus

End-stage renal disease remains a common complication of lupus nephritis, affecting up to 15 % of patients. Clinical symptoms and serologic markers of lupus are usually quiescent once lupus patients reach ESRD. Clinical lupus flares are uncommon post-transplant, perhaps due to the immunosuppressive agents used post-transplant. Recent studies have found a much higher rate of recurrent lupus nephritis, than previously recognized, especially when protocol biopsies are used. Burgos et al. analyzed 177 patients transplanted at a single-center over a 30-year period. Lupus nephritis, as detected by for-cause biopsies, recurred in 11 % of patients, at a mean of 4.5 years post-transplant. The histology of recurrent lupus nephritis was different than that seen in the native kidney biopsies of these patients, with a higher frequency of mesangial lesions and significantly fewer proliferative lesions, perhaps due to earlier diagnosis [52]. Not surprisingly, others have reported lower recurrence rates, between 8.5 and 30 %, when for-cause biopsies are performed. With a single protocol biopsy at a mean of 8 years post-transplant, Norby et al. found histologic evidence of recurrent lupus nephritis in 22 of 41 (54 %) patients, of whom 17 had only mild mesangial findings (WHO class I or II) [53].

The most common clinical presentation of recurrent lupus nephritis is sub-nephrotic proteinuria and graft dysfunction. Extrarenal manifestations are uncommon and tend to be mild. Rapidly progressive GN is rare. While pre-transplant risk factors such as age, ethnicity, gender, native kidney histology type, duration of ESRD, kidney donor source, and post-transplant immunosuppressive regimen do not correlate well with risk of recurrence in case series, registry data have suggested that recurrent disease is more likely in non-Hispanic blacks, women, and patients aged <33 years [54]. Although some authors have recommended that serologic markers of disease activity be normal or stable prior to performing a transplant, there is scant clinical evidence to support this strategy. There are few reports on the treatment of clinically significant recurrent lupus nephritis. In the absence of strong data, treatment of recurrent disease should be similar to native kidney disease.

Despite the risk of recurrent disease, the outcomes with kidney transplant in lupus recipients are excellent. Graft survival after live-donor or deceased-donor transplant is similar to patients with ESRD from other etiologies. However, when recurrent disease does occur, graft survival may be adversely affected. Contreras et al. found a reported rate of recurrent lupus nephritis of 2.44 % when examining registry data over a 20-year period. Although recipients with recurrent lupus nephritis had a fourfold greater risk of graft failure, only 7 % of graft failures in lupus patients were attributable to recurrent disease [54]. Other studies have suggested that recurrent disease has a negligible impact on graft survival [2, 55].

ANCA-Associated Vasculitis

Despite improvements in the treatment of ANCA-associated vasculitis (AAV), up to 20 % of patients will progress to ESRD. Post-transplant disease recurrence has been reported in association with both cANCA and pANCA. Nachman et al. pooled data from 127 recipients with AAV and found a recurrence rate of 17.3 %. The average time to recurrence was 30.9 months, with a range of 4–89 months [56]. Gera et al. reported 35 recipients with AAV in the modern era of immunosuppression and found a clinical recurrence rate of 8.6 %, with an average time to recurrence of 37.1 months [57].

Clinical recurrences of AAV can vary significantly with respect to the severity of disease and the organs involved. Nachman et al. found that 60 % of recurrences were renal in origin (either isolated or in combination with other organ involvement) while 40 % of recurrences were nonrenal in origin [56]. By contrast, all three recurrences reported by Gera et al. were nonrenal in origin [57]. The risk of disease recurrence does not appear to be influenced by the ANCA pattern, ANCA titers at the time of transplant, duration of AAV prior to transplant, time of dialysis prior to transplant, source of donor, or choice of immunosuppression. Once clinical remission is achieved, the continued presence of positive ANCA titers should not preclude or delay transplantation. Although post-transplant ANCA titers are often monitored, data confirming the utility of this practice for predicting disease recurrence are limited.

While recurrent AAV can lead to graft failure, it is not associated with an increased risk of graft loss compared with other forms of GN. In registry data from Australia and New Zealand, 7.7 % of grafts failed over 10 years due to recurrent AAV. However, the hazard ratio for graft failure from recurrent disease was 0.52 [2]. In a pooled analysis of 127 patients, two grafts were lost to recurrent AAV, whereas in a single-center study with a more recent cohort no grafts were lost to recurrent AAV [56, 57]. There are no trials of treatment of AAV in renal transplant recipients. Patients with recurrent disease are typically treated with regimens used for non-transplant patients with AAV, with regimens containing high-dose steroids, cyclophosphamide, and/or rituximab.

Anti-glomerular Basement Membrane Disease

In contrast to AAV, histologic recurrence of anti-GBM disease occurs in 50 % of patients who are transplanted in the presence of circulating anti-GBM antibodies. The risk of recurrence is markedly reduced when transplant is deferred until after anti-GBM antibodies have been undetectable for 6–12 months. With delayed transplantation, clinical recurrence is rare, although late recurrences have been described [58, 59]. Recurrent anti-GBM disease should be managed similar to native kidney disease, with steroids, cyclophosphamide, and plasmapheresis.

De novo anti-GBM disease has been described in patients with Alport's syndrome. Deficiency of the α5 chain of type IV collagen in patients with Alport's syndrome results in the production of antibody in response to neoantigen exposure via the transplant [60]. Despite the presence of anti-GBM antibodies, clinical anti-GBM disease is rare in transplant recipients with Alport's syndrome. De novo anti-GBM disease has been described both in the immediate postoperative period and several years post-transplant [61, 62]. The treatments used for native kidney disease are not as effective in de novo anti-GBM disease, and graft loss is not uncommon. For patients receiving a subsequent transplant after graft failure from de novo disease, anti-GBM disease often occurs at an earlier time post-transplant than in the prior allograft.

Atypical Hemolytic-Uremic Syndrome and Thrombotic Microangiopathy

HUS and TMA may recur or develop de novo following transplant. Approximately 10 % of cases of the HUS are classified as atypical (aHUS), as they are not caused by bacterial infections or Shiga-like toxin. Research has linked aHUS to uncontrolled activation of the complement system. Genetic abnormalities in complement regulatory proteins have been described in aHUS, including factor H, factor I, factor B, membrane cofactor protein, complement C3, and thrombomodulin. In addition, some patients may have antibodies against factor H [63]. aHUS recurs in ~50 % of patients after transplant, and disease recurrence can happen as early as the first week post-transplant. Recurrent aHUS is associated with poor graft survival, with graft failure occurring in 80–90 % of patients with recurrent disease. Graft loss from recurrent disease can occur as early as the first week post-transplant, and more than 80 % of graft losses from recurrent disease occur within the first year post-transplant [64]. The underlying abnormality in the complement system may be predictive of post-transplant outcomes. The recurrence rate is 70–90 % in patients with abnormalities in factor H or factor I, and 40–50 % in patients with abnormalities in C3. By contrast, in patients with abnormalities of membrane cofactor protein, which is highly expressed in the kidney, aHUS recurs in less than 20 % of patients and is associated with similar graft survival to patients transplanted for other causes [64].

Treatment options for recurrent aHUS were historically limited. Factor H is expressed in the liver, and simultaneous liver–kidney transplantation has been performed with the rationale of correcting the underlying genetic defect and treating ESRD [65]. Plasmapheresis has also been tried, with limited success. Eculizumab, a humanized anti-C5 antibody which prevents formation of the membrane attack complex, is now approved as a treatment for aHUS. Since this medication became available, several centers have reported excellent outcomes employing eculizumab either as prophylaxis against recurrent disease or as treatment for recurrent aHUS [66, 67].

Single-center studies have reported de novo TMA rates of 1.5–14 % following kidney transplant. Registry studies have suggested lower rates, with de novo TMA found in only 0.8 % of recipients in an analysis of USRDS data [68, 69]. When de novo TMA occurs, it is most often due to either drug-induced or immunologic injury. Both calcineurin-inhibitors and mTOR inhibitors can cause de novo TMA. TMA may also be a manifestation of antibody-mediated rejection. Rarely, TMA has been described as a complication of infections such as cytomegalovirus. Reported risk factors for de novo TMA include younger age, female recipient, and initial use of sirolimus [69]. De novo TMA presents similar to recurrent disease, with graft dysfunction, hemolytic anemia, and thrombocytopenia. Treatment depends on the etiology. For patients with TMA due to antibody-mediated rejection, plasmapheresis is typically used as first-line therapy. For TMA due to a calcineurin-inhibitor or mTOR inhibitor, the medication should be withdrawn. Plasmapheresis may also be used for drug-induced TMA, although there are no data establishing its efficacy. There are no published data on the use of eculizumab for drug-induced TMA, or on the frequency of complement regulatory abnormalities in this population.

Scleroderma

End-stage renal disease occurs in 20–50 % of patients with scleroderma renal crisis. Data on the risk of recurrent scleroderma in the allograft are scarce. Published reports have suggested recurrence rates of 20–50 %, although a review of UNOS data from 1987 to 2004 found that of 260 transplants performed for ESRD secondary to scleroderma, only five grafts (1.9 %) were lost due to recurrent disease. However, the UNOS data did not report disease recurrence not causing graft failure, so it is possible that clinical or histologic recurrence rates were higher [70]. A review of 11 cases of transplantation in scleroderma found that time from initial presentation of scleroderma renal crisis to development of ESRD in the native kidney was the main risk factor for development of post-transplant disease recurrence. Five of seven patients developing ESRD in less than 1 year developed recurrent disease, compared with 0/4 patients who took more than 1 year to progress to ESRD. Disease recurrence occurred early (4/5 cases within 8 months of transplant) and was associated with a poor prognosis (3/5 allografts lost with 6 months of disease recurrence) [70]. Given the limited data on recurrent scleroderma renal crisis, treatment tends to follow treatment given in native kidney disease.

Fibrillary Glomerulonephritis

Early case reports of renal transplant in patients with fibrillary GN described a high rate of early graft failure due to recurrent disease. However, larger case series noted better graft outcomes despite high rates of clinical recurrence. Pronovost et al. found a 60 % recurrence rate, and noted that the rate of decline in renal function was slower in allografts than in native kidneys [71]. Samaniego et al. found a 50 % recurrence rate (7/14 patients), with the earliest recurrence occurring at 2 years post-transplant. Graft loss from recurrent disease occurred in three patients [72]. Czarnecki et al. reviewed outcomes in 12 patients receiving 15 transplants. Five patients with fibrillary GN without monoclonal gammopathy had no evidence of recurrent disease on protocol biopsy. Seven patients with fibrillary GN with monoclonal gammopathy received ten transplants. Recurrent disease was found in five allografts in four patients, with the earliest recurrence documented at 3 months. Three grafts were lost to recurrent disease, at a mean of 17 months, and two additional patients died of hematologic malignancies [73]. Patients in whom recurrent disease occurs should be evaluated for the presence of a monoclonal gammopathy. In the absence of any studies on treatment of recurrent fibrillary GN, clinical management should be similar to that for native kidney disease.

There are a few reports of de novo fibrillary GN occurring after transplant, though it is also possible that these cases represent recurrence of undiagnosed native kidney disease [74, 75]. Given the dearth of information on de novo fibrillary GN, management of this disease should be similar to management of recurrent fibrillary GN.

Henoch–Schonlein Purpura

Henoch–Schonlein purpura (HSP) is a small-vessel vasculitis characterized by involvement of the joints, skin, gut, and kidneys. HSP is characterized by IgA deposition within tissues, making HSP histologically indistinguishable from primary IgAN. Clinical recurrence of HSP occurs in 15–42 % of transplants, whereas histologic recurrence can be found in up to 78 % of patients [76, 77]. Recurrences are more common and severe in patients who had a rapidly progressive course or necrotizing crescentic GN in their native kidneys [76]. Although recurrence is more common in children, the outcome after recurrence is worse in adults. Clinical recurrence can occur at any time after transplant.

Graft loss from recurrent disease occurs in 0–12 % of patients with HSP. Analysis of registry data showed that 13.6 % of graft losses in HSP patients were attributed to recurrent disease. Despite the risk of allograft failure from recurrent disease, graft outcomes in HSP patients are excellent. Ten-year graft survival is 58.8 %, compared with 54.4 % in the non-HSP population [78]. There are limited data on treatment of recurrent HSP. Pulse-dose steroids and cyclophosphamide have been attempted with limited success. In a single patient, clinical and histologic findings improved in the short term with a course of plasmapheresis.

Metabolic Disease

Diabetes Mellitus

Diabetic nephropathy is the most common cause of ESRD in patients receiving a kidney transplant. Poor glycemic control post-transplant can lead to recurrent diabetic nephropathy. With the improvement in short-term and long-graft survival over the past few decades, recurrent diabetic nephropathy is becoming a more common clinical entity. Recurrent disease was first reported by Mauer et al. in 1976, with diabetic changes found as early as 2.5 years post-transplant [79].

Bhalla et al. reported a histologic recurrence in almost 40 % of diabetic patients at a mean of 6.7 years following transplant [80]. Recurrent diabetic nephropathy has a poor prognosis, with 57 % of recurrences leading to graft failure in one single-center series [6]. Despite the high rate of histologic recurrence, diabetic nephropathy is not a common cause of allograft failure.

De novo post-transplant diabetes can also lead to diabetic nephropathy. Bhalla et al. found that diabetic nephropathy eventually developed in 47 % of patients with new onset post-transplant diabetes, with diabetic changes found in the allograft at a mean of 5.9 years following diagnosis [80]. Miles et al. reported that histologic changes can occur as early as 1 year following the diagnosis of new onset post-transplant diabetes [81]. Burroughs et al. examined Medicare claims data and found that of 4,105 patients who were diagnosed with post-transplant diabetes, 31.3 % were diagnosed with nephropathy over a 3-year period [82]. Thus, the available data suggest that both recurrent and de novo diabetic nephropathy can present earlier and progress more rapidly than in nontransplant patients.

No studies have been performed to address specific preventive measures or treatment strategies for either recurrent or de novo diabetic nephropathy. Extrapolating from the data in native kidney disease, treatment strategies should focus on glycemic control, blood pressure control, and the use of either angiotensin-converting enzyme inhibitors or angiotensin II receptor blockers. The ideal treatment for type 1 diabetes is pancreas transplant, either simultaneous to or following kidney transplant. Successful pancreas transplant can lead to prolonged insulin-independence, and can prevent recurrent diabetic nephropathy. Pancreas transplant may also be a treatment option for some non-obese type 2 diabetics. Islet cell transplant in type 1 diabetics, if able to achieve prolonged insulin-independence, would also be expected to halt or prevent recurrent disease.

Oxalosis

Primary oxalosis occurs as a result of hepatic enzyme deficiency, which causes the accumulation of systemic oxalate and can lead to kidney failure. Primary hyperoxaluria type I is due to alanine:glyoxylate aminotransferase deficiency, while primary hyperoxaluria type II is due to glyoxylate reductase deficiency. Both disorders are rare, with type I being much more common than type II. Renal transplantation without correcting the underlying enzyme deficiency often leads to renal dysfunction and graft failure early after transplant. Aggressive pre-transplant dialysis to lower the serum oxalate concentration, coupled with aggressive diuresis and the administration of pyridoxine, has had limited success in preventing recurrence. The definitive treatment to prevent recurrent oxalosis is to perform liver transplantation to replace the deficient enzyme [83].

Secondary oxalosis, or enteric hyperoxaluria, can result from malabsorption following gastric bypass or in the setting of chronic pancreatitis, and can recur or occur as a de novo disease following kidney transplant. In these patients, pre-transplant management should focus on reducing the circulating oxalate load, including frequent dialysis, maintaining a good urine output to reduce the urinary oxalate concentration, instituting a low-fat and low-oxalate diet, and adding pancreatic enzyme supplements in the setting of pancreatic insufficiency. Recovery of renal function has been reported to occur even in patients who have required dialysis for several months.

Fabry's Disease

Fabry's disease is caused by a deficiency of α-galactosidase A. Accumulation of globotriasosylceramide causes damage in the eyes, autonomic nervous system, cardiovascular system, and kidneys. Enzyme replacement therapy is available for patients with Fabry's disease, and data from case series have suggested that enzyme replacement therapy is safe, effective, and well-tolerated in transplant recipients [84]. Histologic recurrence, as expected, has been described in patients not receiving enzyme replacement therapy. There are no reports of recurrence in patients receiving enzyme replacement therapy [85]. Thus, enzyme replacement treatment should be given to all patients with Fabry's disease following transplant.

References

1. Hariharan S, Adams MB, Brennan DC, Davis CL, First MR, Johnson CP, et al. Recurrent and de novo glomerular disease after renal transplantation: a report from Renal Allograft Disease Registry (RADR). Transplantation. 1999;68(5):635–41. Epub 1999/10/03.
2. Briganti EM, Russ GR, McNeil JJ, Atkins RC, Chadban SJ. Risk of renal allograft loss from recurrent glomerulonephritis. N Engl J Med. 2002;347(2):103–9. Epub 2002/07/12.
3. Andresdottir MB, Hoitsma AJ, Assmann KJ, Koene RA, Wetzels JF. The impact of recurrent glomerulonephritis on graft survival in recipients of human histocompatibility leucocyte antigen-identical living related donor grafts. Transplantation. 1999;68(5):623–7. Epub 1999/10/03.
4. Ponticelli C, Banfi G. Thrombotic microangiopathy after kidney transplantation. Transpl Int. 2006;19(10):789–94. Epub 2006/09/12.
5. Schwimmer J, Nadasdy TA, Spitalnik PF, Kaplan KL, Zand MS. De novo thrombotic microangiopathy in renal transplant recipients: a comparison of hemolytic uremic syndrome with localized renal thrombotic microangiopathy. Am J Kidney Dis. 2003;41(2):471–9. Epub 2003/01/29.
6. Hariharan S, Smith RD, Viero R, First MR. Diabetic nephropathy after renal transplantation. Clinical and pathologic features. Transplantation. 1996;62(5):632–5. Epub 1996/09/15.

7. Ponticelli C, De GRJ. Novo membranous nephropathy (MN) in kidney allografts. A peculiar form of alloimmune disease? Transpl Int. 2012;25(12):1205–10.
8. Mulay AV, van Walraven C, Knoll GA. Impact of immunosuppressive medication on the risk of renal allograft failure due to recurrent glomerulonephritis. Am J Transplant. 2009;9(4):804–11. Epub 2009/04/09.
9. Kukla A, Chen E, Spong R, Weber M, El-Shahawi Y, Gillingham K, et al. Recurrent glomerulonephritis under rapid discontinuation of steroids. Transplantation. 2011;91(12):1386–91. Epub 2011/04/22.
10. Pascual J, Mezrich JD, Djamali A, Leverson G, Chin LT, Torrealba J, et al. Alemtuzumab induction and recurrence of glomerular disease after kidney transplantation. Transplantation. 2007;83(11):1429–34. Epub 2007/06/15.
11. Chang JW, Pardo V, Sageshima J, Chen L, Tsai HL, Reiser J, et al. Podocyte foot process effacement in postreperfusion allograft biopsies correlates with early recurrence of proteinuria in focal segmental glomerulosclerosis. Transplantation. 2012;93(12):1238–44.
12. Cravedi P, Kopp JB, Remuzzi G. Recent progress in the pathophysiology and treatment of FSGS recurrence. Am J Transplant. 2013;13(2):266–74. Epub 2013/01/15.
13. Savin VJ, Sharma R, Sharma M, McCarthy ET, Swan SK, Ellis E, et al. Circulating factor associated with increased glomerular permeability to albumin in recurrent focal segmental glomerulosclerosis. N Engl J Med. 1996;334(14):878–83. Epub 1996/04/04.
14. Wei C, El Hindi S, Li J, Fornoni A, Goes N, Sageshima J, et al. Circulating urokinase receptor as a cause of focal segmental glomerulosclerosis. Nat Med. 2011;17(8):952–60. Epub 2011/08/02.
15. Patrakka J, Ruotsalainen V, Reponen P, Qvist E, Laine J, Holmberg C, et al. Recurrence of nephrotic syndrome in kidney grafts of patients with congenital nephrotic syndrome of the Finnish type: role of nephrin. Transplantation. 2002;73(3):394–403. Epub 2002/03/09.
16. Jungraithmayr TC, Hofer K, Cochat P, Chernin G, Cortina G, Fargue S, et al. Screening for NPHS2 mutations may help predict FSGS recurrence after transplantation. J Am Soc Nephrol. 2011;22(3):579–85. Epub 2011/03/01.
17. Abbott KC, Sawyers ES, Oliver 3rd JD, Ko CW, Kirk AD, Welch PG, et al. Graft loss due to recurrent focal segmental glomerulosclerosis in renal transplant recipients in the United States. Am J Kidney Dis. 2001;37(2):366–73. Epub 2001/02/07.
18. Cibrik DM, Kaplan B, Campbell DA, Meier-Kriesche HU. Renal allograft survival in transplant recipients with focal segmental glomerulosclerosis. Am J Transplant. 2003;3(1):64–7. Epub 2002/12/21.
19. Canaud G, Zuber J, Sberro R, Royale V, Anglicheau D, Snanoudj R, et al. Intensive and prolonged treatment of focal and segmental glomerulosclerosis recurrence in adult kidney transplant recipients: a pilot study. Am J Transplant. 2009;9(5):1081–6. Epub 2009/04/07.
20. Araya CE, Dharnidharka VR. The factors that may predict response to rituximab therapy in recurrent focal segmental glomerulosclerosis: a systematic review. J Transplant. 2011;2011:374213. Epub 2011/12/17.
21. Jhaveri KD, Naber TH, Wang X, Molmenti E, Bhaskaran M, Boctor FN, et al. Treatment of recurrent focal segmental glomerular sclerosis posttransplant with a multimodal approach including high-galactose diet and oral galactose supplementation. Transplantation. 2011;91(6):e35–6. Epub 2011/03/09.
22. Gohh RY, Yango AF, Morrissey PE, Monaco AP, Gautam A, Sharma M, et al. Preemptive plasmapheresis and recurrence of FSGS in high-risk renal transplant recipients. Am J Transplant. 2005;5(12):2907–12. Epub 2005/11/24.
23. Hickson LJ, Gera M, Amer H, Iqbal CW, Moore TB, Milliner DS, et al. Kidney transplantation for primary focal segmental glomerulosclerosis: outcomes and response to therapy for recurrence. Transplantation. 2009;87(8):1232–9. Epub 2009/04/23.
24. Suzuki H, Kiryluk K, Novak J, Moldoveanu Z, Herr AB, Renfrow MB, et al. The pathophysiology of IgA nephropathy. J Am Soc Nephrol. 2011;22(10):1795–803. Epub 2011/09/29.
25. Ortiz F, Gelpi R, Koskinen P, Manonelles A, Raisanen-Sokolowski A, Carrera M, et al. IgA nephropathy recurs early in the graft when assessed by protocol biopsy. Nephrol Dial Transplant. 2012;27(6):2553–8. Epub 2011/12/15.
26. Coppo R, Amore A, Chiesa M, Lombardo F, Cirina P, Andrulli S, et al. Serological and genetic factors in early recurrence of IgA nephropathy after renal transplantation. Clin Transplant. 2007;21(6):728–37. Epub 2007/11/09.
27. Ponticelli C, Traversi L, Feliciani A, Cesana BM, Banfi G, Tarantino A. Kidney transplantation in patients with IgA mesangial glomerulonephritis. Kidney Int. 2001;60(5):1948–54. Epub 2001/11/13.
28. McDonald SP, Russ GR. Recurrence of IgA nephropathy among renal allograft recipients from living donors is greater among those with zero HLA mismatches. Transplantation. 2006;82(6):759–62. Epub 2006/09/29.
29. Moriyama T, Nitta K, Suzuki K, Honda K, Horita S, Uchida K, et al. Latent IgA deposition from donor kidney is the major risk factor for recurrent IgA nephropathy in renal transplantation. Clin Transplant. 2005;19 Suppl 14:41–8. Epub 2005/06/16.
30. Kennoki T, Ishida H, Yamaguchi Y, Tanabe K. Proteinuria-reducing effects of tonsillectomy alone in IgA nephropathy recurring after kidney transplantation. Transplantation. 2009;88(7):935–41. Epub 2009/11/26.
31. Choy BY, Chan TM, Lo SK, Lo WK, Lai KN. Renal transplantation in patients with primary immunoglobulin a nephropathy. Nephrol Dial Transplant. 2003;18(11):2399–404. Epub 2003/10/11.
32. Berthoux F, El Deeb S, Mariat C, Diconne E, Laurent B, Thibaudin L. Antithymocyte globulin (ATG) induction therapy and disease recurrence in renal transplant recipients with primary IgA nephropathy. Transplantation. 2008;85(10):1505–7. Epub 2008/05/24.
33. Clayton P, McDonald S, Chadban S. Steroids and recurrent IgA nephropathy after kidney transplantation. Am J Transplant. 2011;11(8):1645–9. Epub 2011/07/30.
34. Beck Jr LH, Bonegio RG, Lambeau G, Beck DM, Powell DW, Cummins TD, et al. M-type phospholipase A2 receptor as target antigen in idiopathic membranous nephropathy. N Engl J Med. 2009;361(1):11–21. Epub 2009/07/03.
35. Hofstra JM, Beck Jr LH, Beck DM, Wetzels JF, Salant DJ. Anti-phospholipase A(2) receptor antibodies correlate with clinical status in idiopathic membranous nephropathy. Clin J Am Soc Nephrol. 2011;6(6):1286–91. Epub 2011/04/09.
36. Beck Jr LH. Monoclonal anti-PLA2R and recurrent membranous nephropathy: another piece of the puzzle. J Am Soc Nephrol. 2012;23(12):1911–3. Epub 2012/11/10.
37. Dabade TS, Grande JP, Norby SM, Fervenza FC, Cosio FG. Recurrent idiopathic membranous nephropathy after kidney transplantation: a surveillance biopsy study. Am J Transplant. 2008;8(6):1318–22. Epub 2008/05/01.
38. Moroni G, Gallelli B, Quaglini S, Leoni A, Banfi G, Passerini P, et al. Long-term outcome of renal transplantation in patients with idiopathic membranous glomerulonephritis (MN). Nephrol Dial Transplant. 2010;25(10):3408–15. Epub 2010/05/15.
39. Debiec H, Martin L, Jouanneau C, Dautin G, Mesnard L, Rondeau E, et al. Autoantibodies specific for the phospholipase A2 receptor in recurrent and de novo membranous nephropathy. Am J Transplant. 2011;11(10):2144–52. Epub 2011/08/11.
40. Sprangers B, Lefkowitz GI, Cohen SD, Stokes MB, Valeri A, Appel GB, et al. Beneficial effect of rituximab in the treatment of recurrent idiopathic membranous nephropathy after kidney transplantation. Clin J Am Soc Nephrol. 2010;5(5):790–7. Epub 2010/02/27.
41. El-Zoghby ZM, Grande JP, Fraile MG, Norby SM, Fervenza FC, Cosio FG. Recurrent idiopathic membranous nephropathy: early diagnosis by protocol biopsies and treatment with anti-CD20

monoclonal antibodies. Am J Transplant. 2009;9(12):2800–7. Epub 2009/10/23.
42. Honda K, Horita S, Toki D, Taneda S, Nitta K, Hattori M, et al. De novo membranous nephropathy and antibody-mediated rejection in transplanted kidney. Clin Transplant. 2011;25(2):191–200. Epub 2010/03/20.
43. Sethi S, Fervenza FC. Membranoproliferative glomerulonephritis: a new look at an old entity. N Engl J Med. 2012;366(12):1119–31. Epub 2012/03/23.
44. Moroni G, Casati C, Quaglini S, Gallelli B, Banfi G, Montagnino G, et al. Membranoproliferative glomerulonephritis type I in renal transplantation patients: a single-center study of a cohort of 68 renal transplants followed up for 11 years. Transplantation. 2011;91(11):1233–9. Epub 2011/04/20.
45. Lorenz EC, Sethi S, Leung N, Dispenzieri A, Fervenza FC, Cosio FG. Recurrent membranoproliferative glomerulonephritis after kidney transplantation. Kidney Int. 2010;77(8):721–8. Epub 2010/02/05.
46. Little MA, Dupont P, Campbell E, Dorman A, Walshe JJ. Severity of primary MPGN, rather than MPGN type, determines renal survival and post-transplantation recurrence risk. Kidney Int. 2006;69(3):504–11. Epub 2006/01/06.
47. Radhakrishnan S, Lunn A, Kirschfink M, Thorner P, Hebert D, Langlois V, et al. Eculizumab and refractory membranoproliferative glomerulonephritis. N Engl J Med. 2012;366(12):1165–6. Epub 2012/03/23.
48. Appel GB, Cook HT, Hageman G, Jennette JC, Kashgarian M, Kirschfink M, et al. Membranoproliferative glomerulonephritis type II (dense deposit disease): an update. J Am Soc Nephrol. 2005;16(5):1392–403. Epub 2005/04/01.
49. Braun MC, Stablein DM, Hamiwka LA, Bell L, Bartosh SM, Strife CF. Recurrence of membranoproliferative glomerulonephritis type II in renal allografts: The North American Pediatric Renal Transplant Cooperative Study experience. J Am Soc Nephrol. 2005;16(7):2225–33. Epub 2005/05/13.
50. McCaughan JA, O'Rourke DM, Courtney AE. Recurrent dense deposit disease after renal transplantation: an emerging role for complementary therapies. Am J Transplant. 2012;12(4):1046–51. Epub 2012/01/12.
51. Bomback AS, Smith RJ, Barile GR, Zhang Y, Heher EC, Herlitz L, et al. Eculizumab for dense deposit disease and C3 glomerulonephritis. Clin J Am Soc Nephrol. 2012;7(5):748–56. Epub 2012/03/10.
52. Burgos PI, Perkins EL, Pons-Estel GJ, Kendrick SA, Liu JM, Kendrick WT, et al. Risk factors and impact of recurrent lupus nephritis in patients with systemic lupus erythematosus undergoing renal transplantation: data from a single US institution. Arthritis Rheum. 2009;60(9):2757–66. Epub 2009/08/29.
53. Norby GE, Strom EH, Midtvedt K, Hartmann A, Gilboe IM, Leivestad T, et al. Recurrent lupus nephritis after kidney transplantation: a surveillance biopsy study. Ann Rheum Dis. 2010;69(8):1484–7. Epub 2010/05/26.
54. Contreras G, Mattiazzi A, Guerra G, Ortega LM, Tozman EC, Li H, et al. Recurrence of lupus nephritis after kidney transplantation. J Am Soc Nephrol. 2010;21(7):1200–7. Epub 2010/05/22.
55. Moroni G, Tantardini F, Gallelli B, Quaglini S, Banfi G, Poli F, et al. The long-term prognosis of renal transplantation in patients with lupus nephritis. Am J Kidney Dis. 2005;45(5):903–11. Epub 2005/04/30.
56. Nachman PH, Segelmark M, Westman K, Hogan SL, Satterly KK, Jennette JC, et al. Recurrent ANCA-associated small vessel vasculitis after transplantation: a pooled analysis. Kidney Int. 1999;56(4):1544–50. Epub 1999/10/03.
57. Gera M, Griffin MD, Specks U, Leung N, Stegall MD, Fervenza FC. Recurrence of ANCA-associated vasculitis following renal transplantation in the modern era of immunosuppression. Kidney Int. 2007;71(12):1296–301. Epub 2007/04/06.
58. Deegens JK, Artz MA, Hoitsma AJ, Wetzels JF. Outcome of renal transplantation in patients with pauci-immune small vessel vasculitis or anti-GBM disease. Clin Nephrol. 2003;59(1):1–9. Epub 2003/02/08.
59. Khandelwal M, McCormick BB, Lajoie G, Sweet J, Cole E, Cattran DC. Recurrence of anti-GBM disease 8 years after renal transplantation. Nephrol Dial Transplant. 2004;19(2):491–4. Epub 2004/01/23.
60. Kalluri R, Torre A, Shield 3rd CF, Zamborsky ED, Werner MC, Suchin E, et al. Identification of alpha3, alpha4, and alpha5 chains of type IV collagen as alloantigens for Alport posttransplant anti-glomerular basement membrane antibodies. Transplantation. 2000;69(4):679–83. Epub 2000/03/09.
61. Browne G, Brown PA, Tomson CR, Fleming S, Allen A, Herriot R, et al. Retransplantation in Alport post-transplant anti-GBM disease. Kidney Int. 2004;65(2):675–81. Epub 2004/01/14.
62. de Sandes-Freitas TV, Holanda-Cavalcanti A, Mastroianni-Kirsztajn G, Franco MF, Medina-Pestana JO. Late presentation of Alport posttransplantation anti-glomerular basement membrane disease. Transplant Proc. 2011;43(10):4000–1. Epub 2011/12/17.
63. Noris M, Remuzzi G. Atypical hemolytic-uremic syndrome. N Engl J Med. 2009;361(17):1676–87. Epub 2009/10/23.
64. Bresin E, Daina E, Noris M, Castelletti F, Stefanov R, Hill P, et al. Outcome of renal transplantation in patients with non-Shiga toxin-associated hemolytic uremic syndrome: prognostic significance of genetic background. Clin J Am Soc Nephrol. 2006;1(1):88–99. Epub 2007/08/21.
65. Jalanko H, Peltonen S, Koskinen A, Puntila J, Isoniemi H, Holmberg C, et al. Successful liver-kidney transplantation in two children with aHUS caused by a mutation in complement factor H. Am J Transplant. 2008;8(1):216–21. Epub 2007/11/02.
66. Zimmerhackl LB, Hofer J, Cortina G, Mark W, Wurzner R, Jungraithmayr TC, et al. Prophylactic eculizumab after renal transplantation in atypical hemolytic-uremic syndrome. N Engl J Med. 2010;362(18):1746–8. Epub 2010/05/07.
67. Chatelet V, Fremeaux-Bacchi V, Lobbedez T, Ficheux M, Hurault de Ligny B. Safety and long-term efficacy of eculizumab in a renal transplant patient with recurrent atypical hemolytic-uremic syndrome. Am J Transplant. 2009;9(11):2644–5. Epub 2009/09/25.
68. Zarifian A, Meleg-Smith S, O'Donovan R, Tesi RJ, Batuman V. Cyclosporine-associated thrombotic microangiopathy in renal allografts. Kidney Int. 1999;55(6):2457–66. Epub 1999/06/03.
69. Reynolds JC, Agodoa LY, Yuan CM, Abbott KC. Thrombotic microangiopathy after renal transplantation in the United States. Am J Kidney Dis. 2003;42(5):1058–68. Epub 2003/10/29.
70. Pham PT, Pham PC, Danovitch GM, Gritsch HA, Singer J, Wallace WD, et al. Predictors and risk factors for recurrent scleroderma renal crisis in the kidney allograft: case report and review of the literature. Am J Transplant. 2005;5(10):2565–9. Epub 2005/09/16.
71. Pronovost PH, Brady HR, Gunning ME, Espinoza O, Rennke HG. Clinical features, predictors of disease progression and results of renal transplantation in fibrillary/immunotactoid glomerulopathy. Nephrol Dial Transplant. 1996;11(5):837–42. Epub 1996/05/01.
72. Samaniego M, Nadasdy GM, Laszik Z, Nadasdy T. Outcome of renal transplantation in fibrillary glomerulonephritis. Clin Nephrol. 2001;55(2):159–66. Epub 2001/03/28.
73. Czarnecki PG, Lager DJ, Leung N, Dispenzieri A, Cosio FG, Fervenza FC. Long-term outcome of kidney transplantation in patients with fibrillary glomerulonephritis or monoclonal gammopathy with fibrillary deposits. Kidney Int. 2009;75(4):420–7. Epub 2008/11/28.
74. Isaac J, Herrara GA, Shihab FS. De novo fibrillary glomerulopathy in the renal allograft of a patient with systemic lupus erythematosus. Nephron. 2001;87(4):365–8. Epub 2001/04/05.
75. Gough J, Yilmaz A, Yilmaz S, Benediktsson H. Recurrent and de novo glomerular immune-complex deposits in renal transplant

biopsies. Arch Pathol Lab Med. 2005;129(2):231–3. Epub 2005/02/01.

76. Moroni G, Gallelli B, Diana A, Carminati A, Banfi G, Poli F, et al. Renal transplantation in adults with Henoch-Schonlein purpura: long-term outcome. Nephrol Dial Transplant. 2008;23(9):3010–6. Epub 2008/04/22.
77. Han SS, Sun HK, Lee JP, Ha JW, Kim SJ, Kim YS. Outcome of renal allograft in patients with Henoch-Schonlein nephritis: single-center experience and systematic review. Transplantation. 2010;89(6):721–6. Epub 2009/12/17.
78. Samuel JP, Bell CS, Molony DA, Braun MC. Long-term outcome of renal transplantation patients with Henoch-Schonlein purpura. Clin J Am Soc Nephrol. 2011;6(8):2034–40. Epub 2011/06/28.
79. Mauer SM, Barbosa J, Vernier RL, Kjellstrand CM, Buselmeier TJ, Simmons RL, et al. Development of diabetic vascular lesions in normal kidneys transplanted into patients with diabetes mellitus. N Engl J Med. 1976;295(17):916–20. Epub 1976/10/21.
80. Bhalla V, Nast CC, Stollenwerk N, Tran S, Barba L, Kamil ES, et al. Recurrent and de novo diabetic nephropathy in renal allografts. Transplantation. 2003;75(1):66–71. Epub 2003/01/25.
81. Miles AM, Sumrani N, Horowitz R, Homel P, Maursky V, Markell MS, et al. Diabetes mellitus after renal transplantation: as deleterious as non-transplant-associated diabetes? Transplantation. 1998;65(3):380–4. Epub 1998/03/04.
82. Burroughs TE, Swindle J, Takemoto S, Lentine KL, Machnicki G, Irish WD, et al. Diabetic complications associated with new-onset diabetes mellitus in renal transplant recipients. Transplantation. 2007;83(8):1027–34. Epub 2007/04/25.
83. Bergstralh EJ, Monico CG, Lieske JC, Herges RM, Langman CB, Hoppe B, et al. Transplantation outcomes in primary hyperoxaluria. Am J Transplant. 2010;10(11):2493–501. Epub 2010/09/21.
84. Cybulla M, Walter KN, Schwarting A, Divito R, Feriozzi S, Sunder-Plassmann G, et al. Kidney transplantation in patients with Fabry disease. Transpl Int. 2009;22(4):475–81. Epub 2009/02/12.
85. Mosnier JF, Degott C, Bedrossian J, Molas G, Degos F, Pruna A, et al. Recurrence of Fabry's disease in a renal allograft eleven years after successful renal transplantation. Transplantation. 1991;51(4):759–62. Epub 1991/04/01.

Psychosocial Issues in Renal Transplantation

16

Charles Cangro

The early history of hemodialysis and transplantation, the initial limited availability of these lifesaving therapies, and the effect of passage of Public Law 92-603, the End-Stage Renal Disease Program of Medicare, are reviewed. The current success of renal replacement therapies, especially transplantation, and the near universal availability of these therapies in the United States have changed societal expectation. Compared to 50 years ago, ESRD patients expect to receive dialysis, and many seek a better quality of life offered by transplantation. Today transplantation is available to a population of patients who are older, who suffer with more chronic illnesses, and who often have limited financial and psychosocial support.

The influence of psychosocial factors including cognitive deficit, depression, anxiety, psychosis, and psychiatric illness on long-term allograft survival is examined. Risk for nonadherence, the need for social support, and a realistic assessment of the cost of renal transplantation should be a cornerstone of the pre-transplant psychosocial evaluation. The effect of common behaviors such as smoking and tobacco, alcohol, and illicit drug use; lack of exercise; and obesity and the detrimental effect these behaviors can have on recipient and allograft survival must be considered. There is a shortage of donor kidneys, and society is challenged with developing fair and equitable allocation schemes for kidney allografts, a scarce medical resource. As our population ages, lives longer with chronic medical illnesses, the demand for kidneys will only increase.

Just as a thorough evaluation for preexisting medical conditions and appropriate control of these chronic illnesses should be a prerequisite for transplantation, so too a complete psychosocial review of each candidate should be obtained. Actions should be taken before transplantation to address deficiencies in family and social support, individual coping skills, and access to adequate insurance and financial resources.

C. Cangro, M.D., Ph.D. (✉)
University of Maryland School of Medicine,
22 S. Greene Street, N3W143, Baltimore, MD 21201, USA
e-mail: ccangro@medicine.umaryland.edu

There are at least five major factors which interact to determine the success and longevity of a renal transplant: the health of the recipient, the quality of the donor kidney, immunologic factors, the competency of the transplant team, and the psychosocial milieu in which the recipient lives. Specific algorithms have been published to evaluate the medical suitability of an individual to be a transplant recipient. Prospective patients are tested for cardiac reserve and the ability to survive the surgical procedure as well as for the effect of chronic illnesses such as diabetes and hepatic, respiratory, and infectious diseases. Chances for long-term survival are affected by preexisting disease burden. Younger, healthier individuals who do not carry the burden of chronic illness are the best candidates [1–3].

Donor kidneys quality depends not only on whether the donor is living—biologically related or not—or deceased but also on warm and cold ischemia times, donor age and health, and the trauma of organ procurement. Living donor kidneys, from biologically related donors, with shorter cold ischemia times have survival advantage.

Thirdly, immunologic factors play a major role in long-term graft survival. The immunosuppressive medications currently available have, over the past 40 years, diminished the frequency and intensity of rejection episodes. Long-term control of the recipient's immune system remains key to allograft survival.

Yet despite a competent, experienced surgical team transplanting the ideal donor kidney into a healthy recipient, long-term success is not assured. Myriad of psychosocial factors play a significant role in transplantation success.

Historical Perspective: Renal Replacement Therapy for All

The first publications describing extracorporeal dialysis appeared 100 years ago in 1913. In 1924, George Haas in Germany performed the first dialysis treatment involving humans. Jump ahead 20 years to 1945, Willem Kolff of the

M.R. Weir and E.V. Lerma (eds.), *Kidney Transplantation: Practical Guide to Management*,
DOI 10.1007/978-1-4939-0342-9_16, © Springer Science+Business Media New York 2014

Netherlands successfully used a rotating drum kidney to treat a 67-year-old patient with acute kidney injury. The treatment was successful and the patient survived. The Kolff rotating drum kidney became the basis for the Kolff-Brigham rotating drum kidney developed at the Peter Brant Brigham Hospital in Boston. The Kolff-Brigham kidney, developed between 1954 and 1962, became the standard of care for the time and was shipped worldwide. The Kolff-Brigham kidney can be described as the first practical dialysis machine. It was used during the Korean War in MASH units to treat soldiers with acute kidney injury. Before the standardization of this early dialysis technique, patients with severe acute kidney injury and end-stage renal disease routinely died in a number of days to weeks. The rotating drum dialysis machine was a breakthrough. Dialysis machines were expensive however. They were difficult to set up, and the treatments were costly in time and money. Few of the patients who faced end-stage renal disease at that time knew about or had the opportunity to receive dialysis treatment [3, 4].

The first successful renal transplant was performed in 1954 by Joseph Murray, MD at the Peter Brant Brigham Hospital in Boston [5]. The recipient received a kidney from his identical twin brother. The procedure proved that the surgical technique of renal transplantation was possible. However, very few individuals with end-stage renal disease have identical twin siblings. The amazing scope and built-in redundancy of the immune system hampered the expansion of transplantation as a treatment for end-stage kidney disease. Progressive advances using radiation, high dose steroids, and later, Imuran made kidney transplantation possible for a greater number of patients. However, graft survival was still only about 50 % during the 1970s [6]. Some at the time viewed transplantation merely as a bridge or brief reprieve between longer periods of maintenance dialysis for most patients. Between 1954 and 1973, approximately 10,000 kidney transplants were performed. Long-term allograft survival was limited due to suboptimal immunosuppression. Because of medical costs, access to dialysis and transplantation was reserved for a fortunate few with the means, the contacts, and the luck.

A major breakthrough came about in the early 1980s with the discovery of cyclosporine. Now with improved organ preservation, surgical techniques, and this new powerful immunosuppressive medication, 1-year survival of kidney transplants jumped from 65 to 85 % [6]. Options for the patients diagnosed with kidney failure were improving. At the same time advances were made in dialysis. Dialysis machines and membranes were improving.

Patients diagnosed with end-stage renal disease in the 1950s faced near certain imminent death. Dialysis and kidney transplantation were procedures available to very few people at only a few medical centers, and they were medical treatments beyond the financial reach of most patients. Recognizing that the average American could never pay for hemodialysis or a kidney transplantation procedure and the inequality in the access to these lifesaving treatments, the US Congress established an entitlement to the Medicare benefits for people diagnosed with permanent kidney failure in the form of the Social Security Amendment of 1972. This entitlement, which has become known as the End-Stage Renal Disease Program of Medicare, provides medical care to people with the diagnosis of permanent kidney failure who are insured or eligible for coverage under social security. This was the first legislation of its type that provided coverage for a specific health condition to all Medicare-eligible citizens. Under Public Law 92-603, patients with ESRD are entitled to Medicare if they are fully or currently insured for benefits under Social Security or are a spouse or dependent of an insured person. Consequently, entitlement is nearly universal, with 92 % of all persons with ESRD qualifying for Medicare coverage [7, 8].

The End-Stage Renal Disease Program of Medicare made lifesaving renal replacement therapy financially feasible for thousands of Americans providing hope where previously there had been none. The Medicare ESRD Program and subsequent amendments have been extremely successful and are estimated to have prolonged the life of over one million Americans who would have otherwise faced premature death [7]. Life-sustaining dialysis treatment and dialysis as a bridge to transplantation are now available to essentially all individuals in the United States.

The Changing Population of ESRD Patients and the Scope, Cost, and Size of the Medicare End-Stage Renal Disease Program

During the 40-year span of time, 1970 to present, when dialysis and transplant care were improving medicine, other medical advancements have significantly prolonged life expectancy. As a direct result, the ESRD patient population has changed. The median age of ESRD patients and the number of these individuals surviving with concurrent serious chronic medical conditions, such as diabetes, coronary artery disease, hepatitis B, hepatitis C, and HIV, have increased dramatically [9]. Initially diabetes and advanced age were viewed as a contraindication to long-term renal replacement therapy [6]. At present more than 50 % of individuals diagnosed with ESRD who begin renal replacement therapy are over 65 years of age and 45 % have some form of diabetes [6]. Since the medical profession has become so successful in managing chronic conditions in the end-stage renal disease population, now more than ever, many more patients are seeking kidney transplants.

In 1975, when the Medicare End-Stage Renal Disease Program was first available, approximately 16,000 individuals enrolled. By the end of 2009, the most recent year for which accurate figures are available, almost 399,000 patients were being treated for end-stage renal disease, and approximately 172,000 individuals were alive with functioning renal transplants [10]. The cost of providing long-term renal transplant care has grown significantly over the past 40 years. Original annual program expenditures were projected in 1972 to be only 250 million dollars per year [11]. The program has grown far beyond these initial estimates. As of 2009 it had grown to 42 billion dollars per year with 29 billion paid directly by the Medicare program. The reason for this massive balloon in cost is multifactorial. The total number of people who are diagnosed and surviving to reach ERSD annually (incidence) has increased. Over the same time, medicine has become more successful, prolonging life expectancy and keeping individuals with chronic illness healthier longer. Despite caring for a population of patients who are older and afflicted with more chronic illnesses, in terms of cost of care per patient enrolled in the Medicare ESRD Program, the cost has stabilized or decreased [12].

At its inception, the Medicare End-Stage Renal Disease Program was designed to offer a mechanism for individuals with end-stage renal disease to survive. It is estimated that over one million people have benefited from this program. Unfortunately the incidence rate of end-stage renal disease each year has increased progressively over the past 15 years. Although there may be some stabilization in this number, it remains at 350 cases per million per year. Today, in 2013, with more than one in ten Americans—some 20 million people!—having some form of chronic kidney disease, the burden to society of caring for all these patients is increasing [10, 12].

Kidneys Suitable for Transplantation: A Scarce Medical Resource

Society has modified its practices to meet the economic challenges in providing health care to individuals with end-stage renal disease. Under Public Law 92-603, the ESRD Medicare amendment, individuals with renal failure can receive treatment.

The cost per patient of this program is decreasing at the same time that there is greater emphasis on quality initiatives designed to guarantee standard of care treatment. Furthermore, transplantation now makes economic sense to society. The yearly costs for treating a patient on HD are nearly triple the costs of maintaining a transplant patient [13]. Renal transplantation has become so successful that first year graft survival exceeds 90–93 % [14]. Recognizing the improved quality of life and survival benefit of renal transplantation, increasing numbers of individuals are seeking kidney transplants. While a mechanism exists for patients to be maintained on dialysis while awaiting a kidney and funding exists to cover the cost of transplantation, there is a critical shortage of transplantable kidneys.

In 2012 there were over 117,000 patients waiting for a kidney transplant in the United States. During the same time, only 28,000 renal transplants were able to be performed [15]. One in every five individuals on the kidney transplant waiting list will die before they receive a kidney. Who, among the ever-increasing number of patients being evaluated for renal transplantation, should be listed? Can society offer to everyone, regardless of preexisting chronic medical conditions, age, life expectancy, psychosocial support system, competency, and ability to adhere to a complicated medical regimen, the same access and opportunity to receive a kidney transplant?

Can a 68-year-old obese individual with diabetes, hypertension, and coronary artery disease have the same expectation to receive a kidney transplant as a 22-year-old with end-stage renal disease secondary to polycystic kidney disease? Currently organ allocation is based primarily on the length of time on the transplant waiting list.

Several years ago, an effort was made to develop a more equitable distribution of organs to the ever-expanding list of older and more chronically ill patients with renal failure based upon anticipated life years from transplant (LYFT). The concept was that older recipients with a greater burden of chronic illness would be offered kidneys from older donors given the statistically shorter life expectancy. Organs from younger donors would be directed to younger recipients with less burden of chronic disease. In this way society would obtain the maximal number of years of function from the available pool of donated kidneys. In summation it was hoped fewer "years of viable function" would be lost as recipients died with functioning grafts [16]. The proposal was never accepted.

Though dialysis does prolong life, evidence suggests that the quality of life for these patients is poor. The success of transplantation has created an expectation in society that not only can individuals with end-stage renal disease be kept alive on dialysis, but they also can seek a new life with a kidney transplant. Unfortunately, all too often, patients are unaware that transplant recipients face a new chronic illness, one which is often unrecognized pre-transplant, the burden of a life on maintenance immunosuppression.

Evaluation of Potential Renal Transplant Recipients

It has clearly been established that transplantation is the best option for most individuals receiving renal replacement therapy. Quality of life measures, survival, and even medical costs favor transplantation over maintenance hemodialysis. Despite all this, the decision to transplant some candidates is not straightforward. Because in 2013, transplant candidates are often older with concurrent chronic illnesses [16], the medical community needs to understand which medical and psychosocial requirements must be addressed if these transplant patients are to enjoy long-term success.

Specific algorithms have been published to evaluate the medical suitability of an individual to be a transplant recipient. Patients are tested for cardiac reserve and the ability to undergo the surgical procedure. They are examined for the presence and burden of chronic illnesses such as diabetes and hepatic, respiratory, and infectious diseases. Medical decisions are made based upon a patient's chances of surviving the surgery and not being adversely effected by lifelong immunosuppressive therapy. For many medical conditions, published data exists to document and guide the medical decision-making process [1, 2, 17].

For the psychosocial evaluation, the patient's cognition, mental health, psychiatric stability, medical nonadherence, history of substance and tobacco abuse, eating disorders, and presence of obesity are considered. The patient's insurance, finances, and available social support from family and friends are given equal consideration. While the medical selection criteria have been well defined, there has been a paucity of studies that document evidence-based criteria for acceptable psychosocial risks for transplant candidates [18]. The goal of any evaluation is to use evidence-based criteria, whether it be in the medical realm or in the psychosocial realm, to define and identify individuals who have the best opportunity for a successful long life after transplantation. Unfortunately, many psychosocial parameters do not have the same evidence-based absolute contraindications and objective measures available for decision making as in the fields of cardiac medicine, infectious disease, and cancer.

Cognitive Function, Mental Retardation, and Transplantation

Mental retardation is defined as an IQ of less than 70 assessed by the Wechsler Intelligence Scale. A basic intellectual capacity is required if the patient is to learn the skills and knowledge necessary to maintain a healthy lifestyle. Despite this, many mentally retarded individuals have been successfully transplanted and done very well. More than in any other group, however, the success of transplantation in this population has been totally attributed to the social support provided to each of these individuals. The presence of an adequate, committed, and lifelong social support caregiver or group capable of 24/7 monitoring and assistance must be established before mentally retarded patients are transplanted. Without an identified support system willing and capable of giving individualized care, transplantation should not be undertaken.

Ideally every transplant candidate should have the requisite IQ and level of cognitive function to understand why they are being offered a kidney transplant. Severe cognitive defects are most often the result of birth defects, structural brain injury, cerebral palsy, and anoxia. Whenever possible, informed consent for the transplant should be obtained from the patient. If unable to give legal informed consent, assent and acceptance of the procedure should be sought. At minimum, patients with impaired cognition should be willing to accept and not resist the medical care. Posttransplant, those with greater cognitive impairment will require greater supervision and monitoring. This can be provided by a combination of a group home, monitored day care, or devoted social and family support. Even the most challenged individuals with significant cognitive impairment can benefit from renal transplantation. Cognitively impaired patients can be successful transplant recipients if they are cooperative, if adequate support is available to ensure medications are administered on time, and if lab and clinic appointments are kept [19].

Cognitive deficits can develop while waiting for and even after transplantation. With the aging of CKD and ESRD populations, many of whom are now surviving longer, and with more chronic medical illness, the problem of loss of cognitive function and greater dependency on social and family support among the elderly is increasing. Patients now wait an average of 3–5 years for deceased donor kidneys. The elderly can have significant loss in their cognitive ability to care for themselves during this time. Similarly after transplantation, despite having good allograft function, they can experience progressive cognitive losses and loss of ability to follow complex medical regimens [20]. As is the case with many elements of the psychosocial evaluation, cognitive impairment is seldom an absolute contraindication to transplantation. The influence of cognitive function on a patient's candidacy to receive a renal transplant must consider depth and durability of the social support available to help the individual after transplant.

Organic Brain Disorders in Transplantation

Neurocognitive dysfunction that results from metabolic disorders can occur as a result of poor dialysis, liver disease, repeated strokes, intractable seizures, and other metabolic disorders, including alcoholism. Organic brain disorders will impair an individual's ability to adhere to a posttransplant regimen and may make it difficult to establish a therapeutic relationship with the transplant physician. While neurocognitive dysfunction, secondary to uremia, can be improved with adequate dialysis and may improve further with transplantation, such cases must be examined to determine why the patient has uremic organic brain disorder. Adequate dialysis should prevent the development of such a problem. Dialysis that is cut short, not attended on a regular basis, or complicated by nonadherence with diet and food restrictions can contribute to organic brain disorders in ESRD patients. Thus, nonadherence while on dialysis may be a harbinger of later posttransplant nonadherence behavior.

Depression and Anxiety

A patient's mental health is an important predictor of adherence. Depression, anxiety, and adjustment disorder are commonly found during pre-transplant evaluation. As many as one third of ESRD patients report some feelings of depression [21]. Some studies have found that depression and anxiety are a normal condition and response in many individuals who develop end-stage renal disease. Anxiety or depression does not necessarily persist in the posttransplant period. Every patient must be examined closely. Certainly patients who have a history of anxiety and depression before developing end-stage renal disease must be carefully evaluated. While it is nice to believe that a great deal of the anxiety and depression felt by patients awaiting transplantation will disappear with their "cure" after receiving a kidney allograft, this may not occur.

Studies have shown that individuals who are depressed are more likely to suffer with nonadherence. Depression is associated with an increased mortality and morbidity and is considered to be very common among patients with end-stage renal disease. It has been shown in other illnesses that depressed patients are more likely to be nonadherent [22]. Efforts to modify and treat the depression when initially diagnosed with CKD, while on dialysis, and while awaiting transplantation should be made. Early interventions and treatment can have significant beneficial effects upon outcomes both on dialysis and later after transplantation.

The causes of depression in end-stage renal diseases are multifactorial. On dialysis, a loss of control of one's life, being tied to a regular schedule, and dependence upon a machine have all been shown to generate depression over loss of freedom and self-determination. After transplantation, this feeling may continue or may be vastly altered depending upon the perceived relationship between the patient and the posttransplant care providers. Educating patients, involving them in their care, and making them understand that they are able to change their lives all vastly improve a patient's chance for a successful outcome. Feeling better is best achieved with good adherence, participating in care decisions, and exercise. This is an essential point which should be conveyed by the physician to every transplant patient. By empowering the patients to become more involved in their care, but at the same time not overwhelming them, transplant recipients can gain personal satisfaction from their daily achievements and markedly improve their quality of life as a successful transplant patient.

During the pre-transplant evaluation, medical providers who know the patient the best should be asked about the patient's level of depression. Certainly, individuals who have a history of depression before entering end-stage renal disease should be examined closely. Transplantation is not a cure, but rather a prolongation of a different form of chronic disease. While transplant recipients enjoy the end of dialysis treatment three times a week, they must understand they will have to adhere to a medication regimen nearly as time-consuming. For some the structured life on dialysis may be easy compared to the self-discipline and self-motivation needed to take meds on a daily schedule. A patient who misses one or two dialysis sessions quickly becomes symptomatic. Dialysis centers often contact a patient if they fail to attend a dialysis session. In contrast lack of adherence with daily medications after transplantation goes unnoticed for a longer period of time because patients do not immediately become symptomatic. In fact, they often feel better off meds. But nonadherence has catastrophic consequences. Unlike the dialysis attendance record, the only objective measures to monitor nonadherence posttransplant are immunosuppression drug levels, the frequency of routine lab draws, and clinic "no show" rates.

Testing for evidence of depression must be a part of the psychosocial evaluation of a patient seeking transplantation. Screening for depression is a valuable initiative to incorporate into the treatment algorithm of all patients with CKD. Simple tools to evaluate a patient for depression are available to nephrologists as they follow patients through the latter stages of CKD and into ESRD. Early recognition and treatment with counseling and medications during the development of CKD likely will improve the quality of life of patients and promote adherence both before and after transplantation [22].

Psychiatric Illnesses/Psychoses in Transplantation

The major psychiatric illnesses, including schizophrenia and bipolar disease, are less common than depression and anxiety in the ESRD population. Little data exists documenting the success or failure of transplanted patients who suffer schizophrenia, bipolar disease, or similar psychoses. These disorders, if left untreated, likely will increase the risk of poor adherence and make it difficult to establish cooperative treatment relationships between the medical provider and the patient. Appropriate psychiatric treatment and a pre-transplant evaluation by a psychiatrist might justify placing certain psychiatric patients on the transplant waiting list. A common theme throughout the literature on this topic stresses the importance of a patient's social support mechanisms. With good lifelong social support, recipient adherence and allograft survival can be achieved and sustained. The presence of psychoses is not an absolute contraindication to transplantation.

Individuals with personality disorders frequently have difficulty with emotions, social contact, and impulse control. Personality disorders may make it very difficult to establish a working physician/patient relationship. Personality disorders have been reported to be associated with increased noncompliance. Because personality disorders have been clearly shown to be associated with nonadherence, the presence of prior behavior consistent with personality disorder, emotional dysfunction, and maladaptive patterns of social interaction is considered by some to be a contraindication to transplantation. There is limited pharmacologic therapy available for this class of mental illness. Each candidate with evidence of a personality disorder should be evaluated for history of criminal behavior and problems with the law. They should receive a full psychiatric evaluation. Documentation should be obtained from past and present nephrologists and health-care providers demonstrating the ability to maintain long-term medical follow-up.

Nonadherence, Compliance, and Adherence with Medication

Poor adherence to medication regimens has been shown to be a major contributor to suboptimal graft survival. More than a decade ago, it was shown that nonadherence cost the United States over $100,000,000.00 annually. Nonadherence with medications occurs when patients do not take medications as prescribed. Nonadherence also occurs when patients do not have lab work done or fail to show for scheduled appointments. Nonadherence is a primary cause of kidney rejection. Nonadherent patients are seven times more likely to suffer graft failure than are patients who are adherent [23].

Factors known to contribute to nonadherence include the number of medications administered, the complexity of a medication dosing schedule, medications' side effects, palatability, patients' beliefs about the necessity to continue taking the medication, the cost of medication, and the cost to the patient of follow-up care visits. Finally, increased intervals between follow-up encounters, lack of contact with the medical team, and poor reinforcement by health-care providers can increase the risk of nonadherence.

Adherence to medications is only one aspect of the lifestyle change which recipients' of renal allografts must accept and undertake. A strict medicine regimen and diet modification, including salt restriction and heart-healthy foods, are routinely recommended in the posttransplant phase as a mechanism to prolong graft survival and limit patient morbidity and mortality. It would seem only logical, therefore, that pre-transplantation behavior and adherence should be examined to determine if a patient's behavior needs to be addressed before entrusting them with a precious allograft. Currently, adherence with hemodialysis treatments, attendance at dialysis, frequency of early sign-offs, behavioral interactions with the staff at the dialysis center, and compliance with dietary restrictions on phosphorus and salt use are reviewed by some transplant centers to evaluate a patient's suitability for transplantation [24].

Behavior and Kidney Transplantation

Certain behaviors may have detrimental effects on the success of kidney transplantation. These have been hypothesized to include drug and alcohol abuse, smoking, and obesity.

Substance Abuse and Transplantation

Physical dependence and inability to control alcohol use are the hallmarks of alcohol abuse. The effects of alcohol abuse on transplantation had been most widely studied in liver transplant candidates. Most liver transplant programs require a period of abstinence before listing a patient for transplantation. Despite this, there is a lack of scientific evidence to establish that a period of mandated abstinence assures long-term control of alcohol abuse. Alcoholics are frequently found to have polysubstance abuse, including tobacco and illicit drug use. Alcoholism is more common in some psychiatric disorders, including schizophrenia and depression, as well as personality disorders [15]. Alcohol abuse can be associated with the lack of self-care, which by conjecture may lead to posttransplant nonadherence. While data establishing a relationship between prerenal transplant alcohol abuse, nonadherence, and increased graft failure is lacking, a careful assessment of patients with a history of alcoholism, motor vehicle accidents, arrests, and hospitalizations for excessive alcohol use should be undertaken. The greater the number of years without alcohol use pre-transplant, the less the risk of complications resulting from inappropriate alcohol use after transplantation.

Active drug abuse involving opioids, cocaine derivatives, and designer drugs is an absolute contraindication for transplantation. Patients identified as having these substances in their blood at the time of pre-transplant screening should not be allowed to proceed with transplant evaluation until such time they can demonstrate and maintain negative drug screens. Random drug screening samples should be obtained periodically. After discussion, medical assistance and counseling should be made available to interested patients.

While opioids, cocaine, and designer drugs are an absolute contraindication to transplantation, many recent state laws have changed in regard to marijuana. The presence of cannabinoids in a patient's blood at the time of screening should be discussed with the individual along with the consequences of use. Some states allow the use of medical marijuana and the possession of small quantities of cannabis. Responsible use of these may not be an absolute contraindication to listing for transplantation. More research is needed on the effect of cannabis use on renal allograft survival, function, and interaction with other medications. Each patient should be individually assessed as to the effect their drug use has on their ability to comply with posttransplant drug regimens and to adhere to the recommendations provided by the transplant team.

Smoking and Transplantation

Smoking is a form of substance abuse. Practitioners are now required to ask every patient if they smoke and if they want to quit and to direct them towards assistance should they want help with their tobacco abuse. Smoking is associated with decreased longevity, complications with pulmonary function, and premature death and may directly affect renal function [25]. Smoking before transplantation and ongoing tobacco abuse after transplantation definitely increase cardiovascular risks as well as the risk of specific cancers. The cancer risk associated with tobacco abuse is likely increased in the immunosuppressed patient. The deleterious effects of smoking on the vascular system have been confirmed in a large group of renal transplant patients who continue to smoke posttransplant [26].

In the past, patients were required to demonstrate a period of tobacco abstinence before being listed for transplantation. The criteria for listing vary at many institutions. Renal transplant recipients should be encouraged at the time of the initial evaluation to stop tobacco use. Every day without a cigarette will facilitate the respiratory course during the peritransplant period. The longer patients abstain from smoking pre- and posttransplantation, the more beneficial effects they have by limiting organ damage and minimizing cancer risk.

The use of chewing tobacco should likewise be addressed and discouraged. The incidence of oral cancers is significantly higher in patients who chew tobacco. Oral cancers develop and spread more rapidly in individuals on immunosuppressive medications posttransplant [27].

Obesity and Transplantation

Obesity, defined as a body mass index greater then 30, is present in over 40 % of the US population. Obesity is associated with both surgical and postsurgical complications in the transplant population. Obese individuals are at greater risk for wound dehiscence and wound infection. Patients with elevated BMI are at increased risk for cardiovascular disease, decreased pulmonary function, diabetes, and gastrointestinal disorders. In kidney transplant patients, obesity is associated with increased morbidity and mortality [28, 29].

While the immediate postoperative complications from obesity, such as wound dehiscence and infections, can be managed, they prolong hospitalization, lead to a greater need for rehabilitation, and may significantly prolong recovery, especially in the older population. Obesity worsens hypertensive control and predisposes individuals to new-onset diabetes after transplant (NODAT) and worsens diabetic control in individuals already with that diagnosis. While short-term survival of obese patients is comparable to those of nonobese individuals, the 5-year survival of obese transplant patients has been shown to be inferior to that of nonobese controls. Obese individuals have a higher cardiac morbidity and mortality. This finding has led to the realization that individuals being evaluated for transplantation, especially those who are obese and have type 2 diabetes, must receive thorough annual cardiac reevaluations while on the waiting list.

Some programs mandate that patients must demonstrate efforts to lose weight before they are actively listed for transplantation. This demand often will motivate change not previously attempted [30].

Many patients gain weight after transplantation. This puts them at increased risk for diabetes [31]. While the data to encourage exercise among individuals on renal replacement therapy is limited, transplant recipients should be strongly urged to incorporate routine cardiovascular exercise into their posttransplant life. In as little as 3 months postsurgery, the importance of regular cardiovascular exercise should be repeatedly stressed to the patient during every encounter. If patients can be convinced to take up this challenge, they will improve their blood pressure control, improve their diabetic control, and/or limit their risk of developing NODAT. In addition, they will undoubtedly feel better as they take control of another part of their life and feel better for it.

Social Support in Transplantation

Both perceived and received social support play a role in successful medical management of chronically ill patients. Patients who have low perceived support often feel isolated and may experience significantly more depression. The perceived support projected by the transplant team may mitigate the stress, anxiety, and depression associated with renal transplantation. The social support which the transplant recipient receives at home and by those close to him—the spouse, partner, and immediate family—also have beneficial effects on compliance. The clearest example of this is with the older, frail transplant recipient who receives assistance from a social support network in the form of precooked meals, medication timing reminders, transport to and from clinic appointments, and help with various other daily activities that may be difficult to do in the early posttransplant period. The identification of a robust social support team can significantly impact the outcome of not only the transplant surgery itself but also long-term allograft survival [14].

Inadequate identification of social support and, more importantly, the changes that occur in previously identified social support elements as individuals wait for a renal allograft 2, 3, 4, or more years can have significant complicating effects in a transplant patient. Social support is critical to the success of transplantation in the elderly (35). While appropriate elements of the social support structure should be identified during an initial evaluation, they should be reexamined on a periodic basis [32].

Financial Considerations During the Psychosocial Evaluation

At the beginning of this chapter, a historical overview was given on how legislation came about to make dialysis and transplantation available to most people in the United States. The Medicare benefits for maintenance dialysis have no time limitation. When initially proposed, Medicare coverage for transplantation was limited to 12 months. Transplantation was viewed as a cure. The expectation was that patients would be able to return to work and obtain private insurance through their employer. Medicare benefits have since been extended to 36 months posttransplant. Allograft survival posttransplant requires patients to take lifelong maintenance immunosuppression. The average annual cost of immunosuppression is $15,000–$18,000. Unfortunately only one third of transplant recipients return to full-time employment and secure employer-based insurance to cover their medication, lab, and physician costs. One third of transplant recipients qualify for ongoing Medicare coverage based upon having a disability other than ESRD. The remaining one third of individuals can be faced with significant shortfalls in coverage to pay for medications, blood testing, and physician visits after 3 years.

A very important part of the psychosocial evaluation of every transplant candidate is a meeting with a licensed transplant social worker familiar with the time sensitive variation in benefits available to patients after transplantation. For the one third of patients who are not permanently disabled, over 65, unable to return to work, or to find employment with insurance benefits adequate to meet their needs as a transplant recipient, they potentially face the loss of their defined Medicare benefits after 3 years. Such individuals rely heavily on state programs, pharmaceutical sponsored medication supplies and indigent care programs.

Return to Work After Transplantation

The goal of renal transplantation is to provide the patient with a better quality of life, to improve their long-term survival, and ideally to return them to the workforce. But because the population of patients entering end-stage renal disease is older and has more chronic medical conditions than ever before, 82 % will never return to work. While it is unlikely that older individuals will return to the workforce, younger patients should be encouraged to discuss their work expectations early. Receiving a renal allograft is truly a gift meant to improve a patient's quality of life. Since Medicare benefits cover posttransplant care for only 36 months, a patient's quality of life and ability to adhere to the medication regimen will be improved if they can return to work. Given the explosive increase in chronic kidney disease and the aging of the population of the United States, Medicare benefits for those healthy enough to return to work cannot be considered lifelong. New programs aimed at supporting working transplant recipients with their medications and follow-up physician visits would have long-lasting societal benefits [33].

Frequency of Psychosocial Reevaluation

Psychosocial reevaluation should occur at least as often as medical reexamination. Older candidates with limited self-caring skills and support structures liable to change should be flagged for frequent follow-up. Caregivers pass away, suffer their own changes in health, move away, or are deployed. If during the initial evaluation, a transplant candidate is identified as being heavily dependent on a specific support person or group, frequent contact should be maintained. If a change occurs, the support members should be encouraged to call and update the psychosocial information. While they should be reassured it is very unlikely that anyone would be removed for the active waiting list based on a change in a candidate's psychosocial support, knowledge and preparedness will help smooth out postoperative care and improve the likelihood of successful transition into the posttransplant arena.

Long-Term Follow-up Care

Long-term renal allograft and recipient survival require contributions by many individuals. The patient, his or her family, previously identified caregivers, local physicians, and members of the posttransplant team all must maintain a watchful eye on the individual patient's condition. While local nephrologists and primary care physicians are essential to the health maintenance of posttransplant patients, most non-transplant physicians lack the experience and support staff, including posttransplant coordinators, to log, monitor, and maintain immunosuppressive drug levels and allograft function. While community nephrologists may yearn to continue to see and to care for their patients after transplantation, few have the staff, full range of expertise, and resources to follow such patients. An ever-increasing number of private nephrology groups are finding that it is not economically feasible to manage large numbers of posttransplant recipients.

In conclusion, renal transplantation is not a cure, but when well managed, renal transplant patients have a greatly improved quality of life over dialysis patients. Since the medical care of the posttransplant patient is similar to the management of patients with other chronic medical conditions such as heart failure, diabetes, HIV, and cancer, the society and the medical profession must now acknowledge the critical role psychosocial factors can and do play in long-term allograft and patient survival.

References

1. Dudley C, Harden P. Renal Association Clinical Practice Guideline on the assessment of the potential kidney transplant recipient. Nephron Clin Pract. 2011;118 Suppl 1:c209–24.
2. Kasiske BL, Cangro CB, Hariharan S, Hricik DE, Kerman RH, Roth D, Rush DN, Vazquez MA, Weir MR. The evaluation of renal transplantation candidates: clinical practice guidelines. Am J Transplant. 2001;1 Suppl 2:3–95.
3. Peitzman SJ. Chronic dialysis and dialysis doctors in the United States: a nephrologist-historian's perspective. Semin Dial. 2001; 14:200–8.
4. Peitzman SJ. Science, inventors, and the introduction of the artificial kidney in the United States. Semin Dial. 1996;9:276–81.
5. Snyder A. Joseph E. Murray. Lancet. 2013;381:110.
6. Halloran P, Gouriskankar S. Historical overview of pharmacology and immunosuppression. In: Primer of transplantation. 2 ed. Mt. Laurel, NJ: American Society of Transplantation; 2013. p. 73–5.
7. National Research Council. Kidney Failure and the Federal Government. The National Academies Press; 1991.
8. Fetherstonhaugh D. Dialysis: a paradigm case of rationing medical treatment. Renal Soc Australas J. 2009;5:88–94.
9. U.S. Renal Data System. USRDS 2012 annual data report: atlas of chronic kidney disease and end-stage renal disease in the United States. Bethesda, MD: National Institutes of Health, National Institute of Diabetes and Digestive and Kidney Diseases; 2012.
10. National Kidney and Urological Diseases Information Clearinghouse (NKUDIC). Kidney diseases statistics for the United States. Accesses 15 Nov 2012.
11. Klar RM. ESRD program projections and experience. JAMA. 1979;241:239–40.
12. USRDS Annual Data System Report 2012: Atlas of end-stage renal disease in the United States. Am J Kid Dis. 2013;61(Suppl 1):e1-e480.
13. Laupacis A, Keown P, Pus N, Krueger H, Ferguson B, Wong C, Muirhead N. A study of the quality of life and cost-utility of renal transplantation. Kidney Int. 1996;50:235–42.
14. The role of the transplant support person—Iowa City, VA; 2013.
15. Gish RG, Lee A, Brooks L, Leung J, Lau JY, Moore DH. Long-term follow-up of patients diagnosed with alcohol dependence or alcohol abuse who were evaluated for liver transplantation. Liver Transpl. 2001;7:581–7.
16. National Kidney Foundation Presentation at UNOS Kidney Allocation Forum. Kidney Allocation Forum. www.optn.transplant.hrsa.gov/kidneyconceptdocument. Accessed 26 Jan 2009.
17. Steinman TI, Becker BN, Frost AE, Olthoff KM, Smart FW, Suki WN, Wilkinson AH. Guidelines for the referral and management of patients eligible for solid organ transplantation. Transplantation. 2001;71:1189–204.
18. Butler JA, Roderick P, Mullee M, Mason JC, Peveler RC. Frequency and impact of nonadherence to immunosuppressants after renal transplantation: a systematic review. Transplantation. 2004;77: 769–76.
19. Benedetti E, Asolati M, Dunn T, Walczak DA, Papp P, Bartholomew AM, Smith Y, Washington AW, Pollak R. Kidney transplantation in recipients with mental retardation: clinical results in a single-center experience. Am J Kidney Dis. 1998;31:509–12.
20. Madero M, Gul A, Sarnak MJ. Cognitive function in chronic kidney disease. Semin Dial. 2008;21:29–37.
21. Cukor D, Coplan J, Brown C, Friedman S, Cromwell-Smith A, Peterson RA, Kimmel PL. Depression and anxiety in urban hemodialysis patients. Clin J Am Soc Nephrol. 2007;2:484–90.
22. Cukor D, Rosenthal DS, Jindal RM, Brown CD, Kimmel PL. Depression is an important contributor to low medication adherence in hemodialyzed patients and transplant recipients. Kidney Int. 2009;75:1223–9.
23. Dew M, Switzer G, DiMartini A, Matukaitis J, Fitgerald M, Kormos R. Psychosocial assessments and outcomes in organ transplantation. Prog Transplant. 2000;10:239–61.
24. Loghman-Adham M. Medication noncompliance in patients with chronic disease: issues in dialysis and renal transplantation. Am J Manag Care. 2003;9:155–71.
25. Zitt N, Kollerits B, Neyer U, Mark W, Heininger D, Mayer G, Kronenberg F, Lhotta K. Cigarette smoking and chronic allograft nephropathy. Nephrol Dial Transplant. 2007;22:3034–9.
26. Kasiske BL, Klinger D. Cigarette smoking in renal transplant recipients. J Am Soc Nephrol. 2000;11:753–9.
27. Surman OS, Cosimi AB, DiMartini A. Psychiatric care of patients undergoing organ transplantation. Transplantation. 2009;87: 1753–61.
28. Cacciola RA, Pujar K, Ilham MA, Puliatti C, Asderakis A, Chavez R. Effect of degree of obesity on renal transplant outcome. Transplant Proc. 2008;40:3408–12.
29. Meier-Kriesche HU, Arndorfer JA, Kaplan B. The impact of body mass index on renal transplant outcomes: a significant independent risk factor for graft failure and patient death. Transplantation. 2002;73:70–4.
30. Lentine KL, Delos SR, Axelrod D, Schnitzler MA, Brennan DC, Tuttle-Newhall JE. Obesity and kidney transplant candidates: how big is too big for transplantation? Am J Nephrol. 2012;36:575–86.
31. el-Agroudy AE, Wafa EW, Gheith OE, Shehab el-Dein AB, Ghoneim MA. Weight gain after renal transplantation is a risk factor for patient and graft outcome. Transplantation. 2004;77: 1381–5.
32. Batabyal P, Chapman JR, Wong G, Craig JC, Tong A. Clinical practice guidelines on wait-listing for kidney transplantation: consistent and equitable? Transplantation. 2012;94:703–13.
33. Wilkins F, Bozik K, Bennett K. The impact of patient education and psychosocial supports on return to normalcy 36 months post-kidney transplant. Clin Transplant. 2003;17 Suppl 9:78–80.

Risks of Pregnancy in Renal Transplant Recipients

17

Dianne B. McKay and Michelle A. Josephson

History of Pregnancy in Transplant Recipients

Dr. Joseph Murray, who later received the Nobel Prize for performing the first successful kidney transplant, published the first report of pregnancy in transplant recipients in the NEJM [1]. Physicians at that time were worried about the safety of pregnancy in women with kidney transplants and cautioned physicians that there might be significant risks associated with pregnancy in maternal transplant recipients [2, 3]. Despite these early warnings, pregnancy in women with kidney transplants became commonplace. As pregnancy became more common though the care of the pregnant transplant recipient became guided by opinion-based practice, rather than established guidelines [4, 5]. To date we still do not have established guidelines for the care of pregnant transplant recipients or their offspring exposed to immunosuppressive medications in utero.

Sources of Data About Outcomes of Pregnancy in Transplant Recipients

Despite the lack of established guidelines, several registries have evolved to collect outcome data about reproductive issues in renal transplant recipients. These registries have developed both within the United States and throughout the world and provide important information about outcomes for both female and male transplant recipients. The way we manage pregnancy is based on information derived from reports from these voluntary registry data as well as from multi- and single-center reports, many of which rely on retrospective data.

In the United States, the National Transplantation Pregnancy Registry (NTPR) is the predominant source of information on pregnancy outcomes. The registry publishes outcomes on an annual basis and over 2,000 recipients reporting over 3,300 pregnancies have participated in the registry (www.ntpr.giftoflifeinstitute.org). The NTPR relies on voluntary reporting by either the patient or the physician caring for the patient.

Another registry that had previously provided a great deal of information on pregnancy outcomes was the United Kingdom Transplant Pregnancy Registry. This registry directly sought voluntary information from obstetrical units and aggressively collected data from 1992 to 2001. Another voluntary registry that provided important information was the European Dialysis and Transplant Association (EDTA) Registry. The EDTA Registry collected pregnancy data from 1960 to 1992, and recently began to collect data on pregnancies that occurred between 2007 and 2011 through the DIAlysis and Pregnancies in EuRope (DIAPER) study (www.era-edta-reg.org).

Other registries have evolved since these early ones, including registries that continue to provide information about pregnancy collected through the Australia and New Zealand Dialysis and Transplant Registry (www.anzdata.org.au) and several reports have come from centers participating in the Saudi Center for Organ Transplantation (www.scot.org.sa). At this time numerous other registries have developed to study outcomes in maternal transplant recipients and their offspring that are funded by pharmaceutical companies interested in evaluating the short- and long-term risks of their medications during pregnancy.

D.B. McKay, M.D. (✉)
Department of Medicine-Nephrology, University of California, San Diego, 9500 Gilman Drive, La Jolla, CA 92093, USA
e-mail: d1mckay@ucsd.edu

M.A. Josephson, M.D.
Department of Medicine, Section of Nephrology, University of Chicago, Chicago, IL, USA

M.R. Weir and E.V. Lerma (eds.), *Kidney Transplantation: Practical Guide to Management*, DOI 10.1007/978-1-4939-0342-9_17, © Springer Science+Business Media New York 2014

Fertility in Patients with ESRD

Fertility is decreased for both women and men on dialysis [6–8]. Women are often anovulatory, although it is reversed soon after transplantation [9, 10]. Women have been reported to become pregnant soon after transplantation and there are reports of early pregnancy occurring, due to rapid resumption of ovulation in the successfully transplanted patient [11–15]. Men are often infertile as well, due to defects in gonadal function, and their fertility is improved by transplantation [16]. Whether fertility is resumed to normal after transplantation is not known and data on the use of assisted reproduction in transplant recipients is evolving.

As our patients are waiting longer for deceased donor transplants, we are faced with women aging through their ideal reproductive years. In fact women with ESRD reach menopause at an earlier age than women with normal renal function [8]. Since patients are generally waiting longer to receive a deceased donor transplant, women are usually older when they undergo transplantation, and therefore conception can be challenging for the older female transplant recipient. This should be considered in counseling the female transplant recipient considering pregnancy. Men wishing to father children should not be prescribed sirolimus as there are several reports of infertility associated with sirolimus [17–19].

Contraception in Renal Transplant Recipients

Contraception is mandatory in all women of reproductive age and the American Society of Transplantation has recommended that contraception begin before the transplant procedure in women of reproductive age [5]. A report from a single center in Brazil demonstrated that although most female kidney transplant recipients were sexually active before and after transplantation, many were not counseled about the need for contraception and did not use any form of birth control [20]. It is strongly recommended that contraceptive methods be discussed with potential maternal transplant recipients during their pretransplant evaluation [5]. Contraception has not been recommended for male transplant recipients, as data to date suggest that male transplant recipients are not at significant risk of germ cell mutations associated with the use of immunosuppressive medications. There are no recommendations to delay reproduction assigned to male transplant recipients.

Effective contraception requires reliable suppression of fertility. Recommendations do not include the use of single barrier methods—such as condoms or diaphragms, due to the potential unreliability of their use. Reversible contraception methods include intrauterine devices (IUDs), hormonal methods, and barrier methods. The optimal method of contraception depends on several factors, including comorbid diseases that might be impacted by contraceptive hormones (such as liver and bone disease) and interactions with other medications. Although older reports suggested that IUDs were contraindicated in transplant recipients, newer types of IUD formulations appear to be effective without risk of pelvic inflammatory disease [21, 22]. Hormonal agents such as Depo-Provera or Depot medroxyprogesterone acetate are metabolized in the liver and have been associated with bone loss [22]. A recent report suggested efficacy and safety of the contraceptive vaginal ring (NuvaRing) in renal and liver transplant recipients [23]. Recent recommendations of the mycophenolate risk evaluation and mitigation strategies (REMS) program are that transplant recipients at risk of pregnancy either use effective reversible contraception (defined as IUD, combination of one hormone and one barrier method, or simultaneous use of two barrier methods) or consider irreversible contraception (tubal ligation or male vasectomy).

Timing of Pregnancy

The female transplant recipient should become pregnant in a planned manner. The recommendations are that pregnancy is delayed for a year after successful transplantation [5]. This recommendation replaces an earlier one that advised women to wait for 2 years after their transplant to become pregnant. It has now been recognized that newer immunosuppressive medications have decreased the risk of rejection and that allograft function is usually stable by 1 year in the uncomplicated renal transplant recipient. The American Society of Transplantation recommends that pregnancy could be safe in the first year as long as the following caveats were considered: graft function was stable, with no evidence of rejection; allograft function was good (defined as a serum creatinine <1.5 and less than 500 mg protein excreted per 24 h); that the patient was not currently taking teratogenic medications (such as valganciclovir); there were no active infections with agents that could adversely impact the fetus (such as CMV); and that the allograft function was stable. Since the reproductive phase is shortened for women with ESRD, and patients are waiting longer for deceased donor organs, the risk of waiting for 2 years after transplantation to become pregnant is that the patient may no longer be fertile. There are several recent reports that suggest that the rate of spontaneous abortion might be higher in pregnancies planned before 2 years, although this is an area of controversy [24–26].

Risks Associated with Pregnancy for the Mother

There are several risks to consider for pregnancy in the maternal transplant recipient, including the risks of short- and long-term graft function, allograft rejection, acceleration of hypertension, and preeclampsia. Each of these will be discussed under the subheadings below.

Short- and Long-Term Graft Function

The risks of graft loss appear to correlate with allograft function at the time of conception. Hou et al. reported in 1999 that women with graft dysfunction before pregnancy (defined as a serum creatinine >1.5 mg/dL (133 mol/L)) were at increased risk for graft dysfunction during and after pregnancy [27]. The American Society of Transplantation echoed these concerns in their 2008 consensus conference report and stated that maternal transplant recipients with a creatinine <1.5 mg/dL and with minimal proteinuria were at low risk for short- and long-term graft loss, as long as adequate immunosuppression was maintained during the pregnancy (discussed below) [5]. Registry data have subsequently confirmed that women with good graft function at the time of pregnancy did not appear to have an accelerated loss of graft function [28–30]. It is important to realize that assessments of renal function in this population have generally depended on measurements of serum creatinine and protein excretion, and that prospective monitoring of glomerular filtration rates has not been reported in large numbers of patients during and after pregnancy.

Allograft Rejection

Rejection during pregnancy should be prevented if possible, as its detection is more difficult than in the nonpregnant transplant recipient. Creatinine levels normally decrease with the expanding intravascular volume and increased glomerular filtration rate that normally accompanies pregnancy [31]. In fact, two maternal deaths have occurred after discontinuation of immunosuppressive medications during gestation [32]. To avoid rejection, immunosuppressive drug dosing should be watched closely and frequent monitoring of serum drug levels is a must. It is important to monitor calcineurin levels frequently because marked alterations in the volume of drug distribution occur during gestation that affect levels [10]. A recent report though suggests that interpretation of whole blood tacrolimus levels during pregnancy might be challenging, due to variable factors that can increase the unbound fraction of tacrolimus [33].

It is important to realize that the mother is not "naturally" immunosuppressed during her pregnancy and therefore therapeutic immunosuppressive dosing must be maintained [10]. In fact rejection rates in women with solid organ transplants are equivalent to rejection rates in nonpregnant transplant recipients [34]. If rejection does occur, it usually responds to methylprednisolone [35], although antithymocyte globulin and basiliximab have been used successfully based on a registry report [36].

Hypertension

Most transplant recipients have chronic hypertension and maternal transplant recipients are at risk for worsening hypertension during their pregnancy. The NTPR reported hypertension during pregnancy to be at extremely high rates (reported incidence of near 75 %) [37, 38]. The blood pressure varies throughout normal gestation, with the lowest levels during the first trimester, followed by resumption of pre-pregnancy blood pressures late in gestation. A similar, but blunted, pattern is seen in maternal transplant recipients [39]. It is important to try to maintain the blood pressure near normal levels in pregnant recipients to avoid preterm delivery [40]. The preferred agent for blood pressure control during pregnancy is methyldopa, although alpha- and beta-blockers, calcium-channel blockers, alpha-adrenergic blockers, and thiazide diuretics have also been prescribed [41]. Angiotensin-converting-enzyme inhibitors and angiotensin-receptor blockers are associated with fetal death and are therefore contraindicated after the first trimester; and atenolol has been associated with poor fetal growth [41].

Preeclampsia

Preeclampsia occurs commonly in maternal transplant recipients, for reasons that have not yet been clarified. The NTPR reports that up to one third of pregnant transplant recipients develop preeclampsia [42]. The incidence of preeclampsia in patients without hypertension or chronic disease is 5 % [40]. The diagnosis of preeclampsia is challenging because there is often preexisting proteinuria, the blood pressure typically rises in the last trimester in transplant recipients, and uric acid levels are commonly elevated in patients taking calcineurin inhibitors [3, 43]. Whether circulating angiogenic factors will ultimately be used as biomarkers for early detection is too early to tell, but intriguing reports suggest there may be a future role [44]. Close monitoring of the patient by her high-risk obstetrician is mandatory to increase the detection and proper treatment of preeclampsia.

Risks Associated with Pregnancy for the Infant

The developing infant is at risk for several serious complications and these risks have been consistently reported in registry and center publications. The complications reported include preterm birth, low birth weight, intrauterine growth retardation, as well as short-term and long-term defects in immunologic and neurocognitive function.

Preterm Birth

Several recent reports have shown that preterm birth is very common, with an average infant gestational age of 36 weeks [28, 29, 45]. The gestational birth ages seem to be consistent among recipients of other solid organs as well [10].

The reason for early birth rates in maternal transplant recipients is not known, but preterm birth has frequently been seen in maternal patients with chronic kidney disease [46]. The overall risk of preterm delivery is 50 % among all published studies [10]. Data from the NTPR shows a mean gestational age of 36 weeks for maternal transplant recipients taking cyclosporine versus 35 weeks for those prescribed tacrolimus [28]. Whether there are significant differences between preterm birth rates based on immunosuppressive drug regimen is not known at this time.

Low Birth Weight

Approximately 50 % of infants born to transplanted mothers have a birth weight less than 2,500 g (5.5 lbs) [28, 29, 45]. Normal birth weight is approximately 3,400 g (7 lbs, 8 oz). The reason for this low birth is not clear, but may be associated with the high rates of preterm birth. Other reasons for low birth rate in the general population include a young (maternal age under 17) or older (maternal age over 35) mother, a previous history of preterm birth, smoking, high body mass index, uterine infections, and placental growth restriction. The long-term consequences of low birth weight have been reported widely and include a higher likelihood for development of neurocognitive defects and cardiovascular and renal disease later in life, probably related to alterations in organ development during vulnerable times in fetal growth [47]. Pregnancy in women with chronic kidney disease is also highly associated with low birth weight and small gestational age for infants, implying a primary pathological process associated with diminished maternal kidney function [46].

Intrauterine Growth Restriction

Intrauterine growth restriction has been reported to occur in about 20 % of maternal transplant recipients [15, 34]. This syndrome is defined as being less than 10 % for gestational age and is causally associated with low birth weight, preterm delivery, and genetic or chromosomal abnormalities. Women with kidney disease and chronic hypertension have a higher risk for having babies with IUGR. Although there are varied causes it implies placental insufficiency that prevents adequate nutrient delivery to the developing fetus [48]. Whether specific immunosuppressive agents contribute to placental nutrient defects or placental hypoxia is not known. IUGR is strongly associated with decreased cognitive function in adulthood [49].

Immunosuppressive Medications and Short- and Long-Term Outcomes

All immunosuppressive medications cross the maternal–fetal barrier, although they do so variably [38]. There is little information though about the bioavailability of individual immunosuppressive medications in the fetus, although one report showed that levels of calcineurin inhibitors were detectable in the fetal circulation and fetal T cells were as immunosuppressed as well as were maternal T cells [50]. Very little guidance has been provided by the Food and Drug Association safety classification, except for the black box warning for mycophenolate mofetil and mycophenolic acid, which should be avoided in a pregnant patient. Currently there is an REMS program overseeing this issue.

Concerns also involve risks associated with in utero exposure to immunosuppressive medications. During gestation the normal development of an infant requires regulated cell division, cell multiplication, and cell death, processes that occur in a highly regulated manner. Immunosuppressive medications target the very cellular processes that are essential for normal fetal development and therefore many investigators have been concerned that in utero exposure of the developing fetus to immunosuppressive medications might result in aberrant development. Based on extensive animal data, and limited human data, legitimate concerns have been raised that there may be maleffects of gestational immunosuppressive medication use on the developing fetus [10].

Short-term outcomes that have been reported include structural abnormalities and transient immunologic defects. With the exception of mycophenolate, registry reports have not demonstrated a unifying pattern of structural malformations. Gross congenital abnormalities have not been seen at higher levels in infants born to maternal transplant recipients than in the normal population, except in the case of mycophenolate where significant structural abnormalities have been reported [51, 52].

Long-term outcomes are not well defined but there are many reports from animal models of immunologic and neurocognitive defects associated with in utero exposure to immunosuppressive medications. One report in humans suggests that in utero exposure to immunosuppressive medications might increase the offspring's risk for autoimmune disease [53]. Very limited immunologic studies have been conducted in human neonates and these children are not usually recommended to undergo routine immunologic testing. In one study from the NTPR, 24 % of the offspring were reported to have developmental delays [54, 55]. Very limited data is available, as routine neurocognitive testing is not done on infants born to women taking immunosuppressive medications or those with chronic kidney disease.

Delivery

Many women with kidney transplants undergo caesarean delivery [37], but the indications for caesarean delivery should be dictated by obstetrical need. Because the transplanted kidney is in the false pelvis some clinicians have been concerned that vaginal delivery might be impacted. The opinion of consensus experts is that unless there is an obstetrical reason for a caesarean section that the maternal transplant recipient should be delivered vaginally [5].

Breastfeeding

At this time it is not clear whether or not breastfeeding should be recommended for infants of maternal transplant recipients. The infant has been exposed to immunosuppressants throughout gestation, but it is not known whether the bioavailability of immunosuppressive medications is different in breast milk. There are recommendations by the American Association of Pediatrics, which approves the use of breastfeeding in mothers taking prednisone, but not in those taking cyclosporine [56]. They make no recommendations regarding azathioprine or tacrolimus. At this point the data is too limited to make recommendations one way or the other about breastfeeding in maternal transplant recipients. Interestingly, a recent observational study suggested that there were no differences in tacrolimus levels between breast-fed versus bottle-fed infants of maternal transplant recipients [57]. At this point the data are too limited to make recommendations one way or the other about breastfeeding in maternal transplant recipients.

Counseling

Counseling of potential maternal transplant recipients and their partner is essential. This counseling should begin before transplantation, in order to avoid unintended pregnancy. It is important to include the patient's partner in the counseling process, as significant risks exist for maternal morbidity and mortality during the lifetime of her offspring [58]. The parents should be advised of the specific risks of pregnancy for both the mother and her offspring. Recipients should be told that their offspring could suffer from immunologic abnormalities, neurocognitive defects, and malformations (in the case of mycophenolate). We still do not know if there are other malefects of in utero exposure to immunosuppressive medications and therefore patients should also be advised of the limitations of our current knowledge about the safety of pregnancy in renal transplant recipients.

References

1. Murray JE, Reid DE, Harrison JH, Merrill JP. Successful pregnancies after human renal transplantation. N Engl J Med. 1963;269:341–3.
2. Kaufman J, et al. Successful, normal childbirth after kidney homotransplantation. JAMA. 1967;200:338–41.
3. Stratta P, et al. Pregnancy in kidney transplantation: satisfactory outcomes and harsh realities. J Nephrol. 2003;16:792–806.
4. McKay DB, et al. Reproduction and pregnancy in transplant recipients: current practices. Prog Transplant. 2006;16:127–32.
5. McKay D, Josephson M. Reproduction and transplantation: report on the AST consensus conference on reproductive issues and transplantation. Am J Transplant. 2005;5:1–8.
6. Anantharaman P, Schmidt RJ. Sexual function in chronic kidney disease. Adv Chronic Kidney Dis. 2007;14:119–25.
7. Leavey SF, Weitzel WF. Endocrine abnormalities in chronic renal failure. Endocrinol Metab Clin North Am. 2002;31:107–19.
8. Holley JL, Schmidt RJ, Bender FH, Dumler F, Schiff M. Gynecologic and reproductive issues in women on dialysis. Am J Kidney Dis. 1997;29:685–90.
9. de Koning ND, Haagsma EB. Normalization of menstrual pattern after liver transplantation: consequences for contraception. Digestion. 1990;46:239–41.
10. McKay DB, Josephson MA. Pregnancy in recipients of solid organs–effects on mother and child. N Engl J Med. 2006;354:1281–93.
11. Saha MT, Saha HH, Niskanen LK, Salmela KT, Pasternack AI. Time course of serum prolactin and sex hormones following successful renal transplantation. Nephron. 2002;92:735–7.
12. Lim VS, Henriquez C, Sievertsen G, Frohman LA. Ovarian function in chronic renal failure: evidence suggesting hypothalamic anovulation. Ann Intern Med. 1980;93:21–7.
13. Lessan-Pezeshki M, et al. Fertility and contraceptive issues after kidney transplantation in women. Transplant Proc. 2004;36:1405–6.
14. Hou S. Pregnancy in renal transplant recipients. Adv Ren Replace Ther. 2003;10:40–7.
15. Davison JM, Bailey DJ. Pregnancy following renal transplantation. J Obstet Gynaecol Res. 2003;29:227–33.
16. Zeyneloglu HB, Oktem M, Durak T. Male infertility after renal transplantation: achievement of pregnancy after intracytoplasmic sperm injection. Transplant Proc. 2005;37:3081–4.
17. Fritsche L, et al. Testosterone concentrations and sirolimus in male renal transplant patients. Am J Transplant. 2004;4:130–1.
18. Tondolo V, Citterio F, Panocchia N, Nanni G, Castagneto M. Sirolimus impairs improvement of the gonadal function after renal transplantation. Am J Transplant. 2005;5:197.
19. Kaczmarek I, et al. Sirolimus impairs gonadal function in heart transplant recipients. Am J Transplant. 2004;4:1084–8.
20. Guazzelli CA, Torloni MR, Sanches TF, Barbieri M, Pestana JO. Contraceptive counseling and use among 197 female kidney transplant recipients. Transplantation. 2008;86:669–72.
21. Ramhendar T, Byrne P. Use of the levonorgestrel-releasing intrauterine system in renal transplant recipients: a retrospective case review. Contraception. 2012;86:288–9.
22. Krajewski CM, Geetha D, Gomez-Lobo V. Contraceptive options for women with a history of solid-organ transplantation. Transplantation. 2013;95(10):1183–6.
23. Paternoster DM, et al. The contraceptive vaginal ring in women with renal and liver transplantation: analysis of preliminary results. Transplant Proc. 2010;42:1162–5.
24. Gill JS, Zalunardo N, Rose C, Tonelli M. The pregnancy rate and live birth rate in kidney transplant recipients. Am J Transplant. 2009;9:1541–9.
25. Kim HW, et al. The experience of pregnancy after renal transplantation: pregnancies even within postoperative 1 year may be tolerable. Transplantation. 2008;85:1412–9.
26. Xu L, et al. Unwanted pregnancy among Chinese renal transplant recipients. Eur J Contracept Reprod Health Care. 2011;16:270–6.
27. Hou S. Pregnancy in chronic renal insufficiency and end stage renal disease. Am J Kidney Dis. 1999;33:235–52.
28. Armenti VT. Pregnancy after transplantation: milestones and assessments of risk. Am J Transplant. 2011;11:2275–6.
29. Deshpande NA, et al. Pregnancy outcomes in kidney transplant recipients: a systematic review and meta-analysis. Am J Transplant. 2011;11:2388–404.
30. Levidiotis V, Chang S, McDonald S. Pregnancy and maternal outcomes among kidney transplant recipients. J Am Soc Nephrol. 2009;20:2433–40.
31. Davison JM, Milne JEC. Pregnancy and renal transplantation. Br J Urol. 1997;80 Suppl 1:29–32.
32. Sims CJ. Organ transplantation and immunosuppressive drugs in pregnancy. Clin Obstet Gynecol. 1991;34:100–11.

33. Hebert MF, et al. Interpreting tacrolimus concentrations during pregnancy and postpartum. Transplantation. 2013;95:908–15.
34. Armenti VT, et al. Report from the National Transplantation Pregnancy Registry (NTPR): outcomes of pregnancy after transplantation. Clin Transpl. 2003;2002:121–30.
35. Mastrobattista JM, Katz AR. Pregnancy after organ transplant. Obstet Gynecol Clin North Am. 2004;31:415–28.
36. Armenti VT, et al. National transplantation Pregnancy Registry–outcomes of 154 pregnancies in cyclosporine-treated female kidney transplant recipients. Transplantation. 1994;57:502–6.
37. Sibanda N, Briggs JD, Davison JM, Johnson RJ, Rudge CJ. Pregnancy after organ transplantation: a report from the UK Transplant pregnancy registry. Transplantation. 2007;83:1301–7.
38. McKay DB, Josephson MA. Pregnancy after kidney transplantation. Clin J Am Soc Nephrol. 2008;3 Suppl 2:S117–25.
39. del Mar Colon M, Hibbard JU. Obstetric considerations in the management of pregnancy in kidney transplant recipients. Adv Chronic Kidney Dis. 2007;14:168–77.
40. Podymow T, August P. Hypertension in pregnancy. Adv Chronic Kidney Dis. 2007;14:178–90.
41. Umans JG. Medications during pregnancy: antihypertensives and immunosuppressives. Adv Chronic Kidney Dis. 2007;14:191–8.
42. Armenti VT, et al. Report from the National Transplantation Pregnancy Registry (NTPR): outcomes of pregnancy after transplantation. Clin Transpl. 2002;2001:121–30.
43. Morales J, et al. Uric acid handling, pregnancy and cyclosporin in renal transplant women. Nephron. 1990;56:97–8.
44. Levine RJ, et al. Circulating angiogenic factors and the risk of preeclampsia. N Engl J Med. 2004;350:672–83.
45. Bramham K, et al. Pregnancy in renal transplant recipients: a UK national cohort study. Clin J Am Soc Nephrol. 2013;8:290–8.
46. Nevis IF, et al. Pregnancy outcomes in women with chronic kidney disease: a systematic review. Clin J Am Soc Nephrol. 2011;6: 2587–98.
47. Abitbol CL, Rodriguez MM. The long-term renal and cardiovascular consequences of prematurity. Nat Rev Nephrol. 2012;8:265–74.
48. Biswas S, Adhikari A, Chattopadhyay JC, Ghosh SK. Histological changes of placentas associated with intra-uterine growth restriction of fetuses: a case control study. Nepal Med Coll J. 2012;14:18–24.
49. Lohaugen GC, et al. Small for gestational age and intrauterine growth restriction decreases cognitive function in young adults. J Pediatr. 2013;163(2):447–53.
50. Flechner SM, Katz AR, Rogers AJ, Van Buren C, Kahan BD. The presence of cyclosporine in body tissues and fluids during pregnancy. Am J Kidney Dis. 1985;5:60–3.
51. Sifontis NM, et al. Pregnancy outcomes in solid organ transplant recipients with exposure to mycophenolate mofetil or sirolimus. Transplantation. 2006;82:1698–702.
52. LeRay C, Coulomb A, Elefant E, Frydman R, Audibert F. Mycophenolate mofetil in pregnancy after renal transplantation: a case of major fetal malformations. Obstet Gynecol. 2004;103: 1091–4.
53. Scott JR, Branch DW, Holman J. Autoimmune and pregnancy complications in the daughter of a kidney transplant patient. Transplantation. 2002;73:815–6.
54. Nulman I, et al. Long-term neurodevelopment of children exposed in utero to ciclosporin after maternal renal transplant. Paediatr Drugs. 2010;12:113–22.
55. Sgro MD, et al. Pregnancy outcome post renal transplantation. Teratology. 2002;65:5–9.
56. American Academy of Pediatrics Committee on Drugs: the transfer of drugs and other chemicals into human milk. Pediatrics. 1994; 93:137–50.
57. Bramham K, Chusney G, Lee J, Lightstone L, Nelson-Piercy C. Breastfeeding and tacrolimus: serial monitoring in breast-fed and bottle-fed infants. Clin J Am Soc Nephrol. 2013;8:563–7.
58. Ross LF. Ethical considerations related to pregnancy in transplant recipients. N Engl J Med. 2006;354:1313–6.

18 The Prevention and Treatment of Coronary Artery Disease in Kidney Transplant Recipients

Deborah B. Adey

Prevention and Treatment of Cardiovascular Disease in Renal Transplant Recipients

Cardiovascular disease (CVD) is prevalent amongst chronic kidney disease patients, estimated to be 20–1,000-fold increased risk as compared to the general population [1]. The mortality rate of patients with chronic kidney disease on dialysis approaches 20 % per year [2] and is especially high amongst those with underlying diabetes. Chronic kidney disease patients who present for transplant evaluation often undergo extensive pre-transplant evaluation, much of which is focused on detection of underlying CVD. The traditional signs and symptoms of cardiac disease are often masked or altered in chronic kidney disease, making subjective evaluation of underlying cardiac disease challenging. Diabetic patients, who make up 24.9 % [3] of patients on the wait list, are known to have asymptomatic coronary artery disease, likely in part due to their associated autonomic dysfunction [4]. Chest pain, chest discomfort, and other classic symptoms of ischemic heart disease are often absent. Patients on dialysis are often sedentary [5] to a point that they do not exhibit exertional symptoms. This can be further masked by the general sense of fatigue that patients feel with dialysis, especially with in-center intermittent hemodialysis. There is mounting evidence of the benefits of physical activity in the pre-transplant recipient [6, 7]. Patients who are more physically active and have better physical endurance pre-transplant have a more favorable cardiovascular risk post-transplant than do those patients who are more sedentary. Exercise can improve physical endurance in dialysis patients. Encouraging patients with chronic kidney disease to engage in regular physical activity is an important step in the prevention and management of cardiovascular risk.

Upon consideration for transplantation potential candidates are typically evaluated with some degree of cardiovascular testing. Pre-transplant cardiac evaluation remains one of the most controversial topics in making decisions regarding transplant candidacy [8]. At a minimum, all patients undergo an electrocardiogram (ECG) prior to transplant. Intraventricular conduction delays and evidence of prior myocardial infarction may prompt further testing. The extent of cardiac testing is dependent upon the perceived a priori risk for underlying ischemic heart disease. Those patients considered at an unacceptably high risk for perioperative cardiovascular morbidity or mortality may be turned down as candidates for transplantation. Echocardiograms and nuclear medicine myocardial perfusion studies are the predominant modality used in evaluation [9], often on an annual basis. However, how best to evaluate underlying significant coronary artery disease and when to intervene remain controversial [8]. Different centers require different degrees of intervention prior to a patient being listed for transplant. Cardiac catheterization may be performed in those considered high risk for underlying cardiac disease, such as diabetics, and those with a prior history of cardiac events. Those patients with a previous history of CVD (previous myocardial infarction, cardiovascular revascularization, stroke, or claudication) have the highest risk of peri-transplant cardiovascular events [10]. However, presurgical revascularization has not proven to improve postoperative cardiovascular risk [11].

Cardiac function is variably assessed prior to transplant. Impaired cardiac function, systolic and/or diastolic, is often present at the time of transplant. Left ventricular ejection fraction has been shown to be a better predictor [10] of post-transplant outcomes. It is often felt that the uremic milieu, volume overload, and chronic anemia contribute to the underlying dysfunction and that cardiac function may improve with transplantation [12]. Studies by Sharma et al. [13] have suggested that a reliable assessment of preoperative cardiac disease would utilize dobutamine stress echocardiogram. This modality provides information not only on ejection fraction, but the impact of stress on cardiac function.

D.B. Adey (✉)
University of California, Davis, 2233 Stockton Blvd, Housestaff Bldg, Room 2011, Sacramento, CA 95817, USA
e-mail: Deborah.Adey@ucdmc.ucdavis.edu

M.R. Weir and E.V. Lerma (eds.), *Kidney Transplantation: Practical Guide to Management*, DOI 10.1007/978-1-4939-0342-9_18, © Springer Science+Business Media New York 2014

The end result is that patients come to transplant often with some degree of underlying coronary artery disease.

Despite preoperative cardiac evaluation, the most common cause of death amongst kidney transplant recipients is CVD [14]. The incidence of CVD amongst transplant recipients is estimated to be 4.7–40 % at 3 years post-transplant [15, 16]. A long-term study of renal transplant recipients documented a 40 % cumulative incidence of CVD at 10 years post-transplant [17].

Risk Factors for CVD Amongst Renal Transplant Recipients

Traditional risk factors for CVD are prevalent amongst renal transplant recipients. Diabetes is a leading cause of kidney disease and is reflected in the demographics of the transplant population, with 25.7 % [3] of transplant recipients being diabetic. Diabetes is also a primary predictor of macrovascular and microvascular disease, and therefore a predictor of CVD in renal transplant recipients. Hypertension is the second most common listed etiology of end-stage renal disease at 23.5 % [3] and an established risk factor for coronary artery disease. It is estimated that between 75 and 80 % of transplant recipients are hypertensive [18–20] post-transplantation. Though the majority of transplant recipients are on prescribed antihypertensive therapy, many are not adequately controlled [16, 19].

Dyslipidemia is common in the renal transplant population. There appears to be a difference in the lipid profile of patients with chronic kidney disease who are on intermittent dialysis and those post-transplant. Interestingly the lipid profile of the transplant recipient is more similar to that of chronic kidney disease patients on peritoneal dialysis.

Smoking and tobacco abuse is a well-known risk factor for CVD and death. Some programs require smoking cessation prior to proceeding with transplantation [21], especially in diabetics or those with prior cardiac disease. Ninety percent of individuals who smoke pre-transplant continue to smoke post-transplant. Cotinine testing can be used for monitoring adherence to requirements for smoking cessation prior to transplant [22]. Smoking is associated with a cardiovascular event rate of 29.2 % in smokers post-transplant in comparison to a rate of 15.4 % in nonsmokers [23].

Chronic kidney disease is associated with unique cardiovascular risk factors that are carried forward into transplantation. Altered calcium and phosphorus metabolism is associated with increased vascular calcification, and in turn increased risk of CVD. Vascular calcification is common in patients with chronic kidney disease [24, 25]. Calcium and phosphorus management targets minimization of the calcium × phosphorus product to be less than 55 mg^2/dL^2 in an attempt to minimize calciphylaxis and vascular calcification [26].

Hyperhomocysteinemia has been reported to be associated with increased coronary events. Several studies in chronic disease utilizing folic acid replacement to lower homocysteine levels failed to show any cardiovascular benefit. However one meta-analysis of the pooled study did show a 15 % reduction in cardiovascular risk, while another meta-analysis failed to show a significant reduction in cardiovascular risk [27]. Similarly, the FAVORIT study [27] in over 4,000 renal transplant recipients failed to show a difference in cardiovascular outcomes with use of folic acid supplementation to lower homocysteine levels.

There is mounting evidence that chronic inflammation is associated with an increased cardiovascular risk. Chronic inflammation, inherent in dialysis patients, is also associated with increased coronary artery disease [28–30]. The two main sources of inflammation in chronic kidney disease are poor dentition and inflammation related to vascular access for dialysis. Many centers require a dental clearance prior to transplant. Gum inflammation is associated with worse allograft outcomes as well as increased risk of cardiovascular events [31]. Issues related to gingivitis and poor dental health should be addressed prior to transplant. This has become an increasing problem as medical insurance often does not adequately cover the expenses associated with basic dental care. The other major source of inflammation in chronic kidney disease is the vascular access graft or fistula. Infection is common during dialysis, but graft infections can persist or develop post-transplant. Another emerging association with inflammation and elevated C-reactive protein (CRP) is obesity. Obesity is common in chronic kidney disease patients presenting for transplant. The upper limit of body mass index (BMI) acceptable for transplant is gradually increasing but generally around 35 kg/m^2. In addition weight gain is common after transplant. There appears to be a link between obesity, inflammation, and CVD. CRP, driven by IL-6 (a potent inflammatory cytokine), is increased by abdominal adiposity [32]. Winkelmayer has demonstrated an association between increased BMI and elevated CRP, as well as an increased mortality with elevations in CRP [33, 34]. Additionally CRP levels are associated with smoking, diabetes, and hypertriglyceridemia [35]. There is no evidence that CRPs are used routinely as an assessment of underlying inflammation. Interestingly elevations in CRP are not associated with prior cardiovascular events or immunosuppression.

Anemia has been reported to be associated with increased cardiovascular events in chronic kidney disease [36]. The use of erythropoietin has also been reported to exacerbate underlying endothelial dysfunction [37] and promote thrombosis and thus be a contributing factor in cardiovascular events. Correction of anemia with erythropoietin is safe in the immediate perioperative period [38]. The overall benefits of maintaining a hemoglobin of 11–12 g/dL [39] far outweigh the thrombotic risk of erythropoietin agents.

Risks Associated with Transplant

Early Post-transplant (First 90 Days)

This risk of a cardiac event is greatest during the first 3 months post-transplant, with the greatest risk of a post-transplant cardiovascular event being in the first 30 days post-transplant. This is the period of time where volume status is affected by underlying cardiac function, medications, and degree of renal function. The use of perioperative beta-blockade to minimize increased cardiac demands may abrogate these early events. This is especially true for patients who were on beta-blockers prior to admission for transplant. In the current era where delayed graft function may be more common due to the use of more extended criteria kidneys, kidneys with acute kidney injury, and donation after circulatory death kidneys, there needs to be close monitoring of volume status to avoid precipitation of congestive heart failure. In the immediate perioperative period there is increased risk for myocardial infarction due to hemodynamic shifts associated with surgery. Intravenous fluid administration in the operating room and potential volume overload can precipitate atrial fibrillation or congestive heart failure. By definition delayed graft function implies the need for dialysis in the first 7 days post-transplant. In patients requiring dialysis, careful attention needs to be paid to the prescribed ultrafiltration rate. Excessive fluid removal can trigger a reflex tachycardia, increasing myocardial demand, and an increased risk of myocardial ischemia. Excessive ultrafiltration in the immediate perioperative period could also further jeopardize graft function due to hypoperfusion.

Anemia post-transplant has not been well studied with respect to the impact on cardiovascular events. The target hemoglobin in the perioperative period is influenced by the patient's underlying cardiovascular risk, i.e., duration of diabetes and prior history of CVD or known coronary artery disease. Low hemoglobin concentrations can impair oxygen delivery and supply to meet cardiac demands. Transfusions can be associated with volume overload, contributing to congestive heart failure, atrial fibrillation, or other cardiac events. Initiation of erythropoietin agents appears to be safe in the early post-transplant period, though attention to iron deficiency prior to use is important. Doses of erythropoietin should be kept within the recommended guidelines to avoid potential adverse events such as thrombosis.

Long-Term Transplant

The PORT study [40] identified both traditional factors for CVD but more importantly identified factors related to transplant. Transplant-related factors included dialysis vintage, which was associated with an adjusted hazard ratio of 1.41 for major cardiovascular event within 3 years of transplant. Other significant transplant-related factors of note were an acute rejection episode within the prior year with an adjusted HR of 2.21 (1.71–2.86), post-transplant lymphoproliferative disorder aHR of 6.01 (2.03–7.90), and delayed graft function aHR of 1.39 (1.17–1.66). Most of these factors are not modifiable. However awareness of the impact of these factors on the increased risk of a cardiovascular event may help providers better understand this patient population.

New-Onset Diabetes After Transplant

New-onset diabetes after transplantation (NODAT) is a troubling side effect of transplantation. One study reported the development of NODAT in 31.4 % of recipients by the end of the first year post-transplant [41]. Metabolic syndrome is a predictor for the development of NODAT, with the risk correlating with the number of metabolic syndrome characteristics present. Metabolic syndrome is diagnosed when three of the following five characteristics are present: obesity with BMI > 30 kg^2/m^2 or waist circumference >35 in. in women or >40 in. in men, serum triglycerides >150 mg/dL, HDL <50 mg/dL in women or <40 mg/dL in men, fasting blood glucose >110 mg/dL, or a blood pressure >130/85 mmHg. This is similar to type 2 diabetes in that NODAT is a result of a combination of impaired insulin secretion and insulin resistance. NODAT is associated with the use of steroids and the use of calcineurin inhibitors (CNIs), a mainstay of immunosuppression. Glucocorticoids play a role in NODAT by contributing to insulin resistance. Decreased insulin production as a result of islet toxicity can result from the use of CNIs. The general estimate for development of NODAT is 13 % with use of tacrolimus and 8 % with use of cyclosporine-based therapy. The mechanism in which CNIs contribute to NODAT is believed to be a direct toxicity to the islet cells of the pancreas, in part related to the presence of calcineurin in the beta cells of the pancreas. The risk for development of NODAT is highest in those individuals with pre-transplant metabolic syndrome [41], a strong family history of type 2 diabetes, and an elevated BMI. Many patients with type 2 diabetes prior to transplant have lost the need for the use of oral hypoglycemic agents or insulin with the progression of the renal disease to end stage. Once normal renal function is established and clearance of endogenous insulin returns these individuals most likely will need pharmacologic management of glucose control. Post-transplant hyperglycemia and NODAT are independent risk factors for major cardiovascular risk death [42]. The 2012 USRDS [43] data indicates NODAT following transplant remains common, with over 40 % of adult, nondiabetic, Medicare-covered recipients having evidence of diabetes by the end of the third year after transplant. Thirty-one percent of nondiabetic transplant recipients with Medicare Part D coverage have claims for insulin during the first 6 months post-transplant, while 10 % have claims for sulfonylureas.

Medications

Though improved renal function may mitigate some cardiovascular risk, the addition of immunosuppression medications can tip the balance towards increased risk. CNIs (cyclosporine and tacrolimus) may exacerbate hypertension due to vasoconstriction. Chronic exposure to CNIs contributes to intimal hyperplasia of the vasculature and may contribute to hypertension. In addition the CNIs are associated with hyperlipidemia. The mammalian target of rapamycin (mTOR) inhibitors (e.g., sirolimus) can be associated with profound hyperlipidemia. Glucocorticoids contribute to insulin resistance and elevated blood sugars as well as hyperlipidemia.

Hyperlipidemia

Transplant recipients are also classified as having chronic kidney disease, usually stage 2 or 3 at their best post-transplantation. The lipid abnormalities post-transplant are therefore likely a combination of factors related to having chronic kidney disease combined with the adverse effects of immunosuppressive medications. Total cholesterol and LDL are typically elevated in renal transplant recipients as are triglyceride levels. Lipid abnormalities in chronic kidney disease are thought to be in part due to decreased catabolism and clearance of apoB triglyceride-rich lipoproteins, reduced hepatic lipase activity, and impaired lipolysis [44, 45]. Most patients present to transplant with elevated lipid level, and to exacerbate the issue, by 1 year post-transplant, there is a universal increase in all lipid fractions [46]. Several immunosuppressive agents routinely used in transplant recipients can contribute to elevated lipids, including prednisone, CNIs, and mTOR inhibitors. CNIs, cyclosporine more than tacrolimus, are associated with an increase in total cholesterol and LDL [47]. Cyclosporine inhibits 26-hydroxylase, an enzyme in the bile acid pathway [48]. mTOR inhibitors can cause substantial elevations in total cholesterol and triglycerides, possibly through altered hepatic metabolism or alteration in insulin or insulin-like growth factors [49]. In addition, the liberation of dietary restrictions and associated increase in caloric intake may contribute to hyperlipidemia. Hypertriglyceridemia is common in transplant recipients and may reflect poor diabetes control, increased caloric intake, or medication effect. Hypertriglyceridemia is associated with the metabolic syndrome, another risk factor for CVD.

Risk Factor Modification

Care of the transplant recipient is often divided between either a primary care physician or general nephrologist and a transplant physician or team of transplant physicians. The potential for drug interactions and risk of injury to allograft function may make the primary physicians hesitant to prescribe appropriate therapy. Transplant physicians often feel that management of hypertension and hyperlipidemia and counseling on general health issues are in the realm of the primary care physician. The result can be that the patients fall between the cracks of optimal care. On the other hand patients should be held accountable for their health. Excessive weight gains should be discussed with referral to a dietician with knowledge of potential for drug interactions with foods such as grapefruit. Dieticians also should recommend careful washing of fresh fruits and vegetables and avoidance of undercooked or raw meats and fish due to the risk of foodborne illness. This needs to be balanced with recommendations for increased use of properly prepared fruits, vegetables, and whole grains. Participation in regular physical activity should be addressed and discussed at each visit, as should the use of tobacco. Patients who have either continued to smoke, have resumed smoking, or have taken up smoking need to be counseled and if needed be provided information on smoking cessation.

Several papers have documented the inadequacies of management of the cardiovascular risks in transplant recipients [19, 50, 51]. The FAVORIT study [27] evaluated 4,107 transplant recipients over 5 years, 69 % of which had prevalent CVD. In this high-risk group of transplant recipients, it was demonstrated that there was room for improvement in blood pressure and hyperlipidemia management and use of antiplatelet agents. In the Dawson study less than 20 % of transplant recipients considered high cardiovascular risk were receiving optimal medical management with antiplatelet therapy, an angiotensin converting enzyme inhibitor/angiotensin receptor blockers (ACEi/ARB), and a statin at 1 year post-transplant [50]. In a report by Gaston, at 6 months post-transplant less than 60 % of recipients with known cardiac disease were on aspirin, less than 60 % were on a statin, and only 27 % were on an ACEi, but 74 % were on a beta-blocker [52]. Even after an acute myocardial infarction, medical management leaves room for improvement [53]. Use of beta-blockers and statins post-acute myocardial infarction was increased in transplant recipients as compared to the general population, though there is still room for improvement. Of note is that women and the elderly transplant recipients are less likely to receive optimal medical management, as is seen in the general population. The reason for this is not clear. There may be concerns about polypharmacy in the elderly or possibly concerns about side effects from additional medications.

Hypertension Management

Hypertension is prevalent amongst transplant recipients and management of blood pressure is often suboptimal. Approximately 85 % of transplant recipients are reported to be hypertensive [52]. Several studies have indicated that blood pressure is inadequately controlled in the transplant population [19]. Some caution needs to be exercised in interpretation of this data as many patients may not have taken their medications prior to their clinic visit when their blood pressure is checked. Optimally patients need to be educated on home monitoring of blood pressures to assess efficacy and duration of the antihypertensive effect of their medications. Patients' home recordings of blood pressures may help determine if a particular medicine is effective in both degree and duration of blood pressure control. In a study by Fresnedo office blood pressures were compared to ambulatory blood pressures in 868 patients [20]. Though there was correlation, office blood pressures did tend to run higher than ambulatory blood pressures. This raises the question of when the medications were taken in relation to the blood pressure check. The issue of "white coat hypertension" needs to be addressed with the patient. "White coat hypertension" may reflect how the patient responds to and deals with the stresses of life. Target blood pressure should be as the KDIGO recommendations [26], a goal of <130/80 mmHg. Cardiovascular protection with antihypertensive agents has not been well studied in renal transplant recipients. A meta-analysis of antihypertensive agents in renal transplant recipients did not show any specific class of agents to be more cardioprotective than another [54]. However, most studies were of relatively short duration (12 months) and myocardial infarction was not often reported.

In patients with known CVD, beta-blockers should be implemented as per standard guidelines [55]. Perioperative use of beta-blockers may help decrease myocardial demand by controlling tachycardia and therefore minimize early perioperative myocardial infarction. In patients with known CVD or diabetes, it is reasonable to continue beta-blockers, as this is the group of patients at highest risk. The USRDS 2012 [43] data reports that beta-blockers are prescribed for 75 % and 71 % of deceased and living donor recipients, respectively, during the first 6 months post-transplant. In the absence of CVD or diabetes, the adverse side effects of beta-blockers need to be weighed against the benefits. Fatigue, poor physical endurance, and sexual dysfunction are common and may impair the patient's ability to engage in regular physical activity. In addition the side effects of fatigue and sexual dysfunction may result in less patient adherence to the prescribed medications.

Calcium channel blockers, typically the dihydropyridine class of calcium channel blockers, appear to be first-line agents in the control of blood pressure in transplant recipients based on USRDS data. The USRDS [43] reports use of dihydropyridine calcium channel blockers for 65 % and 58 % of deceased donor transplant recipients and living donor transplant recipients respectively. Dihydropyridine calcium channel blockers counteract the vasoconstrictive effect of the CNIs and have no significant drug interactions with the CNIs. In a meta-analysis of antihypertensives [54], the dihydropyridine calcium channel blockers imparted an improvement in estimated glomerular filtration rate by 12 mL/min as compared to ACEi. In addition the use of dihydropyridine calcium channel blockers seemed to favor graft survival. Improved graft survival could be speculated indirectly to impart a benefit in cardiovascular risk and mortality. The non-dihydropyridine calcium channel blockers (verapamil and diltiazem) inhibit the cytochrome P450 system which inhibits the metabolism of the CNIs, potentially resulting in toxic calcineurin inhibitor drug levels. Use of these agents is typically reserved for patients with abnormalities of the atrioventricular conduction pathways who require AV nodal blocking.

The cardiovascular benefits of ACEi and ARBs are well established [56–58]. However, there has not been widespread use in the transplant recipient population due to concerns regarding the effect on the renal allograft. Hyperkalemia can be problematic with the combination of ACEi or ARB and CNIs. This is typically more of an issue in the early weeks to months post-transplant. A rise in creatinine can be observed with initiation of ACEi and ARB, though this is usually a transient phenomenon. However caution is warranted. Patients who have an underlying renal artery stenosis are at risk for a significant elevation in creatinine due to alterations in renal blood flow with use of ACEi or ARB. All patients should be carefully examined and auscultation of the renal allograft performed. The presence of an audible bruit warrants further evaluation of the allograft to rule out an underlying renal artery stenosis that may be contributing to the hypertension. However, the use of ACEi and ARBs is the first-line therapy of post-transplant erythrocytosis and has been safe in that setting [59]. It is common to observe a decrease in hemoglobin after initiation of ACEi or ARB in renal transplant recipients. Discontinuation of the agent typically results in restoration of the hemoglobin to previous levels. No randomized controlled trials have been carried out in renal transplant recipients using ACEi or ARBs. ACE inhibitors are prescribed for 23 % of deceased donor recipients and 22 % of living donor recipients enrolled in Medicare Part D [43]. There are no published studies in the transplant population of the impact of ACEi or ARBs on cardiovascular events. There is one study on the impact of ACEi versus a calcium channel blocker on left ventricular mass, and there was no difference [60]. This result is more likely due to equal efficacy in controlling blood pressure. There is no evidence that once renal function has stabilized, ACEi or ARBs cannot be safely used. Other options for managing blood pressure include central-acting alpha agents such as clonidine and vasodilatory agents such as hydralazine or minoxidil. The goal for blood pressure control should be per the KDIGO guidelines [26].

Table 18.1 Treatment of dyslipidemias in transplant recipients

Dyslipidemia	Goal	Initiate	Increase	Alternative
TG > 500 mg/dL with LDL < 100 mg/dL	TG < 500 mg/dL	TLC	TLC + niacin	Fibrate or statin
LDL 100–129 mg/dL	LDL < 100 mg/dL	TLC	TLC + low-dose statin	Ezetimibe or niacin
LDL > 100 mg/dL	LDL <100	TLC + low-dose statin	TLC + 50 % maximum-dose statin	Ezetimibe or niacin
TG > 200 mg/dL and non-HDL > 130 mg/dL	Non-HDL < 130 mg/dL	TLC + low-dose statin	TLC + 50 % maximum-dose statin	Ezetimibe or niacin

Modified from Kasiske et al. [49]

TG triglycerides, *LDL* low-density lipoproteins, *HDL* high-density lipoproteins, *TLC* therapeutic lifestyle changes

Hyperlipidemia

Approximately 41 % of transplant recipients with Part D coverage have claims for statins during the first 6 months post-transplant, and 90 % of recipients aged 35 or older at transplant have a lipid screening performed during the first year. Management of hyperlipidemia in transplant recipients is also suboptimal [19, 50, 52]. The Assessment of Lescol in Renal Transplantation (ALERT) trial aimed to show an impact of statins on major cardiac events utilizing fluvastatin versus placebo, but failed to do so. One repeated criticism of this study is the relatively low potency of fluvastatin as compared to other available statins. Though the initial trial did show a positive benefit with fluvastatin on combined cardiac death or nonfatal myocardial infarction, it was not until the results of the ALERT-Ext were analyzed was there a positive benefit on major cardiac events [61]. Lentine performed a meta-analysis of available studies of use of statins for the purpose of cardiovascular risk reduction in transplant recipients [62]. Statins lowered total cholesterol by 18–33 %, a 20–43 % reduction in low-density lipoproteins, and 0–23 % reductions in triglycerides. Though not a primary cardiovascular outcome, reduction in lipids serves well as a surrogate marker for risk reduction. Statins are the first-line agents for treatment of hyperlipidemia. However, some caution must be exercised as drug interactions are a potential risk. CNIs can raise the level of statins and increase the risk of rhabdomyolysis, especially if an agent that further inhibits cytochrome P450 is added. Of note is an FDA warning regarding the use of amlodipine with doses of simvastatin greater than 20 mg due to toxicities. Elevation in liver enzymes may occur with use of statins. Monitoring liver enzymes at the initiation of statins or with dose changes is prudent.

Management of hypertriglyceridemia can be challenging, as detailed in Table 18.1. Therapeutic lifestyle changes are the first steps [63]. Dietary changes, exercise, minimization of alcohol, and control of diabetes are recommended. When lifestyle changes are ineffective in bringing triglycerides under control, niacin should be considered as the next-line therapy [63, 64]. Niacin can also be associated with hepatotoxicity but typically at higher doses. Flushing associated with use of niacin can be ameliorated by use of aspirin 30 min prior to taking niacin. Fibrates can be used post-transplant, but with some caution. Gemfibrozil dosing should be reduced by 50 % for an eGFR of less than 60 mL/min. Fenofibrates can cause an elevation in creatinine and therefore need to be used cautiously. Fish oil can also be effective, but the dose required to achieve efficacy is often not well tolerated.

Antiplatelet Agents

The cardioprotective benefit of aspirin is well established. Aspirin is often started or continued in the immediate perioperative period for rheological reasons. This is especially true in patients where the allograft has small vessels or there was a need for vascular reconstruction at the time of surgery. Use of antiplatelet agents is a mainstay of therapy for prevention of cardiovascular events. In the FAVORIT study 38 % of patients greater than 6 years out from transplant were prescribed antiplatelet therapy as compared to 45 % of those less than 6 years since transplant. The increased use of antiplatelet agents in the more recent cohort may reflect an increased level of comfort in transplanting higher risk individuals. Patients are sometimes wary to use aspirin, even at cardioprotective doses, due to admonition from their transplant centers to avoid use of aspirin and nonsteroidal anti-inflammatory agents post-transplant.

Tobacco Use

It is estimated that between 13 and 33 % [65, 66] of kidney transplant recipients smoke. The risk of death is increased approximately 1.5–2.0-fold [67, 68] in recipients who smoke. Smoking cessation should be advised, ideally prior to transplant, but certainly post-transplant. In an analysis of USRDS data it was noted that smoking occurred in an average of 1.20 ± 0.88 years after transplant [68]. Of concern is how infrequently tobacco use is addressed in the primary care setting [69]. Patients are not always forthcoming about tobacco use, and in one assessment of smoking status with cotinine testing, 34 % of individuals who reported not smoking tested positive for cotinine [70]. As smoking is a chemical addiction, it is reasonable to incorporate methods utilizing nicotine replacement therapy with patches or gum during the

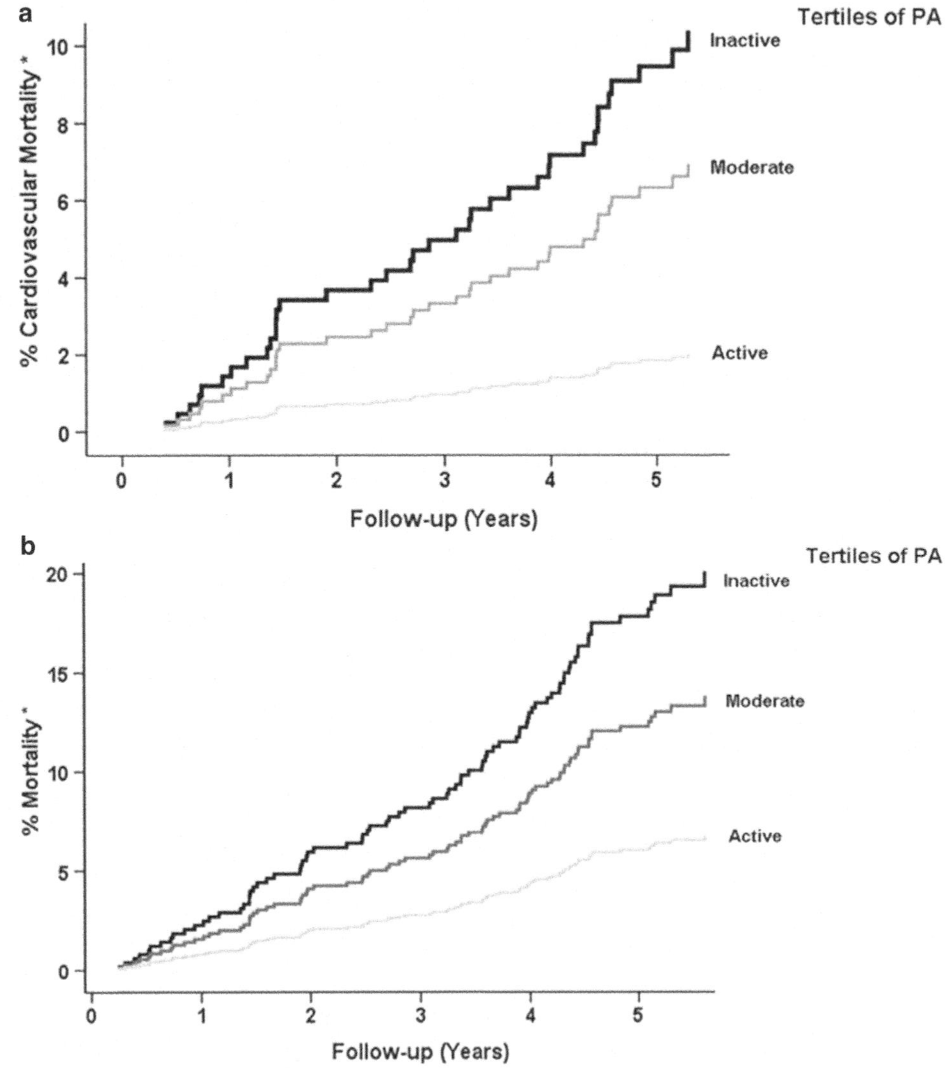

Fig. 18.1 (**a**) Kaplan–Meier curves of cardiovascular mortality according to gender-stratified tertiles of PA. *Adjusted for age ($P<0.001$). (**b**) Kaplan–Meier curves of mortality according to gender-stratified tertiles of PA. *Adjusted for age ($P<0.001$)

cessation process. Pharmacologic therapy with varenicline (Chantix®) [71] is widely advertised and appears to be effective. No reports of use in renal transplant recipients have been published, though experience and personal communications indicate that it appears safe. For some, group therapy provides the best environment for successful smoking cessation. Regardless of the method or methods utilized, tobacco use should be addressed at each clinic visit and recommendations for smoking cessation discussed.

Diet and Exercise

After transplant several dietary restrictions are lifted. High phosphorus and high potassium foods, which were often restricted due to chronic kidney disease, are no longer restricted. Weight gain is typical post-transplant, often as a result of lack of dietary restrictions, improved gustatory satisfaction, and continued relatively sedentary lifestyle. Food may taste better as the often present metallic taste associated with renal failure resolves. Prednisone use is associated with an increase in appetite and many have attributed weight gain to the use of glucocorticoids. In a study by Painter [72], it was observed that the weight gains at 1 year post-transplant of recipients on prednisone were no different than that of those who had been withdrawn from prednisone. In the current era of immunosuppression, steroids are used in only 25–35 % of transplant recipients [3, 73] and it is therefore not as much of an issue.

The benefits of exercise and physical activity have been proven in the general population, as in Fig. 18.1 [74, 75]. A small study of prescribed exercise in renal transplant recipients demonstrated improved cardiorespiratory parameters, such as VO_2max, but no difference in any of the measured biochemical parameters [76]. Of note in this study was a statistically significant decrease in the inflammatory cytokine IL-6 after 30 sessions of exercise training. A 5-year study by Zelle did show significant improvement in cardiovascular and all cause mortality in renal transplant recipients [77]. With reservation the conclusion was that there may be as much as a 40–50 % improvement in cardiovascular risk with increased physical activity in renal transplant recipients. Further support for increased exercise is noted in a study where exercise increased cardiorespiratory fitness [78]. Six months of exercise improved cardiac autonomic parameters as noted in VO_2max, heart rate variability, and baroreflex sensitivity, factors that have been associated with decreased cardiovascular risk in other populations. Whether engagement in physical activity post-transplant confers the same cardiovascular benefits as it does pre-transplant remains controversial. A meta-analysis of 15 randomized controlled trials in solid organ transplant recipients failed to show benefit of exercise [79–81]. There was no demonstrable improvement in lipids, hypertension, post-transplant diabetes, or cardiovascular risk. However, all the trials were small, of relatively short duration, and had variable end points. Despite these controversies, exercise and physical activity should have only a positive impact on renal transplant recipients' risk for heart disease.

In summary, CVD is prevalent in the renal transplant population, less so than in the dialysis population, but more than the general population. Health care providers need to be more aggressive in addressing the risk factors contributing to CVD. Blood pressure should be adequately controlled to achieve a blood pressure ideally less than 130 mmHg systolic and less than 80 mmHg diastolic. Hyperlipidemia needs to be managed with the goal of achieving a total cholesterol of less than 200 mg/dL and an LDL of less than 100 mg/dL, with triglycerides of less than 150 mg/dL. Smoking cessation should be addressed at every visit for patients who are smoking. Weight control, healthy diet, and regular physical activity should be addressed, utilizing the expertise of a dietician and/or exercise physiologist if needed.

References

1. Schiffrin EL, Lipman ML, Mann JFE. Chronic kidney disease: effects on the cardiovascular system. Circulation. 2007;116(1): 85–97.
2. Wolfe RA, Ashby VB, Milford EL, Ojo AO, Ettenger RE, Agodoa LYC, et al. Comparison of mortality in all patients on dialysis, patients on dialysis awaiting transplantation, and recipients of a first cadaveric transplant. N Engl J Med. 1999;341(23):1725–30.
3. Matas AJ, Smith JM, Skeans MA, Lamb KE, Gustafson SK, Samana CJ, et al. OPTN/SRTR 2011 annual data report: kidney. Am J Transplant. 2013;13:11–46.
4. Chico A, Tomás A, Novials A. Silent myocardial ischemia is associated with autonomic neuropathy and other cardiovascular risk factors in type 1 and type 2 diabetic subjects, especially in those with microalbuminuria. Endocrine. 2005;27(3):213–7.
5. Delgado C, Johansen KL. Barriers to exercise participation among dialysis patients. Nephrol Dial Transplant. 2012;27(3):1152–7.
6. Rosas SE, Reese PP, Huan Y, Doria C, Cochetti PT, Doyle A. Pretransplant physical activity predicts all-cause mortality in kidney transplant recipients. Am J Nephrol. 2012;35(1):17–23.
7. Greenwood SA, Lindup H, Taylor K, Koufaki P, Rush R, Macdougall IC, et al. Evaluation of a pragmatic exercise rehabilitation programme in chronic kidney disease. Nephrol Dial Transplant. 2012;27 Suppl 3:iii126–34.
8. Friedman SE, Palac RT, Zlotnick DM, Chobanian MC, Costa SP. A call to action: variability in guidelines for cardiac evaluation before renal transplantation. Clin J Am Soc Nephrol. 2011;6(5):1185–91.
9. Nguyen KN, Patel AM, Weng FL. Ionizing radiation exposure among kidney transplant recipients due to medical imaging during the pre-transplant evaluation. Clin J Am Soc Nephrol. 2013;8(5):833–9.
10. de Mattos AM, Siedlecki A, Gaston RS, Perry GJ, Julian BA, Kew CE, et al. Systolic dysfunction portends increased mortality among those waiting for renal transplant. J Am Soc Nephrol. 2008;19(6):1191–6.
11. McFalls EO, Ward HB, Moritz TE, Goldman S, Krupski WC, Littooy F, et al. Coronary-artery revascularization before elective major vascular surgery. N Engl J Med. 2004;351(27):2795–804.
12. Souza FLD, Bezerra KB, Sousa AR, Ferreira TCA, Oliveira MIG, Martins GP, et al. Estudo das alterações ecocardiográficas nos primeiros seis meses após o transplante renal. Arq Bras Cardiol. 2012;98(6):505–13.
13. Sharma R, Pellerin D, Gaze DC, Gregson H, Streather CP, Collinson PO, et al. Dobutamine stress echocardiography and the resting but not exercise electrocardiograph predict severe coronary artery disease in renal transplant candidates. Nephrol Dial Transplant. 2005;20(10):2207–14.
14. Kasiske BL, Guijarro C, Massy ZA, Wiederkehr MR, Ma JZ. Cardiovascular disease after renal transplantation. J Am Soc Nephrol. 1996;7(1):158–65.
15. Lentine KL, Brennan DC, Schnitzler MA. Incidence and predictors of myocardial infarction after kidney transplantation. J Am Soc Nephrol. 2005;16(2):496–506.
16. U.S. Renal Data System. USRDS 2007 annual data report: atlas of chronic kidney disease and end-stage renal disease in the United States. Bethesda: National Institutes of Health, National Institute of Diabetes and Digestive and Kidney Disease; 2007.
17. Aalten J, Hoogeveen EK, Roodnat JI, Weimar W, Borm GF, De Fijter JW, et al. Associations between pre-kidney-transplant risk factors and post-transplant cardiovascular events and death. Transpl Int. 2008;21(10):985–91.
18. Kasiske BL, Anjum S, Shah R, Skogen J, Kandaswamy C, Danielson B, et al. Hypertension after kidney transplantation. Am J Kidney Dis. 2004;43(6):1071–81.
19. Carpenter MA, Weir MR, Adey DB, House AA, Bostom AG, Kusek JW. Inadequacy of cardiovascular risk factor management in chronic kidney transplantation? Evidence from the FAVORIT study. Clin Transplant. 2012;26(4):E438–46.
20. Fernandez Fresnedo G, Franco Esteve A, Gómez Huertas E, Cabello Chaves V, Díz Gómez JM, Osorio Moratalla JM, et al. Ambulatory blood pressure monitoring in kidney transplant patients: RETENAL study. Transplant Proc. 2012;44(9):2601–2.
21. Levenson JL, Olbrisch ME. Psychosocial evaluation of organ transplant candidates: a comparative survey of process, criteria, and outcomes in heart, liver, and kidney transplantation. Psychosomatics. 1993;34(4):314–23.
22. Pérez-Stable EJ, Marín G, Marín BV, Benowitz NL. Misclassification of smoking status by self-reported cigarette consumption. Am J Respir Crit Care Med. 1992;145(1):53–7.
23. Ponticelli C, Villa M, Cesana B, Montagnino G, Tarantino A. Risk factors for late allograft failure. Kidney Int. 2002;62(5):1848–54.
24. Rosas SE, Mensah K, Weinstein RB, Bellamy SL, Rader DJ. Coronary artery calcification in renal transplant recipients. Am J Transplant. 2005;5:1942–7.
25. Kahn M, Robbins MJ, Kim M, Fuster V. Management of cardiovascular disease in patients with kidney disease. Nat Rev Cardiol. 2013;10(5):261–73.

26. Kidney Disease: Improving Global Outcomes (KDIGO) Transplant Work Group. Special issue: KDIGO clinical practice guideline for the care of kidney transplant recipients. Am J Transplant. 2009;9:S1–155.
27. Bostom AG, Carpenter MA, Kusek JW, Levey AS, Hunsicker L, Pfeffer MA, et al. Homocysteine-lowering and cardiovascular disease outcomes in kidney transplant recipients: primary results from the folic acid for vascular outcome reduction in transplantation trial. Circulation. 2011;123(16):1763–70.
28. Panichi V, Scatena A, Migliori M, Marchetti V, Paoletti S, Beati S. Biomarkers of chronic inflammatory state in uremia and cardiovascular disease. Int J Inflam. 2012;2012:6.
29. Libby P. Inflammation in atherosclerosis. Arterioscler Thromb Vasc Biol. 2012;32(9):2045–51.
30. van Diepen JA, Berbée JFP, Havekes LM, Rensen PCN. Interactions between inflammation and lipid metabolism: relevance for efficacy of anti-inflammatory drugs in the treatment of atherosclerosis. Atherosclerosis. 2013;228(2):306–15.
31. Zwiech R, Bruzda-Zwiech A. Does oral health contribute to post-transplant complications in kidney allograft recipients? Acta Odontol Scand. 2013;71(3–4):756–63.
32. Yudkin JS, Kumari M, Humphries SE, Mohamed-Ali V. Inflammation, obesity, stress and coronary heart disease: is interleukin-6 the link? Atherosclerosis. 2000;148(2):209–14.
33. Winkelmayer WC, Lorenz M, Kramar R, Födinger M, Hörl WH, Sunder-Plassmann G. C-reactive protein and body mass index independently predict mortality in kidney transplant recipients. Am J Transplant. 2004;4(7):1148–54.
34. Winkelmayer WC, Schaeffner ES, Chandraker A, Kramar R, Rumpold H, Sunder-Plassmann G, et al. A J-shaped association between high-sensitivity C-reactive protein and mortality in kidney transplant recipients. Transpl Int. 2007;20(6):505–11.
35. van Ree RM, de Vries APJ, Oterdoom LH, The TH, Gansevoort RT, Homan van der Heide JJ, et al. Abdominal obesity and smoking are important determinants of C-reactive protein in renal transplant recipients. Nephrol Dial Transplant. 2005;20(11):2524–31.
36. Pinto de Carvalho L, McCullough PA, Gao F, Sim LL, Tan HC, Foo D, et al. Renal function and anaemia in acute myocardial infarction. Int J Cardiol. 2013;168(2):1397–401.
37. Fusté B, Serradell M, Escola G, Cases A, Mazzara R, Castillo R, et al. Erythropoietin triggers a signaling pathway in endothelial cells and increases the thrombogenicity of their extracellular matrices in vitro. Thromb Haemost. 2002;88(4):678–85.
38. Van Loo A, Vanholder R, Bernaert P, De Roose J, Lameire N. Recombinant human erythropoietin corrects anaemia during the first weeks after renal transplantation: a randomized prospective study. Nephrol Dial Transplant. 1996;11(9):1815–21.
39. Locatelli F, Aljama P, Canaud B, Covic A, De Francisco A, Macdougall IC, et al. Target haemoglobin to aim for with erythropoiesis-stimulating agents: a position statement by ERBP following publication of the Trial to Reduce Cardiovascular Events with Aranesp® Therapy (TREAT) Study. Nephrol Dial Transplant. 2010;25(9):2846–50.
40. Israni AK, Snyder JJ, Skeans MA, Peng Y, Maclean JR, Weinhandl ED, et al. Predicting coronary heart disease after kidney transplantation: patient outcomes in renal transplantation (PORT) study. Am J Transplant. 2010;10(2):338–53.
41. Bayer ND, Cochetti PT, Anil Kumar M, Teal V, Huan Y, Doria C, et al. Association of metabolic syndrome with development of new-onset diabetes after transplantation. Transplantation. 2010; 90(8):861–6.
42. Wauters RP, Cosio FG, Suarez Fernandez ML, Kudva Y, Shah P, Torres VE. Cardiovascular consequences of new-onset hyperglycemia after kidney transplantation. Transplantation. 2012;94(4): 377–82.
43. United States Renal Data System 2012 Annual Data Report: Atlas of Chronic Kidney Disease & End-Stage Renal Disease in the United States. AJKD 2013;62(6;1023–230.
44. Vaziri ND, Liang K, Parks JS. Down-regulation of hepatic lecithin:cholesterol acyltransferase gene expression in chronic renal failure. Kidney Int. 2001;59:2192–6.
45. Vaziri ND. Dyslipidemia of chronic renal failure: the nature, mechanisms, and potential consequences. Am J Physiol. 2006; 290(2):F262–72.
46. Spinelli GA, Felipe CR, Park SI, Mandia-Sampaio EL, Tedesco-Silva Jr H, Medina-Pestana JO. Lipid profile changes during the first year after kidney transplantation: risk factors and influence of the immunosuppressive drug regimen. Transplant Proc. 2011;43(10):3730–7.
47. Hohage H, Hillebrandt U, Welling U, Zeh M, Heck M, Gerhardt UW, et al. Cyclosporine and tacrolimus: influence on cardiovascular risk factors. Transplant Proc. 2005;37(2):1036–8.
48. deGroen P. Cyclosporine, low-density lipoprotein, and cholesterol. Mayo Clin Proc. 1988;63(10):1012–21.
49. Kasiske B, Cosio FG, Beto J, Bolton K, Chavers BM, Grimm R, et al. Clinical practice guidelines for managing dyslipidemias in kidney transplant patients: a report from the Managing Dyslipidemias in Chronic Kidney Disease Work Group of the National Kidney Foundation Kidney Disease Outcomes Quality Initiative. Am J Transplant. 2004;4:13–53.
50. Dawson KL, Patel SJ, Putney D, Suki WN, Osama Gaber A. Cardioprotective medication use after renal transplantation. Clin Transplant. 2010;24(6):E253–6.
51. Pilmore HL, Skeans MA, Snyder JJ, Israni AK, Kasiske BL. Cardiovascular disease medications after renal transplantation: results from the patient outcomes in renal transplantation study. Transplantation. 2011;91(5):542–51.
52. Gaston RS, Kasiske BL, Fieberg AM, Leduc R, Cosio FC, Gourishankar S, et al. Use of cardioprotective medications in kidney transplant recipients. Am J Transplant. 2009;9(8):1811–5.
53. Lentine KL, Villines TC, Xiao H, Schnitzler MA, Brennan DC, Abbott KC, et al. Cardioprotective medication use after acute myocardial infarction in kidney transplant recipients. Transplantation. 2011;91(10):1120–6.
54. Cross NB, Webster AC, Masson P, O'Connell PJ, Craig JC. Antihypertensives for kidney transplant recipients: systematic review and meta-analysis of randomized controlled trials. Transplantation. 2009;88(1):7–18.
55. Fihn SD, Gardin JM, Abrams J, Berra K, Blankenship JC, Dallas AP, et al. 2012. ACCF/AHA/ACP/AATS/PCNA/SCAI/STS guideline for the diagnosis and management of patients with stable ischemic heart disease: a report of the American College of Cardiology Foundation/American Heart Association Task Force on Practice Guidelines, and the American College of Physicians, American Association for Thoracic Surgery, Preventive Cardiovascular Nurses Association, Society for Cardiovascular Angiography and Interventions, and Society of Thoracic Surgeons. J Am Coll Cardiol. 2012;60(24):e44–164.
56. Weir MR. Effects of renin-angiotensin system inhibition end-organ protection: can we do better? Clin Ther. 2007;29(9):1803–24.
57. Hoogwerf BJ. Renin–angiotensin system blockade and cardiovascular and renal protection. Am J Cardiol. 2010;105(1 Suppl):30a–5.
58. Munger MA. Use of angiotensin receptor blockers in cardiovascular protection. Pharm Ther. 2010;36(1):22–40.
59. Vlahakos D, Marathias K, Agroyannis B, Madias N. Post-transplant erythrocytosis. Kidney Int. 2003;63(4):1187–94.
60. Midtvedt K, Ihlen H, Hartmann A, Bryde P, Bjerkely BL, Foss A, et al. Reduction of left ventricular mass by lisinopril and nifedipine in hypertensive renal transplant recipients: a prospective randomized double-blind study. Transplantation. 2001;72(1):107–14.

61. Holdaas H, Fellström B, Cole E, Nyberg G, Olsson AG, Pedersen TR, et al. Long-term cardiac outcomes in renal transplant recipients receiving fluvastatin: the ALERT extension study. Am J Transplant. 2005;5(12):2929–36.
62. Lentine KL, Brennan DC. Statin use after renal transplantation: a systematic quality review of trial-based evidence. Nephrol Dial Transplant. 2004;19(9):2378–86.
63. Riella LV, Gabardi S, Chandraker A. Dyslipidemia and its therapeutic challenges in renal transplantation. Am J Transplant. 2012; 12(8):1975–82.
64. Brunzell JD. Hypertriglyceridemia. N Engl J Med. 2007; 357(10):1009–17.
65. Sung RS, Althoen M, Howell TA, Ojo AO, Merion RM. Excess risk of renal allograft loss associated with cigarette smoking. Transplantation. 2007;71(12):1752–7.
66. Nogueira JM, Haririan A, Jacobs SC, Cooper M, Weir MR. Cigarette smoking, kidney function, and mortality after live donor kidney transplant. Am J Kidney Dis. 2010;55(5):907–15.
67. Corbett C, Armstrong MJ, Neuberger J. Tobacco smoking and solid organ transplantation. [Editorial]. Transplantation. 2012;94: 979–87.
68. Hurst F, Altieri M, Patel P, Jindal T, Guy S, Sidawy A, et al. Effect of smoking on kidney transplant outcomes: analysis of the United States Renal Data System. Transplantation. 2011;92(10):1101–7.
69. Thorndike AN, Regan S, Rigotti NA. The treatment of smoking by US physicians during ambulatory visits: 1994-2003. Am J Public Health. 2007;97(10):1878–83.
70. Nguyen PTH, Galanti L, Pirson Y, Jadoul M. Identification of current smokers among renal transplant recipients. Nephrol Dial Transplant. 2007;22(7):1974–8.
71. Gonzales D, Rennard SI, Nides M, Oncken C, Azoulay S, Billing CB, et al. Varenicline, an alpha4beta2 nicotinic acetylcholine receptor partial agonist, vs sustained-release bupropion and placebo for smoking cessation: a randomized controlled trial. JAMA. 2006;296(1):47–55.
72. Painter PL, Topp K, Krasnoff J, Adey D, Strasner A, Tomlanovich S, et al. Health-related fitness and quality of life following steroid withdrawal in renal transplant recipients. Kidney Int. 2003; 63(6):2309–16.
73. Kramer BK, Klinger M, Vitko S, Glyda M, Midtvedt K, Stefoni S, et al. Tacrolimus-based, steroid-free regimens in renal transplantation: 3-year follow-up of the ATLAS trial. Transplantation. 2012;94(5):492–8.
74. Kokkinos P, Myers J, Kokkinos JP, Pittaras A, Narayan P, Manolis A, et al. Exercise capacity and mortality in black and white men. Circulation. 2008;117(5):614–22.
75. Ford ES, Bergmann MM, Boeing H, Li C, Capewell S. Healthy lifestyle behaviors and all-cause mortality among adults in the United States. Prev Med. 2012;55(1):23–7.
76. Romano G, Simonella R, Falleti E, Bortolotti N, Deiuri E, Antonutto G, et al. Physical training effects in renal transplant recipients. Clin Transplant. 2010;24(4):510–4.
77. Zelle DM, Corpeleijn E, Stolk RP, de Greef MHG, Gans ROB, van der Heide JJH, et al. Low physical activity and risk of cardiovascular and all-cause mortality in renal transplant recipients. Clin J Am Soc Nephrol. 2011;6(4):898–905.
78. Kouidi E, Vergoulas G, Anifanti M, Deligiannis A. A randomized controlled trial of exercise training on cardiovascular and autonomic function among renal transplant recipients. Nephrol Dial Transplant. 2012;28(5):1294–305.
79. Didsbury M, McGee RG, Tong A, Craig JC, Chapman JR, Chadban S, et al. Exercise training in solid organ transplant recipients: a systematic review and meta-analysis. Transplantation. 2013;95(5):679–87.
80. Jacobson TA, Armani A, McKenney JM, Guyton JR. Safety considerations with gastrointestinally active lipid-lowering drugs. Am J Cardiol. 2007;99(6 Suppl 1):47C–55.
81. Dienz O, Eaton SM, Bond JP, Neveu W, Moquin D, Noubade R, et al. The induction of antibody production by IL-6 is indirectly mediated by IL-21 produced by CD4+ T cells. J Exp Med. 2009;206(1):69–78.

19 Dyslipidemia After Kidney Transplantation

Darshika Chhabra, Anil Vamsi Doppalapudi, Anurag Kumbham, and Edgar V. Lerma

Introduction

Cardiovascular disease (CVD) is a major cause of mortality and graft loss in renal transplantation [1]. Some of the well-established risk factors for CVD are chronic kidney disease (CKD), hypertension, hyperlipidemia, diabetes, obesity, and smoking [2, 3]. Immunosuppressive medications also play a very important role in its pathogenesis. Hypercholesterolemia and hypertriglyceridemia have been reported in as many as 40–80 % and 40–60 % patients post-transplant, respectively [4, 5]. Dyslipidemia is one of the modifiable cardiovascular risk factors and warrants close attention in kidney transplant recipients.

Scope of the Problem and Prevalence

The prevalence of dyslipidemias in kidney transplant recipients is very high (Table 19.1). Particularly common are increases in total cholesterol and low-density lipoprotein (LDL). Forty-four percent of renal transplant recipients tend to have LDL level greater than 100 mg/dL [6]. Triglycerides are often increased, but high-density lipoprotein (HDL) is usually normal.

Etiology of Dyslipidemia in Kidney Transplant Recipients

Many factors influence the prevalence of dyslipidemias in transplant patients.

Potential causes include immunosuppressive medications, diet, obesity, and genetic predisposition.

Some of the primary and secondary causes are summarized below [6, 7]:

1. Male gender
2. Genetic predisposition
3. Increased age
4. Proteinuria, nephritic syndrome, and hypoalbuminemia
5. Kidney dysfunction
   (a) Renin–angiotensin system activity
   (b) Abnormal calcium and phosphorus metabolism
   (c) Renal artery stenosis
6. Immunosuppressive agents
   (a) Calcineurin inhibitors (cyclosporine, tacrolimus)
   (b) Antiproliferative agents (sirolimus)
   (c) Corticosteroids
7. Other medications like atypical antipsychotics, oral estrogen, protease inhibitors, diuretics, and beta-blockers
8. Hypothyroidism
9. Diabetes
10. Excessive alcohol intake
11. Chronic liver disease

Immunosuppressive medications, e.g., prednisone, cyclosporine, and sirolimus, are among the several potential remediable causes of dyslipidemias in kidney transplant patients.

D. Chhabra, M.D., M.P.H. (✉)
Kidney Transplant Program, Advocate Christ Medical Center, 4400 W 95th St, Suite 112, Oak Lawn, IL 60453, USA

Section of Nephrology, University of Illinois at Chicago, Chicago, IL USA
e-mail: darshika.chhabra@advocatehealth.com

A.V. Doppalapudi, M.D.
Internal Medicine, AVD Medical, Sc, 4861 W 95th St, Oak Lawn, IL 60453, USA

A. Kumbham, M.D.
Internal Medicine, Metro Medical Associates, 225 Thamesmar Lane, Suwannee, GA 30024, USA
e-mail: drrahul@gmail.com

E.V. Lerma, M.D.
Department of Medicine, Section of Nephrology, University of Illinois at Chicago, 3543 Wisconsin Avenue, Berwyn, IL 60402, USA
e-mail: edgarvlermamd@pol.net

M.R. Weir and E.V. Lerma (eds.), *Kidney Transplantation: Practical Guide to Management*, DOI 10.1007/978-1-4939-0342-9_19, © Springer Science+Business Media New York 2014

Table 19.1 Prevalence of dyslipidemias in kidney transplant patients

Study	*n*	Age (years)	Cholesterol> 200 mg/dL (%)	LDL> 100 mg/dL (%)	HDL <40 mg/dL (%)	TG mean (mg/dL)
Moore et al. [26]	214	44.7	90	97	48	195
Aakhus et al. [27]	403	47	94		18	
Brown et al. [28]	100	41.8	83	93	30	163

Calcineurin Inhibitors

These medications may produce alterations in lipid profile, as early as 1 month within start of therapy. Cyclosporine may have a higher tendency to cause dyslipidemia than tacrolimus. It inhibits the 26-hydroxylase enzyme, leading to a decrease in bile acid synthesis from cholesterol.

Antiproliferative Agents

Mammalian target of rapamycin (mTOR) inhibitors like sirolimus produce dose-dependent significant increases in total cholesterol and triglyceride levels by various mechanisms. They decrease the catabolism of apolipoprotein B100, inhibit insulin and insulin-like growth factor signals, and/or alter hepatocyte synthesis of lipid moieties.

Corticosteroids

These agents induce increases in total cholesterol with variable effects on triglycerides. They increase the activity of acetyl coenzyme A carboxylase and free fatty acid synthetase, downregulate LDL receptor activity, increase the activity of HMG-CoA reductase, and inhibit lipoprotein lipase. They have been associated with increased levels of very low-density lipoproteins (VLDL), total cholesterol (TC), and triglycerides (TG), as well as a decrease in HDL (high-density lipoproteins) levels. In combination with other agents like cyclosporine, these may have additive effects.

Mycophenolic acid and azathioprine

These agents do not appear to adversely affect the lipid profile.

Transplantation may be associated with other nontraditional CVD risk factors such as acute rejection episodes which cause endothelial damage and require intensification of immunosuppressive regimens.

Assessment of Dyslipidemia

Kidney transplant patients with dyslipidemia require an individualized approach to screening and management, compared to the general population. Recipients should be monitored for development or worsening of already existing hyperlipidemia that may worsen after transplantation. The evaluation should include an assessment for secondary causes as well.

Screening

Target Population

The National Kidney Foundation's Kidney Disease Outcomes Quality Initiative (NKF K/DOQI) and Kidney Disease Improving Global Outcomes (KDIGO) clinical practice guidelines recommend all kidney transplant recipients be screened [4, 8, 8A].

Frequency of Screening

Traditional guidelines were to screen patients prior to transplant and within the first 6 months of kidney transplantation, at 1-year post-transplant, and at least annually thereafter [4]. The more recent 2013 KDIGO guidelines recommend the initial screening in kidney transplantation, however, follow-up measurement may not be required in the majority of patients [8A]. Any modification in therapy or development of a condition which may be associated with dyslipidemia should prompt more frequent testing, starting within 2–3 months of the intervention or status change.

Screening Method

A complete lipid panel after an overnight fast is the preferred method of screening [4]. The panel should include total cholesterol (TC), LDL cholesterol, HDL cholesterol, and triglyceride (TG) levels. Non-HDL cholesterol (calculated as TC minus HDL cholesterol) should also be taken into account.

Treatment

The 2009 Kidney Disease Improving Global Outcomes (KDIGO) clinical practice guidelines are based on the 2004 NKF K/DOQI guidelines for managing dyslipidemias in CKD and provide guidance for managing dyslipidemias in renal transplant patients [4, 8]. KDIGO updated their clinical practice guidelines for lipid management in chronic kidney disease in 2013 [8A]. As in general population, controlling the risk factors leading to CVD should be a major component of post-transplant management strategy.

Treatment Goals

The KDIGO and K/DOQI guidelines [4, 8] consider kidney transplant recipients a high-risk group who should be treated like a CVD risk equivalent, unlike the US National Cholesterol Education Program-Adult Treatment Panel III (NCEP-ATPIII) guidelines [9]. By the traditional 'treat-to-target' approach, goals of dyslipidemia treatment were to lower LDL, non-HDL, and triglyceride levels while improving HDL level. Based on traditional recommendations, these were the target goals:
LDL cholesterol <100 mg/dL
Non-HDL cholesterol <130 mg/dL
TG <150 mg/dL
However, 2013 KDIGO recommendations revised this approach and suggest a 'fire-and-forget' strategy: do not measure LDL unless the results will alter management.

Treatment Strategies

All patients should be counseled about therapeutic lifestyle changes (TLC), which include diet, weight loss, increased physical activity, abstinence from alcohol, and treatment of hyperglycemia, if appropriate. Diet should include <200 mg/day cholesterol, <7 % saturated fat, and increased fiber (10–25 mg/day). Any secondary causes of dyslipidemia should be identified and addressed, if feasible. For example, reducing or eliminating nephritic range proteinuria and treating poorly controlled diabetes or severe hypothyroidism may help with dyslipidemia [8]. Pharmacotherapy plays a major role in the treatment of dyslipidemia, with statins being used the most commonly, based on strong evidence that they reduce LDL cholesterol and cardiovascular events [11].

Table 19.2 Recommended doses (mg/d) of statins in transplant patients [4]

Statin	Recommended dose (mg/day)
Lovastatin	Not done
Fluvastatin	80 mg
Atorvastatin	20 mg
Rosuvastatin	10 mg
Simvastatin/Ezetmibe	20 /10 mg
Pravastatin	40 mg
Simvastatin	40 mg
Pitavastatin	2 mg

The 2013 KDIGO Work Group recommends treatment with a statin [8A]. Other agents used include fibrates (fibric acid derivatives), niacin (nicotinic acid), ezetimibe, and bile acid sequestrants. Table 19.3 summarizes the agents used [6].

Hypertriglyceridemia

Niacin and fibrates have been the first line of therapy in general population to lower triglyceride levels. Due to unfavorable side effect profile and potential interaction with immunosuppressive agents, fibrates should be avoided in post-transplant patients and cautiously used in CKD stage 5 patients. Fibrates, particularly fenofibrate, may be associated with elevated creatinine and with myositis when in combination with a statin (particularly gemfibrozil, which is considered the fibrate of choice) [12]. According to the 2013 KDIGO guidelines, fibric acid derivatives are not recommended to prevent pancreatitis or reduce cardiovascular risk in adults with CKD and hypertriglyceridemia [8A]. They recommend TLC, reserving fibrates for management of patients with TG >1000mg/dl.

Nicotinic acid has not been well studied in advanced CKD and is not recommended for treatment of severe hypertriglyceridemia, given the risk of toxicity (especially flushing and hyperglycemia) [8A]. In patients with normal or mildly elevated TG, statins appear to prevent pancreatitis and may be used along with TLC.

In patient on agents like sirolimus or everolimus, refractory hypertriglyceridemia may necessitate dose lowering or discontinuation of these drugs.

LDL Cholesterol

LDL cholesterol has not been found suitable for assessing coronary risk in persons with CKD [8A]. Higher cardiovascular risk and not elevated LDL is now the primary indication to initiate or adjust lipid-lowering treatment. In kidney transplant patients, coronary risk is sufficiently high to justify the use of statins, irrespective of LDL levels [8A]. The recommended doses of statins in transplant patients is demonstrated in Table 19.2. Contemporary practice emphasizes the use of targets for LDL (e.g. 70 or 100 mg/dl) which requires surveillance of LDL levels and treatment escalation with higher doses of statin or initiation of combination lipid-lowering therapy ("treat-to-target" strategy). However, this has never been proven beneficial in any clinical trial and higher doses of statins have not been proven to be safe in the setting of CKD. Instead, the 2013 KDIGO Work Group recommends a "fire-and-forget" strategy.

Bile acid sequestrants should be avoided in transplant patients as they interfere with absorption of immunosuppressive drugs like mycophenolic acid.

Table 19.3 Review of agents used to manage dyslipidemias [6]

Medication class/ generic name	Typical dosing regimen	Dosing instructions	Major adverse events/drug–drug interactions
Statins (HMG-CoA reductase inhibitors)			
Atorvastatin	10–80 mg/day	Given any time of the day	Headache, nausea, sleep disturbance, elevations in hepatocellular enzymes and alkaline phosphatase. Myositis and rhabdomyolysis, primarily when given with gemfibrozil or cyclosporine; myositis is also seen with severe renal insufficiency (CrCl<30 mL/min). Most statins can also affect digoxin metabolism and levels
Fluvastatin	20–80 mg/day Sustained release = 80 mg/day	Regular release dosed at bedtime or be given twice daily if dose >40 mg/day	
Lovastatin	20–80 mg/day	With the evening meal Should be dosed twice daily if dose >20 mg/day	
Pitavastatin	1–4 mg/day	Any time of the day	
Pravastatin	10–80 mg/day	At bedtime	
Rosuvastatin	5–40 mg/day	Any time of the day	
Simvastatin	10–80 mg/day	At bedtime	
Fibric acid derivatives (fibrates)			
Gemfibrozil	600 mg twice daily	30–60 min before meals	Skin rash, gastrointestinal (nausea, bloating, cramping), myalgia; lowers blood cyclosporine levels; potentially nephrotoxic in cyclosporine-treated patients. Avoid in patients with CrCl <30 mL/min
Fenofibrate	Nanocrystal 145 mg/day Micronized 160–200 mg/day	Micronized taken with meals. Use lower doses with renal insufficiency	
Bile acid sequestrants			
Cholestyramine	4–24 g/day	Take within 30 min of a meal. A double dose with dinner produces same lipid-lowering effect as BID dosing	Nausea, bloating, cramping, and constipation; elevations in LFTs. Impaired absorption of fat soluble vitamins, digoxin, warfarin, thiazides, β-blockers, thyroxine, and phenobarbital. Avoid use with MPA
Colestipol	5–30 g/day	Same as cholestyramine	
Colesevelam	3.75 g/day	Take with meals daily or divided BID	
Cholesterol absorption inhibitors			
Ezetimibe	10 mg/day	Any time of the day	Increased transaminases in combination with statins
Miscellaneous			
Nicotinic acid	1–6 g/day	Given with meals. Start with 100 mg BID and titrate to 500 mg TID. After 6 weeks, check lipids, glucose, liver function, and uric acid. Increase dose as needed	Prostaglandin-mediated cutaneous flushing, headache, warm sensation, and pruritus; hyperpigmentation (particularly in intertriginous regions); dry skin; nausea; vomiting; diarrhea; and myositis
Omega-3-acid ethyl esters	4 g/day (supplement) or 2 servings per week of oily fish	May be given any time of the day	Nausea and GI upset (eructation)

Non-HDL Cholesterol

Low HDL and elevated apolipoprotein B (apoB) or non-HDL is associated with excess risk of future cardiovascular events [8A]. These may be measured in CKD patients, if the results would influence the clinician's decision to prescribe statin treatment, based on estimated cardiovascular risk.

Statins in Transplant Patients

As in the general population, statins need to be monitored for adverse effects such as liver dysfunction and myopathy. An elevation of liver enzymes greater than three times of the upper limit of normal warrants discontinuation or dose reduction. Rechallenging the patient with a different statin at a lower dose is reasonable, once the liver function tests have normalized. Risk of developing myopathy is greater in the elderly, patients with a GFR <30 mL/min, with the use of maximum statin doses and in combination with other cytochrome p450 isoenzyme inhibitors, such as cyclosporine, gemfibrozil, grapefruit, macrolide antibiotics, protease inhibitors, azole antifungals, and non-dihydropyridine calcium channel blockers (diltiazem and verapamil). In general statin doses may need to be reduced by about 50 % in patients on cyclosporine and potentially also in patients on tacrolimus, although data is limited [8]. Amlodipine is a weak inhibitor; however, the Food and Drug Administration (FDA) recommends limiting the dose of simvastatin to 20 mg when used in combination with amlodipine. Table 19.4 provides a comparison of potency and conversion doses of statins.

Discussion

The benefit of aggressive lipid management has been shown to reduce cardiovascular mortality in the general population, in patients without CKD. In the Heart Protection Study, diabetic patients who were randomly allocated to receive

Table 19.4 Statin antilipid strength and conversion doses [6]

Atorvastatin (mg)	Fluvastatin (mg)	Lovastatin (mg)	Pitavastatin (mg)	Pravastatin (mg)	Rosuvastatin (mg)	Simvastatin (mg)	% ↓ in LDL-C (%)
–	40	20	1	20	–	10	30
10	80	40	2	40	–	20	38
20	–	80	4	80	5	40	41
40	–	–	–	–	10	80	47
80	–	–	–	–	20	–	55
–	–	–	–	–	40	–	63

40 mg of simvastatin daily had a reduced rate of first major vascular events compared to placebo, over 5 years of follow-up, even if they did not already have manifest coronary disease or high cholesterol concentrations [13]. Cholesterol-lowering agents have been shown to improve cardiovascular outcomes in both early [14, 15] and advanced CKD [16]. The Study of Heart and Renal Protection (SHARP) trial was a randomized double-blind trial in 9,270 patients with CKD, comparing simvastatin 20 mg plus ezetimibe 10 mg daily with placebo [16]. During a median follow-up of 4.9 years, the lipid-lowering regimen yielded a 17 % overall reduction in first major atherosclerotic events (11.3 % vs. 13.4 % in the placebo group; RR = 0.83, 95 % CI 0.74–0.94), with no benefit on survival. Although the study suggests a benefit in LDL lowering, it does not answer whether statin therapy and/or ezetimibe mediated this effect. Statins in some studies have shown benefits in early CKD by slowing down the progression of renal dysfunction thought to be from anti-inflammatory effects of statins [17]. Conversely, stabilizing renal function may in its turn slow down progression of atherosclerotic disease.

Unlike in the general population, the role of dyslipidemia in post-transplant CVD is not well delineated. However, the only randomized controlled trial to assess statin therapy in kidney transplant recipients suggests that treatment of dyslipidemia could decrease cardiovascular events, including cardiac death post-transplant [18, 19]. The Assessment of Lescol in Renal Transplantation (ALERT) Study demonstrated that kidney transplant recipients randomized to fluvastatin had fewer cardiac deaths or nonfatal myocardial infarctions compared to the placebo group (RR 0.65, 95 % CI 0.48–0.88, $p = 0.005$), over 5.1 years of follow-up [19]. The fluvastatin group had a 32 % reduction in LDL, although no decrease in the rate of coronary intervention procedures or all-cause mortality.

A few observational studies suggest that dyslipidemia may be associated with renal allograft dysfunction, subsequent rejection, and graft loss [20–23]. Two randomized controlled trials did not show any beneficial effect of dyslipidemia treatment on acute rejection episodes [24, 25]. For now, the principal reason to identify and treat dyslipidemia in kidney transplant recipients is to prevent atherosclerotic CVD. According to the 2013 KDIGO guidelines, coronary risk in kidney transplant patients is sufficiently high to justify prescription of statins and to adhere to a fire-and-forget strategy.

Summary

CVD is the leading cause of mortality in kidney transplant recipients and accounts for a significant proportion of death with a functioning allograft. Dyslipidemia is a common modifiable CVD risk factor encountered post-transplant, and efforts should be made to screen all patients and to treat with a statin, to decrease cardiovascular risk. Secondary causes of dyslipidemia should be identified and managed appropriately. Refractory cases of severe lipid abnormalities may warrant changes in immunosuppressive medications known to cause dyslipidemia. Treatment of dyslipidemia with a statin, in an effort to prevent CVD, is an integral part of management of the kidney transplant recipient.

References

1. Kasiske BL, Guijarro C, Massy ZA, Wiederkehr MR, Ma JZ. Cardiovascular disease after renal transplantation. J Am Soc Nephrol. 1996;7(1):158–65.
2. Kasiske BL. Cardiovascular disease after renal transplantation. Semin Nephrol. 2000;20(2):176–87.
3. Ojo AO. Cardiovascular complications after renal transplantation and their prevention. Transplantation. 2006;82(5):603–11.
4. Kasiske B, Cosio FG, Beto J, Bolton K, Chavers BM, Grimm R, et al. Clinical practice guidelines for managing dyslipidemias in kidney transplant patients: a report from the Managing Dyslipidemias in Chronic Kidney Disease Work Group of the National Kidney Foundation Kidney Disease Outcomes Quality Initiative. Am J Transplant. 2004;4 Suppl 7:13–53.
5. Transplantation EEGoR. European best practice guidelines for renal transplantation. Section IV: long-term management of the transplant recipient. IV.5.1. Cardiovascular risks. Cardiovascular disease after renal transplantation. Nephrol Dial Transplant. 2002;17(Suppl 4):24–5.
6. Riella LV, Gabardi S, Chandraker A. Dyslipidemia and its therapeutic challenges in renal transplantation. Am J Transplant. 2012;12(8):1975–82.
7. Zolezzi M. Management of dyslipidemia in renal disease and transplantation. Saudi J Kidney Dis Transpl. 2006;17(2):129–36.

8. KDIGO Transplant Work Group. KDIGO clinical practice guideline for the care of kidney transplant recipients. Am J Transplant. 2009;9 Suppl 3:S1–155.
8A. KDIGO clinical practice guideline for lipid management in chronic kidney disease. Kidney International Supplements. 2013;3(3):259–305.
9. Expert Panel on Detection, Evaluation, and Treatment of High Blood Cholesterol in Adults. Executive summary of the third report of the National Cholesterol Education Program (NCEP) Expert Panel on Detection, Evaluation, And Treatment of High Blood Cholesterol In Adults (Adult Treatment Panel III). JAMA. 2001;285(19):2486–97.
10. National Cholesterol Education Program (NCEP) Expert Panel on Detection Evaluation, and Treatment of High Blood Cholesterol in Adults (Adult Treatment Panel III). Third report of the National Cholesterol Education Program (NCEP) Expert Panel on Detection, Evaluation, and Treatment of High Blood Cholesterol in Adults (Adult Treatment Panel III) final report. Circulation. 2002; 106(25):3143–421.
11. Baigent C, Blackwell L, Emberson J, Holland LE, Reith C, Bhala N, et al. Efficacy and safety of more intensive lowering of LDL cholesterol: a meta-analysis of data from 170,000 participants in 26 randomised trials. Lancet. 2010;376(9753):1670–81. PubMed PMID: 21067804.
12. Davidson MH, Armani A, McKenney JM, Jacobson TA. Safety considerations with fibrate therapy. Am J Cardiol. 2007; 99(6A):3C–18.
13. Collins R, Armitage J, Parish S, Sleigh P, Peto R, Group HPSC. MRC/BHF Heart Protection Study of cholesterol-lowering with simvastatin in 5963 people with diabetes: a randomised placebo-controlled trial. Lancet. 2003;361(9374):2005–16.
14. Tonelli M, Isles C, Curhan GC, Tonkin A, Pfeffer MA, Shepherd J, et al. Effect of pravastatin on cardiovascular events in people with chronic kidney disease. Circulation. 2004;110(12):1557–63.
15. Strippoli GF, Navaneethan SD, Johnson DW, Perkovic V, Pellegrini F, Nicolucci A, et al. Effects of statins in patients with chronic kidney disease: meta-analysis and meta-regression of randomised controlled trials. BMJ. 2008;336(7645):645–51.
16. Baigent C, Landray MJ, Reith C, Emberson J, Wheeler DC, Tomson C, et al. The effects of lowering LDL cholesterol with simvastatin plus ezetimibe in patients with chronic kidney disease (Study of Heart and Renal Protection): a randomised placebo-controlled trial. Lancet. 2011;377(9784):2181–92.
17. Tonelli M, Isles C, Craven T, Tonkin A, Pfeffer MA, Shepherd J, et al. Effect of pravastatin on rate of kidney function loss in people with or at risk for coronary disease. Circulation. 2005;112(2):171–8.
18. Holdaas H, Fellström B, Cole E, Nyberg G, Olsson AG, Pedersen TR, et al. Long-term cardiac outcomes in renal transplant recipients receiving fluvastatin: the ALERT extension study. Am J Transplant. 2005;5(12):2929–36.
19. Holdaas H, Fellström B, Jardine AG, Holme I, Nyberg G, Fauchald P, et al. Effect of fluvastatin on cardiac outcomes in renal transplant recipients: a multicentre, randomised, placebo-controlled trial. Lancet. 2003;361(9374):2024–31.
20. Massy ZA, Kasiske BL. Post-transplant hyperlipidemia: mechanisms and management. J Am Soc Nephrol. 1996;7(7):971–7.
21. Wanner C, Quaschning T, Weingärnter K. Impact of dyslipidaemia in renal transplant recipients. Curr Opin Urol. 2000;10(2):77–80.
22. Wissing KM, Abramowicz D, Broeders N, Vereerstraeten P. Hypercholesterolemia is associated with increased kidney graft loss caused by chronic rejection in male patients with previous acute rejection. Transplantation. 2000;70(3):464–72.
23. Carvalho MF, Soares V. Hyperlipidemia as a risk factor of renal allograft function impairment. Clin Transplant. 2001;15(1):48–52.
24. Holdaas H, Jardine AG, Wheeler DC, Brekke IB, Conlon PJ, Fellstrøm B, et al. Effect of fluvastatin on acute renal allograft rejection: a randomized multicenter trial. Kidney Int. 2001; 60(5):1990–7.
25. Sahu K, Sharma R, Gupta A, Gulati S, Agarwal D, Kumar A, et al. Effect of lovastatin, an HMG CoA reductase inhibitor, on acute renal allograft rejection. Clin Transplant. 2001;15(3):173–5.
26. Moore R, Thomas D, Morgan E, Wheeler D, Griffin P, Salaman J, et al. Abnormal lipid and lipoprotein profiles following renal transplantation. Transplant Proc. 1993;25(1 Pt 2):1060–1.
27. Aakhus S, Dahl K, Widerøe TE. Hyperlipidaemia in renal transplant patients. J Intern Med. 1996;239(5):407–15.
28. Brown JH, Murphy BG, Douglas AF, Short CD, Bhatnagar D, Mackness MI, et al. Influence of immunosuppressive therapy on lipoprotein(a) and other lipoproteins following renal transplantation. Nephron. 1997;75(3):277–82.

Hypertension in the Kidney Transplant Recipient

20

Hani M. Wadei and Stephen C. Textor

Introduction

Hypertension is nearly universal in kidney transplant recipients. Failure to optimally control arterial hypertension remains among the most important non-immunologic factors that directly relate to poor patient and allograft survivals [1–3]. Persistence of hypertension in kidney transplant recipients is associated with increased risk of both fatal and nonfatal cardiovascular events which are already greatly increased in the chronic kidney disease population as compared with the general population [4–8]. Importantly, hypertension is a treatable risk factor. Unfortunately current evidence indicates that arterial blood pressure often remains poorly controlled in kidney transplant recipients [9].

This chapter summarizes the current understanding of the epidemiology, pathophysiology, and management of hypertension in kidney transplant recipients. We propose a time-related treatment strategy based on the basic mechanisms of hypertension in the early and late post-transplant periods, complications of antihypertensive medications, and patient-specific cardiovascular risk factors in the post-transplant period.

Epidemiology of Post-Kidney Transplant Hypertension

Nearly all patients undergoing kidney transplantation have preexisting hypertension and substantial target-organ manifestations. In some cases, the severity of hypertension is reduced after transplantation, particularly after receiving a well-functioning allograft. Rarely do blood pressures fall to normal, particularly during immunosuppression based upon a calcineurin inhibitor (CNI). Epidemiological studies indicate that 50–90 % of kidney transplant recipients have either hypertension (defined as blood pressure higher than 140/90 mmHg) or are taking antihypertensive medications [10, 11]. The prevalence of hypertension following kidney transplantation varies according to multiple factors that include allograft function and time from transplantation. Patients at particular risk are those with preexisting hypertension, elevated body mass index, male gender, African American race, recipients of kidneys from older donors, and those who experience delayed or poor allograft function. The presence of native kidneys, acute rejection episodes, post-transplant proteinuria, recurrent or de novo allograft glomerulonephritis, and the use of CNI and glucocorticoids all have been associated with worsening blood pressure control post-transplantation [10, 12–16].

Diagnosis of Post-transplant Hypertension

Accurate measurement of BP is essential for the diagnosis and management of post-transplant hypertension. Blood pressure levels vary widely depending upon time of day, methods of measurement, and study conditions [17]. Ambulatory blood pressure monitoring (ABPM) has many advantages and is considered the gold standard for assessing blood pressure levels in the kidney transplant population for several reasons. ABPM provides an accurate blood pressure measurement which is the average of multiple readings during the day and nighttime readings; therefore, it is more reliable for diagnosing hypertension than a single-office blood pressure assessment. ABPM also provides better assessment of the level of blood pressure control and detect both "white coat" and "masked" forms of hypertension. For example, in a study that included 119 kidney transplant recipients, ABPM-derived systolic and diastolic BP measurements were

H.M. Wadei, M.D. (✉)
Department of Transplantation, Mayo Clinic College of Medicine, 4500 San Pablo Road, Jacksonville, FL 32224, USA
e-mail: wadei.hani@mayo.edu

S.C. Textor, M.D.
Division of Nephrology and Hypertension, Department of Medicine, Mayo Clinic College of Medicine, 200 First Street SW, Rochester, MN 55905, USA
e-mail: textor.stephen@mayo.edu

M.R. Weir and E.V. Lerma (eds.), *Kidney Transplantation: Practical Guide to Management*, DOI 10.1007/978-1-4939-0342-9_20, © Springer Science+Business Media New York 2014

lower compared to the corresponding office values [18]. Twenty-nine percent had well-controlled hypertension using ABPM criteria compared to 41 % who had office systolic BP (SBP) levels above 140 mmHg indicating that some patients have white coat hypertension [18]. In the kidney transplant population, white coat hypertension is common and studies have demonstrated that the effect of physician presence on arterial blood pressure is more pronounced in the transplant compared to the general population even in recipients suffering from allograft dysfunction and/or proteinuria [19, 20]. Identifying white coat hypertension avoids the cost and adverse effects of unnecessary antihypertensive medications. Masked hypertension is defined as a condition for which office BP measurements indicate adequately controlled BP but BP outside the clinic is elevated. Unlike most forms of essential hypertension, morning office readings in masked hypertension are commonly lower than those obtained during the rest of the day. Using ABPM, masked hypertension has been identified in 15 % of 241 adult kidney transplant recipients [21]. In the pediatric population, masked hypertension is even more common, affecting 30–45 % of studied populations [22, 23]. Although the effects of masked hypertension on allograft function and survival have not been studied in detail, a detrimental effect on the allograft can be inferred from studies of the general and CKD populations that linked masked hypertension with accelerated kidney function loss and increased cardiovascular deaths [24–27].

Evaluation of the diurnal BP variation requires ABPM monitoring. Blood pressure normally follows a diurnal rhythm with higher awake and lower nocturnal periods. On average, mean SBP falls by 10 % or more during the overnight period ("dippers"), even if sleeping is not consistently achieved. Non-dippers fail to achieve a circadian fall in blood pressure, while "reverse dippers" have an actual nocturnal rise in SBP. Figure 20.1 represents different patterns of day–night BP changes. Abnormal day–night BP patterns are associated with more severe target organ damage, including a higher rate of strokes, dementia, left ventricular hypertrophy, and microalbuminuria [27–29]. Even with normal average blood pressure levels, non-dippers with type 1 diabetes are more likely to develop diabetic nephropathy during subsequent years [30]. A non-dipping BP pattern accelerates loss of glomerular filtration rate (GFR) in subjects with and without chronic kidney disease [31, 32]. Disturbance in circadian blood pressure rhythm is common following kidney transplantation [18, 21, 33, 34]. Loss of the nocturnal SBP fall is associated with higher left ventricular mass index, increased cardiovascular events, lower allograft function, and increased risk graft failure following kidney transplantation [18, 34, 35]. In one study, 1-year GFR was higher by 4.5 mL/min/1.73 m^2 for each 10 % drop in nocturnal SBP [18]. In recipients without rejection episodes, non-dippers and reverse dippers at 1 year had lower GFR and more accelerated kidney function loss 3–4 years after transplantation compared to dippers [36] (Fig. 20.2). Other studies have also demonstrated that ABPM values correlate with other manifestations of allograft dysfunction such as proteinuria while office blood pressure had weak or no correlation [33].

When ABPM is not readily available, self-measured blood pressure is a reasonable alternative as home blood pressure readings better correlate with ABPM-derived values than blood pressure obtained in office settings [37]. Therefore, self-measured blood pressure should be encouraged in kidney transplant recipients.

Post-transplant Hypertension: Target Blood Pressure Control

No dedicated studies are available to define the optimal target blood pressure goal in the kidney transplant population, and therefore there is no universal agreement as to the BP goals of these patients. Published recommendations have been inferred from clinical trials in non-transplant populations. The KDIGO Clinical Practice Guidelines for the management of blood pressure in the patients with chronic kidney disease and following kidney transplantation have recently been updated and published [38, 39]. According to these guidelines the target goal in kidney transplant recipients is a blood pressure <130/80 mmHg with lower targets in proteinuric patients [40]. European best practice guidelines specify a target BP <125/75 mmHg in patients with proteinuria [41]. These guidelines emphasize that target BPs in kidney transplant recipients should be similar to the ones provided by the Seventh Report of the Joint National Committee on Prevention, Detection, Evaluation, and Treatment of High Blood Pressure (JNC7) [42]. Importantly, the KDIGO guidelines acknowledge that different targets should be set according to the method of blood pressure readings (office vs. home readings vs. ABPM) (Table 20.1).

BP control remains suboptimal in the kidney transplant population. Results from a multinational study that included 4,107 kidney transplant recipients with stable graft function after a mean of 5 years from kidney transplantation demonstrate that the target goal of BP <130/80 mmHg was not met in 69 % of participants and uncontrolled hypertension defined as BP >140/90 mmHg was present in 44 % of those taking antihypertension medication [9]. Data from the Collaborative Transplant Study that included 29,751 patients indicate that 55 % of kidney transplant patients have SBP higher than 140 mmHg and only 9.8 % have SBP less than 120 mmHg 1 year after transplantation [3]. In another study that used ABPM-derived overall average BP of <130/80 mmHg (which is similar to the target BP advocated by the KDIGO recommendations) to define adequate

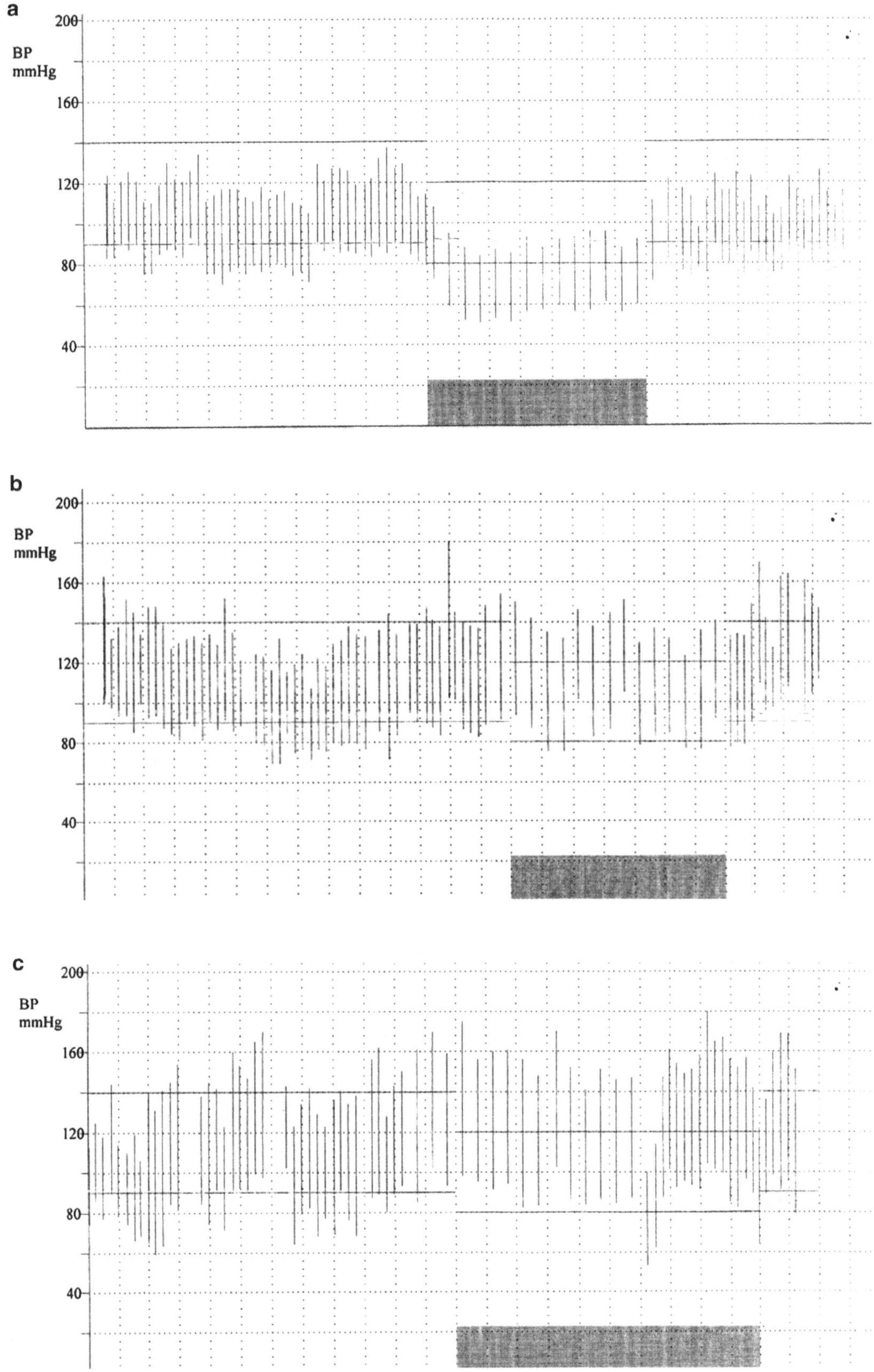

Fig. 20.1 Normal and abnormal 24-h blood pressure monitor tracings (sleep time is designated by the bar at the bottom of each figure). (**a**) Represents a normal 24-h day–night blood pressure change in a healthy person being considered for kidney donation. In this case nocturnal SBP dropped by 22 % compared to the corresponding diurnal value consistent with a dipping pattern. In (**b**), nocturnal BP fails to drop but remains unchanged compared to diurnal value (non-dipper) and in (**c**), nocturnal BP is 7 % higher than daytime SBP (reverse dipper)

Fig. 20.2 Box plots of iothalamate GFR in 36 kidney transplant recipients without rejection at 3 weeks, 1 and 4 years and at last follow-up grouped according to the day–night dipping pattern. Despite similar GFR at 3 weeks and 1 year, non-dipper and reverse dippers had lower GFR at 4 years and at last follow-up compared to dippers ($P=0.04$ and $P=0.05$, respectively). Reprinted with permission [36]

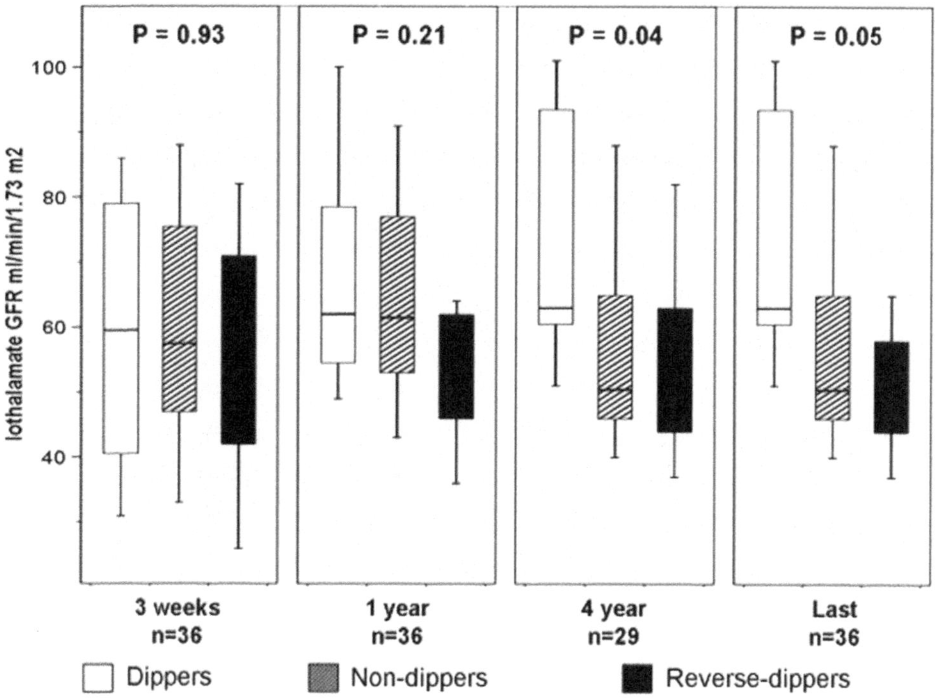

Table 20.1 Adult blood pressure thresholds for defining hypertension

Method of measurement	Threshold (mmHg)
Office or clinic	140/90
Overall ABPM average	125[a]–130/80
ABPM daytime	130[a]–135/85
ABPM nighttime	120/70
Home	130–135/85

Reproduced with permissions from KDIGO Clinical Practice Guidelines for the care of kidney transplant recipients [38]
ABPM ambulatory blood pressure monitoring
[a]According to the European best practice guidelines

BP control found that only 5 % of the studied population had well-controlled hypertension despite the fact that 33 % of this cohort used three or more antihypertensive medications [33]. Some reports indicate that kidney transplant recipients are using more antihypertensive medications and have better BP control in recent years compared to historical controls [10].

Patients' adherence, medication tolerability, medication effect on electrolyte and serum creatinine, and interactions with immunosuppression drugs are potential reasons for the limited use of BP medications that partly explain the suboptimal rate of BP control in the kidney transplant population. Another important factor to consider is the medication cost and the lack of insurance coverage. In one study that surveyed 254 US-based kidney transplant programs, 70 % of the responders reported that their patients have difficulties paying for their immunosuppression medications, reflecting the financial hardships that contribute to the inadequate blood pressure control in kidney transplant recipients [43].

Table 20.2 Mechanisms that contribute to the generation and maintenance of hypertension following kidney transplantation

Pre-transplant factors
Increased vascular stiffness
Vascular calcification
Post-transplant factors
Volume overload
Delayed allograft function
Immunosuppression medications
Calcineurin inhibitors (CNIs)
Corticosteroids
Transplant renal artery stenosis
Poor allograft function
Presence of native kidneys

Pathogenesis of Post-transplant Hypertension

Both recipient- and donor-related factors contribute to the generation and maintenance of post-transplant hypertension. Some recipient-related factors originate before the transplant while others are related to post-transplant immunosuppressive medications, delayed graft function (DGF), and other complications. Some factors that potentiate arterial hypertension differ in the early and late post-transplant periods. These include the effects of volume changes, calcineurin (CNI) inhibitors use and trough level, high-dose steroids, poor or delayed allograft function, development of proteinuria, and transplant renal artery stenosis (TRAS) [14]. Some of the major mechanisms contributing to hypertension following kidney transplantation are summarized in Table 20.2.

ESRD patients have functional and structural alterations in the arterial walls with increased stiffness of large conduit arteries and with evidence of vascular calcification. These changes are present even in the pediatric ESRD population who has been subjected to a short course of dialysis [44, 45]. These pathologic changes persist after transplantation and contribute to post-transplant hypertension following both living and deceased donor kidney transplantation [46, 47]. For example, Bahous and colleagues showed that aortic pulse wave velocity, a correlate of aortic stiffness, is higher in 101 living donor kidney transplant recipients compared to healthy controls and is related to elevated post-transplant mean arterial blood pressure [46]. Similarly, Delahousse demonstrated that aortic stiffness directly correlates with arterial blood pressure at 3 and 12 months from transplantation in 74 cadaveric kidney transplant recipients [47]. Interestingly, aortic stiffness is affected by donor age with kidney transplant patients who receive a kidney from younger donors demonstrating lower aortic stiffness compared to pre-transplant values. The opposite occurs in those who receive a kidney from older donors [47]. This may partially explain why kidneys from older donors are associated with higher risk of post-transplant hypertension [15]. Post-transplant factors also affect arterial stiffness. For example, new-onset diabetes and elevated fasting blood sugar level are related to increased arterial stiffness in kidney transplant recipients [48, 49]. Immunosuppression regimens alter arterial elasticity, and studies indicate that aortic stiffness is lower in kidney transplant recipients maintained on sirolimus compared to those using cyclosporine [50]. Switching from CNI to everolimus is associated with stabilization of arterial stiffness in 17 stable kidney transplant recipients while pulse wave velocity continued to deteriorate in the 10 patients that continued CNI use [51].

Under normal conditions, the kidney itself regulates arterial blood pressure [52]. Multiple mechanisms are involved but reduced GFR is a major factor. Therefore it is not surprising that DGF is an important risk factor for post-transplant hypertension. With DGF, the kidney's ability to excrete sodium is reduced with subsequent lag in daily sodium excretion, salt and water retention, rightward shift of the pressure natriuresis curve, and rise in blood pressure. Management of hypertension associated with DGF ideally would include aggressive fluid removal which in many cases requires dialysis. However, due to concerns regarding hypoperfusion and further aggravation of the existing ischemic injury to the allograft, dialysis is often delayed and if implemented fluid removal is usually limited. As a result kidney transplant recipients experiencing DGF remain in a state of volume overload even in the absence of peripheral edema and their arterial blood pressure is often difficult to control. In many cases, improvement in arterial blood pressure occurs once kidney function starts to recover.

The effects of CNI on arterial blood pressure elevation develop after renal, liver, heart, and bone marrow transplantation as well as in patients using CNI for non-transplant indications [53–56]. The mechanisms involved in CNI-induced hypertension are multifactorial and have recently been reviewed [57]. The primary hemodynamic change attributed to CNI is an increase in systemic vascular resistance due to widespread arterial vasoconstriction [58]. The mechanisms of CNI-induced vasoconstriction are complex. CNI activates the renin–angiotensin–aldosterone system through a direct effect on the juxtaglomerular cells and indirectly through renal vasoconstriction [59–61]. Both human and animal studies document increased intra-renal renin activity with cyclosporine exposure despite low circulating renin and aldosterone levels [62, 63]. Cyclosporine also augments the vasoconstrictive effect of angiotensin II [60]. CNI fosters an imbalance favoring vasoconstrictive factors, such as endothelin-1 and thromboxane A2, over vasodilator compounds, such as prostacyclin and nitric oxide [58]. The fact that experimental administration of endothelin receptor antagonists improves cyclosporine-induced hypertension and renal blood flow in animal models suggests that endothelin plays a role in CNI-induced hypertension [64, 65]. Unfortunately, an important drug interaction develops with concurrent use of cyclosporine and the endothelin receptor blockers bosentan and ambrisentan that interferes delays with hepatic metabolism of both and increases blood levels. Therefore concomitant use of CNI and endothelin receptor blockers is currently contraindicated. CNIs also cause afferent arteriolar vasoconstriction leading to reduction in the GFR and increased tubular reabsorption of sodium even after short-term exposure to the medication [66–69]. Early studies indicated that dietary sodium restriction blunts the BP changes during cyclosporine administration, leading to the designation as "salt-sensitive" hypertension [70]. Recently, mounting evidence indicates that CNI directly activates the renal sodium chloride co-transporter (NCC) inducing hypertension in a mechanism analogous to pseudo-hypoaldosteronism type II (also known as Gordon syndrome) [71, 72]. The mechanism by which CNI activates NCC is still elusive, but in normal mouse distal convoluted tubules, both calcineurin and NCC co-localize, suggesting that calcineurin has a role in regulating the NCC activity [73] (Fig. 20.3). Importantly, CNI-induced activation of the NCC is reversed by hydrochlorothiazide supporting the use of thiazide diuretics in the treatment of CNI-induced hypertension [71]. Known mechanisms involved in CNI-induced hypertension are summarized in Table 20.3.

Although both cyclosporine and tacrolimus cause systemic arterial vasoconstriction, tacrolimus has less severe and more delayed effect on increasing systemic vascular resistance and arterial blood pressure when compared to cyclosporine [55]. Allograft microperfusion visualized by

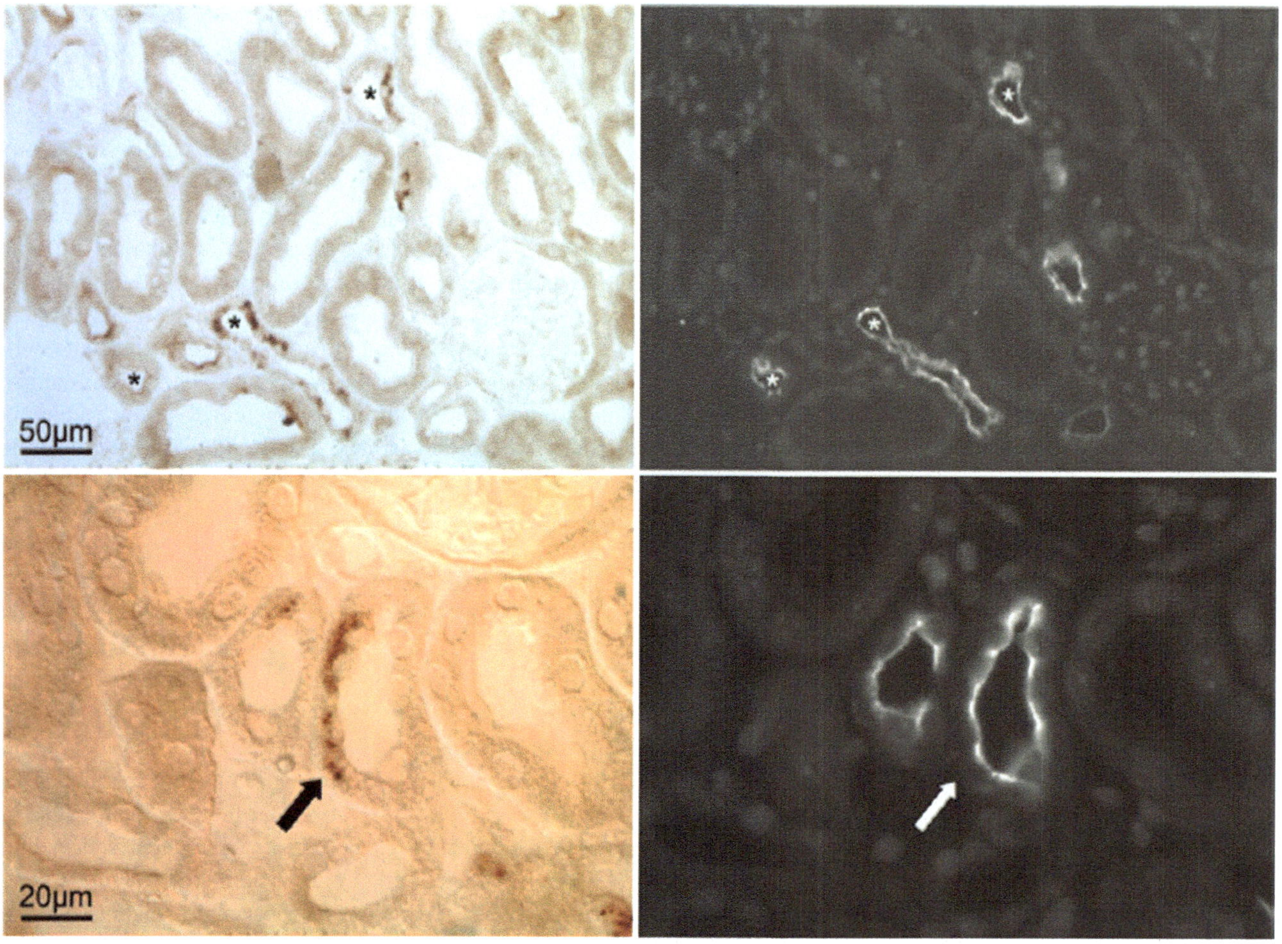

Fig. 20.3 Localization of calcineurin in the mouse kidney. *Upper panel* represents overview images (50 µm) of the distal convoluted tubules. The *(asterisk)* in the left image represents the immunohistochemical detection of calcineurin. *Right image* demonstrates NCC delineating distal convoluted tubules in the same field as calcineurin *(asterisk)*. *Lower panel* is a detailed view (20 µm). The *arrows* point to a site of a partial overexpression of both calcineurin and NCC in a distal convoluted tubule. These observations support a role for facilitated tubular sodium transport as a mechanism by which CNIs such as cyclosporine accelerate hypertension. Reprinted with permission [73]

Table 20.3 Different mechanisms of calcineurin inhibitor (CNI) induced rise in blood pressure

Systemic vasoconstriction
• Imbalance between vasoconstrictive and vasodilators
Increase in vasoconstrictive substance: endothelin-1 and thromboxane A2
Decrease in vasodilator compounds: prostacyclin and nitric oxide
• Increase intra-renal renin activity
• Accentuation of angiotensin II action
• Increase in sympathetic nervous activity[a]
Effect on the renal allograft
• GFR reduction
• Increase tubular sodium reabsorption and activation of NCC

[a]Of questionable significance

contrast-enhanced sonography revealed significant vasoconstriction following cyclosporine intake, an effect that was not observed with tacrolimus and was abrogated following calcium channel medication use [74]. Aortic stiffness by pulse wave velocity is higher in cyclosporine-treated kidney transplant recipients compared to those maintained on tacrolimus [75]. Conversion from cyclosporine to tacrolimus in kidney transplant recipients is associated with modest but measurable reduction in both systolic and diastolic blood pressures which revert to their original values after cyclosporine re-exposure [76, 77]. When used as a primary immunosuppressive agent, results from multicenter studies both from the USA and Europe document a lower incidence of new-onset hypertension and less antihypertensive drug use at 5 years with tacrolimus compared to cyclosporine [78, 79]. These data suggest that tacrolimus has less pronounced effects on blood pressure as compared to cyclosporine.

Both cumulative and daily doses of steroids including bolus steroid treatment for episodes of rejection have been implicated in the rise of blood pressure, especially in the early post-transplant period [80]. Although the mechanism of glucocorticoid-induced hypertension is commonly attributed to the activation of the mineralocorticoid receptor promoting sodium and water retention, recent evidence suggests that glucocorticoid receptor-mediated activation of the vascular smooth muscles plays a role in glucocorticoid-induced hypertension [81].

The reported incidence of TRAS varies widely (from 1 to 25 %) partially due to the reliance on elevated peak systolic velocity at the anastomosis on Doppler ultrasound to diagnose TRAS [82–86]. In one study, the incidence of TRAS increased from 2.4 to 12.4 % after the introduction of Doppler ultrasound [87]. But elevated systolic velocities are not uniformly associated with hemodynamically significant TRAS. For example, only 26 out of 98 (26 %) kidney transplant recipients with elevated systolic velocity on ultrasound had angiographic evidence of TRAS [84]. When severe, TRAS-mediated hypertension can be refractory to medical treatment, can be associated with otherwise unexplained worsening allograft function, and the presence of diuretic-resistant peripheral edema may progress in some cases into pulmonary congestion and/or edema. Despite the activation of the renin–angiotensin–aldosterone system, there is little role for measuring plasma renin activity or aldosterone level since renin can be released from the native kidneys [88]. Even if TRAS is confirmed with angiography and managed with angioplasty with or without stenting, improvement in blood pressure control is not consistently achieved suggesting that TRAS may not be the reason for worsening hypertension. In one study, blood pressure control occurred in 53 % and 75 % of patients 1 and 3 months after angioplasty, respectively [89]. A study by Henning and colleagues showed that despite 93 % technical success rate for angioplasty, the mean dose of antihypertensive medications did not change [90]. Benefit of angioplasty needs also to be weighed against possible complications including immediate renal artery occlusion, dissection, and restenosis which can occur in up to 50 % of cases [83, 84, 91]. Taken together, these data suggest that most TRAS identified on Doppler ultrasound is rarely responsible for the elevated blood pressure in kidney transplant recipients. In some cases, worsening allograft function is the cause of poor blood pressure control and the trigger for Doppler ultrasound examination. Intervention to treat TRAS should be made on a case-by-case basis and should be offered to those with uncontrolled hypertension refractory to medications and those with signs of volume overload [92].

The role of the native kidneys in the overall prevalence of hypertension post-kidney transplantation is unknown. Native kidneys can induce hypertension via a renin-mediated mechanism or through increased sympathetic nerve activity (SNA) [88, 93, 94]. Hausberg and colleagues demonstrated that SNA level remains elevated after successful kidney transplantation and bilateral nephrectomy resulted in reduction in SNA in kidney transplant recipients to a level similar to that of healthy controls [93]. In a study by Huysmans et al., the prevalence of hypertension was lower in 92 recipients with absent native kidneys compared to 237 patients who intact native kidneys (57.8 % vs. 23.9 %, respectively, $P<0.001$) [95]. Bilateral native nephrectomy leads to better blood pressure control in the majority, but not all patients, with resistant hypertension irrespective of whether the nephrectomy is performed before or after kidney transplantation [96–99]. However, native kidney removal has been used less frequently in recent decades, likely due to improved antihypertensive drug therapy and the morbidity associated with surgical nephrectomy. Laparoscopic native nephrectomy has lower rates of surgical complications and is an alternative in selected group of patients who are unresponsive to medical therapy alone [100]. Catheter-based renal denervation has been shown to be effective in controlling hypertension in the general population [101]. Whether catheter-based renal denervation of the native kidneys in transplant recipients will have an effect on arterial blood pressure comparable to the effect of bilateral nephrectomy warrants further study.

Effect of Hypertension on Transplant Outcomes and Cardiovascular Events

Both systolic and diastolic hypertension after kidney transplantation predict reduced patient and allograft survival. Each 10 mmHg increment of SBP above 140 mmHg is associated with an increased relative risk for graft failure (RR: 1.12, CI 1.08–1.15; $P<0.0001$), death-censored graft failure (RR 1.17, CI 1.12–1.22; $P<0.0001$), and patient death (RR 1.18, CI 1.12–1.23; $P<0.0001$) [10]. These risks persist after adjusting for allograft function and rejection episodes [10]. Importantly, uncontrolled hypertension precedes graft failure by several years and the negative impact of post-transplant hypertension on transplant outcomes is evident even in recipients with functioning grafts 5 years from transplantation [10]. Results from a registry study that included 29,751 patients followed for up to 7 years demonstrate that uncontrolled hypertension at 1, 3, and 5 years from transplantation is associated with graded increase in subsequent allograft failure and death-censored graft failure irrespective of rejection episodes and antihypertensive medication use ($P<0.0001$ for all time points) [3]. Single-center studies that included both deceased and living donor kidney transplant recipients confirm the independent, negative impact of uncontrolled hypertension on long-term transplant outcomes [1, 2].

Poor allograft function and uncontrolled hypertension are closely linked, and establishing a cause and an effect relationship of hypertension on poor allograft outcome is difficult in many of the abovementioned studies. However, achieving lower SBP is associated with improved graft and patient survival 7 years after transplantation. In a study that included 24,404 primary deceased donor kidney transplant recipients, patients with uncontrolled hypertension at 1 year who were able to achieve adequate BP control at 3 years had lower risk of subsequent allograft failure than those with sustained hypertension at 3 years (RR 0.79; CI 0.73–0.86; $P<0.001$) [102]. Likewise, better BP control after year 3 was associated with improved 10-year graft survival (RR 0.83; CI 0.72–0.96; $P=0.01$), whereas even a temporary increase in SBP at 3 years was associated with worse graft survival (RR 1.37; CI 1.19–1.58; $P<0.001$) [102].

Uncontrolled hypertension is a potent risk factor for de novo congestive heart failure (CHF) and ischemic heart disease (IHD) in transplant recipients. In a study that included 638 kidney transplant recipients followed for up to 7 years, each 10 mmHg increase in SBP above 128 mmHg was associated with adjusted RR of 1.29 for new IHD (CI 1.1–1.5; $P=001$) and RR of 1.25 for de novo CHF (CI 1.08–1.44; $P<0.001$) [5]. Results from an observational study predict a 2 % increase risk of fatal or nonfatal cardiovascular events for every 1 mmHg increase in SBP [4].

Management of Post-transplant Hypertension: Non-pharmacological Management of Post-transplant Hypertension

Lifestyle modifications including Dietary Approaches to Stop Hypertension (DASH) diet, exercise, moderate alcohol use, weight regulation, and smoking cessation are recommended as a first step in the management of hypertension in the general population [42]. No study yet has tested the efficacy of lifestyle modifications specifically on controlling post-transplant hypertension. Nonetheless, efforts to avoid weight gain, discontinue tobacco use, and increase exercise warrant emphasis for all kidney transplant recipients. Obstructive sleep apnea (OSA) is an underdiagnosed contributor to hypertension in the kidney transplant population. Kidney transplant recipients with OSA have higher levels of SBP despite taking more antihypertensive medications compared to those without OSA (147 ± 21 vs. 139 ± 18 mmHg, $P=0.05$) [103]. Treatment of OSA has been associated with better BP control in the general population but has not been widely studied in kidney transplant recipients [104]. Considering the ubiquitous preexistent risk factors and risks of post-transplant hypertension, lifestyle changes including vigilance in diagnosing and treating OSA ought to be started simultaneously with pharmacological management.

Immunosuppressive Medications Dose Modification

Selection and dosage of immunosuppression after kidney transplantation are rarely determined primarily by BP effects but altering the immunosuppressive regimen can improve arterial blood pressure control. For many reasons, steroid-free protocols are gaining popularity and 23 % of first renal transplants were discharged after transplantation without steroids in 2004 as opposed to 5 % in 2000 [105]. This percentage further increased to 26 % in 2007 (source: www.ustransplant.org). Steroid reduction or withdrawal protocols can be associated with improvement in post-transplant blood pressure control. The results of a meta-analysis that included 34 studies and 5,637 kidney transplant recipients demonstrate that steroid avoidance and steroid withdrawal protocols are associated with somewhat lower risks for hypertension (RR:0.9, CI: 0.85–0.94, $P<0.0001$) compared to patients receiving long-term steroids [106]. This salutary effect of steroid withdrawal on blood pressure control is evident irrespective of race, age, and interval from transplantation to steroid withdrawal with the largest effect on BP observed in those taking the lowest doses of cyclosporin [107–112]. For example, Hocker and colleagues reported lower prevalence of hypertension (50 % vs. 87 %, $P<0.05$) in 23 pediatric kidney transplant recipients following steroid discontinuation 1 year from transplantation compared to 19 well-matched controls [112]. Another study randomized 130 pediatric kidney transplant recipients to complete steroid avoidance versus standard steroid use demonstrated lower SBP over the 3-year follow-up period in the steroid avoidance group ($P=0.017$) [113]. Other studies, however, identify little beneficial effect of steroid withdrawal on post-transplant blood pressure control [114–117] especially with regimens based upon tacrolimus and mycophenolate. Results from a prospective, randomized, double-blind, placebo-controlled study by Woodle et al. that included 386 renal transplant recipients randomized to early corticosteroid elimination versus chronic corticosteroid maintenance (5 mg/day at 6 months) indicate that both systolic and diastolic BP are similar in patient with or without maintenance steroids [114]. The discrepancy in the effect of steroid withdrawal on post-transplant hypertension may be explained by the difference in study designs, lack of adjustment for antihypertensive medication use, variability in kidney function, and the different doses of maintenance steroid used in each study. For example, Savarman and colleagues report a retrospective study of 58 patients followed for 7 years that when prednisone dosage is tapered from 10 mg daily to 10 mg every other day, clinically significant improvements are seen in systolic and diastolic blood pressure and the number of blood pressure medications used but no further benefit is obtained with complete steroid withdrawal [115]. Overall, it appears that a low dose of daily steroids (5 mg/day) has little impact on long-term blood pressure control.

Johnson et al. report the effect of cyclosporine discontinuation on post-transplant hypertension in a multicenter study that included 525 kidney transplant patients on sirolimus and steroids randomized to either continue or withdraw CNI 3 months after transplantation. Blood pressures did not differ between groups at randomization. At 12 months, both systolic (139.8 vs. 133.5 mmHg, $P=0.004$) and diastolic (81.3 vs. 78.6 mmHg, $P=0.027$) blood pressures were lower in the cyclosporine withdrawal arm despite lower doses of antihypertensive medication ($P=0.013$) [118]. Similar effects on BP reduction were evident when CNIs were withdrawn from a mycophenolate mofetil- and steroid-based regimen in patients with stable and dysfunctional allografts [119, 120]. Even 50 % cyclosporine dose reduction led to improvement in BP control and reduction in the number of blood pressure medications in stable kidney transplant recipients [121]. Newer classes of non-CNI immunosuppressive medications such as belatacept are associated with lower number and dose of antihypertensive medications when compared to cyclosporine-based regimens [122]. These studies indicate that CNI withdrawal and minimization protocols are associated with meaningful improvement in blood pressure control. These benefits must be weighed carefully, however, against the increased risk of rejection episodes [123].

Pharmacological Antihypertensive Therapy

Current guidelines do not recommend a particular class of antihypertensive medication to control post-transplant hypertension. Calcium channel blockers (CCBs), diuretics, beta-blockers (BBs), α1-blockers, angiotensin-converting enzyme inhibitors (ACE-I), and angiotensin receptor blockers (ARBs) have all been used to reduce blood pressure after renal transplantation effectively [124, 125]. Recent studies indicate that the utilization of all classes of antihypertensive medications has increased by 2–7-fold over the last decade, reflecting increased commitment by the transplant community to treat hypertension (Fig. 20.4) [126]. Choice of the appropriate antihypertensive medication should therefore be guided by patients' comorbidities, volume status, CNI use, level of kidney function, and the presence of proteinuria. The majority of kidney transplant patients will require 2 or more antihypertensive medications to achieve adequate BP control, and therefore it will be more practical to start with a single antihypertensive medication irrespective of its class and additional medications can be added according to response of therapy and side effects from the initial medication [18, 124]. Clinicians caring for transplant recipients must be particularly aware of potential interactions between antihypertensive agents and immunosuppressives as well as other drugs used in this setting. Table 20.4 summarizes common antihypertensive

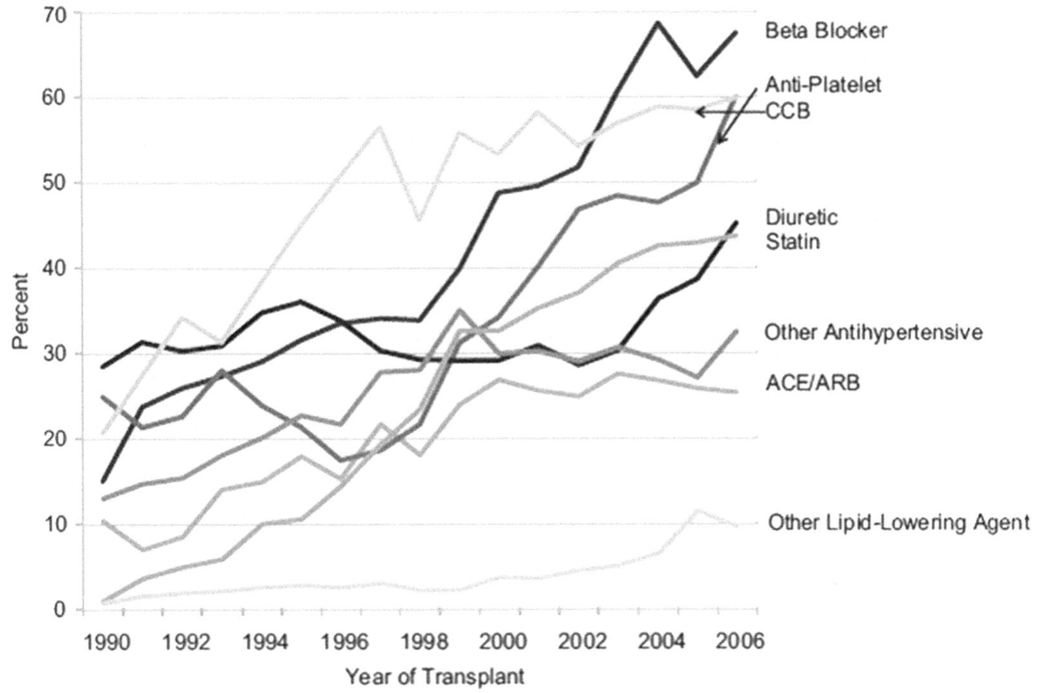

Fig. 20.4 Trend in the utilization of antihypertensive and other cardiovascular medications in the first 4 months from transplantation spanning the period from 1990 to 2006. Utilization of different antihypertensive medications has increased by 2–7-folds over this period. Reprinted with permission [126]

Table 20.4 Antihypertensive medications commonly used in kidney transplant recipients, their potential side effects and their interaction with CNIs

Class of drug	Features	Adverse effects	Effect of renal function on drug excretion	Interaction with CNI and sirolimus
Calcium channel blockers (CCBs)				
Dihydropyridines	Potent vasodilators, antagonizes CNI-mediated vasoconstriction	Edema, headache, gingival hyperplasia, tachycardia		
Nifedipine XL	Rapid onset of action		–	–
Amlodipine	Steady state reached 7–8 days from drug initiation. Long 1/2 life (35 h)		–	+
Non-dihydropyridines				
Diltiazem	Moderate potency	Bradycardia, edema	–	++
Verapamil	Least potent	Constipation, bradycardia	–	++
β-blockers (BBs)				
Atenolol, metoprolol	Less potent antihypertensives, may diminish CNI-related headache	Bradycardia, bronchospasm, potential for rebound tachycardia	–	–
α–β Blockers				
Labetalol	Effective antihypertensives, rapid onset and short duration of action. Multiple daily dosing is required	Bradycardia, postural hypotension	+	–
Central agents				
Clonidine	Rapid onset, effective, short duration of action	Dry mouth, bradycardia, dizziness, rebound hypertension	–	–
Enalapril, lisinopril, ramipril Angiotensin receptor blockers (ARBs) Valsartan, losartan	Limited efficacy and short duration with enalapril. No clear benefit from starting early after transplantation. Especially useful in proteinuric patients	Hyperkalemia, non-anion gap metabolic acidosis, azotemia	++	–
Diuretics				
Thiazides Loop Spironolactone	Potentiate other antihypertensive medications. Effective in volume-dependent hypertension. Spironolactone might have renal protective effects	Prerenal azotemia, electrolyte abnormalities	+	–

– negligible effect, + mild effect, ++ moderate to severe effect

medications used in the management of post-transplant hypertension with reference to potential beneficial and adverse effects.

Calcium Channel Blockers

Dihydropyridine CCBs are the most frequently prescribed antihypertensive class in kidney transplant recipients [124, 126]. As a class, CCBs effectively reduce systemic vascular resistance by acting on the vascular smooth muscle and often control post-transplant hypertension even when prescribed as monotherapy [53]. CCBs are also effective in controlling BP in nonrenal solid organ transplant patients. In a study of 37 hypertensive liver transplant recipients maintained on cyclosporine, 64 % reached goal blood pressure with long-acting nifedipine monotherapy [53]. Importantly, the fall in BP paralleled the fall in the systemic vascular resistance [53].

CCBs in general are well tolerated but commonly magnify CNI-induced gingival hyperplasia and cause lower extremity edema. Drug interactions between CNI and both non-dihydropyridine CCBs (verapamil, diltiazem) and dihydropyridine CCBs (nifedipine, amlodipine, isradipine) are well recognized and require careful monitoring of CNI levels. Non-dihydropyridine CCBs are potent inhibitors of the cytochrome P450 3A4 isoenzyme and co-administration with CNI will increase CNI trough levels [127]. Dihydropyridine CCBs produce modestly an increase in CNI levels and are considered safer than non-dihydropyridine CCBs from a drug interaction prospective [128].

CCBs counteract the systemic and afferent arteriolar vasoconstriction induced by CNI, increase renal blood flow, and increase GFR through an increase in the glomerular hydrostatic pressure and filtration fraction [129–131]. Because of these favorable hemodynamics effects, CCBs have been associated with lower risk of DGF and hyperuricemia which are commonly observed with CNI [132–135].

The effect of CCBs on kidney function and allograft survival has been extensively studied. Midtvedt et al. conducted a randomized, double-blind controlled study with 154 patients randomized to receive either lisinopril or controlled-release nifedipine. BP control was similar in both groups but patients treated with nifedipine had better allograft function that persisted during the 2-year follow-up period [136]. Similarly, results from a retrospective study that included more than 1,600 patients followed for 4 years indicate that CCB use is associated with the lowest risk of graft loss when compared to all other antihypertensive medications [124]. When patients were randomized to receive either the long-acting CCB lacidipine or placebo, lacidipine-treated patients had lower serum creatinine and higher iohexol GFR 1 and 2 years from transplantation despite having similar BP and acute rejection rate compared to the placebo arm [137]. Other randomized studies with isradipine or felodipine showed similar salutary effect of CCBs on kidney function 3–12 months after drug initiation [131, 138]. In a meta-analysis of randomized trials that included 29 studies with more than 2,200 patients randomized to either CCBs or placebo or no treatment, Cross and colleagues demonstrated that CCBs are associated with reduced graft loss (RR: 0.75, CI 0.57–0.99; $P=0.04$) and higher GFR (mean GFR difference 4.5 mL/min, CI 2.2–6.7 mL/min, $P<0.0001$) [139]. Taken together, results of these randomized studies suggest that CCBs may have a salutary effect on post-transplant kidney function and allograft survival as compared to placebo.

Studies demonstrating an increased GFR in cyclosporine-treated patients with CCB use generally reflect vasodilation from dihydropyridine CCB that increased intra-glomerular pressure. The increased pressure is known to increase proteinuria [130]. Whether such afferent vasodilation is beneficial for proteinuric patients over the long term is questionable. Indeed dihydropyridine CCBs accelerate proteinuria and the progression of renal disease in diabetic and nondiabetic proteinuric nephropathies [140]. Therefore caution should be used when dihydropyridine CCBs are prescribed for proteinuric patients and monitoring of urinary protein excretion is recommended in these patients.

In contrast to clear benefits in controlling post-transplant hypertension, observational single-center analyses demonstrate increased risk for ischemic cardiac events occurring beyond the first post-transplant year in kidney recipients maintained on dihydropyridine CCBs (RR, 2.26; CI, 1.24–4.12; $P=0.008$), an association that persisted despite adjusting for other antihypertensive agents and known cardiac risk factors [6]. Prospective trials in other high-risk populations have not confirmed this association, although extrapolation to kidney transplant patients must be done cautiously.

Overall due to their unique properties, proven benefit, and salutary effect on graft function and survival, CCBs are considered by many including transplant work groups as the first-line antihypertensive to be used in kidney transplant recipients [141]. Caution, however, should be implemented for proteinuric patients receiving CCBs.

β-Blockers

BBs are routinely used in kidney transplant recipients with 70 % of patients transplanted in 2006 taking BBs as part of their antihypertensive regimen [126]. Many patients with preexisting cardiovascular disease who were taking BBs prior to transplantation continue taking these medications in the post-transplant period. BBs are also commonly started in the peri-transplant period to reduce the risk of perioperative cardiovascular events. BBs use in the early transplant period has more than quadrupled in recent years [9, 126].

BBs are equally effective to ACE-I in reducing blood pressure but have little impact on albuminuria [142, 143]. The antihypertensive efficacy of BBs may however be limited to patients with preserved native kidneys and was low in nephrectomized patients, attributed to low activity of the renin–angiotensin–aldosterone system in this group [144]. As a class, BBs are associated with bradycardia, fatigue, sexual dysfunction, and hyperlipidemia which are already prevalent in the kidney transplant recipients. Third-generation BBs that combine alpha- and beta-blocking properties such as carvedilol or labetalol are more potent antihypertensive agents and have limited or even beneficial effects on the lipid profile [145]. BBs use may increase the risk for development of post-transplant diabetes and new-onset type 2 diabetes in the general population [146, 147].

Renin–Angiotensin–Aldosterone System Blockers: ACE-I and ARB

Renin–angiotensin–aldosterone system (RAAS) blockers are equally effective to other antihypertensive medications in controlling post-transplant hypertension [148]. The specific potential benefits of ACE-I and ARBs in preserving allograft function in kidney transplant recipients have been the subject of multiple publications. This interest stems from the known beneficial effects of RAAS blockers on delaying the progression of kidney disease in the CKD population [149, 150]. Whether the renoprotective effects of RAAS extend to the kidney transplant population is unclear [142, 143, 151, 152]. A meta-analysis that included 14 studies suggested that use of RAAS blockers is associated with decline in GFR, an effect that persisted even after adjusting for confounding factors and including only studies that utilized RAAS blockers for more than 12 months [148]. This drop in GFR likely is explained by the hemodynamic changes that follow RAAS blockade. However the important question is whether RAAS blockers are associated with long-term protective effect on

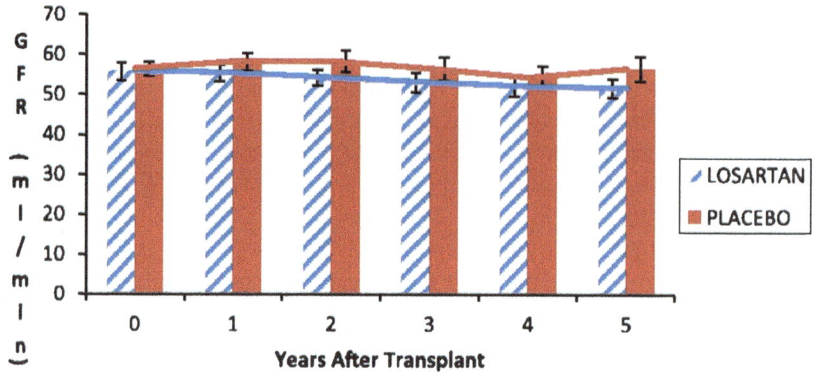

Fig. 20.5 Glomerular filtration rate (GFR) as measured by iothalamate clearance 153 kidney transplant recipients randomized to receive either losartan ($n=77$) or placebo ($n=76$). There was no difference in GFR at any time point between the two groups up to 5 years from transplantation. Reprinted with permission [153]

allograft function and histology. Results of a recently published double-blind randomized placebo-controlled trial that examined the effect of losartan on change in interstitial fibrosis or allograft function over a 5-year period demonstrate that neither the degree of interstitial fibrosis nor GFR was not different at any time point in the ARB compared to the placebo-treated arms (Fig. 20.5) [153]. By contrast, beneficial effects of RAAS blockers regarding limiting proteinuria are well established. Proteinuria declined with RAAS blockers by a mean of −0.47 g/day (95 % CI −0.86 to −0.08, $P=0.02$). The effect of ACE-I and ARB on post-transplant proteinuria has been confirmed in other studies including a recent meta-analysis [124, 139, 142, 154]. Even in recipients without clinically significant proteinuria, ACE-I or ARB use has consistently been associated with lower urinary protein excretion rate compared to patients with similar blood pressure levels who are not taking these medications [155, 156]. Considering the negative impact of proteinuria on post-transplant outcomes, these data suggest that RAAS blockers are particularly beneficial in proteinuric kidney transplant recipients [148, 157, 158].

Whether RAAS blockers have specific benefits regarding patient and graft survivals has also been a matter of debate. In a retrospective study that included more than 2,000 kidney transplant recipients, RAAS blockers at any time point after the transplant were associated with improvement in both 10-year patient and death-censored graft survivals [159]. Other studies that included smaller number of patients but with higher cardiovascular risk profile showed that RAAS blocker used for a median of 14 months was associated with lower mortality but no significant advantage on allograft survival [160]. Data from the collaborative study group that included more than 17,000 patients failed to confirm a beneficial effect of ACE-I or ARB on patient or allograft survivals even when a separate analysis that included patients with increased cardiovascular risk was performed [161]. Importantly, ACE-I or ARB use does not abrogate the negative effect of post-transplant hypertension on allograft survival when graft survival was assessed at different levels of BP readings (Fig. 20.6) [161]. Comparison of RAAS blockers with CCBs in a retrospective study that included 1,662 patients identified no difference in the overall study population, but revealed improved allograft survival with RAAS blockers 4 years after transplantation in recipients with the highest tertiles of both systolic and diastolic blood pressures [124]. In patients with allograft dysfunction, some studies suggest a beneficial effect of RAAS blockers on improving graft in patients with either chronic allograft nephropathy (now identified as interstitial fibrosis/tubular atrophy, IF/TA) or post-transplant glomerular disease [162, 163]. The results of an ongoing randomized study aiming at addressing the effect of RAAS blockers on lowering patients' mortality and prolonging allograft survival in kidney transplant recipients are currently awaited [164].

Cardioprotective benefits of RAAS blockers beyond those associated with reduced blood pressure, especially those of ACE-I, in high-risk patients have been proposed [165]. Although there is no large-scale randomized trial that examined the effect of RAAS blockers on reducing cardiovascular events in kidney transplant recipients, some studies showed a favorable effect of RAAS blockers on mitigating the cardiovascular risk profile and lowering cardiovascular event rates after kidney transplantation. For example, when patients with persistent left ventricular were randomly assigned 3–6 months after transplantation to receive either the ACE-I lisinopril or placebo, regression in the left ventricular mass was observed with lisinopril but not with placebo, an effect that appeared independent of blood pressure control [166]. Another small study found that patients maintained on ACE-I for an average of 10 years had lower risk of the composite of death, major cardiovascular events, doubling of serum creatinine, or allograft loss [156]. On the other hand, the SECRET trial (The Study on Evaluation of Candesartan Cilexetil after Renal Transplantation) which intended to evaluate the effect of the ARB candesartan on reducing the risk of the composite end point of death, graft loss, and cardiovascular event had to be terminated prematurely after enrolling 502 participants due to lower-than-expected

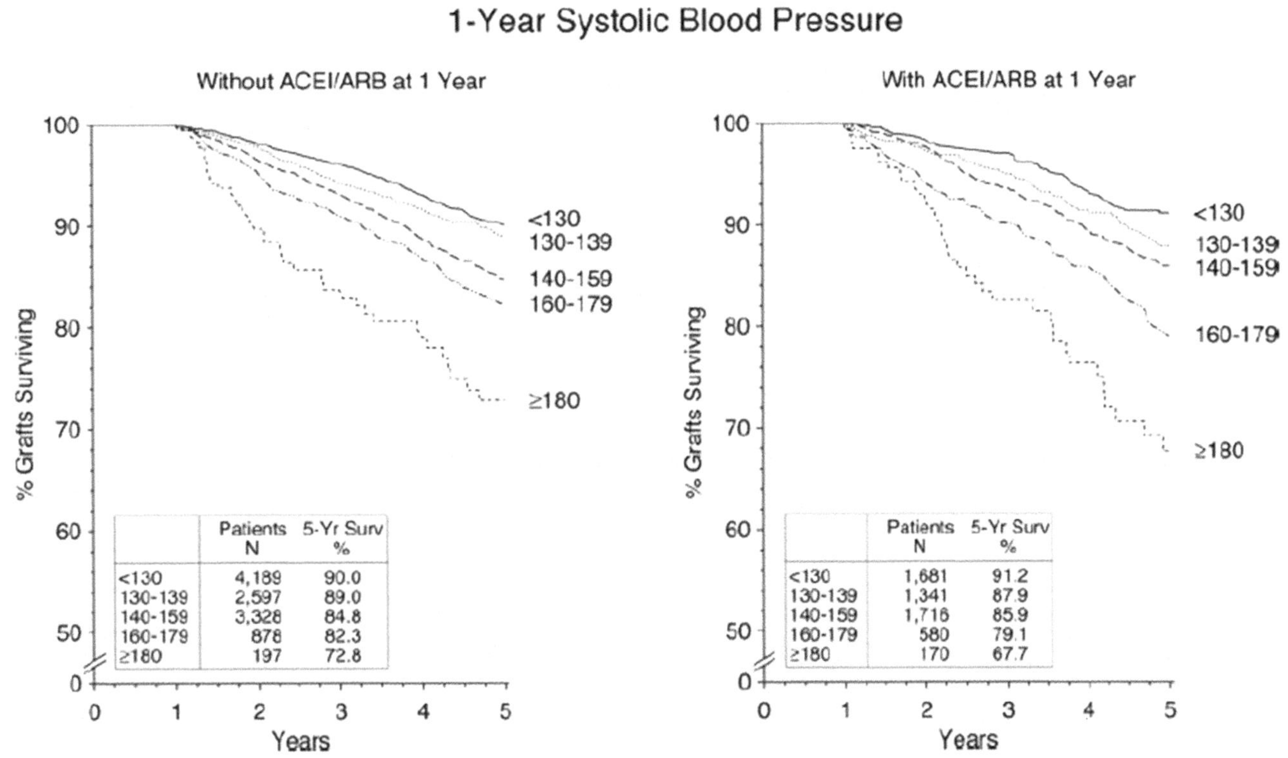

Fig. 20.6 Graft survival rates in 17,209 kidney transplant recipients with or without ACE-I or ARB treatment according to the systolic BP 1 year from transplantation. Kidney allograft survival related primarily to the degree of SBP control and not to the treatment with ACE-I or ARB. At any given level of SBP, there was no difference in allograft survival regardless of ACE-I or ARB use. Reprinted with permission [161]

event rates after enrollment [155]. BP was tightly controlled in both study arms which might have contributed to the low event rate, but there was no benefit of candesartan in lowering cardiovascular event rates [155].

The optimal timing of initiation of RAAS blockers has also been a matter of debate. Early reports of indicate that GFR falls when RAAS blockers are used with cyclosporine and cautioned against the use of ACE-I in the immediate post-transplant period [167]. Current data indicate that transplant centers are cautious in prescribing RAAS blockers in the first 4 months from transplantation even in patients with high cardiovascular risk profile probably for worries related to increased risk of hyperkalemia, fluctuation in serum creatinine, and post-transplant anemia. However, RAAS blocker use increases over time and 24–50 % of kidney recipients are taking RAAS blockers 4–6 months from transplantation [126, 160, 168, 169]. Some studies have addressed the merit of early initiation of RAAS blockers on allograft function. Immediate graft function and/or the occurrence of DGF was compared in 260 patients who either did or did not receive RAAS blockers in the early post-transplant period [170]. Serum creatinine decreased faster and DGF recovered quicker in those receiving RAAS blockers compared to those who did not receive such therapy [170]. A follow-up study by the same group that included 436 patients with DGF concluded that ACE-I and ARB use in the early post-transplant period was associated with higher 10-year actuarial death-censored graft survival and lower all-cause mortality [171]. Whether these outcomes were determined by RAAS blockade or represent selection bias in favor of better allografts for RAAS-blocking therapy cannot be established from these studies.

Hyperkalemia is a known complication of RAAS blockers especially in the early post-transplant period at time when high-dose CNI and sulfamethoxazole–trimethoprim are commonly prescribed. One study showed that 21 % of cases given losartan in the early post-transplant period had to stop this medication for hyperkalemia [152]. When RAAS blockers are utilized after 3 months from transplantation, the rate of hyperkalemia requiring drug discontinuation is remarkably low (2.4–3.4 %) [172, 173]. A meta-analysis of three studies that reported serum potassium levels 12 months from RAAS blocker use concluded that serum potassium level is similar in those receiving RAAS blockers compared to the control arm [148]. These studies suggest that hyperkalemia is common early after transplantation, but the risk of RAAS blocker-induced hyperkalemia declines late after transplantation. Post-transplant anemia, however, has consistently been associated with ACE-I and ARB use [148].

Taken together, physicians taking care of transplant patients should not feel "rushed" in starting RAAS blockers.

Current evidence indicates that RAAS blockers are equally effective to other antihypertensive medications in controlling post-transplant hypertension. There is no clear benefit of RAAS blockers on graft function, patient or graft survival in patients with stable allografts and in those with low cardiovascular risk profile. When prescribed along with other cardioprotective medications, RAAS blockers are associated with better patient survival. RAAS blockers should be encouraged in recipients with proteinuria and those with recurrent glomerular disease. Patients with IF/TA might also benefit from RAAS blockade. Hyperkalemia is a common complication of RAAS blockers especially when these medications are started early after transplantation.

Diuretics

Diuretics are effective antihypertensive medications in the immediate post-transplant period, particularly when hypertension is volume related. Due to their rapid onset of action, loop diuretics are the drug of choice especially with parenteral administration. Thiazide diuretics increase salt and water retention by inhibiting sodium chloride co-transporter (NCC) and therefore can counteract the effects of CNI on NCC activation [73]. Thiazides have longer duration of action and can be given once daily. Thiazides also counteract the effect of CNI on the NCC. Thiazides, however, can precipitate rise in serum creatinine due to their interference with the tubuloglomerular feedback [174]. Spironolactone is a mineralocorticoid receptor antagonist that is effective in controlling arterial hypertension in the general and CKD populations even in patients without laboratory evidence of aldosterone excess [175–177]. Spironolactone has been proposed to have renoprotective and reduced fibrogenic properties in some forms of kidney disease but is associated with elevation [178]. From a cardioprotective standpoint, spironolactone antagonizes cardiac hypertrophy and myocardial fibrosis induced by aldosterone and reduces the risk of death by 30 % over a 2-year follow-up period when added to ACE-I in CGF patients [179]. In the kidney transplant setting, spironolactone induces natriuresis and reduces arterial blood pressure in humans and ameliorates transplant vasculopathy in animal models [180, 181]. Some experimental studies implicate aldosterone in the pathogenesis of CNI-induced nephrotoxicity. Addition of spironolactone limits CNI-induced tubulointerstitial fibrosis and prevents further progression of renal dysfunction and tubulointerstitial fibrosis in rats with preexisting chronic CNI nephrotoxicity [182–184]. However, spironolactone administration can raise serum potassium and creatinine levels, especially when used in the early post-transplant period. Therefore spironolactone is better avoided in this early post-transplant period.

Overall Management Plan for Post-transplant Hypertension

A practical, albeit simplified, management plan for hypertension after kidney transplantation can be based on different time points from transplantation. The time points are arbitrary but coincide generally with changes in the volume status, corticosteroids, and CNI dose requirements in the post-transplant period. This management plan is divided into three phases.

1. *Early post-transplant period* (*the first post-transplant month*): In the first 2–3 weeks after transplantation, hypertension often reflects volume overload and patient's weight may be several kilograms above dialysis dry weight. High-dose CNI and parenteral corticosteroids also contribute to uncontrolled hypertension early after transplantation. Hypertension is best managed by limiting dietary salt intake and initiation of loop diuretics to induce natriuresis. Overly aggressive diuresis should be avoided to prevent acute deterioration in the allograft function. In recipients with delayed allograft function, hemodialysis will remove excess volume and will improve BP control. In this early post-transplant period, we recommend target SBP between 140 and 150 mmHg to ensure adequate allograft perfusion. If hypertension persists despite the above measures especially when hypertension is temporally related to CNI initiation, dihydropyridine CCBs are preferable due to their vasodilator properties that antagonize CNI-induced vasoconstriction and their limited drug to drug interaction. Both amlodipine and long-acting nifedipine are equally effective but the latter has a faster response of action. BBs and the centrally acting agent clonidine can be added as needed. Among BBs, labetalol is associated with less risk of bradycardia and shorter onset of action. ACE-I and ARB should be avoided in this time period due to the increased risk of hyperkalemia and worsening allograft function. In patients with refractory hypertension, especially those with worsening allograft function and diuretic-resistant edema, the possibility of TRAS should be contemplated with Doppler ultrasound with the understanding that elevated peak systolic velocity at the anastomosis is nearly universal in the first 24 h after transplantation.
2. *Intermediate post-transplant period* (*1–4 months*): After 3 weeks, most kidney transplant patients achieve stable trough CNI levels and improved volume status. Achieving lower target blood pressures (<140 mmHg) is warranted both to limit cardiovascular risks and to ensure that blood pressure will remain controlled while patients are under less direct supervision. CCBs, BBs, and central acting agents remain the mainstay of pharmacological therapy in

this period. Selected patients with persistent volume overload may benefit from low-dose loop or thiazide diuretics. Patients with proteinuria can be started on ACE-I or ARB with close monitoring of serum potassium and creatinine levels. Other post-transplant complications that can increase the cardiovascular risks including post-transplant diabetes and hyperlipidemia should be addressed. If TRAS is suggested in this period by Doppler ultrasound examination, pharmacological therapy should be maximized and angioplasty deferred to cases with refractory hypertension, evidence of pulmonary congestion, or worsening kidney function that is related solely to poor renal perfusion.

3. *Late post-transplant period (beyond the fourth post-transplant month)*: Beyond the fourth post-transplant month, efforts should be directed both to reduce cardiovascular risk and to maintain optimal allograft function. Target blood pressure levels should be tailored to each individual patient according to the potential cardiovascular risks. Current guidelines favor lower BP for patients with diabetes, proteinuria, IHD, and CHF (SBP <130/80 mmHg) while a target SBP <140 mmHg is recommended for the rest of the patients. ACE-I and ARB should be used in proteinuric patients and can be considered for the rest of patients as dictated by their comorbidities. Direct aldosterone antagonists may also be beneficial in resistant cases but hyperkalemia should be monitored. ABPM is useful in detecting masked hypertension and assessing the response of antihypertensive medications. Salt restriction should be encouraged and patients should be educated regarding adverse effects of obesity. Attention should be paid to control major additional risks including hyperlipidemia, diabetes, and OSA. In cases with resistant hypertension and allograft dysfunction, TRAS should be excluded, and in refractory cases with no obvious cause of hypertension in patients who are taking maximal medical therapy, bilateral native nephrectomy may be considered.

Conclusion

Hypertension post-kidney transplantation poses a significant management problem and contributes to shortened patient and allograft survivals. Despite awareness of its impact on post-transplant outcomes, published data indicate that the majority of kidney transplant recipients have suboptimal BP control. Management of post-kidney transplant hypertension requires an integrated approach with the initiation of pharmacological and non-pharmacological modalities bearing in mind patient comorbidities and interactions with immunosuppression medications. Current evidence does not dictate any particular class of antihypertensive medications for the treatment of post-transplant hypertension, although CCBs often are well suited to be the initial drug of choice. Modifications of the immunosuppressive medications especially those directed towards CNI dose reduction or elimination have salutary effects on post-transplant BP control but carry an increased risk of rejection. Because long-term graft survival depends heavily on minimizing cardiovascular morbidity and mortality, careful attention to blood pressure control is paramount.

References

1. Mange KC, Cizman B, Joffe M, Feldman HI. Arterial hypertension and renal allograft survival. JAMA. 2000;283:633–8.
2. Mange KC, Feldman HI, Joffe MM, Fa K, Bloom RD. Blood pressure and the survival of renal allografts from living donors. J Am Soc Nephrol. 2004;15:187–93.
3. Opelz G, Wujciak T, Ritz E. Association of chronic kidney graft failure with recipient blood pressure. Collaborative transplant study. Kidney Int. 1998;53:217–22.
4. Aakhus S, Dahl K, Wideroe TE. Cardiovascular disease in stable renal transplant patients in Norway: morbidity and mortality during a 5-yr follow-up. Clin Transplant. 2004;18:596–604.
5. Rigatto C, Parfrey P, Foley R, Negrijn C, Tribula C, Jeffery J. Congestive heart failure in renal transplant recipients: risk factors, outcomes, and relationship with ischemic heart disease. J Am Soc Nephrol. 2002;13:1084–90.
6. Kasiske BL, Chakkera HA, Roel J. Explained and unexplained ischemic heart disease risk after renal transplantation. J Am Soc Nephrol. 2000;11:1735–43.
7. Adams Jr HP, Dawson G, Coffman TJ, Corry RJ. Stroke in renal transplant recipients. Arch Neurol. 1986;43:113–5.
8. Oliveras A, Roquer J, Puig JM, Rodriguez A, Mir M, Orfila MA, Masramon J, Lloveras J. Stroke in renal transplant recipients: epidemiology, predictive risk factors and outcome. Clin Transplant. 2003;17:1–8.
9. Carpenter MA, Weir MR, Adey DB, House AA, Bostom AG, Kusek JW. Inadequacy of cardiovascular risk factor management in chronic kidney transplantation—evidence from the FAVORIT study. Clin Transplant. 2012;26:E438–46.
10. Kasiske BL, Anjum S, Shah R, Skogen J, Kandaswamy C, Danielson B, O'Shaughnessy EA, Dahl DC, Silkensen JR, Sahadevan M, Snyder JJ. Hypertension after kidney transplantation. Am J Kidney Dis. 2004;43:1071–81.
11. Ojo AO. Cardiovascular complications after renal transplantation and their prevention. Transplantation. 2006;82:603–11.
12. Cosio FG, Dillon JJ, Falkenhain ME, Tesi RJ, Henry ML, Elkhammas EA, Davies EA, Bumgardner GL, Ferguson RM. Racial differences in renal allograft survival: the role of systemic hypertension. Kidney Int. 1995;47:1136–41.
13. Cosio FG, Falkenhain ME, Pesavento TE, Henry ML, Elkhammas EA, Davies EA, Bumgardner GL, Ferguson RM. Relationships between arterial hypertension and renal allograft survival in African-American patients. Am J Kidney Dis. 1997;29:419–27.
14. Campistol JM, Romero R, Paul J, Gutierrez-Dalmau A. Epidemiology of arterial hypertension in renal transplant patients: changes over the last decade. Nephrol Dial Transplant. 2004;19 Suppl 3:iii62–6.
15. Ducloux D, Motte G, Kribs M, Abdelfatah AB, Bresson-Vautrin C, Rebibou JM, Chalopin JM. Hypertension in renal transplantation: donor and recipient risk factors. Clin Nephrol. 2002;57: 409–13.

16. Perez Fontan M, Rodriguez-Carmona A, Garcia Falcon T, Fernandez Rivera C, Valdes F. Early immunologic and nonimmunologic predictors of arterial hypertension after renal transplantation. Am J Kidney Dis. 1999;33:21–8.
17. Pickering TG, Shimbo D, Haas D. Ambulatory blood-pressure monitoring. N Engl J Med. 2006;354:2368–74.
18. Wadei HM, Amer H, Taler SJ, Cosio FG, Griffin MD, Grande JP, Larson TS, Schwab TR, Stegall MD, Textor SC. Diurnal blood pressure changes one year after kidney transplantation: relationship to allograft function, histology, and resistive index. J Am Soc Nephrol. 2007;18:1607–15.
19. Prasad GV, Nash MM, Zaltzman JS. A prospective study of the physician effect on blood pressure in renal-transplant recipients. Nephrol Dial Transplant. 2003;18:996–1000.
20. Stenehjem AE, Gudmundsdottir H, Os I. Office blood pressure measurements overestimate blood pressure control in renal transplant patients. Blood Press Monit. 2006;11:125–33.
21. Haydar AA, Covic A, Jayawardene S, Agharazii M, Smith E, Gordon I, O'Sullivan H, Goldsmith DJ. Insights from ambulatory blood pressure monitoring: diagnosis of hypertension and diurnal blood pressure in renal transplant recipients. Transplantation. 2004;77:849–53.
22. Paripovic D, Kostic M, Spasojevic B, Kruscic D, Peco-Antic A. Masked hypertension and hidden uncontrolled hypertension after renal transplantation. Pediatr Nephrol. 2010;25:1719–24.
23. Ferraris JR, Ghezzi L, Waisman G, Krmar RT. ABPM vs office blood pressure to define blood pressure control in treated hypertensive paediatric renal transplant recipients. Pediatr Transplant. 2007;11:24–30.
24. Bangash F, Agarwal R. Masked hypertension and white-coat hypertension in chronic kidney disease: a meta-analysis. Clin J Am Soc Nephrol. 2009;4:656–64.
25. Bobrie G, Chatellier G, Genes N, Clerson P, Vaur L, Vaisse B, Menard J, Mallion JM. Cardiovascular prognosis of "masked hypertension" detected by blood pressure self-measurement in elderly treated hypertensive patients. JAMA. 2004;291:1342–9.
26. Bobrie G, Clerson P, Menard J, Postel-Vinay N, Chatellier G, Plouin PF. Masked hypertension: a systematic review. J Hypertens. 2008;26:1715–25.
27. Clement DL, De Buyzere ML, De Bacquer DA, de Leeuw PW, Duprez DA, Fagard RH, Gheeraert PJ, Missault LH, Braun JJ, Six RO, Van Der Niepen P, O'Brien E. Prognostic value of ambulatory blood-pressure recordings in patients with treated hypertension. N Engl J Med. 2003;348:2407–15.
28. Shimada K, Kawamoto A, Matsubayashi K, Nishinaga M, Kimura S, Ozawa T. Diurnal blood pressure variations and silent cerebrovascular damage in elderly patients with hypertension. J Hypertens. 1992;10:875–8.
29. Verdecchia P, Porcellati C, Schillaci G, Borgioni C, Ciucci A, Battistelli M, Guerrieri M, Gatteschi C, Zampi I, Santucci A, et al. Ambulatory blood pressure. An independent predictor of prognosis in essential hypertension. Hypertension. 1994;24:793–801.
30. Lurbe E, Redon J, Kesani A, Pascual JM, Tacons J, Alvarez V, Batlle D. Increase in nocturnal blood pressure and progression to microalbuminuria in type 1 diabetes. N Engl J Med. 2002; 347:797–805.
31. Agarwal R, Andersen MJ. Prognostic importance of ambulatory blood pressure recordings in patients with chronic kidney disease. Kidney Int. 2006;69:1175–80.
32. Davidson MB, Hix JK, Vidt DG, Brotman DJ. Association of impaired diurnal blood pressure variation with a subsequent decline in glomerular filtration rate. Arch Intern Med. 2006;166:846–52.
33. Paoletti E, Gherzi M, Amidone M, Massarino F, Cannella G. Association of arterial hypertension with renal target organ damage in kidney transplant recipients: the predictive role of ambulatory blood pressure monitoring. Transplantation. 2009;87: 1864–9.
34. Toprak A, Koc M, Tezcan H, Ozener IC, Oktay A, Akoglu E. Night-time blood pressure load is associated with higher left ventricular mass index in renal transplant recipients. J Hum Hypertens. 2003;17:239–44.
35. Ibernon M, Moreso F, Sarrias X, Sarrias M, Grinyo JM, Fernandez-Real JM, Ricart W, Seron D. Reverse dipper pattern of blood pressure at 3 months is associated with inflammation and outcome after renal transplantation. Nephrol Dial Transplant. 2012;27:2089–95.
36. Wadei HM, Amer H, Griffin MD, Taler SJ, Stegall MD, Textor SC. Abnormal circadian blood pressure pattern 1-year after kidney transplantation is associated with subsequent lower glomerular filtration rate in recipients without rejection. J Am Soc Hypertens. 2011;5:39–47.
37. Agena F, Prado Edos S, Souza PS, da Silva GV, Lemos FBC, Mion D, Nahas WC, David-Neto E. Home blood pressure (BP) monitoring in kidney transplant recipients is more adequate to monitor BP than office BP. Nephrol Dial Transplant. 2011; 26:3745–9.
38. Special issue: KDIGO clinical practice guideline for the care of kidney transplant recipients. Am J Transplant. 2009;9:S1–155.
39. Chapter 5: Blood pressure management in kidney transplant recipients (CKD T). Kidney Int Suppl. 2012;2:370–1.
40. K/DOQI. K/DOQI clinical practice guidelines on hypertension and antihypertensive agents in chronic kidney disease. Am J Kidney Dis. 2004;43:S1–290.
41. European best practice guidelines for renal transplantation. Section IV: long-term management of the transplant recipient. Nephrol Dial Transplant. 2002;17 Suppl 4:1–67.
42. Chobanian AV, Bakris GL, Black HR, Cushman WC, Green LA, Izzo Jr JL, Jones DW, Materson BJ, Oparil S, Wright Jr JT, Roccella EJ. The seventh report of the joint national committee on prevention, detection, evaluation, and treatment of high blood pressure: the JNC 7 report. JAMA. 2003;289:2560–72.
43. Evans RW, Applegate WH, Briscoe DM, Cohen DJ, Rorick CC, Murphy BT, Madsen JC. Cost-related immunosuppressive medication nonadherence among kidney transplant recipients. Clin J Am Soc Nephrol. 2010;5:2323–8.
44. Lilien MR, Stroes ES, Op't Roodt J, de Jongh S, Schroder CH, Koomans HA. Vascular function in children after renal transplantation. Am J Kidney Dis. 2003;41:684–91.
45. Litwin M, Wuhl E, Jourdan C, Niemirska A, Schenk JP, Jobs K, Grenda R, Wawer ZT, Rajszys P, Mehls O, Schaefer F. Evolution of large-vessel arteriopathy in paediatric patients with chronic kidney disease. Nephrol Dial Transplant. 2008;23:2552–7.
46. Bahous SA, Stephan A, Blacher J, Safar ME. Aortic stiffness, living donors, and renal transplantation. Hypertension. 2006;47: 216–21.
47. Delahousse M, Chaignon M, Mesnard L, Boutouyrie P, Safar ME, Lebret T, Pastural-Thaunat M, Tricot L, Kolko-Labadens A, Karras A, Haymann JP. Aortic stiffness of kidney transplant recipients correlates with donor age. J Am Soc Nephrol. 2008;19: 798–805.
48. Opazo Saez A, Kos M, Witzke O, Kribben A, Nurnberger J. Effect of new-onset diabetes mellitus on arterial stiffness in renal transplantation. Transplant Int. 2008;21:930–5.
49. Strozecki P, Adamowicz A, Wlodarczyk Z, Manitius J. Factors associated with increased arterial stiffness in renal transplant recipients. Med Sci Monit. 2010;16:CR301–6.
50. Joannidès R, Monteil C, de Ligny BH, Westeel PF, Iacob M, Thervet E, Barbier S, Bellien J, Lebranchu Y, Seguin SG, Thuillez C, Godin M, Etienne I. Immunosuppressant regimen based on sirolimus decreases aortic stiffness in renal transplant recipients in comparison to cyclosporine. Am J Transplant. 2011;11:2414–22.

51. Seckinger J, Sommerer C, Hinkel UP, Hoffmann O, Zeier M, Schwenger V. Switch of immunosuppression from cyclosporine A to everolimus: impact on pulse wave velocity in stable de-novo renal allograft recipients. J Hypertens. 2008;26:2213–9.
52. Wadei HM, Textor SC. The role of the kidney in regulating arterial blood pressure. Nat Rev Nephrol. 2012;8:602–9.
53. Textor SC, Schwartz L, Wilson DJ, Wiesner R, Romero JC, Augustine J, Kos P, Hay E, Gores G, Dickson ER, et al. Systemic and renal effects of nifedipine in cyclosporine-associated hypertension. Hypertension. 1994;23:I220–4.
54. Kone BC, Whelton A, Santos G, Saral R, Watson AJ. Hypertension and renal dysfunction in bone marrow transplant recipients. Q J Med. 1988;69:985–95.
55. Textor SC, Wiesner R, Wilson DJ, Porayko M, Romero JC, Burnett Jr JC, Gores G, Hay E, Dickson ER, Krom RA. Systemic and renal hemodynamic differences between FK506 and cyclosporine in liver transplant recipients. Transplantation. 1993;55:1332–9.
56. Thompson ME, Shapiro AP, Johnsen AM, Itzkoff JM, Hardesty RL, Griffith BP, Bahnson HT, McDonald Jr RH, Hastillo A, Hess M. The contrasting effects of cyclosporin-A and azathioprine on arterial blood pressure and renal function following cardiac transplantation. Int J Cardiol. 1986;11:219–29.
57. Hoorn EJ, Walsh SB, McCormick JA, Zietse R, Unwin RJ, Ellison DH. Pathogenesis of calcineurin inhibitor-induced hypertension. J Nephrol. 2012;25:269–75.
58. Textor SC, Canzanello VJ, Taler SJ, Wilson DJ, Schwartz LL, Augustine JE, Raymer JM, Romero JC, Wiesner RH, Krom RA, et al. Cyclosporine-induced hypertension after transplantation. Mayo Clin Proc. 1994;69:1182–93.
59. Kurtz A, Della Bruna R, Kuhn K. Cyclosporine a enhances renin secretion and production in isolated juxtaglomerular cells. Kidney Int. 1988;33:947–53.
60. Lassila M. Interaction of cyclosporine a and the renin-angiotensin system; new perspectives. Curr Drug Metab. 2002;3:61–71.
61. Mason J, Muller-Schweinitzer E, Dupont M, Casellas D, Mihatsch M, Moore L, Kaskel F. Cyclosporine and the renin-angiotensin system. Kidney Int Suppl. 1991;32:S28–32.
62. Iijima K, Hamahira K, Kobayashi A, Nakamura H, Yoshikawa N. Immunohistochemical analysis of renin activity in chronic cyclosporine nephropathy in childhood nephrotic syndrome. J Am Soc Nephrol. 2000;11:2265–71.
63. Tufro-McReddie A, Gomez RA, Norling LL, Omar AA, Moore LC, Kaskel FJ. Effect of CsA on the expression of renin and angiotensin type 1 receptor genes in the rat kidney. Kidney Int. 1993;43:615–22.
64. Takeda Y, Miyamori I, Wu P, Yoneda T, Furukawa K, Takeda R. Effects of an endothelin receptor antagonist in rats with cyclosporine-induced hypertension. Hypertension. 1995;26:932–6.
65. Siedlecki A, Anderson JR, Jin X, Garbow JR, Lupu TS, Muslin AJ. RGS4 controls renal blood flow and inhibits cyclosporine-mediated nephrotoxicity. Am J Transplant. 2009;10(2):231–41.
66. Ciresi DL, Lloyd MA, Sandberg SM, Heublein DM, Edwards BS. The sodium retaining effects of cyclosporine. Kidney Int. 1992;41:1599–605.
67. Sturrock ND, Lang CC, MacFarlane LJ, Dockrell ME, Ryan M, Webb DJ, Struthers AD. Serial changes in blood pressure, renal function, endothelin and lipoprotein (a) during the first 9 days of cyclosporin therapy in males. J Hypertens. 1995;13:667–73.
68. Textor SC, Burnett Jr JC, Romero JC, Canzanello VJ, Taler SJ, Wiesner R, Porayko M, Krom R, Gores G, Hay E. Urinary endothelin and renal vasoconstriction with cyclosporine or FK506 after liver transplantation. Kidney Int. 1995;47:1426–33.
69. Canzanello VJ, Textor SC, Taler SJ, Wilson DJ, Schwartz L, Wiesner RH, Porayko MK, Krom RA. Renal sodium handling with cyclosporin a and FK506 after orthotopic liver transplantation. J Am Soc Nephrol. 1995;5:1910–7.
70. Curtis JJ, Luke RG, Jones P, Diethelm AG. Hypertension in cyclosporine-treated renal transplant recipients is sodium dependent. Am J Med. 1988;85:134–8.
71. Hoorn EJ, Walsh SB, McCormick JA, Furstenberg A, Yang CL, Roeschel T, Paliege A, Howie AJ, Conley J, Bachmann S, Unwin RJ, Ellison DH. The calcineurin inhibitor tacrolimus activates the renal sodium chloride cotransporter to cause hypertension. Nat Med. 2011;17:1304–9.
72. Melnikov S, Mayan H, Uchida S, Holtzman EJ, Farfel Z. Cyclosporine metabolic side effects: association with the WNK4 system. Eur J Clin Invest. 2011;41:1113–20.
73. Luft FC. How calcineurin inhibitors cause hypertension. Nephrol Dial Transplant. 2012;27:473–5.
74. Kihm LP, Blume C, Seckinger J, Hankel V, Stoffler D, Morath C, Zeier M, Schwenger V. Acute effects of calcineurin inhibitors on kidney allograft microperfusion visualized by contrast-enhanced sonography. Transplantation. 2012;93:1125–9.
75. Strozecki P, Adamowicz A, Wlodarczyk Z, Manitius J. The influence of calcineurin inhibitors on pulse wave velocity in renal transplant recipients. Ren Fail. 2007;29:679–84.
76. Copley JB, Staffeld C, Lindberg J, Hansen A, Bailey C, Anand R, Van Veldhuisen P. Cyclosporine to tacrolimus: effect on hypertension and lipid profiles in renal allografts. Transplant Proc. 1998;30:1254–6.
77. Ligtenberg G, Hene RJ, Blankestijn PJ, Koomans HA. Cardiovascular risk factors in renal transplant patients: cyclosporin a versus tacrolimus. J Am Soc Nephrol. 2001;12:368–73.
78. Vincenti F, Jensik SC, Filo RS, Miller J, Pirsch J. A long-term comparison of tacrolimus (FK506) and cyclosporine in kidney transplantation: evidence for improved allograft survival at five years. Transplantation. 2002;73:775–82.
79. Margreiter R. Efficacy and safety of tacrolimus compared with cyclosporin microemulsion in renal transplantation: a randomised multicentre study. Lancet. 2002;359:741–6.
80. Taler SJ, Textor SC, Canzanello VJ, Schwartz L, Porayko M, Wiesner RH, Krom RA. Role of steroid dose in hypertension early after liver transplantation with tacrolimus (FK506) and cyclosporine. Transplantation. 1996;62:1588–92.
81. Goodwin JE, Zhang J, Geller DS. A critical role for vascular smooth muscle in acute glucocorticoid-induced hypertension. J Am Soc Nephrol. 2008;19:1291–9.
82. Audard V, Matignon M, Hemery F, Snanoudj R, Desgranges P, Anglade MC, Kobeiter H, Durrbach A, Charpentier B, Lang P, Grimbert P. Risk factors and long-term outcome of transplant renal artery stenosis in adult recipients after treatment by percutaneous transluminal angioplasty. Am J Transplant. 2006;6:95–9.
83. Voiculescu A, Schmitz M, Hollenbeck M, Braasch S, Luther B, Sandmann W, Jung G, Mödder U, Grabensee B. Management of arterial stenosis affecting kidney graft perfusion: a single-centre study in 53 patients. Am J Transplant. 2005;5:1731–8.
84. Halimi J-M, Al-Najjar A, Buchler M, Birmele B, Tranquart F, Alison D, Lebranchu Y. Transplant renal artery stenosis: potential role of ischemia/reperfusion injury and long-term outcome following angioplasty. J Urol. 1999;161:28–32.
85. Bruno S, Remuzzi G, Ruggenenti P. Transplant renal artery stenosis. J Am Soc Nephrol. 2004;15:134–41.
86. Ghazanfar A, Tavakoli A, Augustine T, Pararajasingam R, Riad H, Chalmers N. Management of transplant renal artery stenosis and its impact on long-term allograft survival: a single-centre experience. Nephrol Dial Transplant. 2011;26:336–43.
87. Wong W, Fynn SP, Higgins RM, Walters H, Evans S, Deane C, Goss D, Bewick M, Snowden SA, Scoble JE, Hendry BM. Transplant renal artery stenosis in 77 patients–does it have an immunological cause? Transplantation. 1996;61:215–9.
88. Grunfeld JP, Kleinknecht D, Moreau JF, Kamoun P, Sabto J, Garcia-Torres R, Osorio M, Kreis H. Permanent hypertension

after renal homotransplantation in man. Clin Sci Mol Med. 1975;48:391–403.
89. Hagen G, Wadström J, Magnusson M, Magnusson A. Outcome after percutaneous transluminal angioplasty of arterial stenosis in renal transplant patients. Acta Radiol. 2009;50:270–5.
90. Henning BF, Kuchlbauer S, Boger CA, Obed A, Farkas S, Zulke C, Scherer MN, Walberer A, Banas M, Kruger B, Schlitt HJ, Banas B, Kramer BK. Percutaneous transluminal angioplasty as first-line treatment of transplant renal artery stenosis. Clin Nephrol. 2009;71:543–9.
91. Zhang ZF, Liang HM, Feng GS, Zheng CS, Wu HP, Zhou GF. Interventional treatment of transplanted renal artery stenosis. J Interv Radiol. 2008;17:623–6.
92. Hurst FP, Abbott KC, Neff RT, Elster EA, Falta EM, Lentine KL, Agodoa LY, Jindal RM. Incidence, predictors and outcomes of transplant renal artery stenosis after kidney transplantation: analysis of USRDS. Am J Nephrol. 2009;30:459–67.
93. Hausberg M, Kosch M, Harmelink P, Barenbrock M, Hohage H, Kisters K, Dietl KH, Rahn KH. Sympathetic nerve activity in end-stage renal disease. Circulation. 2002;106:1974–9.
94. Curtis JJ, Luke RG, Diethelm AG, Whelchel JD, Jones P. Benefits of removal of native kidneys in hypertension after renal transplantation. Lancet. 1985;2:739–42.
95. Huysmans FT, Hoitsma AJ, Koene RA. Factors determining the prevalence of hypertension after renal transplantation. Nephrol Dial Transplant. 1987;2:34–8.
96. Shoma AM, Eraky I, El-Kappany HA. Pretransplant native nephrectomy in patients with end-stage renal failure: assessment of the role of laparoscopy. Urology. 2003;61:915–20.
97. Sanjeevan KV, Bhat HS, Sudhindran S. Laparoscopic simultaneous bilateral pretransplant nephrectomy for uncontrolled hypertension. Transplant Proc. 2004;36:2011–2.
98. Bales GT, Fellner SK, Chodak GW, Rukstalis DB. Laparoscopic bilateral nephrectomy for renin-mediated hypertension. Urology. 1994;43:874–7.
99. Fornara P, Doehn C, Fricke L, Durek C, Thyssen G, Jocham D. Laparoscopic bilateral nephrectomy: results in 11 renal transplant patients. J Urol. 1997;157:445–9.
100. Fricke L, Doehn C, Steinhoff J, Sack K, Jocham D, Fornara P. Treatment of posttransplant hypertension by laparoscopic bilateral nephrectomy? Transplantation. 1998;65:1182–7.
101. Esler MD, Krum H, Sobotka PA, Schlaich MP, Schmieder RE, Bohm M. Renal sympathetic denervation in patients with treatment-resistant hypertension (the symplicity htn-2 trial): a randomised controlled trial. Lancet. 2010;376:1903–9.
102. Opelz G, Dohler B. Improved long-term outcomes after renal transplantation associated with blood pressure control. Am J Transplant. 2005;5:2725–31.
103. Molnar MZ, Lazar AS, Lindner A, Fornadi K, Czira ME, Dunai A, Zoller R, Szentkiralyi A, Rosivall L, Shapiro CM, Novak M, Mucsi I. Sleep apnea is associated with cardiovascular risk factors among kidney transplant patients. Clin J Am Soc Nephrol. 2010;5:125–32.
104. Marin JM, Agusti A, Villar I, Forner M, Nieto D, Carrizo SJ, Barbe F, Vicente E, Wei Y, Nieto FJ, Jelic S. Association between treated and untreated obstructive sleep apnea and risk of hypertension. JAMA. 2012;307:2169–76.
105. Meier-Kriesche HU, Li S, Gruessner RW, Fung JJ, Bustami RT, Barr ML, Leichtman AB. Immunosuppression: evolution in practice and trends, 1994–2004. Am J Transplant. 2006;6:1111–31.
106. Knight SR, Morris PJ. Steroid avoidance or withdrawal after renal transplantation increases the risk of acute rejection but decreases cardiovascular risk. A meta-analysis. Transplantation. 2010;89: 1–14.
107. Hricik DE, Lautman J, Bartucci MR, Moir EJ, Mayes JT, Schulak JA. Variable effects of steroid withdrawal on blood pressure reduction in cyclosporine-treated renal transplant recipients. Transplantation. 1992;53:1232–5.
108. Vanrenterghem Y, Lebranchu Y, Hene R, Oppenheimer F, Ekberg H. Double-blind comparison of two corticosteroid regimens plus mycophenolate mofetil and cyclosporine for prevention of acute renal allograft rejection. Transplantation. 2000;70:1352–9.
109. Ahsan N, Hricik D, Matas A, Rose S, Tomlanovich S, Wilkinson A, Ewell M, McIntosh M, Stablein D, Hodge E. Prednisone withdrawal in kidney transplant recipients on cyclosporine and mycophenolate mofetil–a prospective randomized study. Steroid withdrawal study group. Transplantation. 1999;68:1865–74.
110. Hricik DE, Knauss TC, Bodziak KA, Weigel K, Rodriguez V, Seaman D, Siegel C, Valente J, Schulak JA. Withdrawal of steroid therapy in African American kidney transplant recipients receiving sirolimus and tacrolimus. Transplantation. 2003;76:938–42.
111. Sarwal MM, Vidhun JR, Alexander SR, Satterwhite T, Millan M, Salvatierra Jr O. Continued superior outcomes with modification and lengthened follow-up of a steroid-avoidance pilot with extended daclizumab induction in pediatric renal transplantation. Transplantation. 2003;76:1331–9.
112. Hocker B, Weber LT, Feneberg R, Drube J, John U, Fehrenbach H, Pohl M, Zimmering M, Frund S, Klaus G, Wuhl E, Tonshoff B. Prospective, randomized trial on late steroid withdrawal in pediatric renal transplant recipients under cyclosporine microemulsion and mycophenolate mofetil. Transplantation. 2009;87:934–41.
113. Sarwal MM, Ettenger RB, Dharnidharka V, Benfield M, Mathias R, Portale A, McDonald R, Harmon W, Kershaw D, Vehaskari VM, Kamil E, Baluarte HJ, Warady B, Tang L, Liu J, Li L, Naesens M, Sigdel T, Waskerwitz J, Salvatierra O. Complete steroid avoidance is effective and safe in children with renal transplants: a multicenter randomized trial with three-year follow-up. Am J Transplant. 2012;12:2719–29.
114. Woodle ESMD, First MRMD, Pirsch JMD, Shihab FMD, Gaber AOMD, Van Veldhuisen PP, for the Astellas Corticosteroid Withdrawal Study Group. A prospective, randomized, double-blind, placebo-controlled multicenter trial comparing early (7 day) corticosteroid cessation versus long-term, low-dose corticosteroid therapy. Ann Surg. 2008;248:564–77.
115. Sivaraman P, Nussbaumer G, Landsberg D. Lack of long-term benefits of steroid withdrawal in renal transplant recipients. Am J Kidney Dis. 2001;37:1162–9.
116. Ronald PP, Baris A, Ronald MF. Prospective, randomized trial of steroid withdrawal in kidney recipients treated with mycophenolate mofetil and cyclosporine. Clin Transplant. 2006;20:10–8.
117. Pelletier RP, Akin B, Ferguson RM. Prospective, randomized trial of steroid withdrawal in kidney recipients treated with mycophenolate mofetil and cyclosporine. Clin Transplant. 2006;20:10–8.
118. Johnson RW, Kreis H, Oberbauer R, Brattstrom C, Claesson K, Eris J. Sirolimus allows early cyclosporine withdrawal in renal transplantation resulting in improved renal function and lower blood pressure. Transplantation. 2001;72:777–86.
119. Schnuelle P, van der Heide JH, Tegzess A, Verburgh CA, Paul LC, van der Woude FJ, de Fijter JW. Open randomized trial comparing early withdrawal of either cyclosporine or mycophenolate mofetil in stable renal transplant recipients initially treated with a triple drug regimen. J Am Soc Nephrol. 2002;13:536–43.
120. Hueso M, Bover J, Seron D, Gil-Vernet S, Sabate I, Fulladosa X, Ramos R, Coll O, Alsina J, Grinyo JM. Low-dose cyclosporine and mycophenolate mofetil in renal allograft recipients with suboptimal renal function. Transplantation. 1998;66:1727–31.
121. Waichi W, Nina T-R, Francis LD, Francesca C, Susan LS, Mary Lin F, Vivian S, Wolfgang CW, Cosimi AB, Manuel P. Analysis of the cardiovascular risk profile in stable kidney transplant recipients after 50 % cyclosporine reduction. Clin Transplant. 2004;18:341–8.

122. Vincenti F, Larsen C, Durrbach A, Wekerle T, Nashan B, Blancho G, Lang P, Grinyo J, Halloran PF, Solez K, Hagerty D, Levy E, Zhou W, Natarajan K, Charpentier B. Costimulation blockade with belatacept in renal transplantation. N Engl J Med. 2005;353: 770–81.
123. Ekberg H, Grinyo J, Nashan B, Vanrenterghem Y, Vincenti F, Voulgari A, Truman M, Nasmyth-Miller C, Rashford M. Cyclosporine sparing with mycophenolate mofetil, daclizumab and corticosteroids in renal allograft recipients: the CAESAR study. Am J Transplant. 2007;7:560–70.
124. Premasathian NC, Muehrer R, Brazy PC, Pirsch JD, Becker BN. Blood pressure control in kidney transplantation: therapeutic implications. J Hum Hypertens. 2004;18:871–7.
125. Martinez-Castelao A, Hueso M, Sanz V, Rejas J, Alsina J, Grinyo JM. Treatment of hypertension after renal transplantation: long-term efficacy of verapamil, enalapril, and doxazosin. Kidney Int Suppl. 1998;68:S130–4.
126. Pilmore HL, Skeans MA, Snyder JJ, Israni AK, Kasiske BL. Cardiovascular disease medications after renal transplantation: results from the patient outcomes in renal transplantation study. Transplantation. 2011;91:542–51.
127. Jones TE, Morris RG. Pharmacokinetic interaction between tacrolimus and diltiazem: dose–response relationship in kidney and liver transplant recipients. Clin Pharmacokinet. 2002;41:381–8.
128. Schrama YC, Koomans HA. Interactions of cyclosporin a and amlodipine: blood cyclosporin a levels, hypertension and kidney function. J Hypertens Suppl. 1998;16:S33–8.
129. Ruggenenti P, Perico N, Mosconi L, Gaspari F, Benigni A, Amuchastegui CS, Bruzzi I, Remuzzi G. Calcium channel blockers protect transplant patients from cyclosporine-induced daily renal hypoperfusion. Kidney Int. 1993;43:706–11.
130. Inigo P, Campistol JM, Lario S, Piera C, Campos B, Bescos M, Oppenheimer F, Rivera F. Effects of losartan and amlodipine on intrarenal hemodynamics and TGF-{beta}1 plasma levels in a crossover trial in renal transplant recipients. J Am Soc Nephrol. 2001;12:822–7.
131. Madsen JK, Sorensen SS, Hansen HE, Pedersen EB. The effect of felodipine on renal function and blood pressure in cyclosporin-treated renal transplant recipients during the first three months after transplantation. Nephrol Dial Transplant. 1998;13:2327–34.
132. Birx DL, Berger M, Fleisher TA. The interference of T cell activation by calcium channel blocking agents. J Immunol. 1984;133:2904–9.
133. Boom H, Mallat MJ, de Fijter JW, Paul LC, Bruijn JA, van Es LA. Calcium levels as a risk factor for delayed graft function. Transplantation. 2004;77:868–73.
134. Palmer BF, Dawidson I, Sagalowsky A, Sandor Z, Lu CY. Improved outcome of cadaveric renal transplantation due to calcium channel blockers. Transplantation. 1991;52:640–5.
135. Chanard J, Toupance O, Lavaud S, Hurault de Ligny B, Bernaud C, Moulin B. Amlodipine reduces cyclosporin-induced hyperuricaemia in hypertensive renal transplant recipients. Nephrol Dial Transplant. 2003;18:2147–53.
136. Midtvedt K, Ihlen H, Hartmann A, Bryde P, Bjerkely BL, Foss A, Fauchald P, Holdaas H. Reduction of left ventricular mass by lisinopril and nifedipine in hypertensive renal transplant recipients: a prospective randomized double-blind study. Transplantation. 2001;72:107–11.
137. Kuypers DR, Neumayer HH, Fritsche L, Budde K, Rodicio JL, Vanrenterghem Y. Calcium channel blockade and preservation of renal graft function in cyclosporine-treated recipients: a prospective randomized placebo-controlled 2-year study. Transplantation. 2004;78:1204–11.
138. van Riemsdijk IC, Mulder PG, de Fijter JW, Bruijn JA, van Hooff JP, Hoitsma AJ, Tegzess AM, Weimar W. Addition of isradipine (Lomir) results in a better renal function after kidney transplantation: a double-blind, randomized, placebo-controlled, multi-center study. Transplantation. 2000;70:122–6.
139. Cross NB, Webster AC, Masson P, O'Connell PJ, Craig JC. Antihypertensives for kidney transplant recipients: systematic review and meta-analysis of randomized controlled trials. Transplantation. 2009;88:7–18.
140. Ruggenenti P, Perna A, Benini R, Remuzzi G. Effects of dihydropyridine calcium channel blockers, angiotensin-converting enzyme inhibition, and blood pressure control on chronic, nondiabetic nephropathies. Gruppo italiano di studi epidemiologici in nefrologia (gisen). J Am Soc Nephrol. 1998;9:2096–101.
141. Knoll GA, Blydt-Hansen TD, Campbell P, Cantarovich M, Cole E, Fairhead T, Gill JS, Gourishankar S, Hebert D, Hodsman A, House AA, Humar A, Karpinski M, Kim SJ, Mainra R, Prasad GVR. Canadian Society of Transplantation and Canadian Society of Nephrology commentary on the 2009 KDIGO clinical practice guideline for the care of kidney transplant recipients. Am J Kidney Dis. 2010;56:219–46.
142. Hausberg M, Barenbrock M, Hohage H, Muller S, Heidenreich S, Rahn KH. Ace inhibitor versus beta-blocker for the treatment of hypertension in renal allograft recipients. Hypertension. 1999;33: 862–8.
143. Suwelack B, Kobelt V, Erfmann M, Hausberg M, Gerhardt U, Rahn KH, Hohage H. Long-term follow-up of ace-inhibitor versus beta-blocker treatment and their effects on blood pressure and kidney function in renal transplant recipients. Transpl Int. 2003;16:313–20.
144. Huysmans FT, van Heusden FH, Wetzels JF, Hoitsma AJ, Koene RA. Antihypertensive effect of beta blockade in renal transplant recipients with or without host kidneys. Transplantation. 1988; 46:234–7.
145. Bell DS, Bakris GL, McGill JB. Comparison of carvedilol and metoprolol on serum lipid concentration in diabetic hypertensive patients. Diabetes Obes Metab. 2009;11:234–8.
146. Roland M, Gatault P, Al-Najjar A, Doute C, Barbet C, Chatelet V, Laouad I, Marlière JF, Nivet H, Büchler M, Lebranchu Y, Halimi JM. Early pulse pressure and low-grade proteinuria as independent long-term risk factors for new-onset diabetes mellitus after kidney transplantation. Am J Transplant. 2008;8:1719–28.
147. Gress TW, Nieto FJ, Shahar E, Wofford MR, Brancati FL. Hypertension and antihypertensive therapy as risk factors for type 2 diabetes mellitus. The Atherosclerosis Risk in Communities Study. N Engl J Med. 2000;342:905–12.
148. Hiremath S, Fergusson D, Doucette S, Mulay AV, Knoll GA. Renin angiotensin system blockade in kidney transplantation: a systematic review of the evidence. Am J Transplant. 2007;7:2350–60.
149. Jafar TH, Schmid CH, Landa M, Giatras I, Toto R, Remuzzi G, Maschio G, Brenner BM, Kamper A, Zucchelli P, Becker G, Himmelmann A, Bannister K, Landais P, Shahinfar S, de Jong PE, de Zeeuw D, Lau J, Levey AS. Angiotensin-converting enzyme inhibitors and progression of nondiabetic renal disease. A meta-analysis of patient-level data. Ann Intern Med. 2001;135:73–87.
150. Brenner BM, Cooper ME, de Zeeuw D, Keane WF, Mitch WE, Parving HH, Remuzzi G, Snapinn SM, Zhang Z, Shahinfar S. Effects of losartan on renal and cardiovascular outcomes in patients with type 2 diabetes and nephropathy. N Engl J Med. 2001;345:861–9.
151. Midtvedt K, Hartmann A, Foss A, Fauchald P, Nordal KP, Rootwelt K, Holdaas H. Sustained improvement of renal graft function for two years in hypertensive renal transplant recipients treated with nifedipine as compared to lisinopril. Transplantation. 2001;72:1787–92.
152. Formica Jr RN, Friedman AL, Lorber MI, Smith JD, Eisen T, Bia MJ. A randomized trial comparing losartan with amlodipine as initial therapy for hypertension in the early post-transplant period. Nephrol Dial Transplant. 2006;21:1389–94.

153. Ibrahim HN, Jackson S, Connaire J, Matas A, Ney A, Najafian B, West A, Lentsch N, Ericksen J, Bodner J, Kasiske B, Mauer M. Angiotensin II blockade in kidney transplant recipients. J Am Soc Nephrol. 2013;24:320–7.
154. Omoto K, Tanabe K, Tokumoto T, Shimmura H, Ishida H, Toma H. Use of candesartan cilexetil decreases proteinuria in renal transplant patients with chronic allograft dysfunction. Transplantation. 2003;76:1170–4.
155. Philipp T, Martinez F, Geiger H, Moulin B, Mourad G, Schmieder R, Lievre M, Heemann U, Legendre C. Candesartan improves blood pressure control and reduces proteinuria in renal transplant recipients: results from secret. Nephrol Dial Transplant. 2010; 25:967–76.
156. Paoletti E, Bellino D, Marsano L, Cassottana P, Rolla D, Ratto E. Effects of ace inhibitors on long-term outcome of renal transplant recipients: a randomized controlled trial. Transplantation. 2013;95(6):889–95.
157. Amer H, Fidler ME, Myslak M, Morales P, Kremers WK, Larson TS, Stegall MD, Cosio FG. Proteinuria after kidney transplantation, relationship to allograft histology and survival. Am J Transplant. 2007;7:2748–56.
158. Roodnat JI, Mulder PG, Rischen-Vos J, van Riemsdijk IC, van Gelder T, Zietse R, JN IJ, Weimar W. Proteinuria after renal transplantation affects not only graft survival but also patient survival. Transplantation. 2001;72:438–44.
159. Heinze G, Mitterbauer C, Regele H, Kramar R, Winkelmayer WC, Curhan GC, Oberbauer R. Angiotensin-converting enzyme inhibitor or angiotensin II type 1 receptor antagonist therapy is associated with prolonged patient and graft survival after renal transplantation. J Am Soc Nephrol. 2006;17:889–99.
160. Hernández D, Muriel A, Abraira V, Pérez G, Porrini E, Marrero D, Zamora J, González-Posada JM, Delgado P, Rufino M, Torres A. Renin–angiotensin system blockade and kidney transplantation: a longitudinal cohort study. Nephrol Dial Transplant. 2012;27: 417–22.
161. Opelz G, Zeier M, Laux G, Morath C, Dohler B. No improvement of patient or graft survival in transplant recipients treated with angiotensin-converting enzyme inhibitors or angiotensin II type 1 receptor blockers: a collaborative transplant study report. J Am Soc Nephrol. 2006;17:3257–62.
162. Pazik J, Ostrowska J, Lewandowski Z, Mroz A, Perkowska-Ptasinska A, Baczkowska T, Durlik M. Renin-angiotensin-aldosterone system inhibitors and statins prolong graft survival in post-transplant glomerulonephritis. Ann Transplant. 2008; 13:41–5.
163. Artz MA, Hilbrands LB, Borm G, Assmann KJ, Wetzels JF. Blockade of the renin-angiotensin system increases graft survival in patients with chronic allograft nephropathy. Nephrol Dial Transplant. 2004;19:2852–7.
164. Knoll GA, Cantarovitch M, Cole E, Gill J, Gourishankar S, Holland D, Kiberd B, Muirhead N, Prasad R, Tibbles LA, Treleaven D, Fergusson D. The Canadian ACE-inhibitor trial to improve renal outcomes and patient survival in kidney transplantation–study design. Nephrol Dial Transplant. 2008;23:354–8.
165. Yusuf S, Sleight P, Pogue J, Bosch J, Davies R, Dagenais G. Effects of an angiotensin-converting-enzyme inhibitor, ramipril, on cardiovascular events in high-risk patients. The Heart Outcomes Prevention Evaluation Study Investigators. N Engl J Med. 2000;342:145–53.
166. Paoletti E, Cassottana P, Amidone M, Gherzi M, Rolla D, Cannella G. Ace inhibitors and persistent left ventricular hypertrophy after renal transplantation: a randomized clinical trial. Am J Kidney Dis. 2007;50:133–42.
167. Curtis JJ, Laskow DA, Jones PA, Julian BA, Gaston RS, Luke RG. Captopril-induced fall in glomerular filtration rate in cyclosporine-treated hypertensive patients. J Am Soc Nephrol. 1993;3:1570–4.
168. Gaston RS, Kasiske BL, Fieberg AM, Leduc R, Cosio FC, Gourishankar S, Halloran P, Hunsicker L, Rush D, Matas AJ. Use of cardioprotective medications in kidney transplant recipients. Am J Transplant. 2009;9:1811–5.
169. Thilly N, Bayat S, Alla F, Kessler M, Briancon S, Frimat L. Determinants and patterns of renin-angiotensin system inhibitors' prescription in the first year following kidney transplantation. Clin Transplant. 2008;22:439–46.
170. Lorenz M, Billensteiner E, Bodingbauer M, Oberbauer R, Horl WH, Haas M. The effect of ace inhibitor and angiotensin II blocker therapy on early posttransplant kidney graft function. Am J Kidney Dis. 2004;43:1065–70.
171. Heinze G, Collins S, Benedict MA, Nguyen LL, Kramar R, Winkelmayer WC, Haas M, Kainz A, Oberbauer R. The association between angiotensin converting enzyme inhibitor or angiotensin receptor blocker use during postischemic acute transplant failure and renal allograft survival. Transplantation. 2006; 82:1441–8.
172. Mitterbauer C, Heinze G, Kainz A, Kramar R, Horl WH, Oberbauer R. ACE-inhibitor or AT2-antagonist therapy of renal transplant recipients is associated with an increase in serum potassium concentrations. Nephrol Dial Transplant. 2008;23:1742–6.
173. Stigant CE, Cohen J, Vivera M, Zaltzman JS. Ace inhibitors and angiotensin ii antagonists in renal transplantation: an analysis of safety and efficacy. Am J Kidney Dis. 2000;35:58–63.
174. Velazquez H. Thiazide diuretics. Ren Physiol. 1987;10:184–97.
175. de Souza F, Muxfeldt E, Fiszman R, Salles G. Efficacy of spironolactone therapy in patients with true resistant hypertension. Hypertension. 2010;55:147–52.
176. Gross E, Rothstein M, Dombek S, Juknis HI. Effect of spironolactone on blood pressure and the renin-angiotensin-aldosterone system in oligo-anuric hemodialysis patients. Am J Kidney Dis. 2005;46:94–101.
177. Lopes R, Lourenco P, Mascarenhas J, Azevedo A, Bettencourt P. Spironolactone therapy in heart failure patients with chronic kidney disease. Clin Cardiol. 2009;32:597.
178. Mehdi UF, Adams-Huet B, Raskin P, Vega GL, Toto RD. Addition of angiotensin receptor blockade or mineralocorticoid antagonism to maximal angiotensin-converting enzyme inhibition in diabetic nephropathy. J Am Soc Nephrol. 2009;20:2641–50.
179. Pitt B, Zannad F, Remme WJ, Cody R, Castaigne A, Perez A, Palensky J, Wittes J. The effect of spironolactone on morbidity and mortality in patients with severe heart failure. Randomized Aldactone Evaluation Study Investigators. N Engl J Med. 1999;341:709–17.
180. Papadimitriou M, Vyzantiadis A, Milionis A, Memmos D, Metaxas P. The effect of spironolactone in hypertensive patients on regular haemodialysis and after renal allotransplantation. Life Support Syst. 1983;1:197–205.
181. Waanders F, Rienstra H, Boer MW, Zandvoort A, Rozing J, Navis G, van Goor H, Hillebrands J-L. Spironolactone ameliorates transplant vasculopathy in renal chronic transplant dysfunction in rats. Am J Physiol Renal Physiol. 2009;296:F1072–9.
182. Feria I, Pichardo I, Juarez P, Ramirez V, Gonzalez MA, Uribe N, Garcia-Torres R, Lopez-Casillas F, Gamba G, Bobadilla NA. Therapeutic benefit of spironolactone in experimental chronic cyclosporine a nephrotoxicity. Kidney Int. 2003;63:43–52.
183. Perez-Rojas J, Blanco JA, Cruz C, Trujillo J, Vaidya VS, Uribe N, Bonventre JV, Gamba G, Bobadilla NA. Mineralocorticoid receptor blockade confers renoprotection in preexisting chronic cyclosporine nephrotoxicity. Am J Physiol Renal Physiol. 2007;292:F131–9.
184. Perez-Rojas JM, Derive S, Blanco JA, Cruz C, de la Maza LM, Gamba G, Bobadilla NA. Renocortical mRNA expression of vasoactive factors during spironolactone protective effect in chronic cyclosporine nephrotoxicity. Am J Physiol Renal Physiol. 2005; 289:F1020–30.

Evaluation and Management of Transplant-Associated Hyperglycemia

21

Roy D. Bloom and Charles Moussallem

Terminology

In addition to those terms introduced above, multiple terms (post-transplant diabetes mellitus (PTDM); new onset diabetes mellitus (NODM); glucose metabolic alterations (GMA); new onset hyperglycemia after transplantation (NOHAT)) have been proposed to describe abnormal glycemic homeostasis in the transplant recipient. Some of this terminology has been confusing in the past due to overlap in the spectrum of glycemic abnormalities they cover. For example, several studies have considered PTDM to reflect any patient that has diabetes after transplantation regardless of whether it predated or only developed after the transplant. Consequently, this term has limited the ability to compare studies that evaluate the impact this disease has on the transplant population and health care resources.

The most contemporary term used in recent consensus guidelines issued by the transplant work group of the Kidney Disease Initiative for Global Outcomes (KDIGO) is NODAT, defined in accordance with either the World Health Organization or American Diabetes Association (ADA) criteria, except specifically referring to kidney transplant recipients [1]. Because this does not cover the prediabetic states, IFG and IGT, also risk factors for cardiovascular disease, we prefer the term transplant-associated hyperglycemia since it is more all encompassing (Fig. 21.1). Further, the fact that the incidence of newly occurring glucose elevation is highest in the first few post-transplant months underscores the *association* between exposures specific to *transplant* and the development of *hyperglycemia*.

R.D. Bloom, M.D. (✉) • C. Moussallem, M.D.
Renal-Electrolyte Division, Department of Medicine,
Perelman School of Medicine, University of Pennsylvania,
One Founders Pavilion, 3400 Spruce Street, Philadelphia,
PA 19104, USA
e-mail: rdbloom@mail.med.upenn.edu

Diagnostic Considerations

While both the World Health Organization and ADA definitions are accepted, we prefer the ADA based on a slightly higher level of stringency regarding IFG (Table 21.1). Utilizing this classification to its maximal extent requires the use of oral glucose tolerance testing (OGTT) which should ideally include both pre- and post-transplant testing. In the early post-transplant period, interpretation of this test may be confounded by hyperglycemia persisting up to 9 h after administration of high-dose steroids [2]. Yates and colleagues have recently proposed the use of hemoglobin A1C (HgbA1C) as an alternative diagnostic test since it can be measured in a non-fasting state, reflects average blood glucose levels over 2–3 months, and correlates well with development of microvascular complications in non-transplant diabetes [3].

While HgbA1C is more biologically stable and has less variability than plasma glucose, it may not be universally available and levels may be affected by the effects of uremia, blood transfusions, erythrocyte-stimulating agent administration, and hemolysis, all factors frequently observed in the perioperative period until the hematocrit stabilizes. A Norwegian study of 929 kidney recipients with nondiabetic FBG at 10 weeks post-transplant found that the combined criterion of fasting blood glucose >90 mg/dL and HgbA1C ≥5.7 % provided a sensitivity of 79 %, from testing only 29 % of the post-transplant population [4]. The KDIGO Guidelines recommend diabetes screening intervals after transplantation as follows: weekly for first 4 weeks; months 3, 6, and 12; and annually after the first year [1].

Incidence and Prevalence

Estimation of the cumulative incidence of TAH depends on the population studied and the surveillance method used. The US registry data analysis suggests that 15 % of kidney

M.R. Weir and E.V. Lerma (eds.), *Kidney Transplantation: Practical Guide to Management*,
DOI 10.1007/978-1-4939-0342-9_21, © Springer Science+Business Media New York 2014

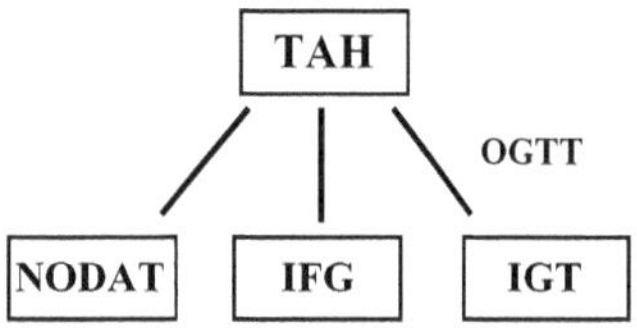

Fig. 21.1 Components of TAH

Table 21.1 American Diabetes Association classification of diabetes mellitus

Criteria	Normal (mg/dL)	IGT/IFG (mg/dL)	Diabetes (mg/dL)
Random plasma glucose with symptoms (polyuria, polydipsia, weight loss)			≥200
Fasting plasma glucose	<100	100–125	≥126
2-h Oral GTT	<140	140–199	≥200

recipients develop clinically diagnosed NODAT by 1 year after transplantation that increases to around 25 % by the end of the third post-transplant year [5]. Single-center reports that have utilized OGTT routinely before and after transplantation indicate that approximately 8 % of patients on the kidney waiting list had undiagnosed diabetes, while at least another one-third had either undiagnosed IFG or IGT [6]. After transplant, in *addition* to kidney recipients classified as having NODAT, the prediabetic states are present in 30–45 % of kidney recipients by 1 year [7]. Sharif and colleagues reported that among 122 patients with fasting plasma glucose 93–125 mg/dL tested by OGTT a median of 5 years post-transplant, over 50 % of patients had TAH, with 10 % meeting criteria for overt NODAT [8]. Evidence from both a meta-analysis and prospective clinical trials confirms that TAH occurs in a substantial proportion of transplant recipients and should be a major cause for concern [9–11].

Transient Versus Persistent TAH

Although reported surprisingly infrequently, transient NODAT in the perioperative phase is a well-recognized post-transplant complication [12]. Accounting for about one-third of NODAT, the transient form is commonly attributed to high steroid dosing and tends to reverse as the glucocorticoid dose diminishes. In a study by Kiberd and colleagues, most transient NODAT developed within the first post-transplant month and had resolved by 12 months after transplant [12]. Most studies suggest that transient NODAT is associated with similar outcomes to nondiabetic recipients unlike in patients that have persistent NODAT where there is an increased risk of cardiovascular adverse events.

Impact of TAH on Outcomes

NODAT is associated with an elevated risk for death, similar to that seen in patients in the general population afflicted with diabetes [5]. Part of the excess mortality in recipients with NODAT may be attributed to infectious complication; however, several studies have now linked NODAT to increased cardiovascular risk as well [5, 13, 14]. Post-transplant follow-up in these studies ranged between 3 and 5 years. Although atherogenesis attributable to hyperglycemia would be expected to develop over a much longer time frame, these previously nondiabetic CKD patients have had a significant cardiovascular risk factor burden for many years.

Hyperglycemia may therefore alter the quantity or quality of established atherosclerosis over a short time frame to promote vascular events. However, it is possible that hyperglycemia per se is not directly responsible for increased cardiovascular disease in patients with NODAT. Rather, NODAT may represent a surrogate of systemic inflammation occurring in a dysregulated post-transplant metabolic milieu characterized not just by abnormal glucose homeostasis but also by deterioration in the lipid profile, higher BP, and elevated inflammatory markers. Even after multivariable adjustment for these other factors, however, Ducloux and co-investigators demonstrated that TAH remains an independent risk factor for cardiovascular events [14]. In a single-center study with similarly detailed information about the metabolic profile of kidney transplant recipients, Cosio et al. reported an adjusted hazard ratio for mortality of 1.80 ($P<0.01$) associated with NODAT [15].

A recent prospective observational study in 1,410 patients investigated the predictive value of a 10-week post-transplant OGTT on the outcomes of kidney recipients with TAH [16]. With a median 6.7 years of follow-up, NODAT was associated with a 1.8-fold increase in cardiovascular mortality and a 1.5-fold increase in overall mortality. Considering the prediabetic states only, IFG was not linked to mortality, while IGT was associated with a 1.4-fold increased death risk, attributable to infection rather than cardiovascular mortality. The increasingly recognized negative impact of NODAT on graft survival is further fuelled in a US registry data study that suggested that for many patients with this complication, mortality becomes an important competing outcome, to the extent that TAH makes it more likely that a patient will die before the allograft fails [17].

Besides the adverse influence of TAH on clinical outcomes, it is widely appreciated that glucose dysregulation after transplant carries with it a substantial economic burden as well. Woodward et al. examined the United States Renal Data System's records for kidney recipients transplanted between 1996 and 1997 and found that by 2 years post-transplant there was an additional $21,500 of cost associated with each patient with NODAT [18]. Because this study relied on Medicare claims data to ascertain a diagnosis of NODAT, it is likely that there was bias towards the affected population having more complicated disease. Therefore, patients with milder forms of NODAT or transient NODAT requiring less intensive treatment may not have been included in the analysis, thereby potentially overestimating the true cost per affected patient.

However, since the publication of this above economic analysis, it is plausible that the effect of recent guidelines and adoption of more stringent diagnostic criteria for TAH may have resulted in greater attention being paid to blood glucose measurement in the perioperative period, thereby leading to fewer readmissions for poorly controlled hyperglycemia. However, it remains to be determined whether this is indeed the case and if so, whether any realized cost saving has been offset by greater expense associated with increased vigilance in glucose management, e.g., use of glucose-lowering therapies, glucose monitoring devices, diabetologist consultation, and education.

The Metabolic Syndrome and Transplant-Associated Hyperglycemia

The metabolic syndrome comprises a constellation of modifiable cardiovascular risk factors that cluster together sharing systemic insulin resistance as a root cause. Metabolic syndrome predisposes to systemic inflammation and cardiovascular disease, while its components (hyperglycemia, hypertension, dyslipidemia, central obesity) are risk factors for progressive kidney disease. Following kidney transplantation, the prevalence of metabolic syndrome increases in conjunction with weight gain [19]. A single-center investigation has shown that, together with obesity, metabolic syndrome is associated with NODAT, as well as inferior patient and graft outcomes [20]. More recently, the multicenter, multinational prospective observational Patient Outcomes in Renal Transplantation (PORT) study comprising 2,253 patients extended these earlier single-center findings by demonstrating that metabolic syndrome was independently associated with subsequent risk of NODAT (hazard ratio 3.46, 95 % CI (2.40–4.98), $p<0.001$) [21]. Examining data from another multicenter observational cohort, Rosas et al. reported that by 1 year post-transplant, there was an incremental growth in the prevalence of NODAT as the number of metabolic syndrome components increased (prevalence at 1 year: 1 component: 24.2 %, 2 components: 29.3 %, 3 components: 31 %, 4 components: 34.8 %, 5 components; $P=0.01$) [22]. We therefore recommend that screening for diabetes and the metabolic syndrome be conducted in concert. It follows that identification, and treatment, of metabolic syndrome in transplant recipients is central to optimizing post-transplant care. While intervention to correct individual components of the metabolic syndrome will be beneficial, recognition of the central pathogenic role of insulin resistance should guide aggressive lifestyle intervention and stimulate clinical investigation of pharmacologic efforts to promote insulin sensitivity and weight loss in the transplant population.

Pathogenesis and Risk Factors

Although the pathogenesis of TAH has similarities with development of hyperglycemia in the general population, kidney recipients have additional distinct pathophysiological mechanisms related to the concomitant generic and transplant-specific risk factors. Glycemic homeostasis is reached by achieving equilibrium between insulin production and bodily needs of insulin. Imbalances arise when pancreatic beta-islet cell insulin production decreases, and insulin need increases or in states of insulin resistance. An extensive literature on TAH has illuminated the many risk factors for development of TAH.

Preexisting risks that predispose individuals to NODAT include increasing age, obesity, male gender, non-Caucasian race, and a family history of diabetes. These traditionally non-modifiable characteristics reflect inherited and acquired defects in insulin sensitivity and β-cell function that contribute to glucose dysregulation. The high incidence of TAH in the months following transplantation reflects superimposition of new, transplant-specific factors on the baseline metabolic milieu of predisposed individuals. The best-elucidated transplant-specific exposures include immunosuppressive agents such as glucocorticoids, calcineurin inhibitors (CNIs) and sirolimus, post-transplant weight gain, and hepatitis C virus (HCV) infection.

Immunosuppression and Transplant-Associated Hyperglycemia

Glucocorticoids

Glucocorticoids impact glucose metabolism by enhancing glucose production in the liver and by reducing peripheral tissue insulin sensitivity. Prior to the introduction of CNIs into the clinical arena, heavy reliance on corticosteroid-based immunosuppression resulted in high rates of NODAT. The supraphysiologic glucocorticoid doses used in early post-transplant induction regimens strongly contribute to very early post-transplant hyperglycemia that may normalize thereafter once steroids are either withdrawn or tapered into the physiologic range.

Calcineurin Inhibitors

The CNIs, tacrolimus and cyclosporine, are strongly associated with development of TAH. Mechanistic clinical and basic science studies demonstrate the critical role of calcineurin in β-cell growth and function. CNIs impair β-cell function by diminishing insulin gene expression, thereby predisposing to TAH [23]. CNIs, especially tacrolimus in the contemporary era, form the foundation of most maintenance immunosuppressive regimens. Most efficacy studies comparing cyclosporine and tacrolimus in kidney recipients have demonstrated higher TAH risk with the latter therapy. The DIRECT trial, a randomized, prospective, multicenter study that compared cyclosporine to tacrolimus, was unique in that the composite of NODAT and IFG within the first six post-transplant months was the primary safety endpoint analyzed [10]. Through the use of sequential OGTT, the study demonstrated rates of abnormal glucose homeostasis of 26 and 33.6 % in cyclosporine- and tacrolimus-treated patients, respectively, with no efficacy difference between the two drugs. NODAT was more frequently transient among cyclosporine- than tacrolimus-treated recipients. The lack of standardization of steroid dosage, open-label design, and enrolment predominantly of Caucasian patients limits generalizability of this study to other populations from either an efficacy or adverse events standpoint. Early clinical studies have more recently indicated that voclosporin, an emerging CNI still in development, has similar efficacy to tacrolimus, but is less diabetogenic [24]. Regardless, studies confirm that CNIs promote TAH and implicate impaired insulin secretion as the etiology.

Target of Rapamycin Inhibitors

The target of rapamycin (TOR) inhibitors, sirolimus and everolimus, inhibit the mammalian target of rapamycin, a widely expressed cellular kinase that mediates cytokine-induced lymphocyte proliferation. Sirolimus, for which there is far more clinical experience, impairs insulin-mediated suppression of hepatic glucose production, causes insulin resistance as a result of ectopic triglyceride deposition, and may exhibit direct β-cell toxicity [25, 26]. In clinical studies, sirolimus in combination with CNI has been associated with higher rates of diabetes than with the CNI alone and use of sirolimus in CNI-elimination regimens has resulted in diminished insulin sensitivity and increased insulin resistance [27, 28]. A recent safety analysis from a randomized controlled trial with everolimus and cyclosporine combination therapy demonstrated a direct relationship between rates of NODAT and increasing everolimus trough concentrations. Thus, although TOR inhibitors are potential therapeutic alternatives to CNIs, their use is unlikely to diminish the incidence of TAH.

Other Immunosuppressive Agents

Other than as isolated reports, the remaining immunosuppressive agents typically used in transplantation have not been associated with NODAT. This includes the antiproliferative agents, mycophenolate mofetil, mycophenolic acid and azathioprine, as well as belatacept.

Obesity

Almost two-thirds of kidney transplant candidates are overweight or obese at the time of transplantation. Shah and colleagues followed patients followed over a mean of 306 days post-transplant and found that the risk of NODAT increased 1.5-fold for overweight and almost twofold for obese individuals [29]. As the optimal criteria for characterizing obesity risk evolve, there is increasing recognition in the general population of the stronger relationship between central obesity, reflected by waist circumference and waist/hip ratio, and cardiovascular disease, rather than traditional BMI measures. To date, one prospective study has extended this observation to kidney transplant recipients as well, where waist circumference was directly related to, while BMI had an inverse association with, all-cause mortality [30].

HCV Infection

Epidemiological studies have strongly associated HCV infection and hyperglycemia in the general population though the pathogenic mechanisms remain to be completely elucidated. Potential mechanisms include increased insulin resistance due to a post-receptor signaling defect induced by HCV infection, diminished hepatic glucose uptake and glycogenesis, as well as a direct cytopathic effect of the virus on β-cells in the pancreas. Growing evidence suggests that a predominant effect of the virus is the induction of insulin resistance and reduced insulin sensitivity, an effect that has been demonstrated in HCV-infected clinically stable kidney transplant recipients [31].

It is likely through this mechanism that HCV infection has also been linked to NODAT in kidney recipients. In one registry study, HCV infection was associated with a 33 % increase in the risk of NODAT [5], while another single-center investigation indicated that the NODAT rate was 40 % among HCV-infected recipients compared to 10 % in uninfected patients [32]. Most of this effect was due to an elevated risk of NODAT among HCV-infected patients treated with tacrolimus. Whether this propensity to NODAT represents exposure to concomitant diabetogenic insults of HCV and tacrolimus versus a more permissive effect of tacrolimus on HCV replication is presently unknown. Taken together, these studies demonstrate that HCV infection predisposes patients to NODAT and that the choice of CNI may have important modifying effects on that risk. Since viral clearance may improve glucose tolerance [33], HCV infection may represent a modifiable risk factor for TAH.

Restoration of Renal Insulin Metabolism

Increased insulin metabolism that occurs concomitantly with restoration of kidney function is an uncommonly cited, but potentially important contributor to TAH. Healthy kidneys contribute significantly to insulin degradation, an effect that is underscored by the marked renal arteriovenous decrease in insulin concentration and the decreased insulin requirements observed clinically as kidney disease progresses in patients with diabetes. Therefore, a functioning kidney transplant unmasks restored insulin metabolism representing is an important, non-modifiable factor that increases post-transplant insulin requirements.

Genetic Polymorphism

Multiple studies have demonstrated that genetic polymorphisms may predispose to diabetes by likely mechanism of apoptosis and beta-cell dysfunction, a key perturbation involved in NODAT pathogenesis. Using a cohort of 306 kidney transplant recipients with no known diabetes mellitus prior to transplant, Kim et al. analyzed a panel of 18 single nucleotide peptides (SNP) within ten genes of the interleukins or their receptors; 53 patients developed NODAT and 11 SNPs were significantly associated with NODAT (IL-7R, IL-17E, IL-17R, and IL-17RB) [34]. Other identified gene polymorphisms associated with NODAT include KNNJ11, a gene leading to impaired β-cell insulin release, and NFATc4.

Other studies have also reported an association between NODAT and specific genes (transcription factor 7-like 2 (TCF7L2), member 8 genes, chemokine ligand 5 gene (CCL5), and vitamin D receptor, KNNJ11).

Further investigations that corroborate and then expand these findings are needed before this technology can be widely utilized in clinical practice. The potential to identify at-risk patients beforehand in order to provide necessary lifestyle modification counseling and to tailor immunosuppression to reduce the risk of NODAT would represent an appealing and substantive advancement to the field.

Detection and Management of NODAT

Detecting and adjusting modifiable risk factors to prevent or minimize the development of TAH is a desirable objective in this patient population. Efforts to accomplish this goal should be initiated in the pre-transplant phase and continue through the early and later post-transplant phases.

Pre-transplant

Identifying at-risk patients in the pre-transplant period may provide the opportunity to actively encourage patient-centered interventions that mitigate later NODAT risk and to facilitate the development of less-diabetogenic immunosuppressive regimens. During this phase, management should focus on risk factor screening (especially for metabolic syndrome and cardiovascular disease), establishing baseline glycemic regulation by checking FPG and 2-h OGTT, counseling and lifestyle modification as well as dietitian referrals as needed. A potential role for bariatric surgery in this setting has not been formally evaluated; however, besides the need to ascertain effectiveness of this treatment for preventing or treating diabetes in this population, an examination of the impact of this surgery on immunosuppressive drug pharmacokinetics and efficacy would be imperative.

For HCV-infected kidney transplant candidates, the induction of a sustained virologic response before transplant is highly desirable. Although interferon may improve glucose tolerance in HCV-infected patients without kidney disease [33], the use of this antiviral therapy is contraindicated after kidney transplantation because of unacceptable rejection risk. However, preliminary evidence suggests that induction of a pre-transplant sustained virologic response by treatment with interferon usually persists after transplantation and may be associated with a reduced incidence of NODAT [35, 36]. Whether the emergence of the new classes of antiviral therapies will supersede the need for pre-transplant interferon remains to be determined.

Immediate Post-transplant

Severe hyperglycemia, requiring high-dose insulin, is common in the immediate postoperative phase due to a combination of factors including surgical stress, medications especially glucocorticoids, and restored insulin metabolism. Timely glycemic control is important to limit postoperative morbidity and complications and per our own center's practice, we recommend liberal consultation with a diabetology service. Fasting and postprandial glucose concentrations should be routinely and closely monitored until corticosteroids have either been withdrawn or tapered to an equivalent of 5 mg of prednisone/day, and the recipient demonstrates euglycemia while eating a full diet. Blood sugars should be checked multiple times during the day (goals are between 90 and 130 mg/dL fasting and less than 180 mg/dL postprandial).

In a recent very interesting randomized controlled trial, Hecking et al. investigated the effect of an aggressive basal insulin regimen, initiated very early post-transplant for blood sugar levels >140 mg/dL, on longer-term glycemic regulation [37]. They demonstrated that recipients treated in this way had a significantly lower HgbA1C concentrations and a 73 % lower odds of developing long-term NODAT than control recipients treated with insulin and/or oral anti-diabetic agents initiated only once blood sugars were consistently in the 180–250 mg/dL range. By the end of the first post-transplant year, all early basal insulin-treated patients were insulin independent whereas 28 % of the control cohort required specific glucose-lowering therapy. The authors attributed this beneficial effect to insulin-mediated pancreatic beta-islet cells protection though further studies are underway to more clearly elucidate the mechanism.

Long-Term Post-transplant

Periodic diabetes screening post-transplant should be done routinely with decreasing frequency as time after transplant increases. International consensus guidelines propose checking FPG weekly for the first month post-transplant with an FPG and then at 3, 6, and 12 months followed by annual surveillance. Many other authors have suggested more frequent screening as well as OGTT screening at 3–6 months post-transplant and then annually. This was supported by an observational study that found OGTT to be more sensitive than FPG for diagnosing NODAT and IGT. After diagnosis of NODAT, treatment should be started to target a fasting glucose of 90–130 mg/dL, a 2-h postprandial BS of <180 mg/dL, and an HbA1C of 7–7.5 %. While HgbA1C <7 % is considered to be reasonable for the majority of diabetic patients in the general population, KDIGO guidelines have opined that the higher target is preferable for transplant patients because of the risks of severe hypoglycemia with more intensive glucose control in this population [1].

The main treatment alternatives after diagnosis of NODAT consist of lifestyle modification, immunosuppression modification, and antidiabetic therapy.

Lifestyle modification: Although seemingly intuitive, data supporting lifestyle modification in this population is quite sparse. One small, single-center, prospective, randomized trial showed that aggressive lifestyle modification improved glycemic control in kidney recipients with NODAT, with resolution of frank diabetes in 4 of 7 patients [38]. In general, appropriate medical nutrition therapy consists of moderate overall carbohydrate intake (130–180 g/day) and calorie reduction along with physical exercise to promote weight loss thus increasing insulin sensitivity.

Immunosuppression modification: Titrating immunosuppression to achieve an optimal balance of efficacy and side effects is an obvious and necessary step when trying to prevent or treat TAH. This can be achieved through minimization, withdrawal, or conversion of potentially diabetogenic immunosuppressive agents.

To limit glucocorticoid-related complications such as hyperglycemia, the use of both steroid avoidance and early withdrawal regimens has been widely embraced by many transplant centers. Current national registry data indicates that glucocorticoids are either completely avoided or withdrawn early post-transplant in about 40 % of new kidney recipients. Multiple uncontrolled or retrospective investigations have suggested that early glucocorticoid withdrawal does not jeopardize allograft or patient outcomes. However, a large, multicenter, randomized, double-blinded, controlled trial demonstrated that early steroid withdrawal under tacrolimus-based maintenance immunosuppression was associated with an increased risk of acute rejection and did not lead to lower rates of NODAT by 5 years post-transplantation [11]. Another prospective study that incorporated protocol kidney biopsy at one year post-transplant demonstrated increased fibrosis in the patients that underwent early steroid withdrawal [39].

Whether elimination of low-dose glucocorticoids (5-mg/day prednisone or equivalent) after chronic use improves glucose metabolism remains a subject of controversy [40, 41]. Using euglycemic, hyperinsulinemic clamp testing, Midvedt examined the impact of prednisolone dose reduction and withdrawal on insulin sensitivity, finding that dose reduction in the supraphysiological range (16 mg/day to 9 mg/day) resulted in a 24 % improvement in insulin sensitivity, while withdrawal of 5 mg/day had no effect [42]. Overall, available studies suggest that, while early steroid withdrawal is safe in many patients in the short to mid-term, it may not be suitable for all patient populations and may not substantially impact long-term glucose metabolism. Based on the above data, our own practice is to rapidly taper the glucocorticoid over 3–4 weeks post-transplant to a minimal maintenance dose below daily physiological requirements, e.g., prednisone 5 mg/day.

The widespread adoption of tacrolimus as the CNI of choice over the past decade has contributed to continued increases in rates of TAH. The reduced diabetogenicity associated with cyclosporine does raise the possibility that conversion to this CNI in tacrolimus-treated patients with NODAT could successfully eliminate hyperglycemia. While supported by small series and anecdotes, this approach is not yet validated in large trials. This practice has to further be balanced against the superior lipid, blood pressure, and kidney function profile observed with tacrolimus as compared to cyclosporine. On the other hand, the routine use of either induction therapy with rabbit antithymocyte globulin or basiliximab or maintenance with antimetabolites allows minimization (as opposed to avoidance) of CNI, thereby leading to lower rates of NODAT compared to CNI alone [43]. It remains to be confirmed whether investigational agents such as voclosporin, an alternative CNI, or the JAK-2 inhibitors will be associated with lower rates of TAH compared to current treatment standards. For future therapies to

Table 21.2 Non-insulin drug treatment options for NODAT

Class	Principle mechanism of action	Example	Side effects	Metabolism/elimination	Altered dosing in CKD
Sulfonylureas	Insulin secretagogue	Glipizide Glyburide Glimepiride	Hypoglycemia	Hepatic	No
Meglitinides	Insulin secretagogue	Repaglinide Nateglinide	Hypoglycemia	CYP2C8/3A4	Yes
Biguanides	↓ Hepatic glucose production	Metformin	Nausea, lactic acidosis	Renal tubular secretion	Yes
TZDs	↑ Insulin sensitivity	Pioglitazone Rosiglitazone	Weight gain, fluid retention	CYP2C8 CYP3A4	No
α-Glucosidase inhibitors	↓ Intestinal glucose absorption	Acarbose	Nausea, flatulence	Major fecal Minor renal	Yes
GLP-1 receptor agonists	(i) ↑ Glucose-mediated insulin secretion (ii) ↓ Glucagon (iii) Weight loss	Exenatide	Nausea, other GI	Major renal	Yes
DPP-4 Inhibitors	↑ GLP-1	Sitagliptin	Minimal	Renal CYP3A4, 2C8	Yes

significantly impact on clinical practice, a more favorable side effect profile including less diabetogenicity, in addition to meeting the high efficacy bar of currently approved treatments, is a prerogative.

Specific glucose-lowering therapies: While insulin is usually the best treatment option for acute hyperglycemia, diabetes-specific agents may be appropriate to use on a longer-term basis in settings where lifestyle and immunosuppression modification alone have failed to correct hyperglycemia. The choice of therapy may be influenced by the circumstances in which hyperglycemia occurred (timing, severity), patient characteristics (weight, immunosuppressive regimen, kidney and liver function, etc.) as well as drug-specific information such as safety, efficacy, potential for interaction, and cost (Table 21.2). Careful monitoring of fasting plasma glucose and potential side effects after initiation or modification of therapy should be carried out. Once specific glucose-lowering therapies are required, we recommend collaborative management with a diabetologist given the ongoing emergence of novel agents with new indications and mechanisms of action.

Although most of the data regarding oral glucose-lowering therapies is anecdotal and limited by observational and/or retrospective methodology, recent years have witnessed the emergence of novel therapies with NODAT-treating potential. The thiazolidinediones promote peripheral insulin sensitivity, enhance pancreatic β-cell function, and exert favorable glucose-independent effects on vascular health, all factors that would favor their use in the kidney transplant population with potential to reduce cardiovascular complications. The currently available thiazolidinediones, rosiglitazone and pioglitazone, have been assessed in NODAT and both appear to be safe and effective, with minimal effect on CNI dosing requirements [44]. Thiazolidinediones have fluid retentive properties and need to be considered in the differential diagnosis of edema in the post-transplant period.

The meglitinides, repaglinide and nateglinide, promote insulin secretion and have lower hypoglycemic potential than sulfonylureas. One observational study has demonstrated that, compared to rosiglitazone, repaglinide had similar effectiveness for treating NODAT and was safe to use in kidney transplant recipients [45].

The final category of glucose-lowering therapies promotes activation of the glucagon-like peptide-1 receptor. The first of these agents, Exenatide, is a subcutaneous injection that lowers fasting and postprandial glucose and promotes weight loss through effects on appetite and gastric emptying. Although not yet formally studied in transplant patients, it appears to have potential. Therapies such as sitagliptin and vildagliptin, dipeptidyl peptidase-4 inhibitors that prevent glucagon-like peptide-1 receptor degradation, have also been developed. The safety and efficacy of these agents have recently been shown in short-term pilot studies [46, 47]. In the sitagliptin investigation, conducted in patients with NODAT, the HgbA1C was lowered after 3 months and the drug was well tolerated and no significant interaction with tacrolimus or sirolimus was observed. The study with vildagliptin was performed in kidney recipients with IGT determined by OGTT, and patients were randomized to one of vildagliptin, a thiazolidinedione, or placebo. After 3 months of follow-up, HgbA1C levels and 2-h glucose levels were lower in the two treatment arms than the placebo group. Whether this biochemical benefit will translate into longer-term clinical benefit remains to be established.

Of the more traditional oral agents used for type 2 diabetes mellitus, metformin, a biguanide that promotes insulin sensitization and reduces hepatic glucose production, has

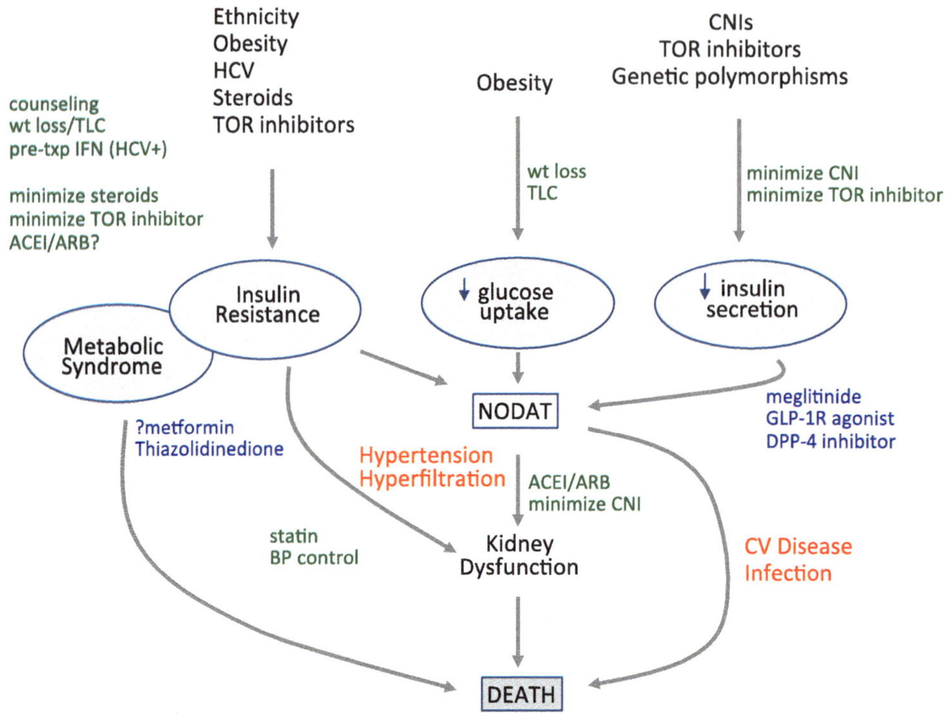

Fig. 21.2 Illustration of the pathogenic mechanisms leading to TAH in kidney recipients. *Red* and *black text* represents disease mechanisms; *blue text* represents potential glucose-lowering therapies targeting specific mechanisms of hyperglycemia; and green text represents other more general therapeutic interventions depicted at sites where their effects may be optimally mediated. *CNI* calcineurin inhibitor, *TOR* target of rapamycin, *HCV* hepatitis C virus, *GLP-1R* glucagon-like peptide-1 receptor, *DPP-4* dipeptidyl peptidase-4, *IFN* interferon, *TLC* therapeutic lifestyle change

remained the most controversial in the kidney transplant arena. Metformin is largely cleared by renal tubular secretion and its exposure increases in the setting of declining kidney function (Metformin package insert). For this reason and because of its rare association with lactic acidosis, use of metformin in men with serum creatinine levels >1.5 mg/dL (1.4 mg/dL in women) is considered a contraindication by the US Food and Drug Administration (http://www.fda.gov/ohrms/dockets/dailys/02/May02/053102/80047964.pdf) and is not recommended by most transplant guideline and consensus groups [1, 48]. Citing the rarity of reported lactic acidosis as a complication of metformin in this population, Sharif has argued that the infinitesimal risk of harm from the drug is strongly outweighed by potential benefits in kidney recipients and has suggested incorporating measurement of drug levels in cases where there may be concern [49]. To date, a single retrospective series of 24 recipients has reported that metformin could be safely used in a carefully monitored setting [50]. Absent a robust clinical trial with metformin in kidney recipients, it is unlikely that this debate will be adequately laid to rest anytime in the near future.

Statins and Lipid-Lowering Therapy

Because statins improve insulin sensitivity, they might be predicted to reduce TAH in kidney recipients. A 70 % reduction in NODAT prevalence was demonstrated in one retrospective analysis of 300 kidney recipients, though this is yet to be validated. Regardless, statin treatment should be prescribed liberally in the transplant population, where dyslipidemia, metabolic syndrome, and high cardiovascular risk are virtually endemic problems. The ALERT study, an underpowered primary intervention randomized controlled trial that evaluated fluvastatin in "relatively low-risk" kidney recipients demonstrated a reduction in major adverse cardiovascular events in statin-treated patients [51]. Since statin bioavailability is markedly elevated by cyclosporine, but not tacrolimus, we recommend that starting doses of this lipid-lowering class of drugs should be lower in transplant patients being treated with cyclosporine maintenance therapy with cautious up-titration.

Renin–Angiotensin System Blockade

A recent meta-analysis of ten large studies, five conducted with angiotensin-converting enzyme inhibitors and five with angiotensin receptor blockers, found that the use of renin–angiotensin system blockade was consistently associated with a reduction in the incidence of diabetes. This finding has not yet been validated either in transplant recipients or in prospective trials in the general population. However, given the potential cardiac, blood pressure-lowering, and renoprotective benefits of these drug classes, we would advocate an extremely low threshold for considering their use.

Conclusion

As the great kidney transplant experiment has evolved into a mature clinical science, TAH has, in contradistinction to other major post-transplant complications such as rejection and opportunistic infection, become an increasingly common and important obstacle to optimal patient and allograft outcomes.

This has been fuelled, in part, by increasingly stringent diagnostic criteria as well as the recognition that the prediabetic states, IFG and IGT, highly prevalent in kidney recipients, bode ominously for cardiovascular disease risk, likely by virtue of their relationship to insulin resistance and the metabolic syndrome. The pathogenic mechanisms linking risk factors for TAH to graft dysfunction and death in kidney recipients are becoming clearer, providing a more rational basis for selecting therapies (Fig. 21.2). Clinical investigation that focuses on the prevention and treatment of TAH with novel strategies and more contemporary agents are emerging, although the impact of these interventions on the clinical endpoints of graft survival, cardiovascular disease, and recipient mortality are not yet established. As the magnitude of the TAH epidemic continues to be progressively inculcated into the consciousness of treating physicians, and as their management philosophies become more proactive, there is a glimmer of hope that kidney recipient outcomes will finally improve.

References

1. Kidney Disease: Improving Global Outcomes (KDIGO) Transplant Work Group. KDIGO clinical practice guidelines for the care of kidney transplant recipients. Am J Transplant. 2009;9 Suppl 3:S1–157.
2. Clore JN, Linda Thurby-Hay L. Glucocorticoid-induced hyperglycemia. Endocr Pract. 2009;15:469–74.
3. Yates CJ, Fourlanos S, Hjelmesæth J, Colman PG, Cohney SJ. New-onset diabetes after kidney transplantation—changes and challenges. Am J Transplant. 2012;12:820–8.
4. Valderhaug TG, Jenssen T, Hartmann A, Midtvedt K, Holdaas H, Reisæter AV, et al. Fasting plasma glucose and glycosylated hemoglobin in the screening for diabetes mellitus after renal transplantation. Transplantation. 2009;88:429–34.
5. Kasiske BL, Snyder JJ, Gilbertson D, Matas AJ. Diabetes mellitus after kidney transplantation in the United States. Am J Transplant. 2003;3:178–85.
6. Bergrem HA, Valderhaug TA, Hartmann A, Hjelmesæth J, Leivestad T, Bergrem H, et al. Undiagnosed diabetes in kidney transplant candidates: a case-finding strategy. Clin J Am Soc Nephrol. 2010;5(4):616–22.
7. Nam JH, Mun JI, Kim SI, Kang SW, Choi KH, Park K, et al. Beta-Cell dysfunction rather than insulin resistance is the main contributing factor for the development of postrenal transplantation diabetes mellitus. Transplantation. 2001;71(10):1417–23.
8. Sharif A, Moore RH, Baboolal K. The use of oral glucose tolerance tests to risk stratify for new-onset diabetes after transplantation: an underdiagnosed phenomenon. Transplantation. 2006; 82(12):1667–72.
9. Montori VM, Basu A, Erwin PJ, Velosa JA, Gabriel SE, Kudva YC. Posttransplantation diabetes: a systematic review of the literature. Diabetes Care. 2002;25(3):583–92.
10. Vincenti F, Friman S, Scheuermann E, Rostaing L, Jenssen T, Campistol JM et al; DIRECT (Diabetes Incidence after Renal Transplantation: Neoral C Monitoring Versus Tacrolimus) Investigators. Results of an international, randomized trial comparing glucose metabolism disorders and outcome with cyclosporine versus tacrolimus. Am J Transplant. 2007;7(6):1506–14.
11. Woodle ES, First MR, Pirsch J, Shihab F, Gaber AO, Van Veldhuisen P. Astellas Corticosteroid Withdrawal Study Group: a prospective, randomized, double-blind, placebo-controlled multicenter trial comparing early (7 day) corticosteroid cessation versus long-term, low-dose corticosteroid therapy. Ann Surg. 2008;248(4):564–77.
12. Kiberd M, Panek R, Kiberd BA. New onset diabetes mellitus post-kidney transplantation. Clin Transplant. 2006;20(5):634–9.
13. Cosio FG, Kudva Y, van der Velde M, Larson TS, Textor SC, Griffin MD, et al. New onset hyperglycemia and diabetes are associated with increased cardiovascular risk after kidney transplantation. Kidney Int. 2005;67(6):2415–21.
14. Ducloux D, Kazory A, Chalopin JM. Posttransplant diabetes mellitus and atherosclerotic events in renal transplant recipients: a prospective study. Transplantation. 2005;79(4):438–43.
15. Cosio FG, Pesavento TE, Kim S, Osei K, Henry M, Ferguson RM. Patient survival after renal transplantation: IV. Impact of post-transplant diabetes. Kidney Int. 2002;62(4):1440–6.
16. Valderhaug TG, Hjelmesæth J, Hartmann A, Røislien J, Bergrem HA, Leivestad T, et al. The association of early post-transplant glucose levels with long-term mortality. Diabetologia. 2011;54(6): 1341–9.
17. Cole EH, Johnston O, Rose CL, Gill JS. Impact of acute rejection and new-onset diabetes on long-term transplant graft and patient survival. Clin J Am Soc Nephrol. 2008;3(3):814–21.
18. Woodward RS, Schnitzler MA, Baty J, Lowell JA, Lopez-Rocafort L, Haider S, et al. Incidence and cost of new onset diabetes mellitus among U.S. wait-listed and transplanted renal allograft recipients. Am J Transplant. 2003;3(5):590–8.
19. Armstrong KA, Campbell SB, Hawley CM, Nicol DL, Johnson DW, Isbel NM. Obesity is associated with worsening cardiovascular risk factor profiles and proteinuria progression in renal transplant recipients. Am J Transplant. 2005;5(11):2710–8.
20. De Vries AP, Bakker SJ, van Son WJ, van der Heide JJ, Ploeg RJ, The HT, et al. Metabolic syndrome is associated with impaired long-term renal allograft function; not all component criteria contribute equally. Am J Transplant. 2004;4(10):1675–83.
21. Israni AK, Snyder JJ, Skeans MA, Kasiske BL, PORT Investigators. Clinical diagnosis of metabolic syndrome: predicting new-onset diabetes, coronary heart disease, and allograft failure late after kidney transplant. Transpl Int. 2012;25(7):748–57.
22. Bayer ND, Cochetti PT, Anil Kumar MS, Teal V, Huan Y, Doria C, et al. Association of metabolic syndrome with development of new-onset diabetes after transplantation. Transplantation. 2010; 90(8):861–6.
23. Redmon JB, Olson LK, Armstrong MB, Greene MJ, Robertson RP. Effects of tacrolimus (FK506) on human insulin gene expression, insulin mRNA levels, and insulin secretion in HIT-T15 cells. J Clin Invest. 1996;98(12):2786–93.
24. Busque S, Cantarovich M, Mulgaonkar S, Gaston R, Gaber AO, Mayo PR, et al. PROMISE Investigators: the PROMISE study: a phase 2b multicenter study of voclosporin (ISA247) versus tacrolimus in de novo kidney transplantation. Am J Transplant. 2011; 11(12):2675–84.
25. Lewis GF, Carpentier A, Adeli K, Giacca A. Disordered fat storage and mobilization in the pathogenesis of insulin resistance and type 2 diabetes. Endocr Rev. 2002;23(2):201–29.
26. Bussiere CT, Lakey JR, Shapiro AM, Korbutt GS. The impact of the mTOR inhibitor sirolimus on the proliferation and function of pancreatic islets and ductal cells. Diabetologia. 2006;49(10):2341–9.
27. Teutonica A, Schena PF, Di Paolo S. Glucose metabolism in renal transplant recipients: effect of calcineurin inhibitor withdrawal and conversion to sirolimus. J Am Soc Nephrol. 2005; 16(10):3128–35.
28. Johnston O, Rose CL, Webster AC, Gill JS. Sirolimus is associated with new-onset diabetes in kidney transplant recipients. J Am Soc Nephrol. 2008;19(7):1411–8.

29. Shah T, Kasravi A, Huang E, Hayashi R, Young B, Cho YW, et al. Risk factors for development of new-onset diabetes mellitus after kidney transplantation. Transplantation. 2006;82(12):1673–6.
30. Kovesdy CP, Czira ME, Rudas A, Ujszaszi A, Rosivall L, Novak M, et al. Body mass index, waist circumference and mortality in kidney transplant recipients. Am J Transplant. 2010;10(12):2644–51.
31. Baid-Agrawal S, Frei U, Reinke P, Schindler R, Kopp MA, Martus P, et al. Impaired insulin sensitivity as an underlying mechanism linking hepatitis C and posttransplant diabetes mellitus in kidney recipients. Am J Transplant. 2009;9(12):2777–84.
32. Bloom RD, Rao V, Weng F, Grossman RA, Cohen D, Mange KC. Association of hepatitis C with posttransplant diabetes in renal transplant patients on tacrolimus. J Am Soc Nephrol. 2002;13(5): 1374–80.
33. Konrad T, Zeuzem S, Vicini P, Toffolo G, Briem D, Lormann J, et al. Evaluation of factors controlling glucose tolerance in patients with HCV infection before and after 4 months therapy with interferon-alpha. Eur J Clin Invest. 2000;30(2):111–21.
34. Kim YG, Ihm CG, Lee TW, Lee SH, Jeong KH, Moon JY, et al. Association of genetic polymorphisms of interleukins with new-onset diabetes after transplantation in renal transplantation. Transplantation. 2012;93(9):900–7.
35. Gursoy M, Koksal R, Karavelioglu D, Colak T, Gur G, Ozdemir N, et al. Pretransplantation alpha-interferon therapy and the effect of hepatitis C virus infection on kidney allograft recipients. Transplant Proc. 2000;32(3):580–2.
36. Kamar N, Toupance O, Buchler M, Sandres-Saune K, Izopet J, Durand D, et al. Evidence that clearance of hepatitis C virus RNA after alpha-interferon therapy in dialysis patients is sustained after renal transplantation. J Am Soc Nephrol. 2003;14(8):2092–8.
37. Hecking M, Haidinger M, Döller D, Werzowa J, Tura A, Zhang J, et al. Early basal insulin therapy decreases new-onset diabetes after renal transplantation. J Am Soc Nephrol. 2012;23(4):739–49.
38. Sharif A, Moore R, Baboolal K. Influence of lifestyle modification in renal transplant recipients with postprandial hyperglycemia. Transplantation. 2008;85(3):353–8.
39. Laftavi MR, Stephan R, Stefanick B, Kohli R, Dagher F, Applegate M, et al. Randomized prospective trial of early steroid withdrawal compared with low-dose steroids in renal transplant recipients using serial protocol biopsies to assess efficacy and safety. Surgery. 2005;137(3):364–71.
40. Sivaraman P, Nussbaumer G, Landsberg D. Lack of long-term benefits of steroid withdrawal in renal transplant recipients. Am J Kidney Dis. 2001;37(6):1162–9.
41. Haririan A, Sillix DH, Morawski K, El-Amm JM, Garnick J, Doshi MD, et al. Short-term experience with early steroid withdrawal in African-American renal transplant recipients. Am J Transplant. 2006;6(10):2396–402.
42. Midtvedt K, Hjelmesaeth J, Hartmann A, Lund K, Paulsen D, Egeland T, et al. Insulin resistance after renal transplantation: the effect of steroid dose reduction and withdrawal. J Am Soc Nephrol. 2004;15(12):3233–9.
43. Vanrenterghem Y, Bresnahan B, Campistol J, Durrbach A, Grinyó J, Neumayer HH, et al. Belatacept-based regimens are associated with improved cardiovascular and metabolic risk factors compared with cyclosporine in kidney transplant recipients (BENEFIT and BENEFIT-EXT studies). Transplantation. 2011;91(9):976–83.
44. Baldwin Jr D, Duffin KE. Rosiglitazone treatment of diabetes mellitus after solid organ transplantation. Transplantation. 2004;77(7): 1009–14.
45. Turk T, Pietruck F, Dolff S, Kribben A, Janssen OE, Mann K, et al. Repaglinide in the management of new-onset diabetes mellitus after renal transplantation. Am J Transplant. 2006;6(4):842–6.
46. Lane JT, Odegaard DE, Haire CE, Collier DS, Wrenshall LE, Stevens RB. Sitagliptin therapy in kidney transplant recipients with new-onset diabetes after transplantation. Transplantation. 2011;92(10):e56–7.
47. Werzowa J, Hecking M, Haidinger M, Lechner F, Döller D, Pacini G, et al. Vildagliptin and pioglitazone in patients with impaired glucose tolerance after kidney transplantation: a randomized, placebo-controlled clinical trial. Transplantation. 2013;95(3):456–62.
48. Davidson J, Wilkinson A, Dantal J, Dotta F, Haller H, Hernandez D, Krentz A, et al., International Expert Panel. New-onset diabetes after transplantation: 2003 International consensus guidelines. Proceedings of an international expert panel meeting. Barcelona, Spain, 19 February 2003. Transplantation. 2003;75(10 Suppl): SS3–24
49. Sharif A. Metformin for patients with diabetes and concomitant renal restrictions—is there an evidence base? Q J Med. 2013;106: 291–4.
50. Kurian B, Joshi R, Helmuth A. Effectiveness and long-term safety of thiazolidinediones and metformin in renal transplant recipients. Endocr Pract. 2008;14(8):979–84.
51. Holdaas H, Fellström B, Jardine AG, Holme I, Nyberg G, Fauchald P, et al. Assessment of LEscol in Renal Transplantation (ALERT) Study Investigators: effect of fluvastatin on cardiac outcomes in renal transplant recipients: a multicentre, randomised, placebo-controlled trial. Lancet. 2003;361(9374):2024–31.

Hematologic Complications of Transplantation

22

Marissa M. Brokhof, David R. Hager, Arjang Djamali, and Vijay Vidyasagar

Anemia

Early Posttransplant Anemia

Anemia (hemoglobin <13 g/dL in males or <12 g/dL in females) is a common complication after transplantation in 20–41 % in renal transplant recipients, with the highest incidence in the immediate 30-day posttransplant period (up to 60 %) [36, 42, 61, 87]. In the early posttransplant period (0–30 days), common nondrug causes of anemia include operative blood loss, phlebotomy, infection and/or sepsis, and low erythropoietin levels from pretransplant chronic kidney disease (CKD) in conjunction with delayed graft function and/or rejection posttransplant. In the perioperative setting, a dilutional anemia must be considered secondary to aggressive volume expansion. The reduced drug clearance from renal insufficiency or with delayed graft function that can be seen posttransplant can escalate the potential for developing anemia. The immediate remedial treatment option is transfusion of blood products, with a goal to maintain a hemoglobin concentration of 8 g/dL [42]. This must be considered if blood loss is evident or in the event that the patient is symptomatic.

Treatment

When possible, the underlying cause of the anemia should be established and treated. Rapid depletion of iron stores occurs posttransplant due to surgical blood loss and increased consumption required for erythropoiesis [97]. Repeated phlebotomy to assess allograft function and immunosuppressant serum concentrations leads to significant blood loss in the acute posttransplant period as well. Peripheral blood smear and iron studies including serum ferritin and transferrin saturation (TSAT) are necessary. Management of posttransplant anemia is based on recommendations from CKD guidelines [42]. Within the posttransplant setting, treatment of iron deficiency is crucial at restoring hemoglobin levels, and replenishment is necessary when serum ferritin is <200 ng/mL and/or transferring saturation is <20 %. Iron replacement through intravenous or oral formulations is usually adequate. Intravenous iron must be avoided in the presence of active infections due to cytokine inhibition that may lead to impaired immunity [67]. Administration of erythropoietin-stimulating agents (ESAs) such as epoetin and the longer-acting darbepoetin is used to maintain hemoglobin to levels of 10–11.5 g/dL. This can minimize the need for frequent blood transfusions and allow management of anemia to take place in an outpatient environment [15, 42]. Normalization of hemoglobin levels with use of ESAs helps to preserve deterioration of kidney function and reduces graft loss [63]. This is due to a reduction in renal oxygen deprivation and hypoxic stress that occurs in the presence of anemia. ESAs should not be used in the setting of active bleeding or in patients with uncontrolled hypertension or stroke.

Nutritional deficiency of folate or vitamin B_{12} stores is a frequent source of both early and late posttransplant anemia and can lead to macrocytosis [42]. Serum folate and B_{12} levels should be evaluated during clinical assessment so that replacement may be initiated [51]. Deficiencies are easily corrected and often oral replacement is all that is needed. Folic acid can be repleted at 1–5 mg daily, with 400 μg daily for maintenance through dietary intake. Supplementation of folate in B_{12}-depleted patients may lead to severe neurological changes, thus B_{12} levels should be assessed and replenished prior to

M.M. Brokhof, Pharm.D., B.C.P.S.
Department of Pharmacy, University of Wisconsin Hospital and Clinics, Madison, WI, USA

D.R. Hager, Pharm.D., B.C.P.S., C.N.S.C. (✉)
University of Wisconsin Hospital and Clinics, 600 Highland Avenue, Madison, WI 53792, USA
e-mail: dhager@uwhealth.org

A. Djamali, M.D., M.S., F.A.S.N. • V. Vidyasagar, M.D., M.P.H.
Division of Nephrology, University of Wisconsin, Madison, WI, USA

M.R. Weir and E.V. Lerma (eds.), *Kidney Transplantation: Practical Guide to Management*,
DOI 10.1007/978-1-4939-0342-9_22,

initiating folate therapy [77]. In B_{12}-deficient patients, B_{12} (cyanocobalamin) 1,000 μg daily is recommended until stores are repleted.

Passenger Lymphocyte Syndrome

In the early posttransplant period, hemolysis should be considered as a possible cause of anemia. A common cause is the passenger lymphocyte syndrome [66]. This occurs when ABO incompatibilities exist (most commonly donor group O and recipient group A) leading to a destruction of red blood cells. Typically, the onset is within 1 week after transplant. Presentation is often with an abrupt and rapid drop in hemoglobin, with an elevated serum bilirubin and lactate dehydrogenase, and a decrease in serum haptoglobin. A Coombs test should be included to detect the presence of autoimmune hemolysis. Hemolysis usually persists for 5–10 days, subsiding gradually, and in most instances can be managed by transfusion of compatible blood products, corticosteroids, and supportive care.

Red Cell Aplasia

Though uncommon, red cell aplasia can occur in the posttransplant patient. Epoetin resistance or hyporesponsiveness can lead to red cell aplasia, with greater epoetin requirements associated with increased age, higher body mass index, iron deficiency anemia, and diabetes [75]. Though rare, infection with parvovirus B19 can result in both acute and chronic anemia in immunosuppressed patients, who can present with reticulocytopenia or a pure red cell aplasia [56]. Diagnosis requires serum PCR testing or ELISA antibody analysis of immunoglobulin (Ig) M and/or IgG antibodies. However, antibodies may not be routinely detected in transplant patients due to immunosuppression. In rare cases, a bone marrow biopsy with histopathological evaluation for the presence of the virus is required. Intravenous immunoglobulin (IVIg 400 mg/kg/day for 5 days) has demonstrated effective treatment response in many cases of parvovirus B19. Infection recurrence rate is greater than 25 % and may require additional courses of IVIg [26, 27, 48].

Medications

Medications are often associated with posttransplant anemia. The antiproliferative agents mycophenolate mofetil, mycophenolate sodium, and azathioprine can lead to a profound bone marrow suppression through direct inhibition of nucleic acid synthesis and by promoting ineffective erythropoiesis [34, 61]. Transplant induction therapy with antithymocyte globulin (ATG) or alemtuzumab can cause an acute drop in hemoglobin levels. This effect may be compounded when used with maintenance immunosuppressants like tacrolimus, sirolimus, and everolimus. Other medications that can lead to anemia include angiotensin-converting enzyme inhibitors (ACEIs), angiotensin receptor blockers (ARBs), and trimethoprim-sulfamethoxazole (TMP-SMX) or dapsone used for infection prophylaxis. When considering dapsone for prophylaxis of *Pneumocystis jiroveci* pneumonia, patients must be evaluated for deficiency of blood glucose-6-phosphate dehydrogenase (G6PD), which often manifests as a hemolytic anemia. Recipients of kidney transplantation commonly receive a combination of the aforementioned agents and are at an increased risk for developing anemia. In most instances, medication-induced anemia is reversible once the dose of the drug is reduced. At times, complete cessation of the offending agent may be required. Management in this setting is similar to that of non-medication-related anemia and may necessitate the administration of ESA therapy if there is no improvement after discontinuing the offending agent [18, 51].

Late Posttransplant Anemia

A strong proportional relationship exists between renal function and hemoglobin levels, with slow or delayed allograft function being one of the most significant factors contributing to late posttransplant anemia. This is due to impairment of erythropoietin production before and after transplant and is worse in the setting of graft rejection [88]. Replenishment of iron stores and ESA supplementation may be necessary to maintain hemoglobin concentrations of 10–11 g/dL [15, 42].

Solid neoplasms are not uncommon in the late (30 days +) posttransplant period and should be considered as a cause of anemia if the above, more frequent causes have been ruled out [51].

Leukopenia

The prevalence of leukopenia (white blood cells $\leq 3.0 \times 10^9$ cells/L) is relatively common in the kidney transplant patient, reported as occurring in 58 % of patients [32]. Opportunistic infections should be considered when any immunosuppressed patient presents with leukopenia or other cytopenias [80]. Cytomegalovirus (CMV) is a frequent cause of infection in the first 6 months of the posttransplant period. Leukopenia is seen in roughly 21 % of patients through direct inhibition of the bone marrow stroma and other hematopoietic precursors [70]. Diagnosis of CMV-related leukopenia is made on routine laboratory analysis by detecting viremia (by plasma CMV DNA PCR) [14, 51]. Prophylaxis against CMV infection for a period of 3–6 months posttransplant with the antiviral valganciclovir is recommended by the International Consensus Guidelines [45]. This prophylaxis when extended to 200 days has demonstrated a sustained reduction in CMV disease for up to 2 years posttransplant, without significant safety concerns or other adverse effects [35]. Intravenous ganciclovir is considered the gold standard for the treatment of CMV but is often associated with leukopenia [45]. However, the International Consensus Guidelines for CMV management stresses upon avoiding dose reductions in ganciclovir and initiating granulocyte colony-stimulating factor (G-CSF) therapy if the absolute neutrophilic count (ANC) drops below 1,000/mm^3.

Medications

Induction and maintenance immunosuppressive agents along with related prophylactics for opportunistic infections have significant hematologic adverse effects and must be recognized as a potential source of leukopenia [51]. A careful review of the transplant patient's medication list in conjunction with the transplant pharmacist is a must in this evaluation process [3]. Rabbit antithymocyte globulin has an established safety and efficacy profile in induction therapy and in the treatment of acute rejection, without the numerous, severe adverse effects of the older induction agents [31]. Nevertheless, it continues to be a common cause of lymphopenia and thrombocytopenia in conjunction with prophylactic antimicrobials, making daily monitoring of white blood cell, lymphocyte, and platelet counts essential. Induction with the monoclonal antilymphocyte antibody alemtuzumab is associated with a more prolonged lymphopenia, with B lymphocytes usually repopulating to normal levels in 3–12 months. Interestingly, CD4+ and CD8+ counts may remain considerably depressed for up to 3 years [10, 55]. Maintenance agents mycophenolate, azathioprine, cyclosporine, and tacrolimus are all associated with significant leukopenia. The antiproliferative agents, azathioprine and mycophenolate, inhibit nucleic acid synthesis, leading to a dose-related decrease in white blood cell proliferation and neutrophil dysplasia [18]. Bone marrow suppression is more profound with azathioprine than mycophenolate [40]. One notable but now less commonly encountered drug–drug interaction, between azathioprine and allopurinol, a xanthine oxidase inhibitor frequently taken for gout, can cause a profound leukopenia and agranulocytosis [22, 69]. Subsequently, azathioprine is not metabolized to mercaptopurine, resulting in increased plasma concentrations and a potentially life-threatening fall in white blood cell counts. Changing the antiproliferative agent from azathioprine to mycophenolate or discontinuation of allopurinol prevents this interaction. Though less common, the calcineurin inhibitors cyclosporine and tacrolimus can decrease white blood cell counts, particularly when used in combination with mycophenolate. Rates of leukopenia are higher with tacrolimus than cyclosporine, with an incidence of neutropenia of about 28 % in the first year, in patients receiving tacrolimus-mycophenolate [20]. The antiviral ganciclovir and its prodrug valganciclovir are commonly used in the treatment and prophylaxis of post-transplant CMV. Leukopenia from valganciclovir is reported to occur in 10–20 % of transplant patients and can be severe in 5–8 %, requiring initiation of G-CSF [11]. Therefore, patients treated with these agents require close surveillance in the immediate and late posttransplant periods [51]. Notably, a dose reduction or discontinuation of mycophenolate is associated with significantly higher rates of acute rejection [44, 65]. When a transplant patient presents with leukopenia, dose reductions of mycophenolate are often considered, rather than a reduction in valganciclovir dosing, thereby increasing the risk of acute rejection and graft loss. In the event that leukopenia occurs, the dose of the antiviral should be reduced or even stopped while cell counts recover. Patients at increased risk for the development of CMV disease should be monitored closely when this is done [32, 73]. Additionally, the use of TMP-SMX for prophylaxis of *Pneumocystis jiroveci* pneumonia may induce leukopenia, though this resolves discontinuation of the drug [51].

Pseudo-Pelger Huet Anomaly

The pseudo-Pelger-Huet anomaly is associated with several medications used in the transplant setting [8, 39]. It is characterized by reduced nuclear segmentation and excessive clumping of chromatin within the neutrophils. Pelger–Huet has been reported with the coadministration of mycophenolate and ganciclovir, likely from the ability of both agents to alter purine utilization within cells. This anomaly frequently resolves after reduction and/or cessation of both drugs.

Treatment

Treatment of leukopenia is based on the absolute neutrophil count (ANC). The threshold at which to treat neutropenia in solid organ transplant patients remains controversial, with ANC <500/mm^3 typically necessitating the use of granulocyte colony-stimulating factors (G-CSF, i.e., filgrastim) [32]. G-CSF acts by stimulating the production, maturation, and activation of immature neutrophils and is invaluable in the management of chronic leukopenia, usually accommodating a lesser need for transfusion of blood products. G-CSF has demonstrated a reversal of neutropenia in 93 % of kidney and liver transplant patients over a mean period of 3.7 days [85].

The rates of infection are significantly higher when neutropenia is not treated [78]. A decline in allograft function has been reported with the administration of G-CSF agents, although the incidence rates vary. Additional studies are urgently needed [54].

Thrombocytopenia

Isolated thrombocytopenia (platelet count <150,000/μL) is relatively uncommon and has limited causes. Medication-induced thrombocytopenia is the most common, so drug profiles should be reviewed carefully for offending agents (Table 22.1). The most clinically significant drug-induced immune thrombocytopenia (DITP) is the development of heparin-induced thrombocytopenia (HIT) which occurs in approximately 1–3 % of patients exposed to heparin products [95]. Heparin is used widely for prevention of deep vein thrombosis, in solutions used for flushing the renal allograft during transplantation, and compounded with other medications to reduce the risk of thrombophlebitis. HIT presents in two subtypes [5]. HIT type 1 is a non-immunologic, transient, self-limiting reduction in platelet counts, and no intervention is necessary. HIT type 2 is a result of the development of IgG and IgM antibodies to platelet factor 4-heparin complex which triggers a hypercoagulable state [4, 7, 38]. Monitoring platelet counts in patients on heparin is critical to identifying patients with HIT. Platelet reductions typically occur between 5 and 10 days following initiation of heparin [5]. Renal transplant patients, however, are likely to have been exposed to heparin previously, i.e., during dialysis, previous hospitalizations, or angio-access procedures, and could potentially develop thrombocytopenia within hours of re-exposure. This is seen commonly in patients exposed to heparin in the previous 100 days [94]. Platelet reductions in excess of 50 % from peak postoperative counts or reductions to less than 150,000/mm^3 should prompt an evaluation [93]. Confirmatory tests include a solid phase platelet factor 4 enzyme-linked immunosorbent assay (PF4) or a ^{14}carbon serotonin release assay (SRA) [92]. Reported sensitivities for the PF4 test range from 75 to 87 % and for the SRA from 59 to 78 %, indicating higher sensitivities for the immunoassay technique. Specificities for these tests range from 86 % for the PF4 to 100 % for the SRA, indicating less false positives with the SRA. Platelet aggregation assays are also available, but less sensitive than either the PF4 or SRA assays. Treatment includes total cessation of all heparin therapies and therapeutic anticoagulation with direct thrombin inhibitors [5, 21]. Currently available alternative therapies include argatroban and lepirudin (FDA approved) and bivalirudin (off label) for use in HIT. Argatroban is preferred at least in theory as dose adjustment is not required

Table 22.1 Medications used in transplant recipients associated with thrombocytopenia

Medication	Mechanism	Incidence	References
mTOR inhibitors	Myelosuppression	10–45 %	[31]
Antithymocyte globulins	Myelosuppression, DITP	10–44 %	[6, 19]
Valproate	DITP, myelosuppression	5–30 %	[55]
Azathioprine	Myelosuppression	10–15 %	[51]
Ganciclovir/valganciclovir	Myelosuppression	5–10 %	[79]
MPA	Myelosuppression	5–10 %	[51]
Linezolid	Myelosuppression	2 % (<14 days); 5 % (15–28 days); 7 % (>28 days)	[9]
Foscarnet	Myelosuppression	1–5 %	[69]
Vancomycin	DITP, unknown secondary mechanism	1–8 % (likely comparable to linezolid)	[62, 74]
Beta-lactam antibiotics (ampicillin, piperacillin, ceftriaxone)	DITP, myelosuppression	1–4 %	[70]
Heparin	DITP	1–3 %	[93]
Acyclovir/valacyclovir	Myelosuppression	<1 %	[69]
Trimethoprim-sulfamethoxazole (TMP-SMX)	DITP, myelosuppression	<1 %	[13]
OKT3	DITP (suggested)	<1 %	[1, 47]
Quinine/quinidine	DITP	<1 %	[35]
Carbamazepine	DITP	<1 %	[80]
Rifampin	DITP	<1 %	[50]
Fluoroquinolones	DITP (probable)	<1 %	[16]
Mirtazapine	DITP	<1 %	[45]
Phenytoin	DITP	<1 %	[60]
H2-receptor antagonists	DITP (probable)	<1 %	[88]

in renal dysfunction. Therapeutic monitoring is required with frequent aPTT measurements (every 6 h) until stable and therapeutic goals are attained.

Other agents causing thrombocytopenia in transplant recipients include antithymocyte globulin (ATG), mammalian target of rapamycin (mTOR) inhibitors, azathioprine, and mycophenolate (Table 22.1). Thrombocytopenia can occur in 37 % of ATG-treated patients and presents with slow, progressive reduction in platelet counts [84]. Coagulopathies are more common with the older, ATGAM equine-based product and were likely the result of antihorse immunoglobulin antibody complexes on the platelet surface [50]. Thrombocytopenia with the more modern rabbit antithymocyte globulin products is the result of Fc domains in the polyclonal product binding to CD32 on platelets, activating aggregation [6]. Dose reduction or discontinuation of therapy usually results in recovered platelet counts [19]. Sirolimus-induced thrombocytopenia, a dose-dependent toxicity resulting from inhibition of interleukin-11 signal transduction, occurs most commonly in the first 1–4 weeks posttransplant and typically resolves spontaneously with dose reduction or temporary discontinuation, required in less than 15 % of patients [33]. Everolimus, another mammalian target of rapamycin inhibitor (mTORi), has similar rates of thrombocytopenia [12].

Other potential causes in the differential should include other medications (Table 22.1), autoimmune thrombocytopenic purpura, thrombotic microangiopathy (TMA), passive immune thrombocytopenia, thrombotic thrombocytopenia purpura (TTP), sepsis, malaria, viral infection (CMV, parvovirus B19), and disseminated intravascular coagulation (in the recipient or donor). These are uncommon and less likely to present as isolated thrombocytopenia [5, 59, 60, 70, 91, 96].

Pancytopenia

Often hematologic complications do not present in isolation but in conjunction with reduced counts across cell lines. These pancytopenias (hemoglobin <13 g/dL in males, <12.0 g/dL in females; neutrophil count <1,500/μL; platelet count <150,000/μL) are most commonly associated with opportunistic infections or medication-related adverse effects.

Opportunistic infections that primarily present as pancytopenias include human herpes virus-6 (HHV-6), human herpes virus-8 (HHV-8), histoplasmosis, and blastomycosis [51]. CMV and parvovirus B19 can present with pancytopenia, but more commonly present with neutropenia and anemia, respectively [25, 70].

HHV-6, the cause of roseola (exanthem subitum), can reactivate in immunocompromised adults or be transmitted via the donor [25]. This often presents 2–4 weeks posttransplant although cases up to 2 years have been described. Clinical presentation can be with pancytopenia, fever, hepatitis, pneumonitis, colitis, and encephalitis. Laboratory investigation should include PCR testing for HHV-6 types A and B or tissue culture. Isolation from BAL fluid or peripheral blood mononuclear cells is unreliable. A positive qualitative test of viral DNA in cerebrospinal fluid is sufficient for the diagnosis of HHV-6 encephalitis [46]. Immunohistochemical stains of tissue biopsies can detect cells with active infection and can allow for differentiation between variants. Variant B is more likely to be resistant to ganciclovir, the preferred therapy. Foscarnet and cidofovir are the most active agents against HHV-6 in vitro, although not preferred given their renal toxicities. Consideration must be given to reduction in immunosuppression. Efficacy monitoring with frequent viral load testing has been suggested [2].

Histoplasma capsulatum often presents in the first year after transplant with fever, night sweats, and weight loss. Though primarily an infection of the lungs, it can also involve the bone marrow causing a pancytopenia [29]. Diagnosis is made via a bone marrow biopsy demonstrating intracellular fungal elements. Treatment includes itraconazole or amphotericin.

Medications, with a particular focus on drug interactions, are a common cause of pancytopenia. This should be evaluated, preferably by enlisting the help of the transplant pharmacist [3]. Common offending agents include mycophenolate, azathioprine (particularly in combination with allopurinol), and TMP-SMX.

Erythrocytosis

Posttransplant erythrocytosis (PTE) is relatively frequent and occurs in 10–15 % of renal transplant recipients [86]. It commonly develops 8–24 months after transplant and is defined as an elevated hematocrit of greater than 51 %, with normal arterial oxygen saturation, along with normal leukocyte and platelet counts. Predisposing factors include male sex, smoking, renal artery stenosis, retention of native kidneys, and adequate erythropoiesis prior to transplantation. It is detected as elevated counts on routine blood tests, concomitantly with hypertension or as the result of a thrombotic event, which can occur in 10–30 % of cases. A large number of patients experience malaise, lethargy, dizziness, and headache, though spontaneous remission of symptoms occurs in approximately 25 % within 2 years from onset [89]. While the pathogenesis of PTE remains uncertain, excessive production of erythropoietin (EPO) due to unrestrained stimulation of the retained native kidneys has been theorized. As PTE may occur with low or even undetectable levels of EPO, its pathogenesis is likely multifactorial. Several other hormonal systems, specifically, the renin-angiotensin system (RAS) and endogenous androgens, likely play a role. Angiotensin II may be responsible for inappropriately enhancing and sustaining erythropoietin levels directly or indirectly via stimulation of adrenal cortical androgen production. This supports the use of an ACEI or an ARB to reduce EPO production via inactivation of the RAS [42]. Inactivation of the RAS leads to a dose-dependent decrease in hematocrit in over 90 % of patients within the first month of treatment. Nadir hematocrit may be reached within 3 months, with stable levels for a period of 1–3 years [89]. A lack of response to these agents may require a trial of alternative therapies like theophylline or serial phlebotomy [51]. Less frequent causes of PTE include ureteral stenosis and hydronephrosis and renal cell carcinoma (RCC) of the native kidney(s), particularly in the presence of cystic disease. In the setting of renal carcinoma or polycystic kidney disease, erythrocytosis is common due to excess and/or uncontrolled production of erythropoietin from the cysts [74]. This often mandates nephrectomy for RCC or placement of ureteral stents if stenosis or hydronephrosis is present.

Leukocytosis

Fluctuations in white blood cell counts are common in the immediate postoperative period after kidney transplantation. Daily monitoring is frequently warranted [51]. Leukocytosis is defined as a white blood cell count $\geq 11.0 \times 10^9$ cells/L and is most often caused by an increase in mature neutrophils. Surgical inflammation, infection, and the use of corticosteroids posttransplant are prominent sources of leukocytosis. Acute inflammation from the transplant stimulates granulocyte production and stimulates numerous proinflammatory cytokines including tumor necrosis factor-α. The acute leukocytosis demonstrated in the setting of infection results from the rapid release of neutrophils. In the setting of sepsis and septic shock, systemic endotoxin production and inflammation lead to a potentially rapid rise or fall in white blood cell counts. Corticosteroids reduce neutrophil adhesion, inducing migration from the bone marrow into the circulation, with prednisone doses of 40–80 mg/day leading to a mean increase in absolute neutrophil count (ANC) of 4,000/μL [17].

Certain Unique Conditions in Transplant Patients

Renal transplant recipients are at risk for conditions peculiar to transplantation (Table 22.2) either through calcineurin toxicity resulting in renal endothelial injury (TMA), exposure to foreign immune cells in a state of immunosuppression (graft-versus-host disease), or immunosuppression-related infection or reactivation (posttransplant lymphoproliferative disorder and hemophagocytic syndrome (HPS)).

TMA presents early posttransplant as a thrombocytopenia and hemolytic anemia, the result of intraluminal platelet thrombosis and obstruction in the lumina of arterioles and capillaries [59]. Histologic changes include glomerular and arteriolar thrombosis with intracapillary accumulation of erythrocytes. Risk factors for TMA include use of calcineurin inhibitors (incidence 4–15 % with cyclosporine, 1 % with tacrolimus) and mTOR inhibitors, acute antibody-mediated rejection (AMR), CMV infection, donation after cardiac death organ, recipient scleroderma, or antiphospholipid antibody syndrome. Treatment should include withdrawal or reduction in CNI therapy in conjunction with plasma exchange therapy, with consideration for use of eculizumab particularly in those with recurrent TMA or those with known risk factors, including mutations in complement factor H or the presence of antiphospholipid antibodies [30, 98, 99]. When associated with AMR, graft loss is common, and treatment with bortezomib and eculizumab has been attempted [59]. Plasma exchange combined with co-stimulation blockade has also been suggested as an alternative to CNIs and has been reasonably successful. Eculizumab may have a role in prevention of TMA in patients receiving grafts for atypical hemolytic uremic syndrome [98].

HPS is an uncommon complication where nonneoplastic macrophages consume leukocytes, erythrocytes, and platelets as a result of uncontrolled stimulation by tumor necrosis factor-α and IL-2. HPS is diagnosed by meeting five of eight clinical criteria: (1) fever, (2) cytopenia of two lines, (3) hypertriglyceridemia and/or hypofibrinogenemia, (4) hyperferritinemia, (5) hemophagocytosis, (6) elevated soluble interleukin-2 receptor, (7) decreased natural killer cell activity, and (8) splenomegaly [68]. Bone marrow biopsy can confirm the diagnosis in 70 % of cases, demonstrating proliferation of mature histiocytes actively consuming other blood cells. Reactive or acquired HPS in transplant recipients occurs in the setting of opportunistic infection (most typically viral, e.g., Epstein–Barr virus (EBV)), mycobacterial or malignancy [80]. Prognosis is poor with a reported mortality rate of 53 % in the small number of reported cases; graft loss rates are high from a combination of rejection, septic shock, and nephrectomy as rescue treatment. Case reports favor the use of IVIg for treatment; however, therapy is mostly supportive—treating the underlying infection, reduction in immunosuppression (RI), and consideration for the use of pulse steroids and plasma exchange.

Posttransplantation lymphoproliferative disorder (PTLD) is a spectrum of polyclonal and monoclonal lymphoid proliferations seen in transplant recipients [58]. Commonly, these present as polyclonal B-cell proliferations from EBV-infected, EBV-transformed, and EBV-immortalized B cells [26]. These cells, in the presence of immunosuppression, can undergo unregulated proliferation as a result of increased pro-replication cytokines like interleukin-10 (IL-10), IL-6, and tumor necrosis factor-β. Given this risk, an ongoing program of EBV

Table 22.2 Etiologies and descriptions of unique causes of pancytopenia

Complication	Incidence (%)	Primary causative factors	Presentation	Time to onset posttransplant	Diagnosis	Treatment
TMA	1–5	CNIs, mTORi, AMR, CMV	1. Fever 2. Neurologic abnormalities 3. Renal dysfunction 4. Thrombocytopenia 5. Hemolytic anemia	Immediate period to 3 months	Renal biopsy	Withdrawal of CNI, plasma exchange
PTLD	1–2	EBV	1. Fever 2. Night sweats 3. Weight loss/anorexia 4. Abdominal pain	EBV (+)<1 year; EBV (−)>1 year	Tissue biopsy	Rituximab, RI
Kaposi's sarcoma	0.50	HHV-8	1. Skin lesions (red to purple to dark blue) 2. Fever 3. Splenomegaly 4. Lymphadenopathy	Variable (2 months to 10 years)	Tissue biopsy	RI, change to mTORI, chemotherapy (vinblastine, bleomycin, taxanes)
HPS	0.40	EBV, CMV, HHV-6, HHV-8, mycobacteria infection	1. Fever 2. Hepatosplenomegaly 3. Pancytopenia 4. Weight loss 5. Night sweats 6. Splenomegaly	<1 year	Bone marrow biopsy	IVIg, RI
CML	0.2–2	AZA	1. Abdominal pain 2. Fatigue 3. Pruritus 4. Splenomegaly	2–10 years	Bone marrow biopsy	Imatinib, INF-alpha
AML	0.2–2	AZA	1. Fatigue 2. Dyspnea 3. Angina 4. Purpura 5. Bleeding 6. Fever 7. Skin and soft tissue inflammation	5 to >15 years	Bone marrow biopsy	Chemotherapy (daunorubicin, cytarabine, etoposide)
GVHD	Rare	Dose of graft lymphocytes, 1-way HLA-matched donor	1. Fever 2. Rash 3. Diarrhea 4. Liver dysfunction	<1 year	HLA typing	Unknown; RI? Steroids? IL-2 RA?
HSGDTCL	Rare	CSA, AZA	1. Hepatosplenomegaly with abdominal discomfort 2. Fever 3. Night sweats 4. Cachexia	>10 years	Bone marrow biopsy	Chemotherapy (CHOP, alemtuzumab, hyperCVAD)

AML acute myeloid leukemia; *AZA* azathioprine; *AMR* antibody-mediated rejection: *CHOP* cyclophosphamide, doxorubicin, vincristine, prednisone: *CML* chronic myeloid leukemia: *CMV* cytomegalovirus: *CNI* calcineurin inhibitor: *CSA* cyclosporine: *EBV* Epstein-Barr virus: *GVHD* graft-versus-host disease: *HHV* human herpes virus: *HLA* human leukocyte antigen: *HPS* hemophagocytic syndrome: *HSGDTCL* hepatosplenic gamma-delta T-cell lymphoma: *hyperCVAD* cyclophosphamide, vincristine, doxorubicin, dexamethasone, methotrexate, cytarabine: *IL-2 RA* interleukin 2 receptor antagonist: *INF* interferon: *IVIg* intravenous immunoglobulin: *mTORI* mammalian target of rapamycin inhibitor: *PTLD* posttransplant lymphoproliferative disorder: *RI* reduction of immunosuppression: *TMA* thrombotic microangiopathy

viral load monitoring, particularly in EBV-seronegative recipients, is necessary [41]. Diagnosis is made by tissue biopsy and often includes immunohistochemical analysis, flow cytometry, and molecular studies [28]. EBV-encoded RNA in situ hybridization can be utilized to identify EBV-transformed cells as the cause. Treatment has dramatically improved with the addition of rituximab (progression-free survival and overall survival at 3 years >70 %), but also typically involves reduction of immunosuppression with consideration for chemotherapy, surgery, or radiation [23]. The role of antiviral therapy is debated in either the prevention or treatment of PTLD, but reducing immunosuppression is prudent and typically required for these patients [28]. Hematologic malignancies can also present as cytopenias or leukemias (Table 22.2). Other less common hematologic malignancies include hepatosplenic gamma-delta T-cell lymphoma (HSGDTCL) and Kaposi's sarcoma (likely related to HHV-8 infection) [51].

Evaluation of Cytopenias After SOT

Anemia Workup (Fig. 22.1)

Initial analysis should include a peripheral blood smear, hemoglobin, hematocrit, mean corpuscular volume (MCV), serum erythropoietin, iron studies including ferritin, TSAT, reticulocyte count, serum B12, and erythrocyte folate levels. If hemolysis is suspected, haptoglobin, lactate dehydrogenase, reticulocyte count, and indirect bilirubin should be analyzed. Additional blood analysis includes G6PD evaluation for potential deficiency-related anemia.

Workup of anemia in the immediate post-surgery setting should include a serum creatinine, a 24-h urine collection if possible (identification of allograft dysfunction, EPO deficiency), a renal ultrasound to evaluate for potential hematoma or blood loss, and possibly a renal biopsy [51, 80, 83]. Bone marrow aspiration and biopsy may be necessary if an immediate cause of anemia is not found. Hematology consultation may then be warranted.

Leukopenia Workup

Workup of posttransplant leukopenia should include peripheral blood smear (leukocyte/neutrophil paucity, psudeo-Pelger-Huet cells, or immature cells). If leukopenia is

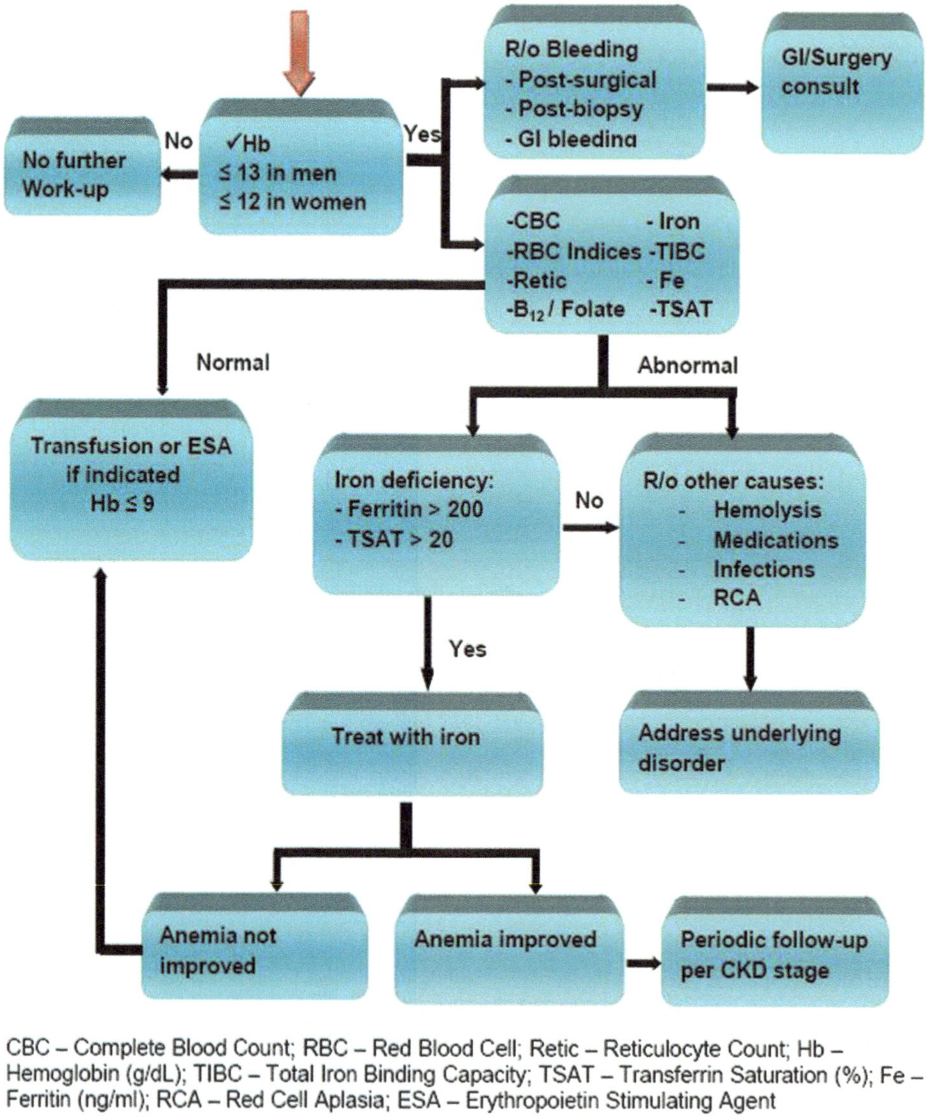

Fig. 22.1 Flowchart of anemia workup and management

confirmed, an evaluation for opportunistic infections should be considered, particularly for CMV and EBV DNA by plasma PCR. A Pelger-Huet anomaly may be detected with coadministration of mycophenolate and ganciclovir (coarse clumping of nuclear chromatin on blood smear). A complete review of the patient's medication list is required, with reasonable modifications in pharmacological management (dose reduction, drug discontinuation). Therapeutic drug monitoring utilizing serum trough concentrations of immunosuppressant agents (cyclosporine, tacrolimus) should be undertaken to assess for supratherapeutic blood levels and dose adjustments made accordingly. A bone marrow biopsy and hematology consultation may be warranted to evaluate cytogenetics and hypocellularity if an immediate cause of leukopenia is not ascertained.

Thrombocytopenia Workup

Workup is dependent on the severity of thrombocytopenia and the presentation of the patient [79]. Platelet transfusion should be considered for patients with platelet counts <10,000/μL as the risk for spontaneous bleeding is increased. In asymptomatic patients, in vitro clumping or pseudothrombocytopenia must be excluded, usually by examination of a peripheral blood smear. A sample should then be recollected with an appropriately citrated container. If thrombocytopenia is confirmed, a detailed history to identify any source of bleeding, infectious symptomatology, medication use, and social history (HIV and alcohol use) should be completed. Initial laboratory workup should include a peripheral blood smear, serum creatinine, DIC panel, LDH, and liver function tests including a total and direct bilirubin. If hemolysis is suspected, direct antiglobulin testing (Coombs test), reticulocyte count, and haptoglobin should additionally be analyzed. Bone marrow biopsy should be reserved for patients with a suspected myelosuppressive condition.

Conclusion

Kidney transplant recipients are at increased risk for the development of a variety of hematologic abnormalities. A wide spectrum of anomalies can be detected both in the immediate and late posttransplant period. This may include an easily treatable condition like anemia or a more life-threatening process like PTLD or HPS. Medications and infections are the usual culprits, with immunosuppressant and antimicrobial agents playing an important role in the development of cytopenias. A thorough review of all medications in the transplant recipient is therefore required. Additionally, analysis and replenishment of deficient nutrient stores is very important. Viral and fungal infections are common in the posttransplant patient and must be aggressively pursued and treated, with dose adjustments to immunosuppression and anti-infectives when available.

To sum up, hematologic complications can be complex, can occur with a wide clinical spectrum, and can present unique challenges in the posttransplant patient. Therefore, a comprehensive management plan involving multiple health care specialties is often necessary to optimize patient outcomes.

References

1. Abramowicz D, Pradier O, Marchant A, Florquin S, De Pauw L, Vereerstraeten P, et al. Induction of thromboses within renal grafts by high-dose prophylactic OKT3. Lancet. 1992;339:777–8.
2. Agut H. Deciphering the clinical impact of acute human herpesvirus 6 (HHV-6) infections. J Clin Virol. 2011;52:164–71.
3. Alloway RR, Dupuis R, Gabadi S, Kaiser TE, Taber DJ, Tichy EM, et al. Evolution of the role of the transplant pharmacist on the multidisciplinary transplant team. Am J Transplant. 2011;11:1576–83.
4. Amiral J, Bridey F, Dreyfus M, Vissoc AM, Fressinaud E, Wolf M, et al. Platelet factor 4 complexed to heparin is the target for antibodies generated in heparin-induced thrombocytopenia. Thromb Haemost. 1992;68:95–6.
5. Aneregg BA, Baillie GM, Lin A, Lazarachick J. Heparin-induced thrombocytopenia in a renal transplant recipient. Am J Transplant. 2005;5:1537–40.
6. Ankersmit HJ, Roth GA, Zuckermann A, Brunner M, Rosin C, Buchta C, et al. CD32-mediated platelet aggregation in vitro by anti-thymocyte globulin: implication of therapy-induced in vivo thrombocytopenia. Am J Transplant. 2003;3:754–9.
7. Arnold DM, Kukaswadia S, Nazi I, Esmail A, Dewar L, Smith JW, et al. A systematic evaluation of laboratory testing for drug-induced immune thrombocytopenia. J Thromb Haemost. 2013;11(1):169–76. doi:10.1111/jth.12052.
8. Best S, Salvati F, Kallo J, et al. Lamin B-receptor mutations in Pelger-Huët anomaly. Br J Haematol. 2003;123(3):542.
9. Birmingham MC, Rayner CR, Meagher AK, Flavin SM, Batts DH, Schentag JJ. Linezolid for the treatment of multidrug resistant, gram-positive infections: experience from a compassionate-use program. Clin Infect Dis. 2003;36:159–68.
10. Bloom DD, Hu H, Fechner JH, et al. T-lymphocyte alloresponses of Campath-1H-treated kidney transplant patients. Transplantation. 2006;81(1):81–7.
11. Brum S, Nolasco F, Sousa J, et al. Leukopenia in kidney transplant patients with the association of valganciclovir and mycophenolate mofetil. Transplant Proc. 2008;40:752–4.
12. Budde K, Becker T, Arns W, Sommerer C, Reinke P, Eisenberger U, et al. Everolimus-based, calcineurin-inhibitor-free regimen in recipients of de-novo kidney transplants: an open-label, randomised, controlled trial. Lancet. 2011;377:837–47.
13. Caluwe R, Van Laecke S, Emonds MP, Peeters P, Vanholder R. Immediate posttransplant cotrimoxazole-induced immune thrombocytopenia. Am J Transplant. 2010;10:943–6.
14. Carstens J, Andersen HK, Spencer E, et al. Cytomegalovirus infection in renal transplant recipients. Transpl Infect Dis. 2006;8:203–12.
15. Centers for Disease Control and Prevention. National chronic kidney disease fact sheet: general information and national estimates on chronic kidney disease in the United States, 2010. Atlanta, GA: U.S. Department of Health and Human Services, CDC; 2010.
16. Cheah CY, De Keulenaer B, Leahy MF. Fluoroquinolone-induced immune thrombocytopenia: a report and review. Intern Med J. 2009;39:619–23.
17. Dale DC, Fauci AS, Guerry IV D, et al. Comparison of agents producing a neutrophilic leukocytosis in man. Hydrocortisone,

prednisone, endotoxin, and etiocholanolone. J Clin Invest. 1975;56(4):808.
18. Danesi R, Del Tacca M. Hematologic toxicity of immunosuppressive treatment. Transplant Proc. 2004;36:703–4.
19. Deeks ED, Keating GM. Rabbit antithymocyte globulin (Thymoglobulin®): a review of its use in the prevention and treatment of acute renal allograft rejection. Drugs. 2009;69:1483–512.
20. De Rycke A, Dierickx D, Kuypers DR. Tacrolimus-induced neutropenia in renal transplant recipients. Clin J Am Soc Nephrol. 2011;6(3):690–4.
21. Dracopoulos S, Vougas V, Kassimatis TI, Theodoridis T, Ali ME, Apostolou T. Heparin-induced thrombocytopenia type II: a serious hazard in preemptive renal transplantation: a case report. Transplant Proc. 2007;39:3481–4.
22. Elion GB, Callahan S, Nathan H. Potentiation by inhibition of drug degradation: 6-substituted purines and xanthine oxidase. Biochem Pharmacol. 1963;12:85–93.
23. Evens AM, David KA, Helenowski I, Nelson B, Kaufman D, Kircher SM, et al. Multicenter analysis of 80 solid organ transplantation recipients with post-transplantation lymphoproliferative disease: outcomes and prognostic factors in the modern era. J Clin Oncol. 2010;28:1038–46.
24. Everly MJ, Bloom RD, Tsai De, Trofe J. Posttransplant lymphoproliferative disorder. Ann Pharmacother. 2007;11:1850–8.
25. Fischer SA. Emerging viruses in transplantation: there is more to infection after transplant than CMV and EBV. Transplantation. 2008;86:1327–39.
26. Garewal G, Ahluwalia J, Varma N, et al. Parvovirus B19 infection-associated red-cell aplasia in renal-transplant recipients: clues from the bone marrow. Transplantation. 2004;77:320–1.
27. Gosset C, Viglietti D, Hue K, et al. How many times can parvovirus B19-related anemia recur in solid organ transplant recipients? Transpl Infect Dis. 2012;14(5):E64–70.
28. Green M. Management of Epstein-Barr virus-induced post-transplant lymphoproliferative disease in recipients of solid organ transplantation. Am J Transplant. 2001;1:103–8.
29. Grim SA, Proia L, Miller R, Alhyraba M, Costas-Chavarri A, Oberholzer J. A multicenter study of histoplasmosis and blastomycosis after solid organ transplantation. Transpl Infect Dis. 2012; 14:17–23.
30. Hadaya K, Ferrari-Lucraz S, Fumeaux D, Boehlen F, Toso C, Moll S, et al. Eculizumab in acute recurrence of thrombotic microangiopathy after renal transplantation. Am J Transplant. 2011;11: 2523–7.
31. Hardinger KL. Rabbit antithymocyte globulin induction therapy in adult renal transplantation. Pharmacotherapy. 2006;26:1771–83.
32. Hartmann EL, Gatesman M, Roskopf-Somerville J, et al. Management of leukopenia in kidney and pancreas transplant recipients. Clin Transplant. 2008;22:822–8.
33. Hong JC, Kahan BD. Sirolimus-induced thrombocytopenia and leucopenia in renal transplant recipients: risk factors, incidence, progression, and management. Transplantation. 2000;69:2085–90.
34. Howarth JE, Waters HM, Shanks D, et al. Effects of azathioprine on response on renal anemia to subcutaneous recombinant human erythropoietin. Am J Clin Pathol. 1993;46:41–4.
35. Humar A, Limaye AP, Blumberg EA, et al. Extended valganciclovir prophylaxis in D+/R− kidney transplant recipients is associated with long-term reduction in cytomegalovirus disease: two-year results of the IMPACT study. Transplantation. 2010;90(12):1427–31.
36. Karakus S, Kanbay M, Koseoglu HK, et al. Causes of anemia in renal transplant recipients. Transplant Proc. 2004;36:164–5.
37. Kaufman DW, Kelly JP, Johannes CB, Sandler A, Harmon D, Stolley PD, et al. Acute thrombocytopenic purpura in relation to the use of drugs. Blood. 1993;82:2714–8.
38. Kelton JG, Sheridan D, Santos A, Smith J, Steeves K, Smith C, et al. Heparin-induced thrombocytopenia: laboratory studies. Blood. 1988;72:925–30.
39. Kennedy GA, Kay TD, Johnson DW, et al. Neutrophil dysplasia characterized by pseudo-Pelger-Huet anomaly occurring with the use of mycophenolate mofetil and ganciclovir following renal transplantation: a report of five cases. Pathology. 2002;34:263–6.
40. Khosroshahi HT, Asghari A, Estakhr R, et al. Effects of azathioprine and mycophenolate mofetil-immunosuppressive regimens on the erythropoietic system of renal transplant recipients. Transplant Proc. 2006;38:2077–9.
41. Kidney Disease: Improving Global Outcomes (KDIGO) Transplant Work Group. KDIGO clinical practice guideline for the care of kidney transplant recipients. Am J Transplant. 2009;9:S1–157.
42. Kidney Disease: Improving Global Outcomes (KDIGO) Transplant Work Group. KDIGO clinical practice guideline for anemia in chronic kidney disease. Kidney Int. 2012;2:279–335.
43. Klaassen RJ, van Gelder T, Rischen-Vos J, et al. Losartan, an angiotensin-II receptor antagonist, reduces hematocrits in kidney transplant recipients with posttransplant erythrocytosis. Transplantation. 1997;64:780–2.
44. Knoll GA, MacDonald I, Khan A, et al. Mycophenolate mofetil dose reduction and the risk of acute rejection after renal transplantation. J Am Soc Nephrol. 2003;14:2381.
45. Kotton CN, Kumar D, Caliendo AM, et al. International consensus guidelines on the management of cytomegalovirus in solid organ transplantation. Transplantation. 2010;89(7):779–95.
46. Lautenschlager I, Razonable RR. Human herpesvirus-6 infections in kidney, liver, lung and heart transplantation: review. Transpl Int. 2012;25:493–502.
47. Liu X, Sahud MA. Glycoprotein IIB/IIIA complex is the target in mirtazapine-induced immune thrombocytopenia. Blood Cells Mol Dis. 2003;30:241–5.
48. Lui SL, Luk WK, Cheung CY, et al. Nosocomial outbreak of parvovirus B19 infection in a renal transplant unit. Transplantation. 2001;71:59–64.
49. Mackie F, Verran D, Horvath J, Teller D. Severe thrombocytopenia with OKT3 use for steroid-resistant rejection in a cadaveric renal transplant recipient. Nephrol Dial Transplant. 1996;11:2378.
50. Madaio MP, Spiegel JE, Levey AS. Life-threatening thrombocytopenia complicating antithymocyte globulin therapy for acute kidney transplant rejection. Transplantation. 1988;45:647–9.
51. Marinella MA. Hematologic abnormalities following renal transplantation. Int Urol Nephrol. 2010;42:151–64.
52. Martínez E, Collazos J, Mayo J. Hypersensitivity reactions to rifampin: pathogenetic mechanisms, clinical manifestations, management strategies, and review of the anaphylactic-like reactions. Medicine (Baltimore). 1999;78:361–9.
53. Mathew TH. A blinded, long-term, randomized multicenter study of mycophenolate mofetil in cadaveric renal transplantation: results at three years. Tricontinental Mycophenolate Mofetil Renal Transplantation Study Group. Transplantation. 1998;65:1450–4.
54. Minguez C, Mazuecos A, Ceballos A, et al. Worsening of renal function in a renal transplant patient treated with granulocyte colony-stimulating factor. Nephrol Dial Transplant. 1995;10:2166–7.
55. Morris PJ, Russell NK. Alemtuzumab (Campath-1H): a systematic review in organ transplantation. Transplantation. 2006;81(10):1361.
56. Musiani M, Zerbini M, Gentilomi G, et al. Parvovirus B19 clearance from peripheral blood after acute infection. J Infect Dis. 1995;172:1360–3.
57. Nasreddine W, Beydoun A. Valproate-induced thrombocytopenia: a prospective monotherapy study. Epilepsia. 2008;49:438–45.
58. Newstead CG. Lymphoproliferative disease post-renal transplantation. Nephrol Dial Transplant. 2000;15:1913–6.

59. Noris M, Remuzzi G. Thrombotic microangiopathy after kidney transplantation. Am J Transplant. 2010;10:1517–23.
60. Nuesch R, Cynke E, Jost MC, Zimmerli W. Thrombocytopenia after kidney transplantation. Am J Kidney Dis. 2000;35:537–8.
61. Ourahma S, Mercadai L, Tezenas du Montcel S, et al. Anemia in the period immediately following renal transplantation. Transplant Proc. 2007;39:1446–50.
62. Pandey M, Yarlagadda L. Drug-induced thrombocytopenia: a less known interaction. Blood Coagul Fibrinolysis. 2012;23:778–80.
63. Pallet N, Rabant M, Legendre C, et al. The nephroprotective properties of recombinant human erythropoietin in kidney transplantation: experimental facts and clinical proofs. Am J Transplant. 2012;12(12):3184–90.
64. Patel N, VanDeWall H, Tristani L, Rivera A, Woo B, Dihmess A, et al. A comparative evaluation of adverse platelet outcomes among Veterans' Affairs patients receiving linezolid or vancomycin. J Antimicrob Chemother. 2012;67:727–35.
65. Pelletier RP, Akin B, Henry ML, et al. The impact of mycophenolate mofetil dosing patterns on clinical outcome after renal transplantation. Clin Transplant. 2003;17:200.
66. Petz LD. Immune hemolysis associated with transplantation. Semin Hematol. 2005;42:145–55.
67. Pieracci FM, Barie PS. Iron and the risk of infection. Surg Infect (Larchmt). 2005;6 Suppl 1:S41–6.
68. Ponticelli C, Alberighi OD. Haemophagocytic syndrome—a life-threatening complication of renal transplantation. Nephrol Dial Transplant. 2009;24:2623–7.
69. Ragab AH, Gilkerson E, Myers M. The effect of 6-mercaptopurine and allopurinol on granulopoiesis. Cancer Res. 1974;34:2246–9.
70. Razeghi E, Hadadi A, Mansor-Kiaei M, Molavi M, Khashasyar P, Pourmand G. Clinical manifestation, laboratory findings, and the response of treatment in kidney transplant recipients with CMV infection. Transplant Proc. 2007;39:993–6.
71. Razonable RR. Antiviral drugs for viruses other than human immunodeficiency virus. Mayo Clin Proc. 2011;86:1009–26.
72. Reichardt P, Handrick W, Linke A, Schille R, Kiess W. Leukocytopenia, thrombocytopenia and fever related to piperacillin/tazobactam treatment—a retrospective analysis in 38 children with cystic fibrosis. Infection. 1999;27:355–6.
73. Rerolle JP, Szelag JC, LeMeur Y. Unexpected rate of severe leukopenia with the association of mycophenolate mofetil and valganciclovir in kidney transplant recipients. Nephrol Dial Transplant. 2007;22:671–2.
74. Rosse WF, Waldmann TA, Cohen P. Renal cysts and erythropoietin and polycythemia. Am J Med. 1963;34:76–81.
75. Rossert J, Gassmann-Mayer C, Frei D, et al. Prevalence and predictors of epoetin hyporesponsiveness in chronic kidney disease patients. Nephrol Dial Transplant. 2007;22(3):794–800.
76. Ruggero MA, Abdelghany O, Topal JE. Vancomycin-induced thrombocytopenia without isolation of a drug-dependent antibody. Pharmacotherapy. 2012;32:e321–5.
77. Schaefer RM, Teschner M, Kosch M. Folate metabolism in renal failure. Nephrol Dial Transplant. 2002;17(5):24–7.
78. Schmaldienst S, Bekesi G, Deicher R, et al. Recombinant human granulocyte colony-stimulating factor after kidney transplantation: a retrospective analysis to evaluate the benefit or risk of immunostimulation. Transplantation. 2000;69(4):527–31.
79. Sekhon SS, Roy V. Thrombocytopenia in adults: a practical approach to evaluation and management. South Med J. 2006;6:491–8.
80. Smith EP. Hematologic disorders after solid organ transplantation. Hematology Am Soc Hematol Educ Program. 2010;2010:281–6.
81. Taber DJ, Ashcraft E, Baillie GM, Berkman S, Rogers J, Baliga PK, et al. Valganciclovir prophylaxis in patients at high risk for development of cytomegalovirus disease. Transpl Infect Dis. 2004;6:101–9.
82. Taher AT, Arabi M, Sibai H, Nasreddine W, Otrock ZK, Musallam KM, et al. Carbamazepine-induced thrombocytopenia. Blood Cells Mol Dis. 2012;48:197–8.
83. Tefferi A, Hanson CA, Inwards DJ. How to interpret and pursue an abnormal complete blood cell count in adults. Mayo Clin Proc. 2005;80:923–36.
84. Thymoglobulin®[package insert]. Cambridge, MA: Genzyme Corporation; 2004.
85. Turgeon N, Hovingh GK, Fishman JA, et al. Safety and efficacy of granulocyte colony-stimulating factor in kidney and liver transplant recipients. Transpl Infect Dis. 2000;2:15–21.
86. Usalan C, Erdem Y, Caglar M, et al. Effect of enalapril on exaggerated erythropoietin response to phlebotomy in erythrocytosic renal transplant patients. Nephrol Dial Transplant. 1998;13:2884–9.
87. Vanrenterghem Y, Ponticelli C, Morales JM, et al. Prevalence and management of anemia in renal transplant recipients: a European survey. Am J Transplant. 2003;3:835–45.
88. Vanrenterghem Y. Anaemia after renal transplantation. Nephrol Dial Transplant. 2004;19 Suppl 5:54–8.
89. Vlahakos DV, Marathias KP, Agroyannis B, et al. Posttransplant erythrocytosis. Kidney Int. 2003;63:1187–94.
90. Wade EE, Rebuck JA, Healey MA, Rogers FB. H_2 antagonist-induced thrombocytopenia: is this a real phenomenon? Intensive Care Med. 2002;28:459–65.
91. Waldman M, Kopp JB. Parvovirus-B19-associated complications in renal transplant recipients. Nat Clin Pract Nephrol. 2007;3:540–50.
92. Walenga JM, Jeske WP, Fasanella AR, Wood JJ, Bakhos M. Laboratory tests for the diagnosis of heparin-induced thrombocytopenia. Semin Thromb Hemost. 1999;25:43–9.
93. Warkentin TE. Clinical picture of heparin-induced thrombocytopenia. In: Warkentin TE, Greinacher A, editors. Heparin-induced thrombocytopenia. New York: Marcel Dekker; 2004. p. 53.
94. Warkentin TE, Kelton JG. Temporal aspects of heparin induced thrombocytopenia. N Engl J Med. 2001;344:1286–92.
95. Warkentin TE, Levine MN, Hirsh J, Horsewood P, Roberts RS, Gent M, et al. Heparin-induced thrombocytopenia in patients treated with low-molecular weight heparin or unfractionated heparin. N Engl J Med. 1995;332:1330–5.
96. West KA, Anderson DR, McAlister VC, Hewlett TJ, Belitsky P, Smith JW, et al. Alloimmune thrombocytopenia after organ transplantation. N Engl J Med. 1999;341:1504–7.
97. Zheng S, Coyne DW, Joist H, et al. Iron deficiency anemia and iron losses after renal transplantation. Transpl Int. 2009;22(4):434.
98. Zimmerhackl LB, Hofer J, Cortina G, Mark W, Wurzner R, Jungraithmayer TC, et al. Prophylactic eculizumab after renal transplantation in atypical hemolytic-uremic syndrome. N Engl J Med. 2010;362:1746–8.
99. Zuber J, Le Quintrec ML, Sberro-Soussan R, Loirat C, Fremeaux-Bacchi V, Legendre C. New insights into postrenal transplant hemolytic uremic syndrome. Nat Rev Nephrol. 2011;7:23–35.

Liver Disease in Renal Transplant Recipients

23

Andres F. Carrion, Fabrizio Fabrizi, and Paul Martin

Liver failure is responsible for 8–28 % of all deaths in renal transplant recipients [1, 2]. Several diseases are prevalent in this immunosuppressed population and a variety of hepatic insults occurring during the intra- and postoperative periods contribute to this. These include comorbid conditions such as diabetes mellitus with associated nonalcoholic fatty liver disease (NAFLD), drug-induced liver injury (DILI), hepatic involvement in multisystem disorders such as systemic lupus erythematosus, and viral hepatitis B and C with long-term hemodialysis implicated in their acquisition [3]. Fortunately, the incidence and prevalence of viral hepatitis has decreased in individuals on maintenance hemodialysis, but obesity and metabolic disorders such as dyslipidemia, insulin resistance, and overt diabetes mellitus are common in this population. The differential diagnosis of hepatic dysfunction in a renal transplant recipient therefore includes preexisting liver disease, newly acquired viral hepatitis, opportunistic infections such as cytomegalovirus (CMV), and DILI (Table 23.1). Management of hepatic dysfunction in a renal transplant recipient includes evaluation of the cause, intervention with specific therapy such as antiviral agents if indicated, and exclusion of DILI. It is also important to identify renal transplant candidates at risk for worsening liver disease posttransplant due to viral hepatitis so that antiviral therapy can be initiated to preempt progression once therapeutic immunosuppression is introduced.

A.F. Carrion, M.D.
Division of Gastroenterology, University of Miami Miller School of Medicine, Miami, FL, USA

F. Fabrizi, M.D.
Division of Nephrology and Dialysis, Maggiore Hospital, IRCCS Foundation, Milan, Italy

P. Martin, M.D., F.R.C.P., F.R.C.P.I. (✉)
Division of Hepatology, University of Miami Miller School of Medicine, 1500 Northwest 12 Avenue, Jackson Medical Tower E-1101, Miami, FL 33136, USA
e-mail: PMartin2@med.miami.edu

Approach to the Renal Transplant Recipient with Hepatic Dysfunction

Evaluation of hepatic dysfunction in a renal transplant recipient is guided, in part, by its onset in relation to transplant, pattern, and duration (Fig. 23.1). In the immediate postoperative period, considerations include hepatic dysfunction due to intraoperative events. An abrupt rise in serum aminotransferases with a lesser elevation in bilirubin, alkaline phosphatase, and the international normalized ratio (INR) may reflect intraoperative hypotension and associated hepatic hypoperfusion, which can be confirmed by review of the operative records. If no additional insults contributed to hepatic dysfunction, prompt resolution can be anticipated. Currently favored anesthetic agents have a low rate of hepatotoxicity in contrast to halothane. Some anesthetics such as halothane undergo extensive hepatic metabolism, and in some susceptible individuals, immune-mediated hepatic injury may occur, which typically manifests with elevated serum aminotransferases within several days of surgery [4]. Although newer anesthetic agents are safer and less hepatotoxic than halothane, there have been case reports of significant hepatotoxicity associated with sevoflurane, desflurane, and isoflurane [5–7].

The differential diagnosis for hepatic dysfunction shifts beyond the immediate postoperative period. Generally, immunosuppressive drugs are not particularly hepatotoxic, but freshly transplanted recipients may be prescribed other medications such as antibiotics that may cause DILI. Immunosuppressive regimens used in renal transplant recipients vary considerably by transplant center. The following agents are currently used in various combination regimens: glucocorticoids, azathioprine, mycophenolate mofetil, mycophenolic acid, cyclosporine, tacrolimus, everolimus, and sirolimus [8]. Most transplant centers favor combination of a calcineurin inhibitor (cyclosporine or tacrolimus), an antimetabolite (azathioprine, mycophenolate mofetil, or mycophenolic acid), and prednisone (for different lengths of time) [9].

M.R. Weir and E.V. Lerma (eds.), *Kidney Transplantation: Practical Guide to Management*,
DOI 10.1007/978-1-4939-0342-9_23, © Springer Science+Business Media New York 2014

Table 23.1 Differential of hepatic dysfunction in renal transplant recipients

Type of liver insult	Setting	Characteristic findings
Ischemic hepatic injury	Hypotension during surgery but may also occur with severe volume depletion and hepatic hypoperfusion at any time posttransplant	Marked but transient elevation of aminotransferases within 48–72 h, followed by mild transient cholestasis
DILI	One or multiple drugs with hepatotoxic potential or drug–drug interactions. Idiosyncratic or drug-dependent toxicity	Variable presentation, from asymptomatic elevation of liver enzymes to acute liver failure. Pattern of hepatic injury varies by drug (hepatocellular, cholestatic, mixed)
NAFLD	Metabolic syndrome, new-onset diabetes after transplantation	Mild elevation of aminotransferases, imaging studies or biopsy demonstrating fatty infiltration of the liver
De novo acute HBV or HCV infection	Traditional risk factors for infection with HBV and HCV: drug use, tattoos, unprotected sex, hemodialysis, transfusion of blood products	Marked elevation of aminotransferases with or without cholestasis. Positive HBc-IgM or HBV-DNA for acute HBV, HCV-RNA for acute HCV
Chronic HBV or HCV infection	HBV or HCV infection pre-transplant	Progression of liver disease with signs of hepatocellular dysfunction
CMV hepatitis	CMV-seropositive donor and CMV-seronegative recipient. Antirejection agents: antilymphocyte antibodies, muromonab, alemtuzumab	Wide spectrum of disease, from asymptomatic infection to acute and fulminant hepatitis. Positive PCR, CMV-pp65 antigenemia, immunohistochemistry

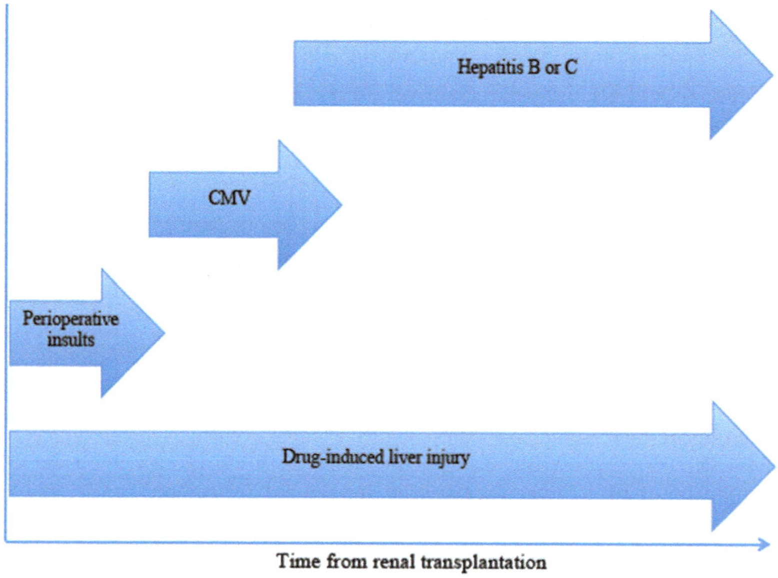

Fig. 23.1 Timeline of different liver diseases post-renal transplantation

Mild, and typically transient, elevations of serum aminotransferases are commonly seen in renal transplant recipients receiving calcineurin inhibitors such as cyclosporine or tacrolimus and often do not require further evaluation. However, a thorough workup including liver biopsy is indicated when persistent elevation occurs and no other plausible explanations for abnormal liver chemistries exist. If the postoperative course is complicated, for instance, by a wound infection, hepatic dysfunction may result due to the cholestatic effect of sepsis. In addition to surgical complications, therapeutic immunosuppression conveys a risk of opportunistic infections. The risk of CMV infection is greatest in CMV naïve recipients and those who receive additional immunosuppression for graft rejection. Hepatic involvement with hepatocellular dysfunction may be a feature of CMV disease [10]. Fibrosing cholestatic hepatitis, a severe and rapidly progressing form of liver injury typically resulting in devastating hepatic failure, described in individuals with hepatitis B or C, has also been reported in renal transplant recipients with CMV infection [11].

Elevations of serum aminotransferases and/or gamma-glutamyl transpeptidase may be due to ingestion of alcohol and/or hepatotoxic products including herbal remedies and health supplements; therefore, a detailed history is needed to elucidate consumption of these products in renal transplant recipients. The growing epidemic of obesity and the metabolic syndrome with associated detrimental effects on health and overall survival has not spared renal transplant candidates or recipients. NAFLD is the hepatic component of the metabolic syndrome with a disease spectrum ranging from simple hepatic steatosis to nonalcoholic steatohepatitis (NASH) and cirrhosis [12]. Accumulating evidence supports common comorbid risk factors for NAFLD and chronic kidney disease (CKD). In addition, epidemiologic studies show an increased incidence and prevalence of CKD in individuals with NAFLD, an association that appears to be independent of common risk factors such as obesity, diabetes mellitus, and hypertension [13, 14]. There are no data, however, about the incidence or prevalence of NAFLD in renal transplant recipients.

Widespread use of erythroid-stimulating agents such as erythropoietin and darbopoetin-α for treatment of chronic anemia has paralleled a lowered requirement for blood products with a decreased incidence and prevalence of iron overload syndromes in individuals undergoing dialysis and renal transplant recipients. Quantitative determination of iron in liver biopsy specimens and testing for genetic mutations responsible for hereditary hemochromatosis (C282Y and H63D) may be occasionally necessary to confidently distinguish primary hemochromatosis from secondary iron overload.

Hepatitis B in Renal Transplant Candidates and Recipients

The incidence and prevalence of hepatitis B virus (HBV) infection has markedly decreased over the past few decades in individuals with CKD as result of immunization, routine testing, reduced need for transfusion of blood products, awareness and enforcement of infection control precautions, and availability of effective antiviral agents [15]. There is, however, significant variation in prevalence of HBV infection in hemodialysis populations by country: 1 % in the United States, 5.9 % in Italy, 12 % in Brazil, and 1.3–14.6 % in Asian Pacific countries [15–18].

Liver biopsy has a valuable role in the evaluation of potential renal transplant candidates with HBV infection, as it is often difficult to estimate the severity of liver disease in this population based only on clinical data [19]. Assessment of fibrosis extent by noninvasive methods such as transient elastography (i.e., FibroScan®) may be another option in the future [20]. Elevations of serum aminotransferases are typically modest in HBV-infected individuals undergoing maintenance hemodialysis or with advanced CKD [21]. The histologic finding of cirrhosis on liver biopsy raises concern about hepatic decompensation after isolated renal transplantation. Combined liver–kidney transplantation should be considered if no clinical improvement is apparent after several months of treatment with suppressive antiviral therapy, especially in individuals with decompensated cirrhosis [22]. Milder liver disease on histology does not preclude isolated renal transplantation; however, accelerated progression may occur posttransplant if effective antiviral therapy is not used concomitantly with immunosuppression [19]. Endoscopy should be performed to detect gastroesophageal varices, which reflect more advanced liver disease. Determining the presence of markers of viral replication (hepatitis B e antigen [HBeAg] and HBV-deoxyribonucleic acid [DNA]) is key in potential renal transplant recipients; however, their absence does not preclude HBV reactivation posttransplant [19].

The effects of immunosuppressive therapy on HBV have been well characterized in several clinical settings including transplant recipients and individuals receiving systemic chemotherapy [23, 24]. The overwhelming majority of cases of HBV reactivation occur in hepatitis B surface antigen (HBsAg)-positive individuals; however, HBV reactivation has also been observed in renal transplant recipients with serological evidence of remote resolved infection manifest by absent HBsAg and positive total anti-hepatitis B core (HBc) pre-transplant (referred to as an "isolated core antibody"), and importantly is not a pattern induced by vaccination which results only in HBV surface antibody production [25]. Virologic and serologic markers, as well as the immunosuppressive regimen used, determine the risk of HBV reactivation in renal transplant recipients. The serologic and virologic statuses of the donor are important risk factors for de novo HBV infection in renal transplant recipients. HBV-naïve recipients of an allograft from an HBsAg-positive donor are predictably at highest risk. In contrast, the risk of de novo HBV infection from HBsAg-negative/anti-HBc-positive donors to HBsAg-negative/anti-HBc-negative recipients is very low [26]. HBV reactivation is accompanied by increased or reappearance of HBV-DNA in an individual with previously undetectable HBV-DNA. Increased HBV-DNA levels in renal transplant recipients with HBV reactivation typically precede elevations in alanine-aminotransferase (ALT). Reappearance of serum HBsAg in a recipient who only had total ("isolated") anti-HBc, as evidence of remote resolved HBV infection, is well recognized and can be prevented by an oral antiviral HBV agent.

Renal transplant recipients with HBV infection have had poorer outcomes compared to noninfected controls. For instance, data from a meta-analysis demonstrate that HBsAg seropositivity is associated with 2.5-fold higher risk of death and 1.5-fold higher risk of renal allograft loss compared to HBsAg-negative controls [27]. The presence of HBsAg and either HBV-DNA or HBeAg is associated with increased posttransplant mortality from liver disease compared to renal transplant recipients with positive HBsAg but negative HBV-DNA and HBeAg [28]. A recent report from the United Network for Organ Sharing (UNOS) database suggests, however, that in recent years decreased survival is no longer occurring in HBV-infected renal transplant recipients, presumably reflecting the use of oral antiviral therapy, although liver failure is still more common than in uninfected controls [29].

The cornerstone of preventing HBV infection in renal transplant recipients is effective immunization of HBsAg-negative individuals with CKD, ideally during early stages of renal disease before immune function is compromised. All nonimmune individuals with CKD undergoing hemodialysis require hepatitis B vaccine. Following completion of the vaccination series, immunity should be verified with quantitative determination of hepatitis B surface antibody (anti-HBs) [30]. Importantly, individuals with CKD undergoing hemodialysis develop adequate immune response after HBV immunization at a much lower rate compared to the general population (40–50 % versus >95 %, respectively) [3]; therefore, in this population, it is recommended to administer four double doses (40 μg intramuscularly each dose) at 0, 1, 2, and 6 months [31]. Annual quantitative determination of anti-HBs is recommended in renal transplant candidates successfully immunized (anti-HBs titers above 10 mIU/mL) [19]. In addition, antiviral prophylaxis depending upon donor/recipient status is also important [32]. In the absence of antiviral prophylaxis against HBV, approximately 2–10 % of renal transplant recipients with HBV infection pre-transplant will develop reactivation [33]. Administration of antiviral agents to individuals at increased risk for HBV reactivation either prior to or immediately after renal transplantation is considered prophylaxis [34]. Several issues, however, remain unsettled about using prophylactic antiviral agents including the optimal length of therapy, efficacy in renal transplantation (as prophylactic approaches were derived from bone marrow transplant protocols), and the efficacy in HBeAg-negative or HBV-DNA-negative renal transplant candidates. In contrast to the prophylactic approach, a preemptive strategy implies routine testing of renal transplant recipients for HBV-DNA and initiation of antiviral therapy for individuals with newly detected HBV-DNA or marked increased HBV-DNA (i.e., ≥1 log) [35]. There are no data comparing one strategy over the other in renal transplant recipients, and decisions should be based on resource availability and local expertise. Importantly, either strategy results in better outcomes, including patient survival, compared to initiation of antiviral therapy once clinically significant HBV reactivation occurs [35].

Multiple agents are available for the treatment of HBV infection in the non-transplant setting: interferon alfa-2b, pegylated interferon alfa-2a, lamivudine, adefovir, entecavir, telbivudine, and tenofovir. The use of interferons (either standard or pegylated) has significantly decreased with the advent of potent oral antiviral agents with less frequent and more tolerable side effects, as well as low rates of resistance, resulting in effective viral suppression [36–38]. In addition, interferon is contraindicated in renal transplant recipients as it may precipitate severe and often irreversible graft dysfunction. All five oral anti-HBV agents are renally excreted and dose adjustments must be anticipated in individuals with CKD (Table 23.2). Experience with lamivudine for the treatment of HBV is the most extensive; however, mutations in the YMDD motif of the DNA polymerase commonly occur resulting in drug resistance that limits the use of this agent in clinical practice [39]. Entecavir and tenofovir are currently the mainstay therapies against HBV, primarily because of their high potency and low risk of resistance; however, data on the efficacy and safety of these agents in renal transplant recipients is scarce [40]. The standard dose of tenofovir is 300 mg once daily and reduced frequency instead of decreased dose is needed in individuals with impaired renal function (Table 23.2). Although the optimal frequency has not been established for individuals with creatinine clearance less than 10 mL/min, a weekly dose of 300 mg is recommended for individuals undergoing hemodialysis [40]. Entecavir is the agent of choice for individuals with impaired renal function; however, dose reductions should also be anticipated (Table 23.2). The dose of entecavir for individuals with normal renal function is 0.5 mg once daily [40]. All HBV-infected individuals are at increased risk of hepatocellular carcinoma, even in the absence of cirrhosis, and need to be screened with twice yearly ultrasound and alpha-fetoprotein.

Table 23.2 Dose adjustments of anti-HBV agents in individuals with impaired renal function [40]

Agent	CrCl	Recommended dose
Entecavir (lamivudine naïve)	≥50	0.5 mg QD
	30–49	0.25 mg QD or 0.5 mg Q48 h
	10–29	0.15 mg QD or 0.5 mg Q72 h
	<10	0.05 mg QD or 0.5 mg Q7 days
	HD	0.05 mg QD or 0.5 mg Q7 days
Entecavir (lamivudine resistant)	≥50	1 mg QD
	30–49	0.5 mg QD or 1 mg Q48 h
	10–29	0.3 mg QD or 1 mg Q72 h
	<10	0.1 mg QD or 1 mg Q7 days
	HD	0.1 mg QD or 1 mg Q7 days
Tenofovir	≥50	300 mg QD
	30–49	300 mg Q48 h
	10–29	300 mg Q72–96 h
	<10	300 mg Q7 days
	HD	No recommendation available
Telbivudine	≥50	600 mg QD
	30–49	600 mg Q48 h
	<30	600 mg Q72 h
	HD	600 mg Q96 h (after HD)
Adefovir	≥50	10 mg QD
	30–49	10 mg Q48 h
	10–29	10 mg Q72 h
	HD	10 mg Q7 days (after HD)
Lamivudine	≥50	100 mg QD
	30–49	100 mg × 1, then 50 mg QD
	15–29	100 mg × 1, then 25 mg QD
	5–14	35 mg × 1, then 15 mg QD
	<5	35 mg × 1, then 10 mg QD

CrCl creatinine clearance, *HD* hemodialysis, *QD* once daily

Hepatitis C in Renal Transplant Candidates and Recipients

Hepatitis C virus (HCV) infection is a frequent problem in individuals with CKD [41]. Similar to HBV infection, the seroprevalence of anti-HCV antibodies in individuals undergoing maintenance hemodialysis varies by country: 2.7–3.9 % in the United Kingdom and Germany, 7.8 % in the United States, 16.4 % in Brazil, 22.2 % in Italy and Spain, and as high as 75–80 % in Morocco and Egypt [15, 42–44]. In the United States, the seroprevalence of HCV infection is approximately fivefold higher in individuals undergoing maintenance hemodialysis compared to the general population (7.8 % versus 1.6 %, respectively) [15, 45]. Nosocomial transmission within hemodialysis units is the most important risk factor and is proportional to the prevalence of HCV within individual hemodialysis units and time on hemodialysis [46].

HCV infection is associated with a 57 % higher risk of death in individuals with CKD undergoing hemodialysis compared to HCV-negative hemodialysis controls [47]. The increased mortality reflects not only a higher incidence of hepatic dysfunction but also faster progression to cirrhosis and frequent coinfection with other viruses that share common routes of transmission (i.e., HBV and human immunodeficiency virus [HIV]) as well as higher incidence and prevalence of cardiovascular diseases, anemia, hepatocellular carcinoma, and essential mixed (type II) cryoglobulinemia [48–50].

Routine testing for HCV is recommended in individuals with CKD regardless of the severity of kidney disease (Table 23.3). Screening with third-generation enzyme immunoassay (EIA) is accurate in individuals with CKD, and the polymerase chain reaction (PCR) assay for HCV-ribonucleic acid (RNA) is used to detect viremia in seropositive individuals and to exclude false negative EIA results if suspicion of HCV infection remains (i.e., individuals undergoing hemodialysis in units with high prevalence of HCV or renal transplant recipients with unexplained hepatic dysfunction). Individuals undergoing maintenance hemodialysis should have monthly screening for HCV with ALT. Importantly, ALT levels may remain within the so called "normal" range in HCV viremic individuals on hemodialysis; therefore, biannual or yearly testing with EIA or PCR is also recommended [42, 51].

Important advances in HCV therapy have occurred recently with substantial improvement in rates of sustained virological response (SVR), typically defined as a negative HCV-RNA level 6 months after completion of therapy, although recent data support the use of shorter interval following therapy to confirm SVR (12 weeks) with comparable outcomes. The recent licensing of direct-acting antiviral agents (DAA), notably sofosbuvir, a polymerase inhibitor, and simeprevir, a protease inhibitor, offers the possibility of interferon free regimens, although clinical studies in renal populations need to be performed to confirm safety. The absence of interferon will allow use of these regimens in renal transplant recipients. Previously HCV genotype 1, the commonest genotype, had been least responsive to interferon based regimens (Table 23.4) [52]. Individuals with

Table 23.4 Suggested anti-HCV regimens for patients with different stages of CKD [42]

CKD stage	CrCl (mL/min)	Anti-HCV therapy
1	≥90	PEG-IFN and ribavirin + DAA agents (for HCV genotypes 1, 2, and 3)
2	60–90	
3	30–59	PEG-IFN alpha-2b (1 μg/kg) or PEG-IFN alpha-2a (135 μg) subcutaneously once a week plus ribavirin 200–800 mg/day divided in two doses (consider adding a DAA, if tolerated)
4	15–29	
5	<15 non-dialysis	
5 dialysis	<15 on dialysis	*Preferred regimen*: standard IFN (alpha-2a or 2b) 3 mU subcutaneously thrice weekly
		Alternative regimen: PEG-IFN alpha-2b (1 μg/kg/week) or PEG-IFN alpha-2a (135 μg/week) subcutaneously ± very low dose ribavirin

CKD chronic kidney disease, *CrCl* creatinine clearance, *DAA* direct-acting antiviral, *IFN* interferon, *HCV* hepatitis C virus, *PEG-IFN* pegylated interferon

Table 23.3 Diagnostic recommendations for HCV in patients with CKD [42, 51]

Patient groups	Recommended tests
Non-dialysis CKD patients	Test all patients, regardless of CKD stage, with third-generation EIA
Initiation of HD or transfer from HD unit with low prevalence of HCV	Third-generation EIA, followed by PCR assay if positive
Transfer from HD unit with high prevalence of HCV	PCR assay
Maintenance HD at units with low prevalence of HCV	Test every 6–12 months with third-generation EIA. Test monthly for ALT
Maintenance HD at HD units with high prevalence of HCV	Test every 6–12 months with PCR. Test monthly for ALT
HD patients with unexplained abnormal ALT levels	PCR assay
Pre- and post-RT periods	PCR assay
Possible nosocomial infection or HCV outbreak at HD unit	PCR assay and consider repeating in 2–12 weeks if negative

HCV hepatitis C virus, *CKD* chronic kidney disease, *HD* hemodialysis, *ALT* alanine-aminotransferase, *RT* renal transplant, *EIA* enzyme immunoassay, *PCR* polymerase chain reaction

HCV genotypes 1, 2, and 3, increased toxicity of multidrug regimens may occur. Of major concern, individuals with CKD have a high prevalence of anemia at baseline which correlates with the severity of renal dysfunction: 1.3 % in CKD stage 2, 5.2 % in CKD stage 3, 44.1 % in CKD stage 4, and greater than 70 % in CKD stage 5 [53, 54]. Tolerability of interferon-based regimens in individuals with impaired renal function and high prevalence of anemia at baseline had been a major challenge [52]. Ribavirin causes hemolytic anemia in a dose-dependent fashion and erythroid-stimulating agents such as erythropoietin or darbepoetin alfa are commonly used in clinical practice to improve hemoglobin levels during treatment [55].

Current practice guidelines suggest consideration of anti-HCV therapy in renal transplant candidates with an estimated survival of at least 5 years [42, 51]. It may also be appropriate to consider treatment in renal transplant candidates with CKD with less severe histological hepatic injury than the recommended criteria used for the general population (i.e., a METAVIR score ≥2/4 or an Ishak score ≥3/6) [42]. Antiviral treatment should ideally be offered to individuals with CKD during the earlier stages of renal disease to abort progression of liver disease. The major limitation for the use of interferon-based therapy to treat HCV in renal transplant recipients is the risk of inducing acute graft rejection; therefore, interferon is in general, contraindicated in renal transplant recipients [42]. Current guidelines had suggested considering interferon-based therapy only for selected cases of fibrosing cholestatic hepatitis in an effort to prevent hepatocellular failure [51]. The new oral regimens described above will obviate this concern.

HCV infection is also a major problem in renal transplant recipients resulting in diminished patient and graft survival compared to HCV-negative controls. Data from a meta-analysis show 79 % and 56 % higher relative risks of death and graft failure, respectively, in HCV-infected renal transplant recipients compared to HCV-negative controls [56]. The increased mortality in HCV-infected renal transplant recipients is largely attributed to an increased incidence of hepatic dysfunction and hepatocellular carcinoma [57, 58]. In addition, HCV is associated with various complications in renal transplant recipients including de novo and recurrent allograft nephropathy, new-onset diabetes after transplantation (NODAT), and sepsis [56, 59]. Post-renal transplant outcomes do not appear to vary among individuals infected with different HCV genotypes [60].

The most common manifestations of kidney disease in renal transplant recipients with HCV infection are proteinuria, membranoproliferative glomerulonephritis, and membranous nephropathy [61, 62]. Less commonly observed diseases include renal thrombotic microangiopathy and acute or chronic transplant glomerulopathies [61, 63]. HCV-infected individuals have a fivefold higher incidence of proteinuria following renal transplantation compared to HCV-negative controls [64]. Recurrent and de novo glomerular disease in renal allografts also occur more commonly in HCV-positive renal transplant recipients and immunosuppression has been implicated as an important risk factor [65]. The incidence of de novo glomerulonephritis varies significantly depending on the recipient's HCV status (34 % versus 6.6 % for HCV-positive and HCV-negative recipients, respectively) [66]. Results from a small uncontrolled clinical trial showed that successful pre-transplant anti-HCV therapy (defined as achievement of SVR) significantly decreases the incidence of de novo posttransplant glomerulonephritis [67]. The prognosis of de novo glomerulonephritis is worse in HCV-positive than in HCV-negative renal transplant recipients and HCV infection also increases the risk of allograft failure and return to dialysis [68]. Some data suggest that successful treatment of HCV in renal transplant candidates may result in up to 50 % reduction of episodes of acute graft rejection posttransplantation, although confirmation of these findings is needed [69].

HCV infection is associated with higher prevalence of diabetes mellitus pre- and post-renal transplantation [70, 71]. Although the exact mechanisms responsible for abnormal glycemic control in HCV-infected individuals remain unclear, evidence suggest that HCV induces insulin resistance by downregulation of insulin receptors and beta-cell dysfunction [72–74]. Data from a meta-analysis demonstrate a fourfold higher incidence of NODAT in HCV-infected renal transplant recipients compared to HCV-negative controls [71]. Importantly, renal transplant recipients with NODAT have increased all-cause mortality and higher incidence of major cardiovascular events (i.e., cardiac death or nonfatal acute myocardial infarction) compared to nondiabetic renal transplant recipients (20 % versus 37 %, respectively, after 8 years of follow-up) [75]. NODAT has been associated with the use of glucocorticoids and tacrolimus in renal transplant recipients and decreased incidence of this complication has been reported with other immunosuppressive regimens including cyclosporine and mycophenolate mofetil [76, 77]. Pre-transplant antiviral therapy may decrease the prevalence of NODAT from 25 to 7 %; however, it is unclear if the benefit reflects fewer episodes of acute graft rejection requiring glucocorticoids or if it is directly associated with virological response because SVR rates were not reported and subgroup analyses were not done [69].

Conclusions

Hepatic dysfunction is commonly encountered in renal transplant candidates and recipients and is an important risk factor for morbidity and mortality. Posttransplant immunosuppression is implicated in more rapid progression to fibrosis in viral hepatitis with a high risk for reactivation of hepatitis B. Metabolic disturbances such as established diabetes mellitus or NODAT, hypertension, and dyslipidemia are also common in renal transplant recipients and may increase the risk of NAFLD. Therefore, comprehensive and interdisciplinary care of individuals with kidney and liver disease should be directed to control modifiable risk factors, prevent HBV infection through immunization, and treatment of HBV and HCV to diminish progression of liver disease and prevent hepatic decompensation. If an initial noninvasive workup with serologies and abdominal ultrasound does not provide an obvious explanation and hepatic dysfunction persists, evaluation with liver biopsy is indicated. In transplant candidates with chronic HBV and HCV, liver biopsy is appropriate to exclude cirrhosis, which should prompt consideration of combined liver-kidney transplant if there is evidence of portal hypertension or marked synthetic impairment. Antiviral therapy for HCV continues to rapidly evolve with availability of potent agents that allow shorter duration of treatment, reduced toxicity, and high SVR rates. In addition, combination regimens of new agents will allow interferon-free/ribavirin-free all-oral therapy.

References

1. Gheith OA, Saad MA, Hassan AA, A-Eldeeb S, Agroudy AE, Sheashaa H, et al. Hepatic dysfunction in kidney transplant recipients: prevalence and impact on graft and patient survival. Clin Exp Nephrol. 2007;11(4):309–15. Epub 2007/12/19.
2. Pereira BJ, Levey AS. Hepatitis C virus infection in dialysis and renal transplantation. Kidney Int. 1997;51(4):981–99. Epub 1997/04/01.
3. Papafragkakis H, Fabrizi F, Martin P. Viral hepatitis in renal transplantation. Clin Nephrol. 2011;76(1):29–39. Epub 2011/07/05.
4. Martin JL. Volatile anesthetics and liver injury: a clinical update or what every anesthesiologist should know. Can J Anaesth. 2005;52(2):125–9.
5. Anderson JS, Rose NR, Martin JL, Eger EI, Njoku DB. Desflurane hepatitis associated with hapten and autoantigen-specific IgG4 antibodies. Anesth Analg. 2007;104(6):1452–3. Table of contents. Epub 2007/05/22.
6. Nishiyama T, Yokoyama T, Hanaoka K. Liver function after sevoflurane or isoflurane anaesthesia in neurosurgical patients. Can J Anaesth. 1998;45(8):753–6.
7. Alotaibi WM. Severe hepatic dysfunction after sevoflurane exposure. Saudi Med J. 2008;29(9):1344–6. Epub 2008/09/25.
8. Halloran PF. Immunosuppressive drugs for kidney transplantation. N Engl J Med. 2004;351(26):2715–29. Epub 2004/12/24.
9. Wong W, Venetz JP, Tolkoff-Rubin N, Pascual M. 2005 Immunosuppressive strategies in kidney transplantation: which role for the calcineurin inhibitors? Transplantation. 2005;80(3):289–96. Epub 2005/08/06.
10. Ljungman P, Griffiths P, Paya C. Definitions of cytomegalovirus infection and disease in transplant recipients. Clin Infect Dis. 2002;34(8):1094–7. Epub 2002/03/27.
11. Agarwal SK, Kalra V, Dinda A, Gupta S, Dash SC, Bhowmik D, et al. Fibrosing cholestatic hepatitis in renal transplant recipient with CMV infection: a case report. Int Urol Nephrol. 2004; 36(3):433–5. Epub 2005/03/24.
12. Vuppalanchi R, Chalasani N. Nonalcoholic fatty liver disease and nonalcoholic steatohepatitis: selected practical issues in their evaluation and management. Hepatology. 2009;49(1):306–17. Epub 2008/12/10.
13. Targher G, Chonchol M, Zoppini G, Abaterusso C, Bonora E. Risk of chronic kidney disease in patients with non-alcoholic fatty liver disease: is there a link? J Hepatol. 2011;54(5):1020–9. Epub 2010/12/15.
14. Chang Y, Ryu S, Sung E, Woo HY, Oh E, Cha K, et al. Nonalcoholic fatty liver disease predicts chronic kidney disease in nonhypertensive and nondiabetic Korean men. Metabolism. 2008;57(4):569–76. Epub 2008/03/11.
15. Finelli L, Miller JT, Tokars JI, Alter MJ, Arduino MJ. National surveillance of dialysis-associated diseases in the United States, 2002. Semin Dial. 2005;18(1):52–61. Epub 2005/01/25.
16. Mioli VA, Balestra E, Bibiano L, Carletti P, Della Bella S, Fanciulli E, et al. Epidemiology of viral hepatitis in dialysis centers: a national survey. Nephron. 1992;61(3):278–83. Epub 1992/01/01.
17. Oguchi H, Miyasaka M, Tokunaga S, Hora K, Ichikawa S, Ochi T, et al. Hepatitis virus infection (HBV and HCV) in eleven Japanese hemodialysis units. Clin Nephrol. 1992;38(1):36–43. Epub 1992/07/01.
18. Teles SA, Martins RM, Vanderborght B, Stuyver L, Gaspar AM, Yoshida CF. Hepatitis B virus: genotypes and subtypes in Brazilian hemodialysis patients. Artif Organs. 1999;23(12):1074–8. Epub 2000/01/05.
19. Kalia H, Fabrizi F, Martin P. Hepatitis B virus and renal transplantation. Transplant Rev (Orlando). 2011;25(3):102–9. Epub 2011/05/03.
20. Liu CH, Liang CC, Huang KW, Liu CJ, Chen SI, Lin JW, et al. Transient elastography to assess hepatic fibrosis in hemodialysis chronic hepatitis C patients. Clin J Am Soc Nephrol. 2011;6(5):1057–65. Epub 2011/03/12.
21. Fabrizi F, Lunghi G, Finazzi S, Colucci P, Pagano A, Ponticelli C, et al. Decreased serum aminotransferase activity in patients with chronic renal failure: impact on the detection of viral hepatitis. Am J Kidney Dis. 2001;38(5):1009–15. Epub 2001/10/31.
22. Baccaro ME, Pepin MN, Guevara M, Colmenero J, Torregrosa JV, Martin-Llahi M, et al. Combined liver-kidney transplantation in patients with cirrhosis and chronic kidney disease. Nephrol Dial Transplant. 2010;25(7):2356–63. Epub 2010/02/09.
23. Tsai MC, Chen YT, Chien YS, Chen TC, Hu TH. Hepatitis B virus infection and renal transplantation. World J Gastroenterol. 2010;16(31):3878–87. Epub 2010/08/17.
24. Liu CJ, Chen PJ, Chen DS, Kao JH. Hepatitis B virus reactivation in patients receiving cancer chemotherapy: natural history, pathogenesis, and management. Hepatol Int. 2013;7(2):316–22. Epub 2011/06/15.
25. Fabrizi F, Bunnapradist S, Martin P. HBV infection in patients with end-stage renal disease. Semin Liver Dis. 2004;24 Suppl 1:63–70. Epub 2004/06/12.
26. Wachs ME, Amend WJ, Ascher NL, Bretan PN, Emond J, Lake JR, et al. The risk of transmission of hepatitis B from HBsAg(-), HBcAb(+), HBIgM(-) organ donors. Transplantation. 1995;59(2): 230–4. Epub 1995/01/27.
27. Fabrizi F, Martin P, Dixit V, Kanwal F, Dulai G. HBsAg seropositive status and survival after renal transplantation: meta-analysis of observational studies. Am J Transplant. 2005;5(12):2913–21. Epub 2005/11/24.

28. Fairley CK, Mijch A, Gust ID, Nichilson S, Dimitrakakis M, Lucas CR. The increased risk of fatal liver disease in renal transplant patients who are hepatitis Be antigen and/or HBV DNA positive. Transplantation. 1991;52(3):497–500. Epub 1991/09/01.
29. Reddy PN, Sampaio MS, Kuo HT, Martin P, Bunnapradist S. Impact of pre-existing hepatitis B infection on the outcomes of kidney transplant recipients in the United States. Clin J Am Soc Nephrol. 2011;6(6):1481–7. Epub 2011/05/14.
30. Recommendations for preventing transmission of infections among chronic hemodialysis patients. MMWR Recomm Rep. 2001;50(RR-5):1–43. Epub 2001/05/15.
31. Rangel MC, Coronado VG, Euler GL, Strikas RA. Vaccine recommendations for patients on chronic dialysis. The Advisory Committee on Immunization Practices and the American Academy of Pediatrics. Semin Dial. 2000;13(2):101–7. Epub 2000/05/05.
32. Lau DT, Hewlett AT. Screening for hepatitis A and B antibodies in patients with chronic liver disease. Am J Med. 2005;118(Suppl 10A):28S–33. Epub 2005/11/08.
33. Weikert BC, Blumberg EA. Viral infection after renal transplantation: surveillance and management. Clin J Am Soc Nephrol. 2008;3 Suppl 2:S76–86. Epub 2008/03/20.
34. Marzano A, Angelucci E, Andreone P, Brunetto M, Bruno R, Burra P, et al. Prophylaxis and treatment of hepatitis B in immunocompromised patients. Dig Liver Dis. 2007;39(5):397–408. Epub 2007/03/27.
35. Chan TM, Fang GX, Tang CS, Cheng IK, Lai KN, Ho SK. Preemptive lamivudine therapy based on HBV DNA level in HBsAg-positive kidney allograft recipients. Hepatology. 2002;36(5):1246–52. Epub 2002/10/24.
36. Lai CL, Shouval D, Lok AS, Chang TT, Cheinquer H, Goodman Z, et al. Entecavir versus lamivudine for patients with HBeAg-negative chronic hepatitis B. N Engl J Med. 2006;354(10):1011–20. Epub 2006/03/10.
37. Chang TT, Gish RG, de Man R, Gadano A, Sollano J, Chao YC, et al. A comparison of entecavir and lamivudine for HBeAg-positive chronic hepatitis B. N Engl J Med. 2006;354(10):1001–10. Epub 2006/03/10.
38. Marcellin P, Heathcote EJ, Buti M, Gane E, de Man RA, Krastev Z, et al. Tenofovir disoproxil fumarate versus adefovir dipivoxil for chronic hepatitis B. N Engl J Med. 2008;359(23):2442–55. Epub 2008/12/05.
39. Fontaine H, Thiers V, Chretien Y, Zylberberg H, Poupon RE, Brechot C, et al. HBV genotypic resistance to lamivudine in kidney recipients and hemodialyzed patients. Transplantation. 2000;69(10):2090–4. Epub 2000/06/14.
40. Lok AS, McMahon BJ. Chronic hepatitis B: update 2009. Hepatology. 2009;50(3):661–2. Epub 2009/08/29.
41. Johnson DW, Dent H, Yao Q, Tranaeus A, Huang CC, Han DS, et al. Frequencies of hepatitis B and C infections among haemodialysis and peritoneal dialysis patients in Asia-Pacific countries: analysis of registry data. Nephrol Dial Transplant. 2009;24(5):1598–603. Epub 2008/12/20.
42. Ghany MG, Strader DB, Thomas DL, Seeff LB. Diagnosis, management, and treatment of hepatitis C: an update. Hepatology. 2009;49(4):1335–74. Epub 2009/03/31.
43. Fissell RB, Bragg-Gresham JL, Woods JD, Jadoul M, Gillespie B, Hedderwick SA, et al. Patterns of hepatitis C prevalence and seroconversion in hemodialysis units from three continents: the DOPPS. Kidney Int. 2004;65(6):2335–42. Epub 2004/05/20.
44. Martin P, Fabrizi F. Hepatitis C virus and kidney disease. J Hepatol. 2008;49(4):613–24. Epub 2008/07/30.
45. Armstrong GL, Wasley A, Simard EP, McQuillan GM, Kuhnert WL, Alter MJ. The prevalence of hepatitis C virus infection in the United States, 1999 through 2002. Ann Intern Med. 2006;144(10):705–14. Epub 2006/05/17.
46. Fabrizi F, Poordad FF, Martin P. Hepatitis C infection and the patient with end-stage renal disease. Hepatology. 2002;36(1):3–10. Epub 2002/06/27.
47. Fabrizi F, Martin P, Dixit V, Bunnapradist S, Dulai G. Meta-analysis: effect of hepatitis C virus infection on mortality in dialysis. Aliment Pharmacol Ther. 2004;20(11–12):1271–7. Epub 2004/12/21.
48. Fabrizi F, Takkouche B, Lunghi G, Dixit V, Messa P, Martin P. The impact of hepatitis C virus infection on survival in dialysis patients: meta-analysis of observational studies. J Viral Hepat. 2007; 14(10):697–703. Epub 2007/09/19.
49. Kalantar-Zadeh K, McAllister CJ, Miller LG. Clinical characteristics and mortality in hepatitis C-positive haemodialysis patients: a population based study. Nephrol Dial Transplant. 2005;20(8):1662–9. Epub 2005/05/21.
50. Butt AA, Khan UA, Skanderson M. Comorbidities and their impact on mortality in HCV and HCV-HIV-coinfected persons on dialysis. J Clin Gastroenterol. 2008;42(9):1054–9. Epub 2008/11/18.
51. Kidney Disease: Improving Global Outcomes. KDIGO clinical practice guidelines for the prevention, diagnosis, evaluation, and treatment of hepatitis C in chronic kidney disease. Kidney Int Suppl. 2008;(109):S1–99. Epub 2008/05/03.
52. Ghany MG, Nelson DR, Strader DB, Thomas DL, Seeff LB. An update on treatment of genotype 1 chronic hepatitis C virus infection: 2011 practice guideline by the American Association for the Study of Liver Diseases. Hepatology. 2011;54(4):1433–44. Epub 2011/09/08.
53. Astor BC, Muntner P, Levin A, Eustace JA, Coresh J. Association of kidney function with anemia: the Third National Health and Nutrition Examination Survey (1988-1994). Arch Intern Med. 2002;162(12):1401–8. Epub 2002/06/22.
54. Hsu CY, McCulloch CE, Curhan GC. Epidemiology of anemia associated with chronic renal insufficiency among adults in the United States: results from the Third National Health and Nutrition Examination Survey. J Am Soc Nephrol. 2002;13(2):504–10. Epub 2002/01/24.
55. Deltenre P, Moreno C, Tran A, Ollivier I, Provot F, Stanke F, et al. Anti-viral therapy in haemodialysed HCV patients: efficacy, tolerance and treatment strategy. Aliment Pharmacol Ther. 2011;34(4):454–61. Epub 2011/06/21.
56. Fabrizi F, Martin P, Dixit V, Bunnapradist S, Dulai G. Hepatitis C virus antibody status and survival after renal transplantation: meta-analysis of observational studies. Am J Transplant. 2005;5(6):1452–61. Epub 2005/05/13.
57. Mahmoud IM, Sobh MA, El-Habashi AF, Sally ST, El-Baz M, El-Sawy E, et al. Interferon therapy in hemodialysis patients with chronic hepatitis C: study of tolerance, efficacy and post-transplantation course. Nephron Clin Pract. 2005;100(4):c133–9. Epub 2005/04/28.
58. Toth CM, Pascual M, Chung RT, Graeme-Cook F, Dienstag JL, Bhan AK, et al. Hepatitis C virus-associated fibrosing cholestatic hepatitis after renal transplantation: response to interferon-alpha therapy. Transplantation. 1998;66(9):1254–8. Epub 1998/11/24.
59. Bruchfeld A, Wilczek H, Elinder CG. Hepatitis C infection, time in renal-replacement therapy, and outcome after kidney transplantation. Transplantation. 2004;78(5):745–50. Epub 2004/09/17.
60. Natov SN, Lau JY, Ruthazer R, Schmid CH, Levey AS, Pereira BJ. Hepatitis C virus genotype does not affect patient survival among renal transplant candidates. The New England Organ Bank Hepatitis C Study Group. Kidney Int. 1999;56(2):700–6. Epub 1999/08/05.
61. Cosio FG, Sedmak DD, Henry ML, Al Haddad C, Falkenhain ME, Elkhammas EA, et al. The high prevalence of severe early post-transplant renal allograft pathology in hepatitis C positive recipients. Transplantation. 1996;62(8):1054–9. Epub 1996/10/27.

62. Terrault NA, Adey DB. The kidney transplant recipient with hepatitis C infection: pre- and posttransplantation treatment. Clin J Am Soc Nephrol. 2007;2(3):563–75. Epub 2007/08/19.
63. Baid S, Pascual M, Williams Jr WW, Tolkoff-Rubin N, Johnson SM, Collins B, et al. Renal thrombotic microangiopathy associated with anticardiolipin antibodies in hepatitis C-positive renal allograft recipients. J Am Soc Nephrol. 1999;10(1):146–53. Epub 1999/01/16.
64. Hestin D, Guillemin F, Castin N, Le Faou A, Champigneulles J, Kessler M. Pretransplant hepatitis C virus infection: a predictor of proteinuria after renal transplantation. Transplantation. 1998;65(5):741–4. Epub 1998/04/01.
65. Burstein DM, Rodby RA. Membranoproliferative glomerulonephritis associated with hepatitis C virus infection. J Am Soc Nephrol. 1993;4(6):1288–93. Epub 1993/12/01.
66. Ozdemir BH, Ozdemir FN, Sezer S, Colak T, Haberal M. De novo glomerulonephritis in renal allografts with hepatitis C virus infection. Transplant Proc. 2006;38(2):492–5. Epub 2006/03/22.
67. Cruzado JM, Casanovas-Taltavull T, Torras J, Baliellas C, Gil-Vernet S, Grinyo JM. Pretransplant interferon prevents hepatitis C virus-associated glomerulonephritis in renal allografts by HCV-RNA clearance. Am J Transplant. 2003;3(3):357–60. Epub 2003/03/05.
68. Cruzado JM, Carrera M, Torras J, Grinyo JM. Hepatitis C virus infection and de novo glomerular lesions in renal allografts. Am J Transplant. 2001;1(2):171–8. Epub 2002/07/09.
69. Gursoy M, Guvener N, Koksal R, Karavelioglu D, Baysal C, Ozdemir N, et al. Impact of HCV infection on development of posttransplantation diabetes mellitus in renal allograft recipients. Transplant Proc. 2000;32(3):561–2. Epub 2000/05/17.
70. Bloom RD, Rao V, Weng F, Grossman RA, Cohen D, Mange KC. Association of hepatitis C with posttransplant diabetes in renal transplant patients on tacrolimus. J Am Soc Nephrol. 2002;13(5): 1374–80. Epub 2002/04/19.
71. Fabrizi F, Martin P, Dixit V, Bunnapradist S, Kanwal F, Dulai G. Post-transplant diabetes mellitus and HCV seropositive status after renal transplantation: meta-analysis of clinical studies. Am J Transplant. 2005;5(10):2433–40. Epub 2005/09/16.
72. Delgado-Borrego A, Casson D, Schoenfeld D, Somsouk M, Terella A, Jordan SH, et al. Hepatitis C virus is independently associated with increased insulin resistance after liver transplantation. Transplantation. 2004;77(5):703–10. Epub 2004/03/17.
73. Shintani Y, Fujie H, Miyoshi H, Tsutsumi T, Tsukamoto K, Kimura S, et al. Hepatitis C virus infection and diabetes: direct involvement of the virus in the development of insulin resistance. Gastroenterology. 2004;126(3):840–8. Epub 2004/02/28.
74. Kawaguchi T, Yoshida T, Harada M, Hisamoto T, Nagao Y, Ide T, et al. Hepatitis C virus down-regulates insulin receptor substrates 1 and 2 through up-regulation of suppressor of cytokine signaling 3. Am J Pathol. 2004;165(5):1499–508. Epub 2004/10/29.
75. Hjelmesaeth J, Hartmann A, Leivestad T, Holdaas H, Sagedal S, Olstad M, et al. The impact of early-diagnosed new-onset post-transplantation diabetes mellitus on survival and major cardiac events. Kidney Int. 2006;69(3):588–95. Epub 2006/01/06.
76. Deol HS, Tuch BE. Effect of interleukin-10 on human anti-porcine xenogeneic cellular response in vitro. Transplantation. 2000;69(1):112–9. Epub 2000/02/01.
77. Miller J, Mendez R, Pirsch JD, Jensik SC. Safety and efficacy of tacrolimus in combination with mycophenolate mofetil (MMF) in cadaveric renal transplant recipients. FK506/MMF Dose-Ranging Kidney Transplant Study Group. Transplantation. 2000;69(5):875–80.

Management of Transplantation Renal Bone Disease: Interplay of Bone Mineral Density and Decisions Regarding Bisphosphonate Use

24

Hala M. Alshayeb, Stuart M. Sprague, and Michelle A. Josephson

Introduction of Post-transplant Bone Loss

The pathogenesis of post-transplant bone disease is multifactorial (Fig. 24.1). Bone mineral density (BMD) loss is common after kidney transplantation, particularly in the first post-transplant year [1–3] and is more pronounced in the lumbar spine than the femoral neck [50]. The rate of decline in BMD during the first 6–12 months post-transplantation ranges between 3 and 9 % [8–11, 45, 46]. The diminished degree of bone loss observed in some of the more recent studies may be a consequence of the use of lower glucocorticoid doses [10, 45, 46, 51]. However, bone loss persists after the first-year post-transplant as BMD reductions continue at rates of 1–2 % per year [52, 53]. Kidney transplant recipients are at 4.5-fold greater risk of fractures in comparison to the general population [4, 5, 7]. They have a 30 % higher risk of hip fracture during the first 3 years post-transplantation in comparison to dialysis patients on the waiting list for kidney transplant [54]. Post-kidney transplant fractures tend to occur more commonly in cortical bone with lower extremity fractures accounting for approximately 35 %, followed by fractures in the ribs, upper extremities, and vertebrae [4]. Unfortunately, measurements of BMD or trends of decreasing BMD have not been predictive of fractures [55, 56].

H.M. Alshayeb, M.D.
Department of Internal Medicine—Nephrology, Joan C. Edwards School of Medicine, Marshall University, 1249 15th Street, Huntington, WV 25701, USA
e-mail: Halamalshayeb@gmail.com

S.M. Sprague, D.O.
Department of Medicine, Section of Nephrology and Hypertension, NorthShore University Health System, 2650 Ridge Avenue, Evanston, IL 60201, USA
e-mail: stuartmsprague@gmail.com

M.A. Josephson, M.D. (✉)
Department of Medicine, Section of Nephrology, University of Chicago Medicine, Suite S-512, MC 5100, 5841 South Maryland Avenue, Chicago, IL 60637, USA
e-mail: mjosephs@medicine.bsd.uchicago.edu

Osteonecrosis is another major debilitating bone complication seen in transplant patients that is associated with chronic glucocorticoid use [6]. Osteonecrosis generally occurs in weight-bearing bones like the femoral head and knees. Most cases of osteonecrosis occur in the first year following transplant [6]. The reported incidence of osteonecrosis in the femoral head among kidney transplant recipients ranges between 4 and 25 % [57–60], with lower occurrences associated with decreased cumulative glucocorticoid use [61].

Screening Diagnosis and Monitoring of Post-transplant Bone Disease

Biochemical Evaluation

Determinations of calcium, phosphate, vitamin D (25-hydroxycholecalciferol), and parathyroid hormone (PTH) concentrations are used to define, monitor, and target treatment of post-transplant CKD-mineral bone disorders (CKD-MBD) [62, 63]. Table 24.1 provides recommendations on the frequency of monitoring biochemical parameters of post-transplant CKD-MBD (based on KDIGO and KDOQI guidelines) with more frequent monitoring advised during the first 12 weeks [12, 56, 64]. Additionally, serum vitamin D should be checked in the early post-transplant period [64]. Unfortunately, the biochemical targets representing optimal management of post-transplant bone CKD-MBD have not yet been defined. In the absence of studies specific to transplant patients, targets tailored to the degree of renal impairment seem reasonable. Though it has been recognized that PTH concentrations are a poor discriminator of bone turnover in CKD, they are even less reliable in the transplant patient [65].

Bone Biomarkers: Biomarkers of bone formation (bone-specific alkaline phosphatase, osteocalcin, procollagen C-terminal propeptide (PICP), and procollagen N-terminal

M.R. Weir and E.V. Lerma (eds.), *Kidney Transplantation: Practical Guide to Management*, DOI 10.1007/978-1-4939-0342-9_24, © Springer Science+Business Media New York 2014

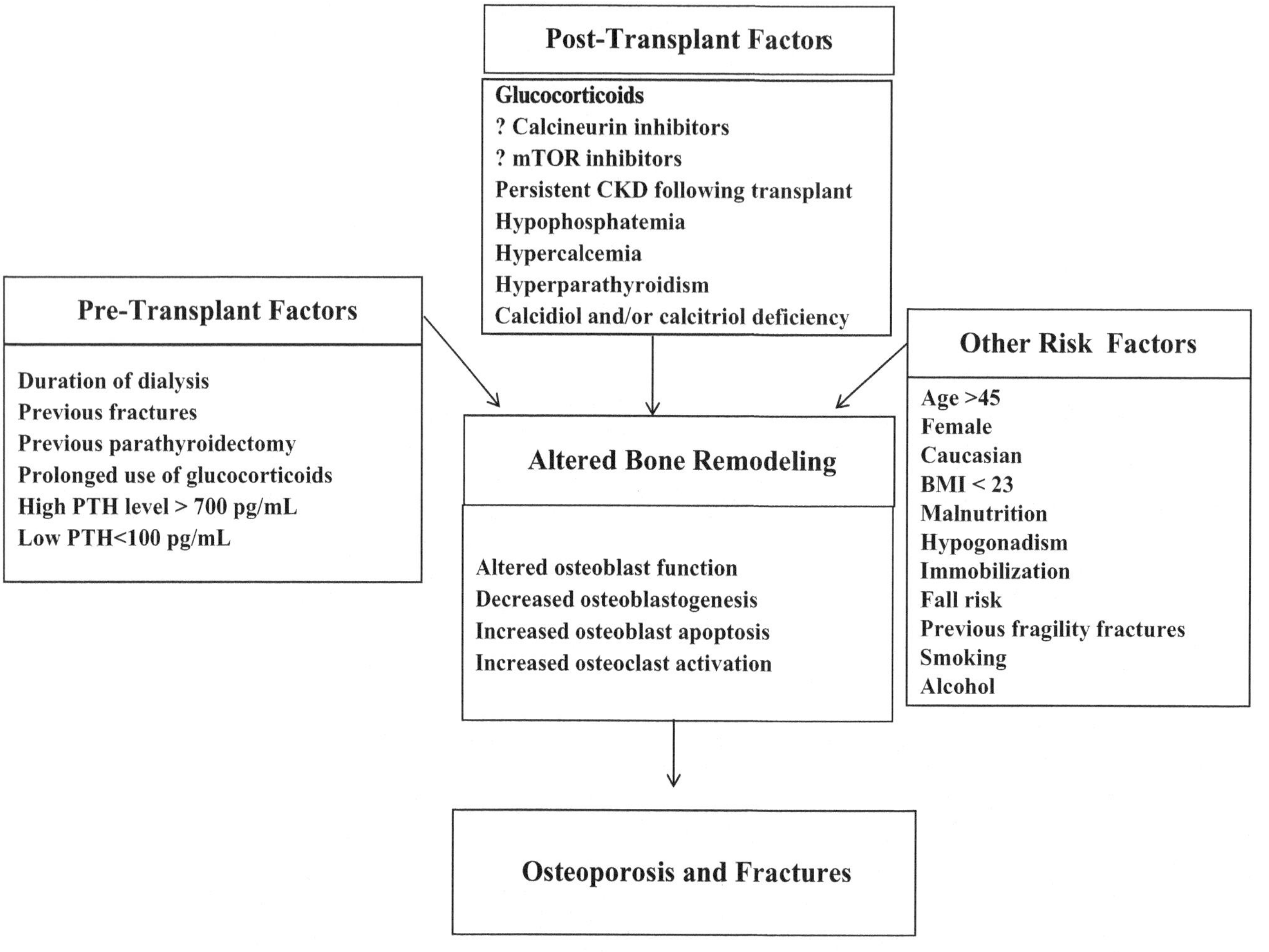

Fig. 24.1 The risk factors and pathogenesis of post-transplant bone loss and post-transplant fracture: the pathogenesis of post-transplant bone disease is multifactorial including but not limited to pre-transplant-related factors, transplant-related factors, and factors that increase the risk of osteoporosis and fractures. All these factors result in uncoupling bone formation and bone resorption with higher rate of the latter and subsequently increase bone loss and bone fractures. *CKD* chronic kidney disease, *PTH* parathyroid hormone, *BMI* body mass index [9–29]

Table 24.1 Combined KDIGO and KDOQI CKD-MBD monitoring guidelines for serum calcium, phosphorus, and intact PTH

Monitoring frequency guidelines				
CKD stage	GFR range (mL/min/1.73 m^2)	PTH (pg/mL)	Alkaline phosphatase (U/L)	Calcium and phosphorus (mg/dL)
CKD1 T	>90	Once in the first 3 months and then every 12 months	–	Weekly in the first 3 months till levels are normal and then every 6–12 months
CKD2 T	60–90		–	
CKD3 T	30–59		Every 12 months	
CKD4 T	15–29	Once in the first 3 months and then every 6–12 months	Every 12 months	Weekly in the first 3 months till levels are normal and then every 3–6 month
CKD5 T	<15	Once in the first 3 months and then every 3–6 months	Every 12 months	Weekly in the first 3 months till levels are normal and then every 1–3 months

Note. Conversion factors for units: eGFR in mL/min/1.73 m^2 to mL/s/1.73 m^2, ×0.01667; serum calcium in mg/dL to mmol/L, ×0.2495; serum phosphorus in mg/dL to mmol/L, ×0.323
eGFR estimated glomerular filtration rate, *PTH* intact parathyroid hormone

PINP) and bone resorption (urinary collagen breakdown products, TRAP5b) have been used to predict osteoporosis and fractures in the normal population. However, these biomarkers correlate poorly with bone loss as measured by densitometry and bone histology in the transplant patient and have not been shown to predict fracture risk. Until further information is available, there is probably no utility to measure these markers in the post-transplant patient.

Radiographic Evaluation

Densitometry

Bone densitometry, most commonly performed by dual-energy X-ray absorptiometry (DXA), is a readily available, noninvasive, rapid, cost-effective, and relatively precise method of screening BMD with low radiation exposure. However, the usefulness of DXA scans in patients with CKD and post-transplantation is limited because they do not reflect bone quality, turnover, or architecture [66]. The scans do not distinguish the underlying cause of bone loss. Low BMD measurements in post-kidney transplant recipients may be a consequence of osteoporosis and/or osteodystrophic bone disease [67]. The World Health Organization (WHO) [68] criteria defining fracture risk for osteopenia and osteoporosis are based on studies performed in normal postmenopausal Caucasian populations, thus limiting their applicability to kidney transplant recipients. Furthermore, there is no proven predictive relationship between BMD and fracture risk in kidney transplant recipients; in fact at least one study demonstrated that BMD did not distinguish those who went on to experience a fracture from those who did not [55]. BMD measurements in kidney transplant patients should not be looked at in isolation but should be analyzed and considered in the setting of a clinical assessment with biochemical data and possibly bone histology. However despite all of these limitations, BMDs may have a role in the transplant population. Sequential measurements of BMD may be helpful to guide antiresorptive therapy. KDIGO guidelines recommend measuring BMD at the time of transplantation or within the first 3 months after transplantation [23, 56, 69] when estimated GFR is >30 mL/min/m^2, particularly in patients with risk factors for rapid bone loss. However, KDIGO does not recommend DXA scans in patients with eGFR < 30 mL/min/1.73 m^2 as they are of no proven benefit in predicting fracture risk or the type of post-transplant bone disease [56]. DXA scans can be repeated at 12-month intervals if BMD decreases by greater than 5 % or half of a standard deviation; otherwise, DXA scan can be obtained every 2 years [70] to monitor response to therapy or to help decide whether therapy should be continued.

Conventional Radiographic Studies

Conventional radiography is helpful in identifying fractures, however is of limited value in distinguishing the different bone lesions of renal osteodystrophy. Lateral spine radiographs may be obtained to screen for asymptomatic spinal fragility fractures.

High-Resolution Quantitative Computed Tomography

High-resolution quantitative computed tomography (HR-QCT) is an accurate, noninvasive method of measuring volumetric BMD. It provides high-resolution three-dimensional images with information about volumetric BMD and microarchitecture with separation between cortical and trabecular bone [71]. Changes in volumetric vertebral BMD were found to correlate with changes detected in trabecular bone volume by bone biopsy [71]. Additionally, the trabecular microarchitecture in the radius and tibia using HR-QCT appears to better predict fracture risk in postmenopausal women [72] and is better than DXA in determining risk of fracture in patients with CKD [73, 74]. Unfortunately, this technology is not yet widely available, is costly, and has the disadvantage of high radiation exposure. The utility of this technique in the evaluation of post-transplant bone disease needs to be further evaluated before used outside of the research environment.

Magnetic Resonance Imaging

Magnetic resonance imaging (MRI) is a noninvasive screening and diagnostic modality for the early detection of osteonecrosis [75]. The newest generation of high-resolution MRI scanners can also be used to evaluate bone microarchitecture, resulting in images that may represent a "virtual bone biopsy" [76]. A pilot study of micro-MRI in 17 young adults on maintenance hemodialysis compared with healthy controls demonstrated cortical thinning and disruption of the trabecular architecture in the former [77]. Two other preliminary studies have demonstrated that transplant recipients had significantly lower MRI measurements of bone volume and microarchitecture compared with controls; however, spine QCT, trabecular BMD, and DXA hip and spine BMD did not differ between transplant recipients and controls [78, 79] Micro-MRI appears to be a promising tool; however, more data are required to determine its utility in assessing bone disease in the post-transplant patient.

General Measures

The goals of therapy for post-transplant bone disease include increasing bone mass to avoid fractures, normalizing bone turnover, minimizing the risk of osteonecrosis, and optimizing calciotropic and phosphotropic mineral metabolism. Prevention and treatment of post-transplant bone loss and fracture reduction should begin in the pre-transplant period by following preventive measures that are of proven benefit in both the CKD and general population [80], such as limiting the use of steroids, engaging in 30 min of daily vigorous physical exercise, avoiding nicotine and alcohol consumption, and fall risk reduction. Management of the disorders associated with CKD-MBD including hyperparathyroidism, calcium and phosphorus derangements, and treatment of vitamin D insufficiency and deficiency is appropriate.

In the post-transplant period, calcium and vitamin D supplementation can be considered in all kidney transplant recipients who do not have hypercalcemia; however, the effects of vitamin D on BMD in post-transplant recipients are still controversial [51, 81]. Although short-term use of gonadal hormone therapy in solid organ transplant recipients with hypogonadism may slow bone loss, this therapy may increase the risk of coronary artery disease, cancer, and thrombotic events and should not be used routinely [82]. Therapy of post-transplant hypophosphatemia should be considered only in symptomatic patients or patients with serum levels below 1–1.5 mg/dL, given the risk of hypocalcemia, nephrocalcinosis [83], and persistent hyperparathyroidism [84]. When used phosphate supplementation should be closely monitored.

Glucocorticoids Minimizing Protocols

The use of high steroid doses in the early post-transplant period has been associated with a substantial and accelerated bone loss in the first 6–12 months post-kidney transplant [1–3, 69, 85]. In the short term, glucocorticoids profoundly inhibit bone formation and increase bone resorption. With long-term exposure, steroids are associated with low bone turnover and increased apoptosis of both osteoblasts and osteoclasts [86] (Fig. 24.2). The increasing use of steroid-free immunosuppression [87] with steroid withdrawal initiated at a variety of post-transplant time points including 4 days, 3 or 12 months has been associated with preserved and improved BMD at the femoral neck and lumbar spine [88–90]. In addition, minimizing steroid therapy has resulted in less osteonecrosis [61]. To date, there are no data linking the improvement in BMD observed in transplant patients withdrawn from steroids with a reduction in fracture risk. Some observational studies suggest that steroid-free regimens [87] and early steroid withdrawal (discharge from the hospital off steroids after renal transplantation) [88] are associated with decreased incident fractures after the first-year post-transplantation. This finding is not uniform as at least one observational study demonstrated that steroid withdrawal 2–6 months after solid organ transplantation did not result in decreased fractures [91]. Prospective randomized controlled trials are needed to evaluate the role of steroid free regimens or the timing of steroid free regimens withdrawal on fracture risk reduction.

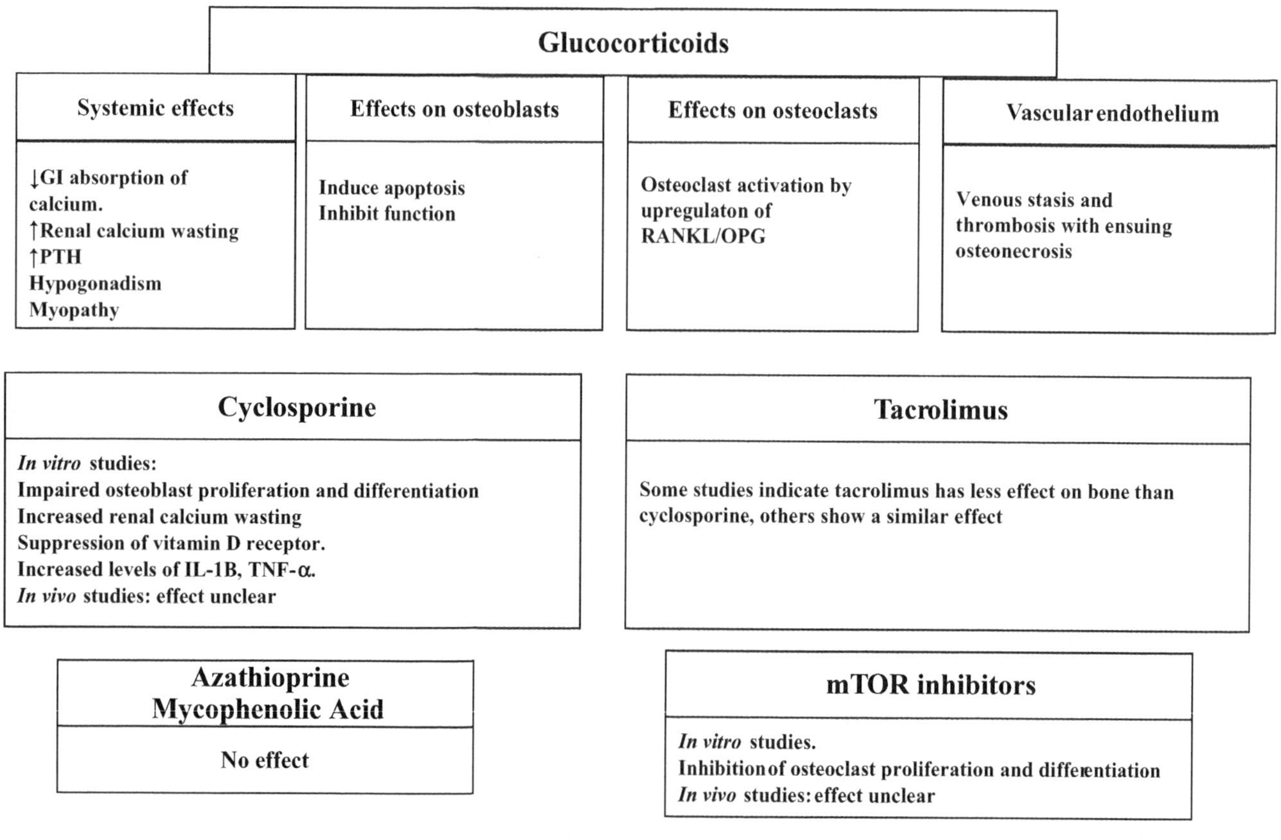

Fig. 24.2 Mechanisms underlying immunosuppressive medication's effect on bone. *GI* gastrointestinal, *PTH* parathyroid hormone, *RANKL* receptor activator of nuclear factor kappa-B ligand, *OPG* osteoprotegerin, *IL-1B* interleukin 1B, *TNF-a* tumor necrosis factor-a [27–32]

Antiresorptive Therapy

Antiresorptive therapy may be indicated for patients with osteopenia or osteoporosis, who have no evidence of low bone turnover or refractory hyperparathyroidism, and preserved renal function (eGFR > 35 mL/min) in the first post-transplant year [56]. Consideration of antiresorptive therapy use is warranted if the patient is on a steroid-based immunosuppression protocol and/or has a history of fragility fractures [23].

Bisphosphonates

Bisphosphonates are synthetic analogues of pyrophosphates that bind to hydroxyapatite in the bone and directly inhibit osteoclastic bone resorption [92–94]. Bisphosphonates also reduce osteoclastic activity by decreasing osteoclast progenitor development and recruitment and by promoting osteoclast apoptosis [92–94]. As well bisphosphonates prevent osteocyte and osteoblast apoptosis [95]. Data from clinical trials show that both oral and intravenous bisphosphonates prevent bone loss in the lumbar spine and femoral neck in the first post-transplant year [33–43] and beyond [55]. There is a lack of evidence, however, that bisphosphonate use has any beneficial effect on bone strength or fracture prevention in the kidney transplant population. This lack of supporting data may be because of the underpowered nature of studies undertaken to examine this issue. When dosed appropriately in properly selected patients and used for limited periods of time, bisphosphonate therapy is well tolerated, safe, and effective for the prevention and management of post-transplant bone loss. Intravenous zoledronic acid or ibandronate can be an alternative to oral bisphosphonates in patients who cannot tolerate the oral formulation or have difficulty with the dosing requirements. Bisphosphonates should be used with caution in patients with reduced kidney function and their use should be avoided in patients with eGFR of less than 30–35 mL/min, given the prolonged duration of action and accumulation in bone resulting in the possibility of inducing or perpetuating adynamic bone disease [40, 96]. To reiterate, though bisphosphonates have been demonstrated to attenuate bone loss following transplantation, they have not been shown to reduce fractures. In fact, one study demonstrated increased fractures in patients receiving bisphosphonate therapy [55]. Bisphosphonate therapy is generally contraindicated in patients with evidence of low bone turnover [40], and obtaining a bone biopsy before institution of bisphosphonate therapy is the most accurate means of characterizing bone turnover and avoiding its use in adynamic bone states.

A Cochrane review of 24 trials, including 1,209 kidney transplant recipients, evaluating the risks and benefits of bisphosphonates, vitamin D analogues, and calcitonin versus no treatment found that all of the interventions provided clinically significant prevention of bone loss in both the femoral neck and lumbar spine, with the exception of calcitonin [38] which did not improve femoral neck BMD [33]. Bisphosphonates were superior to calcitriol in preserving BMD. No single therapy was found to prevent fractures; however, lack of demonstration does not necessarily mean they do not reduce fractures, because as noted earlier, none of these trials were powered to detect a reduction in fracture risk. However, combining the effect of all therapies versus no intervention, there was a 49 % reduction in the relative fracture risk (confidence interval 0.27–0.99). In another meta-analysis by Stein et al., 11 trials evaluated fracture incidence in 780 solid organ transplant recipients (4 of the 11 trials and 42 % of the patients had kidney transplants) that received either bisphosphonates or vitamin D receptor agonists (VDRAs) within the first-year post-transplant [97]. There were 134 reported fractures in these studies. The use of bisphosphonates or VDRAs was associated with a reduced number of subjects with any fracture and vertebral fractures specifically. The discordance in findings between the Cochrane review and the meta-analysis by Stein et al. may be attributable to discrepancies in the methodology of the analyses, differences between the study populations, the timing of initiation of therapy and most importantly that not all studies included reported on fractures. Specifically in the Palmer et al. review, only 11/24 studies (34/514 patients) had reported fracture data [33], while in the Stein et al. review, 134 incident fractures were reported in the 659 subjects who had follow-up information [97]. These data suggest that preventive therapy including bisphosphonates or VDRAs is likely better than no therapy or calcium alone in preventing post-transplant bone loss and perhaps even fractures. In summary, bisphosphonates may have a role in select patient populations: specifically those at risk for fracture but without evidence for low turnover bone disease. The appropriate duration of therapy is not known; however, a maximum of 12–18 months of therapy immediately post-transplantation may be sufficient. Prospective appropriately controlled studies are required to determine the optimal role of bisphosphonate therapy.

Vitamin D Receptor Agonists

VDRAs can preserve and improve BMD by several mechanisms. VDRAs promote differentiation of osteoblast precursors into mature cells, significantly suppress osteoclastic bone activity, and maintain trabecular bone volume and wall thickness [98, 99]. In addition VDRAs can reverse glucocorticoid-induced decreases in intestinal calcium absorption and mitigate against secondary hyperparathyroidism [99].

Some studies demonstrate that oral calcitriol lowers PTH in patients with persistent post-transplant hyperparathyroidism [100, 101]. Several placebo controlled clinical trials demonstrate that active vitamin D preserves and improves BMD at both the lumbar spine and femoral neck in renal allograft recipients [45–49]. None of these studies show that VDRAs have any deleterious effects on renal allograft function. Clinically important outcomes such as mortality, hospitalizations, or fractures were not evaluated in these studies. Although, bisphosphonates have been shown to be superior to VDRAs in preserving and improving BMD in clinical trials [33, 102, 103], there is emerging evidence that suggests the use of either bisphosphonates or VDRAs in solid organ transplant recipients prevents fractures in the first post-transplant year [97]. Table 24.2 summarizes the indications, risks, and contraindications of VDRA therapy.

Calcimimetics

The calcimimetic cinacalcet functions as an allosteric activator of the calcium-sensing receptor (CaSR), the molecular mechanism that mediates calcium-regulated PTH secretion by parathyroid glands. It has been shown to be effective in the treatment of persistent post-transplant hyperparathyroidism and hypercalcemia [104–109]. However, data regarding the influence of cinacalcet on BMD in renal allograft recipients are scarce. Small observational studies [110] and case reports [111] demonstrate that cinacalcet therapy for post-transplant hyperparathyroidism is associated with improved BMD, a finding that needs to be further evaluated in a well-designed prospective study. Table 24.2 summarizes the indications, risks, and contraindications of cinacalcet therapy.

Teriparatide

Teriparatide is a recombinant human PTH (1-34) that has anabolic bone effects in both glucocorticoid-induced [112] and postmenopausal osteoporosis [113]. Its use has been shown to reduce fracture rates in postmenopausal females. Teriparatide, however, did not improve BMD in a small randomized controlled trial in renal transplant recipients [114].

Denosumab and Odanacatib

Denosumab is a fully humanized monoclonal antibody that blocks the receptor activator of nuclear factor kappa-B (RANK) and subsequently inhibits the formation, function, and survival of osteoclasts. Odanacatib (ODN) is a selective, potent, and reversible inhibitor of cathepsin K (CatK). Both of these agents have been shown to improve BMD in postmenopausal women in clinical trials [115–117], and denosumab is currently FDA approved for postmenopausal osteoporosis. Clinical studies evaluating the potential effects of these agents in the prevention of post-transplant BMD loss and fracture reduction have not been performed.

Parathyroidectomy

The surgical correction of hyperparathyroidism remains indicated for persistent post-transplant hyperparathyroidism that cannot be controlled by medical management with VDRAs or cinacalcet. Approximately 0.5–5 % of kidney transplant recipients ultimately require surgical parathyroidectomy (PTX) [118, 119]. There is a paucity of data available on the effects of PTX on bone histology, BMD, and fracture risk reduction.

General indications for PTX for post-transplant hyperparathyroidism are listed in Table 24.2.

Summary of Take-Home Points

- Post-transplant osteopenia and osteoporosis are very common in kidney transplant recipients.
- Kidney allograft recipients are at an increased risk of fractures.
- Post-transplant BMDs do not predict fracture risk.
- The pathogenesis of post-transplant bone disease is multifactorial resulting from the interactions of complex abnormalities in pre-transplant CKD-MBD and renal osteodystrophy, the degree of kidney dysfunction post-transplant, peri-transplant disturbances in vitamin D-FGF-23-PTH access, and the deleterious skeletal effects of immunosuppressive therapy.
- Bisphosphonate therapy in selected patients with high bone turnover and preserved eGFR (>35 mL/min/1.73 m^2) is associated with improved BMDs and may reduce post-transplant fractures when given during the first-year post-transplantation.
- VDRA therapy may be useful to preserve BMD as well as to treat patients with hyperparathyroidism without hypercalcemia.
- Steroid-sparing and steroid withdrawal immunosuppressive protocols have been shown to improve BMD; however, any beneficial effect on post-transplant fractures is unproven.
- Cinacalcet is the drug of choice for persistent post-transplant hyperparathyroidism with hypercalcemia.
- PTX is indicated for patients who fail medical therapy and develop complications of hyperparathyroidism.

Table 24.2 Therapies for post-transplant bone disease

Therapy	Indications	Effect on BMD	Effect on bone fracture	Side effects	Contraindications	Monitoring of therapy
Bisphosphonates	1. Improvement of BMD in kidney transplant recipients with eGFR > 30 mL/min/1.73 m^2 who have osteopenia or osteoporosis in the first 12 months post-transplant, after excluding low turnover bone disease	Improve femoral neck and lumbar spine BMD[a]	May decrease fracture risk[b]	Risk of adynamic bone disease and subsequent fractures, especially if used in patients with low eGFR	1. Low turnover bone disease	Bone biomarkers may be helpful
	2. Prevention of bone loss in kidney transplant recipients who have normal BMD but are at high risk of fractures after excluding low bone turnover				2. eGFR < 30 mL/min/1.73 m^2	Serum calcium levels
VDRAs	1. Persistent post-transplant hyperparathyroidism with relatively low calcium levels	Improve femoral neck and lumbar spine BMD[a]	May decrease fracture risk[b]	Risk of hypercalcemia	Hypercalcemia	Serum calcium, phosphorus, and PTH
	2. Prevention of bone loss in kidney transplant recipients with eGFR < 30 mL/min/1.73 m^2 who have hyperparathyroidism without hypercalcemia			Hyperphosphatemia	Hyperphosphatemia	Bone biomarkers may be helpful
	3. Kidney transplant recipients with eGFR > 30 mL/min/1.73 m^2 who have osteopenia or osteoporosis in the first 12 months post-transplant and who have low turnover bone disease confirmed by biopsy or suggested by trend of bone biomarkers			Oversuppression of parathyroid gland and decrease bone turnover	Calciphylaxis	
Calcimimetics	Persistent post-transplant hyperparathyroidism with hypercalcemia (off-label use)	Improve BMD[c]	Unknown	Hypocalcemia Gastrointestinal side effects	Hypocalcemia	Periodic monitoring of serum calcium, phosphorus, and PTH
Parathyroidectomy	Persistent post-transplant hyperparathyroidism with	Improve BMD[c]	Unknown	Hungry bone syndrome	Anatomical	Serum calcium, phosphorus, magnesium, and potassium in the immediate postsurgical period
	1. Parathyroid hyperplasia			Possible acute worsening in eGFR with subsequent improvement	Hypoparathyroidism	
	2. Hypercalcemia			Long-term effects on allograft function unclear	Hypocalcemia	
	3. Unexplained or worsening allograft function					
	4. Symptomatic bone disease, spontaneous fracture, vascular calcification, and/or calciphylaxis in the presence of hyperparathyroidism					

eGFR estimated glomerular filtration rate, *iPTH* intact parathyroid hormone, *VDRA* vitamin D receptor agonist
[a]Evidence from randomized trials
[b]Based on meta-analysis
[c]Based on observational descriptive study

References

1. Brandenburg VM, Politt D, Ketteler M, Fassbender WJ, Heussen N, Westenfeld R, et al. Early rapid loss followed by long-term consolidation characterizes the development of lumbar bone mineral density after kidney transplantation. Transplantation. 2004;77(10):1566–71. Epub 2004/07/09.
2. Brandenburg VM, Westenfeld R, Ketteler M. The fate of bone after renal transplantation. J Nephrol. 2004;17(2):190–204. Epub 2004/08/06.
3. Stein E, Ebeling P, Shane E. Post-transplantation osteoporosis. Endocrinol Metab Clin North Am. 2007;36(4):937–63, viii. Epub 2007/11/07.
4. Vautour LM, Melton 3rd LJ, Clarke BL, Achenbach SJ, Oberg AL, McCarthy JT. Long-term fracture risk following renal transplantation: a population-based study. Osteoporos Int. 2004;15(2):160–7. Epub 2003/12/11.
5. Nisbeth U, Lindh E, Ljunghall S, Backman U, Fellstrom B. Fracture frequency after kidney transplantation. Transplant Proc. 1994;26(3):1764. Epub 1994/06/01.
6. Paydas S, Balal M, Demir E, Sertdemir Y, Erken U. Avascular osteonecrosis and accompanying anemia, leucocytosis, and decreased bone mineral density in renal transplant recipients. Transplant Proc. 2011;43(3):863–6. Epub 2011/04/14.
7. Abbott KC, Oglesby RJ, Hypolite IO, Kirk AD, Ko CW, Welch PG, et al. Hospitalizations for fractures after renal transplantation in the United States. Ann Epidemiol. 2001;11(7):450–7. Epub 2001/09/15.
8. Julian BA, Laskow DA, Dubovsky J, Dubovsky EV, Curtis JJ, Quarles LD. Rapid loss of vertebral mineral density after renal transplantation. N Engl J Med. 1991;325(8):544–50. Epub 1991/08/22.
9. Horber FF, Casez JP, Steiger U, Czerniak A, Montandon A, Jaeger P. Changes in bone mass early after kidney transplantation. J Bone Miner Res. 1994;9(1):1–9. Epub 1994/01/01.
10. Mikuls TR, Julian BA, Bartolucci A, Saag KG. Bone mineral density changes within six months of renal transplantation. Transplantation. 2003;75(1):49–54. Epub 2003/01/25.
11. Almond MK, Kwan JT, Evans K, Cunningham J. Loss of regional bone mineral density in the first 12 months following renal transplantation. Nephron. 1994;66(1):52–7. Epub 1994/01/01.
12. Kidney Disease: Improving Global Outcomes (KDIGO) CKD-MBD Work Group. KDIGO clinical practice guideline for the diagnosis, evaluation, prevention, and treatment of chronic kidney disease-mineral and bone disorder (CKD-MBD). Kidney Int Suppl. 2009;(113):S1–130. Epub 2009/08/01.
13. Ramsey-Goldman R, Dunn JE, Dunlop DD, Stuart FP, Abecassis MM, Kaufman DB, et al. Increased risk of fracture in patients receiving solid organ transplants. J Bone Miner Res. 1999;14(3):456–63. Epub 1999/02/23.
14. Van Staa TP, Leufkens HG, Abenhaim L, Zhang B, Cooper C. Use of oral corticosteroids and risk of fractures. J Bone Miner Res. 2000;15(6):993–1000. Epub 2000/06/07.
15. Unal A, Kocyigit I, Sipahioglu MH, Tokgoz B, Kavuncuoglu F, Oymak O, et al. Loss of bone mineral density in renal transplantation recipients. Transplant Proc. 2010;42(9):3550–3. Epub 2010/11/26.
16. Ozel L, Ata P, Ozel MS, Toros AB, Kara M, Unal E, et al. Risk factors for osteoporosis after renal transplantation and effect of vitamin D receptor Bsm I polymorphism. Transplant Proc. 2011;43(3):858–62. Epub 2011/04/14.
17. Nikkel LE, Hollenbeak CS, Fox EJ, Uemura T, Ghahramani N. Risk of fractures after renal transplantation in the United States. Transplantation. 2009;87(12):1846–51. Epub 2009/06/23.
18. Kanaan N, Claes K, Devogelaer JP, Vanderschueren D, Depresseux G, Goffin E, et al. Fibroblast growth factor-23 and parathyroid hormone are associated with post-transplant bone mineral density loss. Clin J Am Soc Nephrol. 2010;5(10):1887–92. Epub 2010/07/17.
19. Dolgos S, Hartmann A, Bonsnes S, Isaksen GA, Godang K, Ueland T, et al. Early changes in bone mass, biochemical bone markers and fibroblast growth factor 23 after renal transplantation. Scand J Clin Lab Invest. 2009;69(2):161–7. Epub 2008/10/31.
20. Braga Junior JW, Neves RM, Pinheiro MM, Frisoli Junior A, Castro CH, Szejnfeld VL, et al. Prevalence of low trauma fractures in long-term kidney transplant patients with preserved renal function. Braz J Med Biol Res. 2006;39(1):137–47. Epub 2006/01/10.
21. Marcen R, Caballero C, Uriol O, Fernandez A, Villafruela JJ, Pascual J, et al. Prevalence of osteoporosis, osteopenia, and vertebral fractures in long-term renal transplant recipients. Transplant Proc. 2007;39(7):2256–8. Epub 2007/09/25.
22. Opelz G, Dohler B. Association of mismatches for HLA-DR with incidence of posttransplant hip fracture in kidney transplant recipients. Transplantation. 2011;91(1):65–9. Epub 2011/04/01.
23. Mainra R, Elder GJ. Individualized therapy to prevent bone mineral density loss after kidney and kidney-pancreas transplantation. Clin J Am Soc Nephrol. 2010;5(1):117–24. Epub 2009/12/08.
24. Rojas E, Carlini RG, Clesca P, Arminio A, Suniaga O, De Elguezabal K, et al. The pathogenesis of osteodystrophy after renal transplantation as detected by early alterations in bone remodeling. Kidney Int. 2003;63(5):1915–23. Epub 2003/04/05.
25. Lehmann G, Ott U, Stein G, Steiner T, Wolf G. Renal osteodystrophy after successful renal transplantation: a histomorphometric analysis in 57 patients. Transplant Proc. 2007;39(10):3153–8. Epub 2007/12/20.
26. Sprague SM, Belozeroff V, Danese MD, Martin LP, Olgaard K. Abnormal bone and mineral metabolism in kidney transplant patients—a review. Am J Nephrol. 2008;28(2):246–53. Epub 2007/11/09.
27. Maalouf NM, Shane E. Osteoporosis after solid organ transplantation. J Clin Endocrinol Metab. 2005;90(4):2456–65. Epub 2004/12/30.
28. Adachi JD, Bensen WG, Hodsman AB. Corticosteroid-induced osteoporosis. Semin Arthritis Rheum. 1993;22(6):375–84. Epub 1993/06/01.
29. Weinstein RS, Jilka RL, Parfitt AM, Manolagas SC. Inhibition of osteoblastogenesis and promotion of apoptosis of osteoblasts and osteocytes by glucocorticoids. Potential mechanisms of their deleterious effects on bone. J Clin Investig. 1998;102(2):274–82. Epub 1998/07/17.
30. Schlosberg M, Movsowitz C, Epstein S, Ismail F, Fallon MD, Thomas S. The effect of cyclosporin A administration and its withdrawal on bone mineral metabolism in the rat. Endocrinology. 1989;124(5):2179–84. Epub 1989/05/01.
31. Moreira RO, Thiago LS, Oliveira FL, Balduino A, Borojevic R, Duarte ME, et al. Cyclosporine A, but not tacrolimus, is associated with impaired proliferation and differentiation of human osteoblast-like cells in vitro. Med Sci Monit. 2009;15(3):BR65–70. Epub 2009/02/28.
32. Stewart PJ, Stern PH. Cyclosporines: correlation of immunosuppressive activity and inhibition of bone resorption. Calcif Tissue Int. 1989;45(4):222–6. Epub 1989/10/01.
33. Palmer SC, McGregor DO, Strippoli GF. Interventions for preventing bone disease in kidney transplant recipients. Cochrane Database Syst Rev. 2007;(3):CD005015. Epub 2007/07/20.
34. Grotz W, Nagel C, Poeschel D, Cybulla M, Petersen KG, Uhl M, et al. Effect of ibandronate on bone loss and renal function after kidney transplantation. J Am Soc Nephrol. 2001;12(7):1530–7. Epub 2001/06/26.
35. Mitterbauer C, Schwarz C, Haas M, Oberbauer R. Effects of bisphosphonates on bone loss in the first year after renal transplan-

tation—a meta-analysis of randomized controlled trials. Nephrol Dial Transplant. 2006;21(8):2275–81. Epub 2006/04/01.
36. Fan SL, Almond MK, Ball E, Evans K, Cunningham J. Pamidronate therapy as prevention of bone loss following renal transplantation. Kidney Int. 2000;57(2):684–90. Epub 2000/01/29.
37. Jeffery JR, Leslie WD, Karpinski ME, Nickerson PW, Rush DN. Prevalence and treatment of decreased bone density in renal transplant recipients: a randomized prospective trial of calcitriol versus alendronate. Transplantation. 2003;76(10):1498–502. Epub 2003/12/06.
38. El-Agroudy AE, El-Husseini AA, El-Sayed M, Ghoneim MA. Preventing bone loss in renal transplant recipients with vitamin D. J Am Soc Nephrol. 2003;14(11):2975–9. Epub 2003/10/22.
39. Nowacka-Cieciura E, Cieciura T, Baczkowska T, Kozinska-Przybyl O, Tronina O, Chudzinski W, et al. Bisphosphonates are effective prophylactic of early bone loss after renal transplantation. Transplant Proc. 2006;38(1):165–7. Epub 2006/03/01.
40. Coco M, Glicklich D, Faugere MC, Burris L, Bognar I, Durkin P, et al. Prevention of bone loss in renal transplant recipients: a prospective, randomized trial of intravenous pamidronate. J Am Soc Nephrol. 2003;14(10):2669–76. Epub 2003/09/30.
41. Haas M, Leko-Mohr Z, Roschger P, Kletzmayr J, Schwarz C, Mitterbauer C, et al. Zoledronic acid to prevent bone loss in the first 6 months after renal transplantation. Kidney Int. 2003;63(3):1130–6. Epub 2003/03/13.
42. Abediazar S, Nakhjavani MR. Effect of alendronate on early bone loss of renal transplant recipients. Transplant Proc. 2011;43(2):565–7. Epub 2011/03/29.
43. Torregrosa JV, Fuster D, Pedroso S, Diekmann F, Campistol JM, Rubi S, et al. Weekly risedronate in kidney transplant patients with osteopenia. Transpl Int. 2007;20(8):708–11. Epub 2007/06/09.
44. Torregrosa JV, Fuster D, Monegal A, Gentil MA, Bravo J, Guirado L, et al. Efficacy of low doses of pamidronate in osteopenic patients administered in the early post-renal transplant. Osteoporos Int. 2011;22(1):281–7. Epub 2010/03/17.
45. Josephson MA, Schumm LP, Chiu MY, Marshall C, Thistlethwaite JR, Sprague SM. Calcium and calcitriol prophylaxis attenuates posttransplant bone loss. Transplantation. 2004;78(8):1233–6. Epub 2004/10/27.
46. El-Agroudy AE, El-Husseini AA, El-Sayed M, Mohsen T, Ghoneim MA. A prospective randomized study for prevention of postrenal transplantation bone loss. Kidney Int. 2005;67(5):2039–45. Epub 2005/04/21.
47. El-Husseini AA, El-Agroudy AE, El-Sayed M, Sobh MA, Ghoneim MA. A prospective randomized study for the treatment of bone loss with vitamin d during kidney transplantation in children and adolescents. Am J Transplant. 2004;4(12):2052–7. Epub 2004/12/04.
48. Torres A, Garcia S, Gomez A, Gonzalez A, Barrios Y, Concepcion MT, et al. Treatment with intermittent calcitriol and calcium reduces bone loss after renal transplantation. Kidney Int. 2004;65(2):705–12. Epub 2004/01/14.
49. De Sevaux RG, Hoitsma AJ, Corstens FH, Wetzels JF. Treatment with vitamin D and calcium reduces bone loss after renal transplantation: a randomized study. J Am Soc Nephrol. 2002;13(6):1608–14. Epub 2002/06/01.
50. Kodras K, Haas M. Effect of kidney transplantation on bone. Eur J Clin Invest. 2006;36 Suppl 2:63–75. Epub 2006/08/04.
51. Wissing KM, Broeders N, Moreno-Reyes R, Gervy C, Stallenberg B, Abramowicz D. A controlled study of vitamin D3 to prevent bone loss in renal-transplant patients receiving low doses of steroids. Transplantation. 2005;79(1):108–15. Epub 2005/02/17.
52. Cruz DN, Wysolmerski JJ, Brickel HM, Gundberg CG, Simpson CA, Mitnick MA, et al. Parameters of high bone-turnover predict bone loss in renal transplant patients: a longitudinal study. Transplantation. 2001;72(1):83–8. Epub 2001/07/27.
53. Pichette V, Bonnardeaux A, Prudhomme L, Gagne M, Cardinal J, Ouimet D. Long-term bone loss in kidney transplant recipients: a cross-sectional and longitudinal study. Am J Kidney Dis. 1996;28(1):105–14. Epub 1996/07/01.
54. Ball AM, Gillen DL, Sherrard D, Weiss NS, Emerson SS, Seliger SL, et al. Risk of hip fracture among dialysis and renal transplant recipients. JAMA. 2002;288(23):3014–8. Epub 2002/12/17.
55. Conley E, Muth B, Samaniego M, Lotfi M, Voss B, Armbrust M, et al. Bisphosphonates and bone fractures in long-term kidney transplant recipients. Transplantation. 2008;86(2):231–7. Epub 2008/07/23.
56. Kidney Disease: Improving Global Outcomes Transplant Work Group. KDIGO clinical practice guideline for the care of kidney transplant recipients. Am J Transplant. 2009;9 Suppl 3:S1–155. Epub 2009/10/23.
57. Tang S, Chan TM, Lui SL, Li FK, Lo WK, Lai KN. Risk factors for avascular bone necrosis after renal transplantation. Transplant Proc. 2000;32(7):1873–5. Epub 2000/12/20.
58. Celik A, Tekis D, Saglam F, Tunali S, Kabakci N, Ozaksoy D, et al. Association of corticosteroids and factor V, prothrombin, and MTHFR gene mutations with avascular osteonecrosis in renal allograft recipients. Transplant Proc. 2006;38(2):512–6. Epub 2006/03/22.
59. Hedri H, Cherif M, Zouaghi K, Abderrahim E, Goucha R, Ben Hamida F, et al. Avascular osteonecrosis after renal transplantation. Transplant Proc. 2007;39(4):1036–8. Epub 2007/05/26.
60. Lausten GS, Lemser T, Jensen PK, Egfjord M. Necrosis of the femoral head after kidney transplantation. Clin Transplant. 1998;12(6):572–4. Epub 1998/12/16.
61. Marston SB, Gillingham K, Bailey RF, Cheng EY. Osteonecrosis of the femoral head after solid organ transplantation: a prospective study. J Bone Joint Surg Am. 2002;84-A(12):2145–51. Epub 2002/12/11.
62. Fernandez-Fresnedo G, Rodrigo E, Ruiz JC, Martin de Francisco AL, Arias M. Bone metabolism according to chronic kidney disease stages in patients undergoing kidney transplantation: a 5-year database analysis. Transplant Proc. 2009;41(6):2403–5. Epub 2009/09/01.
63. Ambrus C, Molnar MZ, Czira ME, Rosivall L, Kiss I, Remport A, et al. Calcium, phosphate and parathyroid metabolism in kidney transplanted patients. Int Urol Nephrol. 2009;41(4):1029–38. Epub 2009/08/25.
64. Kasiske BL, Zeier MG, Chapman JR, Craig JC, Ekberg H, Garvey CA, et al. KDIGO clinical practice guideline for the care of kidney transplant recipients: a summary. Kidney Int. 2010; 77(4):299–311. Epub 2009/10/23.
65. Cruz EA, Lugon JR, Jorgetti V, Draibe SA, Carvalho AB. Histologic evolution of bone disease 6 months after successful kidney transplantation. Am J Kidney Dis. 2004;44(4):747–56. Epub 2004/09/24.
66. Bates DW, Black DM, Cummings SR. Clinical use of bone densitometry: clinical applications. JAMA. 2002;288(15):1898–900. Epub 2002/10/17.
67. Grotz WH, Mundinger FA, Gugel B, Exner V, Kirste G, Schollmeyer PJ. Bone fracture and osteodensitometry with dual energy X-ray absorptiometry in kidney transplant recipients. Transplantation. 1994;58(8):912–5. Epub 1994/10/27.
68. Kanis JA. Assessment of fracture risk and its application to screening for postmenopausal osteoporosis: synopsis of a WHO report. WHO Study Group. Osteoporos Int. 1994;4(6):368–81. Epub 1994/11/01.
69. Huang M, Sprague SM. Bone disease in kidney transplant patients. Semin Nephrol. 2009;29(2):166–73. Epub 2009/04/18.
70. Sprague SM, Josephson MA. Bone disease after kidney transplantation. Semin Nephrol. 2004;24(1):82–90. Epub 2004/01/20.

71. Genant HK, Engelke K, Prevrhal S. Advanced CT bone imaging in osteoporosis. Rheumatology (Oxford). 2008;47 Suppl 4:iv9–16. Epub 2008/07/02.
72. Liu XS, Stein EM, Zhou B, Zhang CA, Nickolas TL, Cohen A, et al. Individual trabecula segmentation (ITS)-based morphological analyses and micro finite element analysis of HR-pQCT images discriminate postmenopausal fragility fractures independent of DXA measurements. J Bone Miner Res. 2012;27:263–72. Epub 2011/11/11.
73. Nickolas TL, Cremers S, Zhang A, Thomas V, Stein E, Cohen A, et al. Discriminants of prevalent fractures in chronic kidney disease. J Am Soc Nephrol. 2011;22(8):1560–72. Epub 2011/07/26.
74. Nickolas TL, Stein E, Cohen A, Thomas V, Staron RB, McMahon DJ, et al. Bone mass and microarchitecture in CKD patients with fracture. J Am Soc Nephrol. 2010;21(8):1371–80. Epub 2010/04/17.
75. Sugano N, Kubo T, Takaoka K, Ohzono K, Hotokebuchi T, Matsumoto T, et al. Diagnostic criteria for non-traumatic osteonecrosis of the femoral head. A multicentre study. J Bone Joint Surg Br. 1999;81(4):590–5. Epub 1999/08/27.
76. Wehrli FW, Saha PK, Gomberg BR, Song HK, Snyder PJ, Benito M, et al. Role of magnetic resonance for assessing structure and function of trabecular bone. Top Magn Reson Imaging. 2002;13(5):335–55. Epub 2002/12/05.
77. Wehrli FW, Leonard MB, Saha PK, Gomberg BR. Quantitative high-resolution magnetic resonance imaging reveals structural implications of renal osteodystrophy on trabecular and cortical bone. J Magn Reson Imaging. 2004;20(1):83–9. Epub 2004/06/29.
78. Link TM, Saborowski, Kisters K, Kempkes M, Kosch M, Newitt D, et al. Changes in calcaneal trabecular bone structure assessed with high-resolution MR imaging in patients with kidney transplantation. Osteoporos Int. 2002;13(2):119–29. Epub 2002/03/22.
79. Rajapakse CS, Leonard MB, Bhagat YA, Sun W, Magland JF, Wehrli FW. Micro-MR imaging-based computational biomechanics demonstrates reduction in cortical and trabecular bone strength after renal transplantation. Radiology. 2012;262(3):912–20. Epub 2012/02/24.
80. Sperschneider H, Stein G. Bone disease after renal transplantation. Nephrol Dial Transplant. 2003;18(5):874–7. Epub 2003/04/11.
81. Sahin G, Yasar NS, Sirmagul B, Bal C, Yalcin AU. The effect of low-dose cholecalciferol and calcium treatment on posttransplant bone loss in renal transplant patients: a prospective study. Ren Fail. 2008;30(10):992–9. Epub 2008/11/19.
82. Isoniemi H, Appelberg J, Nilsson CG, Makela P, Risteli J, Hockerstedt K. Transdermal oestrogen therapy protects postmenopausal liver transplant women from osteoporosis. A 2-year follow-up study. J Hepatol. 2001;34(2):299–305.
83. Evenepoel P, Lerut E, Naesens M, Bammens B, Claes K, Kuypers D, et al. Localization, etiology and impact of calcium phosphate deposits in renal allografts. Am J Transplant. 2009;9(11):2470–8. Epub 2009/08/18.
84. Caravaca F, Fernandez MA, Ruiz-Calero R, Cubero J, Aparicio A, Jimenez F, et al. Effects of oral phosphorus supplementation on mineral metabolism of renal transplant recipients. Nephrol Dial Transplant. 1998;13(10):2605–11. Epub 1998/10/30.
85. Kulak CA, Borba VZ, Kulak Junior J, Campos DJ, Shane E. Posttransplantation osteoporosis. Arq Bras Endocrinol Metabol. 2010;54(2):143–9. Epub 2010/05/21.
86. Weisinger JR, Carlini RG, Rojas E, Bellorin-Font E. Bone disease after renal transplantation. Clin J Am Soc Nephrol. 2006;1(6):1300–13. Epub 2007/08/21.
87. Pereira S, Pedroso S, Martins L, Santos P, Almeida M, Freitas C, et al. Bone mineral density after simultaneous kidney-pancreas transplantation: four years follow-up of 57 recipients. Transplant Proc. 2010;42(2):555–7. Epub 2010/03/23.
88. Nikkel LE, Mohan S, Zhang A, McMahon DJ, Boutroy S, Dube G, et al. Reduced fracture risk with early corticosteroid withdrawal after kidney transplant. Am J Transplant. 2012;12(3):649–59. Epub 2011/12/14.
89. Hazzan M, Glowacki F, Lionet A, Provot F, Noel C. [Weaning from corticosteroid therapy after kidney transplantation]. Nephrol Ther. 2009;5 Suppl 6:S355–8. Epub 2010/02/05. Sevrage de la corticotherapie apres transplantation renale.
90. Ing SW, Sinnott LT, Donepudi S, Davies EA, Pelletier RP, Lane NE. Change in bone mineral density at one year following glucocorticoid withdrawal in kidney transplant recipients. Clin Transplant. 2011;25(2):E113–23. Epub 2010/10/22.
91. Edwards BJ, Desai A, Tsai J, Du H, Edwards GR, Bunta AD, et al. Elevated incidence of fractures in solid-organ transplant recipients on glucocorticoid-sparing immunosuppressive regimens. J Osteoporos. 2011;2011:591793. Epub 2011/09/17.
92. Rodan GA, Fleisch HA. Bisphosphonates: mechanisms of action. J Clin Invest. 1996;97(12):2692–6. Epub 1996/06/15.
93. Sato M, Grasser W, Endo N, Akins R, Simmons H, Thompson DD, et al. Bisphosphonate action. Alendronate localization in rat bone and effects on osteoclast ultrastructure. J Clin Invest. 1991;88(6):2095–105. Epub 1991/12/01.
94. Colucci S, Minielli V, Zambonin G, Cirulli N, Mori G, Serra M, et al. Alendronate reduces adhesion of human osteoclast-like cells to bone and bone protein-coated surfaces. Calcif Tissue Int. 1998;63(3):230–5. Epub 1998/08/14.
95. Plotkin LI, Lezcano V, Thostenson J, Weinstein RS, Manolagas SC, Bellido T. Connexin 43 is required for the anti-apoptotic effect of bisphosphonates on osteocytes and osteoblasts in vivo. J Bone Miner Res. 2008;23(11):1712–21. Epub 2008/07/04.
96. Coco M, Pullman J, Cohen HW, Lee S, Shapiro C, Solorzano C, et al. Effect of risedronate on bone in renal transplant recipients. J Am Soc Nephrol. 2012;23(8):1426–37. Epub 2012/07/17.
97. Stein EM, Ortiz D, Jin Z, McMahon DJ, Shane E. Prevention of fractures after solid organ transplantation: a meta-analysis. J Clin Endocrinol Metabol. 2011;96(11):3457–65. Epub 2011/08/19.
98. Cueto-Manzano AM, Konel S, Freemont AJ, Adams JE, Mawer B, Gokal R, et al. Effect of 1,25-dihydroxyvitamin D3 and calcium carbonate on bone loss associated with long-term renal transplantation. Am J Kidney Dis. 2000;35(2):227–36. Epub 2000/02/17.
99. Sambrook P. Alfacalcidol and calcitriol in the prevention of bone loss after organ transplantation. Calcif Tissue Int. 1999;65(4):341–3. Epub 1999/09/15.
100. Steiner RW, Ziegler M, Halasz NA, Catherwood BD, Manolagas S, Deftos LJ. Effect of daily oral vitamin D and calcium therapy, hypophosphatemia, and endogenous 1-25 dihydroxycholecalciferol on parathyroid hormone and phosphate wasting in renal transplant recipients. Transplantation. 1993;56(4):843–6. Epub 1993/10/01.
101. Lobo PI, Cortez MS, Stevenson W, Pruett TL. Normocalcemic hyperparathyroidism associated with relatively low 1:25 vitamin D levels post-renal transplant can be successfully treated with oral calcitriol. Clin Transplant. 1995;9(4):277–81. Epub 1995/08/01.
102. Koc M, Tuglular S, Arikan H, Ozener C, Akoglu E. Alendronate increases bone mineral density in long-term renal transplant recipients. Transplant Proc. 2002;34(6):2111–3. Epub 2002/09/25.
103. Nam JH, Moon JI, Chung SS, Kim SI, Park KI, Song YD, et al. Pamidronate and calcitriol trial for the prevention of early bone loss after renal transplantation. Transplant Proc. 2000;32(7):1876. Epub 2000/12/20.
104. Serra AL, Wuhrmann C, Wuthrich RP. Phosphatemic effect of cinacalcet in kidney transplant recipients with persistent hyperparathyroidism. Am J Kidney Dis. 2008;52(6):1151–7. Epub 2008/10/28.

105. Serra AL, Schwarz AA, Wick FH, Marti HP, Wuthrich RP. Successful treatment of hypercalcemia with cinacalcet in renal transplant recipients with persistent hyperparathyroidism. Nephrol Dial Transplant. 2005;20(7):1315–9. Epub 2005/06/09.
106. Copley JB, Germain M, Stern L, Pankewycz O, Katznelson S, Shah T, et al. Evaluation of cinacalcet HCl treatment after kidney transplantation. Transplant Proc. 2010;42(7):2503–8. Epub 2010/09/14.
107. Gomez Marques G, Obrador Mulet A, Vilar Gimeno A, Pascual Felip MJ, Alarcon Zurita A, Molina Guasch M, et al. Treatment with cinacalcet of secondary hyperparathyroidism after renal transplantation. Transplant Proc. 2009;41(6):2139–43. Epub 2009/09/01.
108. Serra AL, Savoca R, Huber AR, Hepp U, Delsignore A, Hersberger M, et al. Effective control of persistent hyperparathyroidism with cinacalcet in renal allograft recipients. Nephrol Dial Transplant. 2007;22(2):577–83. Epub 2006/09/29.
109. El-Amm JM, Doshi MD, Singh A, Migdal S, Morawski K, Sternbauer D, et al. Preliminary experience with cinacalcet use in persistent secondary hyperparathyroidism after kidney transplantation. Transplantation. 2007;83(5):546–9. Epub 2007/03/14.
110. Bergua C, Torregrosa JV, Fuster D, Gutierrez-Dalmau A, Oppenheimer F, Campistol JM. Effect of cinacalcet on hypercalcemia and bone mineral density in renal transplanted patients with secondary hyperparathyroidism. Transplantation. 2008;86(3):413–7. Epub 2008/08/14.
111. Decleire PY, Devogelaer JP, Goffin E. Cinacalcet improves bone mineral density in a renal transplant recipient with persistent hyperparathyroidism. Clin Nephrol. 2008;69(3):231–2. Epub 2008/04/10.
112. Saag KG, Shane E, Boonen S, Marin F, Donley DW, Taylor KA, et al. Teriparatide or alendronate in glucocorticoid-induced osteoporosis. N Engl J Med. 2007;357(20):2028–39. Epub 2007/11/16.
113. Finkelstein JS, Wyland JJ, Lee H, Neer RM. Effects of teriparatide, alendronate, or both in women with postmenopausal osteoporosis. J Clin Endocrinol Metab. 2010;95(4):1838–45. Epub 2010/02/19.
114. Cejka D, Benesch T, Krestan C, Roschger P, Klaushofer K, Pietschmann P, et al. Effect of teriparatide on early bone loss after kidney transplantation. Am J Transplant. 2008;8(9):1864–70. Epub 2008/09/13.
115. Jamal SA, Ljunggren O, Stehman-Breen C, Cummings SR, McClung MR, Goemaere S, et al. Effects of denosumab on fracture and bone mineral density by level of kidney function. J Bone Miner Res. 2011;26(8):1829–35. Epub 2011/04/15.
116. Papapoulos S, Chapurlat R, Libanati C, Brandi M, Brown J, Czerwinski E, et al. Five years of denosumab exposure in women with postmenopausal osteoporosis: results from the first two years of the FREEDOM extension. J Bone Miner Res. 2012;27(3):694–701. Epub 2011/11/25.
117. Bone HG, McClung MR, Roux C, Recker RR, Eisman JA, Verbruggen N, et al. Odanacatib, a cathepsin-K inhibitor for osteoporosis: a two-year study in postmenopausal women with low bone density. J Bone Miner Res. 2010;25(5):937–47. Epub 2009/10/31.
118. Evenepoel P, Claes K, Kuypers D, Maes B, Vanrenterghem Y. Impact of parathyroidectomy on renal graft function, blood pressure and serum lipids in kidney transplant recipients: a single centre study. Nephrol Dial Transplant. 2005;20(8):1714–20. Epub 2005/05/28.
119. Drakopoulos S, Koukoulaki M, Apostolou T, Pistolas D, Balaska K, Gavriil S, et al. Total parathyroidectomy without autotransplantation in dialysis patients and renal transplant recipients, long-term follow-up evaluation. Am J Surg. 2009;198(2):178–83. Epub 2009/02/17.

25 Malignancies After Transplantation and Posttransplant Lymphoproliferative Disorder

Ahmed I. Kamal and Roslyn B. Mannon

Abbreviations

ADPKD	Autosomal dominant polycystic kidney disease
BCC	Basal cell cancer
CNI	Calcineurin inhibitor
CT	Computerized tomography
EAR	Excess absolute risk
EBV	Epstein-Barr virus
HBV	Hepatitis B
HCV	Hepatitis C
HPV	Human papillomavirus
IPTTR	Israel Penn Transplant Tumor Registry
MRI	Magnetic resonance imaging
mTORi	mTOR inhibitor
NMSC	Nonmelanoma skin cancer
PCR	Polymerase chain reaction
PSA	Prostate-specific antigen
PTLD	Posttransplant lymphoproliferative disorder
SCC	Squamous cell cancer
SIR	Standardized incidence ratio
SRTR	Scientific Registry of Transplant Recipients

The Epidemiology of Posttransplant Malignancy

Cancer occurrence after solid organ transplant is higher than in the general public. A limitation in our full understanding of this issue comes from the lack of national data registry for cancer after transplantation. Valuable insights have been made in this area utilizing data from the Israel Penn Transplant Tumor Registry (IPTTR), a voluntary cancer registry [1], but due to the voluntary nature of these data, the registry data are incomplete. Recent analysis linking data from the Scientific Registry of Transplant Recipients (SRTR) to state and center registries has provided much larger numbers of affected recipients, with much more significant understanding about the role of transplantation on tumor occurrence in the end-stage renal disease population. With over 175,000 solid organ recipients transplanted from 1997 to 2008 included in an analysis of which more than half are kidney transplant recipients, the incidence of cancer was 1,375 per 100,000 person-years equating to a standardized incidence ratio (SIR) of 2.10 [95 % CI, 2.06–2.14] and excess absolute risk (EAR) of 719.3 [95 % CI, 693.3–745.6] per 100,000 person-years [2]. The most common cancers that had significantly elevated risk compared to the general population were non-Hodgkin's lymphoma (SIR 7.54 [95 % CI, 7.17–7.93]) and cancers of the lung (SIR, 1.97 [95 % CI, 1.86–2.08]), liver (SIR, 11.56 [95 % CI, 10.83–12.33]), and kidney (SIR, 4.65 [95 % CI, 4.32–4.99]).

In analysis of kidney recipient-specific data, Vadjic and colleagues performed a population-based cohort study of over 28,000 individuals with end-stage renal disease who underwent renal replacement therapy from 1982 to 2003, using linkage with the Australia and New Zealand Dialysis and Transplant Registry and the Australian National Cancer Statistics Clearing House [3]. In this patient population, the overall incidence of cancer, when excluding nonmelanoma skin cancers (NMSC) and cancers associated with ESRD, was markedly increased after transplantation (SIR, 3.27 [95 % CI, 3.09–3.46]) compared to a slight increase of cancer in dialysis patients (SIR, 1.35 [95 % CI, 1.27–1.45]), as well as prior to renal replacement therapy (SIR, 1.16 [95 % CI, 1.08–1.25]). The average time of onset was 9.4 years, and SIR increased over time post transplant. In transplant recipients, SIRs were significantly elevated for melanoma, Kaposi's sarcoma, non-Hodgkin's and Hodgkin's

A.I. Kamal
Department of Medicine and Transplantation, Mansoura University, Mansoura, Egypt

R.B. Mannon (✉)
Division of Nephrology, Department of Medicine, University of Alabama at Birmingham, 1900 University Boulevard, THT 643, Birmingham, AL 35233, USA
e-mail: rmannon@uab.edu

M.R. Weir and E.V. Lerma (eds.), *Kidney Transplantation: Practical Guide to Management*,
DOI 10.1007/978-1-4939-0342-9_25, © Springer Science+Business Media New York 2014

disease as well as leukemia, and for cancers of the lip, salivary gland, esophagus, lung, stomach, and colon compared to either dialysis patients or those prior to dialysis replacement. SIRs ranged from 2.35 (colon) up to 41.6 (lip), with the exception of thyroid cancer, and all SIRs were greatest following transplantation and none had a lower incidence post transplantation. Cancers associated with ESRD such as renal cell, urinary tract, and myeloma had higher incidences before replacement therapy, during dialysis, as well as post transplantation. These data suggest that preexisting cancer risk, the factors related to ESRD, and dialysis are not the major contributors of posttransplant malignancy, where the use of immunosuppression is the key risk. The risk factors are elaborated further below.

Risk Factors for Posttransplant Malignancy

Viral infection: A number of factors are associated with tumor genesis and they are listed in Table 25.1. These include both modifiable and non-modifiable risk factors. Viral infection has been strongly linked to cancer in the transplant recipient. Infection-associated cancers include the following: non-Hodgkin's lymphoma, Hodgkin's lymphoma, and nasopharyngeal cancer (due to *Epstein-Barr virus*); Kaposi's sarcoma (*human herpesvirus* 8); cancers of the cervix, vulva, vagina, penis, anus, and oropharynx including tonsil (*human papillomavirus* (*HPV*)) [4]; liver cancer (*hepatitis B and C viruses*); and stomach cancer (*Helicobacter pylori*). A variety of subtypes of HPV have also been identified in biopsies of NMSC (HPV 8, 19) [5] and Bowen's disease (HPV 16, 73) [6]. These viruses may remain dormant but, in the immunocompromised host, support malignant transformation. In general, tumors such as posttransplant lymphoproliferative disorder (PTLD) or Kaposi's sarcoma often respond to reduction in immunosuppression. As shown in Table 25.2, SIR incidence varies in posttransplant recipients significantly except for tumors of the cervix, nasopharynx, and vagina. The overall risk for all infection-related cancers is substantial. Interestingly, the HIV-positive transplant recipient appears to be at no further risk of malignancy after transplant than the uninfected renal transplant recipient [7].

Immunosuppression: A critical and obvious risk factor in this patient population is the use of immunosuppression. This includes not only the maintenance therapies but also induction strategies such as T cell depletion that add to the overall suppressive burden. Indeed, the level and intensity of immunosuppression have been correlated to higher rates of cancer in solid organ transplant recipients that have greater exposures [8]. Immunosuppression may also have untoward effects on innate and adaptive immunity in the context of tumor surveillance [9, 10]. Additionally, the class of agent also has specific impact on cancer development. Depletional induction therapies have been associated with EBV-mediated PTLD [11]. The use of belatacept, the costimulatory inhibitor, is also associated with a higher risk of PTLD, particularly in EBV-naïve recipients who received EBV-seropositive organs. Calcineurin inhibitors, both cyclosporine A and tacrolimus, may promote cancer formation by stimulating transforming growth factor beta (TGFβ) with enhanced small vessel growth [12, 13]. Clinical evidence is not conclusive, however, of a direct relationship between CNI use and higher rates of malignancy [14, 15].

The antimetabolite azathioprine is known to sensitize skin to UV light-mediated damage. However, the mycophenolate mofetil may lower cancer development [16, 17] through its primary inhibition of inosine monophosphate dehydrogenase, an enzyme elevated in a number of malignancies [18, 19].

Table 25.1 Risk factors for developing cancer after renal transplantation

Modifiable risk factors
1. Smoking
2. Sun exposure
3. Geographical location
4. Immunosuppressive drug therapy
Non-modifiable risk factors
1. Age
2. Male gender
3. White ethnicity
4. Genetic disposition
5. Oncogenic viruses
6. Chronic renal disease/dialysis duration
7. Posttransplant life span
8. Presence of cystic kidney disease
9. History of previous malignancy

Table 25.2 Incidence of infection-related malignancies after transplantation [2, 3, 60, 127]

Cancer site	Virus	SIR (95 % CI)	*P* value
Non-Hodgkin's lymphoma	EBV	7.54 (7.17–7.93)	<0.001
Liver	Hepatitis C and hepatitis B	11.56 (10.83–12.33)	<0.001
Stomach	*H. pylori*	1.67 (1.42–1.96)	<0.001
Kaposi sarcoma	HHV8	61.46 (50.96–73.49)	<0.001
Oropharynx including tonsil	HPV	2.01(1.64–2.43)	<0.001
Anus	HPV	5.84 (4.70–7.18)	<0.001
Hodgkin's lymphoma	EBV	3.58 (2.86–4.43)	<0.001
Vulva	HPV	7.60 (5.77–9.83)	<0.001
Cervix	HPV	1.03 (0.75–1.38)	0.88
Penis	HPV	4.13 (2.59–6.26)	<0.001
Nasopharynx	EBV	0.96 (0.42–1.90)	>0.99
Vagina	HPV	2.35 (0.94–4.84)	0.07
Total		2.10 (2.06–2.14)	<0.001

There are insufficient data, however, to support this notion as a preventive therapy.

Of significant interest this decade has been the growing number of reports using inhibitors of mammalian target of rapamycin (mTORi). This class of agents has antiproliferative and inhibitory properties for a variety of other solid tumors [20] through inhibition of VEGF. In kidney transplant recipients converted to mTORi [21] or on mTORi-based maintenance therapy [22], the incidence of cancers was reduced compared to CNI-based regimens, particularly NMSC, although these are retrospective studies and with limited follow-up. More recent prospective studies converting to mTORi have shown slower rates of skin cancer growth and prevention of further recurrences as demonstrated in a recent clinical trial [23]. The use of mTORi for maintenance immunosuppression in recipients with prior cancer and for those in whom cancer develops has been advocated by some in the field [24]. However, the relative lack of prospective, well-controlled studies using mTORi for prevention of all malignancies makes this strategy difficult to recommend in all situations.

Preexisting cancer: A critical risk to posttransplant disease is cancer prior to transplantation. Recurrence risk is dependent on the type of tumor, stage [25], management, and the interval between treatment of the tumor and a subsequent renal transplant. High rates of recurrence have been observed with multiple myeloma [26], suggesting a critical treatment plan prior to considering transplantation. Consequently, malignancy-free waiting periods are recommended for each cancer type in order to alleviate the morbidity of cancer recurrence after transplantation (Table 25.3) [27, 28].

Table 25.3 Proposed waiting times for kidney transplant after malignancy [27]

Cancer	Recommended pre-transplant waiting time (year)
Breast	
• Carcinoma in situ	2
• Cancer	5
Lung cancer	2
Colon cancer	
• Stage 1	2
• Stage 2 or greater	5
Renal cell cancer	
• Small, low grade	2
• Large, high grade	5
Prostate	2
Liver	Not recommended
Multiple myeloma	Not recommended
Lymphoma	2
• CNS lymphoma HIV	Not recommended
Leukemia	2
Skin cancer	
• Malignant melanoma (in situ)	5
• Squamous cell	2
• Basal cell	No wait
Testicular	2
Cervical/uterine	2
Bladder	
• Noninvasive	2
• Noninvasive	5
Kaposi's sarcoma	
• Limited	2
• Diffuse, disseminated in HIV	Not recommended

Donor-derived transmitted tumors: Prior to 2000, cancer transmission from deceased donor organs was thought to be relatively uncommon with a rate of 0.017 % [29], but a relatively high mortality when they occur. These rates, however, were based on registry data that were incomplete [30]. Further reports from the IPTTR suggested that transmission rates for donors with malignancy were substantially higher at 42 %, with the highest rate of transmission from known cancer-bearing donors to be in renal transplant recipients [31]. CNS tumors were the most commonly identified in donors, and the highest transmission rates were for choriocarcinoma and melanoma. These data support the need for better assessment of donor malignancy history and risk of transmission. Recognizing the limitations of this voluntary registry, analysis of donor OPTN/UNOS data from 2000 to 2005 indicated that only 2 % of deceased donor organs came from donors with history of malignancy [32]. In this series, nonmelanoma squamous cell cancers of the skin, CNS tumors, and uterine cancer were the most common cancers noted in donors. Recently, a malignancy subcommittee for the OPTN/UNOS Disease Transmission Advisory Committee analyzed current literature and created levels of risk from 0 (no risk) to 4 (high risk) and also a category for unknown risk [33]. Additionally, all possible cancers were classified by this scheme based on clinical behavior of the tumor, cure probability, and time to metastasize (Table 25.4). These guidelines provide a basis to the donor surgeon in terms of appropriate utilization of donor organs and allow the informed risk assessment to the recipient who may succumb to their end-stage disease prior to transplantation.

Cancer After Renal Transplantation: De Novo Cancers

The relative incidences of cancers after kidney transplantation have already been defined above. We will now explore the key common posttransplant malignancies, their management, and outcomes.

Table 25.4 Donor transmission risk categorization for specific tumors after transplantation [33]

Risk category (% transmission)	Tumor
No significant risk	• Benign tumors
Minimal risk (<0.1 %)	• Basal cell skin cancer • Squamous cell skin cancer without metastases • Carcinoma in situ, skin • In situ cervical carcinoma • In situ vocal cord carcinoma • Superficial papillary carcinoma of the bladder • Solitary papillary thyroid carcinoma, ≤0.5 cm • Minimally invasive follicular thyroid carcinoma (≤1.0 cm) • Resected solitary renal cell carcinoma ≤1.0 cm, well differentiated (Fuhrman 1–2)
Low risk (0.1–1 %)	• Resected solitary renal cell carcinoma ≥1.0 cm ≤2.5 cm, well differentiated (Fuhrman 1–2) • Low-grade CNS tumor (WHO grade I or II) • Primary CNS teratoma • Solitary papillary thyroid carcinoma 0.5–2.0 cm • Minimally invasive follicular carcinoma thyroid 1.0–2.0 cm • History of treated non-CNS malignancy (≥5 years prior) with >99 % probability of cure
Intermediate risk (1–10 %)	• Breast carcinoma in situ (Stage 0) • Colon carcinoma in situ (Stage 0) • History of treated non-CNS malignancy (≥5 years prior) with probability of cure 90–99 % • Resected solitary renal cell carcinoma T1b (4–7 cm), well differentiated (Fuhrman 1–2) stage 1
High risk (>10 %)	• Malignant melanoma • Breast carcinoma > stage 0 (active) • Colon carcinoma > stage 0 (active) • Choriocarcinoma • CNS tumor (any) with ventriculoperitoneal or atrial shunt, surgery, irradiation or extra-CNS manifestations • CNS tumor WHO grade III or IV • Leukemia or lymphoma • History of melanoma, leukemia, lymphoma, small cell lung/neuroendocrine carcinoma • Any other history of treated non-CNS malignancy either (a) insufficient follow-up to predict behavior, (b) considered incurable, or (c) with probability of cure <90 % • Metastatic carcinoma • Sarcoma • Lung cancer (stages I–IV) • Renal cell carcinoma >7 cm or stage II–IV • Small cell/neuroendocrine carcinoma, any site of origin • Active cancer not listed elsewhere

Skin cancer: NMSC is the most commonly occurring post kidney transplant cancer. Squamous cell carcinoma (SCC) and basal cell carcinoma (BCC) account for 95 % of post-transplant NMSC [34]. Interestingly, compared to the general public, SCC is far more frequent than BCC at an incidence of 4:1 [35]. The incidence of NMSC increases steadily with time post transplantation with an incidence of 5 % at 2 years, 10–27 % at 10 years, and up to 60 % at 20 years in the United States and western Europe [36–38] and a mean time of development of 8–10 years post transplantation. These are aggressive tumors, recurring locally in 13 % of patients with metastases in 5–8 %. Moreover, and the presence of one is predictive of multiple subsequent lesions and these recipients have frequent second primary cancers.

Disease results from both skin exposure and reduced immune surveillance in the context of the overall burden of immunosuppression. A lower incidence of skin cancer has been seen in living donor transplant recipients who require less overall immunosuppression. Azathioprine has been associated with higher rates of skin cancer by sensitization to UVA-induced skin damage [39]. Several studies have shown patients on three-drug immunosuppressive regimens had a threefold increased risk of NMSC compared to patients taking two-drug regimens [3, 21, 40, 41]. Note, however, that low-dose cyclosporine has been shown to confer a lower risk of NMSC than standard-dose cyclosporine [42]. As previously discussed, recent studies with mTORi demonstrate beneficial effects on slowing growth rates and the development of new lesions [23].

Other risk factors for NMSC include male gender and age, such that patients who received their transplant after the age of 55 have a 12-fold higher risk for development of skin cancer compared to patients who received grafts before the age of 34 [43]. In renal transplant recipients, HPV 8 DNA has been detected in 80 % of precancerous lesions such as Bowen's disease compared with only 30 % of the general population, again supporting the notion that viral-related mechanisms are important in NMSC development post transplantation [44, 45].

Treatment of transplant-related skin cancer requires a multidisciplinary effort particularly in the context of multiple lesions, their size, and location. Annual evaluation by a dermatologist is recommended, with more frequent visits for high-risk patients. Education before and after transplantation covering skin cancer prevention, detection, and treatment is essential. This includes discussion of avoidance of sun exposure, the use of protective clothing, and the appropriate application of UVB-retarding sunscreen. Compliance in this area can be difficult, as this is not covered by insurance or Medicare. Lesions such as actinic keratoses, keratoacanthomas, and Bowen's disease (SCC in situ) should be followed closely and treated as those lesions are associated with potential for SCC development [46].

With suspected or proven squamous cell lesions, surgical excision with clear margins is the standard of care. Superficial lesions may be managed with cryotherapy or electrocautery and curettage. Invasive squamous cell cancers require more aggressive management due to the higher risk of recurrence and metastasis. Local regional lymph node may be curable by lymphadenectomy alone, but may require adjuvant treatment with chemotherapy or radiation. BCC generally do not metastasize and do not require care beyond the standard used for the general public, but the treatment of specific lesions, however, does not prevent recurrence or the development of new cancers.

For larger treatment areas, additional therapy may include topical imiquimod, 5-fluorouracil, photodynamic therapy, and 3 % diclofenac gel. Systemic retinoids have been shown to slow the development of new lesions, and topical retinoids reduce actinic keratoses. Clearly, immunosuppressive modification is needed, but there is no consensus on specific agent reduction or approach. As already noted, the use of mTORi shows promise as an alternative strategy both to avoid rejection and limit disease progression.

Melanoma is a less frequent cause of skin cancer, but with a fourfold higher incidence than in the general population [3]. Disease may be due to donor transmission or from prior disease or developed de novo post transplantation. Posttransplant outcomes, as demonstrated by a recent retrospective analysis of European transplant centers, showed a 27 % mortality rate. However, recipients with T1 and T2 lesions have similar results to otherwise age- and sex-matched individuals with melanomas [47]. However, with more advanced disease (T3 and T4), the hazard ratio for death was 11.49 ($p < 0.001$) compared to non-transplanted individuals. Thus, treatment of melanoma requires an aggressive management plan, with wide local excision and/or sentinel lymphadenectomy. Reduction in immunosuppression is recommended but there are insufficient data with regard to specific strategies in this group [48].

Kaposi's sarcoma: As in other skin cancers, this vascular tumor is markedly more frequent in posttransplant recipients compared to non-immunosuppressed individuals [49]. Presenting as a dark red or blue nodular or maculopapular cutaneous lesion, it more commonly affects the skin of the lower limbs, although the trunk and arms may be affected [50]. It is more frequently seen in men than women [51]. Visceral organs may be affected in 10 % of cases and carry a more severe prognosis. Notably, allograft involvement is extremely rare [52]. HHV 8 infection at time of transplantation is a critical risk factor; incidence rate varies from 5 % in Mediterranean and African descent population to 0.5 % in western and northern countries reflecting specific geographic distribution [51, 53]. Hence, donor screening for HHV 8 virus may be useful in areas with considerable rate of infection to avoid posttransplant transmission. This of course has to be weighed into the need and benefit for transplantation compared to dialysis and the opportunity for available organs. A key management strategy is to reduce or discontinue immunosuppression and typically the lesions will regress [54]. The introduction of mTORi has been associated with dramatic reduction in lesions [55] and a reduction in recipient mortality after disease diagnosis [56].

Renal cell and genitourinary tract cancers: The incidence of renal cell carcinoma is nearly 100 times greater in end-stage renal disease and transplant patients than the general population [3, 57]. Disease presentation is often aggressive with median survival of 17 months post diagnosis [58]. Most cancers arise in the native kidneys rather than the renal allograft and are more aggressive than in non-immunocompromised hosts. There are no recommended guidelines for use of urinalysis or urine cytology. Routine ultrasonographic surveillance of the native kidneys is not recommended and there are no prospective data to determine if such a screening strategy is cost-effective. In general, patients with or without ADPKD who have Bosniak I (simple benign cysts) or II cysts (one or two septations, fine-wall calcifications, non-enhancing hyper dense cysts) should undergo renal ultrasonography twice yearly, followed by CT or MRI for suspicious lesions. Bosniak IIF patients should have ultrasound every 3 months and annual CT or MRI. Nephrectomy is indicated for progressive lesions or Bosniak III or IV lesions [59]. The presence of unexplained hematuria should prompt evaluation to exclude renal or bladder lesions. There is an increased risk of developing neoplasms of the native urinary tract especially in patients with a history of analgesic nephropathy, prolonged exposure to cyclophosphamide, and those with a history of Chinese Herb exposure [60]. Urine cytology is not a reliable diagnostic tool. In addition to radiologic imaging as recommended above, serum BK and adenovirus PCR [61] and PSA are recommended. Patients with non-glomerular hematuria should also undergo cystoscopy.

Colon cancer: Though a common tumor in the non-immunosuppressed population, colorectal cancer is *not* seen at a higher frequency post kidney transplantation [62, 63]. However, in a recent study of age 50 and older kidney transplant recipients screened with fecal occult blood testing and colonoscopy, advanced colorectal disease was found in 13 % [64], and such data support the need for the standard use of screening colonoscopy.

Anogenital cancer: While these cancers occur in about 2–3 % of recipients, this is significantly more frequent than in the general population. The association with HPV has been identified over the last decade and is nearly uniform in anogenital cancers [65]. This association, especially with HPV 16 and 18, has provided additional incentive to vaccinate the pre-transplant patient, although recipients already infected may make vaccination futile [66]. The role of vaccination post transplantation is more controversial as it may be ineffective due to a delayed antibody response, with lower seroconversion rate and more rapid decline of antibody level compared to the general population [4]. Disease may be multifocal, and gynecologic exams should be performed regularly.

Cervical cancer: There is a marked increase risk of cervical cancer in the posttransplant patient population compared to the general population, although many of these lesions are in situ [67]. Standard treatment applies in this population as well. Screening through Pap smear has been extremely effective in the general population, and again, there is no justification to alter this screening post transplantation [4]. While the role of colposcopy has been debated, there is a lack of evidence to suggest employing this in kidney transplant recipients [68]. The strong association with HPV has been discussed above, supporting appropriate screening post transplantation. The effective role of vaccination remains to be fully determined [69].

Breast cancer: Compared to the general population, the incidence of breast cancer is not increased in the post kidney transplant recipient [3]. Mortality in this disease is high in the general population, based on stage of disease. In transplant recipients, outcomes are comparable to the general population although survival is worse with more advanced disease [70]. Standard management includes surgery, chemotherapy, and/or radiation. Screening reduces mortality in the general population and there are no data to suggest additional screening is necessary in the kidney transplant population [4]. A further discussion regarding appropriate cancer prevention screening is given below.

Hepatobiliary cancer: Hepatocellular cancer is primarily associated with hepatitis B and C infections and incidence varies depending on the prevalence of these infections which varies with geography. However, the risk of cancer is significantly higher in this population with an SIR of 11.56 [2]. Disease prevalence in this population is such that it argues for appropriate antiviral treatment prior to transplantation [71]. Most recipients have advanced disease when they present, making effective therapy less likely. The role of screening for all transplant recipients is questionable and may not be cost-effective [4, 69]. However, in high-risk recipients, the use of hepatic ultrasound as a sensitive tool to detect small hepatocellular cancers is meaningful and is recommended to occur at 6-month intervals in those with long-standing liver disease and hepatitis [72].

Lung cancer: While lung cancer is more common in post-transplant recipients, the difference is not as dramatic as that of other tumors with an SIR of 1.46 [2]. Cigarette use clearly increases the risk of cancer in the renal transplant recipient [73], and hence cessation should be encouraged and emphasized. Outcomes are similar to the general population. There are no supportive data to engage in routine screening using radiography or sputum sampling [69]. The use of chest CT for high-risk patients that smoke following transplantation is similarly unknown.

Prostate cancer: The risk of this cancer is not elevated post transplantation, but it is a prevalent cancer in the older population [2]. Survival rates are relatively better than other cancers due to the slow growing nature and local spread of disease, followed by metastasis to bone. Regular screening methods have been advocated using digital rectal exam and prostate-specific antigen testing [74], although this is not uniformly accepted as the magnitude of benefit of screening is estimated as smaller in the kidney transplant recipient [74]. While the incidence is low, the aging recipient population may result in a higher than expected frequency of cases over time.

Posttransplant Lymphoproliferative Disorder

PTLD is a major cause of morbidity and mortality after solid organ transplantation [75]. The incidence of PTLD differs according to the type of the transplanted organ, being lowest among renal transplant recipients at 1–2 % [76] and highest for intestinal transplant recipients ranging from 19 to 30 % [77, 78]. The risk in renal transplant recipients should not be understated and represents a 20–50-fold higher risk of lymphoma compared to the general population [2]. Most PTLDs are B cell, large non-Hodgkin's lymphomas but those of T cell in origin confer a more dismal prognosis. Greater than 50 % of PTLDs present in extra-nodal sites and involve the gastrointestinal tract, lungs, liver, mucosal tissue, skin, and CNS. In the renal allograft recipient, PTLD is more likely to develop in the renal allograft, while in heart transplant recipients, lymphoma typically presents in the heart allograft. This predilection of the transplanted organ for subsequent development of PTLD may be attributed to local immune response to foreign tissue. Presentation may be bimodal in fashion with prevalence in the early posttransplant period at 1–2 years and another peak at 4–5 years after transplantation [77].

Pathogenesis: More than 90 % of recipients have been previously infected with EBV and are lifelong carriers of the virus [78]. Among immunocompetent hosts, control of virally infected B cell proliferation is maintained by the development of host antiviral immune response. In a persistent infection, EBV antigen-specific T cells are maintained at a frequency of 1–5 % of peripheral blood T cells that eliminate reactivating and proliferating infected B cells. In contrast, in transplant recipients, 60–70 % of PTLD cases are associated with EBV infection due to unrestrained growth of EBV-infected B cells [79]. The transformation of EBV-infected memory B cells into malignant tissue involves the production of latent viral proteins related to EBV nuclear antigen 2 (EBNA-2). Activation of this transcription factor initiates B cell proliferation. B cells containing these viral particles are normally recognized and destroyed by cytotoxic T cells. In immunosuppressed patients, when T cell functions are impaired, uncontrolled proliferation of EBV-infected B cells will lead to the development of PTLD [80].

EBV-negative PTLD incidence is estimated at 30–40 % [81] and typically presents later within 3–5 years after transplantation with monomorphic pathology and carries worse prognosis [82, 83]. The mechanism of EBV-negative PTLD development is not clear. Some reports suggest a role of HHV8 [84], or possible chronic antigenic stimulation of the immune system [85]. The existence of EBV-unrelated PTLD strengthens the theory of multifactorial pathogenic process involving the interaction between viral oncogenes, impaired immunity, genetic actors, and chronic antigen stimulation [86].

Epidemiology and risk factors: A number of risk factors have been identified. These include recipient EBV seronegativity at the time of transplantation [76, 77, 87] and, in particular, those receiving an EBV-seropositive donor organ. The cumulative burden of immunosuppression [88] and the use of T cell depletional induction therapy have also been associated with disease [76]. Interestingly, induction with alemtuzumab appears to confer a more "protective" effect against PTLD, with significantly lower incidence of PTLD compared to rabbit antithymocyte globulin [89]. Diseases are more commonly seen in non-Hispanic white recipients [77, 87], children and typically adolescents [90], and in those recipients over the age of 65 [76, 87]. Finally, greater HLA mismatch between donor and recipient has been noted, as well as simultaneous kidney-pancreas transplantation compared to solitary kidney transplantation, perhaps related to overall immunosuppressive strategy [76, 87].

It is not clear what the effect of maintenance immunosuppression has on PTLD incidence. The role of CNI has been debated and may be related to the extent of monitored drug levels [88, 91]. Similarly the possibly protective role of mTORi [22] is now debated as a number of studies have been associated with increased incidence with the use of the agent [89, 92, 93]. Belatacept, an antibody that blocks costimulatory signaling in T cells, has been found to be associated with increased incidence of central nervous system PTLD when compared to a maintenance regimen with cyclosporine, and this was seen particularly in EBV-seronegative recipients of seropositive organs and frequently in those that rejected and required additional T cell depletional therapy [94].

Pathology: The remarkable pathologic diversity of PTLD makes its classification complicated. The most recent and widely used classification is the World Health Organization classification of hematopoietic disorders [95] that includes early lesions, polymorphic PTLD, monomorphic PTLD which includes B and T cell neoplasm, and classical Hodgkin's lymphoma. The terminology polymorphic refers to the heterogeneous nature of the lesions, with a variable degree of cytologic atypia, that include atypical immunoblasts and Reed-Sternberg-like cells, with destruction of the underlying architecture [96]. Monomorphic PTLD are composed of plasma cells or lymphocytes with a uniform appearance and are most frequently B cell in origin. Ninety percent of PTLD are of host origin [97]; donor-derived PTLD tend to be localized to the graft and frequently carry a better prognosis [98].

Diagnosis: Typically, patients present with nonspecific symptoms such as localized pain, fever, weight loss, anorexia, and lymphadenopathy [99]. Graft involvement after renal transplantation is fairly common, but disease may also be disseminated affecting lymph nodes, graft, gastrointestinal tract, lung, or liver. Evaluation and diagnosis of PTLD requires a high index of suspicion and tissue confirmation is the gold standard. CT scan [100], positive emission tomography (PET) scan [101, 102], quantitative EBV PCR, and increasing LDH are useful adjunctive tests. The diagnosis of CNS PTLD requires confirmation of malignant cells in CSF or from tissue biopsy. Positive MRI with gadolinium [103], positive CSF for EBV, and positive quantitative EBV PCR in serum are also highly suggestive of a diagnosis of PTLD. Some advocate for preemptive monitoring of EBV PCR in high-risk groups [104, 105].

Prognosis: At 1 and 5 years, survival rates for adults are reported at 93 % and 86 % and 80 % and 60 % for allograft survival, respectively [8]. Mortality related to PTLD reaches 40–60 % with a number of negative prognostic factors including multiple site involvement [106], CNS involvement [107], non-B cell tumor [108], EBV-negative disease [109], coinfection with hepatitis B or C [110], and elevated LDH at the time of diagnosis [106, 111].

Management: Prevention and recognition of risk is a key consideration often outweighed by the necessity for transplantation [112]. The efficacy of EBV vaccine remains uncertain [113], and standard antiviral prophylaxis lacks impact as the thymidine kinase which activates these drugs is not present in a dormant infected B cell [114]. Immunosuppression reduction is a mainstay of initial management, and response should be relatively immediate [106]. In EBV-driven PTLD, reducing immunosuppression allows the host cytotoxic T cell function to be at least partially restored, with the goal of increasing host EBV-specific CTLs and elimination of virally infected lymphocytes. The approach to reducing immunosuppressive therapy needs to be carefully managed and will depend on the nature and extent of the disease and the type of transplant recipient. Response can be determined in part with serial quantitation of EBV genome in the patient's serum and serial radiologic measurements. Rituximab, an anti-CD20, therapy is a first step in treatment and may be used as monotherapy in mild cases of immunosuppressive reduction although disease relapse is more common [115]. Anthracycline-based chemotherapy with cyclophosphamide, doxorubicin, vincristine, and prednisolone (CHOP) is the most commonly used combination in the treatment of PTLD with a 5-year disease-free survival >60 % [116]. Recent data suggested better results and survival with rituximab plus CHOP (R-CHOP) [117]. Combination therapy is indicated with clinically aggressive disease or failure of other lines of treatment. CNS PTLD carries high mortality up to 88 %, for which local radiotherapy and methotrexate should be used as it crosses the blood-brain barrier [118]. In an unrelenting disease, experimental approaches have included the use of a recipient's cytotoxic T cells or partially HLA-matched cells directed against EBV-infected cells taking the advantage of treating EBV without increased risk of graft rejection [119]. There are promising data using ganciclovir with arginine butyrate which induces thymidine kinase and activates the antiviral drugs [120]. Finally, should graft loss be experienced, successful re-transplantation has been reported, typically waiting at least 2 years as a disease-free period [121].

Prevention and Surveillance for Posttransplant Cancers

Critical to prevention of posttransplant cancer is appropriate pre-transplant screening. Recipient evaluation should always include an extensive history and physical and radiologic exam that includes chest X-ray and native renal ultrasound [27] and age-appropriate screening such as mammography and pap smear, prostate antigen testing, and colonoscopy using standard guidelines, although substantial debate exists in the transplant community regarding uniform practices [122].

Post transplantation, systematic screening for malignancy is recommended for early detection and intervention [123]. A number of screening guidelines exist [122, 124], and some of these recommendations have already been noted above. However, it is important to identify the differences between the general population and those with chronic kidney disease population who undergo transplantation [125]. Importantly, assay ranges and radiologic findings appropriate for non-transplant patients may be different from those applicable to the transplant population. Specific principles of cancer screening in the transplant population have not been fully and consistently defined. The screening process requires that early detection and recognition of a particular disease is of value with improved health outcomes including quality and quantity of life and that the screening procedure and societal treatment costs be economically balanced. Benefits of screening to detect early cancer must be weighed against the costs of screening and potential harm to the individual. This is even more relevant for transplant patients where an individual's life expectancy is lower than that of the general population. It remains uncertain whether current screening guidelines for the general population are wholly applicable to transplant patients, not just because of expected survival differences, but because of screening test performance and interpretation, response to treatment, and the existence of comorbid diseases [126]. Thus, detection of a disease by routine screening and the associated subsequent treatment and morbidity that might not otherwise have manifest in the course of the patient's lifetime may be undesirable medically, psychologically, and financially. Further consideration is being given in the transplant community in this regard.

Summary

Posttransplant malignancy is a major cause of morbidity and mortality in the kidney transplant recipient. Cancer risk exceeds that in the general population, and a number of tumors are associated with oncogenic viruses. A variety of risk factors exist including long-term exposure to immunosuppression coupled with lifestyle-associated risks. Prevention is key and includes specified waiting times for those with prior cancers to remain tumor free. Controversy exists with regard to appropriate screening and follow-up. Immunosuppression reduction may be effective in those with infection-related tumors. Recent data has demonstrated that mTORi may be an appropriate management strategy in NMSC of the skin. The judicious use of long-term immunosuppression continues to be a critical question in the kidney transplant recipient to maximize long-term outcome and balance over immunosuppression with the risks of kidney allograft rejection.

References

1. Miao Y, Everly JJ, Gross TG, Tevar AD, First MR, Alloway RR, et al. De novo cancers arising in organ transplant recipients are associated with adverse outcomes compared with the general population. Transplantation. 2009;87(9):1347–59. Epub 2009/05/09.
2. Engels EA, Pfeiffer RM, Fraumeni Jr JF, Kasiske BL, Israni AK, Snyder JJ, et al. Spectrum of cancer risk among US solid organ transplant recipients. JAMA. 2011;306(17):1891–901.
3. Vajdic CM, McDonald SP, McCredie MR, van Leeuwen MT, Stewart JH, Law M, et al. Cancer incidence before and after kidney transplantation. JAMA. 2006;296(23):2823–31.
4. Webster AC, Wong G, Craig JC, Chapman JR. Managing cancer risk and decision making after kidney transplantation. Am J Transplant. 2008;8(11):2185–91.
5. Dubina M, Goldenberg G. Viral-associated nonmelanoma skin cancers: a review. Am J Dermatopathol. 2009;31(6):561–73. Epub 2009/07/11.
6. Grundmeier N, Hamm H, Weissbrich B, Lang SC, Brocker EB, Kerstan A. High-risk human papillomavirus infection in Bowen's disease of the nail unit: report of three cases and review of the literature. Dermatology. 2011;223(4):293–300. Epub 2012/01/25.
7. Nissen NN, Barin B, Stock PG. Malignancy in the HIV-infected patients undergoing liver and kidney transplantation. Curr Opin Oncol. 2012;24(5):517–21. Epub 2012/07/05.
8. Shapiro R, Nalesnik M, McCauley J, Fedorek S, Jordan ML, Scantlebury VP, et al. Posttransplant lymphoproliferative disorders in adult and pediatric renal transplant patients receiving tacrolimus-based immunosuppression. Transplantation. 1999;68(12):1851–4. Epub 2000/01/11.
9. Thibaudin D, Alamartine E, Mariat C, Absi L, Berthoux F. Long-term kinetic of T-lymphocyte subsets in kidney-transplant recipients: influence of anti-T-cell antibodies and association with posttransplant malignancies. Transplantation. 2005;80(10):1514–7. Epub 2005/12/13.
10. Morteau O, Blundell S, Chakera A, Bennett S, Christou CM, Mason PD, et al. Renal transplant immunosuppression impairs natural killer cell function in vitro and in vivo. PLoS One. 2010;5(10):e13294. Epub 2010/10/23.
11. Cherikh WS, Kauffman HM, McBride MA, Maghirang J, Swinnen LJ, Hanto DW. Association of the type of induction immunosuppression with posttransplant lymphoproliferative disorder, graft survival, and patient survival after primary kidney transplantation. Transplantation. 2003;76(9):1289–93. Epub 2003/11/25.
12. Hojo M, Morimoto T, Maluccio M, Asano T, Morimoto K, Lagman M, et al. Cyclosporine induces cancer progression by a cell-autonomous mechanism. Nature. 1999;397(6719):530–4. Epub 1999/02/24.
13. Maluccio M, Sharma V, Lagman M, Vyas S, Yang H, Li B, et al. Tacrolimus enhances transforming growth factor-beta1 expression and promotes tumor progression. Transplantation. 2003;76(3):597–602. Epub 2003/08/19.
14. Gallagher MP, Kelly PJ, Jardine M, Perkovic V, Cass A, Craig JC, et al. Long-term cancer risk of immunosuppressive regimens after kidney transplantation. J Am Soc Nephrol. 2010;21(5):852–8. Epub 2010/05/01.
15. Shuttleworth D, Marks R, Griffin PJ, Salaman JR. Epidermal dysplasia and cyclosporine therapy in renal transplant patients: a comparison with azathioprine. Br J Dermatol. 1989;120(4):551–4. Epub 1989/04/01.
16. O'Neill JO, Edwards LB, Taylor DO. Mycophenolate mofetil and risk of developing malignancy after orthotopic heart transplantation: analysis of the transplant registry of the International Society for Heart and Lung Transplantation. J Heart Lung Transplant. 2006;25(10):1186–91. Epub 2006/10/19.
17. Robson R, Cecka JM, Opelz G, Budde M, Sacks S. Prospective registry-based observational cohort study of the long-term risk of malignancies in renal transplant patients treated with mycophenolate mofetil. Am J Transplant. 2005;5(12):2954–60.
18. Buell JF, Gross TG, Woodle ES. Malignancy after transplantation. Transplantation. 2005;80(2 Suppl):S254–64. Epub 2005/10/28.
19. Engl T, Makarevic J, Relja B, Natsheh I, Muller I, Beecken WD, et al. Mycophenolate mofetil modulates adhesion receptors of the beta1 integrin family on tumor cells: impact on tumor recurrence and malignancy. BMC Cancer. 2005;5:4. Epub 2005/01/13.
20. Wang X, Sun SY. Enhancing mTOR-targeted cancer therapy. Expert Opin Ther Targets. 2009;13(10):1193–203. Epub 2009/08/22.
21. Campistol JM, Eris J, Oberbauer R, Friend P, Hutchison B, Morales JM, et al. Sirolimus therapy after early cyclosporine withdrawal reduces the risk for cancer in adult renal transplantation. J Am Soc Nephrol. 2006;17(2):581–9. Epub 2006/01/26.
22. Kauffman HM, Cherikh WS, Cheng Y, Hanto DW, Kahan BD. Maintenance immunosuppression with target-of-rapamycin inhibitors is associated with a reduced incidence of de novo malignancies. Transplantation. 2005;80(7):883–9.
23. Euvrard S, Morelon E, Rostaing L, Goffin E, Brocard A, Tromme I, et al. Sirolimus and secondary skin-cancer prevention in kidney transplantation. N Engl J Med. 2012;367(4):329–39. Epub 2012/07/27.
24. Monaco AP. The role of mTOR inhibitors in the management of posttransplant malignancy. Transplantation. 2009;87(2):157–63. Epub 2009/01/22.
25. Woodle ES, Gupta M, Buell JF, Neff GW, Gross TG, First MR, et al. Prostate cancer prior to solid organ transplantation: the Israel Penn International Transplant Tumor Registry experience. Transplant Proc. 2005;37(2):958–9.
26. Penn I. Evaluation of transplant candidates with pre-existing malignancies. Ann Transplant. 1997;2(4):14–7.
27. The Evaluation of the Renal Transplant Candidates. Clinical practice guidelines. Am J Transplant. 2001;1:1–95.
28. Pham PT, Pham PA, Pham PC, Parikh S, Danovitch G. Evaluation of adult kidney transplant candidates. Semin Dial. 2010;23(6):595–605.
29. Myron Kauffman H, McBride MA, Cherikh WS, Spain PC, Marks WH, Roza AM. Transplant tumor registry: donor related malignancies. Transplantation. 2002;74(3):358–62. Epub 2002/08/15.
30. Kauffman HM, McBride MA, Delmonico FL. First report of the United Network for Organ Sharing Transplant Tumor Registry: donors with a history of cancer. Transplantation. 2000;70(12):1747–51. Epub 2001/01/11.
31. Buell JF, Beebe TM, Trofe J, Gross TG, Alloway RR, Hanaway MJ, et al. Donor transmitted malignancies. Ann Transplant. 2004;9(1):53–6.

32. Kauffman HM, Cherikh WS, McBride MA, Cheng Y, Hanto DW. Deceased donors with a past history of malignancy: an organ procurement and transplantation network/united network for organ sharing update. Transplantation. 2007;84(2):272–4. Epub 2007/08/02.
33. Nalesnik MA, Woodle ES, Dimaio JM, Vasudev B, Teperman LW, Covington S, et al. Donor-transmitted malignancies in organ transplantation: assessment of clinical risk. Am J Transplant. 2011;11(6):1140–7.
34. Harwood CA, Proby CM, McGregor JM, Sheaff MT, Leigh IM, Cerio R. Clinicopathologic features of skin cancer in organ transplant recipients: a retrospective case-control series. J Am Acad Dermatol. 2006;54(2):290–300.
35. Euvrard S, Kanitakis J, Claudy A. Skin cancers after organ transplantation. N Engl J Med. 2003;348(17):1681–91.
36. Kasiske BL, Snyder JJ, Gilbertson DT, Wang C. Cancer after kidney transplantation in the United States. Am J Transplant. 2004;4(6):905–13.
37. Bordea C, Wojnarowska F, Millard PR, Doll H, Welsh K, Morris PJ. Skin cancers in renal-transplant recipients occur more frequently than previously recognized in a temperate climate. Transplantation. 2004;77(4):574–9.
38. Ramsay HM, Reece SM, Fryer AA, Smith AG, Harden PN. Seven-year prospective study of nonmelanoma skin cancer incidence in U.K. renal transplant recipients. Transplantation. 2007;84(3):437–9.
39. O'Donovan P, Perrett CM, Zhang X, Montaner B, Xu YZ, Harwood CA, et al. Azathioprine and UVA light generate mutagenic oxidative DNA damage. Science. 2005;309(5742):1871–4.
40. Otley CC, Maragh SL. Reduction of immunosuppression for transplant-associated skin cancer: rationale and evidence of efficacy. Dermatol Surg. 2005;31(2):163–8. Epub 2005/03/15.
41. Ulrich C, Kanitakis J, Stockfleth E, Euvrard S. Skin cancer in organ transplant recipients—where do we stand today? Am J Transplant. 2008;8(11):2192–8. Epub 2008/09/11.
42. Dantal J, Hourmant M, Cantarovich D, Giral M, Blancho G, Dreno B, et al. Effect of long-term immunosuppression in kidney-graft recipients on cancer incidence: randomised comparison of two cyclosporin regimens. Lancet. 1998;351(9103):623–8. Epub 1998/03/21.
43. Otley CC, Cherikh WS, Salasche SJ, McBride MA, Christenson LJ, Kauffman HM. Skin cancer in organ transplant recipients: effect of pretransplant end-organ disease. J Am Acad Dermatol. 2005;53(5):783–90. Epub 2005/10/26.
44. Berkhout RJ, Bouwes Bavinck JN, ter Schegget J. Persistence of human papillomavirus DNA in benign and (pre)malignant skin lesions from renal transplant recipients. J Clin Microbiol. 2000;38(6):2087–96.
45. Harwood CA, Surentheran T, McGregor JM, Spink PJ, Leigh IM, Breuer J, et al. Human papillomavirus infection and non-melanoma skin cancer in immunosuppressed and immunocompetent individuals. J Med Virol. 2000;61(3):289–97.
46. Pedotti P, Cardillo M, Rossini G, Arcuri V, Boschiero L, Caldara R, et al. Incidence of cancer after kidney transplant: results from the North Italy transplant program. Transplantation. 2003;76(10):1448–51.
47. Matin RN, Mesher D, Proby CM, McGregor JM, Bouwes Bavinck JN, Del Marmol V, et al. Melanoma in organ transplant recipients: clinicopathological features and outcome in 100 cases. Am J Transplant. 2008;8(9):1891–900.
48. Otley CC, Berg D, Ulrich C, Stasko T, Murphy GM, Salasche SJ, et al. Reduction of immunosuppression for transplant-associated skin cancer: expert consensus survey. Br J Dermatol. 2006;154(3):395–400.
49. Sampaio MS, Cho YW, Qazi Y, Bunnapradist S, Hutchinson IV, Shah T. Posttransplant malignancies in solid organ adult recipients: an analysis of the U.S. national transplant database. Transplantation. 2012;94(10):990–8.
50. Zmonarski SC, Boratynska M, Puziewicz-Zmonarska A, Kazimierczak K, Klinger M. Kaposi's sarcoma in renal transplant recipients. Ann Transplant. 2005;10(2):59–65.
51. Campistol JM, Schena FP. Kaposi's sarcoma in renal transplant recipients—the impact of proliferation signal inhibitors. Nephrol Dial Transplant. 2007;22 Suppl 1:i17–22.
52. Dudderidge TJ, Khalifa M, Jeffery R, Amlot P, Al-Akraa M, Sweny P. Donor-derived human herpes virus 8-related Kaposi's sarcoma in renal allograft ureter. Transpl Infect Dis. 2008;10(3):221–6.
53. Bergallo M, Costa C, Margio S, Sidoti F, Re D, Segoloni GP, et al. Human herpes virus 8 infection in kidney transplant patients from an area of northwestern Italy (Piemonte region). Nephrol Dial Transplant. 2007;22(6):1757–61. Epub 2007/03/14.
54. Razonable RR, Zerr DM, Practice ASTIDCo. HHV-6, HHV-7 and HHV-8 in solid organ transplant recipients. Am J Transplant. 2009;9 Suppl 4:S97–100.
55. Stallone G, Schena A, Infante B, Di Paolo S, Loverre A, Maggio G, et al. Sirolimus for Kaposi's sarcoma in renal-transplant recipients. N Engl J Med. 2005;352(13):1317–23. Epub 2005/04/01.
56. Yaich S, Charfeddine K, Zaghdane S, El Aoud N, Jarraya F, Kharrat M, et al. Sirolimus for the treatment of kaposi sarcoma after renal transplantation: a series of 10 cases. Transplant Proc. 2012;44(9):2824–6. Epub 2012/11/14.
57. Denton MD, Magee CC, Ovuworie C, Mauiyyedi S, Pascual M, Colvin RB, et al. Prevalence of renal cell carcinoma in patients with ESRD pre-transplantation: a pathologic analysis. Kidney Int. 2002;61(6):2201–9. Epub 2002/05/25.
58. Bokemeyer C, Thon WF, Brunkhorst T, Kuczyk MA, Pichlmayr R, Kleim V. High frequency of urothelial cancers in patients with kidney transplantations for end-stage analgesic nephropathy. Eur J Cancer. 1996;32A(1):175–6. Epub 1996/01/01.
59. Israel GM, Bosniak MA. An update of the Bosniak renal cyst classification system. Urology. 2005;66(3):484–8. Epub 2005/09/06.
60. Morath C, Mueller M, Goldschmidt H, Schwenger V, Opelz G, Zeier M. Malignancy in renal transplantation. J Am Soc Nephrol. 2004;15(6):1582–8. Epub 2004/05/22.
61. Randhawa P, Mannon RB. A case of late kidney allograft failure: a clinical pathological conference from American society of nephrology kidney week 2011. Clin J Am Soc Nephrol. 2012;7(11):1884–9. Epub 2012/08/04.
62. Hibberd AD, Trevillian PR, Wlodarczyk JH, Kemp DG, Stein AM, Gillies AH, et al. Effect of immunosuppression for primary renal disease on the risk of cancer in subsequent renal transplantation: a population-based retrospective cohort study. Transplantation. 2013;95(1):122–7. Epub 2012/12/15.
63. Aigner F, Boeckle E, Albright J, Kilo J, Boesmueller C, Conrad F, et al. Malignancies of the colorectum and anus in solid organ recipients. Transpl Int. 2007;20(6):497–504. Epub 2007/03/09.
64. Collins MG, Teo E, Cole SR, Chan CY, McDonald SP, Russ GR, et al. Screening for colorectal cancer and advanced colorectal neoplasia in kidney transplant recipients: cross sectional prevalence and diagnostic accuracy study of faecal immunochemical testing for haemoglobin and colonoscopy. BMJ. 2012;345:e4657. Epub 2012/07/27.
65. Meeuwis KA, Melchers WJ, Bouten H, van de Kerkhof PC, Hinten F, Quint WG, et al. Anogenital malignancies in women after renal transplantation over 40 years in a single center. Transplantation. 2012;93(9):914–22. Epub 2012/03/02.
66. FUTURE II Study Group. Quadrivalent vaccine against human papillomavirus to prevent high-grade cervical lesions. N Engl J Med. 2007;356(19):1915–27. Epub 2007/05/15.
67. Fairley CK, Sheil AG, McNeil JJ, Ugoni AM, Disney AP, Giles GG, et al. The risk of ano-genital malignancies in dialysis and

transplant patients. Clin Nephrol. 1994;41(2):101–5. Epub 1994/02/01.

68. ter Haar-van Eck SA, Rischen-Vos J, Chadha-Ajwani S, Huikeshoven FJ. The incidence of cervical intraepithelial neoplasia among women with renal transplant in relation to cyclosporine. Br J Obstet Gynaecol. 1995;102(1):58–61. Epub 1995/01/01.
69. Wong G, Howard K, Webster A, Chapman JR, Craig JC. The health and economic impact of cervical cancer screening and human papillomavirus vaccination in kidney transplant recipients. Transplantation. 2009;87(7):1078–91. Epub 2009/04/09.
70. Barrett WL, First MR, Aron BS, Penn I. Clinical course of malignancies in renal transplant recipients. Cancer. 1993;72(7):2186–9.
71. Hoffmann CJ, Subramanian AK, Cameron AM, Engels EA. Incidence and risk factors for hepatocellular carcinoma after solid organ transplantation. Transplantation. 2008;86(6):784–90. Epub 2008/09/25.
72. Zhang BH, Yang BH, Tang ZY. Randomized controlled trial of screening for hepatocellular carcinoma. J Cancer Res Clin Oncol. 2004;130(7):417–22. Epub 2004/03/26.
73. Danpanich E, Kasiske BL. Risk factors for cancer in renal transplant recipients. Transplantation. 1999;68(12):1859–64. Epub 2000/01/11.
74. Breyer BN, Whitson JM, Freise CE, Meng MV. Prostate cancer screening and treatment in the transplant population: current status and recommendations. J Urol. 2009;181(5):2018–25; discussion 25–6. Epub 2009/03/17.
75. Webber SA, Naftel DC, Fricker FJ, Olesnevich P, Blume ED, Addonizio L, et al. Lymphoproliferative disorders after paediatric heart transplantation: a multi-institutional study. Lancet. 2006;367(9506):233–9.
76. Caillard S, Lamy FX, Quelen C, Dantal J, Lebranchu Y, Lang P, et al. Epidemiology of posttransplant lymphoproliferative disorders in adult kidney and kidney pancreas recipients: report of the French registry and analysis of subgroups of lymphomas. Am J Transplant. 2012;12(3):682–93.
77. Quinlan SC, Pfeiffer RM, Morton LM, Engels EA. Risk factors for early-onset and late-onset post-transplant lymphoproliferative disorder in kidney recipients in the United States. Am J Hematol. 2011;86(2):206–9.
78. Cohen JI. Epstein-Barr virus infection. N Engl J Med. 2000;343(7):481–92.
79. Loren AW, Porter DL, Stadtmauer EA, Tsai DE. Post-transplant lymphoproliferative disorder: a review. Bone Marrow Transplant. 2003;31(3):145–55.
80. Thorley-Lawson DA, Gross A. Persistence of the Epstein-Barr virus and the origins of associated lymphomas. N Engl J Med. 2004;350(13):1328–37.
81. Nelson BP, Nalesnik MA, Bahler DW, Locker J, Fung JJ, Swerdlow SH. Epstein-Barr virus-negative post-transplant lymphoproliferative disorders: a distinct entity? Am J Surg Pathol. 2000;24(3):375–85.
82. Dotti G, Fiocchi R, Motta T, Mammana C, Gotti E, Riva S, et al. Lymphomas occurring late after solid-organ transplantation: influence of treatment on the clinical outcome. Transplantation. 2002;74(8):1095–102.
83. Swerdlow SH. T-cell and NK-cell posttransplantation lymphoproliferative disorders. Am J Clin Pathol. 2007;127(6):887–95.
84. Kapelushnik J, Ariad S, Benharroch D, Landau D, Moser A, Delsol G, et al. Post renal transplantation human herpesvirus 8-associated lymphoproliferative disorder and Kaposi's sarcoma. Br J Haematol. 2001;113(2):425–8.
85. Birkeland SA, Hamilton-Dutoit S. Is posttransplant lymphoproliferative disorder (PTLD) caused by any specific immunosuppressive drug or by the transplantation per se? Transplantation. 2003;76(6):984–8.
86. Nourse JP, Jones K, Gandhi MK. Epstein-Barr virus-related post-transplant lymphoproliferative disorders: pathogenetic insights for targeted therapy. Am J Transplant. 2011;11(5):888–95.
87. Kasiske BL, Kukla A, Thomas D, Wood Ives J, Snyder JJ, Qiu Y, et al. Lymphoproliferative disorders after adult kidney transplant: epidemiology and comparison of registry report with claims-based diagnoses. Am J Kidney Dis. 2011;58(6):971–80.
88. Opelz G, Dohler B. Lymphomas after solid organ transplantation: a collaborative transplant study report. Am J Transplant. 2004;4(2):222–30.
89. Kirk AD, Cherikh WS, Ring M, Burke G, Kaufman D, Knechtle SJ, et al. Dissociation of depletional induction and posttransplant lymphoproliferative disease in kidney recipients treated with alemtuzumab. Am J Transplant. 2007;7(11):2619–25.
90. Smith JM, Corey L, Healey PJ, Davis CL, McDonald RA. Adolescents are more likely to develop posttransplant lymphoproliferative disorder after primary Epstein-Barr virus infection than younger renal transplant recipients. Transplantation. 2007; 83(11):1423–8. Epub 2007/06/15.
91. Dharnidharka VR, Tejani AH, Ho PL, Harmon WE. Post-transplant lymphoproliferative disorder in the United States: young Caucasian males are at highest risk. Am J Transplant. 2002;2(10):993–8.
92. Nee R, Hurst FP, Dharnidharka VR, Jindal RM, Agodoa LY, Abbott KC. Racial variation in the development of posttransplant lymphoproliferative disorders after renal transplantation. Transplantation. 2011;92(2):190–5.
93. McDonald RA, Smith JM, Ho M, Lindblad R, Ikle D, Grimm P, et al. Incidence of PTLD in pediatric renal transplant recipients receiving basiliximab, calcineurin inhibitor, sirolimus and steroids. Am J Transplant. 2008;8(5):984–9. Epub 2008/04/18.
94. Grinyo J, Charpentier B, Pestana JM, Vanrenterghem Y, Vincenti F, Reyes-Acevedo R, et al. An integrated safety profile analysis of belatacept in kidney transplant recipients. Transplantation. 2010;90(12):1521–7. Epub 2010/11/20.
95. Swerdlow S, Harris NL. WHO classification of tumours of the haematopoietic and lymphoid tissues. 4th ed. Lyon: International Agency for Research on Cancer; 2008.
96. Evens AM, Roy R, Sterrenberg D, Moll MZ, Chadburn A, Gordon LI. Post-transplantation lymphoproliferative disorders: diagnosis, prognosis, and current approaches to therapy. Curr Oncol Rep. 2010;12(6):383–94. Epub 2010/10/22.
97. Larson RS, Scott MA, McCurley TL, Vnencak-Jones CL. Microsatellite analysis of posttransplant lymphoproliferative disorders: determination of donor/recipient origin and identification of putative lymphomagenic mechanism. Cancer Res. 1996;56(19):4378–81.
98. Olagne J, Caillard S, Gaub MP, Chenard MP, Moulin B. Post-transplant lymphoproliferative disorders: determination of donor/recipient origin in a large cohort of kidney recipients. Am J Transplant. 2011;11(6):1260–9.
99. Morgans AK, Reshef R, Tsai DE. Posttransplant lymphoproliferative disorder following kidney transplant. Am J Kidney Dis. 2010;55(1):168–80.
100. Pickhardt PJ, Siegel MJ. Posttransplantation lymphoproliferative disorder of the abdomen: CT evaluation in 51 patients. Radiology. 1999;213(1):73–8.
101. Bakker NA, Pruim J, de Graaf W, van Son WJ, van der Jagt EJ, van Imhoff GW. PTLD visualization by FDG-PET: improved detection of extranodal localizations. Am J Transplant. 2006;6(8):1984–5.
102. von Falck C, Maecker B, Schirg E, Boerner AR, Knapp WH, Klein C, et al. Post transplant lymphoproliferative disease in pediatric solid organ transplant patients: a possible role for [18F]-FDG-PET(/CT) in initial staging and therapy monitoring. Eur J Radiol. 2007;63(3):427–35.

103. Kwee TC, Kwee RM, Nievelstein RA. Imaging in staging of malignant lymphoma: a systematic review. Blood. 2008;111(2): 504–16.
104. Humar A, Michaels M, Monitoring AIWGoID. American Society of Transplantation recommendations for screening, monitoring and reporting of infectious complications in immunosuppression trials in recipients of organ transplantation. Am J Transplant. 2006;6(2):262–74.
105. Martin SI, Dodson B, Wheeler C, Davis J, Pesavento T, Bumgardner GL. Monitoring infection with Epstein-Barr virus among seromismatch adult renal transplant recipients. Am J Transplant. 2011;11(5):1058–63.
106. Tsai DE, Hardy CL, Tomaszewski JE, Kotloff RM, Oltoff KM, Somer BG, et al. Reduction in immunosuppression as initial therapy for posttransplant lymphoproliferative disorder: analysis of prognostic variables and long-term follow-up of 42 adult patients. Transplantation. 2001;71(8):1076–88.
107. Nalesnik MA. Clinicopathologic characteristics of post-transplant lymphoproliferative disorders. Recent Results Cancer Res. 2002;159:9–18.
108. Ghobrial IM, Habermann TM, Maurer MJ, Geyer SM, Ristow KM, Larson TS, et al. Prognostic analysis for survival in adult solid organ transplant recipients with post-transplantation lymphoproliferative disorders. J Clin Oncol. 2005;23(30):7574–82.
109. Vegso G, Hajdu M, Sebestyen A. Lymphoproliferative disorders after solid organ transplantation-classification, incidence, risk factors, early detection and treatment options. Pathol Oncol Res. 2011;17(3):443–54.
110. Dominguez-Gil B, Morales JM. Transplantation in the patient with hepatitis C. Transpl Int. 2009;22(12):1117–31. Epub 2009/08/07.
111. Trofe J, Buell JF, Beebe TM, Hanaway MJ, First MR, Alloway RR, et al. Analysis of factors that influence survival with post-transplant lymphoproliferative disorder in renal transplant recipients: the Israel Penn International Transplant Tumor Registry experience. Am J Transplant. 2005;5(4 Pt 1):775–80.
112. Lazda VA. Evaluation of Epstein-Barr virus (EBV) antibody screening of organ donors for allocation of organs to EBV serostatus matched recipients. Transplant Proc. 2006;38(10):3404–5.
113. Posfay-Barbe KM, Siegrist CA. Immunization and transplantation—what is new and what is coming? Pediatr Transplant. 2009;13(4):404–10.
114. Opelz G, Daniel V, Naujokat C, Fickenscher H, Dohler B. Effect of cytomegalovirus prophylaxis with immunoglobulin or with antiviral drugs on post-transplant non-Hodgkin lymphoma: a multicentre retrospective analysis. Lancet Oncol. 2007;8(3):212–8.
115. Choquet S, Leblond V, Herbrecht R, Socie G, Stoppa AM, Vandenberghe P, et al. Efficacy and safety of rituximab in B-cell post-transplantation lymphoproliferative disorders: results of a prospective multicenter phase 2 study. Blood. 2006;107(8): 3053–7.
116. Taylor AL, Bowles KM, Callaghan CJ, Wimperis JZ, Grant JW, Marcus RE, et al. Anthracycline-based chemotherapy as first-line treatment in adults with malignant posttransplant lymphoproliferative disorder after solid organ transplantation. Transplantation. 2006;82(3):375–81.
117. Trappe R, Oertel S, Leblond V, Mollee P, Sender M, Reinke P, et al. Sequential treatment with rituximab followed by CHOP chemotherapy in adult B-cell post-transplant lymphoproliferative disorder (PTLD): the prospective international multicentre phase 2 PTLD-1 trial. Lancet Oncol. 2012;13(2):196–206.
118. Nabors LB, Palmer CA, Julian BA, Przekwas AM, Kew CE. Isolated central nervous system posttransplant lymphoproliferative disorder treated with high-dose intravenous methotrexate. Am J Transplant. 2009;9(5):1243–8.
119. Haque T, Wilkie GM, Jones MM, Higgins CD, Urquhart G, Wingate P, et al. Allogeneic cytotoxic T-cell therapy for EBV-positive posttransplantation lymphoproliferative disease: results of a phase 2 multicenter clinical trial. Blood. 2007;110(4): 1123–31.
120. Perrine SP, Hermine O, Small T, Suarez F, O'Reilly R, Boulad F, et al. A phase 1/2 trial of arginine butyrate and ganciclovir in patients with Epstein-Barr virus-associated lymphoid malignancies. Blood. 2007;109(6):2571–8.
121. Karras A, Thervet E, Le Meur Y, Baudet-Bonneville V, Kessler M, Legendre C. Successful renal retransplantation after post-transplant lymphoproliferative disease. Am J Transplant. 2004;4(11):1904–9.
122. Batabyal P, Chapman JR, Wong G, Craig JC, Tong A. Clinical practice guidelines on wait-listing for kidney transplantation: consistent and equitable? Transplantation. 2012;94(7):703–13. Epub 2012/09/06.
123. Ajithkumar TV, Parkinson CA, Butler A, Hatcher HM. Management of solid tumours in organ-transplant recipients. Lancet Oncol. 2007;8(10):921–32.
124. Kasiske BL, Zeier MG, Chapman JR, Craig JC, Ekberg H, Garvey CA, et al. KDIGO clinical practice guideline for the care of kidney transplant recipients: a summary. Kidney Int. 2010;77(4):299–311.
125. Wong G, Webster AC, Chapman JR, Craig JC. Reported cancer screening practices of nephrologists: results from a national survey. Nephrol Dial Transplant. 2009;24(7):2136–43. Epub 2009/02/04.
126. Wong G, Chapman JR, Craig JC. Cancer screening in renal transplant recipients: what is the evidence? Clin J Am Soc Nephrol. 2008;3 Suppl 2:S87–100. Epub 2008/03/20.
127. Bouvard V, Baan R, Straif K, Grosse Y, Secretan B, El Ghissassi F, et al. A review of human carcinogens—part B: biological agents. Lancet Oncol. 2009;10(4):321–2.

Antibody-Mediated Rejection in Kidney Transplantation

26

Richard Ugarte, Boonsong Kiangkitiwan, and Abdolreza Haririan

Introduction

Hyperacute rejection was a major hurdle to successful outcomes in early years of organ transplantation. Shortly after vascular anastomosis of the organ, the graft would mottle and fail. The histological characteristics of this phenomenon were well recognized. These included accumulation of numerous polymorphonuclear leukocytes in peritubular and glomerular capillaries, extensive microvascular thrombosis, and cortical necrosis [1]. It was quickly recognized that preexisting antibodies in recipient serum reacting with donor human leukocyte antigens (HLA) were responsible for this phenomenon. Eluates from rejected kidneys were shown to have activity against HLA, and in some cases, IgG deposits were shown in immunofluorescence (IF) microscopy. Development of crossmatch testing was a breakthrough that provided a tool to almost completely eliminate hyperacute rejection in kidney transplantation. Leukocytes from 10 to 40 randomly selected individuals were exposed to sera from the recipients in the presence of complement [2]. It was shown that with cytotoxicity in >20 % of the cells in the panel, 80 % of the recipients lost their grafts shortly after transplantation, in contrast to 4.1 % failure among those with negative crossmatch. This simple assay, complement-dependent cytotoxicity (CDC), greatly prevented early poor outcomes in the following years. The percentage of panel cells that died was named panel-reactive antibodies (PRA). Technical advancements improved the sensitivity and specificity of the PRA and crossmatch assays [3]. Addition of antihuman globulin (AHG) was an improvement, but more recently these cell-based assays were replaced by solid-phase assays, where isolated HLA antigens placed on synthetic surface were exposed to patient sera. Enzyme-linked immunoadsorption assay (ELISA) was soon replaced by flow cytometry and a small footprint fluoroanalyzer (Luminex) [4]. Although the latter techniques have improved the sensitivity and specificity for detection of HLA antigens, they cannot detect non-HLA antigens that cell-based assays might have shown. Advances in HLA typing have significantly contributed to the improvement in HLA antibody detection. While serologic method and low-resolution DNA typing can identify 88 class I and 65 class II antigens, high-resolution DNA typing discriminates between more than 4,600 class I and more than 1,000 class II alleles [5].

With the widespread use of crossmatch assays and dramatic reduction in poor outcomes early after transplantation, the focus of attention was turned towards T cell-mediated graft injury and rejection in the following years. Histological characteristics of acute cellular rejection (ACR) were well defined, and specific criteria for grading the severity of rejection were described and widely adopted [6]. In parallel, immunosuppressive agents to prevent and treat ACR were developed. With the availability of cyclosporine in the early 1980s, short-term transplant outcomes significantly improved [7–10]. With the improvement in its formulation and development of tacrolimus and mycophenolate mofetil (MMF) and reduction in incidence of ACR, these outcomes were further improved [11–14]. However, the role of antibody-mediated graft injury was to a large extent overlooked. An important limiting factor was the lack of specific diagnostic histological changes to identify this type of injury. A major breakthrough occurred when Feucht et al. applied complement-split product, C4d staining that they had developed earlier for study of glomerulonephritides, to renal allografts with rejection [15]. They showed that a significant number of patients with cellular rejection demonstrate strong deposition of C4d in peritubular capillaries (PTC). The importance of this finding was not appreciated for several years until Colvin and colleagues demonstrated the significance of PTC C4d deposits in diagnosis of antibody-mediated

R. Ugarte, M.D., M.H.S. • B. Kiangkitiwan, M.D.
A. Haririan, M.D., M.P.H. (✉)
Division of Nephrology, Department of Medicine, University of Maryland School of Medicine, 22 South Greene Street, N3W143, Baltimore, MD 21201, USA
e-mail: ahariria@medicine.umaryland.edu

M.R. Weir and E.V. Lerma (eds.), *Kidney Transplantation: Practical Guide to Management*,
DOI 10.1007/978-1-4939-0342-9_26, © Springer Science+Business Media New York 2014

rejection (AMR) [16]. Since then, a great deal of attention has been paid to the role of AMR in organ transplantation, including its diagnostic features and therapeutic options.

In this chapter, we will examine the pathogenesis, clinical manifestations, and histological characteristics of AMR and discuss the available diagnostic tools and therapeutic strategies.

Pathogenesis

The principal targets for B cell-mediated alloimmune response are class I and class II HLA antigens. Class I antigens are composed of a variable chain (α chain) and a constant chain of β2-microglobulin, and class II antigens are made of two variable polypeptide chains (α and β) [17]. The peptide binding groove is formed by three-dimensional interaction of two peptide domains on both antigen classes. The B-cells recognize short stretches of 3–8 amino acids on the surface of the donor HLA molecules (epitopes) [18–20]. These epitopes can be shared between different antigens of the same class. Therefore, sensitization against a single epitope could cause alloantibody response against multiple HLA antigens. After recognition of alloantigen on HLA molecule, B cells proliferate and transform into plasma cells, and these cells mass produce monoclonal antibodies against the donor [21]. This donor-specific antibody (DSA) then binds to the respective HLA antigen on the endothelial cells of the allograft and through complement-dependent and complement-independent mechanisms can cause endothelial injury that leads to acute or chronic graft injury. Figure 26.1 is schematic of how DSA affects the organ.

Activation of complement system plays a major role in antibody-mediated graft injury. After the binding of DSA to and cross-linking of target epitopes on the surface of endothelial cells, this system becomes activated through classical pathway (Fig. 26.2). With final activation of C5, membrane attack complex (MAC) will form by assembly of C5b-C9, which can cause cell apoptosis and death. The by-product of activation of complement system is the formation of anaphylatoxins (C3a, C5a) that cause chemotaxis and activation of inflammatory cells [21]. C4d is the breakdown product of C4b, with unclear biological function that can bind covalently to the surface of endothelial cells and basement membrane. In normal kidneys, C4d can be found in the glomerular vascular pole and mesangium, due to the high complement turnover.

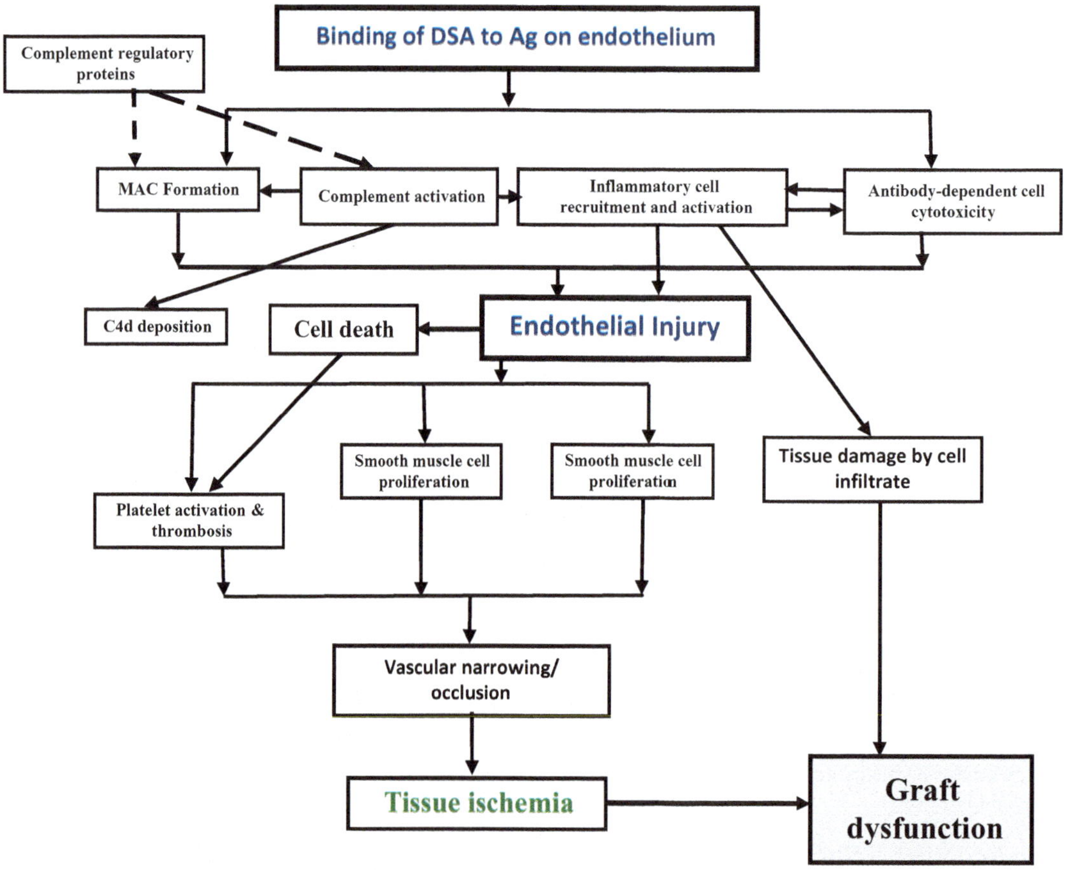

Fig. 26.1 Mechanisms of allograft injury by donor-specific antibody

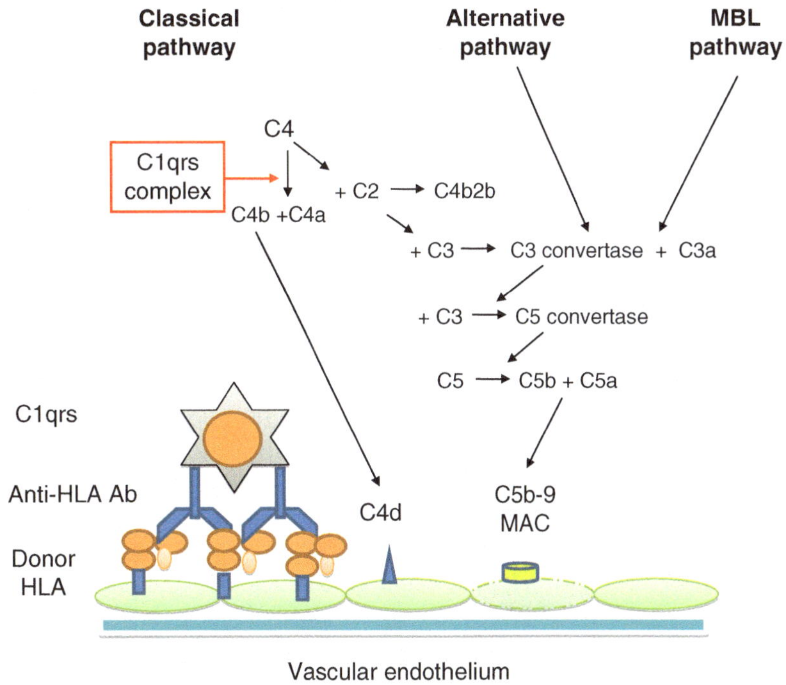

Fig. 26.2 Schematic of different pathways of complement activation [29]

In cases of immune-mediated glomerulopathies, C4d deposition can extend into the glomerular capillaries, but only rarely into the PTC [22, 23]. Its detection in PTC generally indicates antibody-mediated activation of complement system; therefore, it is considered the "fingerprint" telltale sign of the antibody action. However, not all cases with AMR demonstrate PTC C4d deposition. Halloran and colleagues have provided evidence for C4d-negative AMR [24–26]. Complement-independent antibody-mediated endothelial injury has been clearly shown in animal models [27]. Recent experimental evidence suggests the important role of natural killer (NK) cells, independent of complement, in antibody-mediated chronic allograft vasculopathy in murine heart allografts [28]. Histological and gene expression profiling of renal allograft biopsies also support the role of NK cells in pathogenesis of AMR [26].

The endothelial response to DSA depends on different factors including density of the antigen on the cells, affinity of the antibody for the target, its complement-activating ability, concentration of antibody, synergy between antibodies against different epitopes [30], and presence of complement regulatory proteins. IgG3 and IgG1 strongly activate complement, while IgG2 is a weak and IgG4 is a poor complement activator [31, 32].

At higher concentrations, DSA binding can lead to lytic lesions and apoptosis of the cells with denudation of the underlying matrix and subsequent platelet activation and thrombosis in the microvasculature [33–36]. The lytic changes are generally found in the early posttransplant period [33, 37–39] and can vary in severity from mild to severe [40]. However, at lower concentrations, antibody ligation of HLA molecules on the endothelial cells stimulates cell proliferation, with upregulation of fibroblast growth factor receptor and activation of mTOR pathway playing important roles [41, 42]. The resultant endothelial cell activation is accompanied by increased expression of adhesion molecules VCAM-1 and ICAM-1 and release of von Willebrand factor and P-selectin, leading to adherence and activation of inflammatory cells and platelets [42]. Sublytic levels of DSA can cause rearrangement of the actin cytoskeleton leading to change in endothelial cell morphology from polygonal and flat to contracted and rounded. This transformation opens gaps between the cells to expose the underlying matrix, triggering activation of the coagulation cascade and platelet aggregation, resulting in formation of microthrombi [37, 43]. The activated platelets in turn recruit inflammatory cells by expressing thromboxanes and RANTES [44, 45] and cause the expression of P-selectin and integrins that aid leukocyte trafficking [46, 47].

Presence of anti-graft antibody without functional injury has been postulated (accommodation). This phenomenon is more common with ABO antibodies [48–52]. Upregulation of complement regulatory proteins, decay accelerating factor, complement receptor-related protein, and CD59 is one of the hypothesized mechanisms of accommodation. Increased expression of pro-survival genes such as Bcl-2, Bcl-xL, and cytoprotective heme oxygenase and nitric oxide could also be involved [25, 42, 48, 53–58].

Study of gene expression patterns in the biopsies has shown that grafts with AMR have increased expression of endothelial cell transcripts [26, 59]. The presence of this expression pattern in biopsy along with DSA is significantly associated with higher risk of graft failure.

DSA: Epidemiology and Impact on Outcome

Sensitization to HLA antigens and other non-HLA antigens can happen with pregnancy, previous organ transplantation, blood transfusion, or through cross-reactivity with infectious agents or allergens. The degree of sensitization is assessed pre-transplant by using PRA assay. Rising PRA value indicates that the recipient has antibodies against larger number of HLA antigens, either from prior direct exposure or through epitope sharing. Currently, 34.6 % of patients on the US transplant wait list are sensitized to HLA antigens, 15.5 % with peak PRA >80 % (Table 5.1a, US Registry of Transplant Recipients 2010) [60]. Crossmatch testing prevents transplanting an organ in a recipient with DSA at a high enough titer and affinity to make the assay positive that could lead to hyperacute rejection. However, low level DSA could be unrecognized or even accepted for transplantation. In addition, the recipients may develop DSA de novo or by anamnestic response from prior exposure.

There are a number of studies that have examined the impact of pre-transplant and de novo DSA on long-term outcome. The available data suggest that DSA is generally predictive of worse results, including graft function, proteinuria, and graft failure.

In a study on 402 patients with negative CDC crossmatch at transplant, 8-year graft survival was significantly worse (61 %) among patients with preexisting HLA-DSA compared with both sensitized patients without HLA-DSA (93 %) and nonsensitized patients (84 %) [61]. Close to 40 % of those with pre-transplant DSA experienced AMR. The peak HLA-DSA Luminex mean fluorescence intensity (MFI) predicted AMR better than current HLA-DSA MFI ($P=0.028$). Amico et al. showed a significantly higher risk of AMR or ACR in patients with pre-transplant DSA [62]. However, only those experiencing AMR had worse graft survival. In another study, Couzi et al. reported that the presence of HLA-DSA detected only by the single antigen bead (SAB) assay in the context of a negative flow cytometry (FC) crossmatch was not associated with increased risk of acute rejection [63]. In a cohort of 54 patients with preformed DSA who received adjunctive IVIG with or without rituximab and plasma exchange, 80 % experienced subclinical AMR at 3 months; this group had a higher rate of interstitial fibrosis and tubular atrophy (IFTA) (100 % vs. 33.3 %, $P<0.01$) and a higher rate of transplant glomerulopathy (TG) (43 % vs. 0 %, $P=0.02$) compared to patients without subclinical AMR at 3 months [64]. More recently, in a systematic review and meta-analysis, Mohan et al. concluded that the presence of preformed DSA, despite a negative FC crossmatch, nearly doubles the risk of AMR (RR: 1.98, $P<0.001$, 95% CI: 1.36–2.89) and increases the risk of graft failure by 76 % ($P=0.01$, 95% CI: 1.13–2.74) [65].

As noted previously, DSA can develop de novo. In a prospective study of more than 1,200 patients, 5.5 % developed donor-specific HLA and 11.3 % developed non-donor-specific HLA antibodies de novo [66]. In a smaller cohort of 249 recipients, 11.2 % developed HLA antibodies, and 4.4 % had DSA [67]. HLA antibody in this cohort was associated with higher serum creatinine. In a report from a UK center, among patients transplanted between 1985 and 2006 in those who developed DSA, 3-year graft survival after antibody detection was worse (69.5 % vs. 91.1 %, $P=0.035$) [68]. Graft failure was more likely in patients with DSA with excess of 0.2 g/L proteinuria at antibody detection (42 % vs. 0 %, $P=0.008$). In a cohort of 244 consecutively transplanted kidney and kidney/pancreas recipients without pre-transplant DSA transplanted between 2007 and 2009 and screened for de novo DSA at 1, 6, 12, and 24 months and when clinically indicated, DSA was detected in 27 % of all patients, all during the first year posttransplant [69]. DSA-positive patients were significantly more likely to have acute rejection (both AMR/ACR) compared with no DSA (29 % vs. 9.5 %, $P<0.001$) and lower estimated 2-year graft survival (83 % vs. 98 %, $P<0.001$). Ntokou et al. demonstrated de novo DSA in 15.4 % and third party HLA antibody in 32.8 % of the patients in Greece [70]. Presence of HLA antibody was an independent predictor of graft failure: for class I (HR: 31.8), class II (HR: 20.9), and non-DSA HLA antibody (HR: 5.9).

Detection of DSA with graft dysfunction or for-cause biopsies also has been shown to be associated with worse graft outcome. Our group analyzed 297 patients who underwent for-cause biopsies; 31.3 % were DSA-positive, 58 (19.5 %) with class I, 68 (22.9 %) with class II DSA, and 33 (11.1 %) with both class I and class II DSA [71]. Those with class I only DSA did not have higher risk of graft failure from the time of sampling compared with DSA-negative patients, while those with class II DSA alone or in combination with class I DSA had worse graft survival (adjusted HR: 2.5, $P=0.001$, 95% CI: 1.4–4.3 for class II only and HR: 2.7, $P<0.001$, 95% CI: 1.6–4.7 for class I/II DSA). Examining the time of testing posttransplant, during the first year, any form of DSA, including class I alone, was predictive of worse graft survival. However, after the first year, only class II DSA was associated with higher risk of graft failure. Lee et al. in a case-control study also showed that those with HLA antibody in first year had higher risk of graft loss (adjusted HR: 7.8, $P<0.001$, 95% CI: 3.0–20.1) [72].

Despite all these reports, the presence of DSA is not always associated with poor outcome. There are reports of patients with de novo DSA who maintain stable, good graft function with no significant proteinuria for years, without obvious adverse clinical consequences [73].

Non-HLA-DSA

Clinical and histological features of AMR occur in association with circulating HLA-DSA. However, there are patients with similar presentation, but HLA-DSA cannot be identified, even using SAB assay [74]. We have previously reported that in patients with diffuse PTC C4d staining, 31.1 % did not have detectable HLA-DSA [71].

In a subset of these patients, low concentration of circulating antibody and absorption of the DSA in the allograft could explain the negative test results. It has been shown that after nephrectomy in patients with failed organ and negative DSA in the blood, the antibody can be eluted from the tissue and detected in the blood after removal of the allograft [75]. Marrari and Duquesnoy used micro bead-based Luminex antibody-binding assay in 65 cases that underwent transplant nephrectomy following rejection, before and after surgical removal of the allograft [76]. The incidence of DSA reactivity pre- and post-nephrectomy for HLA-A,B and HLA-DRB1 mismatch categories were 64 % vs. 87 % ($P=0.003$) and 57 % vs. 86 % ($P<0.0001$), respectively.

HLA typing for non-ABC/DR loci has not been routine. Therefore, HLA-DSA targeting DQ, DP, or DRB3-4 antigens cannot be discovered, unless the typing is performed. In a study of 138 patients with functioning grafts, DP antibody was detected in 5.1 % of the patients [77]. In contrast, among 185 patients with rejection, this frequency was 19.5 %. Jolly et al. reported two cases with pre-transplant HLA-DP DSA who after transplantation experienced recurrent acute AMR and graft failure [78]. Zhu et al. conducted a case-control study comparing 29 patients with graft failure and 25 controls with functioning grafts [79]. In the former group, out of 17 patients who received DQ-mismatched organs, 13 (76 %) had DSA against HLA-DQ antigen, compared with 1 of 11 (9 %) in the control group ($P<0.001$).

Non-HLA antigens could also be the target of humoral alloimmune response. Major histocompatibility complex class I chain-related gene (MICA) DSA and anti-angiotensin receptor I (AT1) antibody are two major examples of such antibodies [80–82]. In a study of 39 rejected compared with 26 functioning grafts, IgG HLA plus MICA antibodies were found in 77 % of the former, as compared with 42 % of the latter group ($P<0.01$); IgG/IgM HLA antibodies were detected in 72 % and 46 %, respectively [83]. Among 185 consecutive renal transplant patients, Panigrahi et al. detected MICA antibodies in 16 %, which was associated with worse graft survival compared to those with negative testing (60 % vs. 86 %, $P=0.001$) [84]. Among the HLA antibody-negative patients, 82 % of the former and 21.4 % of the latter groups had MICA antibody. Amico et al. described ten patients with early AMR due to non-HLA-DSA; only in three, the antibody could be identified as MICA-DSA [85]. Dragun et al. for the first time reported 16 patients with refractory vascular rejection and malignant hypertension without anti-HLA antibody who had activating IgG antibodies targeting angiotensin receptor 1 (AT1) [80]. Interestingly, AT1 antagonist losartan blocked the agonistic effects of the antibodies. Other allo- or autoantibodies described as targets of antibody response in AMR causing graft injury include vimentin, agrin, collagen V, K-α1-tubulin, and nucleolin, among others [86–90]. Despite these identified targets, in some cases with clinical and pathological manifestation of AMR, the target antigen cannot be identified [34].

Regardless of the target, development of DSA is usually associated with graft injury. When this injury is acute and associated with acute rise in serum creatinine, the resultant syndrome is called acute AMR, which is associated with certain histological features. However, the antibody-mediated effect can cause slow histological changes presenting with slowly worsening graft function and proteinuria. This clinical syndrome, chronic AMR, has certain histological characteristics that separate it from acute AMR. In the next sections, we will discuss the clinical presentation, histological features, and treatment of these two syndromes.

Acute Antibody-Mediated Rejection

Introduction

Acute AMR is a clinical syndrome defined by acute graft dysfunction resulting from the effect of DSA on the allograft. This dysfunction could be in the form of acute rise in serum creatinine or undeclining serum creatinine in early posttransplant period. The extreme form of this syndrome is hyperacute rejection, in which the transplanted kidney becomes ischemic and necrotic immediately or shortly after implantation. Histologically, the allograft shows platelet aggregation along the glomerular and peritubular capillary microcirculation, leading to occlusive microthrombi and renal cortical necrosis [35, 91]. There is also pronounced neutrophilic margination and inflammation resulting in glomerulitis and peritubular capillaritis [1, 2, 92, 93]. This catastrophic event occurs as a result of high levels of undetected DSA or blood group (ABO) isoagglutinins at the time of transplantation [71, 94]. With the introduction and advances in crossmatch assays, this phenomenon has been effectively eliminated.

In 1990, Halloran et al. described a form of AMR that was different from hyperacute and typical acute rejection [40]. They described seven pre-sensitized patients with class I HLA-DSA in association with atypical but distinctive patterns of rejection. The clinical presentation was rapid onset of oliguria and deterioration of graft function, with histological picture of acute tubular necrosis. Renal histology showed granular complement deposition, polymorphonuclear infiltration, and endothelial injury in the microvasculature.

In three patients, the glomerular capillaries showed fibrin thrombi and widening of the subendothelial space, similar to hemolytic uremic syndrome. They hypothesized that anti-class I antibody appearing or persisting in the early posttransplant period can cause a unique form of acute rejection characterized by prominent microvascular injury, ATN, PMN infiltration, and complement staining. During the subsequent years, this pattern of acute rejection was better characterized, and the time course of the cellular and molecular events was delineated [16]. The prominent microvascular inflammation has been consistently associated with AMR [36, 41, 56, 95–102]. Unlike hyperacute rejection, acute AMR causes a slower vascular compromise to the allograft microcirculation, hence does not present as catastrophic graft failure and loss; although uninterrupted acute AMR can progress to graft loss within a short period of time [103–105].

With better understanding of the biology and histology of acute AMR, its diagnostic criteria have transformed over the past two decades. The Banff working group has revised these criteria a few times and is in the process of refining them further following the recent meeting in 2013 [106–112].

Clinical Presentation and Histology

Acute AMR typically presents in early posttransplant period, either as delayed or slow graft function or acute deterioration of graft function after initial improvement and stabilization. The DSA is generally anti-donor HLA antibody, but it can have a non-HLA target, as described previously. The former can be against class I or class II HLA antigen(s). In early acute AMR, class I antigens are more commonly involved. The early cases are generally the result of low DSA titers that do not cause positive crossmatch testing at the time of surgery or are undetectable at the time. Later cases are more often the result of de novo DSA.

The true incidence of acute AMR varies depending on the characteristics of the patient population, with reported rates from 5 to 23 % in unselected recipients and 12–37 % of biopsies taken for acute rejection and up to 60 % in desensitized patients with positive crossmatch or ABO-incompatible transplantation [112–118]. Histological features of AMR in the presence of DSA can be found in surveillance biopsies in the absence of graft dysfunction. These subclinical cases will increase the true rate of acute AMR after kidney transplantation.

The risk factors for acute AMR include previous transplantation, particularly those with early graft loss, multiple repeat mismatches, multiple preformed DSA, multiple sensitizing events, and high-risk combinations (husband-to-wife and child-to-mother) [119, 120].

Acute AMR as a pathological diagnosis was formally recognized in the Banff working group has revised these criteria a few times and is in the process of refining them further following the recent meeting in 2013 [106–112]. Diagnosis of acute AMR requires both morphologic evidence of graft injury and immunohistologic evidence of antibody effect. In the presence of serologic evidence, circulating DSA, this constellation can be called acute AMR (Table 26.1). According to the Banff criteria, the histological evidence can be one of the three types:

Table 26.1 Banff criteria for diagnosis of acute AMR

1. Morphologic evidence
   - Acute tubular injury (type I)
   - Neutrophils and/or monocytes/macrophages in PTC and/or glomeruli (type II)
   - Thrombi in glomerular capillaries, arterioles, and/or small arteries (type II)
   - Arterial fibrinoid necrosis (type III)
2. Immunohistologic evidence
   - Diffuse C4d in PTC
   - Ig and/or complement in arterial fibrinoid necrosis
3. Serologic evidence
   - Circulating DSA to donor HLA or other targets

Type I, acute tubular injury; type II, neutrophils and/or monocytes/macrophages in PTC and/or glomeruli or thrombi in glomerular capillaries, arterioles, and/or small arteries; and type III, arterial fibrinoid necrosis. It is clear that when AMR is characterized with only acute tubular injury in the biopsy, in the absence of other supportive evidence, its distinction from other forms of tubular injury would be impossible. In other words, in patients with delayed graft function, which is generally associated with tubular injury attributed to ischemia/reperfusion injury, diagnosis of acute AMR can be missed if screening for serologic and immunohistologic markers of AMR is not carried out.

The immunohistologic evidence of AMR is documented by demonstration of C4d deposition in PTC or Ig or complement in fibrinoid necrosis. C4d can be detected either by immunofluorescence (IF) or immunohistochemistry (IHC). IF is performed on frozen tissue section using a monoclonal antibody against C4d. For IHC paraffin-embedded tissue section is stained with tagged polyclonal anti-C4d antibody [121]. For diagnosis of AMR diffuse (>50 %) PTC staining is required (Banff C4d3). Since IHC is less sensitive than IF, in more than half of the biopsies with focal pattern (10–50 % of PTC, Banff C4d2) with IHC, the pattern is diffuse using the latter [111, 121, 122]. Our group, along with others, has shown that focal staining with IHC has an association with graft survival similar to diffuse pattern [71].

The Banff classification recognizes the intensity of peritubular capillaritis (ptc) and glomerulitis (g) by scoring them from 0 to 3, based on the extent of capillaries and number of luminal inflammatory cells involved [107, 111]. ptc/g score >0 is indicative of histological evidence of AMR. Acute AMR often occurs in combination with features of ACR, including interstitial inflammation and tubulitis. Therefore, screening for DSA and C4d staining are essential for complete evaluation of an allograft biopsy.

Management

Despite the great progress that has been made in prevention and treatment of cell-mediated rejection, the treatment of AMR remains for the most part nonspecific and suboptimal. The proposed treatment strategies are mostly based on retrospective data in small cohort of patients, often with variable diagnostic criteria and with relatively short follow-up periods [123]. Diagnosis of acute AMR is based on graft dysfunction associated with histological and immunohistologic evidence of demonstrable circulating DSA. Treatment protocols for these cases are based on three basic concepts:

1. Suppression of T-cell function to decrease/eliminate T cell-mediated B-cell activation
2. Removal or neutralization of circulating DSA and complement components
3. Prevention of DSA formation through depletion or suppression of antibody-forming plasma cells or their precursor B cells

The B lymphocytes function as antigen-presenting cells (APC) to T cells; on the other hand, the process of B-cell activation is dependent on T lymphocytes. Antibody response to protein antigens requires CD4+ helper T lymphocytes that recognize the antigen [21]. Moreover, T cell-mediated acute rejection often accompanies AMR in the biopsy. Therefore, targeting T lymphocytes has become a part of the therapeutic protocols in treatment of acute AMR. Different centers use intravenous methylprednisolone or thymoglobulin for this purpose. Although the latter may have additional effects on AMR effector cells, as discussed later. In the following section, we will concentrate on more specific treatment modalities.

Intravenous Immunoglobulin

Intravenous immunoglobulin (IVIG) has been used for treatment of various autoimmune diseases [124]. A number of different mechanisms have been suggested for its action. Anti-idiotypic activity with neutralization of the noxious antibodies, suppression and neutralization of cytokines and activated complement components, blockade of leukocyte adhesion molecules, upregulation of inhibitory Fcγ receptor IIB, blockade of FcRn receptors and hence shortening the half-life of targeted antibodies, and blockade of activating Fcγ receptor, immunomodulation by sialylated IgG, which also promotes B-cell apoptosis, are among the proposed properties of IVIG [124–132]. IVIG effects extend beyond the half-life and presence of IVIG in circulation, attributed to its ability to modulate cell-mediated immunity through Fc receptors [133]. The different IVIG preparations differ from each other in concentration of Ig, type and content of sugar, sodium concentration, and osmotic load [123]. In addition, the anti-HLA antibody inhibitory effect of these preparations may also vary [134]. Adverse effects of IVIG occur in less than 5 % of the patients. The serious adverse reaction include aseptic meningitis, anaphylactic reaction, hypercoagulability resulting in deep venous thrombosis, pulmonary embolism, retinal vein thrombosis, stroke, myocardial infarction, clotting of dialysis access, and acute kidney injury.

For treatment of acute AMR, IVIG has been generally used with two different dosing regimens; high dose (2 g/kg), administered as a single or in split doses, and low dose (100 mg/kg), which is administered along with plasmapheresis, after each exchange treatment. The efficacy of high-dose IVIG in treatment of acute AMR was first reported by Jordan et al. [135]. They described their experience in ten patients with severe rejection, four with high levels of DSA. All the rejection episodes were reversed, and DSA titers rapidly dropped. This group have reported efficacy of high-dose IVIG in desensitization of high-PRA recipients or those with positive crossmatch [115, 136–138].

Plasmapheresis

Removing the DSA from circulation is an important component of treatment of acute AMR. Plasmapheresis provides the fastest and most effective method of achieving this goal. The modalities include removing the whole plasma and replacing the equivalent volume with albumin or fresh frozen plasma (plasma exchange) or selective removal of Ig, using double-filtration plasmapheresis [26, 139–141]. The alternative method is immunoadsorption using staphylococcal protein A column or sheep anti-IgG antibody column to remove IgG component of the plasma [142–147]. Plasma exchange is currently the only modality available in the United States. Considering the volume of distribution and rebound of the antibody, several 1–1.5 volume exchanges are required for reducing the antibody titer. Generally, one immunoadsorption treatment is equivalent to three plasma exchanges regarding the antibody removal efficacy.

The major side effects of plasma exchange include coagulopathy and bleeding diathesis, volume contraction, and potential transmission of pathogens.

Since plasmapheresis only removes the circulating DSA and does not affect the antibody-producing plasma cells or their precursor B cells, reappearance of the DSA even after several treatments is expected. Therefore, this modality is used in combination with other agents that decrease antibody production. In two small case series, combination of plasma exchange or immunoadsorption and rescue immunosuppression with tacrolimus (TAC) and MMF resulted in excellent outcome in patients with AMR [116, 148]. Abraham et al. reported their experience in 20 patients with acute AMR early posttransplant [149]. Eighteen patients with viable grafts received plasma exchanges in conjunction with replacement of azathioprine with MMF and intensification of cyclosporine with or without conversion to TAC. They reported reversal of AMR in 78 % of the cases. The responders had received more intense plasmapheresis (median of 0.9 exchanges/patient/day) compared with nonresponders (0.5 exchanges/patient/day, $P=0.0053$).

On the other hand, Shah et al. reported their experience using plasmapheresis in conjunction with thymoglobulin (0.75 mg/kg/day 5–10 days) in treatment of acute AMR in seven renal transplant recipients [118]. There was one graft loss; however, the other six patients had 1-year graft survival similar to recipients without AMR. This group has shown a concentration-dependent apoptosis in plasma cells and naïve or stimulated B cells in vivo after exposure to thymoglobulin [118, 150]. This effect also has been demonstrated with myeloma cells [151].

Majority of the centers, including ours, currently use plasmapheresis in combination with low-dose IVIG after each treatment, either for desensitization or for treatment of acute AMR. With this method, removal of the circulating DSA is accompanied with supposedly antibody/complement neutralization and its reduced production. Montgomery et al. first presented the efficacy of this combination therapy in reversal of acute AMR in seven cases, three as rescue therapy and four in the setting of desensitized positive crossmatch transplants [119]. Rocha et al. treated 14 patients with early acute AMR with plasmapheresis/IVIG and reported 1-year graft survival (81 %) similar to patients treated for ACR (84 %) [117]. In another study of nine patients with acute AMR, eight responded to combination therapy with 1-year serum creatinine of 1.8 mg/dL [152]. Lehrich et al. reported their experience with this method in 22 patients and showed a significant improvement in graft survival compared to historical controls [153]. We recently reviewed the results of plasmapheresis/IVIG therapy in 47 patients with strict diagnosis of acute AMR in our center (unpublished data). The half-life of the grafts after diagnosis was 26 months, and graft survival by 4 years was only 33 %. Presence of acute ACR in the index biopsy was a poor prognostic factor.

Rituximab

CD20 is an activated-glycosylated transmembrane phosphoprotein expressed on the majority of stages of B-cell development; it is present from late pro-B cells through memory cells, but not on either early pro-B cells or plasmablasts and plasma cells [154]. It is suspected that it acts as a calcium channel in the cell membrane. Therefore, it has become a target for therapy in B-cell lymphomas. Rituximab, a chimeric murine/human monoclonal antibody, is approved in the United States for this indication. This antibody after binding to CD20 molecule on the surface of B cells leads to elimination of the cell through three proposed mechanisms, complement-dependent cytotoxicity, antibody-dependent cellular cytotoxicity (ADCC), and stimulation of apoptosis [155]. B-cell depletion may also impair the expansion of effector T cells after antigen exposure and increase the regulatory T cells [156]. These properties have made rituximab an attractive choice for including in the acute AMR treatment regimen. The dose used in treatment of lymphoma is usually weekly infusion of 375 mg/m^2 for 4 consecutive weeks. However, in patients with rheumatoid arthritis, two doses of 1 g 2 weeks apart have been used [157]. Although a lower dose of 500 mg has been reported to be effective in salvage therapy for acute AMR [158]. Rituximab causes a profound and prolonged depletion of B cells in the periphery and secondary lymphoid organs. In a phase one dose escalation trial of rituximab in dialysis patients, Vieira et al. showed similarly extensive depletion of CD19+ cells after a single dose of 50, 150, and 375 mg/m^2. This severe depletion persisted until about 3 months later, and by 1 year only partial recovery was observed [159]. Genberg et al. studied 43 kidney transplant recipients who received a single dose of rituximab, 91 % had complete depletion of the B lymphocytes, and in 78 % of the patients with late samples, CD19+ cells remained <5 cells/mL for as long as 14–16 months [160]. They also demonstrated significant reduction of these cells in lymph nodes and the allografts. Zarkhin et al. examined the B-cell phenotype before and after treatment of rejection with rituximab and showed that in patients with rejection naïve/memory B-cell ratio is reduced compared to stable patients, and after rituximab therapy this ratio recovers back to the level seen in stable recipients by 1 year [161].

Potential acute adverse effects of rituximab include acute bronchospasm, angioedema, respiratory distress, cardiogenic shock, and anaphylaxis, particularly in patient with high pretherapy leukocyte counts [162]. It may cause reactivation of hepatitis B or C, CMV, and mycobacterium tuberculosis, and cases of Progressive multifocal leukoencephalopathy (PML) caused by JC virus have been reported.

Becker et al. used a single dose of rituximab as rescue therapy in 27 sensitized patients with refractory acute rejection (no testing for DSA or C4d) and observed significant improvement in graft function and 85 % graft survival at 2 years [163]. Faguer et al. reported their experience in eight patients with acute AMR who received 4 weekly doses of rituximab in addition to plasma exchange [164]. Graft survival after a median of 10 months was 75 % and mean serum creatinine was 1.7 mg/dL. Kaposztas et al. retrospectively compared 26 patients who received plasmapheresis and rituximab for treatment of acute AMR with 28 who only received plasmapheresis [165]. Although patient survival was similar between the two groups, 2-year graft survival was significantly better with rituximab (90 % vs. 60 %, $P=0.005$). Jordan et al. have used a combination of high-dose IVIG and rituximab for desensitizing highly sensitized renal transplant candidates [166]. In 76 patients who were transplanted after receiving this regimen, 22 (29 %) experienced acute AMR early posttransplant and were treated with the same combination. Six cases lost their grafts due to AMR, with 2-year graft survival of 84 % [167]. Mulley et al. reported their experience with a single low-fixed dose of 500 mg rituximab in seven patients with acute AMR unresponsive to plasmapheresis/IVIG [158].

After a mean follow-up of 21 months, graft survival was 100 % and serum creatinine levels were significantly lower than the time of diagnosis. Lefaucheur et al. compared the efficacy of 2 weekly doses of rituximab 375 mg/m^2 after plasmapheresis and high-dose IVIG in treatment of acute AMR in 12 patients to historical controls treated only with high-dose IVIG [168]. Graft survival at 3 years was 91.7 % in the rituximab group and 50 % in the control group ($P=0.02$), and DSA levels were significantly lower 3 months post-rejection in the former group.

Bortezomib

As discussed previously, plasma cells that are the producers of the antibodies are not affected by rituximab and the other modalities discussed. Bortezomib is a proteasome inhibitor that is widely used for treatment of multiple myeloma. By reversibly inhibiting 26S proteasome with high affinity and specificity, it disrupts degradation of ubiquitinylated, abnormal, and misfolded proteins, leading to cell apoptosis [169]. Studies, in vitro and in vivo, have shown that this drug has a propensity to cause apoptosis in CD138+ plasma cells [141, 170, 171]. In addition, bortezomib may cause apoptosis of T_H cells and reduction in B cells [172]. The regimen for treatment of multiple myeloma includes cycles of four doses at 1.3 mg/m^2 on days 1, 4, 7, and 11.

Idica et al. demonstrated the ability of this drug in reversal of DSA in kidney transplant patients [173]. They showed that in 10 out of 13 patients (77 %), DSA disappeared and in the other three the titer was significantly reduced. This group then reported the use of bortezomib in six patients experiencing eight episodes of mixed AMR and ACR [174]. In all cases, the rejection was reversed and graft function improved, and there was a profound and prolonged reduction in DSA. The major side effects including thrombocytopenia, gastrointestinal toxicity, and paresthesias were transient. Perry et al. compared the activity of four agents, rituximab, thymoglobulin, IVIG, and bortezomib, on plasma cells and antibody production [170]. They showed that in vitro only bortezomib caused plasma cell apoptosis and blocked anti-HLA antibody secretion. In two patients treated with this agent for acute AMR, they demonstrated a transient decrease in plasma cells in the bone marrow and a significant reduction in DSA. Trivedi et al. used this drug in conjunction with intravenous methylprednisolone and plasmapheresis among 11 patients with anti-HLA antibodies (eight with DSA), in the absence of acute AMR, and observed successful reduction in antibody MFI to less than 1,000 in 9 within a median of 22 days after initiation of treatment [175]. The largest experience has been reported by Flechner et al. in a series of 20 patients with AMR diagnosed 19.8 months (mean) post-transplant who received a single dose of bortezomib in addition of plasmapheresis and high-dose IVIG [176]. After a mean follow-up of 9.8 months, graft survival was 85 %, estimated glomerular filtration rate was 41.9 ± 16.8 mL/min, and 59 % had significant proteinuria.

Sureshkumar et al. described disappearance of DSA and improved renal function in two patients with early acute AMR after addition of bortezomib to plasmapheresis and IVIG [177]. We observed disappearance of DSA in a patient with early AMR who was treated with plasmapheresis, IVIG, and rituximab after receiving bortezomib. But in two cases with late AMR, this agent was not effective in achieving significant reduction in dominant DSAs [178].

Complement Blockers

As discussed previously, complement activation is a major mechanism of DSA-induced graft injury, and C5 component plays a central role by releasing C5a and formation of MAC with other components (C6-9). Therefore, C5 seems to be a good target for abrogating DSA effect on the organ. Eculizumab is a humanized monoclonal antibody directed against complement protein C5, inhibiting conversion of C5 to C5b that is approved for use in paroxysmal nocturnal hemoglobinuria and atypical hemolytic uremic syndrome [179]. Locke et al. presented a single case of severe AMR in a young recipient with previous history of failed renal allograft and autologous bone marrow transplant for Hodgkin's lymphoma, who received a kidney from his mother with positive crossmatch [180]. Despite plasmapheresis and IVIG, he remained anuric. After receiving eculizumab, rituximab, and IVIG, his crossmatch became negative and ultimately his creatinine improved to 1.1 mg/dL. However, 4 months after transplant, the patient died of pulmonary hemorrhage due to veno-occlusive disease. This group later reported a highly sensitized recipient who had received bortezomib, plasmapheresis, and rituximab preconditioning and underwent a flow-positive crossmatch transplantation and experienced early AMR [181]. Eculizumab was started and the rejection was reversed, with normal serum creatinine at 6 months and negative flow crossmatch. Stegall et al. examined the efficacy of eculizumab at the time of transplant and postoperatively up to 13 weeks in living donor kidney recipients with positive crossmatch who received thymoglobulin induction with or without plasma exchange [39]. The incidence of acute AMR in the first 3 months posttransplant was 7.7 % (2/26) compared with 41.2 % in the historical control ($P=0.003$). Similar numbers for development of transplant glomerulopathy at 1 year were 6.7 % (1/15) vs. 35.7 % (15/42) ($P=0.044$).

Patients who are considered for this therapy should receive prior vaccination against meningococcus and pneumococcus.

The other complement target that has been studied in animal models is the C1 complex. Use of recombinant C1-inhibitor that disengages C1r and C1s in primate kidney transplant model has been effective in preventing acute AMR in sensitized animals [182]. This protein also inhibits the lectin pathway, kallikrein, and the coagulation components, factors XIIa and XIa. The potential advantage of this protein compared to eculizumab is that it does not affect the alternate pathway of complement activation, hence decreases the risk of certain infections [29].

Splenectomy

Splenectomy that has been mostly used in desensitization for ABO-incompatible transplantation has been used as rescue therapy in cases with persistent acute AMR. By substantial and immediate reduction in B-cell and plasma cell mass, splenectomy could lead to a reduction in DSA production to an extent that other adjunctive therapies could control the AMR [183] Locke et al. reported five patients experiencing severe AMR after positive crossmatch transplantation, unresponsive to plasmapheresis/IVIG and rituximab who underwent splenectomy and experienced reversal of rejection [183, 184]. Kaplan et al. reported four cases with acute AMR unresponsive to plasmapheresis/IVIG and rituximab or alemtuzumab, in the setting of ABO-incompatible transplantation in two and positive crossmatch in one, who underwent splenectomy and showed rapid decline in serum creatinine and reduction in antibody levels [185]. Others have also reported successful results after splenectomy for refractory acute AMR, unresponsive to standard therapy [186, 187].

Treatment Summary and Recommendation

Optimal treatment of acute AMR remains unclear. The treatment modalities reviewed have been used by extrapolation from other clinical conditions and supportive experimental data. The clinical experience with these options individually or in combination has been reported only in small cohorts and by retrospective comparisons. Randomized clinical trials have not been feasible. Therefore, adopting a treatment strategy can only be based on available literature and local experience in the patient population treated in the center. The following regimen is a reasonable approach to treatment of acute AMR based on the presented data and our own experience.

With biopsy-proven acute AMR, in conjunction with documented DSA and graft dysfunction, treatment can be started with steroid pulse and initiation of alternate day plasmapheresis (plasma exchange or immunoadsorption) with low-dose IVIG after each treatment. In cases with concomitant moderate to severe ACR, thymoglobulin can replace steroid pulse. If the graft dysfunction and histological evidence of AMR persist after 2 weeks of treatment in addition to continuation of plasmapheresis/IVIG, a single dose of rituximab or a cycle of bortezomib could be added. Failure to control AMR may warrant addition of eculizumab and in extreme cases splenectomy.

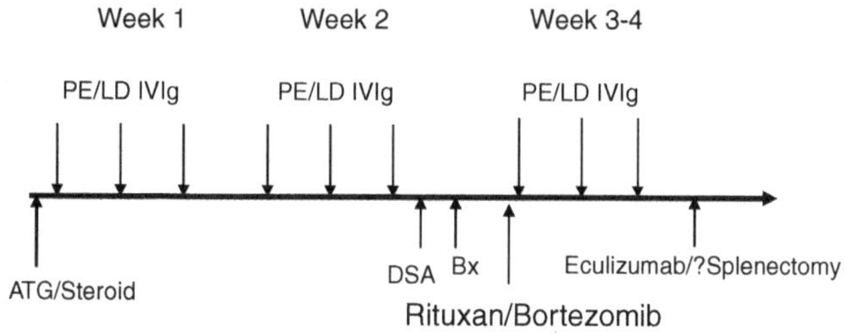

Chronic Antibody-Mediated Rejection

Introduction

Chronic AMR is a clinicopathological manifestation of chronic active graft injury as a result of donor-directed antibody. The dominant histological manifestation of this process is transplant glomerulopathy (TG). It is typically accompanied by various degrees of IFTA, multilayering of the PTC basement membrane, or arterial fibrous intimal thickening [110]. In the presence of these histological findings, presence of circulating DSA and footprint of its action in the tissue, i.e., PTC C4d, are required to label this syndrome as chronic AMR. However, an increasing number of studies point to cases with negative C4d in the biopsy [59, 71, 100, 188]. In this section, we will focus our discussion on TG as the main manifestation of chronic AMR.

Epidemiology

TG is characterized by double contours in more than 10 % of glomerular capillary loops. The reported incidence and prevalence of this entity varies. Using only for-cause biopsies, the estimated prevalence of TG was approximately 3 % of the patients at a median of 6 years posttransplant [189, 190]. Gloor et al. examined both protocol and for-cause biopsies and observed that 9.5 % of the patients with a mean follow-up of 41 ± 17 months had TG at a median of 21 ± 14 months (range 4–61) after transplant [191]. Interestingly, almost half of the patients were diagnosed based on the protocol biopsies in well-functioning grafts, this suggests that the clinical presentation of TG can lag behind the histological changes, and using only indication biopsies can underestimate its true prevalence. In this study, the overall cumulative incidence of TG increased from 4 % at 1 year to 20 % at 5 years, whereas the respective incidences in surveillance biopsies were 2.8 and 11.5 % [191].

TG is strongly and independently associated with poor graft survival [191]. In the Mayo Clinic experience, graft survival was 62 % with TG compared with 95 % without TG

($P<0.0001$). Mean graft survival after the diagnosis of TG was 43±7 months. The variables associated with reduced graft survival in TG cases included graft function and proteinuria at diagnosis, the severity of PTC-itis, total interstitial inflammation, the severity of interstitial fibrosis, and cg score [190, 192–194]. PTC basement membrane multilayering (PTCBMML) and arterial hyalinosis were also significant predictors of graft survival in TG [192]. The presence of any grade TG and chronic allograft vasculopathy is poor prognostic factor [195].

The association of PTC C4d staining and graft outcome in TG is controversial. Some studies have shown no association [190, 194], whereas others have documented a negative impact of late C4d positivity on graft survival [193]. C4d positivity was associated with a more rapid rate in functional decline [192]. In another study, C4d alone did not independently predict graft loss but the combined presence of C4d positivity, TG, and serum creatinine of >2.3 mg/dL at biopsy was a poor prognostic factor [196]. In the report from the Edmonton group, the cumulative death-censored graft survival was 40 % in TG with anti-HLA antibodies/C4d compared with 35 % in TG without anti-HLA antibodies/C4d at 15-year posttransplant, with no significant statistical difference [189]. We examined the outcome in 145 patients with TG at our center (unpublished data). Graft survival at 66 months of diagnosis was only 10 %. Diffuse PTC C4d by IHC was predictive of worse graft survival.

Pathogenesis

The role of donor-directed alloantibody in pathogenesis of graft in TG injury has been clearly demonstrated. Different animal models have been used to demonstrate its pathogenicity and the time course of events in TG. In a T-cell-deficient rat model, Koch et al. showed that injecting a monoclonal antibody against a mismatched nonclassical major histocompatibility complex (MHC), Ib antigen caused massive proteinuria and severe glomerulopathy [197]. de Heer et al. found that Lewis rats carrying a Fisher 344 renal allograft with TG produce antibodies against one or more novel antigen(s) of donor glomerular and tubular basement membranes [198]. In a cynomolgus monkey model, Colvin et al. described the natural history of chronic AMR [22, 199]. The authors proposed that the process starts with development of DSA followed by appearance of C4d in the biopsy leading to histological changes of TG and later graft dysfunction.

In the cohort reported from Mayo Clinic, 76 % of TG cases had detectable anti-HLA antibodies. Of those, 71 % were against class I, 90 % were against class II, and 61 % were against both [191]. TG cases with detectable HLA antibodies were more likely to be women, younger, and recipients of second transplants [193]. The incidence of TG was significantly higher among patients with anti-class II antibodies than among patients with anti-class I antibodies [193]. Examining biopsies for cause, we observed that DSA alone or in combination with C4d positivity was predictive of TG (OR: 5.8, $P=0.02$, 95% CI: 1.3–25.4 for C4d–/DSA+ and OR: 17.9, $P<0.001$, 95% CI: 4.9–65.2 for C4d+/DSA+ group). Furthermore, TG was associated only with class II DSA, either alone or with class I (OR: 8.3, $P<0.001$, 95% CI: 2.8–24.8 for class II only and OR: 14.1, $P<0.001$, 95% CI: 4.9–40.0 for class I/II DSA). In patients with DSA and positive crossmatch prior to transplant, the 1-year incidence of TG is increased to 22 % [200]. Sis et al. reported that 70 % of the patients with TG had detectable anti-HLA antibodies, 61 % class I, 91 % class II, and 52 % both [189]. DSA was present in 85 % of those with positive antibodies, 50 % class I, 86 % II, and 36 % both. The risk of TG is even significantly higher in patients with non-DSA-HLA class II antibody compared to those with no antibodies [191]. This could be due to limitations in detecting HLA-DSA with current techniques, association with non-HLA-DSA that are not assayed, cross-reactivity due to shared epitopes, or low levels of DSA, all absorbed in the graft [22, 90, 103, 200–202]. The risk of TG is not different between patients with antibodies against DR or DQ antigens [22, 193, 201].

The following steps in pathogenesis of TG are plausible, supported by available data. The initial phase is binding of the DSA, particularly class II antibodies, to allograft endothelial cells (EC). Through complement-dependent and complement-independent mechanisms, as described previously, the antibodies cause phenotypic changes in EC, presenting as cell swelling in the initial phases. Inflow of inflammatory cells especially monocytes ensue [99, 203]. With ongoing EC injury, diminished patency of the capillary loops and progression to reduplication of the glomerular basement membrane occurs. It is unclear how DSA-induced EC injury results in this reduplication and what role the recruited inflammatory cells play. Over time, EC injury may evolve into pancapillary multilayering of basement membranes and obliteration of PTC, leading to IFTA, likely secondary to ischemia [204]. Although it seems that TG develops as a result of ongoing endothelial cell activation and injury by the humoral response, it has been hypothesized that in some cases, it may occur following a period of accommodation, broken by an acute injury [103].

PTC deposition of complement-split product C4d is present in a subgroup of TG cases, supporting the participation of the classical pathway of complement activation in the pathogenesis of chronic AMR [205]. However, some TG cases have negative C4d staining, suggesting involvement of complement-independent mechanisms. Fahim et al. have reported a predominance of monocytes compared with T cells in PTC and glomeruli in C4d-positive biopsies [96]. Our group has shown the strong association of glomerular CD 68-positive cells (macrophages) with TG and as the only independent predictor of graft survival [99]. One can hypothesize that after initial stages of injury that are DSA-dependent, the subsequent stages of establishment and progression of TG and nephron mass loss are mediated by the recruited inflammatory cells, particularly monocyte/macrophages. The presence of cellular infiltrates in glomeruli (glomerulitis) is currently not considered as one of the diagnostic criteria for TG by the Banff classification, but this requires revisiting.

Proinflammatory cytokines including interleukin (IL)-1β, IL-6, and TNF-α, secreted by activated monocytes in peripheral blood, have been associated with TG, with ex vivo data supporting the role of regulatory T cells in downregulating these cytokines [91].

Elster et al. using low-density arrays identified increased expression of 57 individual genes in TG compared with stable function biopsies [206]. The Bayesian analysis identified association between ICAM-1, IL-10, CCL3, CD86, VCAM-1, MMP-9, MMP-7, and LAMC2 and allograft pathology.

Emerging tools such as C1q-SAB Luminex assay or C4d-Flow PRA beads with Luminex that can detect complement-fixing IgG antibodies, protein microarray technology, and biomarkers such as CRP expression in renal allograft biopsies may provide more insights into the pathogenesis of TG [207–210].

Clinical Manifestation

The clinical manifestation of TG is generally insidious and nonspecific, consisting of proteinuria, unexplained loss of allograft function, and hypertension. Proteinuria is typically minor, but it can be in the nephrotic range. TG biopsies with proteinuria had more severe glomerular double contours (cg score) and increase in mesangial matrix (mm score) in comparison to TG without proteinuria [189].

At the time of 1-year protocol biopsies, patients with TG, when compared to non-TG cases, had no difference in serum creatinine concentration or estimated GFR but had a marginal increase in proteinuria [191]. Although poorer graft function and increased proteinuria were associated with the severity of TG classified by cg scores, the association was not statistically significant [191].

A great majority of cases with TG are diagnosed after the first year posttransplant. However, TG can be seen as early as 2–3 months after transplantation.

Histology

According to Banff criteria, the morphologic characteristics of chronic AMR include glomerular double contours in more than 10 % of glomerular capillary loops and/or peritubular basement membrane multilayering and/or interstitial fibrosis/tubular atrophy and/or fibrous intimal thickening in arteries [22] (Table 26.2, Fig. 26.3).

Table 26.2 Banff criteria for diagnosis of chronic AMR

Morphological features
• Transplant glomerulopathy (double contours) *and/or*
• PTC BM multilayering *and/or*
• IF/TA *and/or*
• Arterial fibrous intimal thickening
Diffuse PTC C4d deposition
DSA

In the early phase, the pathological pattern of TG is focal, affecting only a few glomeruli [6]. But the number of involved glomeruli progressively increases, with increasing percentage of capillary loops affected in subsequent biopsies [191]. TG may develop independently from interstitial fibrosis, tubular atrophy, and/or transplant arteriopathy [189, 191].

The severity of TG is graded by the extent of double contours affecting peripheral capillary loops in the most affected, nonsclerotic glomeruli, "cg" score [107]. Most TG lesions at 1 year are mild [191]. In another series, 40 % of cases were severe, with double contours in more than 50 % of the loops [190]. The "cg" score is associated with the incidence and severity of glomerulitis ("g" score) but not with interstitial inflammation ("i" score), tubulitis ("t" score), interstitial fibrosis ("ci"), and tubular atrophy ("ct") [191]. When compared to non-TG biopsies, interstitial inflammation, tubulitis, interstitial fibrosis, and arteriolar hyalinosis, but not tubular atrophy, were significantly increased in TG in protocol biopsies at 1-year posttransplant [191].

Glomerular inflammation may play a role in the development of TG [99, 195, 211]. Our group has shown the predominance of CD68+ cells in the glomeruli found in TG and glomerulitis [99]. Infiltrating CD68+ cells may help to differentiate chronic active humoral rejection from other types of chronic injury [195]. In our study, the presence of CD68+ cells more than 12 in the most inflamed glomerulus was strongly associated with TG, DSA, Banff g score, and C4d staining [99]. High levels of macrophages were the only independent predictor of graft failure among different histological changes. The intensity of mononuclear cell infiltration within fibrotic areas was reported to be strongly correlated with the extent of future tubulointerstitial injury, and more intense mononuclear cell inflammation within areas of tubulointerstitial damage predicted subsequent progression of tubular damage [211]. Batal et al. evaluated three grading systems to define glomerulitis, including percentage of glomerular involvement, peak inflammation in the most severely affected glomerulus, and the presence of endocapillary occlusion by inflammatory cells. Glomerulitis defined by the presence of ≥5 leukocytes/glomerulus was the best predictor of features

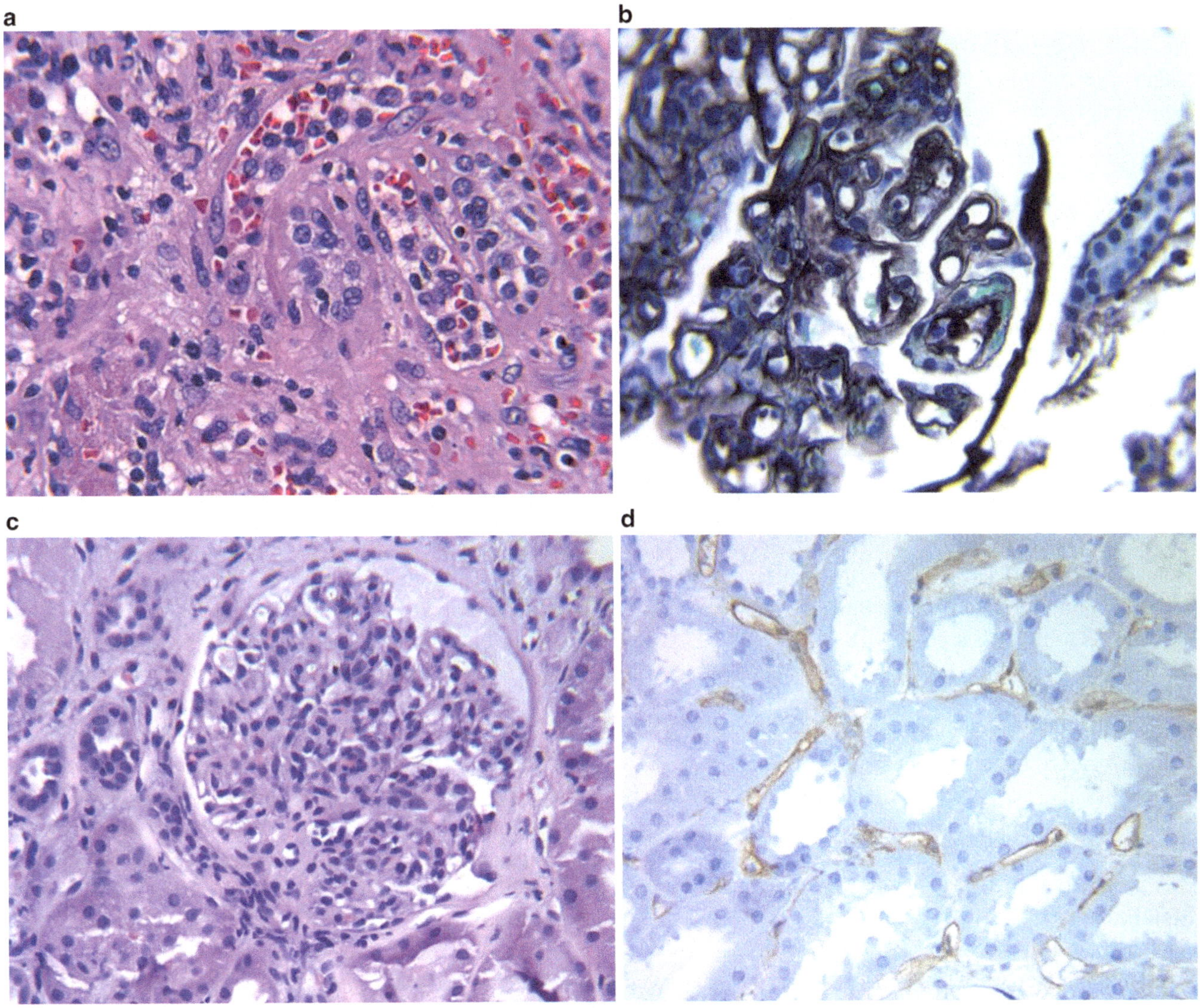

Fig. 26.3 Features of chronic AMR, (**a**) peritubular capillaritis, (**b**) double contouring of glomerular basement membrane, (**c**) peritubular capillary C4d deposition by immunohistochemistry, and (**d**) glomerulitis. Courtesy of Dr. C. Drachenberg

of AMR and graft outcome [212]. Nair et al. proposed that endotheliosis (occlusive EC swelling in glomerular capillary loops) is a more accurate and specific precursor of TG than mere glomerulitis and when detected as early as few weeks posttransplant could predict the development of features of TG within the subsequent few months [213].

Biopsies with TG can also show secondary focal and segmental glomerulosclerosis (FSGS). This has been attributed to decreased expression of hepatocyte growth factor (HGF), which probably through Met signaling has antiapoptotic effects on podocytes [214].

C4d deposition in PTC has been reported in 36–46 % of TG cases, along with deposition in glomerular capillaries in 42 % [71, 111, 190]. In our previous study, DSA alone or in combination with C4d positivity by IHC was predictive of TG [71]. The odds of TG was 4.6-fold higher for focal C4d staining compared to negative/minimal staining ($P=0.003$, 95% CI: 1.7–12.6) and 6.8-fold for diffuse C4d ($P<0.001$, 95% CI: 2.5–18.3) [71]. C4d positivity in PTC and/or glomeruli has been associated with young age at biopsy and minimization of immunosuppression within 3–6 months preceding the biopsy, due to either drug withdrawal or suboptimal drug dose/blood levels [190].

About one third of TG biopsies may have negative C4d [190]. C4d negativity could be explained by complement-independent antibody-mediated mechanisms, undetectable C4d due to technical shortcomings, or dynamic nature of C4d deposition before and after the establishment of TG and in response to treatment in acute AMR [22, 122, 190, 215].

In the cohort reported by Sis et al., about 90 % of biopsies with TG also showed PTCBMML [189]. The degree of PTCBMML did not correlate with cg score or other Banff scores, C4d deposition, presence of anti-HLA antibody, time posttransplant, serum creatinine at biopsy, proteinuria, HLA mismatch, recipient age, donor age, and prior acute rejection [189]. When compared to non-TG biopsies, the extent of

PTCBMML and vascular fibrous intimal thickening (cv score) in TG biopsies was not different, indicating that both lesions are common in late allograft biopsies for cause. Roufosse et al. have suggested that with three or more layers in early biopsies, the risk of future TG increases by 40 %, and with five or more layers this risk increases by 60 %; therefore, PTCBMML in early biopsy is a useful marker of early chronic AMR [216]. Liapis et al. reported that although severe PTCBMML is a helpful finding for diagnosis of rejection-induced graft injury, it cannot precisely predict the Banff rejection category. In contrast, its absence is useful in excluding chronic AMR [217].

In the report by the Alberta group, all cases with TG had glomerular capillary loop double contours, 70 % had HLA antibodies, 90 % were with PTCBMML, and 40 % with C4d [189]. The most common phenotypes were positivity of all four components and the first three. Most had either antibodies or C4d. Only 26 % had no detectable antibodies and C4d.

In a study of serial biopsies with a mean follow-up of 15 ± 14.7 months (range: 1–59) following diagnosis, 35 % of cg1 lesions at diagnosis progressed to cg2 and cg3, while 56 % with cg2 progressed to cg3 [191]. In 24 % of the patients, follow-up biopsies failed to show TG. Interstitial fibrosis, tubular atrophy, and chronic vasculopathy significantly worsened in subsequent biopsies. The mechanism of TG progression has not been well understood, but it could be due to persistent inflammation and ischemia [194].

Risk Factors of TG

A number of studies have identified risk factors for development of TG. In a multivariate analysis, acute rejection, hepatitis C, transplant number, and anti-HLA antibodies present at transplant were independently associated with the development of TG [191]. In this study, 33 % of patients with acute rejection developed TG. Among cases of TG with anti-HLA antibodies and/or C4d, 43 % had no prior rejection [189]. The TG cases with anti-HLA antibodies or C4d had more AMR episodes in the past, but this was not statistically significant. The median interval between the diagnosis of TG and prior AMR was 12.1 ± 10 months [189]. Thirty-one percent of patients with hepatitis C antibody prior to transplant may develop TG, compared to 9 % hepatitis C antibody-negative patients [191].

Differential Diagnosis

The clinical and pathological presentation of chronic AMR overlaps with that of a number of other causes of chronic allograft dysfunction [218]. Recurrent or de novo immune complex glomerulopathy and chronic thrombotic microangiopathy (TMA) can cause reduplication of GBM, with findings in light microscopy similar to TG. Cell-mediated TG has the same features as antibody-mediated TG with absence of DSA and C4d. Obstructive nephropathy, radiation nephritis, TMA, and glomerulonephritides can cause PTCBMML. IFTA as the only morphologic manifestation of chronic AMR is nonspecific and can be seen with all causes of chronic allograft dysfunction. Clinical history, serologies, electron microscopy, detection of DSA, and PTC C4d staining will usually discriminate between these entities and chronic AMR.

Management

Current therapies for chronic AMR are likely of limited value. There is no clear evidence for a safe and effective therapeutic approach. Various immunosuppressive regimens have been suggested, but none are known to be very effective. Progressive graft failure and return to dialysis is the common outcome. Theruvath et al. switched four patients with DSA and TG with widespread PTC C4d deposits and declining graft function from a predominantly cyclosporine-based regimen to tacrolimus and MMF [219]. In two patients, DSA became undetectable after 9 months, and a repeat biopsy performed after 12 months revealed a decrease in C4d deposition in PTC. However, another study of 11 patients argued against the efficacy of tacrolimus/MMF rescue therapy [220]. Despite the conflicting evidence and lack of a robust study, conversion to tacrolimus and mycophenolate is considered by many clinicians to be an appropriate step.

Strategies to treat acute AMR are overall more effective; therefore, in a subset of patients, acute AMR is considered a treatable lesion. As discussed in previous section, currently there is no effective therapy to reduce anti-HLA Ab levels to reduce the risk of TG and improve graft survival. In the case of TG, class II DSA is more involved, and complete disappearance of HLA antibodies using plasma exchange is generally unsuccessful (personal experience). Rituximab, an anti-CD20 monoclonal antibody, can cause B-cell depletion, hence decrease the activation and transformation of new donor-reactive B lymphocytes, but cannot impact long-lived plasma cells that produce the antibodies. Bortezomib can cause plasma cell death and decrease the antibody level, but it has not been effective in eliminating the DSA and is associated with significant side effects.

Billing et al. initiated a pilot study on treatment of chronic AMR in six pediatric renal transplant patients with 4 weekly doses of IVIG (1 g/kg/dose) followed by a single dose of anti-CD20 (375 mg/m^2) 1 week after the last IVIG infusion. Four patients had improved or stable GFR during follow-up [221]. More recently, this group published their extended experience in 20 pediatric patients with this regimen [222].

Loss of eGFR decreased from 7.6 mL/min/1.73 m^2 during 6 months prior to therapy to 2.1 mL/min/1.73 m^2 during 6 months following the treatment ($P=0.0013$). All nine patients without TG compared with only 5 of 11 (45 %) with TG responded to treatment ($P=0.014$). The degree of TG, cg score, was associated with response to therapy (OR: −0.49, $P=0.042$). However, larger studies are required to evaluate effectiveness of this regimen.

Smith et al. reported their experience with addition of 3–5 doses of rituximab, alone or in combination with other therapies, including solumedrol, thymoglobulin, plasmapheresis, or IVIG, to maintenance immunosuppression in 14 patients with chronic AMR, in comparison to 17 controls [223]. The median allograft survival time was 685 days in rituximab group and 439 days in control group. The survival time was significantly better in responders compared with nonresponders and controls. No pathological parameters predicted response to therapy.

Vogelbacher et al. used an experimental rat model and showed that combination of bortezomib and sirolimus can inhibit chronic AMR [224].

Supportive care for proteinuric chronic kidney disease, including tight blood pressure control and blockage of the renin–angiotensin system, is strongly recommended. Although treatment with an angiotensin-converting enzyme inhibitor or angiotensin receptor blocker can decrease proteinuria, currently there is no evidence that this strategy improves patient or graft survival in those with chronic AMR [225].

Preventing TG in patients at risk and its early detection are very important. Scheduled screening for DSA and protocol biopsies, particularly in patients at higher risk, could identify early stages of chronic AMR. Optimization of maintenance immunosuppressive regimen, including conversion from cyclosporine to tacrolimus, in conjunction with maximizing MMF and addition of steroid, in those on dual therapy, would be advisable. Based on very limited data, trial of rituximab and high-dose IVIG could be considered, especially at early stages of the process. Better understanding of the pathogenesis of TG will help discover safer and more effective therapies. Development or trial of newer agent targeting specific B-cell or plasma cell pathways could increase the efficacy and limit the adverse effects of therapy [154, 226].

References

1. Williams GM, Hume DM, Hudson Jr RP, et al. "Hyperacute" renal-homograft rejection in man. N Engl J Med. 1968;279: 611–8.
2. Patel R, Terasaki PI. Significance of the positive crossmatch test in kidney transplantation. N Engl J Med. 1969;280:735–9.
3. Tait BD, Susal C, Gebel HM, et al. Consensus guidelines on the testing and clinical management issues associated with HLA and non-HLA antibodies in transplantation. Transplantation. 2013;95: 19–47.
4. Fuggle SV, Martin S. Tools for human leukocyte antigen antibody detection and their application to transplanting sensitized patients. Transplantation. 2008;86:384–90.
5. Anthony Nolan Research Institute. HLA nomenclature. London, UK; 2013. www.hla.alleles.org.
6. Racusen LC, Solez K, Colvin RB, et al. The Banff 97 working classification of renal allograft pathology. Kidney Int. 1999;55: 713–23.
7. Cho SI, Bradley JW, Monaco AP, et al. Comparison of kidney transplant survival between patients treated with cyclosporine and those treated with azathioprine and antithymocyte globulin. Am J Surg. 1984;147:518–23.
8. Cohen DJ, Loertscher R, Rubin MF, et al. Cyclosporine: a new immunosuppressive agent for organ transplantation. Ann Intern Med. 1984;101:667–82.
9. Gordon RD, Iwatsuki S, Shaw Jr BW, et al. Cyclosporine-steroid combination therapy in 84 cadaveric renal transplants. Am J Kidney Dis. 1985;5:307–12.
10. Margreiter R, Huber C, Spielberger M, et al. Cyclosporine in the treatment of acute cadaveric kidney graft rejection refractory to high-dose methylprednisolone. Transplantation. 1983;36:203–4.
11. Gonwa T, Johnson C, Ahsan N, et al. Randomized trial of tacrolimus + mycophenolate mofetil or azathioprine versus cyclosporine + mycophenolate mofetil after cadaveric kidney transplantation: results at three years. Transplantation. 2003;75:2048–53.
12. Johnson C, Ahsan N, Gonwa T, et al. Randomized trial of tacrolimus (Prograf) in combination with azathioprine or mycophenolate mofetil versus cyclosporine (Neoral) with mycophenolate mofetil after cadaveric kidney transplantation. Transplantation. 2000;69:834–41.
13. Sollinger HW. Mycophenolate mofetil for the prevention of acute rejection in primary cadaveric renal allograft recipients. U.S. Renal Transplant Mycophenolate Mofetil Study Group. Transplantation. 1995;60:225–32.
14. Starzl TE, Fung J, Jordan M, et al. Kidney transplantation under FK 506. JAMA. 1990;264:63–7.
15. Feucht HE, Felber E, Gokel MJ, et al. Vascular deposition of complement-split products in kidney allografts with cell-mediated rejection. Clin Exp Immunol. 1991;86:464–70.
16. Collins AB, Schneeberger EE, Pascual MA, et al. Complement activation in acute humoral renal allograft rejection: diagnostic significance of C4d deposits in peritubular capillaries. J Am Soc Nephrol. 1999;10:2208–14.
17. Klein J, Sato A. The HLA system. First of two parts. N Engl J Med. 2000;343:702–9.
18. Dankers MK, Witvliet MD, Roelen DL, et al. The number of amino acid triplet differences between patient and donor is predictive for the antibody reactivity against mismatched human leukocyte antigens. Transplantation. 2004;77:1236–9.
19. Duquesnoy RJ, Marrari M. HLAMatchmaker: a molecularly based algorithm for histocompatibility determination. II. Verification of the algorithm and determination of the relative immunogenicity of amino acid triplet-defined epitopes. Hum Immunol. 2002;63:353–63.
20. Duquesnoy RJ, Marrari M, Mulder A, et al. Structural aspects of human leukocyte antigen class I epitopes detected by human monoclonal antibodies. Hum Immunol. 2012;73:267–77.
21. Abbas AK, Lichtman AH. Cellular and molecular immunology. 5th ed. Philadelphia: Elsevier Saunders; 2005.
22. Colvin RB. Antibody-mediated renal allograft rejection: diagnosis and pathogenesis. J Am Soc Nephrol. 2007;18:1046–56.
23. Feucht HE. Complement C4d in graft capillaries—the missing link in the recognition of humoral alloreactivity. Am J Transplant. 2003;3:646–52.
24. Mengel M, Husain S, Hidalgo L, Sis B. Phenotypes of antibody-mediated rejection in organ transplants. Transpl Int. 2012;25(6): 611–22.

25. Sis B, Halloran PF. Endothelial transcripts uncover a previously unknown phenotype: C4d-negative antibody-mediated rejection. Curr Opin Organ Transplant. 2010;15(1):42–8.
26. Hidalgo LG, Sis B, Sellares J, et al. NK cell transcripts and NK cells in kidney biopsies from patients with donor-specific antibodies: evidence for NK cell involvement in antibody-mediated rejection. Am J Transplant. 2010;10:1812–22.
27. Hirohashi T, Uehara S, Chase CM, et al. Complement independent antibody-mediated endarteritis and transplant arteriopathy in mice. Am J Transplant. 2010;10:510–7.
28. Hirohashi T, Chase CM, Della PP, et al. A novel pathway of chronic allograft rejection mediated by NK cells and alloantibody. Am J Transplant. 2012;12:313–21.
29. Heeger PS. A complementary approach to treating antibody-mediated transplant rejection. Kidney Int. 2010;78:125–7.
30. Murata K, Fox-Talbot K, Qian Z, et al. Synergistic deposition of C4d by complement-activating and non-activating antibodies in cardiac transplants. Am J Transplant. 2007;7:2605–14.
31. Honger G, Hopfer H, Arnold ML, et al. Pretransplant IgG subclasses of donor-specific human leukocyte antigen antibodies and development of antibody-mediated rejection. Transplantation. 2011;92:41–7.
32. Stegall MD, Chedid MF, Cornell LD. The role of complement in antibody-mediated rejection in kidney transplantation. Nat Rev Nephrol. 2012;8:670–8.
33. Gloor J, Cosio F, Lager DJ, Stegall MD. The spectrum of antibody-mediated renal allograft injury: implications for treatment. Am J Transplant. 2008;8(7):1367–73.
34. Grafft CA, Cornell LD, Gloor JM, Cosio FG, Gandhi MJ, Dean PG, Stegall MD, Amer H. Antibody-mediated rejection following transplantation from an HLA-identical sibling. Nephrol Dial Transplant. 2010;25(1):307–10.
35. Halloran PF, Schlaut J, Solez K, et al. The significance of the anti-class I response. II. Clinical and pathologic features of renal transplants with anti-class I-like antibody. Transplantation. 1992;53:550–5.
36. Trpkov K, Campbell P, Pazderka F, Cockfield S, Solez K, Halloran PF. Pathologic features of acute renal allograft rejection associated with donor-specific antibody, analysis using the Banff grading schema. Transplantation. 1996;61(11):1586–92.
37. Racusen LC, Haas M. Antibody-mediated rejection in renal allografts: lessons from pathology. Clin J Am Soc Nephrol. 2006;1:415–20.
38. Stegall MD, Gloor JM. Deciphering antibody-mediated rejection: new insights into mechanisms and treatment. Curr Opin Organ Transplant. 2010;15(1):8–10.
39. Stegall MD, Diwan T, Raghavaiah S, Cornell LD, Burns J, Dean PG, Cosio FG, Gandhi MJ, Kremers W, Gloor JM. Terminal complement inhibition decreases antibody-mediated rejection in sensitized renal transplant recipients. Am J Transplant. 2011;11(11):2405–13.
40. Halloran PF, Wadgymar A, Ritchie S, Falk J, Solez K, Srinivasa NS. The significance of the anti-class I antibody response. I. Clinical and pathologic features of anti-class I-mediated rejection. Transplantation. 1990;49(1):85–91.
41. Jindra PT, Jin YP, Rozengurt E, Reed EF. HLA class I antibody-mediated endothelial cell proliferation via the mTOR pathway. J Immunol. 2008;180(4):2357–66.
42. Zhang X, Reed EF. Effect of antibodies on endothelium. Am J Transplant. 2009;9:2459–65.
43. Saadi S, Wrenshall LE, Platt JL. Regional manifestations and control of the immune system. FASEB J. 2002;16:849–56.
44. Kuo HH, Morrell CN, Baldwin III WM. Alloantibody induced platelet responses in transplants: potent mediators in small packages. Hum Immunol. 2012;73:1233–8.
45. Morrell CN, Murata K, Swaim AM, et al. In vivo platelet-endothelial cell interactions in response to major histocompatibility complex alloantibody. Circ Res. 2008;102:777–85.
46. Tedesco F, Pausa M, Nardon E, et al. The cytolytically inactive terminal complement complex activates endothelial cells to express adhesion molecules and tissue factor procoagulant activity. J Exp Med. 1997;185:1619–27.
47. Yamakuchi M, Kirkiles-Smith NC, Ferlito M, et al. Antibody to human leukocyte antigen triggers endothelial exocytosis. Proc Natl Acad Sci U S A. 2007;104:1301–6.
48. Koch CA, Khalpey ZI, Platt JL. Accommodation: preventing injury in transplantation and disease. J Immunol. 2004;172:5143–8.
49. Lynch RJ, Platt JL. Escaping from rejection. Transplantation. 2009;88:1233–6.
50. Lynch RJ, Platt JL. Accommodation in renal transplantation: unanswered questions. Curr Opin Organ Transplant. 2010;15:481–5.
51. Park WD, Grande JP, Ninova D, et al. Accommodation in ABO-incompatible kidney allografts, a novel mechanism of self-protection against antibody-mediated injury. Am J Transplant. 2003;3:952–60.
52. Platt JL. Accommodation: how you see it, how you don't. Am J Transplant. 2011;11:2007–8.
53. Blume OR, Yost SE, Kaplan B. Antibody-mediated rejection: pathogenesis, prevention, treatment, and outcomes. J Transplant. 2012;2012:201754.
54. Colvin RB, Smith RN. Antibody-mediated organ-allograft rejection. Nat Rev Immunol. 2005;5(10):807–17.
55. Delikouras A, Hayes M, Malde P, et al. Nitric oxide-mediated expression of Bcl-2 and Bcl-xl and protection from tumor necrosis factor-alpha-mediated apoptosis in porcine endothelial cells after exposure to low concentrations of xenoreactive natural antibody. Transplantation. 2001;71:599–605.
56. Einecke G, Sis B, Reeve J, Mengel M, Campbell PM, Hidalgo LG, Kaplan B, Halloran PF. Antibody-mediated microcirculation injury is the major cause of late kidney transplant failure. Am J Transplant. 2009;9(11):2520–31.
57. Saadi S, Platt JL. Humoral rejection and endothelial cell activation, 2001. Xenotransplantation. 2002;9:239–41.
58. Tegla CA, Cudrici C, Patel S, et al. Membrane attack by complement: the assembly and biology of terminal complement complexes. Immunol Res. 2011;51:45–60.
59. Sis B, Jhangri GS, Bunnag S, et al. Endothelial gene expression in kidney transplants with alloantibody indicates antibody-mediated damage despite lack of C4d staining. Am J Transplant. 2009;9:2312–23.
60. US Department of Health and Human Services. Scientific registry of transplant recipients; 2013. http://www.srtr.org/.
61. Lefaucheur C, Loupy A, Hill GS, et al. Preexisting donor-specific HLA antibodies predict outcome in kidney transplantation. J Am Soc Nephrol. 2010;21:1398–406.
62. Amico P, Honger G, Mayr M, et al. Clinical relevance of pretransplant donor-specific HLA antibodies detected by single-antigen flow-beads. Transplantation. 2009;87:1681–8.
63. Couzi L, Araujo C, Guidicelli G, et al. Interpretation of positive flow cytometric crossmatch in the era of the single-antigen bead assay. Transplantation. 2011;91:527–35.
64. Loupy A, Suberbielle-Boissel C, Hill GS, et al. Outcome of subclinical antibody-mediated rejection in kidney transplant recipients with preformed donor-specific antibodies. Am J Transplant. 2009;9:2561–70.
65. Mohan S, Palanisamy A, Tsapepas D, et al. Donor-specific antibodies adversely affect kidney allograft outcomes. J Am Soc Nephrol. 2012;23:2061–71.
66. Hourmant M, Cesbron-Gautier A, Terasaki PI, et al. Frequency and clinical implications of development of donor-specific and non-donor-specific HLA antibodies after kidney transplantation. J Am Soc Nephrol. 2005;16:2804–12.
67. Cardarelli F, Pascual M, Tolkoff-Rubin N, et al. Prevalence and significance of anti-HLA and donor-specific antibodies long-term after renal transplantation. Transpl Int. 2005;18:532–40.

68. Fotheringham J, Angel C, Goodwin J, et al. Natural history of proteinuria in renal transplant recipients developing de novo human leukocyte antigen antibodies. Transplantation. 2011;91: 991–6.
69. Cooper JE, Gralla J, Cagle L, et al. Inferior kidney allograft outcomes in patients with de novo donor-specific antibodies are due to acute rejection episodes. Transplantation. 2011;91: 1103–9.
70. Ntokou IS, Iniotaki AG, Kontou EN, et al. Long-term follow up for anti-HLA donor specific antibodies postrenal transplantation: high immunogenicity of HLA class II graft molecules. Transpl Int. 2011;24:1084–93.
71. Haririan A, Kiangkitiwan B, Kukuruga D, et al. The impact of c4d pattern and donor-specific antibody on graft survival in recipients requiring indication renal allograft biopsy. Am J Transplant. 2009;9:2758–67.
72. Lee PC, Zhu L, Terasaki PI, et al. HLA-specific antibodies developed in the first year posttransplant are predictive of chronic rejection and renal graft loss. Transplantation. 2009;88:568–74.
73. Bartel G, Regele H, Wahrmann M, et al. Posttransplant HLA alloreactivity in stable kidney transplant recipients-incidences and impact on long-term allograft outcomes. Am J Transplant. 2008;8:2652–60.
74. Zhang Q, Reed EF. Non-MHC antigenic targets of the humoral immune response in transplantation. Curr Opin Immunol. 2010;22:682–8.
75. Martin L, Guignier F, Mousson C, et al. Detection of donor-specific anti-HLA antibodies with flow cytometry in eluates and sera from renal transplant recipients with chronic allograft nephropathy. Transplantation. 2003;76:395–400.
76. Marrari M, Duquesnoy RJ. Detection of donor-specific HLA antibodies before and after removal of a rejected kidney transplant. Transpl Immunol. 2010;22:105–9.
77. Qiu J, Cai J, Terasaki PI, et al. Detection of antibodies to HLA-DP in renal transplant recipients using single antigen beads. Transplantation. 2005;80:1511–3.
78. Jolly EC, Key T, Rasheed H, et al. Preformed donor HLA-DP-specific antibodies mediate acute and chronic antibody-mediated rejection following renal transplantation. Am J Transplant. 2012;12:2845–8.
79. Zhu L, Lee PC, Everly MJ, et al. Detailed examination of HLA antibody development on renal allograft failure and function. Clin Transpl. 2008:171–87.
80. Dragun D, Muller DN, Brasen JH, et al. Angiotensin II type 1-receptor activating antibodies in renal-allograft rejection. N Engl J Med. 2005;352:558–69.
81. Morales-Buenrostro LE, Alberu J. Anti-major histocompatibility complex class I-related chain A antibodies in organ transplantation. Transplant Rev (Orlando). 2008;22:27–38.
82. Reinsmoen NL, Lai CH, Heidecke H, et al. Anti-angiotensin type 1 receptor antibodies associated with antibody mediated rejection in donor HLA antibody negative patients. Transplantation. 2010;90:1473–7.
83. Mizutani K, Terasaki P, Rosen A, et al. Serial ten-year follow-up of HLA and MICA antibody production prior to kidney graft failure. Am J Transplant. 2005;5:2265–72.
84. Panigrahi A, Gupta N, Siddiqui JA, et al. Post transplant development of MICA and anti-HLA antibodies is associated with acute rejection episodes and renal allograft loss. Hum Immunol. 2007;68:362–7.
85. Amico P, Honger G, Bielmann D, et al. Incidence and prediction of early antibody-mediated rejection due to non-human leukocyte antigen-antibodies. Transplantation. 2008;85:1557–63.
86. Azimzadeh AM, Pfeiffer S, Wu GS, Schröder C, Zhou H, Zorn III GL, Kehry M, Miller GG, Rose ML, Pierson III RN. Humoral immunity to vimentin is associated with cardiac allograft injury in nonhuman primates. Am J Transplant. 2005;5(10):2349–59.
87. Mahesh B, Leong HS, McCormack A, et al. Autoantibodies to vimentin cause accelerated rejection of cardiac allografts. Am J Pathol. 2007;170:1415–27.
88. Nath DS, Tiriveedhi V, Basha HI, et al. A role for antibodies to human leukocyte antigens, collagen-V, and K-alpha1-Tubulin in antibody-mediated rejection and cardiac allograft vasculopathy. Transplantation. 2011;91:1036–43.
89. Qin Z, Lavingia B, Zou Y, et al. Antibodies against nucleolin in recipients of organ transplants. Transplantation. 2011;92:829–35.
90. Joosten SA, Sijpkens YW, van Ham V, et al. Antibody response against the glomerular basement membrane protein agrin in patients with transplant glomerulopathy. Am J Transplant. 2005;5:383–93.
91. De Serres SA, Vadivel N, Mfarrej BG, et al. Monocyte-secreted inflammatory cytokines are associated with transplant glomerulopathy in renal allograft recipients. Transplantation. 2011;91:552–9.
92. Colvin RB, Nickeleit V. Renal transplant pathology. In: Charles JJ, Olsen JL, Schwarz MM, et al., editors. Heptinstall's pathology of the kidney. Philadelphia: Lippincott Williams & Wilkins; 2007. p. 1347–490.
93. Hamdy AF, Bakr MA, Ghoneim MA. Proteinuria among primarily sirolimus treated live-donor renal transplant recipients' long-term experience. Exp Clin Transplant. 2010;8:283–91.
94. Hood B, Olander R, Nagy Z, et al. Glomerulopathy in the transplanted kidney. Scand J Urol Nephrol. 1970;4:135–42.
95. Cosio FG, Lager DJ, Lorenz EC, Amer H, Gloor JM, Stegall MD. Significance and implications of capillaritis during acute rejection of kidney allografts. Transplantation. 2010;89(9):1088–94.
96. Fahim T, Böhmig GA, Exner M, Huttary N, Kerschner H, Kandutsch S, Kerjaschki D, Bramböck A, Nagy-Bojarszky K, Regele H. The cellular lesion of humoral rejection: predominant recruitment of monocytes to peritubular and glomerular capillaries. Am J Transplant. 2007;7(2):385–93.
97. Gibson IW, Gwinner W, Bröcker V, Sis B, Riopel J, Roberts IS, Scheffner I, Jhangri GS, Mengel M. Peritubular capillaritis in renal allografts: prevalence, scoring system, reproducibility and clinicopathological correlates. Am J Transplant. 2008;8(4):819–25.
98. Haas M. Pathologic features of antibody-mediated rejection in renal allografts: an expanding spectrum. Curr Opin Nephrol Hypertens. 2012;21(3):264–71.
99. Papadimitriou JC, Drachenberg CB, Munivenkatappa R, Ramos E, Nogueira J, Sailey C, Klassen DK, Haririan A. Glomerular inflammation in renal allografts biopsies after the first year: cell types and relationship with antibody-mediated rejection and graft outcome. Transplantation. 2010;90(12):1478–85.
100. Papadimitriou JC, Drachenberg CB, Ramos E, et al. Antibody-mediated allograft rejection: morphologic spectrum and serologic correlations in surveillance and for cause biopsies. Transplantation. 2013;95(1):128–36.
101. Wavamunno MD, O'Connell PJ, Vitalone M, Fung CL, Allen RD, Chapman JR, Nankivell BJ. Transplant glomerulopathy: ultrastructural abnormalities occur early in longitudinal analysis of protocol biopsies. Am J Transplant. 2007;7(12):2757–68.
102. Wood KJ, Goto R. Mechanisms of rejection: current perspectives. Transplantation. 2012;93(1):1–10.
103. Fotheringham J, Angel CA, McKane W. Transplant glomerulopathy: morphology, associations and mechanism. Nephron Clin Pract. 2009;113:c1–7.
104. Kooijmans-Coutinho MF, Hermans J, Schrama E, et al. Interstitial rejection, vascular rejection, and diffuse thrombosis of renal allografts. Predisposing factors, histology, immunohistochemistry, and relation to outcome. Transplantation. 1996;61:1338–44.
105. Lobo PI, Spencer CE, Stevenson WC, et al. Evidence demonstrating poor kidney graft survival when acute rejections are associated with IgG donor-specific lymphocytotoxin. Transplantation. 1995;59:357–60.

106. Elloso MM, Azrolan N, Sehgal SN, et al. Protective effect of the immunosuppressant sirolimus against aortic atherosclerosis in apo E-deficient mice. Am J Transplant. 2003;3:562–9.
107. Racusen LC, Colvin RB, Solez K, et al. Antibody-mediated rejection criteria—an addition to the Banff 97 classification of renal allograft rejection. Am J Transplant. 2003;3:708–14.
108. Sis B, Mengel M, Haas M, et al. Banff '09 meeting report: antibody mediated graft deterioration and implementation of Banff working groups. Am J Transplant. 2010;10:464–71.
109. Solez K, Axelsen RA, Benediktsson H, et al. International standardization of criteria for the histologic diagnosis of renal allograft rejection: the Banff working classification of kidney transplant pathology. Kidney Int. 1993;44:411–22.
110. Solez K, Colvin RB, Racusen LC, et al. Banff '05 meeting report: differential diagnosis of chronic allograft injury and elimination of chronic allograft nephropathy ('CAN'). Am J Transplant. 2007;7:518–26.
111. Solez K, Colvin RB, Racusen LC, et al. Banff 07 classification of renal allograft pathology: updates and future directions. Am J Transplant. 2008;8:753–60.
112. Takemoto SK, Zeevi A, Feng S, et al. National conference to assess antibody-mediated rejection in solid organ transplantation. Am J Transplant. 2004;4:1033–41.
113. Crespo M, Pascual M, Tolkoff-Rubin N, et al. Acute humoral rejection in renal allograft recipients: I. Incidence, serology and clinical characteristics. Transplantation. 2001;71:652–8.
114. Gloor JM, DeGoey SR, Pineda AA, et al. Overcoming a positive crossmatch in living-donor kidney transplantation. Am J Transplant. 2003;3:1017–23.
115. Jordan SC, Vo A, Bunnapradist S, et al. Intravenous immune globulin treatment inhibits crossmatch positivity and allows for successful transplantation of incompatible organs in living-donor and cadaver recipients. Transplantation. 2003;76:631–6.
116. Pascual M, Saidman S, Tolkoff-Rubin N, et al. Plasma exchange and tacrolimus-mycophenolate rescue for acute humoral rejection in kidney transplantation. Transplantation. 1998;66:1460–4.
117. Rocha PN, Butterly DW, Greenberg A, et al. Beneficial effect of plasmapheresis and intravenous immunoglobulin on renal allograft survival of patients with acute humoral rejection. Transplantation. 2003;75:1490–5.
118. Shah A, Nadasdy T, Arend L, et al. Treatment of C4d-positive acute humoral rejection with plasmapheresis and rabbit polyclonal antithymocyte globulin. Transplantation. 2004;77:1399–405.
119. Montgomery RA, Zachary AA, Racusen LC, et al. Plasmapheresis and intravenous immune globulin provides effective rescue therapy for refractory humoral rejection and allows kidneys to be successfully transplanted into cross-match-positive recipients. Transplantation. 2000;70:887–95.
120. Montgomery RA, Zachary AA. Transplanting patients with a positive donor-specific crossmatch: a single center's perspective. Pediatr Transplant. 2004;8:535–42.
121. Seemayer CA, Gaspert A, Nickeleit V, et al. C4d staining of renal allograft biopsies: a comparative analysis of different staining techniques. Nephrol Dial Transplant. 2007;22:568–76.
122. Nadasdy GM, Bott C, Cowden D, et al. Comparative study for the detection of peritubular capillary C4d deposition in human renal allografts using different methodologies. Hum Pathol. 2005;36: 1178–85.
123. Singh N, Pirsch J, Samaniego M. Antibody-mediated rejection: treatment alternatives and outcomes. Transplant Rev (Orlando). 2009;23:34–46.
124. Gelfand EW. Intravenous immune globulin in autoimmune and inflammatory diseases. N Engl J Med. 2012;367:2015–25.
125. Anthony RM, Nimmerjahn F, Ashline DJ, et al. Recapitulation of IVIG anti-inflammatory activity with a recombinant IgG Fc. Science. 2008;320:373–6.
126. Kaneko Y, Nimmerjahn F, Ravetch JV. Anti-inflammatory activity of immunoglobulin G resulting from Fc sialylation. Science. 2006;313:670–3.
127. Kazatchkine MD, Kaveri SV. Immunomodulation of autoimmune and inflammatory diseases with intravenous immune globulin. N Engl J Med. 2001;345:747–55.
128. Muta T, Kurosaki T, Misulovin Z, et al. A 13-amino-acid motif in the cytoplasmic domain of Fc gamma RIIB modulates B-cell receptor signalling. Nature. 1994;368:70–3.
129. Seite JF, Cornec D, Renaudineau Y, et al. IVIg modulates BCR signaling through CD22 and promotes apoptosis in mature human B lymphocytes. Blood. 2010;116:1698–704.
130. Semple JW, Kim M, Lazarus AH, et al. Gamma-globulins prepared from sera of multiparous women bind anti-HLA antibodies and inhibit an established in vivo human alloimmune response. Blood. 2002;100:1055–9.
131. Watanabe J, Scornik JC. IVIG and HLA antibodies. Evidence for inhibition of complement activation but not for anti-idiotypic activity. Am J Transplant. 2005;5:2786–90.
132. Yu Z, Lennon VA. Mechanism of intravenous immune globulin therapy in antibody-mediated autoimmune diseases. N Engl J Med. 1999;340:227–8.
133. Reinsmoen NL, Lai CH, Vo A, et al. Acceptable donor-specific antibody levels allowing for successful deceased and living donor kidney transplantation after desensitization therapy. Transplantation. 2008;86:820–5.
134. Wassmuth R, Hauser IA, Schuler K, et al. Differential inhibitory effects of intravenous immunoglobulin preparations on HLA-alloantibodies in vitro. Transplantation. 2001;71:1436–42.
135. Jordan SC, Quartel AW, Czer LS, et al. Posttransplant therapy using high-dose human immunoglobulin (intravenous gammaglobulin) to control acute humoral rejection in renal and cardiac allograft recipients and potential mechanism of action. Transplantation. 1998;66:800–5.
136. Jordan SC, Vo AA, Nast CC, et al. Use of high-dose human intravenous immunoglobulin therapy in sensitized patients awaiting transplantation: the Cedars-Sinai experience. Clin Transpl. 2003: 193–8.
137. Jordan SC, Tyan D, Stablein D, et al. Evaluation of intravenous immunoglobulin as an agent to lower allosensitization and improve transplantation in highly sensitized adult patients with end-stage renal disease: report of the NIH IG02 trial. J Am Soc Nephrol. 2004;15:3256–62.
138. Tyan DB, Li VA, Czer L, et al. Intravenous immunoglobulin suppression of HLA alloantibody in highly sensitized transplant candidates and transplantation with a histoincompatible organ. Transplantation. 1994;57:553–62.
139. Ahmed T, Senzel L. The role of therapeutic apheresis in the treatment of acute antibody-mediated kidney rejection. J Clin Apher. 2012;27:173–7.
140. Tanabe K. Double-filtration plasmapheresis. Transplantation. 2007;84:S30–2.
141. Tyden G, Kumlien G, Efvergren M. Present techniques for antibody removal. Transplantation. 2007;84:S27–9.
142. Bartel G, Wahrmann M, Regele H, et al. Peritransplant immunoadsorption for positive crossmatch deceased donor kidney transplantation. Am J Transplant. 2010;10:2033–42.
143. Bohmig GA, Regele H, Exner M, et al. C4d-positive acute humoral renal allograft rejection: effective treatment by immunoadsorption. J Am Soc Nephrol. 2001;12:2482–9.
144. Bosch T. Therapeutic apheresis—state of the art in the year 2005. Ther Apher Dial. 2005;9:459–68.
145. Lorenz M, Regele H, Schillinger M, et al. Peritransplant immunoadsorption: a strategy enabling transplantation in highly sensitized crossmatch-positive cadaveric kidney allograft recipients. Transplantation. 2005;79:696–701.

146. Pretagostini R, Berloco P, Poli L, et al. Immunoadsorption with protein A in humoral rejection of kidney transplants. ASAIO J. 1996;42:M645–8.
147. Schwenger V, Morath C. Immunoadsorption in nephrology and kidney transplantation. Nephrol Dial Transplant. 2010;25:2407–13.
148. Liu M, Ji SM, Tang Z, et al. C4d-positive acute humoral renal allograft rejection: rescue therapy by immunoadsorption in combination with tacrolimus and mycophenolate mofetil. Transplant Proc. 2004;36:2101–3.
149. Abraham KA, Brown C, Conlon PJ, et al. Plasmapheresis as rescue therapy in accelerated acute humoral rejection. J Clin Apher. 2003;18:103–10.
150. Zand MS. B-cell activity of polyclonal antithymocyte globulins. Transplantation. 2006;82:1387–95.
151. Timm MM, Kimlinger TK, Haug JL, et al. Thymoglobulin targets multiple plasma cell antigens and has in vitro and in vivo activity in multiple myeloma. Leukemia. 2006;20:1863–9.
152. White NB, Greenstein SM, Cantafio AW, et al. Successful rescue therapy with plasmapheresis and intravenous immunoglobulin for acute humoral renal transplant rejection. Transplantation. 2004;78:772–4.
153. Lehrich RW, Rocha PN, Reinsmoen N, et al. Intravenous immunoglobulin and plasmapheresis in acute humoral rejection: experience in renal allograft transplantation. Hum Immunol. 2005;66:350–8.
154. Barnett N, Dorling A, Mamode N. B cells in renal transplantation: pathological aspects and therapeutic interventions. Nephrol Dial Transplant. 2011;26:767–74.
155. Reff ME, Carner K, Chambers KS, et al. Depletion of B cells in vivo by a chimeric mouse human monoclonal antibody to CD20. Blood. 1994;83:435–45.
156. Lund FE, Randall TD. Effector and regulatory B cells: modulators of CD4(+) T cell immunity. Nat Rev Immunol. 2010;10:236–47.
157. Pescovitz MD. Rituximab, an anti-cd20 monoclonal antibody: history and mechanism of action. Am J Transplant. 2006;6:859–66.
158. Mulley WR, Hudson FJ, Tait BD, et al. A single low-fixed dose of rituximab to salvage renal transplants from refractory antibody-mediated rejection. Transplantation. 2009;87:286–9.
159. Vieira CA, Agarwal A, Book BK, et al. Rituximab for reduction of anti-HLA antibodies in patients awaiting renal transplantation: 1. Safety, pharmacodynamics, and pharmacokinetics. Transplantation. 2004;77:542–8.
160. Genberg H, Hansson A, Wernerson A, et al. Pharmacodynamics of rituximab in kidney allotransplantation. Am J Transplant. 2006;6:2418–28.
161. Zarkhin V, Lovelace PA, Li L, et al. Phenotypic evaluation of B-cell subsets after rituximab for treatment of acute renal allograft rejection in pediatric recipients. Transplantation. 2011;91:1010–8.
162. Genentech I. RITUXAN_(RITUXIMAB): highlights of prescription information. San Francisco: Genentech, Inc.; 2012.
163. Becker YT, Becker BN, Pirsch JD, et al. Rituximab as treatment for refractory kidney transplant rejection. Am J Transplant. 2004;4:996–1001.
164. Faguer S, Kamar N, Guilbeaud-Frugier C, et al. Rituximab therapy for acute humoral rejection after kidney transplantation. Transplantation. 2007;83:1277–80.
165. Kaposztas Z, Podder H, Mauiyyedi S, et al. Impact of rituximab therapy for treatment of acute humoral rejection. Clin Transplant. 2009;23:63–73.
166. Vo AA, Lukovsky M, Toyoda M, et al. Rituximab and intravenous immune globulin for desensitization during renal transplantation. N Engl J Med. 2008;359:242–51.
167. Vo AA, Peng A, Toyoda M, et al. Use of intravenous immune globulin and rituximab for desensitization of highly HLA-sensitized patients awaiting kidney transplantation. Transplantation. 2010;89:1095–102.
168. Lefaucheur C, Nochy D, Andrade J, et al. Comparison of combination plasmapheresis/IVIg/anti-CD20 versus high-dose IVIg in the treatment of antibody-mediated rejection. Am J Transplant. 2009;9:1099–107.
169. Voorhees PM, Dees EC, O'Neil B, et al. The proteasome as a target for cancer therapy. Clin Cancer Res. 2003;9:6316–25.
170. Perry DK, Burns JM, Pollinger HS, et al. Proteasome inhibition causes apoptosis of normal human plasma cells preventing alloantibody production. Am J Transplant. 2009;9:201–9.
171. Neubert K, Meister S, Moser K, et al. The proteasome inhibitor bortezomib depletes plasma cells and protects mice with lupus-like disease from nephritis. Nat Med. 2008;14:748–55.
172. Raghavan R, Jeroudi A, Achkar K, et al. Bortezomib in kidney transplantation. J Transplant. 2010;1–6.
173. Idica A, Kaneku H, Everly MJ, et al. Elimination of post-transplant donor-specific HLA antibodies with bortezomib. Clin Transpl. 2008:229–39.
174. Everly MJ, Everly JJ, Susskind B, et al. Bortezomib provides effective therapy for antibody- and cell-mediated acute rejection. Transplantation. 2008;86:1754–61.
175. Trivedi HL, Terasaki PI, Feroz A, et al. Abrogation of anti-HLA antibodies via proteasome inhibition. Transplantation. 2009;87:1555–61.
176. Flechner SM, Fatica R, Askar M, et al. The role of proteasome inhibition with bortezomib in the treatment of antibody-mediated rejection after kidney-only or kidney-combined organ transplantation. Transplantation. 2010;90:1486–92.
177. Sureshkumar KK, Hussain SM, Marcus RJ, et al. Proteasome inhibition with bortezomib: an effective therapy for severe antibody mediated rejection after renal transplantation. Clin Nephrol. 2012;77:246–53.
178. Manitpisitkul W, Wilson NS, Philosophe B, et al. Rescue therapy for acute antibody mediated rejection with a proteosome inhibitor after kidney transplantation. Clin Transpl. 2010:421–8.
179. FDA. Eculizumab (Soliris). 2013. http://www.fda.gov/.
180. Locke JE, Magro CM, Singer AL, et al. The use of antibody to complement protein C5 for salvage treatment of severe antibody-mediated rejection. Am J Transplant. 2009;9:231–5.
181. Lonze BE, Dagher NN, Simpkins CE, et al. Eculizumab, bortezomib and kidney paired donation facilitate transplantation of a highly sensitized patient without vascular access. Am J Transplant. 2010;10:2154–60.
182. Tillou X, Poirier N, Le Bas-Bernardet S, et al. Recombinant human C1-inhibitor prevents acute antibody-mediated rejection in alloimmunized baboons. Kidney Int. 2010;78:152–9.
183. Locke JE, Zachary AA, Haas M, et al. The utility of splenectomy as rescue treatment for severe acute antibody mediated rejection. Am J Transplant. 2007;7:842–6.
184. Locke JE, Zachary AA, Mohammed BS, et al. Rescue splenectomy for severe acute antibody-mediated rejection. Clin Transpl. 2006:518–20.
185. Kaplan B, Gangemi A, Thielke J, et al. Successful rescue of refractory, severe antibody mediated rejection with splenectomy. Transplantation. 2007;83:99–100.
186. Tzvetanov I, Spaggiari M, Jeon H, et al. The role of splenectomy in the setting of refractory humoral rejection after kidney transplantation. Transplant Proc. 2012;44:1254–8.
187. Roberti I, Geffner S, Vyas S. Successful rescue of refractory acute antibody-mediated renal allograft rejection with splenectomy—a case report. Pediatr Transplant. 2012;16:E49–52.
188. Loupy A, Hill GS, Suberbielle C, et al. Significance of C4d Banff scores in early protocol biopsies of kidney transplant recipients with preformed donor-specific antibodies (DSA). Am J Transplant. 2011;11:56–65.
189. Sis B, Campbell PM, Mueller T, Hunter C, Cockfield SM, Cruz J, Meng C, Wishart D, Solez K, Halloran PF. Transplant glomeru-

lopathy, late antibody-mediated rejection and the ABCD tetrad in kidney allograft biopsies for cause. Am J Transplant. 2007;7(7): 1743–52.
190. Perkowska-Ptasinska A, Ciszek M, Chmura A, et al. Transplant glomerulopathy: clinical and pathological correlations. Transplant Proc. 2009;41:141–9.
191. Gloor JM, Sethi S, Stegall MD, et al. Transplant glomerulopathy: subclinical incidence and association with alloantibody. Am J Transplant. 2007;7:2124–32.
192. John R, Konvalinka A, Tobar A, et al. Determinants of long-term graft outcome in transplant glomerulopathy. Transplantation. 2010;90:757–64.
193. Issa N, Cosio FG, Gloor JM, Sethi S, Dean PG, Moore SB, DeGoey S, Stegall MD. Transplant glomerulopathy: risk and prognosis related to anti-human leukocyte antigen class II antibody levels. Transplantation. 2008;86(5):681–5.
194. Cosio FG, Gloor JM, Sethi S, et al. Transplant glomerulopathy. Am J Transplant. 2008;8:492–6.
195. Divella C, Rossini M, Loverre A, et al. Immunohistochemical characterization of glomerular and tubulointerstitial infiltrates in renal transplant patients with chronic allograft dysfunction. Nephrol Dial Transplant. 2010;25:4071–7.
196. Kieran N, Wang X, Perkins J, et al. Combination of peritubular c4d and transplant glomerulopathy predicts late renal allograft failure. J Am Soc Nephrol. 2009;20:2260–8.
197. Koch M, Broecker V, Heratizadeh A, et al. Induction of chronic renal allograft injury by injection of a monoclonal antibody against a donor MHC Ib molecule in a nude rat model. Transpl Immunol. 2008;19:187–91.
198. de Heer E, Davidoff A, van der Wal A, et al. Chronic renal allograft rejection in the rat. Transplantation-induced antibodies against basement membrane antigens. Lab Invest. 1994;70: 494–502.
199. Smith RN, Kawai T, Boskovic S, et al. Four stages and lack of stable accommodation in chronic alloantibody-mediated renal allograft rejection in Cynomolgus monkeys. Am J Transplant. 2008;8:1662–72.
200. Gloor JM, Cosio FG, Rea DJ, et al. Histologic findings one year after positive crossmatch or ABO blood group incompatible living donor kidney transplantation. Am J Transplant. 2006;6:1841–7.
201. Cai J, Terasaki PI, Mao Q, et al. Development of nondonor-specific HLA-DR antibodies in allograft recipients is associated with shared epitopes with mismatched donor DR antigens. Am J Transplant. 2006;6:2947–54.
202. Dinavahi R, George A, Tretin A, et al. Antibodies reactive to non-HLA antigens in transplant glomerulopathy. J Am Soc Nephrol. 2011;22:1168–78.
203. Mengel M, Gwinner W, Schwarz A, et al. Infiltrates in protocol biopsies from renal allografts. Am J Transplant. 2007;7: 356–65.
204. Lipták P, Kemény E, Morvay Z, Szederkényi E, Szenohradszky P, Marofka F, Toldi J, Exner M, Iványi B. Peritubular capillary damage in acute humoral rejection: an ultrastructural study on human renal allografts. Am J Transplant. 2005;5(12):2870–6.
205. Feucht HE, Schneeberger H, Hillebrand G, et al. Capillary deposition of C4d complement fragment and early renal graft loss. Kidney Int. 1993;43:1333–8.
206. Elster EA, Hawksworth JS, Cheng O, et al. Probabilistic (Bayesian) modeling of gene expression in transplant glomerulopathy. J Mol Diagn. 2010;12:653–63.
207. Jabs WJ, Meier M, Lamprecht P, et al. Local expression of C-reactive protein is associated with deteriorating graft function in acute and chronic failure of kidney transplants. Nephron Clin Pract. 2011;117:c390–7.
208. Le RS, Devys A, Girard C, et al. Biomarkers for the diagnosis of the stable kidney transplant and chronic transplant injury using the ProtoArray® technology. Transplant Proc. 2010;42:3475–81.
209. Yabu JM, Higgins JP, Chen G, et al. C1q-fixing human leukocyte antigen antibodies are specific for predicting transplant glomerulopathy and late graft failure after kidney transplantation. Transplantation. 2011;91:342–7.
210. Bohmig GA, Bartel G, Wahrmann M. Antibodies, isotypes and complement in allograft rejection. Curr Opin Organ Transplant. 2008;13:411–8.
211. Nankivell BJ, Borrows RJ, Fung CL, et al. Delta analysis of post-transplantation tubulointerstitial damage. Transplantation. 2004;78:434–41.
212. Batal I, Lunz III JG, Aggarwal N, et al. A critical appraisal of methods to grade transplant glomerulitis in renal allograft biopsies. Am J Transplant. 2010;10:2442–52.
213. Nair R, Fraer M, Agrawal N, et al. Acute transplant glomerulopathy is associated with antibody-mediated rejection and poor graft outcome. Transplant Proc. 2010;42:3507–12.
214. Agustian PA, Schiffer M, Gwinner W, et al. Diminished met signaling in podocytes contributes to the development of podocytopenia in transplant glomerulopathy. Am J Pathol. 2011;178:2007–19.
215. Regele H, Bohmig GA, Habicht A, et al. Capillary deposition of complement split product C4d in renal allografts is associated with basement membrane injury in peritubular and glomerular capillaries: a contribution of humoral immunity to chronic allograft rejection. J Am Soc Nephrol. 2002;13:2371–80.
216. Roufosse CA, Shore I, Moss J, et al. Peritubular capillary basement membrane multilayering on electron microscopy: a useful marker of early chronic antibody-mediated damage. Transplantation. 2012;94:269–74.
217. Liapis G, Singh HK, Derebail VK, et al. Diagnostic significance of peritubular capillary basement membrane multilaminations in kidney allografts: old concepts revisited. Transplantation. 2012;94:620–9.
218. Haas M. Transplant glomerulopathy: it's not always about chronic rejection. Kidney Int. 2011;80:801–3.
219. Theruvath TP, Saidman SL, Mauiyyedi S, et al. Control of antidonor antibody production with tacrolimus and mycophenolate mofetil in renal allograft recipients with chronic rejection. Transplantation. 2001;72:77–83.
220. Schwarz C, Regele H, Huttary N, et al. Rescue therapy with tacrolimus and mycophenolate mofetil does not prevent deterioration of graft function in C4d-positive chronic allograft nephropathy. Wien Klin Wochenschr. 2006;118:397–404.
221. Billing H, Rieger S, Ovens J, et al. Successful treatment of chronic antibody-mediated rejection with IVIG and rituximab in pediatric renal transplant recipients. Transplantation. 2008;86:1214–21.
222. Billing H, Rieger S, Susal C, et al. IVIG and rituximab for treatment of chronic antibody-mediated rejection: a prospective study in paediatric renal transplantation with a 2-year follow-up. Transpl Int. 2012;25:1165–73.
223. Smith RN, Malik F, Goes N, et al. Partial therapeutic response to rituximab for the treatment of chronic alloantibody mediated rejection of kidney allografts. Transpl Immunol. 2012;27:107–13.
224. Vogelbacher R, Meister S, Guckel E, et al. Bortezomib and sirolimus inhibit the chronic active antibody-mediated rejection in experimental renal transplantation in the rat. Nephrol Dial Transplant. 2010;25:3764–73.
225. Knoll GA. Proteinuria in kidney transplant recipients: prevalence, prognosis, and evidence-based management. Am J Kidney Dis. 2009;54:1131–44.
226. Vincenti F, Kirk AD. What's next in the pipeline. Am J Transplant. 2008;8:1972–81.

Prevention and Management of Infectious Complications in Kidney Transplant Recipients

27

Rowena Delos Santos and Daniel C. Brennan

Abbreviations

BAL	Bronchoalveolar lavage
BCG	Bacillus Calmette–Guerin
CMV	Cytomegalovirus
CNIs	Calcineurin inhibitors
CNS	Central nervous system
CSF	Cerebral spinal fluid
EBV	Epstein–Barr virus
HAART	Highly active antiretroviral therapy
HBcAb+	Hepatitis B core antibody positive
HBV	Hepatitis B
HBVsAg+	Hepatitis B surface antigen positive
HCV	Hepatitis C virus
HIV	Human immunodeficiency virus
HSV	Herpes simplex virus
HTLV	Human T-lymphotropic virus
INH	Isoniazid
KS	Kaposi's sarcoma
MRSA	Methicillin-resistant *Staphylococcus aureus*
NAT	Nucleic acid testing
PCR	Polymerase chain reaction
PTLD	Posttransplantation lymphoproliferative disease
RPR	Rapid plasma regain testing
SVR	Sustained viral response
TMP–SMX	Trimethoprim–sulfamethoxazole
UTIs	Urinary tract infections
VZV	Varicella zoster virus

R. Delos Santos, M.D. (✉) • D.C. Brennan, M.D., F.A.C.P. (✉)
Washington University in St. Louis, 660 S. Euclid Avenue,
St. Louis, MO 63110, USA
e-mail: rdelossa@dom.wustl.edu; brennan@wudosis.wustl.edu

Introduction

Kidney transplantation is the treatment of choice for those with stage 5 chronic kidney disease and end-stage renal disease because it improves the quality and extends the quantity of life for these patients [1]. Despite improvements in both patient and kidney allograft survival over the last several years, this population continues to have significant morbidity and mortality from infectious complications. Infectious complications are currently the second most common cause of hospital admissions among kidney transplant patients in the first year posttransplant [2]. The United States Renal Data System annual data report from 2011 reports a hospital admission rate of 40.6 per 100 patient-years at risk for complications related to the kidney transplant over the first year and 32.2 admissions per 100 patient-years at risk for infections over the first year [2]. By 2-years posttransplantation, infections are the leading cause of hospitalizations in this population, with 17.5 admits per 100 patient-years at risk, while admissions for complications related to kidney transplant decrease to 11.7 admits per 100 patient-years at risk [2]. The most common infections leading to hospitalizations include urinary tract infections (UTIs), septicemia, and pneumonia (USRDS, ADR 2011) [2]. Infection is the second leading cause of death in patients who die with a functioning allograft, comprising 20% of all deaths [2]. Thus, transplantation attempts to reach the balance between prevention of allograft rejection and maintenance of immune integrity against pathogens.

Apart from immunosuppressants, several factors, including age, nutrition, diabetes, uremia, dialysis, and malnutrition related to ESRD, contribute to the depressed immune state [3]. In addition to this, some infections such as cytomegalovirus (CMV) and hepatitis C virus (HCV) can predispose to other infections. Posttransplant patients are continually exposed to both hospital and community organisms. All these factors affect the overall immune state of transplant patients, resulting in a "net state" of immunosuppression [4]. Thus, transplant practitioners require an understanding of the

M.R. Weir and E.V. Lerma (eds.), *Kidney Transplantation: Practical Guide to Management*,
DOI 10.1007/978-1-4939-0342-9_27, © Springer Science+Business Media New York 2014

complex interactions between the immune system and patients' preexisting conditions and exposures to provide the appropriate preventative and active treatments to kidney transplant patients.

Pre-transplant Recipient and Donor Evaluation

Prior to transplantation, recipients undergo an extensive evaluation to determine whether they have predisposing conditions or exposures requiring treatment prior to transplantation or prophylaxis after transplant. A thorough history and tests for exposures to viruses such as CMV, herpes, hepatitis, human immunodeficiency virus (HIV), human papillomavirus, and exposure to endemic mycoses and tuberculosis, are included in the evaluation. The medical history also contains inquiries into pet and occupational exposures, as well as a review of systems that may lead to the discovery of active infections. For instance, a history of chronic obstructive pulmonary disease, tuberculosis or positive purified protein derivative test, diabetes mellitus, hepatitis, diverticulosis or diverticulitis, sinusitis, chronic UTIs, prostatitis, dental caries, a history of blood transfusions, and drug or alcohol abuse would be important to identify during the initial medical history and review. All this information could lead to different management, testing, and treatment required prior to transplantation. In addition, the primary etiology for end-stage renal disease in patients may lead to investigation into whether pre-transplant nephrectomy is necessary, particularly for polycystic kidney disease, reflux nephropathy, and infected nephrolithiasis. Pre-transplant screening tests for potential kidney recipients are listed in Table 27.1.

In addition to these screening tests, a vaccination history is obtained for tetanus, diphtheria, pertussis, polio, influenza, pneumococcus, hepatitis A and B, and *Haemophilus influenzae* type B, measles, mumps, and rubella [5, 6]. The different immunizations that should be questioned for in the initial evaluation of a potential transplant recipient and antibody titers quantified are listed in Table 27.2. Testing titers should be done prior to transplantation because some vaccinations, namely, the live-attenuated viral vaccines including oral polio (no longer available in the United States), nasal influenza and varicella zoster virus (VZV), measles, mumps, rubella, and bacillus Calmette–Guerin (BCG) are contraindicated after transplantation [7]. These vaccines should be given several months prior to transplantation. Varicella vaccine can be given to children safely in pediatric pre-transplant patients and should be given to adults who have low titers prior to transplant [8].

Kidney transplant donors also undergo several tests prior to donation. Donors may harbor infectious diseases that can be transmitted to the recipient through the donated organ.

Table 27.1 Pre-transplant screening tests

Serologies
Cytomegalovirus
Herpes simplex virus 1 and 2
Hepatitis A, B, and C viruses
Epstein–Barr virus (EBV)
Varicella zoster virus
Human immunodeficiency virus
Rapid plasma regain
Tuberculin skin test or QuantiFERON-TB Gold or T-SPOT.TB test
Endemic fungi
Non-serologic tests
Urinalysis with culture
Pap-smear with pelvic exam
Prostate exam
Dental evaluation
Chest radiograph
Tests to consider after thorough history
Toxoplasma serology
Human T-cell leukemia virus
Colonoscopy
Ultrasound of the gallbladder
Stool culture, test for ova and parasite

There have been reports of viral transmission of adenovirus, West Nile, parvovirus, hepatitis B and C, herpes simplex, HIV, human T-lymphotropic virus, influenza, parainfluenza, rabies, polyomaviruses, and lymphocytic choriomeningitis virus through the transplanted organ [9]. In addition, bacterial, mycobacterial, fungal, and parasitic infections have also been transmitted from a donor to recipient. These include *Enterococcus, Acinetobacter, Ehrlichia, E. coli, Klebsiella, Legionella, Listeria,* Lyme disease, *Nocardia, Serratia, Staphylococcus aureus, Streptococcus*, Rocky Mountain spotted fever, Syphilis, *Candida, Coccidioides, Cryptococcus*, histoplasmosis, *Aspergillus*, Tuberculosis, *Trypanosoma cruzi*, Schistosomiasis, *Strongyloides*, malaria, and *Balamuthia* [9]. Despite the various numbers of possible transmitted infections from organ donor to recipient, transmission is reported in <1 % of donors [9].

Current recommendations for pre-transplant testing in living donors include tests for CMV, HIV 1 and 2, hepatitis B surface antigen and surface antibody, hepatitis B core antibody, HCV antibody and nucleic acid testing (NAT), rapid plasma regain (RPR) testing, human T-lymphotropic virus (HTLV), tuberculosis testing, and Epstein–Barr virus (EBV) [10]. Screening urinalyses with cultures are performed on living donors. For deceased donors, blood cultures are typically obtained to rule out a systemic bacterial infection. Systemic infections are generally a contraindication to accepting a deceased donor organ. Prior to organ procurement, deceased donors are given antibiotics, usually a cephalosporin. At the time of organ transplantation, a recipient

Table 27.2 Immunizations

Name	Immunization type	Re-immunization	Contraindications
Influenza	Inactivated, component (IM)	Yearly	Intranasal formulation as this is live-attenuated virus
Pneumococcal	Component	Second dose 5 years after initial	_
Tetanus-diphtheria	Toxoid	Every 10 years, booster at 5 years if deep puncture wound	Neurological reaction or anaphylaxis after previous dose
Varicella	Live attenuated	Second dose after 1–2 months	Immunosuppressed; only given prior to transplantation; not given to those who have received blood products in the previous 6 months
Meningococcal	Component	3–5 years if antibody titers decline	_
Haemophilus Influenza type B	Conjugated	Second dose after 2 months	_
Hepatitis A	Formalin-inactivated	Booster at 6–12 months (Havrix), booster 6 months (Vaqta)	_
Hepatitis B	Recombinant	Repeat 1 and 2 months. Check titer 1 month after last shot and if <10, give booster	_
Measles, Mumps, Rubella	Live attenuated	Second dose 4–6 years after	Anaphylaxis to first dose of vaccine, pregnancy, immunosuppressed

Table 27.3 Donor evaluation and testing

Serologies
Cytomegalovirus
EBV
Human immunodeficiency virus 1 and 2
Hepatitis B virus surface antigen and surface antibody
Hepatitis B virus core antibody
Hepatitis C virus antibody
Hepatitis C and HIV nucleic acid testing
Rapid plasma reagin
Human T-lymphotropic virus
Tuberculin skin test
Non-serologic tests
Urinalysis with culture
Blood and sputum culture (if deceased donor)
Pregnancy test for premenopausal donors
PSA for men >50 years
Consider ANA if family history of lupus
If recipient of the donor has polycystic kidney disease, obtain US kidneys if >30 years old, CT if less than 30 years old

will also receive prophylactic antibiotics, with or without placement of antibiotics intravesically during the transplant surgery [11, 12]. The various tests that potential kidney donors undergo prior to donation are listed in Table 27.3.

Posttransplantation Infections

Timing of Posttransplant Infections

Historically, posttransplant infections have been described according to the length of time from transplant: 1 month, second through 6 months, and greater than 6 months. A timeline with various possible infectious organisms that can affect post-kidney transplant recipients are shown in Fig. 27.1. The differences in infection types seen during these periods are due to the decreasing amounts of immunosuppressants needed after transplant and the different exposures that patients experience after their transplant. There are instances, however, where patients will have significant increases in their net immunosuppression, such as during episodes of acute and/or chronic rejection which require pulse steroids or increases in their overall immunosuppressant doses. The infectious risk again increases during this time period, similar to the early transplant period when patients' immunosuppression doses were higher. The timeline is not rigid as patients receive antibiotic and antiviral medications that may change the time at which infections occur in the absence of prophylaxis or treatment.

In the first month posttransplant, most infections are nosocomial and related to the surgical procedure. Relatively few are due to occult infections in the transplant recipient or transmitted from the donor. Common infections occurring within the first month of transplant include surgical wound infections, UTIs, pneumonia, and catheter-related blood stream infections from indwelling central venous catheters. Methods for decreasing infectious risk include meticulous observation of sterile conditions during surgery and removal of foreign bodies such as central lines, urinary catheters, ureteral stents, drainage tubes, and endotracheal tubes as soon as feasibly possible. Early ambulation and pulmonary care can help reduce the risk of pneumonia. Isolation of the patient and use of gowns, masks, and gloves for health-care personnel or visitors, even if the patient is neutropenic, has been shown to be unnecessary [13]. Several viral infections may reactivate in the first month, including herpes simplex virus (HSV) 1 and 2, human herpes virus (HHV)-6, EBV, CMV, and VZV in the absence of prophylaxis.

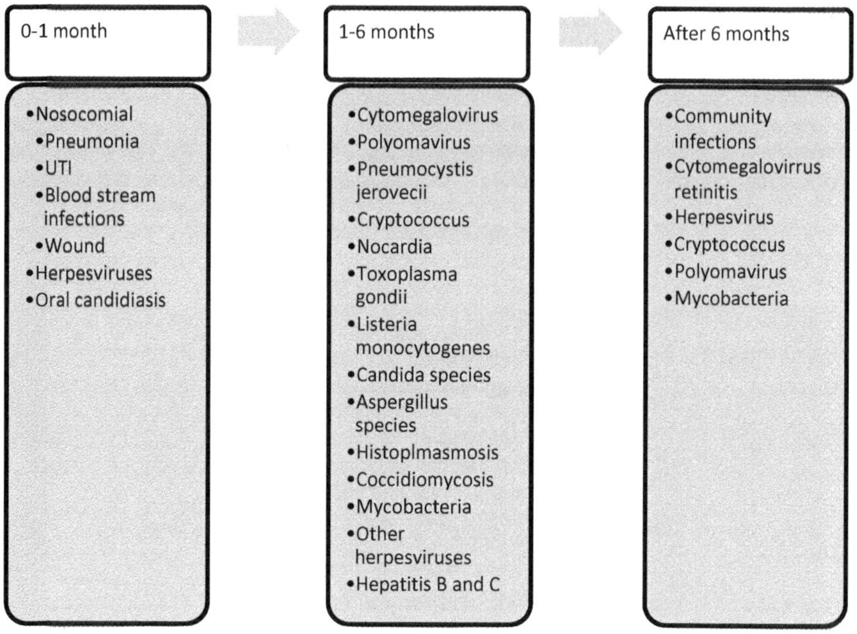

Fig. 27.1 Timeline and infectious organisms after kidney transplant

By the second to sixth month after transplantation, the nosocomial infections have historically been replaced by infections from opportunistic and reactivated organisms due to the relatively high doses of immunosuppressants that patients receive in the early posttransplant period. These infections included CMV, *Pneumocystis jirovecii*, *Cryptococcus neoformans*, *Nocardia* species, *Toxoplasma gondii*, *Listeria monocytogenes*, and *Candida* and *Aspergillus* species. With steroid avoidance and minimization, these opportunistic infections, except for CMV, are not commonly seen. However, EBV, CMV (in the absence of adequate prophylaxis), herpes viruses such as HSV 1 and 2, HHV-6, HHV-7, HBV, HCV, polyomavirus, *Mycobacteria*, histoplasmosis, and coccidiomycosis can reactivate during months 2–6 or later.

By 6 months posttransplantation, most centers have decreased immunosuppression to lower maintenance doses, and the antilymphocyte antibody induction effects have diminished. Consequently, patients will then usually suffer from similar infections affecting the general population including UTI's, influenza, diarrhea, cold sores, and pneumonia. A few notable exceptions to this include viral infections, including CMV retinitis that can occur late and herpes or zoster lesions which may be sentinel lesions for CMV. Several infections paired with prophylaxis medications that can help prevent disease are listed in Table 27.4.

Table 27.4 Prophylaxis use in transplant recipients

Infectious agent	Prophylaxis
Wound infections	Perioperative antibiotics
Urinary tract infections	Trimethoprim–sulfamethoxazole, ciprofloxacin
Herpes simplex viruses	Acyclovir
Varicella zoster virus	Acyclovir, immune globulin
EBV	Acyclovir, valganciclovir, ganciclovir
Cytomegalovirus	Ganciclovir, valganciclovir
Pneumocystis jiroveci	Trimethoprim–sulfamethoxazole
Oral candidiasis	Nystatin swish and swallow, clotrimazole troche

Bacterial Infections

Notable posttransplant bacterial infections include those that affect immune-competent patients and those that do not usually affect non-immunosuppressed patients. Bacterial infections commonly seen during the immediate posttransplant surgical period include those related to the surgery. These include infections of the blood stream due to central lines, lungs, surgical site, and urinary tract.

UTIs commonly occur in transplant patients who do not receive antibiotic prophylaxis, with an incidence of 29–79% [14, 15]. Symptoms for UTI include dysuria, frequency, and urgency. Some patients may not experience symptoms, and the only evidence of infection would be through routine urinalysis and culture. Risk factors for UTIs include female gender, recurrent UTI's pre-transplant, prolonged duration of dialysis after surgery, diabetes, neurogenic bladder, prolonged use of bladder catheters postsurgery, allograft trauma, polycystic kidney disease, and ureteral anastomotic complications [14, 16, 17]. Empiric treatment for UTIs should cover the most common organisms but should be tailored to the organism once culture and specificities return. Common pathogens leading to UTIs include bacteria in the *Enterobacteriaceae* family (*Escherichia coli*, *Proteus*, *Citrobacter*, *Enterobacter*, *and Klebsiella*), *Pseudomonas aeruginosa*, *Enterococci*, and *Staphylococci* [18]. Due to the high rates of urinary infections, vigilance in implementing preventative measures is important. It has been shown that the early removal of a urinary catheter decreases the incidence of UTIs [19]. Many centers prescribe antibiotic prophylaxis for their posttransplant patients. One randomized study showed the beneficial effects of prophylactic use of double strength trimethoprim–sulfamethoxazole (TMP–SMX) 320 mg/1,600 mg) [18]. In this study, patients had no difference in the rate of UTIs with a catheter in place; however, after catheter removal the overall risk of bacterial UTI was <10 % [18]. Though there was not an increased rate of resistant bacterial infections in the treated group, patients who had bacterial infections were more likely caused by resistant bacteria [18]. An additional benefit in using TMP–SMX as antibiotic prophylaxis for UTIs is its effectiveness as prophylaxis for *Pneumocystis jirovecii* (formally known as *Pneumocystis carinii*).

Patients may also have persistent bacteriuria posttransplant, which should be evaluated further with ultrasound or computed tomography (CT) for a nidus of infection such as an abscess. Early detection and treatment of UTIs is important, as these infections can lead to more serious infections, including bacteremia and pyelonephritis. Pyelonephritis with bacteremia will present with fevers, pain or tenderness over the allograft, and usually allograft dysfunction. The urinary tract is the most common source for bacteremia in transplant patients, with a reported 2-week mortality of 11 % [20].

Pneumonia

Pneumonias are also a common cause of infections and hospitalization in post-kidney transplant patients. Prior to transplant, the incidence of pneumonias in these patients is 37 episodes per 100 patient-years, then sharply increases in the first month post-kidney transplant to 216 episodes per 100 patient-years, then declines to approximately 60 episodes per 100 patient-years by the end of the first year, and remains steady thereafter [21]. Overall, patients are 3.62 times more likely to have pneumonia in the first 12 months after transplant than after 12 months [22]. Cough, fever, shortness of breath, evidence of oxygen desaturation, and pulmonary physical findings are important signs and symptoms in the initial evaluation. Diagnostic tests include blood and sputum gram stain and culture, chest X-ray and computed tomography, and bronchoscopy or open lung biopsy with cultures are done. Despite testing, however, the etiology of the pneumonia is not found in a significant proportion of patients, between 23 and 31 % from two studies [22, 23]. Organisms found on testing in one study include bacteria (mostly *S. aureus*, *S. pneumonia*, *P. aeruginosa*, *K. pneumonia*, *Acinetobacter*, *Haemophilus*, *Enterobacter*, *E. coli*, *and Nocardia*), *Tuberculosis*, mixed bacteria, fungus, *Pneumocystis*, atypical organisms, CMV, and other viruses [22, 23].

Due to the relatively high mortality rates (12.5–40 % in some studies) associated with pneumonia, broad-spectrum antibiotics usually in the form of a third-generation cephalosporin, a β-lactam with β-lactamase inhibitor, or a quinolone are initiated [24, 25]. Some will add vancomycin depending on the clinical situation and local methicillin-resistant *Staphylococcus aureus* (MRSA) resistance rates. Consideration should be made for adding an antifungal if there is no improvement. Once the etiologic factor has been found, therapy can be directed and simplified to the specific organism.

Wound Infections

The incidence of wound infections after kidney transplantation has decreased from 25 to 56% in earlier studies to 4.8% in a more recent study [26, 27]. Risks for wound infections include increased body mass index, urine leak, need for reoperation through the primary incision, immunosuppressants (particularly use of Mycophenolate Mofetil), and diabetes [26]. Improvements in the incidence of wound infections in kidney transplantation are due to the use of prophylactic antibiotics and bladder irrigation with antibiotic solution.

Nocardiosis

Nocardia species is a ubiquitous organism in the environment usually inhaled or directly inoculated through soil particles [28]. The most common species found are *N. asteroides*, *N. farcinica*, and *N. brasiliensis*. Disease presentation varies in the immunocompromised host. Most infections caused by *Nocardia* are primarily pulmonary, manifesting with fever, chills, cough, and dyspnea. *Nocardia* will also commonly disseminate to other organ systems in nearly half of affected patients, including central nervous and integumentary system involvement [28]. Patients with central nervous system (CNS) involvement may present with confusion, fevers, headache, vision changes, weakness, and lethargy from brain abscesses. Skin findings include subcutaneous nodules, abscesses, swelling, and cellulitis. Diagnostic methods for Nocardiosis include skin, sputum or bronchoalveolar lavage (BAL) culture, X-ray or computed tomography of the lungs, and MRI of the brain [29]. Treatment for Nocardiosis usually includes TMP–SMX for a prolonged course. Other treatments include third-generation cephalosporins, aminoglycosides, minocycline, and amoxicillin-clavulanate [28–30].

Legionella

Legionella usually presents as pneumonia with a peripheral patchy infiltrate or consolidation on CXR. *Legionella pneumophila* is the most common *Legionella* species causing infection and is associated with epidemics from contaminated respiratory equipment and contaminated heating and cooling systems and drinking water. Diagnostic testing for this condition includes a urine antigen for *Legionella*, which identifies serogroup 1, and culture. Other tests used for diagnosis are the direct fluorescent antibody (DFA) test in BAL or sputum specimens [31]. The treatment of choice for Legionnaires' disease is azithromycin, fluoroquinolones, followed by doxycycline and TMP–SMX. Rifampin is not used for monotherapy but is used in combination therapy. Azithromycin has no interaction with calcineurin inhibitors (CNIs), while rifampin increases the cytochrome P-450 activity, leading to significantly lower CNI levels and adjustment in dosing while on this medication.

Listeriosis

Listeriosis is a disease caused by *Listeria monocytogenes*, an organism that can contaminate meats, vegetables, and dairy products through soil and water contact and enter the gastrointestinal tract to cause disease. Most infections will occur early in the posttransplant period, and usually in the summer months, with one study showing that some transplant patients' fecal matter can contain *Listeria* [32]. Patients may present with gastroenteritis, CNS infection, and meningitis, with up to a 33% mortality [33]. Diagnosis of CNS disease requires a lumbar puncture, which reveals polymorphonuclear monocytes and low glucose. There may or may not be Gram-positive bacilli on smear/culture and should be repeated if no bacteria are seen on the initial test. Ampicillin is the first-line treatment for this infection, followed by TMP–SMX.

Viral Infections

Herpes Viral Infections

The herpes family includes eight herpes viruses including HSV 1 and 2, VZV, EBV, CMV, and HHV-6, 7, and 8. Each can cause significant reactivation in patients taking immunosuppressants. The different HHVs and the disease associated with each virus are listed in Table 27.5.

Table 27.5 Human Herpes viruses and resultant diseases

HHV-1 Herpes simplex 1 (HSV 1)	Herpes labialis
HHV-2 Herpes simplex 2 (HSV 2)	Herpes genitalis
HHV-3 Varicella zoster virus (VZV)	Chicken pox
	Shingles
HHV-4 EBV	Mononucleosis
	Burkitt's lymphoma
	Posttransplant lymphoproliferative disorder (PTLD)
	Nasopharyngeal carcinoma
	Oral hairy leukoplakia
HHV-5 Cytomegalovirus (CMV)	Cytomegalovirus viremia, syndrome, disease
	Salivary gland virus disease
HHV-6 Human herpes virus 6	Roseola subitum
HHV-7 Human herpes virus 7	Roseola subitum
	Pityriasis rosea
HHV-8 Human herpes virus 8	Kaposi's sarcoma
	Castleman's disease
	Effusion lymphoma

Cytomegalovirus

CMV is the most common herpes virus affecting post-kidney transplant recipients with significant morbidity. CMV may be detected in urine, blood, or saliva in 50–75 % of renal transplant recipients after transplant, but only 8–32% of recipients will experience symptoms related to CMV disease [34]. Factors affecting the development of clinical disease include the serostatus of both the donor and recipient at the time of transplant, with the highest risk of developing symptomatic disease in D+/R− patients, and less risk in D−/R+, D+/R+ D−/R− Other factors affecting the development of CMV symptoms and disease include induction with antilymphocyte antibody, other active viral infections, and the strength and amount of maintenance immunosuppressants [35]. Allograft rejection treatment can increase the rate of CMV infection, while CMV infection and the required reduction in maintenance immunosuppression as part of treatment for CMV can predispose patients to allograft rejection and chronic allograft dysfunction [34, 36]. New infections can occur in seronegative recipients from their seropositive donor or from an exposure, while previously seropositive recipients can have a new infection from their donor or from reactivation of latent disease in the recipient.

Symptoms and signs of CMV disease usually appear as fever, malaise, diarrhea, thrombocytopenia, neutropenia, and transaminitis. Recipients can also present with symptoms related to involvement of the pulmonary, hepatic, gastrointestinal, nervous, retinal, renal, and cardiac systems [34, 36]. CMV is also associated with acceleration of coronary artery disease. Diagnosis of CMV viremia requires evaluation of the peripheral blood for viral load using several possible methods such as pp65 antigenemia assay, amplification of CMV DNA or RNA, shell vial, and hybridization [36]. The nucleic acid-based tests are preferred for accuracy and quantification. In some cases, tissue invasive disease may not have a detectable viral level, making a tissue biopsy necessary for diagnosis.

Due to significant morbidity and mortality related to CMV infection, several different strategies have emerged: general prophylaxis, selective prophylaxis, preemptive, and deferred methods of management [37]. Selective prophylaxis entails providing prophylaxis specifically to recipients who are D+/R− and at highest risk of developing symptomatic disease. General prophylaxis provides antiviral prophylaxis to all recipients regardless of CMV serostatus.

Preemptive therapy refers to monitoring CMV viral load, and treating viremia prior to the development of symptoms. The deferred approach to CMV viremia is where patients with viremia undergo treatment only when they manifest symptoms. These strategies differ significantly, with no uniformly agreed upon approach.

Prophylactic therapy is effective in decreasing CMV disease, infection, and mortality [38]. Medications used primarily for CMV prophylaxis are ganciclovir and valganciclovir. Although acyclovir, valacyclovir, and CMV immune globulin have been used in some centers, these have been shown to have limited efficacy [38–40].

There are a few issues that arise from following the prophylactic approach. Ganciclovir-resistant CMV develops in 7% of recipients who receive this antiviral, largely due to the viral kinase UL97 gene responsible for phosphorylating ganciclovir and making it an active drug [41]. Second, prophylaxis is expensive [42]. Third, the use of prophylaxis may only lead to later onset of CMV disease after the completion of the prophylactic antivirals [43, 44]. Of note, there is no consensus on the number of months of prophylactic therapy for patients after transplantation. Some studies advocate approximately 3 months with close monitoring for the development of CMV viremia while others advocate a longer course of 6 months due to the emergence of late onset CMV disease and the cost-effectiveness of a longer course compared to a shorter course [43, 45–48].

Doses for prophylaxis are oral ganciclovir 1,000 mg three times daily or valganciclovir 900 mg daily. One study showed no significant differences between using either drug, and valganciclovir has better bioavailability compared to oral ganciclovir (70% vs. 7%) [49, 50]. Of note, both drugs require dose adjustment for those with renal insufficiency. The different CMV risk categories, prophylaxis medications, and medications used for treatment of CMV are listed in Table 27.6.

The preemptive approach may be associated with decreased development of late onset CMV disease, but the cost of weekly or bimonthly viral load assessments may not be more cost-effective compared to prophylaxis [37, 51]. The deferred strategy of treating CMV disease when symptoms develop usually requires intravenous ganciclovir 5 mg/kg every 12 h or oral valganciclovir 900 mg twice a day for 2–3 weeks or until symptoms abate. One study has shown no difference in outcomes between the oral valganciclovir and IV ganciclovir in the treatment of CMV disease [52]. In addition to antiviral treatment, reduction in mycophenolate and azathioprine may be required. Cidofovir and foscarnet can also be used to treat symptomatic CMV disease, but their use is limited by nephrotoxicity. If treated inadequately, CMV may develop resistance to ganciclovir and other medications used to treat the disease. Two prominent genes, UL97 and UL54, encoding the viral protein kinase and DNA polymerase respectively, confer resistance to ganciclovir (UL97/UL54) and foscarnet and cidofovir (UL54) [53]. Leflunomide and maribavir may prove useful in treating patients with ganciclovir-resistant CMV strains [54].

Table 27.6 CMV risk, prophylaxis, and treatment

CMV risk categories
High risk
CMV D+/R–
Intermediate risk
CMV D+/R+ or CMV D–/R+
Low risk
CMV D–R–
Prophylaxis medications
Ganciclovir 1,000 mg oral three times daily Valganciclovir 900 mg oral daily
Treatment medications
Ganciclovir intravenous 5 mg/kg every 12 h
Valganciclovir 900 mg oral twice daily
Cidofovir
Foscarnet
Leflunomide

D = donor, R = recipient, (+) = positive serology, (–) = negative serology

Herpes Simplex Virus

HSV 1 and 2 are associated with herpes labialis and genitalis, respectively. Initially patients will have acute infections followed by a period of dormancy within the sensory nerve ganglia. In the first several months posttransplant, patients may experience reactivation of their latent disease. This manifests as ulcerations of the mucus membranes or herpetiform skin lesions. Others can present with more serious complications such as esophagitis, hepatitis, encephalitis, pneumonitis, and disseminated disease. Diagnosis is achieved by lab tests including the Tzanck smear and culture. Polymerase chain reaction (PCR) testing in the cerebral spinal fluid (CSF) is preferred for the evaluation of possible CNS disease. Treatment for simple oral or genital lesions is acyclovir 200 mg orally 4–5 times daily. Other antiviral medications include valacyclovir and famciclovir. Serious infections require intravenous acyclovir dosed at 5–15 mg/kg every 8 h. The resistance of HSV to acyclovir is 4–7 % in immunocompromised hosts [55].

Varicella Zoster Virus

Reactivation of VZV is a concern in renal transplant recipients, as over 90% have been exposed to the virus prior to transplant. The diagnosis is made with the discovery of pain, shingles, or vesicles in a dermatomal distribution with confirmation through Tzanck smear, DFA, or PCR. Like HSV, VZV can present with hepatitis, encephalitis, pneumonia, and disseminated disease. Treatment for a zoster outbreak is acyclovir 800 mg orally five times daily. Alternatives are famciclovir and valacyclovir. Those with disseminated disease should be treated with intravenous acyclovir 10 mg/kg every 8 h for 7 days. In addition to this, patients should be placed in negative pressure rooms until all lesions have dried to prevent the spread to individuals who have never been exposed to VZV. If exposed, these seronegative individuals should receive varicella immune globulin within 72 h and oral acyclovir 200 mg five times daily. Up to 25% of patients with zoster will have post-herpetic neuralgia, which can be treated using tricyclic antidepressants, narcotics, gabapentin, pregabalin, and tramadol [56].

Epstein–Barr virus

EBV is a virus which most adults have been exposed to previously, with a 95% seropositive prevalence among adults. Kidney transplant recipients who are seronegative or seropositive collectively have a 20% rate of new infection or reactivation within the first year posttransplant [57]. Diagnostic testing includes plasma PCR testing for viral DNA to detect new or reactive disease. EBV can cause symptoms of fatigue, mononucleosis-like syndrome, Burkitt's lymphoma, nasopharyngeal carcinoma and, in posttransplant patients, posttransplantation lymphoproliferative disease (PTLD), which is potentially fatal. The risks of developing PTLD include EBV seronegative status, immunosuppressants, and youth. The long-term incidence of PTLD is 1–2 % in kidney transplant recipients [58]. In addition, the use of one of the newer immunosuppressants, belatacept, is associated with a higher risk of PTLD than conventional immunosuppression including antilymphocyte therapy [59].

The majority of PTLD is due to B-cell proliferation of affected EBV cells that normally remain dormant under T-cell control but proliferate after T-cell suppression with immunosuppressants. Prophylaxis used to prevent CMV viremia can also be used to prevent EBV viremia. Some centers have employed a monitoring strategy to detect viremia early in seronegative recipients and have treated these patients with rituximab to help prevent the development of PTLD [60]. Studies have also shown that administration of EBV-specific cytotoxic T-lymphocytes to seronegative recipients can be used as prophylaxis for EBV [61, 62].

Human Herpes Virus 6, 7, 8

HHV-6 is a beta herpes virus that causes roseola infantum, or exanthema subitum in children. Most people have had the infection prior to adulthood, and transplant recipients can experience reactivation of their disease, with similar symptoms to CMV. Other potential complications of reactivation are hepatitis, encephalitis, and hemophagocytic syndrome [63]. Antiviral treatment for HHV-6 is similar to that used for CMV, although it is controversial whether HHV-6 is susceptible to ganciclovir [64]. HHV-7 is another HHV that many have been previously exposed and is associated with roseola and pityriasis rosea in children. Reactivation of this infection can also be associated with CMV disease [65]. Unlike HHV-6, ganciclovir is clearly inadequate to treat HHV-7, and affected transplant recipients may require cidofovir [66]. HHV-8 is the etiologic virus of Kaposi's sarcoma (KS), Castleman's disease, and primary effusion lymphoma [67]. Less than 3% of the population are seropositive for HHV-8, with pockets of higher prevalence >25 % in parts of Italy, Greece, and Africa [67]. Though the virus is sexually transmitted, HHV-8 can be acquired from the donated kidney [68]. The incidence of KS among transplant recipients is 0.1–5 % and tends to present within the first 3 years after transplantation in an aggressive manner [69]. Treatment usually involves decreasing immunosuppression, radiation, and chemotherapy, although some cases may regress with the use of rapamycin [70].

Prophylaxis used for CMV may also decrease the incidence of KS in transplant recipients indirectly by preventing CMV reactivation [71].

Hepatitis Viruses

The prevalence of chronic hepatitis B surface antigen positive (HBVsAg+) carriers is between 10 and 25% [72]. The presence of chronic liver disease in renal transplant recipients is associated with an increased risk of sepsis and liver failure [73]. The viruses affect the immune response by suppressing the immune system, which has a twofold effect of decreasing the likelihood of allograft rejection but also increasing the risk for infection [74].

Hepatitis B (HBV) is a DNA virus that can cause significant liver disease in kidney transplant recipients, including hepatitis and cirrhosis. Disease can result from worsening of previously controlled disease, new infection, or transmission through the donor allograft. The possibility of worsening or reactivated disease in those who are HBV+ underscores the need to obtain a baseline liver biopsy prior to renal transplantation. Concern for reactivation or seroconversion arises from data that recipients who are HBsAg− and HBsAb+ (hepatitis B core antibody positive (HBcAb+) have progressed to reactivation of their disease and disease progression [75]. In a meta-analysis performed to evaluate studies of lamivudine for treatment of HBV, the overall estimate for clearance of HBV using lamivudine was 91%; however, the estimate for development of lamivudine resistance was 18% [72]. Adefovir, tenofovir, entecavir, and emtricitabine are other antivirals that are useful to treat HBV. Entecavir is less nephrotoxic than tenofovir.

HCV is a single-stranded RNA virus with a prevalence of 10–41 % among transplant recipients [76]. Transmission of the virus is hematologic, thus making HCV transmissible through renal allografts from donors with HCV, though there is rare transmission if the donor is anti-HCV antibody positive and HCV RNA negative. In renal allograft recipients with HCV, chronic hepatitis develops in more than 60% [77]. Both recipient and allograft survivals decrease in HCV-positive recipients (65 and 49%) compared to HCV negative recipients (80 and 63%) [78]. Unfortunately, recipients with HCV can develop cirrhosis, hepatocellular carcinoma, membranous glomerulonephritis, membranoproliferative glomerulonephritis, cryoglobulinemia, and thrombotic microangiopathy. As a result of the complexities of HCV infection long term in the kidney transplant recipient, the pre-transplant evaluation is extensive, including liver biopsy, HCV genotyping, and RNA quantification.

Treatment using pegylated-interferon alpha, ribavirin, and amantadine can be offered prior to transplantation, as treatment with interferon can lead to acute rejection. Over the last decade, there have been strides in the treatment of hepatitis C, particularly in patients who are infected with genotype 1. Two new direct-acting antivirals in a class of protease inhibitors have been developed and tested for the treatment of hepatitis C. Their mechanism of action is to inhibit the action of NS3/NS4A HCV serine protease, effectively preventing the formation of important nonstructural proteins of HCV [79]. The first is telaprevir which has been studied in a population of patients with hepatitis C genotype 1 who had not previously been treated. In phase I and II trials, the use of this oral drug for 12 weeks with peg-interferon and ribavirin for 24 weeks led to the sustained viral response (SVR) of 69% [80, 81]. Genotype 1b responds better to telaprevir than genotype 1a [82]. In phase III studies of previously treated or treatment naïve HCV genotype I infected individuals, investigators found significant SVR in those treated with telaprevir (70–80 % SVR) compared to those who received standard therapy with pegylated-interferon alfa-2b and ribavirin (20–40 % SVR) [83, 84]. The medication has side effects, making it difficult to tolerate, including pruritus, anemia, and rash.

Another serine protease inhibitor that has proven effective in clinical trials is boceprevir. In phase III studies, in patients previously treated for HCV genotype I, the rate of SVR was 59–66 % in those patients treated with boceprevir compared to those who received standard therapy with pegylated-interferon alpha 2a and ribavirin 21% [85]. Because of the previously found difference in response rates between blacks and whites, investigators sought to differentiate the SVR in a non-black cohort and black cohort of patients using boceprevir [86, 87]. For the non-black cohort, the SVR was 67–68 % in those receiving boceprevir compared to those who received standard therapy (40%) [87]. For the black cohort, the use of boceprevir led to a 42–53 % SVR compared to those treated with pegylated-interferon alpha 2a and ribavirin (23 %) [87]. Boceprevir was associated with anemia requiring erythropoietin-stimulating agents during therapy.

There are concerns for the use of triple therapy for HCV genotype 1 treatment in the posttransplant population. Most concerning is the interaction between the protease inhibitors and CNIs [88]. Both telaprevir and boceprevir inhibit cytochrome P450 3A4, which is involved in the metabolism of CNIs. It has been shown in healthy volunteers that the trough levels of cyclosporine and tacrolimus increase by 4.6-fold and 70-fold, respectively, in the presence of steady-state telaprevir [89]. They also found that the half-life of both cyclosporine and tacrolimus increased significantly with telaprevir [89]. Use of the protease inhibitor drugs requires close monitoring in the presence of CNI use. These serine protease inhibitors have not yet been approved in transplanted patients, though several studies are currently ongoing in cohorts of liver transplant recipients to determine their efficacy and safety in this population of patients.

Influenza

Influenza viral infections affect posttransplantation recipients similar to those who are not immunosuppressed, manifesting with fevers, myalgias, headache, and cough. However, more serious presentations may occur in immunosuppressed patients, including primary viral and secondary bacterial pneumonias, rhabdomyolysis, and encephalitis. Due to the potential seriousness of the disease, transplant recipients and their close contacts should receive the influenza vaccine yearly. At the time of the H1N1 pandemic of 2009, transplant recipients safely received the injectable version of the regular and H1N1 vaccine, with better immune response when the two were given simultaneously [90, 91]. Recipients should not, however, receive the live-attenuated version of the vaccine, as this could lead to active disease. Anyone with an egg allergy or not able to receive the vaccine should receive alternative medications for prophylaxis, if exposed or for treatment. These include the M2 blockers amantadine and rimantadine and the viral neuraminidase inhibitors, zanamivir and oseltamivir. The M2 blockers are only effective against influenza A, while the neuraminidase inhibitors have activity against both influenza A and B. Influenza A can develop resistance to the M2 blockers, and the antiviral resistance of the circulating influenza strain should be taken into consideration. Adjustments for renal function must be made as these drugs are renally cleared.

Risk of Allosensitization with Vaccination

There has been some discussion over the risk of allosensitization after immunizations. It has previously been shown that anti-HLA antibodies are found at very low levels in healthy males after influenza vaccination, likely as a result of natural antibody production to cross-reactive epitopes from infectious organisms or perhaps through vaccinations [92, 93]. Anti-HLA antibodies have been discovered after non-allogeneic stimulus in healthy adults after immunization with hepatitis B vaccine by 2 months postvaccination in 9/20 patients [94]. There are mixed results from investigators who have evaluated allosensitization after influenza vaccinations. Two studies found that a certain small number of patients (5.6–17.3 %) develop new de novo anti-HLA antibodies directed against both donor and non-donor HLA after receiving the influenza vaccine [95, 96]. One criticism to the study by Katerinis is that the influenza vaccine was an adjunctive vaccine which could potentiate the development of anti-HLA antibodies [97]. Another study found augmented cellular immunity after influenza vaccination, but not in the humoral response in transplanted patients, while the non-transplanted individuals experienced an enhanced cellular immune response, with a few developing new alloantibodies [98]. There are several studies that did not observe development of HLA antibodies in stable posttransplant patients after administration of influenza vaccine [90, 99–101]. Overall, it is still considered safe to administer the influenza vaccine to transplanted patients 3 months posttransplantation, with a very small likelihood of development of anti-donor-specific antibodies. The risks of the development of donor-specific antibodies must be weighed against the benefit of vaccination and prevention of an influenza infection in transplant recipients.

Human Immunodeficiency Virus

Until more recently, an infection with HIV was considered a contraindication to transplantation. Prior to effective highly active antiretroviral therapy (HAART), there were concerns related to uncontrolled HIV disease and the risk for opportunistic infections with an increased immunocompromised state from the combination of both HIV infection and immunosuppressants. However, with effective HAART medications and the ability to achieve undetectable viral loads and CD4+ counts of >500 on therapy, patient survival with HIV has increased. Consequently, some centers in the United States and Europe have been transplanting HIV-infected patients, with 1- and 3-year patient survival rates of 85%–94% and 64%–88%, respectively [102–105]. The 1- and 3-year allograft survival rates are 75–90% and 74%. The cumulative incidence of rejection rates varies widely among studies, with 1- and 3-year rates of 29%–52% and 41%–70%, respectively [102–105]. Compared to non-HIV-infected recipients, the acute rejection rates are to two- to threefold higher in HIV-infected individuals, for unclear reasons [105]. Difficulties may arise in these patients when dosing and maintaining immunosuppressant drug levels, as some HAART medications (protease inhibitors such as ritonavir, saquinavir, indinavir, nelfinavir) inhibit the cytochrome P-450 system, severely slowing the metabolism of some immunosuppressants, namely, cyclosporine, tacrolimus, and sirolimus so that these medications are dosed only once daily or once weekly at times [106, 107].

Polyomaviruses

Polyomaviruses (JC virus, Simian virus, or BK virus) are DNA viruses that can cause significant disease in renal transplant recipients. Of particular interest in kidney allograft patients is BK virus, which can reactivate posttransplant and lead to allograft nephropathy. These viruses will not be discussed in this chapter, as a separate chapter is dedicated to this topic (Chap. 28).

Fungal Infections

Fungal infections are a significant cause of morbidity and mortality in the renal transplant population, with infections occurring in approximately 1–14% of patients and a mortality rate of 59–75% depending on which fungus or mold is involved [108–110]. Risk factors for developing fungal infections include age, corticosteroid use, diabetes, liver disease, CMV disease, use of broad-spectrum antibiotics, and the presence of indwelling catheters and derangements in mucosal barriers [110, 111]. The symptomatology and presentation for disease can be subtle and masked by the presence of immunosuppressants, requiring practitioners' vigilance in keeping these diseases in the differential, and obtaining cultures of the suspected site(s) of infection. Systemic treatment for fungal infections can be given orally or intravenously, however, most critically ill patients receive amphotericin B. Other antifungal medications include the azoles (fluconazole, etc.), triazoles (voriconazole, posaconazole), and echinocandins (micafungin, caspofungin, and anidulafungin) [112]. Many antifungals will interfere with the metabolism of cyclosporine, tacrolimus, and sirolimus, requiring close monitoring of levels for these drugs. The most potent of these are ketoconazole, itraconazole, voriconazole, and posaconazole with less interference by fluconazole. Empiric reduction of the dose of cyclosporine, tacrolimus, and sirolimus is usually initiated at the time the azole is commenced. The different fungi, tissues that manifest disease, diagnostic tests, and antifungal therapies are summarized in Table 27.7.

Candida

Candida species (*C. albicans, C. glabrata, C. parapsilosis, C. krusei, and C. tropicalis*) cause the most disease among all disease-causing fungi. *Candida* infections lead to mucocutaneous lesions such as thrush, onychomycosis, intertrigo, vaginitis, and esophagitis. They can also cause urinary catheter funguria as well as significant systemic diseases, with catheter-related candidemia. Candidemia can develop into candidal endophthalmitis, endocarditis, arteritis, mycotic aneurysms,

Table 27.7 Fungal infections, diagnosis, and treatment options

			Treatment options	
Fungus	Organ system disease manifestation	Diagnostic test	Primary treatment	Secondary/ salvage treatment
Candida	Urinary tract infection Surgical site infection Mucocutaneous Pneumonitis Pyelonephritis Fungus ball Abscesses Vaginitis Intertrigo Esophagitis	Culture of suspected tissue Blood culture	Oral, cutaneous, vaginal Clotrimazole Nystatin swish and swallow Fluconazole Mild illness Fluconazole Severe illness or azole resistant strain Amphotericin B Echinocandin	Itraconazole Posaconazole Voriconazole
Cryptococcus	Pneumonia Skin/soft tissue infection Meningitis Fungemia	Culture of suspected tissue CSF for cryptococcal antigen Serum cryptococcal antigen Histopathology	Fluconazole if less severe More severe infection Amphotericin B 5-Flucytosine	Itraconazole Posaconazole Voriconazole
Aspergillosis	Pneumonia Aspergilloma with cavitary lesions Sinusitis CNS infection Dissemination	Culture of suspected tissue Galactomannan assay Histopathology	Amphotericin B Voriconazole	Itraconazole Posaconazole Echinocandin
Mucormycosis	Pneumonia Cavitary lesion Rhino-orbital-cerebral Cutaneous infection Sinusitis Gastrointestinal tract Central nervous system Renal system	Culture of suspected tissue Histopathology	Amphotericin B	Posaconazole
Histoplasmosis	Skin/soft tissue infection Pneumonia/pulmonary granuloma Rheumatologic disease Disseminated disease	Culture of suspected tissue (includes bone marrow) Blood cultures for fungi Urine and serum histoplasma antigen Immunodiffusion and complement fixation	Mild/moderate disease Itraconazole Severe illness Amphotericin B followed by itraconazole suppressive therapy	Posaconazole Fluconazole Voriconazole
Coccidiomycosis	Skin/soft tissue Rheumatologic disease Pneumonia/cavitary lesions Renal disease Central nervous system Disseminated disease	Culture of suspected tissue Histopathology Complement fixation	Mild/moderate disease Fluconazole Itraconazole Severe disease Amphotericin B followed by fluconazole or itraconazole suppressive therapy	Posaconazole Voriconazole

osteomyelitis, pneumonitis, pyelonephritis, fungus balls, intra-abdominal lesions, meningitis and brain abscesses, and skin abscesses. To diagnose an infection, a stain and culture for fungal elements is performed from the affected tissue.

Treating candidal fungal infections can be straightforward or very difficult. Oral, cutaneous, and vaginal infections can be treated with a course of oral antifungals such as fluconazole, nystatin, and clotrimazole. Candiduria, even if asymptomatic in renal transplant recipients, should be treated because many have diabetes, bladder dysfunction, and high-dose immunosuppressants that increase the risk for development of invasive disease [113]. Invasive disease requires intravenous treatment and should be accompanied by an evaluation for resistance and other complications related to systemic infection [114].

Cryptococcus

Cryptococcus neoformans is an organism that is found in soil with bird excrements, usually acquired through inhalation. Another emerging species of *Cryptococcus* is *C. gattii*, which is common in the Pacific Northwest [115–117]. Infection occurs in 2.8–4% of renal transplant recipients in America and Asia [118]. Presentation of cryptococcosis can be in the pulmonary (6%), skin and soft tissue (13%), and in the CNS (55%) [119]. Symptoms include skin lesions such as cellulitis, pneumonia, and CNS findings such as fever, headache, focal neurologic deficits, and mental status changes. Mortality has been reported to range from 42 to 63% [119, 120]. Cryptococcus neoformans infections can be treated with a 6-month course of fluconazole in less severe cases but, for significantly ill patients, will require treatment with amphotericin B and 5-flucytosine.

Posaconazole, itraconazole, and voriconazole all have comparable in vitro activity against *Cryptococcus* species [112].

Aspergillosis

Aspergillosis is caused mostly by *Aspergillus fumigatus*, which is a common mold in the environment and enters the body through inhalation of mold spores. Other species in the genus *Aspergillus* are capable of causing disease. Two studies found that *Aspergillus* species was one of the leading causes of fungal infections in post-kidney transplant patients, usually presenting in the first 6 months posttransplantation [108, 109]. Symptoms of infection include fever, cough, hemoptysis, and pleuritic chest pain where a pulmonary infection or aspergilloma is concerned. If the mold disseminates throughout the body, it can affect all body systems, including the CNS, and carries a 36–45% or higher mortality [121, 122].

Risk factors for infection include immunosuppressant therapy (corticosteroid and antilymphocyte antibody), antibiotic use and neutropenia, and underlying pulmonary disease [108, 121–123].

Diagnosis requires demonstrating the presence of *Aspergillus* in tissue through sampling the respiratory tract, which is highly suggestive of disease in high-risk patients [122]. The galactomannan assay is a test that detects an *Aspergillus*-specific cell wall polysaccharide which is released into the bloodstream with infections and can be used to help in diagnosis and correlates with outcomes, though it has its limitations with a significant false positive and false negative rate with a sensitivity of 81% and specificity of 89% [124, 125]. Thus, a high index for suspicion and thorough evaluation is paramount for diagnosis.

For decades the treatment of choice for disseminated aspergillosis was amphotericin B, with the now newer lipid soluble formulation of amphotericin B being less nephrotoxic [121]. Now, first-line treatment for invasive aspergillosis is voriconazole, which was shown in a randomized study to have a better survival (70.8% vs. 57.9%) and response rate (52.8% vs. 31.6%) compared to amphotericin B [126].

Mucormycosis

Mucormycosis is caused by fungi of the *Mucor*, *Rhizopus*, *Cunninghamella,* and *Absidia* species. These fungi are ubiquitous and uncommonly cause disease with an incidence in kidney transplant patients of 0.4–0.5 %, though when it does cause disease can have a 50–93 % mortality [127].

Risk factors for disease include diabetes, an immunocompromised state, immunosuppressant use, neutropenia, deferoxamine treatment for iron overload states, and treatment for allograft rejection [127].

Disease manifestations usually involve the rhino-orbital-cerebral area, pulmonary system, renal system, cutaneous changes, gastrointestinal tract, and CNS. Signs and symptoms include fever, headache, rhinosinusitis pain, orbit pain and swelling, eschar formation on the skin surrounding the nasosinus area, skin swelling, ophthalmoplegia, respiratory difficulties, and GI bleeding [127, 128].

Diagnosis usually involves evaluation with CT scan, culture, BAL, and pathologic evaluation of the affected tissue. Treatment usually includes extensive debridement of the affected and necrotic tissues, as well as intravenous lipid formulation of amphotericin B, while posaconazole is used as salvage therapy [127, 128].

Histoplasmosis/Coccidiomycosis

The endemic mycoses are histoplasmosis and coccidiomycosis. Histoplasmosis is caused by *Histoplasma capsulatum* and is found along the Ohio and Mississippi River Valleys with an incidence of symptomatic infection of 1 per 1,000 patient-years [129].

Disease can be a primary infection, reactivation, or acquired from the allograft [130]. Disease can be self-limited, causing findings such as fevers, pulmonary granulomas, rheumatologic findings, or skin cellulitis [131–133]. Histoplasmosis can present as disseminated disease involving multiple organ systems and cause disease of the liver, hematologic system, CNS, musculoskeletal system, and urinary system. It can lead to urinary tract obstruction, thrombotic microangiopathy, hepatitis, myofasciitis, meningitis, and cranial nerve palsies [131–133].

A diagnosis of histoplasmosis can be made through laboratory testing including the *Histoplasma* urine antigen testing, serology testing with complement and immunodiffusion, culture of affected tissue including possible BAL or bone marrow biopsy. Computed tomography (CT) scan may be useful and suggestive [129, 132]. Treatment for disseminated disease is with amphotericin B, followed by voriconazole or itraconazole for a prolonged course and for some, lifelong therapy [129].

Coccidiomycosis is caused by *Coccidioides immitis*, which is found in the Southwestern United States, Arizona, San Joaquin valley, northern Mexico, and some regions in South America. In areas where the Coccidioides is endemic, and if renal transplant recipients do not receive prophylaxis with an antifungal, the incidence of infection is 4–8 % [134, 135]. Infections can result from reactivation within the first year or new infection at any time after transplant.

Patients who have coccidiomycosis will have disseminated disease with several affected organ systems, including the skin, soft tissue and joints, pulmonary, renal, and CNS. Unlike histoplasmosis, coccidiomycosis carries a 22–72% mortality rate among findings from several studies [134, 136, 137].

Diagnosis of coccidiomycosis includes serologic testing and cultures from affected tissue.

Treatment for this disease is usually with amphotericin B, followed by long-term suppressive therapy with itraconazole, fluconazole, or ketoconazole [134, 136, 137].

Pneumocystis

Pneumocystis jirovecii is a fungus that causes pneumonia in those who are immunosuppressed with corticosteroids, HIV-infected patients, those with cancer or undergoing chemotherapy, and those with impaired cellular immunity. It will lead to disease in approximately 6–20 % of transplanted patients who do not receive prophylaxis after transplantation [23, 138].

Risk factors for infection include a history of allograft rejection, infection with CMV, tuberculosis, immunomodulating viruses, and immunosuppressant use [139, 140]. Of note, there has also been interhuman transmission of *Pneumocystis*, causing outbreaks of the disease [141–143].

The presentation of *P. jirovecii* usually includes a nonproductive cough, fever, and dyspnea, and findings on physical exam include hypoxia. Laboratory and imaging that will assist in the diagnosis of the infection include an elevated lactate dehydrogenase, infiltrate on chest X-ray or CT, and BAL or sputum showing the organisms on silver stain or antibody testing.

Treatment for the disease includes TMP–SMX or primaquine/clindamycin or atovaquone and steroids if needed to decrease inflammation [144]. Prophylaxis medications include low dose TMP–SMX, atovaquone, or inhaled pentamidine [145, 146]. Dapsone may be used for prophylaxis but is not effective for treatment.

Mycobacterium Tuberculosis

Mycobacterium tuberculosis infection ranges from 1.2 to 15 % among transplant recipients [147]. The disease usually occurs through reactivation within the first year posttransplantation, however, can occur at any time posttransplant and can occur through allograft transmission [147].

Risk factors for the development of disease include travel to or living in endemic areas, extremes of age, previous gastrointestinal surgery, diabetes, CMV, kidney or liver disease, and immunosuppressant therapy.

The most common presentations for *M. tuberculosis* are pulmonary infection with fever, cough, weight loss and focal (40%) or miliary pattern (22%) on chest X-ray, or disseminated disease involving the gastrointestinal, musculoskeletal, integumentary, renal, and CNS [147]. Mortality for patients with TB is 30%, higher for disseminated disease.

The pre-transplant time period should focus on questioning recipients and donors on risk factors, exposures, prior positive PPD, and any previous treatment. A positive PPD in patients with CKD/ESRD prior to transplant is >5 mm of induration and evidence of disease on CXR or close contact with TB. If a PPD is positive prior to transplantation, these patients should undergo treatment for latent TB [148].

The evaluation of a patient suspected of TB includes three induced sputum collected in the morning and sent for acid fast bacilli and culture. If these patients are unable to provide adequate samples, a bronchoscopy with BAL fluid can be sent. Other bodily fluids or tissue, if suspected of being infected, can be sent for stain and culture. The QuantiFERON-TB Gold test and T-SPOT.TB test can be used to help in the diagnosis of latent and active TB infection in lieu of the tuberculin skin test, along with radiographic, history, and other diagnostics [149]. The advantage of these tests is that they are not affected by a previous immunization with the BCG [149].

Pre-transplant patients who are diagnosed with latent TB should receive either treatment with isoniazid (INH) for 6–9 months or rifampin for 4 months. The shorter courses are usually due to concerns for compliance or drug–drug interaction, cost, or adverse side effects [148]. Active TB is treated with a directly observed four drug combination of INH, rifampin, pyrazinamide, and ethambutol. After the first 2 months, the treatment lasts for another 4–7 months [150]. Due to the risk of drug interactions and liver abnormalities with some of these medications, posttransplant patients receiving active treatment should be followed closely. For instance, rifampin and INH will induce hepatic cytochrome P450 enzyme, resulting in increased metabolism of cyclosporine, tacrolimus, and sirolimus.

Evaluation of Fevers

Transplant patients commonly develop fevers. In cases where transplant recipients present with significant graft dysfunction and fever, one should consider rejection as a possibility. Due to more potent immunosuppressive agents, the presentation of acute rejection with fever is less common. As a result of the masking ability of immunosuppressants, kidney transplant recipients may not present with typical symptoms and signs of infection. A high index of suspicion combined with knowledge of the environmental exposures, risk, and potential infections that occur during specific times after transplantation will assist transplant practitioners in their evaluation and diagnostic testing. Cultures of blood and urine, as well as chest X-ray, are obtained. Depending on the presence or absence of previous exposure, a CMV and EBV PCR should be sent. BK uncommonly causes fever. Sputum gram stain and culture are obtained if possible, but if patients are unable to produce sputum and have evidence of an infiltrate, bronchoscopy with BAL may be required. For those with pneumonia, evaluation for active TB is needed if there is an exposure history or previous treatment for latent TB, and evaluation may be needed for *P. jirovecii* if patients only have a limited duration of prophylaxis with TMP–SMX.

Empiric broad-spectrum antibiotic therapy is started in patients until an infectious etiology is discovered and antibiotics can be tailored to the specific organism. Fluoroquinolones and azithromycin may be used for outpatients as initial therapy. Doses for fluoroquinolones may require adjustment, and azithromycin is the only macrolide antibiotic that does not inhibit the cytochrome P450 system and cause elevations in CNI levels. For patients who are hospitalized, it is customary to begin empiric antibiotics with ceftazidime or cefepime with vancomycin for the first 48–72 h pending the results of cultures.

Conclusions

In conclusion, infections continue to be a source of significant morbidity and mortality among kidney transplant recipients. This chapter has provided a summary of the most common non-opportunistic and opportunistic infections that afflict the posttransplant population. The practitioners who care for these patients must remain vigilant and pursue an infectious work-up whenever there is a possibility of infection.

References

1. Wolfe RA, Ashby VB, Milford EL, Ojo AO, Ettenger RE, Agodoa LY, et al. Comparison of mortality in all patients on dialysis, patients on dialysis awaiting transplantation, and recipients of a first cadaveric transplant. N Engl J Med. 1999;341(23):1725–30.
2. U.S. Renal Data System, USRDS 2011 Annual data report: atlas of chronic kidney disease and end-stage renal disease in the United States, National Institutes of Health, National Institute of Diabetes and Digestive and Kidney Diseases, Bethesda, MD, 2011
3. Vanholder R, Van Loo A, Dhondt AM, De Smet R, Ringoir S. Influence of uraemia and haemodialysis on host defence and infection. Nephrol Dial Transplant. 1996;11(4):593–8.
4. Fishman JA. Infection in solid-organ transplant recipients. N Engl J Med. 2007;357(25):2601–14.
5. Huzly D, Neifer S, Reinke P, Schroder K, Schonfeld C, Hofmann T, et al. Routine immunizations in adult renal transplant recipients. Transplantation. 1997;63(6):839–45.
6. Kazancioglu R, Sever MS, Yuksel-Onel D, Eraksoy H, Yildiz A, Celik AV, et al. Immunization of renal transplant recipients with pneumococcal polysaccharide vaccine. Clin Transplant. 2000;14(1):61–5.
7. Guidelines for vaccination of solid organ transplant candidates and recipients. Am J Transplant. 2004;4 Suppl 10:160–3.
8. Furth SL, Fivush BA. Varicella vaccination in pediatric kidney transplant candidates. Pediatr Transplant. 2002;6(2):97–100.
9. Ison MG, Nalesnik MA. An update on donor-derived disease transmission in organ transplantation. Am J Transplant. 2011; 11(6):1123–30.
10. Scientific Registry of Transplant Recipients (SRTR). 2009.
11. Midtvedt K, Hartmann A, Midtvedt T, Brekke IB. Routine perioperative antibiotic prophylaxis in renal transplantation. Nephrol Dial Transplant. 1998;13(7):1637–41.
12. Salehipour M, Salahi H, Fathikalajahi A, Mohammadian R, Emadmarvasti V, Bahador A, et al. Is perioperative intravesically applied antibiotic solution effective in the prophylaxis of urinary tract infections after renal transplantation? Urol Int. 2010;85(1):66–9.
13. Nauseef WM, Maki DG. A study of the value of simple protective isolation in patients with granulocytopenia. N Engl J Med. 1981;304(8):448–53.
14. Tolkoff-Rubin NE, Rubin RH. Urinary tract infection in the immunocompromised host. Lessons from kidney transplantation and the AIDS epidemic. Infect Dis Clin North Am. 1997;11(3): 707–17.
15. Trzeciak S, Sharer R, Piper D, Chan T, Kessler C, Dellinger RP, et al. Infections and severe sepsis in solid-organ transplant patients admitted from a university-based ED. Am J Emerg Med. 2004;22(7):530–3.
16. Alangaden GJ, Thyagarajan R, Gruber SA, Morawski K, Garnick J, El-Amm JM, et al. Infectious complications after kidney transplantation: current epidemiology and associated risk factors. Clin Transplant. 2006;20(4):401–9.
17. Vidal E, Torre-Cisneros J, Blanes M, Montejo M, Cervera C, Aguado JM, et al. Bacterial urinary tract infection after solid organ transplantation in the RESITRA cohort. Transpl Infect Dis. 2012;14(6):595–603.
18. Fox BC, Sollinger HW, Belzer FO, Maki DG. A prospective, randomized, double-blind study of trimethoprim-sulfamethoxazole for prophylaxis of infection in renal transplantation: clinical efficacy, absorption of trimethoprim-sulfamethoxazole, effects on the microflora, and the cost-benefit of prophylaxis. Am J Med. 1990;89(3):255–74.
19. Rabkin DG, Stifelman MD, Birkhoff J, Richardson KA, Cohen D, Nowygrod R, et al. Early catheter removal decreases incidence of urinary tract infections in renal transplant recipients. Transplant Proc. 1998;30(8):4314–6.
20. Wagener MM, Yu VL. Bacteremia in transplant recipients: a prospective study of demographics, etiologic agents, risk factors, and outcomes. Am J Infect Control. 1992;20(5):239–47.
21. Kutinova A, Woodward RS, Ricci JF, Brennan DC. The incidence and costs of sepsis and pneumonia before and after renal transplantation in the United States. Am J Transplant. 2006;6(1): 129–39.
22. Chang GC, Wu CL, Pan SH, Yang TY, Chin CS, Yang YC, et al. The diagnosis of pneumonia in renal transplant recipients using invasive and noninvasive procedures. Chest. 2004;125(2): 541–7.
23. Reichenberger F, Dickenmann M, Binet I, Soler M, Bolliger C, Steiger J, et al. Diagnostic yield of bronchoalveolar lavage following renal transplantation. Transpl Infect Dis. 2001;3(1):2–7.
24. Mermel LA, Maki DG. Bacterial pneumonia in solid organ transplantation. Semin Respir Infect. 1990;5(1):10–29.
25. Sileri P, Pursell KJ, Coady NT, Giacomoni A, Berliti S, Tzoracoleftherakis E, et al. A standardized protocol for the treatment of severe pneumonia in kidney transplant recipients. Clin Transplant. 2002;16(6):450–4.
26. Humar A, Ramcharan T, Denny R, Gillingham KJ, Payne WD, Matas AJ. Are wound complications after a kidney transplant more common with modern immunosuppression? Transplantation. 2001;72(12):1920–3.
27. Koyle MA, Ward HJ, Twomey PA, Glassock RJ, Rajfer J. Declining incidence of wound infection in cadaveric renal transplant recipient. Urology. 1988;31(2):103–6.
28. Yu X, Han F, Wu J, He Q, Peng W, Wang Y, et al. Nocardia infection in kidney transplant recipients: case report and analysis of 66 published cases. Transpl Infect Dis. 2011;13(4):385–91.
29. Horl MP, Schmitz M, Ivens K, Grabensee B. Opportunistic infections after renal transplantation. Curr Opin Urol. 2002;12(2): 115–23.
30. Wilson JP, Turner HR, Kirchner KA, Chapman SW. Nocardial infections in renal transplant recipients. Medicine (Baltimore). 1989;68(1):38–57.
31. Waterer GW, Baselski VS, Wunderink RG. Legionella and community-acquired pneumonia: a review of current diagnostic tests from a clinician's viewpoint. Am J Med. 2001;110(1): 41–8.
32. MacGowan AP, Marshall RJ, MacKay IM, Reeves DS. Listeria faecal carriage by renal transplant recipients, haemodialysis patients and patients in general practice: its relation to season, drug therapy, foreign travel, animal exposure and diet. Epidemiol Infect. 1991;106(1):157–66.

33. Stamm AM, Dismukes WE, Simmons BP, Cobbs CG, Elliott A, Budrich P, et al. Listeriosis in renal transplant recipients: report of an outbreak and review of 102 cases. Rev Infect Dis. 1982;4(3):665–82.
34. Sia IG, Patel R. New strategies for prevention and therapy of cytomegalovirus infection and disease in solid-organ transplant recipients. Clin Microbiol Rev. 2000;13(1):83–121; table of contents.
35. Bataille S, Moal V, Gaudart J, Indreies M, Purgus R, Dussol B, et al. Cytomegalovirus risk factors in renal transplantation with modern immunosuppression. Transpl Infect Dis. 2010;12(6):480–8.
36. Preiksaitis JK, Brennan DC, Fishman J, Allen U. Canadian society of transplantation consensus workshop on cytomegalovirus management in solid organ transplantation final report. Am J Transplant. 2005;5(2):218–27.
37. Khoury JA, Storch GA, Bohl DL, Schuessler RM, Torrence SM, Lockwood M, et al. Prophylactic versus preemptive oral valganciclovir for the management of cytomegalovirus infection in adult renal transplant recipients. Am J Transplant. 2006;6(9):2134–43.
38. Hodson EM, Barclay PG, Craig JC, Jones C, Kable K, Strippoli GF, et al. Antiviral medications for preventing cytomegalovirus disease in solid organ transplant recipients. Cochrane Database Syst Rev. 2005;4, CD003774.
39. Jassal SV, Roscoe JM, Zaltzman JS, Mazzulli T, Krajden M, Gadawski M, et al. Clinical practice guidelines: prevention of cytomegalovirus disease after renal transplantation. J Am Soc Nephrol. 1998;9(9):1697–708.
40. Snydman DR, Werner BG, Heinze-Lacey B, Berardi VP, Tilney NL, Kirkman RL, et al. Use of cytomegalovirus immune globulin to prevent cytomegalovirus disease in renal-transplant recipients. N Engl J Med. 1987;317(17):1049–54.
41. Limaye AP, Corey L, Koelle DM, Davis CL, Boeckh M. Emergence of ganciclovir-resistant cytomegalovirus disease among recipients of solid-organ transplants. Lancet. 2000;356(9230):645–9.
42. Geddes CC, Church CC, Collidge T, McCruden EA, Gillespie G, Matthews E, et al. Management of cytomegalovirus infection by weekly surveillance after renal transplant: analysis of cost, rejection and renal function. Nephrol Dial Transplant. 2003;18(9):1891–8.
43. Kidney Disease: Improving Global Outcomes (KDIGO) Transplant Work Group. KDIGO clinical practice guideline for the care of kidney transplant recipients. Am J Transplant. 2009;9 Suppl 3:S1–155.
44. Emery VC. Prophylaxis for CMV should not now replace preemptive therapy in solid organ transplantation. Rev Med Virol. 2001;11(2):83–6.
45. Blumberg EA, Hauser IA, Stanisic S, Mueller E, Berenson K, Gahlemann CG, et al. Prolonged prophylaxis with valganciclovir is cost effective in reducing posttransplant cytomegalovirus disease within the United States. Transplantation. 2010;90(12):1420–6.
46. Boillat Blanco N, Pascual M, Venetz JP, Nseir G, Meylan PR, Manuel O. Impact of a preemptive strategy after 3 months of valganciclovir cytomegalovirus prophylaxis in kidney transplant recipients. Transplantation. 2011;91(2):251–5.
47. Humar A, Lebranchu Y, Vincenti F, Blumberg EA, Punch JD, Limaye AP, et al. The efficacy and safety of 200 days valganciclovir cytomegalovirus prophylaxis in high-risk kidney transplant recipients. Am J Transplant. 2010;10(5):1228–37.
48. Humar A, Limaye AP, Blumberg EA, Hauser IA, Vincenti F, Jardine AG, et al. Extended valganciclovir prophylaxis in D+/R− kidney transplant recipients is associated with long-term reduction in cytomegalovirus disease: two-year results of the IMPACT study. Transplantation. 2010;90(12):1427–31.
49. Paya C, Humar A, Dominguez E, Washburn K, Blumberg E, Alexander B, et al. Efficacy and safety of valganciclovir vs. oral ganciclovir for prevention of cytomegalovirus disease in solid organ transplant recipients. Am J Transplant. 2004;4(4):611–20.
50. Pescovitz MD. Absence of teratogenicity of oral ganciclovir used during early pregnancy in a liver transplant recipient. Transplantation. 1999;67(5):758–9.
51. Small LN, Lau J, Snydman DR. Preventing post-organ transplantation cytomegalovirus disease with ganciclovir: a meta-analysis comparing prophylactic and preemptive therapies. Clin Infect Dis. 2006;43(7):869–80.
52. Asberg A, Humar A, Rollag H, Jardine AG, Mouas H, Pescovitz MD, et al. Oral valganciclovir is noninferior to intravenous ganciclovir for the treatment of cytomegalovirus disease in solid organ transplant recipients. Am J Transplant. 2007;7(9):2106–13.
53. Baldanti F, Lurain N, Gerna G. Clinical and biologic aspects of human cytomegalovirus resistance to antiviral drugs. Hum Immunol. 2004;65(5):403–9.
54. Drew WL, Miner RC, Marousek GI, Chou S. Maribavir sensitivity of cytomegalovirus isolates resistant to ganciclovir, cidofovir or foscarnet. J Clin Virol. 2006;37(2):124–7.
55. Bacon TH, Levin MJ, Leary JJ, Sarisky RT, Sutton D. Herpes simplex virus resistance to acyclovir and penciclovir after two decades of antiviral therapy. Clin Microbiol Rev. 2003;16(1):114–28.
56. Hempenstall K, Nurmikko TJ, Johnson RW, A'Hern RP, Rice AS. Analgesic therapy in postherpetic neuralgia: a quantitative systematic review. PLoS Med. 2005;2(7):e164.
57. Khameneh ZR, Soin J, Durlik M, Lao M, Paczek L, Gaciong Z. Factors affecting reactivation of Epstein-Barr virus infection after kidney allograft transplantation. Ann Transplant. 1999;4(2):18–22.
58. Comoli P, Maccario R, Locatelli F, Valente U, Basso S, Garaventa A, et al. Treatment of EBV-related post-renal transplant lymphoproliferative disease with a tailored regimen including EBV-specific T cells. Am J Transplant. 2005;5(6):1415–22.
59. Larsen CP, Grinyo J, Medina-Pestana J, Vanrenterghem Y, Vincenti F, Breshahan B, et al. Belatacept-based regimens versus a cyclosporine A-based regimen in kidney transplant recipients: 2-year results from the BENEFIT and BENEFIT-EXT studies. Transplantation. 2010;90(12):1528–35.
60. Martin SI, Dodson B, Wheeler C, Davis J, Pesavento T, Bumgardner GL. Monitoring infection with Epstein-Barr virus among seromismatch adult renal transplant recipients. Am J Transplant. 2011;11(5):1058–63.
61. Comoli P, Labirio M, Basso S, Baldanti F, Grossi P, Furione M, et al. Infusion of autologous Epstein-Barr virus (EBV)-specific cytotoxic T cells for prevention of EBV-related lymphoproliferative disorder in solid organ transplant recipients with evidence of active virus replication. Blood. 2002;99(7):2592–8.
62. Khanna R, Bell S, Sherritt M, Galbraith A, Burrows SR, Rafter L, et al. Activation and adoptive transfer of Epstein-Barr virus-specific cytotoxic T cells in solid organ transplant patients with posttransplant lymphoproliferative disease. Proc Natl Acad Sci U S A. 1999;96(18):10391–6.
63. Rossi C, Delforge ML, Jacobs F, Wissing M, Pradier O, Remmelink M, et al. Fatal primary infection due to human herpes virus 6 variant A in a renal transplant recipient. Transplantation. 2001;71(2):288–92.
64. Yoshida M, Yamada M, Tsukazaki T, Chatterjee S, Lakeman FD, Nii S, et al. Comparison of antiviral compounds against human herpes virus 6 and 7. Antiviral Res. 1998;40(1–2):73–84.
65. Kidd IM, Clark DA, Sabin CA, Andrew D, Hassan-Walker AF, Sweny P, et al. Prospective study of human betaherpesviruses after renal transplantation: association of human herpesvirus 7 and cytomegalovirus co-infection with cytomegalovirus disease and increased rejection. Transplantation. 2000;69(11):2400–4.

66. Zhang Y, Schols D, De Clercq E. Selective activity of various antiviral compounds against HHV-7 infection. Antiviral Res. 1999;43(1):23–35.
67. Schulz TF, Moore PS. Kaposi's sarcoma-associated herpesvirus: a new human tumor virus, but how? Trends Microbiol. 1999;7(5): 196–200.
68. Regamey N, Tamm M, Wernli M, Witschi A, Thiel G, Cathomas G, et al. Transmission of human herpesvirus 8 infection from renal-transplant donors to recipients. N Engl J Med. 1998; 339(19):1358–63.
69. Antman K, Chang Y. Kaposi's sarcoma. N Engl J Med. 2000;342(14):1027–38.
70. Hosseini-Moghaddam SM, Soleimanirahbar A, Mazzulli T, Rotstein C, Husain S. Post renal transplantation Kaposi's sarcoma: a review of its epidemiology, pathogenesis, diagnosis, clinical aspects, and therapy. Transpl Infect Dis. 2012;14(4):338–45.
71. Martin DF, Kuppermann BD, Wolitz RA, Palestine AG, Li H, Robinson CA. Oral ganciclovir for patients with cytomegalovirus retinitis treated with a ganciclovir implant. Roche Ganciclovir Study Group. N Engl J Med. 1999;340(14):1063–70.
72. Fabrizi F, Dulai G, Dixit V, Bunnapradist S, Martin P. Lamivudine for the treatment of hepatitis B virus-related liver disease after renal transplantation: meta-analysis of clinical trials. Transplantation. 2004;77(6):859–64.
73. Rao KV, Kasiske BL, Anderson WR. Variability in the morphological spectrum and clinical outcome of chronic liver disease in hepatitis B-positive and B-negative renal transplant recipients. Transplantation. 1991;51(2):391–6.
74. Rao KV, Ma J. Chronic viral hepatitis enhances the risk of infection but not acute rejection in renal transplant recipients. Transplantation. 1996;62(12):1765–9.
75. Roberts RC, Lane C, Hatfield P, Clutterbuck E, Atkins M, Brown A, et al. All anti-HBc-positive, HBsAg-negative dialysis patients on the transplant waiting list should be regarded as at risk of hepatitis B reactivation post-renal transplantation—report of three cases from a single centre. Nephrol Dial Transplant. 2006;21(11): 3316–9.
76. Boletis JN. Epidemiology and mode of transmission of hepatitis C virus infection after renal transplantation. Nephrol Dial Transplant. 2000;15 Suppl 8:52–4.
77. Kallinowski B, Hergesell O, Zeier M. Clinical impact of hepatitis C virus infection in the renal transplant recipient. Nephron. 2002;91(4):541–6.
78. Mathurin P, Mouquet C, Poynard T, Sylla C, Benalia H, Fretz C, et al. Impact of hepatitis B and C virus on kidney transplantation outcome. Hepatology. 1999;29(1):257–63.
79. Perni RB, Almquist SJ, Byrn RA, Chandorkar G, Chaturvedi PR, Courtney LF, et al. Preclinical profile of VX-950, a potent, selective, and orally bioavailable inhibitor of hepatitis C virus NS3-4A serine protease. Antimicrob Agents Chemother. 2006;50(3): 899–909.
80. Hezode C, Forestier N, Dusheiko G, Ferenci P, Pol S, Goeser T, et al. Telaprevir and peginterferon with or without ribavirin for chronic HCV infection. N Engl J Med. 2009;360(18):1839–50.
81. McHutchison JG, Lawitz EJ, Shiffman ML, Muir AJ, Galler GW, McCone J, et al. Peginterferon alfa-2b or alfa-2a with ribavirin for treatment of hepatitis C infection. N Engl J Med. 2009;361(6): 580–93.
82. Legrand-Abravanel F, Colson P, Leguillou-Guillemette H, Alric L, Ravaux I, Lunel-Fabiani F, et al. Influence of the HCV subtype on the virological response to pegylated interferon and ribavirin therapy. J Med Virol. 2009;81(12):2029–35.
83. Jacobson IM, McHutchison JG, Dusheiko G, Di Bisceglie AM, Reddy KR, Bzowej NH, et al. Telaprevir for previously untreated chronic hepatitis C virus infection. N Engl J Med. 2011; 364(25):2405–16.
84. Zeuzem S, Andreone P, Pol S, Lawitz E, Diago M, Roberts S, et al. Telaprevir for retreatment of HCV infection. N Engl J Med. 2011;364(25):2417–28.
85. Bacon BR, Gordon SC, Lawitz E, Marcellin P, Vierling JM, Zeuzem S, et al. Boceprevir for previously treated chronic HCV genotype 1 infection. N Engl J Med. 2011;364(13):1207–17.
86. Muir AJ, Bornstein JD, Killenberg PG. Peginterferon alfa-2b and ribavirin for the treatment of chronic hepatitis C in blacks and non-Hispanic whites. N Engl J Med. 2004;350(22):2265–71.
87. Poordad F, McCone Jr J, Bacon BR, Bruno S, Manns MP, Sulkowski MS, et al. Boceprevir for untreated chronic HCV genotype 1 infection. N Engl J Med. 2011;364(13):1195–206.
88. Charlton M. Telaprevir, boceprevir, cytochrome P450 and immunosuppressive agents—a potentially lethal cocktail. Hepatology. 2011;54(1):3–5.
89. Garg V, van Heeswijk R, Lee JE, Alves K, Nadkarni P, Luo X. Effect of telaprevir on the pharmacokinetics of cyclosporine and tacrolimus. Hepatology. 2011;54(1):20–7.
90. Broeders NE, Hombrouck A, Lemy A, Wissing KM, Racape J, Gastaldello K, et al. Influenza A/H1N1 vaccine in patients treated by kidney transplant or dialysis: a cohort study. Clin J Am Soc Nephrol. 2011;6(11):2573–8.
91. Esposito S, Meregalli E, Daleno C, Ghio L, Tagliabue C, Valzano A, et al. An open-label, randomized clinical trial assessing immunogenicity, safety and tolerability of pandemic influenza A/H1N1 MF59-adjuvanted vaccine administered sequentially or simultaneously with seasonal virosomal-adjuvanted influenza vaccine to paediatric kidney transplant recipients. Nephrol Dial Transplant. 2011;26(6):2018–24.
92. Morales-Buenrostro LE, Terasaki PI, Marino-Vazquez LA, Lee JH, El-Awar N, Alberu J. "Natural" human leukocyte antigen antibodies found in nonalloimmunized healthy males. Transplantation. 2008;86(8):1111–5.
93. Roddy M, Clemente M, Poggio ED, Bukowski R, Thakkar S, Waxenecker G, et al. Heterogeneous alterations in human alloimmunity associated with immunization. Transplantation. 2005; 80(3):297–302.
94. Alberu J, Morales-Buenrostro LE, de Leo C, Vargas-Rojas MI, Marino-Vazquez LA, Crispin JC. A non-allogeneic stimulus triggers the production of de novo HLA antibodies in healthy adults. Transpl Immunol. 2007;18(2):166–71.
95. Brakemeier S, Schweiger B, Lachmann N, Glander P, Schonemann C, Diekmann F, et al. Immune response to an adjuvanted influenza A H1N1 vaccine (Pandemrix((R))) in renal transplant recipients. Nephrol Dial Transplant. 2012;27(1):423–8.
96. Katerinis I, Hadaya K, Duquesnoy R, Ferrari-Lacraz S, Meier S, van Delden C, et al. De novo anti-HLA antibody after pandemic H1N1 and seasonal influenza immunization in kidney transplant recipients. Am J Transplant. 2011;11(8):1727–33.
97. Kumar D, Campbell P, Humar A. Donor-specific alloantibody upregulation after influenza vaccination in transplant recipients. Am J Transplant. 2011;11(11):2538; author's reply 9–40.
98. Danziger-Isakov L, Cherkassky L, Siegel H, McManamon M, Kramer K, Budev M, et al. Effects of influenza immunization on humoral and cellular alloreactivity in humans. Transplantation. 2010;89(7):838–44.
99. Candon S, Thervet E, Lebon P, Suberbielle C, Zuber J, Lima C, et al. Humoral and cellular immune responses after influenza vaccination in kidney transplant recipients. Am J Transplant. 2009;9(10):2346–54.
100. Kumar D, Blumberg EA, Danziger-Isakov L, Kotton CN, Halasa NB, Ison MG, et al. Influenza vaccination in the organ transplant recipient: review and summary recommendations. Am J Transplant. 2011;11(10):2020–30.
101. Manuel O, Humar A, Chen MH, Chernenko S, Singer LG, Cobos I, et al. Immunogenicity and safety of an intradermal boosting

strategy for vaccination against influenza in lung transplant recipients. Am J Transplant. 2007;7(11):2567–72.
102. Mazuecos A, Fernandez A, Andres A, Gomez E, Zarraga S. Kidney transplantation outcomes in HIV infection: the European experience. Am J Transplant. 2011;11(3):635–6.
103. Qiu J, Terasaki PI, Waki K, Cai J, Gjertson DW. HIV-positive renal recipients can achieve survival rates similar to those of HIV-negative patients. Transplantation. 2006;81(12):1658–61.
104. Roland ME, Barin B, Carlson L, Frassetto LA, Terrault NA, Hirose R, et al. HIV-infected liver and kidney transplant recipients: 1- and 3-year outcomes. Am J Transplant. 2008;8(2):355–65.
105. Stock PG, Barin B, Murphy B, Hanto D, Diego JM, Light J, et al. Outcomes of kidney transplantation in HIV-infected recipients. N Engl J Med. 2010;363(21):2004–14.
106. Frassetto LA, Browne M, Cheng A, Wolfe AR, Roland ME, Stock PG, et al. Immunosuppressant pharmacokinetics and dosing modifications in HIV-1 infected liver and kidney transplant recipients. Am J Transplant. 2007;7(12):2816–20.
107. Kumar MS, Sierka DR, Damask AM, Fyfe B, McAlack RF, Heifets M, et al. Safety and success of kidney transplantation and concomitant immunosuppression in HIV-positive patients. Kidney Int. 2005;67(4):1622–9.
108. Altiparmak MR, Apaydin S, Trablus S, Serdengecti K, Ataman R, Ozturk R, et al. Systemic fungal infections after renal transplantation. Scand J Infect Dis. 2002;34(4):284–8.
109. Pappas PG, Alexander BD, Andes DR, Hadley S, Kauffman CA, Freifeld A, et al. Invasive fungal infections among organ transplant recipients: results of the Transplant-Associated Infection Surveillance Network (TRANSNET). Clin Infect Dis. 2010; 50(8):1101–11.
110. Tharayil John G, Shankar V, Talaulikar G, Mathews MS, Abraham Abraham M, Punnakuzhathil Thomas P, et al. Epidemiology of systemic mycoses among renal-transplant recipients in India. Transplantation. 2003;75(9):1544–51.
111. Howard RJ, Simmons RL, Najarian JS. Fungal infections in renal transplant recipients. Ann Surg. 1978;188(5):598–605.
112. Sabatelli F, Patel R, Mann PA, Mendrick CA, Norris CC, Hare R, et al. In vitro activities of posaconazole, fluconazole, itraconazole, voriconazole, and amphotericin B against a large collection of clinically important molds and yeasts. Antimicrob Agents Chemother. 2006;50(6):2009–15.
113. Edwards Jr JE, Bodey GP, Bowden RA, Buchner T, de Pauw BE, Filler SG, et al. international conference for the development of a consensus on the management and prevention of severe candidal infections. Clin Infect Dis. 1997;25(1):43–59.
114. Pappas PG, Rex JH, Sobel JD, Filler SG, Dismukes WE, Walsh TJ, et al. Guidelines for treatment of candidiasis. Clin Infect Dis. 2004;38(2):161–89.
115. Datta K, Bartlett KH, Baer R, Byrnes E, Galanis E, Heitman J, et al. Spread of Cryptococcus gattii into Pacific Northwest region of the United States. Emerg Infect Dis. 2009;15(8):1185–91.
116. Kidd SE, Hagen F, Tscharke RL, Huynh M, Bartlett KH, Fyfe M, et al. A rare genotype of Cryptococcus gattii caused the cryptococcosis outbreak on Vancouver Island (British Columbia, Canada). Proc Natl Acad Sci U S A. 2004;101(49):17258–63.
117. MacDougall L, Kidd SE, Galanis E, Mak S, Leslie MJ, Cieslak PR, et al. Spread of Cryptococcus gattii in British Columbia, Canada, and detection in the Pacific Northwest, USA. Emerg Infect Dis. 2007;13(1):42–50.
118. John GT, Mathew M, Snehalatha E, Anandi V, Date A, Jacob CK, et al. Cryptococcosis in renal allograft recipients. Transplantation. 1994;58(7):855–6.
119. Husain S, Wagener MM, Singh N. Cryptococcus neoformans infection in organ transplant recipients: variables influencing clinical characteristics and outcome. Emerg Infect Dis. 2001;7(3): 375–81.
120. Chugh KS, Sakhuja V, Jain S, Talwar P, Minz M, Joshi K, et al. High mortality in systemic fungal infections following renal transplantation in third-world countries. Nephrol Dial Transplant. 1993;8(2):168–72.
121. Bowden R, Chandrasekar P, White MH, Li X, Pietrelli L, Gurwith M, et al. A double-blind, randomized, controlled trial of amphotericin B colloidal dispersion versus amphotericin B for treatment of invasive aspergillosis in immunocompromised patients. Clin Infect Dis. 2002;35(4):359–66.
122. Perfect JR, Cox GM, Lee JY, Kauffman CA, de Repentigny L, Chapman SW, et al. The impact of culture isolation of Aspergillus species: a hospital-based survey of aspergillosis. Clin Infect Dis. 2001;33(11):1824–33.
123. Gustafson TL, Schaffner W, Lavely GB, Stratton CW, Johnson HK, Hutcheson Jr RH. Invasive aspergillosis in renal transplant recipients: correlation with corticosteroid therapy. J Infect Dis. 1983;148(2):230–8.
124. Miceli MH, Grazziutti ML, Woods G, Zhao W, Kocoglu MH, Barlogie B, et al. Strong correlation between serum Aspergillus galactomannan index and outcome of aspergillosis in patients with hematological cancer: clinical and research implications. Clin Infect Dis. 2008;46(9):1412–22.
125. Wheat LJ. Rapid diagnosis of invasive aspergillosis by antigen detection. Transpl Infect Dis. 2003;5(4):158–66.
126. Herbrecht R, Denning DW, Patterson TF, Bennett JE, Greene RE, Oestmann JW, et al. Voriconazole versus amphotericin B for primary therapy of invasive aspergillosis. N Engl J Med. 2002;347(6): 408–15.
127. Almyroudis NG, Sutton DA, Linden P, Rinaldi MG, Fung J, Kusne S. Zygomycosis in solid organ transplant recipients in a tertiary transplant center and review of the literature. Am J Transplant. 2006;6(10):2365–74.
128. Aslani J, Eizadi M, Kardavani B, Khoddami-Vishteh HR, Nemati E, Hoseini SM, et al. Mucormycosis after kidney transplantations: report of seven cases. Scand J Infect Dis. 2007;39(8):703–6.
129. Cuellar-Rodriguez J, Avery RK, Lard M, Budev M, Gordon SM, Shrestha NK, et al. Histoplasmosis in solid organ transplant recipients: 10 years of experience at a large transplant center in an endemic area. Clin Infect Dis. 2009;49(5):710–6.
130. Limaye AP, Connolly PA, Sagar M, Fritsche TR, Cookson BT, Wheat LJ, et al. Transmission of Histoplasma capsulatum by organ transplantation. N Engl J Med. 2000;343(16):1163–6.
131. Davies SF, Sarosi GA, Peterson PK, Khan M, Howard RJ, Simmons RL, et al. Disseminated histoplasmosis in renal transplant recipients. Am J Surg. 1979;137(5):686–91.
132. Wheat LJ, Kohler RB, Tewari RP. Diagnosis of disseminated histoplasmosis by detection of Histoplasma capsulatum antigen in serum and urine specimens. N Engl J Med. 1986;314(2):83–8.
133. Wheat LJ, Smith EJ, Sathapatayavongs B, Batteiger B, Filo RS, Leapman SB, et al. Histoplasmosis in renal allograft recipients. Two large urban outbreaks. Arch Intern Med. 1983;143(4): 703–7.
134. Braddy CM, Heilman RL, Blair JE. Coccidioidomycosis after renal transplantation in an endemic area. Am J Transplant. 2006;6(2):340–5.
135. Cohen IM, Galgiani JN, Potter D, Ogden DA. Coccidioidomycosis in renal replacement therapy. Arch Intern Med. 1982;142(3): 489–94.
136. Blair JE. Coccidioidal pneumonia, arthritis, and soft-tissue infection after kidney transplantation. Transpl Infect Dis. 2004;6(2): 74–6.
137. Blair JE, Logan JL. Coccidioidomycosis in solid organ transplantation. Clin Infect Dis. 2001;33(9):1536–44.
138. Neff RT, Jindal RM, Yoo DY, Hurst FP, Agodoa LY, Abbott KC. Analysis of USRDS: incidence and risk factors for Pneumocystis jiroveci pneumonia. Transplantation. 2009;88(1):135–41.

139. Arend SM, Westendorp RG, Kroon FP, van't Wout JW, Vandenbroucke JP, van Es LA, et al. Rejection treatment and cytomegalovirus infection as risk factors for Pneumocystis carinii pneumonia in renal transplant recipients. Clin Infect Dis. 1996;22(6):920–5.
140. Radisic M, Lattes R, Chapman JF, del Carmen RM, Guardia O, Seu F, et al. Risk factors for Pneumocystis carinii pneumonia in kidney transplant recipients: a case–control study. Transpl Infect Dis. 2003;5(2):84–93.
141. Gianella S, Haeberli L, Joos B, Ledergerber B, Wuthrich RP, Weber R, et al. Molecular evidence of interhuman transmission in an outbreak of Pneumocystis jirovecii pneumonia among renal transplant recipients. Transpl Infect Dis. 2010;12(1):1–10.
142. Phipps LM, Chen SC, Kable K, Halliday CL, Firacative C, Meyer W, et al. Nosocomial Pneumocystis jirovecii pneumonia: lessons from a cluster in kidney transplant recipients. Transplantation. 2011;92(12):1327–34.
143. Yazaki H, Goto N, Uchida K, Kobayashi T, Gatanaga H, Oka S. Outbreak of Pneumocystis jiroveci pneumonia in renal transplant recipients: P. jiroveci is contagious to the susceptible host. Transplantation. 2009;88(3):380–5.
144. Goto N, Oka S. Pneumocystis jirovecii pneumonia in kidney transplantation. Transpl Infect Dis. 2011;13(6):551–8.
145. Gabardi S, Millen P, Hurwitz S, Martin S, Roberts K, Chandraker A. Atovaquone versus trimethoprim-sulfamethoxazole as Pneumocystis jirovecii pneumonia prophylaxis following renal transplantation. Clin Transplant. 2012;26(3):E184–90.
146. Saukkonen K, Garland R, Koziel H. Aerosolized pentamidine as alternative primary prophylaxis against Pneumocystis carinii pneumonia in adult hepatic and renal transplant recipients. Chest. 1996;109(5):1250–5.
147. Singh N, Paterson DL. Mycobacterium tuberculosis infection in solid-organ transplant recipients: impact and implications for management. Clin Infect Dis. 1998;27(5):1266–77.
148. Targeted tuberculin testing and treatment of latent tuberculosis infection. This official statement of the American Thoracic Society was adopted by the ATS Board of Directors, July 1999. This is a Joint Statement of the American Thoracic Society (ATS) and the Centers for Disease Control and Prevention (CDC). This statement was endorsed by the Council of the Infectious Diseases Society of America (IDSA), September 1999, and the sections of this statement. Am J Respir Crit Care Med. 2000;161(4 Pt 2):S221–47.
149. Mazurek GH, Jereb J, Vernon A, LoBue P, Goldberg S, Castro K. Updated guidelines for using interferon gamma release assays to detect Mycobacterium tuberculosis infection—United States, 2010. MMWR Recomm Rep. 2010;59(5):1–25.
150. Blumberg HM, Burman WJ, Chaisson RE, Daley CL, Etkind SC, Friedman LN, et al. American Thoracic Society/Centers for Disease Control and Prevention/Infectious Diseases Society of America: treatment of tuberculosis. Am J Respir Crit Care Med. 2003;167(4):603–62.

Human Polyomavirus (HPyV) and Organ Transplantation

28

Sabine Karam and Ravinder Wali

Human Polyomaviruses

Polyomaviruses are ubiquitous in nature. Human polyomaviruses (HPyV) are known for their high prevalence and long dormancy in the general population and risk of reactivation with immunological perturbations. Polyomavirus infects up to 90 % of the general population [1].

Polyomaviruses are small (30–45 nm), nonenveloped, circular double-stranded DNA viruses, with the genomic structure consisting early genes encoding the regulatory large T and small t antigens, the late genes encoding three viral capsid proteins (VP1, VP2, and VP3), and the agnoprotein. Agnoprotein plays a critical role in the assembly of viral particles. Viral gene expression is controlled by the noncoding control region (NCCR). After initial infection, host immune response consists of developing neutralizing antibodies that have been demonstrated to be targeted against the major capsid protein VP1, and these antibodies are closely correlated with antibody titers measured by hemagglutination inhibition titers [1]. VP1 is characterized by the presence of external loops, BC, DE, EF, GH, and HI, which are involved in receptor binding. Two of these loops (BC and EF) are prone to develop mutations [2]; however, the role of these mutations in the development of clinical disease is not well defined.

Different types of polyomaviruses have been reported during the past decade. Polyomaviral infection in humans was first reported from England and named BK virus (Patient initials; B.K.) and another type of polyomavirus was isolated from oligodendrocytes of a patient with human immunodeficiency virus (HIV) disease, named JC virus (patient initials: J.C.), each group reported the existence of these polymaviruses in humans independently of each other in 1971 [3, 4].

BKPyV and JCPyV circulate independently at both the individual and population levels. Individuals that have antibodies against BKPyV are often seronegative to JCPyV and vice versa [5].

BKPyV is highly prevalent as more than 85 % of the general population is seropositive after adulthood. BKPyV is divided into four different subtypes—I, II, III, and IV—additionally, subtype I has other subgroups (Ia, Ib-1, Ib-2, and Ic).

During the past several years, seven other novel polyomaviruses have been detected in various specimen types. However, only two of these recently identified viruses have been specifically implicated in human diseases:

MCPyV is associated with Merkel cell carcinoma [6].

TSPyV causes trichodysplasia spinulosa [7].

Both of these polyomaviral diseases were diagnosed in people with different degrees of immunocompromised state [6, 7].

Five other PyVs have not been associated with any particular disease patterns as yet, and these include:

Polyomaviruses KIPyV and WUPyV were isolated from respiratory secretions of pediatric patients with acute respiratory disease [8–10].

Other three polyomaviruses labeled as HPyV6, HPyV7, and HPyV9 were detected in urine, blood, or both in healthy population [11].

Prevalence in the General Population

BKPyV as well as JCPyV infection usually occurs in childhood without specific symptoms, followed by a non-replicative state primarily in the urogenital tract or oligodendrocytes, respectively. Among all the polyomaviruses, asymptomatic reactivation and low-level replication of BKPyV with viruria have been reported in 5 % of healthy individuals. A population-based study in Taiwan demonstrated that asymptomatic viruria was present in nearly 19 % of the general

S. Karam, M.D.
Balamand University, Faculty of Medicine, Beirut, Lebanon

R. Wali, M.D. (✉)
University of Maryland School of Medicine, Baltimore, MD, USA

Inova Health System, 3300 Gallows Road, Falls Church, VA 22042-9937, USA
e-mail: ravinder.wali@inova.org

M.R. Weir and E.V. Lerma (eds.), *Kidney Transplantation: Practical Guide to Management*,
DOI 10.1007/978-1-4939-0342-9_28,

population [12]. Study of healthy blood donors by Egli et al. in Swiss population demonstrated that higher percentage of young adults are seropositive of BKPyV compared to JCPyV (>80 % vs. 58 %), respectively. With advancing age, antibody titers wane for BK but not for JC virus. Asymptomatic JC viruria in this population based study was more common than BK viruria (19 % vs. 7 %), respectively [13]. It is possible that both BK and JC viruria may develop in the aging population without iatrogenic immunosuppression [14].

The incidence of asymptomatic activation increases exponentially with the advent of immune dysregulation, as has been observed in patients with SLE with or without the use of immunomodulatory therapy [15].

Life Cycle of Polyomaviruses (Different from Other Viruses)

Siminan vacuolating virus-40 (SV40) is the prototype polyomavirus, it remains dormant in rhesus monkeys, macaque, and hamsters. SV40 has nearly 70 % genetic homology to other types of polyomaviruses such as BK and JC viruses [16]. SV40 first binds to major histocompatibility class 1 antigens on the cell surface. Unlike other viral entry into the cell, SV40 is endocytosed via caveolae and not by clathrin-coated vesicles. Caveolae are microindentations in the plasma membrane and are involved in transcytosis, signal transduction, and the uptake of membrane components and other ligands [17]. Once the single virus particle is trapped in caveola, it is separated from the cell wall as a vesicle, and these vesicles then fuse with larger, preexisting cell structures, caveosomes, from which viruses are formed in larger vesicular structures and carried to the smooth endoplasmic reticulum (ER). ER thus is a predefined and natural pathway that allows the virus to integrate with the nucleus of the cell [18]. However, it is interesting to note that JC virus tissue invasion follows clathrin-dependent receptor pathway [19].

Magnitude of the Problem

Primary infection with HPyV is followed by long-term latency through the life of the host. BKPyV particularly remains dormant in the urogenital epithelial cells; intermittent reactivation has been reported in up to 40 % of healthy individuals along with low-grade viruria without symptoms or adverse events and with spontaneous resolution [20].

Following the isolation of BKPyV from ureteric stenosis in a recipient of kidney transplant [3] and JCPyV from a patient with progressive multifocal leukoencephalopathy (PML) [4], for the past three decades, it became clear that under conditions of immunosuppression, these HPyV can undergo reactivation, from mild subclinical replication to a severe lytic infection of the host cells, and it has been demonstrated that 30–50 % of recipients of organ transplants may develop viruria, with progression to viremia, that can occur in up to 25 % of the recipients of kidney transplants.

Spectrum of Diseases Associated with Reactivation of Human Polyomaviruses

1. Asymptomatic viruria
2. Asymptomatic viremia almost always in combination with viruria
3. Human polyomavirus-associated nephropathy (HPyVAN) in kidney transplant recipients or native kidney dysfunction in recipients of other solid organ transplants
4. Polyomaviral-associated hemorrhagic cystitis in bone marrow transplant (BMT) recipients
5. PML due to JC viral reactivation syndrome
6. Vasculopathy due invasive polyomaviral invasion of the endothelial cells
7. Polyomavirus-associated hemophagocytic syndrome
8. Merkel cell carcinoma of skin
9. Trichodysplasia spinulosa-associated skin disease (alopecia and polyomavirus (TSPyV))
10. Bladder cancer
11. Atypical retinitis: anterior uveitis and blindness following treatment for polyomaviral disease
12. Asymptomatic pyuria or hematuria in pregnancy

Mechanisms of Cell Injury Following Polyomavirus Reactivation

During the replication cycle of the viruses in general and polyomaviruses in particular, double-stranded RNA (dsRNA) is generated, which represents the genome of these viruses, that allows the cell's innate system to be activated by germ line-encoded pattern recognition receptors (PRR) [21]; these are potent inducers of antiviral defense mechanisms to allow innate immune recognition and control of the infection [22]. Among the groups of PRR are different isoforms of Toll-like receptors (TLR) especially TLR3, melanoma differentiation-associated gene 5 (MDA5) and retinoic acid-inducible gene-1 (RIG-1). Activation of these receptors results in the production of pro-inflammatory cytokines and interferon-regulating factors, which in turn promotes the production of type 1 IFN to activate the innate immunity to clear viral infection. Viruses have developed various mechanisms to evade the human immune system, including the suppression of type I IFN responses and translation of host genes [23, 24].

BK virus (BKV) infection promotes transcription of TLR3, RIG-I, and inflammatory mediators in renal collecting duct cells [25] suggesting that the virus can trigger one or more dsRNA receptors as well. Furthermore, dsRNA receptor activation results in activation of both intrinsic and extrinsic apoptotic pathways which ultimately lead to cell death [26, 27].

Polyomaviral Latency to Reactivation

During the past decade, it became apparent that the use of immunosuppression therapy is a strong risk factor for reactivation of these dormant viruses. However, this reactivation can initially be asymptomatic, but the degree of viremia at a particular threshold of viral load may be a potential risk factor for tissue-invasive disease [28], for example, BKPyV nephropathy (BKPyN) or ureteric stenosis in kidney transplant recipients, hemorrhagic cystitis in BMTs, and other rare manifestations such as vasculopathy, pneumonitis, encephalitis, retinitis, and even multiple organ failure [29, 30].

Considering that tissue diagnosis is a gold standard for the diagnosis of polyoma-related end-organ damage, therefore screening tests for early detection of reactivation syndrome have been evaluated. Table 28.1 describes the limitations of different modalities of screening tests for risk stratification of patients at risk of developing polyomavirus-related complications [31–33].

It is not clear whether the use of immunosuppression therapy is associated with mutations, deletions, or rearrangements in the NCCR region of polyomaviruses which leads to aggressive disease from these dormant viruses [41].

Due to spontaneous deletions, rearrangements, and amplifications in the polyoma NCCR regions, different quasispecies have been identified. Architectural rearrangements in the NCCRs of BKV do not appear to be a prerequisite for development of hemorrhagic cystitis in hematopoietic stem cell transplant recipients [42]. Analysis of BKV TCR sequences at times demonstrated substitution or insertion, but no specific pattern has been recognized that could be responsible for the aggressiveness of this virus in a cohort of kidney transplant recipients induced with basiliximab [43]. Moreover, it might be clinically useful to know whether specific BKV subtypes or rearrangements could be linked to a particular disease state such as polyomavirus-associated nephropathy or hemorrhagic cystitis in renal or bone marrow transplant patients, respectively.

Advances in Immunosuppression Therapy as a Risk Factor for Polyomaviral Disease

Cyclosporine vs. Tacrolimus: Risk Factors for BKPyV Reactivation

While BKV nephropathy was relatively rare in the cyclosporine era, increased use of tacrolimus- and mycophenolic acid (MPA)-based therapy has been associated with a resurgence of this disease [29, 44, 45]. A recently published study (RCT) lends some support to the long-held notion that following induction with basiliximab and maintenance IS therapy with CsA-MPA resulted in lower incidence as well lesser degree of BK viremia compared to the use of tacrolimus-MPA combination therapy [46]. However, these short-term results may not portend a benefit for long-term graft function and graft survival.

Quadruple IS Therapy

During the past decade, acute T cell-mediated rejection has decreased to as low as 20 % as the majority of centers use quadruple immunosuppression including induction therapy with depleting antibodies [47]. This accomplishment, however, has been confounded by increasing trends in post-transplant infections, particularly increased incidence of BKPyV reactivation syndrome in the post-transplant period. Although no universal pattern of its emergence has been recognized, reports for the past decade suggest that polyomaviral reactivation develops in 30–40 % of recipients of kidney trans-

Table 28.1 Different screening tests for the detection of polyomaviral reactivation in the blood and urine

Screening test	Sensitivity (%)	Specificity (%)	PPV (%)	NPV (%)
BK viremia[a]	100	96	50	100
BK viruria[b]	100	92	31	100
Decoy cells[c]	25	84	5	97
Urinary capsid protein (VP1)[d]	93.8	93.9		
Haufen cells[e]	100	99	97	100

[a]BK viremia at viral load threshold >1.6E+04 copies/mL [28, 34]
[b]BK viruria at viral load threshold >2.5E+07 copies/mL. The degree and intensity of BKPyV-related viruria have been correlated with the degree of viremia [35, 36]
[c]Decoy cells [37, 38]
[d]Urinary VP1: cutoff value of 6.5 × 10 BKV VP1 mRNA copy number per nanogram of total RNA [39]
[e]Haufen cells: the use of negative staining electron microscopy to detect the cast-like three-dimensional polyomaviral aggregates (Haufen) in urine [40]

plant and 5–10 % of heart, lung, and pancreas transplants. It can progress to the development of polyomaviral-associated nephropathy (PyVAN) in approximately 1–10 % of post-transplant population. PyVAN develops as a consequence of BKV reactivation in more than 95 % of cases and less than 5 % of cases are attributed to reactivation of JC virus, but none so far reported due to SV40.

Before the year 2000, PyVAN was usually diagnosed after the onset of allograft dysfunction and was associated with very high allograft attrition rate (50–70 %) [48].

Polyomaviral-Associated Nephropathy

Histopathological evaluation of allograft biopsies in recipients of kidney transplants demonstrated that interstitial nephritis is the leading lesion due to BKPyV or JCPyV reactivation [38, 44, 49].

Diagnosis of polyomavirus nephropathy (PyVAN) is established on the evaluation of biopsy specimens. The histological diagnosis is confirmed by the presence of staining for SV40 antibodies that cross-react with BKPyV or JCPyV due to more than 70 % genomic overlap [49]. Histological changes include renal tubular damage, interstitial fibrosis, and inflammatory reactions in the presence of SV40 antigen positive staining by immunohistochemistry or immunohybridization techniques. Additionally, PyV DNA can be demonstrated in the allograft biopsy specimens [50]. Drachenberg et al. have described various stages of PVAN, allowing to stratify the degree of allograft damage and helping in determining the prognosis of the allograft survival. However, during early stages of the PyV reactivation, histology could be normal, and hence it is of limited sensitivity in the early stage of disease [51, 52].

The definitive diagnosis of PyVAN requires a renal biopsy, ideally containing two cores of cortex and medulla obtained with a 15-gauge needle. Diagnostic confirmation of PyVAN can easily be achieved by immunohistochemistry using commercially available antibodies to detect the simian virus 40 T antigen or the BKV T antigen. In addition to immunohistochemistry, in situ hybridization and electron microscopy can be used to confirm the diagnosis of PyVAN [38, 49, 53, 54], and fluorescein in situ hybridization (FISH) is considered to be a sensitive marker for the detection of polyomavirus [55]. However, they can only serve as confirmatory adjunct diagnostic tools in cases when PyVAN is already suspected histologically. Since BKV affects the kidney in a random, multifocal manner, false-negative biopsy results may occur, especially in an early stage of disease.

Morphologically, PyVAN is characterized by viral replication in tubular epithelial cells showing typical intranuclear viral inclusion bodies of different phenotypes [51]. Viral cytopathic changes are often seen in small groups of cells located in distinct nephrons. The renal medulla is preferentially affected during the early stages of the disease before viral replication spreads to the renal cortex and cytopathic changes become apparent in proximal tubules [38, 49, 56]. The main feature of the polyomavirus inclusions is the presence of enlarged nuclei with smudgy, ground-glass, basophilic inclusions that completely replace the nuclear chromatin. The electron microscopy analysis shows clusters of intranuclear, rounded, electron-dense virions measuring 40–45 nm in diameter and arranged in parallel linear arrays inside the infected tubular epithelial cells. PyVAN shows varying degrees of tubular epithelial cell injury ranging from occasional intranuclear viral inclusion bodies to widespread tubular epithelial cell necrosis with denudation of basement membranes. The interstitium is typically infiltrated by mononuclear leukocytes with active tubulitis, and this form of tubulointerstitial nephritis closely mimics acute cellular rejection [51, 57].

A histological grading system has been proposed in 2004 to correlate the extent of tissue damage with clinical graft outcome [51, 57]. The histological PVAN-A pattern is characterized by mild to moderate viral cytopathogenic changes accompanied by only minimal interstitial inflammation, fibrosis, and tubular atrophy ($\leq$10 %). In PVAN-B, cytopathogenic changes vary from moderate to extensive, together with mild (11–25 %), moderate (26–50 %), and severe (>50 %) interstitial inflammation, the latter designating the subtypes PVAN-B1, PVAN-B2, and PVAN-B3, respectively. Tubular atrophy and interstitial fibrosis are minimal, mild (11–25 %), and moderate (26–50 %) in PVAN-B1, PVAN-B2, and PVAN-B3, respectively. In PVAN-C, severe interstitial fibrosis and tubular atrophy (>50 %) indicate irreversible chronic allograft damage associated with variable degrees of (residual) interstitial inflammation and viral cytopathogenic alterations.

A revised classification schema that includes three stages was proposed in the report of the 2009 Banff meeting: stage A (early changes, without tubular epithelial cell necrosis), stage B (active nephropathy with virally induced tubular necrosis), and stage C (late sclerosing changes) [58].

This pathological classification is reliable from the viewpoint of interobserver reproducibility; however, its clinical significance is less clear with only stage C showing a significantly poorer prognosis compared with stages A and B in a clinicopathological study [51, 52, 57–59]. Further prospective analyses are necessary.

Concomitant diagnosis of acute allograft rejection in the presence of PyVAN should be considered if one finds endarteritis, fibrinoid vascular necrosis, glomerulitis, or C4d deposits along peritubular capillaries [38, 58, 60, 61].

JCV-mediated PyVAN should be considered in kidney transplant patients with histological signs of PyVAN, declining renal function, and the absence of BKV in blood, urine, and graft tissue [53, 59, 62].

Risk Factors for Progression in BKPyN

Different studies demonstrated that very high viral load, treatment with tacrolimus vs. cyclosporine or mTOR inhibitors, delayed diagnosis, and slow rate of decay in viremia after modifications in baseline immunosuppression therapy are predictors of poor outcome following the diagnosis of PyVAN [63].

Treatment Strategies Following Detection of PyV Reactivation Syndrome After Organ Transplantation

Reduction or modification of baseline immunosuppression therapy continues to remain the mainstay of treatment for patients with different types of polyomaviral reactivation in solid organ transplant recipients. This is particularly well studied now for BKPyV viremia with or without the onset of BK viral nephritis [64–66].

Preemptive reduction in immunosuppression therapy is most effective in presumptive PVAN as defined by surrogate markers (i.e., high BKV viremia) [45]. In this setting, preservation of allograft function remains the most important outcome.

It is believed that reduction in the intensity of IS therapy allows the recovery of BKV-specific T cell immunity, though the time needed for the immunological recovery remains unknown; certainly during that period, cytopathic changes in the allograft may continue to progress. Despite remarkable progress in our understanding of the natural history of polyomaviral reactivation during the past decade, important challenges remain, such as the rare patient with PVAN refractory to any intervention intervention, the newly recognized the newly recognized association of PVAN with urogenital tumors [67, 68] and now recently developed evidence of Merkel cell canner of the skin.

There are no specific guidelines for reduction in IS therapy after detecting BK viremia. Due to the lack of standardized tools to measure the level and magnitude of IS at the point-of-care makes it difficult to individualize this strategy; obviously, the concerns are that (a) too little reduction may trigger further replication and increase the magnitude of viremia, (b) too much reduction in IS therapy is a risk factor of the development of T cell- as well as B cell-mediated organ rejection, and (c) too rapid reduction in IS therapy could result in immune reconstitution syndrome (IRS) which per se is a risk factor for the development of organ transplant rejection or worsening viral infection [69].

- Small case series, mostly retrospective in design, showed that elimination of one agent or reduction in the doses of the all three IS agents was associated with similar outcomes for graft failure as well as acute rejection [70].
- Replacement of CNI or antiproliferative agents with mTOR-I: the use of mTOR-I in place of CNI could be at times advantageous for faster and more efficacious BKV clearance in plasma and urine and may be associated with a steady improvement in allograft function and without acute rejection [71, 72].

In addition to modifications of baseline IS therapy, which has not been standardized (as different centers use different approaches to modify the baseline IS therapy), the use of other adjunctive therapies, such as the use of leflunomide, cidofovir, fluoroquinolones, intravenous immunoglobulins (IVIgs), and immunomodulatory immunotherapy, has been studied. These adjunctive therapies in the absence of well-defined clinical studies continue to remain elusive in their efficacy for the treatment of polyomaviral reactivation syndromes.

Adjunctive Therapies Following HPyV Reactivation Syndrome

Leflunomide

The immunomodulatory drug leflunomide is used for the treatment of rheumatoid arthritis. It has been used off-label in patients with PyVAN, yet its antiviral mechanism is not very well established other than it has the ability to induce the depletion of pyrimidine in the virion as well as host cell. Bernhoff et al. using PRTEC (proximal tubular epithelial cells) showed that LEF-A (leflunomide metabolite) at 10 μg/mL reduced the extracellular BKV load by 90 %. This level of leflunomide, however, was associated with marked degree of cytostatic effects [73].

Leflunomide was used in 17 patients with biopsy-confirmed BKPvN, and after discontinuing mycophenolate mofetil, patients who had blood levels of A77 1726 (metabolite of leflunomide) above 40 μg/mL above 40Ug/ml had a significant decrease in the plasma viral load [74]. However, the long-term graft outcome and drug-related toxicity were not reported.

Evaluation of T cell functions (intralymphocyte cytokine expression for IL-2 and TNF-alpha), T cell activation (transferring receptor (CD71) and IL-2 alpha-chain (CD25) expression), and T cell proliferation after initiating treatment with leflunomide did not demonstrate any changes in T cell function despite potential benefit of treatment in the form of decrease in viral load with the use of leflunomide-based therapy following discontinuation of mycophenolate mofetil [75]. Other studies have demonstrated limited efficacy and increased potential of side effects with leflunomide use in recipients of kidney transplants [75, 76].

Pharmacodynamic study by Krisl et al. correlated blood A77 1726 concentration of leflunomide and BK viral load reduction ($n=52$) in comparison to similar degree of BK viral disease without the use of leflunomide ($n=24$) and demonstrated that the use of leflunomide did not reduce BKPy viremia [77].

A recent literature review by Wu and Harris [78] regarding the off-label use of leflunomide for refractory BKPyAN showed there were a total of two in vitro culture studies, five case reports/series, two retrospective cohort studies, and three prospective observational trials which had used leflunomide as an adjunctive therapy along with reduction in maintenance IS therapy. This analysis suggested that leflunomide at target blood concentrations of around 40 mg/L reduces BK viremia/viruria. It is indeed associated with dose-limiting adverse events.

The use of leflunomide should include careful monitoring of blood cell counts, hepatic functions, and drug concentrations to prevent the drug-related adverse events. Due to the lack of controlled randomized trials, however, the use of leflunomide as first-line treatment should not be routinely recommended.

The clinical correlation between leflunomide levels and its efficacy in clearing viremia remains debatable. But the toxicity profile such as anemia, hemolysis, thrombotic microangiopathy, and neuropathy remains a major concern especially at leflunomide at target blood concentrations of greater than 40 mg/L levels [79].

Cidofovir

Cidofovir is a nucleoside analogue, has been demonstrated to inhibit BKV replication in vitro, and has been explored in observational studies in the treatment of refractory BKPyAN. However, its efficacy has never been demonstrated in randomized controlled trials. Several case reports have demonstrated that treatment with low-dose cidofovir can ameliorate BK viremia/viruria along with recovery of graft function particularly if BKPyVAN continues to progress despite modification and reduction in the intensity of baseline IS therapy [80].

Recent analysis by probabilistic modeling demonstrated that treatment with cidofovir in combination with immunosuppression reduction can lead to cost savings and improved graft survival, BKPyAN, and improved health outcomes in patients with BKPyVAN [81].

A small series of pediatric patients, age range from 5 to 21 years, were treated with cidofovir (0.25–1 mg/kg/dose) every 2–3 week. Total number of cidofovir doses ranged from 1 to 18 (mean 8) for a total of eight patients after confirming the diagnosis of BKPyAN with clearance of viremia as well as preservation of allograft function [82].

Different studies have reported that cidofovir dose ranges from 0.25 to 1 mg/kg every 1–3 weeks, depending on renal function [80, 83]. The treatment duration ranged from 6 weeks to 6 months and is usually monitored by temporal trends in viremia and viruria [68].

A recent systematic review identified 21 publications reporting the use of cidofovir for the treatment of BKPyVAN; most of these were in the form of case reports or small series. The efficacy of cidofovir therapy could not be assessed in 17 of these publications because of lack of surrogate end points or long-term follow-up data or because it was used with concomitant reduction of immunosuppressive drugs; hence, it was concluded that cidofovir alone may not lead to beneficial effect on BK viremia [84].

Clearly, there is an absolute lack of comparative effectiveness studies in the treatment of BK viral disease; therefore, risks associated with the use of cidofovir should be carefully evaluated [85].

Fluoroquinolones

Fluoroquinolones have the ability to inhibit BK DNA topoisomerases II and IV as well as large T-antigen (LT-ag) helicase and DNA gyrase activities. The effects of ofloxacin and levofloxacin on BKPyV replication were analyzed in vitro on renal proximal tubular epithelial cells. BK replication was arrested in a dose-dependent manner and without complete eradication of the infection. The use of these agents has the potential to abrogate the cell injury by decreasing the viral load. However, safety and efficacy including the doses of the drug to achieve in vivo therapeutic concentration akin to in vitro levels remain to be established [86].

Patients who had been exposed to levofloxacin or ciprofloxacin for more than a month in the immediate post-transplant period were less likely to develop BK reactivation syndrome during the first post-transplant year compared to those without such exposure [87]. Another study demonstrated that the use of ciprofloxacin prophylaxis during first 30 days after transplantation leads to a lower rate of BKV infection at 3 months but not at 12 months [88].

The long-term effectiveness and optimal duration and type of fluoroquinolone for prophylaxis against BKV reactivation remain unknown. Antipolyomaviral activity of different fluoroquinolones is currently under investigation [89].

Intravenous Immunoglobulin Therapy

IVIg therapy has been used for the rescue therapy of those patients who failed to show declining trend in viremia following modification of IS therapy [90]. Efficacy and safety of IVIg therapy in polyomaviral disease remain unknown; it is possible that amelioration of viremia with the use of IVIg therapy could be related to immunomodulatory effects of such therapy [91].

In vitro studies show that human IVIgs at concentrations within the range 10–100 μg/mL cause 95.8–98.7 % inhibition of BKV DNA loads after 7 days in cell cultures, provided that the IVIgs and BKV are co-incubated for at least 2 h prior to infection [91–93]. However, clinical experience with IVIgs in PyVAN is limited with sparse evidence of any benefit [94]. In the absence of controlled studies, the high costs associated with adjuvant IVIg treatment make it even a less attractive option [95].

In summary: Detailed systematic review of the therapeutic modalities used in the prevention and treatment of BKPyV disease [96] that included published reports in MEDLINE, EMBASE, and Cochrane databases (1950–2008) as well as published abstracts from the American Transplant Congress (2005–2008) identified more than 500 publications, and review of these published reports did not suggest that addition of cidofovir, leflunomide, IVIg, or ciprofloxacin had a benefit on death-censored graft failure compared to IS reduction alone.

PyV-Specific Immunotherapy

All five BKV antigens are immunogenic and elicit T cell elicit T cell responses of varying degrees in different patients. Using novel approach of a mixture of overlapping peptide pools encompassing all five BKV antigens (viral protein [VP] 1, VP2, VP3, large tumor antigen, and small tumor antigen). Patients who had rapid clearance of BK viremia had polyfunctional T cells polyfunctional T-Cells such as interferon gamma-and IL-2 producing CD4-positive T cells [97]. This observation is particularly important as it may allow to develop polyomaviral immunotherapy.

Immunotherapy by adoptive transfer of cellular effectors can help to abrogate the clinical symptoms associated with opportunistic infections in the post-transplant period. Such therapy has been demonstrated to control some virus-related diseases in transplant recipients, particularly Epstein–Barr virus and cytomegalovirus. Infusion of BKV-specific T cells may potentially reconstitute functional BKV immunity and reduce clinical complications of BKV infection. After monocyte-derived dendritic cells were pulsed with a peptide pool of all the five BKV proteins VP1, VP2, VP3, large T antigen, and small T antigen, it resulted in the generation of BKV-specific T cells, can be used to induce adaptive immunity against the BKV-specific T cells, that can be a goal-directed immunotherapy particularly in patients who develop BKPyVAN as well as acute allograft rejection [98]. It is not used in the realms of clinical practice as yet.

Monitoring of IS Therapy Using Cylex Immune Cell Function Assay

Recently, the Cylex immune cell function assay (ICFA) (ImmuKnow; Cylex, Inc., Columbia, MD) was approved by the U.S. Food and Drug Administration (FDA) to measure global immune response in solid organ transplant patients receiving immunosuppressive therapy.

Current monitoring systems of immunosuppression in solid organ transplant recipients are typically focused on prevention of clinical toxicities of immunosuppressive drugs. We lack the ability to determine the optimal level of immunosuppression at individual basis. It is being postulated that ImmuKnow assay results can reveal either overimmunosuppression with individuals at risk of infection or bone marrow suppression or underimmunosuppression with individuals at risk of organ rejection.

The Cylex ImmuKnow test (Cylex, Columbia, MD) measures immune cell function (ICF) and is based on the amount of adenosine triphosphate (ATP) released when T cells are stimulated by phytohemagglutinin. Low levels of ICFA have been associated with BK viremia in small sample studies [99, 100]; these observations support the notion that overimmunosuppression could be a major risk factor for polyoma viral reactivation syndrome. Similarly, very low values on ICF test correlated with viruria in kidney transplant recipients [101].

Allograft Rejection Vs. Polyomaviral Nephritis on Histological Examination

BKPyVAN along with graft dysfunction often times produces a daunting task of identifying the concomitant presence of T cell-mediated acute rejection. It is being postulated that IS modification or reduction should be undertaken only when the presence of concomitant rejection has been excluded. However, in the presence of significant inflammatory reaction in the biopsy specimen, it becomes a very challenging task for the renal pathologist as well as for the clinician. Studies have suggested that histological features of acute cellular rejection as well as polyoma nephritis could be very similar as demonstrated by immunohistological analysis and gene expression profile [102].

Similarly, Masutani et al. [103] reported single-center retrospective study of the natural history of polyomaviruria in a cohort of patients when more than 80 % were induced with single-dose alemtuzumab, followed by tacrolimus-based monotherapy along with early steroid discontinuation in 70 % of the cohort. Viruria developed in 43 %, and combination of viruria and viremia was noted in 10 %. Nearly 21 % developed biopsy-proven BKPyV-associated nephropathy.

Surprisingly, patients with persistent viruria had very high acute rejection rate (36.7 %) compared to 28 % in those without viruria. However, the grade of rejection was not elaborated. Treatment refractory rejection was more common in patients with viruria vs. without viruria (36.2 % vs. 19.6 %).

Masutani et al. [103] as well others have demonstrated that during BKPyV reactivation there is an increased upregulation of plethora of inflammatory markers including interleukin (IL)-6, IL-3, and granzyme b in the urine [104, 105]. In the presence of BKPyV reactivation, at times it could be difficult to differentiate inflammatory changes that could accompany the viral-induced CD8+ cell response in the graft and different grades of T cell-mediated rejection [102]. However, the use of other techniques such as immunophenotyping of the allograft biopsy may yield helpful information for clinical decision making [60].

Genomic biomarkers in the near future may help to make this distinction without ambiguity, since treatment of concomitant T cell-mediated rejection could practically lead to more immunosuppression, hence fostering BKPyV replication, thus a vicious cycle.

Type of Polyoma Viral Reactivation in the Post-transplant Period

Is It BKPyV or JC PyV Reactivation?

Several studies have demonstrated that JCPyV viral reactivation can happen in the recipients of kidney and other organ transplants. JC reactivation is less common than BK viral reactivation, usually has a benign clinical course, and responds briskly to modification of IS therapy, without jeopardizing the graft survival [62, 106].

Urinary shedding of BKPyV and JCPyV (viruria) was studied in a small but a longitudinal study of 41 kidney and 33 liver transplant recipients. Polyomaviral shedding was more common in liver than kidney recipients. Among these, JCV was more common in liver recipients, and JCV viral loads were much higher than those of BK viruria in both the liver and kidney recipients [106]. The role of JC viruria in recipients of kidney transplants is more often associated with better outcomes than either BK or combination of BK and JC viruria [62].

HLA Mismatch and HPyV Disease

Risk of HLA mismtach (HLA-MM) and HLA mismatch (MM) and BKPyV disease, Drachenberg et al. correlated the relationship of HLA mismatch (MM) and BKPyN and graft loss; those with higher degrees of HLA-MM with polyoma disease were at increased risk for graft loss compared to those with lower degrees of HLA-MM [107]. The exact impact of this correlation has not been well established, but raises an intriguing question, if HLA-MM [108, 109] and ABO incompatibility [110] may be associated with more severe form of BK disease as a consequence of more intense IS therapy or is it that HLA-MM exposes tubular cells to immune damage by innate immunity and thereby tubular epithelial cell injury triggers intense BKPy viral replication and intense epithelial cell inflammation [111]. The association of HLA-MM and the development of BK- or JCPyV need more evaluation.

Retransplantation and Role of Transplant Nephrectomy Following Graft Failure Due to BKPyN

Retransplantation following graft loss due to BKPyV disease remains a cause for concern due to the anxiety related to the potential possibility of recurrence of PyV disease in the new graft. Retrospective study compiled data on adult patients undergoing repeat transplantation after previous loss of allograft to PyBKVN from six US centers. A total of 31 patients underwent retransplantation after a median of 6 months after failure of the first allograft, 10 of these underwent preemptive retransplantation. Twenty-six patients had documented clearance of viremia. Only 13 underwent transplant nephrectomy before the retransplantation. Following repeat transplant, 11 (35 %) had BKV replication in urine and plasma with two patients experiencing BKVN. Seven patients developed acute rejection [112].

Other reports also support the notion that retransplantation can be successfully performed following loss of allograft due to PyV disease but with a caution that such patients should have undetectable or very low viremia/viruria at the time of retransplantation. Viremia should be monitored more frequently in the post-transplant period [113, 114].

The use of interventions designed to reduce active viral replication, including preemptive nephrectomy of the failed graft, could be considered [115] but may not be necessary for the successful outcome of retransplantation [116].

Nonrenal Solid Organ Transplantation and BKPyV Disease

BKPyV replication may occur anytime in the post-transplant period; recent studies have demonstrated that a trend peaks during the first 3–6 months post-transplantation, though it is not unusual to develop late reactivation past first year after transplantation. On the contrary, BKPyV reactivation in recipients of other solid organ transplants usually develops in the later years after transplantation.

The overall frequency of BKV viruria, in non-kidney SOT recipients, is variable at rates, and even in those SOT recipients such as lung recipients, the frequency of activation is far lower than recipients of kidney transplants [117]. Studies in recipients of other solid organ transplants such as the liver, heart, and pancreas alone demonstrated a lack of correlation between viremia, viruria, and renal dysfunction [118–121]. Therefore, general screening is not recommended. Biopsy-confirmed PyV disease affecting the native kidneys is based on a few case reports [106, 122, 123].

In summary, BK or JC viruria may develop in more than 10 % of recipients with nonrenal solid organ transplantation (NRSOT); its impact on the development of renal dysfunction in such patients is far from proven [124]. Hence screening for PyV reactivation should be limited to those who have new-onset renal dysfunction following SOT.

Other Systemic Diseases Associated with HPyV Reactivation

Progressive Multifocal Leukoencephalopathy

It is a demyelinating disease of the central nervous system caused by the neurotropic human polyomavirus (JCPyV) that results in lytic infection of oligodendrocytes. PML was first described as a complication of lymphoproliferative disorders more than 50 years ago and emerged as a major complication of HIV infection in the 1970s [4].

Despite the ubiquity of this virus, PML is rare and always seen in association with an underlying immunosuppressive state, such as HIV infection, autoimmune diseases, cancer, and organ transplantation. JCV remains quiescent in the kidneys as well as oligodendrocytes, where it displays a stable archetypal noncoding control region (NCCR). Conversely, rearranged JCV NCCRs, including tandem repeat patterns found in the brain of PML patients, have been associated with neurovirulence. The specific sites and specific sites and mechanisms of JCV NCCR transformation remain yet to be explored. PML has been reported among the heart, kidney, and liver transplant recipients, but its true incidence in these patient groups is not known [125, 126].

The major risk factor for the development of PML is indeed the presence of immunocompromised state; accordingly, PML has been increasingly diagnosed in patients treated with biological therapies such as monoclonal antibodies (mAbs) called biologics [127, 128].

Skin Manifestations

Trichodysplasia Spinulosa

Trichodysplasia spinulosa (TS) is a skin disease due to TSPyV reactivation. It is characterized by (1) history of organ transplantation and/or drug-induced immunosuppression, (2) eruptive follicular papules with spiny excrescences concentrated in the central face with spread to trunk and extremities, and (3) alopecia of varying degrees.

The histopathologic findings are distinctive and include distended hair follicles containing sheets of eosinophilic cells and the presence of viral inclusions on ultrastructural examination, along with molecular confirmation of polyomavirus in the lesions of trichodysplasia spinulosa [129]. Treatment includes supportive therapy along with the general principle of reduction in maintenance IS therapy and careful monitoring of allograft function and skin lesions.

Merkel Cell Skin Cancer (Merkel Cell Cancer)

Merkel cell cancer (MCC) in the immunocompromised host is invariably due to reactivation of MCPyV [6, 106]. MCC arises most often on sun-exposed areas and is more common in fair-skinned people, but not uncommon in other colored people especially if immunocompromised.

It derives its name from the similarity of these cancer cells to normal Merkel cells in the skin that were first described over 100 years ago by Friedrich Sigmund Merkel. MCC in the immunocompromised host is more often due to MCPyV infection [130]. It is now diagnosed more easily due to the availability of special stain (CK20) that differentiates it from other types of skin cancers.

Merkel cell carcinoma usually appears as a firm, painless lesion on a sun-exposed area. These tumors are typically red, blue, or skin-colored and vary greatly in size at the time of first presentation. The major challenge of MCC is that it oftentime presents with spread to local lymph nodes; therefore, sentinel node biopsy is an essential part of diagnosis and management.

Treatment is mostly along the principles that include reduction in the intensity of IS therapy, surgical excision of the primary lesion along with any nodes that are involved with MCC, radiation therapy, as well as chemotherapy if nodes are positive. Overall, the 5-year survival rate is about 60 %, though it can be higher if MCC is diagnosed before local invasion.

BKPyV-Associated Hemophagocytic Syndrome

Hemophagocytic syndrome is a rare symptom complex that can develop due to PyV reactivation. Constellation of signs and symptoms of hemophagocytic syndrome includes fever of unknown origin, pancytopenia, and increased levels of lactate dehydrogenase, ferritin, triglycerides, and alanine aminotransferase in the setting of negative bacterial or viral etiology. Several case series of hemophagocytic syndrome due to PyV reactivation have been described by several authors [131,

132]. Early diagnosis is critical since management is simply supportive in combination with early withdrawal of IS therapy and careful monitoring for allograft rejection. If recognized early, it is often associated with resolution of symptoms with prompt discontinuation of IS therapy.

BKPyV-Associated Multisystem Disease

Single case report illustrates that reactivation of HPyV can result in systemic illness, leading to multiorgan failure. During the epidemic of AIDS, BKPyV reactivation was demonstrated with the development of nephritis, retinitis, as well as meningoencephalitis [133, 134]. Additionally, BKPyV reactivation was associated with development of life-threatening pneumonia following bone marrow transplantation [135]. Although tissue tropism is well defined for different types of polyomavirus, a recent report of endothelial invasion with BKPyV illustrates that polyomaviruses in the immunocompromised host could lead to fatal dissemination [136]. Whether changes in tissue tropism is due to mutational changes in BKPyV remains to be proven.

BKPyV-Associated Hemorrhagic Cystitis

Hemorrhagic cystitis (HC) is a well-known complication after allogeneic BMT as well as hematopoietic stem cell transplantation (HSCT). It can develop in up to 70 % of hematopoietic stem cell transplant recipients and is associated with prolonged hospitalization [137]. Mutations in the noncoding control region (NCCR) and specific BKV subtypes defined by sequence analysis of major capsid protein VP1 have been associated with development of hemorrhagic cystitis in hematopoietic stem cell transplant recipients [42]. Early bleeding (occurring 24–72 h after transplant) is usually as a consequence of toxic effects of the drugs used for the induction therapy [138]. Non-chemotherapy-induced hemorrhagic cystitis is usually documented later after hematopoietic stem cell transplants (more than 2 weeks in the allogeneic setting), often due to reactivation of BKPyV in the bladder [139]. However, the precise role of BKV in the etiology of hemorrhagic cystitis in hematopoietic stem cell transplant recipients remains unclear, since approximately 50 % of all such adult transplant recipients develop viruria, yet do not develop symptoms of HC.

Predisposing factors for HC include allogeneic transplant, advanced age at transplantation, possibly graft-versus-host disease (GVHD), thrombocytopenia, coagulopathy, and viral infections (polyoma BKV, cytomegalovirus, and adenovirus). The most common factor however is rapid replication of HPyV-related cystitis [139, 140], and it is clear that polyoma reactivation is in fact directly related to the intensity of the conditioning regimen [139–143].

BKV-associated hemorrhagic cystitis (HC) mild hematuria with or without dysuria to life-threatening bleeding and clots that may cause urinary obstruction and renal failure. It is often associated with significant morbidity and mortality in hematopoietic stem cell transplantation (HSCT) patients [139–143]. Unfortunately, its development is difficult to predict since BK viruria is very common after HSCT and can be present in patients with and without HC. In the past, it was thought that HC could be due to the use of cyclophosphamide or due to adenoviral invasion of the bladder mucosa. Recent studies have demonstrated that the most common cause of HC is in fact reactivation of BKPyV; the use of RFLP (restriction fragment length polymorphism assay) showed the presence of BKV subtypes I and IV, with the prevalence of subtype I (4/5).

One of the treatments that has been recently tried is the use of fluoroquinolones for prophylaxis as well as treatment of BKPyV disease. It has been shown that fluoroquinolones have the ability to inhibit cellular topoisomerases II and IV as well as large T-antigen (LT-ag) helicase activity. In vitro studies have shown that fluoroquinolones inhibit BK viral replication by direct inhibition of the BK-encoded DNA gyrase.

The effects of ofloxacin and levofloxacin on BKPyV replication were analyzed in vitro on renal proximal tubular epithelial cells. BKPyV replication was arrested in a dose-dependent manner, without complete eradication of the infection. The use of these agents has the potential to abrogate the cell injury by decreasing the viral load. However, safety and efficacy including the doses of different quinolones to achieve in vivo therapeutic concentration akin to in vitro levels remain to be established [86].

The use of ciprofloxacin prophylaxis from the outset was demonstrated to be safe and effective in reducing the incidence of severe BKPyV-related HC after allogeneic HSCT [144, 145].

Currently, the mainstay of treatment for polyomavirus-associated hemorrhagic cystitis includes symptomatic treatment, pain relief, hydration, and continuous bladder irrigation. Other strategies that have been used for palliative treatment in cases of severe hemorrhagic cystitis include the use of fibrin glue, intravesicular sodium hyaluronate, and prostaglandin E2 bladder instillation.

Attempts to eradicate viruria, with the use of intravesical cidofovir [146], have been reported. However, resolution of symptoms may not be universal.

Others have shown an association between plasma viral load and development of hemorrhagic cystitis, and it is possible that measuring both viremia and viruria can help to predict the development of HC and preemptive therapy can prevent the complications of hematuria [147, 148]. The use of intravenous low-dose cidofovir has been used at the risk of developing therapy-related acute kidney injury, as well as metabolic acidosis [149, 150].

Bladder Cancer

Several case reports have demonstrated that chronic reactivation of polyomavirus in recipients of kidney transplants could lead to the development of bladder cancer [67, 151].

Summary

Human polyomaviruses (HPyVs) after primary infection remain latent in more than 90 % of the general population. Viral reactivation—as evidenced by the presence of viral DNA in urine or rarely blood—can occur intermittently throughout the life of the host but rarely causing disease in an apparently healthy immunocompetent host. This chapter focused on four major HPyVs such as BKPyV, JCPyV, MCPyV, and TSPyV and their disease associations in immunocompromised host. Other types of HPyV that have been typed but are still not associated with any disease pattern include HPyVs 3, 4, 6, 9, and 10. Increased recognition of BKPyV in recipients of kidney transplants, JCPyV-associated PML in immunocompromised patients due to HIV, patients treated with biologics, and hemorrhagic cystitis in recipients of bone marrow or stem cell transplant unraveled the critical importance of host immune effector mechanisms in the control of these latent infections. The most common type of HPyV reactivation is BKPyV reactivation in recipients of kidney transplants leading to viruria and viremia, and if viremia reaches a particular threshold, the host will develop nephropathy, which increases the risk for graft failure. Active surveillance to detect viremia and/or viruria following kidney transplantation is worthwhile as it allows early and stepwise reduction in maintenance IS therapy to arrest the viral replication. However, difficult-to-treat cases may need adjunctive therapy, though there is a lack of safe and effective antipolyomaviral agents. Most of these adjunctive therapies are empirical in nature, and risk-benefits are certainly unknown given the lack of robust controlled studies. Reduction in IS therapy should be followed with caution as such patients can be at risk for the development of T cell- as well as B cell-mediated immune injury of the allograft. The most challenging task is identification of those recipients at risk of reactivation at a stage that is early enough to facilitate treatment intervention to prevent the development of PyVAN. In cases of multisystem disease or those who continue to show progression in viremia following judicious modifications in IS therapy, such patients may be candidates for HPyV-specific immunotherapy. Future challenges include early identification of other disease states that could develop due to recent identification of KIPyV and WUPyV from respiratory secretions of pediatric patients with acute respiratory illnesses and other polyomaviruses such as HPyV3, HPyV7, and HPyV9 isolated from urine as well as blood in healthy populations; these may portend a potential threat to immunocompromised host if these undergo reactivation like BK-, JC-, MC-, and TS-PyVs.

References

1. Knowles WA, Pipkin P, Andrews N, Vyse A, Minor P, Brown DW, et al. Population-based study of antibody to the human polyomaviruses BKV and JCV and the simian polyomavirus SV40. J Med Virol. 2003;71(1):115–23.
2. Tremolada S. Mutations in the external loops of BK virus VP1 and urine viral load in renal transplant recipients. J Cell Physiol. 2010;222:195–9.
3. Gardner SD, Field AM, Coleman DV, Hulme B. New human papovavirus (B.K.) isolated from urine after renal transplantation. Lancet. 1971;1(7712):1253–7.
4. Padgett BL, Walker DL, ZuRhein GM, Eckroade RJ, Dessel BH. Cultivation of papova-like virus from human brain with progressive multifocal leucoencephalopathy. Lancet. 1971;1(7712):1257–60.
5. Taguchi F, Kajioka J, Miyamura T. Prevalence rate and age of acquisition of antibodies against JC virus and BK virus in human sera. Microbiol Immunol. 1982;26(11):1057–64.
6. Feng H, Shuda M, Chang Y, Moore PS. Clonal integration of a polyomavirus in human Merkel cell carcinoma. Science. 2008;319(5866):1096–100.
7. van der Meijden E, Janssens RW, Lauber C, Bouwes Bavinck JN, Gorbalenya AE, Feltkamp MC. Discovery of a new human polyomavirus associated with trichodysplasia spinulosa in an immunocompromised patient. PLoS Pathog. 2010;6(7):e1001024.
8. Allander T, Andreasson K, Gupta S, Bjerkner A, Bogdanovic G, Persson MA, et al. Identification of a third human polyomavirus. J Virol. 2007;81(8):4130–6.
9. Gaynor AM, Nissen MD, Whiley DM, Mackay IM, Lambert SB, Wu G, et al. Identification of a novel polyomavirus from patients with acute respiratory tract infections. PLoS Pathog. 2007;3(5):e64.
10. Payungporn S, Chieochansin T, Thongmee C, Samransamruajkit R, Theamboolers A, Poovorawan Y. Prevalence and molecular characterization of WU/KI polyomaviruses isolated from pediatric patients with respiratory disease in Thailand. Virus Res. 2008;135(2):230–6.
11. Babakir-Mina M, Ciccozzi M, Perno CF, Ciotti M. The novel KI, WU, MC polyomaviruses: possible human pathogens? New Microbiol. 2011;34(1):1–8.
12. Ming F, Eisenthal R, Whish WJ, Hubble J. The kinetics of affinity-mediated cell-surface attachment. Enzyme Microb Technol. 2000;26(2–4):216–21.
13. Egli A. Prevalence of polyomavirus BK and JC infection and replication in 400 healthy blood donors. J Infect Dis. 2009;199: 837–46.
14. Zhong S. Age-related urinary excretion of BK polyomavirus by nonimmunocompromised individuals. J Clin Microbiol. 2007;45: 193–8.
15. Sundsfjord A, Osei A, Rosenqvist H. BK and JC viruses in patients with systemic lupus erythematosus: prevalent and persistent BK viruria, sequence stability of the viral regulatory regions, and nondetectable viremia. J Infect Dis. 1999;180:1–9.
16. Bollag B, Chuke WF, Frisque RJ. Hybrid genomes of the polyomaviruses JC virus, BK virus, and simian virus 40: identification of sequences important for efficient transformation. J Virol. 1989;63:863–72.
17. Pelkmans L, Kartenbeck J, Helenius A. Caveolar endocytosis of simian virus 40 reveals a new two-step vesicular-transport pathway to the ER. Nat Cell Biol. 2001;3(5):473–83.

18. Pelkmans L, Puntener D, Helenius A. Local actin polymerization and dynamin recruitment in SV40-induced internalization of caveolae. Science. 2002;296(5567):535–9.
19. Pho MT, Ashok A, Atwood WJ. JC virus enters human glial cells by clathrin-dependent receptor-mediated endocytosis. J Virol. 2000;74(5):2288–92.
20. Polo C, Perez JL, Mielnichuck A, Fedele CG, Niubo J, Tenorio A. Prevalence and patterns of polyomavirus urinary excretion in immunocompetent adults and children. Clin Microbiol Infect. 2004;10(7):640–4.
21. Thompson MR, Kaminski JJ, Kurt-Jones EA, Fitzgerald KA. Pattern recognition receptors and the innate immune response to viral infection. Viruses. 2011;3(6):920–40.
22. Takeuchi O, Akira S. Pattern recognition receptors and inflammation. Cell. 2010;140(6):805–20.
23. Bowie AG, Unterholzner L. Viral evasion and subversion of pattern-recognition receptor signalling. Nat Rev Immunol. 2008;8(12):911–22.
24. Trinchieri G. Type I, interferon: friend or foe? J Exp Med. 2010;207(10):2053–63.
25. Ribeiro A, Wornle M, Motamedi N, Anders HJ, Grone EF, Nitschko H, et al. Activation of innate immune defense mechanisms contributes to polyomavirus BK-associated nephropathy. Kidney Int. 2012;81(1):100–11.
26. Abend JR, Low JA, Imperiale MJ. Global effects of BKV infection on gene expression in human primary kidney epithelial cells. Virology. 2010;397:73–9.
27. Heutinck KM, Rowshani AT, Kassies J, Claessen N, van Donselaar-van der Pant KA, Bemelman FJ, et al. Viral double-stranded RNA sensors induce antiviral, pro-inflammatory, and pro-apoptotic responses in human renal tubular epithelial cells. Kidney Int. 2012;82(6):664–75.
28. Hirsch HH, Knowles W, Dickenmann M. Prospective study of polyomavirus type BK replication and nephropathy in renal-transplant recipients. N Engl J Med. 2002;347:488–96.
29. Hirsch HH, Steiger J, Polyomavirus BK. Lancet Infect Dis. 2003;3(10):611–23.
30. Reploeg MD, Storch GA, Clifford DB. Bk virus: a clinical review. Clin Infect Dis. 2001;33(2):191–202.
31. Chakera A. Detection of polyomavirus BK reactivation after renal transplantation using an intensive decoy cell surveillance program is cost-effective. Transplantation. 2011;92:1018–23.
32. Viscount HB. Polyomavirus polymerase chain reaction as a surrogate marker of polyomavirus-associated nephropathy. Transplantation. 2007;84:340–5.
33. Nickeleit V, True K, Detwiler R, Kozlowski T, Singh H. Risk assessment for polyomavirus nephropathy using urine cytology and the detection of decoy cells: cheap and efficient. Transplantation. 2012;94(7):e42–4.
34. Nickeleit V, Klimkait T, Binet IF. Testing for polyomavirus type BK DNA in plasma to identify renal-allograft recipients with viral nephropathy. N Engl J Med. 2000;342:1309–15.
35. Bressollette-Bodin C. A prospective longitudinal study of BK virus infection in 104 renal transplant recipients. Am J Transplant. 2005;5:1926–33.
36. Nickeleit V. BK-virus nephropathy in renal transplants-tubular necrosis, MHC-class II expression and rejection in a puzzling game. Nephrol Dial Transplant. 2000;15:324–32.
37. Boldorini R. Genomic mutations of viral protein 1 and BK virus nephropathy in kidney transplant recipients. J Med Virol. 2009;81:1385–93.
38. Drachenberg CB. Human polyoma virus in renal allograft biopsies: morphological findings and correlation with urine cytology. Hum Pathol. 1999;30:970–7.
39. Ding R, Medeiros M, Dadhania D. Noninvasive diagnosis of BK virus nephritis by measurement of messenger RNA for BK virus VP1 in urine. Transplantation. 2002;74:987–94.
40. Singh HK. Presence of urinary Haufen accurately predicts polyomavirus nephropathy. J Am Soc Nephrol. 2009;20:416–27.
41. Memon IA, Parikh BA, Gaudreault-Keener M, Skelton R, Storch GA, Brennan DC. Progression from sustained BK viruria to sustained BK viremia with immunosuppression reduction is not associated with changes in the noncoding control region of the BK virus genome. J Transplant. 2012;2012:761283.
42. Carr MJ, McCormack GP, Mutton KJ, Crowley B. Unique BK virus non-coding control region (NCCR) variants in hematopoietic stem cell transplant recipients with and without hemorrhagic cystitis. J Med Virol. 2006;78(4):485–93.
43. Anzivino E, Bellizzi A, Mitterhofer AP, Tinti F, Barile M, Colosimo MT, et al. Early monitoring of the human polyomavirus BK replication and sequencing analysis in a cohort of adult kidney transplant patients treated with basiliximab. Virol J. 2011;8:407.
44. Binet I. Polyomavirus disease under new immunosuppressive drugs: a cause of renal graft dysfunction and graft loss. Transplantation. 1999;67:918–22.
45. Brennan DC. Incidence of BK with tacrolimus versus cyclosporine and impact of preemptive immunosuppression reduction. Am J Transplant. 2005;5:582–94.
46. Hirsch HH, Vincenti F, Friman S, Tuncer M, Citterio F, Wiecek A, et al. Polyomavirus BK replication in de novo kidney transplant patients receiving tacrolimus or cyclosporine: a prospective, randomized, multicenter study. Am J Transplant. 2013;13(1):136–45.
47. Hanaway MJ, Woodle ES, Mulgaonkar S, Peddi VR, Kaufman DB, First MR, et al. Alemtuzumab induction in renal transplantation. N Engl J Med. 2011;364(20):1909–19.
48. Ramos E, Drachenberg CB, Papadimitriou JC. Clinical course of polyoma virus nephropathy in 67 renal transplant patients. J Am Soc Nephrol. 2002;13:2145–51.
49. Randhawa PS, Finkelstein S, Scantlebury V. Human polyoma virus-associated interstitial nephritis in the allograft kidney. Transplantation. 1999;67:103–9.
50. Randhawa P, Shapiro R, Vats A. Quantitation of DNA of polyomaviruses BK and JC in human kidneys. J Infect Dis. 2005;192(3):504–9.
51. Drachenberg CB. Histological patterns of polyomavirus nephropathy: correlation with graft outcome and viral load. Am J Transplant. 2004;4:2082–92.
52. Gaber LW, Egidi MF, Stratta RJ, Lo A, Moore LW, Gaber AO. Clinical utility of histological features of polyomavirus allograft nephropathy. Transplantation. 2006;82(2):196–204.
53. Hirsch HH, Randhawa P. BK polyomavirus in solid organ transplantation. Am J Transplant. 2013;13 Suppl 4:179–88.
54. Nickeleit V. Polyomavirus infection of renal allograft recipients: from latent infection to manifest disease. J Am Soc Nephrol. 1999;10:1080–9.
55. Wang Z, Portier BP, Hu B, Chiesa-Vottero A, Myles J, Procop GW, et al. Diagnosis of BK viral nephropathy in the renal allograft biopsy: role of fluorescence in situ hybridization. J Mol Diagn. 2012;14(5):494–500.
56. Randhawa PS, Demetris AJ. Nephropathy due to polyomavirus type BK. N Engl J Med. 2000;342(18):1361–3.
57. Hirsh HH, Randhawa P. BK virus in solid organ transplant recipients. Am J Transplant. 2009;9 Suppl 4:S136–46.
58. Masutani K, Shapiro R, Basu A, Tan H, Wijkstrom M, Randhawa P. The Banff 2009 working proposal for polyomavirus nephropathy: a critical evaluation of its utility as a determinant of clinical outcome. Am J Transplant. 2012;12(4):907–18.
59. Celik B, Shapiro R, Vats A, Randhawa PS. Polyomavirus allograft nephropathy: sequential assessment of histologic viral load, tubulitis, and graft function following changes in immunosuppression. Am J Transplant. 2003;3(11):1378–82.
60. Ahuja M, Cohen EP, Dayer AM. Polyoma virus infection after renal transplantation. Use of immunostaining as a guide to diagnosis. Transplantation. 2001;71:896–9.

61. Randhawa P, Shapiro R. Conceptual problems in the diagnosis and therapy of acute rejection in patients with polyomavirus nephropathy. Am J Transplant. 2004;4(5):840.
62. Drachenberg CB, Hirsch HH, Papadimitriou JC, Gosert R, Wali RK, Munivenkatappa R, et al. Polyomavirus BK versus JC replication and nephropathy in renal transplant recipients: a prospective evaluation. Transplantation. 2007;84(3):323–30.
63. Schwarz A, Linnenweber-Held S, Heim A, Brocker V, Rieck D, Framke T, et al. Factors influencing viral clearing and renal function during polyomavirus BK-associated nephropathy after renal transplantation. Transplantation. 2012;94(4):396–402.
64. Hariharan S. BK virus nephritis after renal transplantation. Kidney Int. 2006;69(4):655–62.
65. Saad ER. Successful treatment of BK viremia using reduction in immunosuppression without antiviral therapy. Transplantation. 2008;85:850–4.
66. Sood P, Senanayake S, Sujeet K, Medipalli R, Zhu YR, Johnson CP, et al. Management and outcome of BK viremia in renal transplant recipients: a prospective single-center study. Transplantation. 2012;94(8):814–21.
67. Geetha D, Tong BC, Racusen L, Markowitz JS, Westra WH. Bladder carcinoma in a transplant recipient: evidence to implicate the BK human polyomavirus as a causal transforming agent. Transplantation. 2002;73(12):1933–6.
68. Ramos E, Drachenberg CB, Wali R, Hirsch HH. The decade of polyomavirus BK-associated nephropathy: state of affairs. Transplantation. 2009;87:621–30.
69. Ginevri F. Prospective monitoring of polyomavirus BK replication and impact of pre-emptive intervention in pediatric kidney recipients. Am J Transplant. 2007;7:2727–35.
70. Geetha D, Parkhie S, Nadkarni GN, He C, Shafi T. Polyomavirus-associated nephropathy: a comparison of 2 different strategies for immunosuppression reduction. Medicine (Baltimore). 2011;90(5):296–302.
71. Sanchez Fructuoso AI, Calvo N, Perez-Flores I, Valero R, Rodriguez-Sanchez B, García de Viedma D, et al. Mammalian target of rapamycin signal inhibitors could play a role in the treatment of BK polyomavirus nephritis in renal allograft recipients. Transpl Infect Dis. 2011;13(6):584–91.
72. Wali RK, Drachenberg C, Hirsch HH, Papadimitriou J, Nahar A, Mohanlal V, et al. BK virus-associated nephropathy in renal allograft recipients: rescue therapy by sirolimus-based immunosuppression. Transplantation. 2004;78(7):1069–73.
73. Bernhoff E. Leflunomide inhibition of BK virus replication in renal tubular epithelial cells. J Virol. 2010;84:2150–6.
74. Williams JW, Javaid B, Kadambi PV. Leflunomide for polyomavirus type BK nephropathy. N Engl J Med. 2005;352:1157–8.
75. Canivet C. Polyoma BK, virus-associated nephropathy in kidney-transplant patients: effects of leflunomide on T-cell functions and disease outcome. Int Immunopharmacol. 2009;9:1131–6.
76. Faguar S. Leflunomide treatment for polyomavirus BK-associated nephropathy after kidney transplantation. Transpl Int. 2007;20:962–9.
77. Krisl JC, Taber DJ, Pilch N, Chavin K, Bratton C, Thomas B, et al. Leflunomide efficacy and pharmacodynamics for the treatment of BK viral infection. Clin J Am Soc Nephrol. 2012;7(6):1003–9.
78. Wu JK, Harris MT. Use of leflunomide in the treatment of polyomavirus BK-associated nephropathy. Ann Pharmacother. 2008;42(11):1679–85.
79. Leca N. Higher levels of leflunomide are associated with hemolysis and are not superior to lower levels for BK virus clearance in renal transplant patients. Clin J Am Soc Nephrol. 2008;3:829–35.
80. Kadambi PV, Josephson MA, Williams J. Treatment of refractory BK virus-associated nephropathy with cidofovir. Am J Transplant. 2003;3:186–91.
81. Hua DK, Howard K, Craig JC, Chapman JR, Wong G. Cost-effectiveness of cidofovir treatment of polyomavirus nephropathy in kidney transplant recipients. Transplantation. 2012;93(2):188–94.
82. Araya CE, Lew JF, Fennell RS, Neiberger RE, Dharnidharja VR. Intermediate dose cidofovir does not cause additive nephrotoxicity in BK virus allograft nephropathy. Pediatr Transplant. 2008;12:790–5.
83. Kuypers DR. Adjuvant low-dose cidofovir therapy for BK polyomavirus interstitial nephritis in renal transplant recipients. Am J Transplant. 2005;5:1997–2004.
84. Lamoth F, Pascual M, Erard V, Venetz JP, Nseir G, Meylan P. Low-dose cidofovir for the treatment of polyomavirus-associated nephropathy: two case reports and review of the literature. Antivir Ther. 2008;13(8):1001–9.
85. Hakeem A, Sharma H, Sharma A. Cidofovir may be deleterious in BK virus-associated nephropathy. Transplantation. 2011;91(2):e11–2.
86. Sharma BN, Li R, Bernhoff E, Gutteberg TJ, Rinaldo CH. Fluoroquinolones inhibit human polyomavirus BK (BKV) replication in primary human kidney cells. Antiviral Res. 2011;92(1):115–23.
87. Gabardi S. Evaluation of fluoroquinolones for the prevention of BK viremia after renal transplantation. Clin J Am Soc Nephrol. 2010;5:1298–304.
88. Wojciechowski D, Chanda R, Chandran S, Lee B, Webber A, Macaraig M, et al. Ciprofloxacin prophylaxis in kidney transplant recipients reduces BK virus infection at 3 months but not at 1 year. Transplantation. 2012;94(11):1117–23.
89. Randhawa PS. Anti-BK virus activity of ciprofloxacin and related antibiotics. Clin Infect Dis. 2005;41:1366–7.
90. Anyaegbu EI, Almond PS, Milligan T, Allen WR, Gharaybeh S, Al-Akash SI. Intravenous immunoglobulin therapy in the treatment of BK viremia and nephropathy in pediatric renal transplant recipients. Pediatr Transplant. 2012;16(1):E19–24.
91. Dalianis T. Immunotherapy for polyomaviruses: opportunities and challenges. Immunotherapy. 2012;4(6):617–28.
92. Randhawa PS, Schonder K, Shapiro R, Farasati N, Huang Y. Polyomavirus BK neutralizing activity in human immunoglobulin preparations. Transplantation. 2010;89:1462–5.
93. Sener A. Intravenous immunoglobulin as a treatment for BK virus associated nephropathy: one-year follow-up of renal allograft recipients. Transplantation. 2006;81:117–20.
94. Maggiore U, Medici MC, Vaglio A, Buzio C. Increased viral load after intravenous immunoglobulin therapy for BK virus-associated nephropathy. Transpl Infect Dis. 2010;12(5):470–2.
95. Kuypers DR. Management of polyomavirus-associated nephropathy in renal transplant recipients. Nat Rev Nephrol. 2012;8(7):390–402.
96. Johnston O. Treatment of polyomavirus infection in kidney transplant recipients: a systematic review. Transplantation. 2010;89:1057–70.
97. Trydzenskaya H, Sattler A, Muller K, Schachtner T, Dang-Heine C, Friedrich P, et al. Novel approach for improved assessment of phenotypic and functional characteristics of BKV-specific T-cell immunity. Transplantation. 2011;92(11):1269–77.
98. Blyth E, Clancy L, Simms R, Gaundar S, O'Connell P, Micklethwaite K, et al. BK virus-specific T cells for use in cellular therapy show specificity to multiple antigens and polyfunctional cytokine responses. Transplantation. 2011;92(10):1077–84.
99. Gralla J, Huskey J, Wiseman AC. Trends in immune function assay (ImmuKnow; Cylex) results in the first year post-transplant and relationship to BK virus infection. Nephrol Dial Transplant. 2012;27(6):2565–70.
100. Helantera I, Koskinen P. Association of immune cell function assay with protocol biopsy findings and viral infections in well matched kidney transplant recipients. Clin Nephrol. 2010;74(2):123–31.

101. Batal I. Measurements of global cell-mediated immunity in renal transplant recipients with BK virus reactivation. Am J Clin Pathol. 2008;129:587–91.
102. Mannon RB, Hoffmann SC, Kampen RL. Molecular evaluation of BK polyomavirus nephropathy. Am J Transplant. 2005;5:2883–93.
103. Masutani K, Shapiro R, Basu A, Tan H, Ninomiya T, Randhawa P. Putative episodes of T-cell-mediated rejection in patients with sustained BK viruria but no viremia. Transplantation. 2012;94(1):43–9.
104. Kim SH, Ahn HJ, Kim YS, Kim SI, Kim HS, Jeong HJ. Urinary HLA-DR and CD54 expression—indicators for inflammatory activity in decoy cell shedding patients. Nephrol Dial Transplant. 2006;21(9):2601–6.
105. Sadeghi M. Urinary proinflammatory cytokine response in renal transplant recipients with polyomavirus BK viruria. Transplantation. 2009;88:1109–16.
106. Kusne S, Vilchez RA, Zanwar P, Quiroz J, Mazur MJ, Heilman RL, et al. Polyomavirus JC urinary shedding in kidney and liver transplant recipients associated with reduced creatinine clearance. J Infect Dis. 2012;206(6):875–80.
107. Drachenberg CB, Papadimitriou JC, Mann D, Hirsch HH, Wali R, Ramos E. Negative impact of human leukocyte antigen matching in the outcome of polyomavirus nephropathy. Transplantation. 2005;80(2):276–8.
108. Awadalla Y. HLA mismatching increases the risk of BK virus nephropathy in renal transplant recipients. Am J Transplant. 2004;4:1691–6.
109. Awadallah Y, Duquesnoy R, Randhawa P, Shapiro R. HLA susceptibility to BKV infection. Am J Transplant. 2006;6:640.
110. Sharif A, Alachkar N, Bagnasco S, Geetha D, Gupta G, Womer K, et al. Incidence and outcomes of BK virus allograft nephropathy among ABO- and HLA-incompatible kidney transplant recipients. Clin J Am Soc Nephrol. 2012;7(8):1320–7.
111. Hammer MH. HLA type-independent method to monitor polyoma BK virus-specific CD4 and CD8 T-cell immunity. Am J Transplant. 2006;6:625–31.
112. Geetha D, Sozio SM, Ghanta M, Josephson M, Shapiro R, Dadhania D, et al. Results of repeat renal transplantation after graft loss from BK virus nephropathy. Transplantation. 2011;92(7):781–6.
113. Ramos E, Vincenti F, Lu WX. Retransplantation in patients with graft loss caused by polyoma virus nephropathy. Transplantation. 2004;77:131–3.
114. Womer KL, Patton PR, Kaplan B. Aggressive post-transplant monitoring of more importance to successful outcome following re-transplantation for BK virus nephropathy than absence of pre-transplant viremia. Transpl Int. 2008;21:1103–4.
115. Mindlova M, Boucek P, Saudek F, Jedinakova T, Voska L, Honsova E, et al. Kidney retransplantation following graft loss to polyoma virus-associated nephropathy: an effective treatment option in simultaneous pancreas and kidney transplant recipients. Transpl Int. 2008;21(4):353–6.
116. Hirsh HH, Ramos E. Retransplantation after polyomavirus-associated nephropathy: just do it? Am J Transplant. 2006;6:7–9.
117. Egli A, Helmersen DS, Taub K, Hirsch HH, Johnson A. Renal failure five years after lung transplantation due to polyomavirus BK-associated nephropathy. Am J Transplant. 2010;10(10):2324–30.
118. Barton TD, Blumberg EA, Doyle A, Ahya VN, Ferrenberg JM, Brozena SC, et al. A prospective cross-sectional study of BK virus infection in non-renal solid organ transplant recipients with chronic renal dysfunction. Transpl Infect Dis. 2006;8(2):102–7.
119. Munoz P. Prevalence of BK virus replication among recipients of solid organ transplants. Clin Infect Dis. 2005;41:1720–5.
120. Razonable RR, Brown RA, Humar A, Covington E, Alecock E, Paya CV. A longitudinal molecular surveillance study of human polyomavirus viremia in heart, kidney, liver, and pancreas transplant patients. J Infect Dis. 2005;192(8):1349–54.
121. Salama M, Boudville N, Speers D, Jeffrey GP, Ferrari P. Decline in native kidney function in liver transplant recipients is not associated with BK virus infection. Liver Transpl. 2008;14(12):1787–92.
122. Haririan A, Hamze O, Drachenberg CB, Ramos E, Weir MR, Klassen DK. Polyomavirus reactivation in native kidneys of pancreas alone allograft recipients. Transplantation. 2003;75(8):1186–90.
123. Vilchez RA, Kusne S. Molecular and clinical perspectives of polyomaviruses: emerging evidence of importance in non-kidney transplant populations. Liver Transpl. 2006;12(10):1457–63.
124. Doucette KE, Pang XL, Jackson K, Burton I, Carbonneau M, Cockfield S, et al. Prospective monitoring of BK polyomavirus infection early posttransplantation in nonrenal solid organ transplant recipients. Transplantation. 2008;85(12):1733–6.
125. Shitrit D, Lev N, Bar-Gil-Shitrit A, Kramer MR. Progressive multifocal leukoencephalopathy in transplant recipients. Transpl Int. 2005;17(11):658–65.
126. Verhelst X, Vanhooren G, Vanopdenbosch L, Casselman J, Laleman W, Pirenne J, et al. Progressive multifocal leukoencephalopathy in liver transplant recipients: a case report and review of the literature. Transpl Int. 2011;24(4):e30–4.
127. Bellizzi A, Nardis C, Anzivino E, Rodio D, Fioriti D, Mischitelli M, et al. Human polyomavirus JC reactivation and pathogenetic mechanisms of progressive multifocal leukoencephalopathy and cancer in the era of monoclonal antibody therapies. J Neurovirol. 2012;18(1):1–11.
128. Carson KR, Focosi D, Major EO, Petrini M, Richey EA, West DP, et al. Monoclonal antibody-associated progressive multifocal leucoencephalopathy in patients treated with rituximab, natalizumab, and efalizumab: a review from the research on adverse drug events and reports (RADAR) project. Lancet Oncol. 2009;10(8):816–24.
129. Elaba Z, Hughey L, Isayeva T, Weeks B, Solovan C, Solovastru L, et al. Ultrastructural and molecular confirmation of the trichodysplasia spinulosa-associated polyomavirus in biopsies of patients with trichodysplasia spinulosa. J Cutan Pathol. 2012;39(11):1004–9.
130. Sihto H, Kukko H, Koljonen V, Sankila R, Bohling T, Joensuu H. Clinical factors associated with Merkel cell polyomavirus infection in Merkel cell carcinoma. J Natl Cancer Inst. 2009;101(13):938–45.
131. Esposito L, Hirsch H, Basse G, Fillola G, Kamar N, Rostaing L. BK virus-related hemophagocytic syndrome in a renal transplant patient. Transplantation. 2007;83(3):365.
132. Karras A, Thervet E, Legendre C. Hemophagocytic syndrome in renal transplant recipients: report of 17 cases and review of literature. Transplantation. 2004;77(2):238–43.
133. Bratt G, Hammarin AL, Grandien M, Hedquist BG, Nennesmo I, Sundelin B, et al. BK virus as the cause of meningoencephalitis, retinitis and nephritis in a patient with AIDS. AIDS. 1999;13(9):1071–5.
134. Hedquist BG, Bratt G, Hammarin AL, Grandien M, Nennesmo I, Sundelin B, et al. Identification of BK virus in a patient with acquired immune deficiency syndrome and bilateral atypical retinitis. Ophthalmology. 1999;106(1):129–32.
135. Sandler ES, Aquino VM, Goss-Shohet E, Hinrichs S, Krisher K. BK papova virus pneumonia following hematopoietic stem cell transplantation. Bone Marrow Transplant. 1997;20(2):163–5.
136. Petrogiannis-Haliotis T, Sakoulas G, Kirby J. BK-related polyomavirus vasculopathy in a renal-transplant recipient. N Engl J Med. 2001;345:1250–5.
137. Sencer SF, Haake RJ, Weisdorf DJ. Hemorrhagic cystitis after bone marrow transplantation. Risk factors and complications. Transplantation. 1993;56(4):875–9.
138. Santos GW, Tutschka PJ, Brookmeyer R, Saral R, Beschorner WE, Bias WB, et al. Marrow transplantation for acute nonlymphocytic leukemia after treatment with busulfan and cyclophosphamide. N Engl J Med. 1983;309(22):1347–53.

139. Silva LP, Patah PA, Saliba RM, Szewczyk NA, Gilman L, Neumann J, et al. Hemorrhagic cystitis after allogeneic hematopoietic stem cell transplants is the complex result of BK virus infection, preparative regimen intensity and donor type. Haematologica. 2010;95(7):1183–90.
140. Leung AY, Suen CK, Lie AK, Liang RH, Yuen KY, Kwong YL. Quantification of polyoma BK viruria in hemorrhagic cystitis complicating bone marrow transplantation. Blood. 2001;98(6): 1971–8.
141. Dalianis T, Ljungman P. Full myeloablative conditioning and an unrelated HLA mismatched donor increase the risk for BK virus-positive hemorrhagic cystitis in allogeneic hematopoietic stem cell transplanted patients. Anticancer Res. 2011;31(3):939–44.
142. Giraud G, Bogdanovic G, Priftakis P, Remberger M, Svahn BM, Barkholt L, et al. The incidence of hemorrhagic cystitis and BK-viruria in allogeneic hematopoietic stem cell recipients according to intensity of the conditioning regimen. Haematologica. 2006;91(3):401–4.
143. Giraud G, Priftakis P, Bogdanovic G, Remberger M, Dubrulle M, Hau A, et al. BK-viruria and haemorrhagic cystitis are more frequent in allogeneic haematopoietic stem cell transplant patients receiving full conditioning and unrelated-HLA-mismatched grafts. Bone Marrow Transplant. 2008;41(8):737–42.
144. Leung AY. Ciprofloxacin decreased polyoma BK virus load in patients who underwent allogeneic hematopoietic stem cell transplantation. Clin Infect Dis. 2005;40:528–37.
145. Miller AN, Glode A, Hogan KR, Schaub C, Kramer C, Stuart RK, et al. Efficacy and safety of ciprofloxacin for prophylaxis of polyomavirus BK virus-associated hemorrhagic cystitis in allogeneic hematopoietic stem cell transplantation recipients. Biol Blood Marrow Transplant. 2011;17(8):1176–81.
146. Bridges B, Donegan S, Badros A. Cidofovir bladder instillation for the treatment of BK hemorrhagic cystitis after allogeneic stem cell transplantation. Am J Hematol. 2006;81(7):535–7.
147. Erard V, Kim HW, Corey L, Limaye A, Huang ML, Myerson D, et al. BK DNA viral load in plasma: evidence for an association with hemorrhagic cystitis in allogeneic hematopoietic cell transplant recipients. Blood. 2005;106(3):1130–2.
148. Leung AY, Yuen KY, Kwong YL. Polyoma BK virus and haemorrhagic cystitis in haematopoietic stem cell transplantation: a changing paradigm. Bone Marrow Transplant. 2005;36(11):929–37.
149. Cesaro S, Hirsch HH, Faraci M, Owoc-Lempach J, Beltrame A, Tendas A, et al. Cidofovir for BK virus-associated hemorrhagic cystitis: a retrospective study. Clin Infect Dis. 2009;49(2):233–40.
150. Savona MR, Newton D, Frame D, Levine JE, Mineishi S, Kaul DR. Low-dose cidofovir treatment of BK virus-associated hemorrhagic cystitis in recipients of hematopoietic stem cell transplant. Bone Marrow Transplant. 2007;39(12):783–7.
151. Alexiev BA, Randhawa P, Vazquez ME, Zeng G, Luo C, Ramos E, et al. BK virus-associated urinary bladder carcinoma in transplant recipients: report of 2 cases, review of the literature, and proposed pathogenetic model. Hum Pathol. 2013;44(5):908–17.

Post-transplant Proteinuria: Differential Diagnosis and Management

29

Ayub Akbari and Greg A. Knoll

Proteinuria is a common problem in kidney transplant recipients. It occurs in up to 45 % of patients, depending on the definition of proteinuria. Proteinuria arising from native kidneys declines rapidly after transplantation. Persistent or new onset of proteinuria in renal transplant recipients is associated with worse outcomes. The etiology of proteinuria in transplant recipients includes transplant-specific kidney diseases as well as those affecting the general population. This chapter will review measurement issues, prevalence, etiology, prognosis, and management of proteinuria in renal transplant recipients.

Measurement of Proteinuria

Quantification of proteinuria is standard practice in patients with a transplanted kidney. In the general population, 40–80 mg of protein is excreted in the urine each day. Most of this is low molecular weight protein with very small amounts of albumin (approximately 10 mg/day). The upper limit of normal protein excretion in the general population is 150 mg/day and for albumin is 30 mg/day. It is not clear if these same thresholds should be used given that renal transplant recipients have a single functioning kidney and there may be residual proteinuria from the native kidneys. Given the lack of transplant-specific data and the fact that small amounts of proteinuria have been associated with worse patient and allograft survival, the KDIGO transplant guidelines recommend using the same cutoffs as in the general population (Table 29.1).

Although 24-h urine collection is the gold standard for measurement of protein excretion, it is cumbersome for patients and prone to collection errors. Moreover, daily creatinine excretion is not reliable in determining completeness of the urine collection as creatinine excretion falls after transplantation. Since spot urine measurements are easier to perform and convenient, many transplant centers routinely perform spot measurements of proteinuria (or albuminuria) instead of the 24-h collection. In order to account for the dilution of protein in the urine, spot measurements of proteinuria (albuminuria) must be corrected for spot creatinine excretion giving a ratio of protein:creatinine (PCR) or albumin:creatinine (ACR). The KDIGO transplant guideline suggests that PCR and ACR are alternatives for 24-h urine collection in kidney transplant recipients. PCR and ACR thresholds are shown in Table 29.1.

Studies conducted in renal transplant population indicate the correlation of PCR to 24-h urine protein excretion to be in the range of 0.75–0.98 and the sensitivity and specificity to be 74–99 % and 73–99 %, respectively, using different cutoffs for proteinuria. Although correlation is important, it measures relative agreement and not the absolute agreement and thus it ignores bias. Although PCR may be strongly correlated to 24-h protein excretion, it may substantially over- or underestimate total protein excretion. Similarly, sensitivity and specificity provide useful information but do not inform the clinician about the quantitative accuracy of the test. Measurements of bias and accuracy are better measures of agreement than correlation, specificity, and sensitivity. In a study involving 192 kidney transplant recipients, the accuracy of spot urine measurements was modest. Only 47 % of PCR estimates were within 30 % of the 24-h value for those with proteinuria >1,000 mg/day. The results were marginally better for those with lesser amounts of proteinuria. Similarly, 38–80 % of ACR estimates (depending on the degree of albuminuria) were within 30 % of 24-h urine collection.

A. Akbari M.D., M.Sc.
Division of Nephrology, Kidney Research Centre, Ottawa Hospital Research Institute, Riverside Campus, 1967 Riverside Drive, Ottawa, ON, Canada K1H 7W9

G.A. Knoll, M.D., M.Sc. (✉)
Division of Nephrology, Kidney Research Centre, Ottawa Hospital Research Institute, Riverside Campus, 1967 Riverside Drive, Ottawa, ON, Canada K1H 7W9

Clinical Epidemiology Program, Ottawa Hospital Research Institute, Ottawa, ON, Canada
e-mail: gknoll@ottawahospital.on.ca

M.R. Weir and E.V. Lerma (eds.), *Kidney Transplantation: Practical Guide to Management*,
DOI 10.1007/978-1-4939-0342-9_29, © Springer Science+Business Media New York 2014

Table 29.1 Thresholds for proteinuria and albuminuria

	Albumin		Total protein	
	24-h (mg/day)	ACR (mg/g)	24-h (mg/day)	PCR (mg/g)
Normal	<30	<17 (men) <25 (women)	<300	<200
Microalbuminuria	30–300	17–250 (men) 25–355 (women)	NA	NA
Albuminuria	>300	>250 (men) >355 (women)	NA	NA
Proteinuria	NA	NA	>300	>200

Reproduced with permission from Shamseddin MK, Knoll GA. Posttransplantation proteinuria: an approach to diagnosis and management. Clin J Am Soc Nephrol 6: 1786–1793, 2011
24-h 24-h urine collection (mg/day), *ACR* albumin–creatinine ratio (mg/g), *PCR* protein–creatinine ratio (mg/g), *NA* not applicable

In view of this data, we recommend using a 24-h measurement of protein excretion before making any major clinical decisions (e.g., need for biopsy) based on the presence of proteinuria.

Prevalence of Proteinuria

The cutoff used for diagnosis of proteinuria has a major impact on its prevalence. In kidney transplant studies the prevalence has varied from 7.5 to 45 % depending on the threshold used (Table 29.2). When proteinuria is defined as greater than 150 mg/day (as in nontransplant population), the prevalence of proteinuria at 12 months post-transplantation is as high as 45 %. With a higher cutoff of 1 g/day, the prevalence has ranged from 7.5 to 40 % with an average of 19 % (Table 29.2). Even nephrotic range proteinuria has been reported in the transplant population with a prevalence of 13 %. These data suggest that proteinuria is just as common a problem in the renal transplant population as it is in the nontransplant chronic kidney disease (CKD) population.

Source and Causes of Proteinuria in Renal Transplant Recipients

Transplant recipients with considerable residual urine output, such as those who undergo preemptive transplantation or kidney transplantation soon after starting renal replacement therapy, may be quite proteinuric initially because of proteinuria from native kidneys. Although the mechanism remains unknown, native kidney proteinuria usually resolves at about 1 month post-transplantation. In a small study involving 14 live donor recipients, PCR was measured pretransplant and then weekly in the postoperative period. The PCR ranged from 0.5 to 9.2 (average = 2.9) pretransplant but normalized to <0.2 in all patients by 10 weeks post-transplantation. The average time to resolution of proteinuria was 4.5 weeks. Similar findings were seen in a larger prospective study involving 115 kidney transplant recipients. In this study, proteinuria fell from 3,650 ± 3,702 to 550 ± 918 mg/day at 3 weeks post-transplantation. There were 61 patients with pretransplant proteinuria values greater than 1.5 g/day and by 3 weeks post-transplantation only eight patients had this level of proteinuria. These studies suggest that proteinuria from the native kidneys resolves early post-transplantation and that persistent or increasing amounts of proteinuria should be assumed to be from the allograft.

There have been several studies that have examined the histological lesions in kidney transplant patients with proteinuria. Similar to what was seen with the prevalence data, histological diagnosis varied depending on the degree of proteinuria at the time of biopsy (Table 29.3). For patients with significant proteinuria (e.g., >1.5 or 2 g/day), glomerular pathology (e.g., recurrent and de novo glomerulonephritis and transplant glomerulopathy) seems most common. In a study involving 276 kidney transplant patients, the average proteinuria was 2.7 g/day for those with glomerular pathology compared to <500 mg/day for all other diagnoses including acute rejection and interstitial fibrosis/tubular atrophy. In fact, for patients with >1.5 g/day of proteinuria, 80 % have been found to have glomerular diseases. Transplant-specific diagnoses are more common than native kidney disease such as glomerulonephritis in renal transplant recipients with proteinuria. In the largest and most recent study to date, 58 % of transplant patients with proteinuria >150 mg/day had a transplant-specific diagnosis. The histological lesions included allograft nephropathy (also called chronic rejection or interstitial fibrosis/tubular atrophy) in 45 %, transplant glomerulopathy in 8 %, and acute rejection in 5 %. This compared to only 11 % with glomerulonephritis (Table 29.3).

Of the immunosuppressive medications used in kidney transplantation, only the mTOR inhibitors (sirolimus and everolimus) have been associated with proteinuria. Worsening of preexisting proteinuria and de novo proteinuria have both been described with these medications. Calcineurin inhibitor avoidance and calcineurin inhibitor withdrawal regimens using mTOR inhibitors have both reported proteinuria. Sirolimus and everolimus should be avoided in patients with

Table 29.2 Prevalence of proteinuria in kidney transplant recipients

References	Sample size	Definition of proteinuria	Time post-transplantation	Prevalence of proteinuria (%)
Fernandez (2002), Spain	532	>3 g/day	>12 months	13.7
Yakupoglu (2004), USA	570	>3 g/day	>1 week	13.0
First (1984), USA	639	>2 g/day	>1 month	12.1
Vathsala (1990), USA	704	>1 g/day	>1 month	12.8
Kim (1994), South Korea	204	>1 g/day	>1 month	27.9
Chung (2000), South Korea	197	>1 g/day	>3 months	12.5
Park (2000), South Korea	884	>1 g/day	>6 months	40.0
Karthikeyan (2003), Canada	459	>1 g/day	>6 months	12.0
Halimi (2005), France	484	>1 g/day	12 months	20.4
Fernandez (2004), Spain	3,365	>1 g/day	12 months	7.5
Chung (2000), South Korea	197	>0.5 g/day	>3 months	13.2
Fernandez (2002), Spain	532	>0.5 g/day	>12 months	36.4
Fernandez (2004), Spain	3,365	>0.5 g/day	12 months	15.3
Halimi (2005), France	484	>0.5 g/day	12 months	35.2
Sancho (2007), Spain	337	>0.5 g/day	>3 months	20.2
Amer (2007), USA	613	>0.5 g/day	12 months	15.3
Ibis (2007), Turkey	130	>0.3 g/day	12 months	34.3
Roodnat (2001), The Netherlands	722	>0.2 g/L	12 months	31.0
Amer (2007), USA	613	>0.15 g/day	12 months	45.0

Table 29.3 Allograft histology in kidney transplant recipients with proteinuria

References	Proteinuria at time of biopsy	Sample size with biopsy	Allograft nephropathy[a] (%)	Transplant glomerulopathy (%)	Glomerular disease[b] (%)	Acute rejection (%)	Other (%)
Yakupoglu (2004), USA	>3 g/day	73	18	16	66[c]	0	0
First (1984), USA	>2 g/day	77	27	39	29	0	5
Park (2000), South Korea	>1 g/day	81	54	0	27	7	11
Kim (1994), South Korea	>1 g/day	44	20	14	41	14	11
Vathsala (1990), USA	>1 g/day	63	49	24	12	15	0
Chung (2000), South Korea	>0.5 g/day	26	8	8	73	0	12
Amer (2007), USA	>0.15 g/day	276	45	8	11	5	31

Reproduced with permission from Proteinuria in Kidney Transplant Recipients: Prevalence, Prognosis, and Evidence-Based Management, *Am J Kidney Dis* 54:1131–1144, 2009

[a]Allograft nephropathy includes the following diagnoses: chronic allograft nephropathy, chronic rejection, interstitial fibrosis and tubular atrophy

[b]Glomerular disease includes recurrent and de novo glomerulonephritis and diabetic nephropathy

[c]Sixty-five percent had superimposed chronic allograft nephropathy

significant proteinuria and consideration should be given to stopping these medications in those who develop significant proteinuria as it is potentially reversible.

Prognosis

Proteinuria and albuminuria in transplant recipients have been associated with progressive kidney disease, graft loss, and mortality. In a study involving 722 renal transplant recipients with proteinuria >0.2 g/L, the risk of transplant failure as well as patient death was approximately twofold higher compared to those without proteinuria. In a large study involving 3,365 kidney transplant patients, the risk of graft loss (adjusted relative risk 2.33) and mortality (adjusted relative risk 2.05) was significantly increased for patients with >0.5 g/day of proteinuria. There have been several other studies linking proteinuria with death and graft loss. In these analyses, the adjusted relative risk for allograft loss has ranged from 1.15 to 5.34 with an average value of 2.7. Similarly, the adjusted risk of death for patients with proteinuria has ranged from 1.20 to 8.60 with a median value of 1.98. Most studies have also shown a consistent association between worsening proteinuria and cardiovascular events as well as cardiovascular cause of death.

Increasing levels of proteinuria are also associated with worsening graft survival. As shown in Fig. 29.1, even relatively mild proteinuria <500 mg/day is associated with a

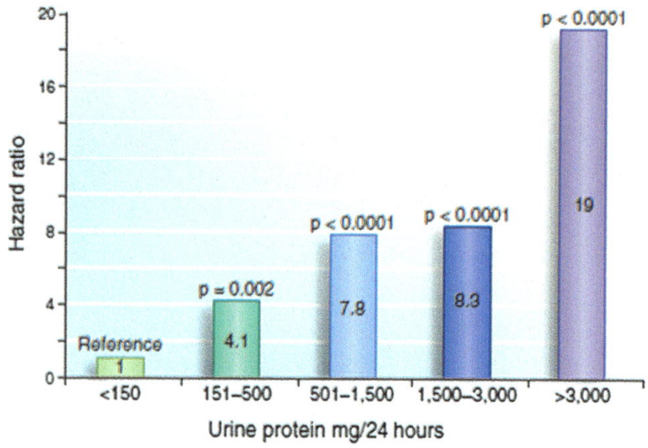

Fig. 29.1 The relationship between proteinuria at 1-year post-transplant and subsequent graft loss. Even small amounts of proteinuria (151–500 mg/day) are associated with a significant increase in allograft failure compared to those without proteinuria. Reproduced with permission from Amer H, and Cosio FG. Significance and Management of Proteinuria in Kidney Transplant Recipients. J Am Soc Nephrol 20: 2490–2492, 2009

fourfold increased risk of graft loss. Patients with nephrotic range proteinuria have a risk of graft loss that is nearly 20 times higher compared to those without proteinuria (Fig. 29.1). Most studies have assessed prognosis using the 24-h urine protein measurement. In a study involving 500 renal transplant recipients, the ACR and PCR were shown to be predictive of death-censored graft loss. Using receiver operating characteristic curves, the *c*-statistic for PCR was 0.82 (95 % CI 0.75–0.90) and for ACR it was 0.83 (95 % CI 0.76–0.90) indicating quite excellent discrimination. This study suggests that both the ACR and PCR can be used instead of the 24-h urine collection to assess prognosis in the kidney transplant population.

Management of Proteinuria

New and unexplained proteinuria (as defined in Table 29.1) in a kidney transplant recipient is an indication for kidney biopsy. Although the KDIGO transplant guidelines recommend kidney biopsy for unexplained proteinuria >3 g/day, others suggest a lower biopsy threshold of >1.5 g/day. Given the important prognostic information gained and the potential for therapeutic intervention we recommend proceeding with biopsy at the lower threshold of >1.5 g/day of proteinuria as outlined in Fig. 29.2. Treatment for specific histological lesions (e.g., plasmapheresis for recurrent focal segmental glomerulosclerosis) will not be discussed in this chapter but rather the approach to the nonspecific reduction in proteinuria.

In *nontransplant* patients, therapies for proteinuria reduction have been assessed in many randomized controlled trials. Tested interventions include dietary protein restriction, sodium restriction, blood pressure control, renin–angiotensin system blockade, non-dihydropyridine calcium channel blocker use, aldosterone antagonists, and pentoxyfylline. Evidence in *nontransplant* patients suggests that angiotensin converting enzyme (ACE) inhibitors and angiotensin receptor blockers (ARB) are the preferred agents since they not only reduce proteinuria but also retard progression of CKD and delay the need for dialysis and transplantation. Strategies to reduce proteinuria in the renal transplant recipient will be reviewed in the following section.

While it seems obvious that blood pressure control would reduce proteinuria and improve outcomes in kidney transplant recipients, there have been no randomized trials addressing this question. In the absence of specific data, it seems reasonable to follow the KDIGO Clinical Practice Guideline for the Management of Blood Pressure in Chronic Kidney Disease published in 2012. In this guideline it is suggested that blood pressure be controlled to a target <130/80 irrespective of the level of urine albumin excretion. In addition, no statement is made recommending one antihypertensive agent over another but they do suggest that clinicians take into account the time after transplantation, use of calcineurin inhibitors, the presence or absence of persistent albuminuria, and other comorbid conditions before selecting an agent. Unfortunately both of these recommendations are very weak due to the lack of data (Grade 2D and "Not Graded").

Two randomized crossover studies performed more than 10 years ago have addressed the use of protein-restricted diet in renal transplant recipients. Protein restriction of 0.55 or 0.7 g/kg/day resulted in a statistically significant decrease in proteinuria but progression of CKD was not assessed. It is not known if similar effects would be seen today in the era of better blood pressure control. In any event, because of risk of malnutrition, such intervention should only be carried out with close follow-up arranged by a renal dietician.

There are compelling theoretical reasons to believe that blocking the renin–angiotensin system in transplant recipients would be beneficial. These include a high prevalence of CKD with reduced GFR and proteinuria; high risk of cardiovascular mortality and morbidity including left ventricular dysfunction; large proportion of patients with diabetes; high prevalence of hypertension; and constant hyperfiltration in the setting of a solitary kidney. Unlike the nontransplant CKD setting, it is still not known whether renin–angiotensin system blockade in renal transplant recipients leads to better long-term outcomes such as improved patient and graft survival.

In 2007, a systematic review of 21 randomized trials ($n=1,549$) evaluating ACE-inhibitor and ARB use in kidney transplantation was published. ACE-inhibitor and/or ARB use was associated with a decline in proteinuria in all four trials that reported this outcome; however, the overall change was not statistically different from the comparator group (weighted mean difference −0.23 g/day; 95 % CI −0.52 to 0.06; $P=0.12$). When the analysis was restricted to trials with at least 12 months of follow-up ($n=2$ trials), the change

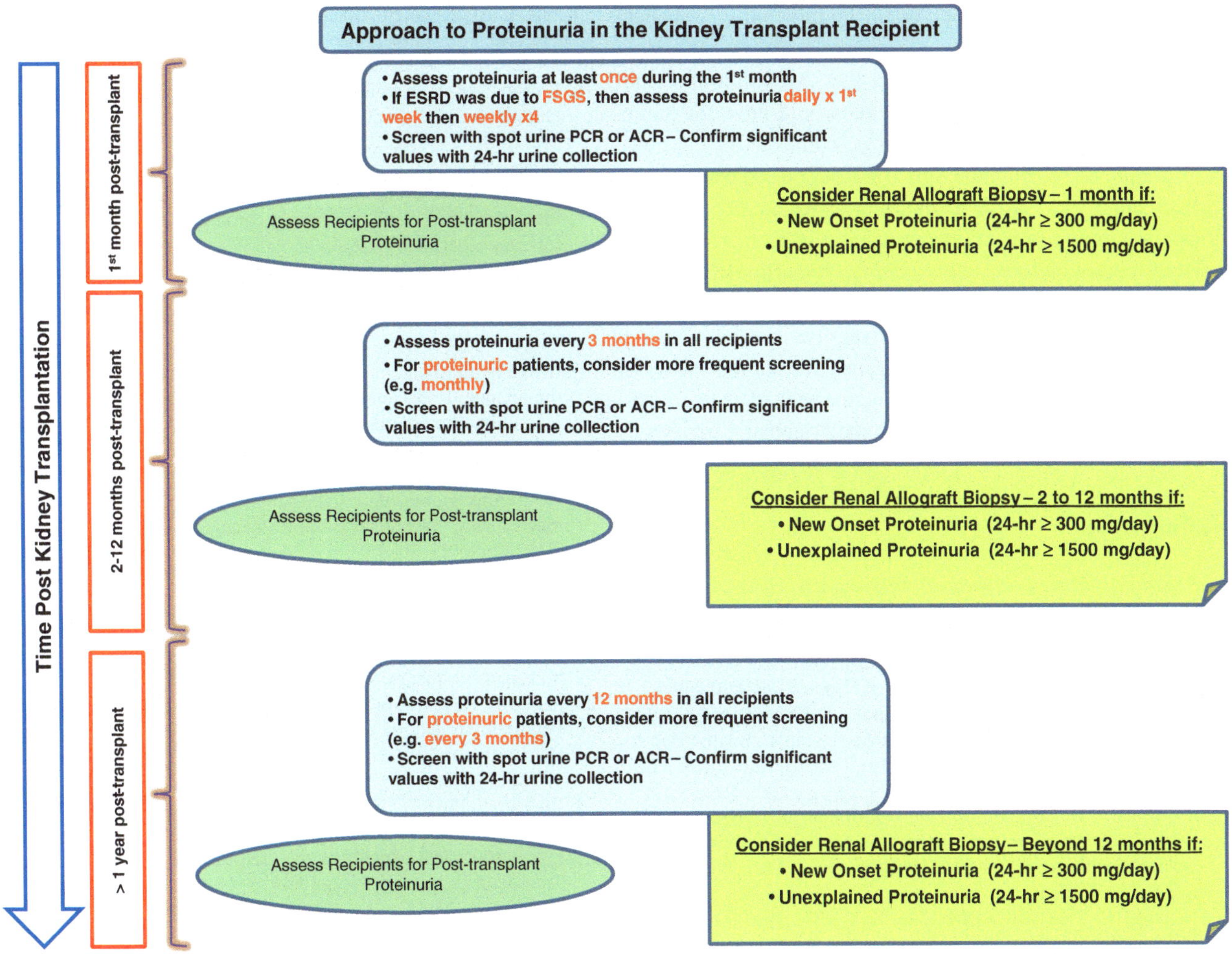

Fig. 29.2 Approach to proteinuria in the kidney transplant patient at different times post-transplantation. Reproduced with permission from Shamseddin MK, Knoll GA. Posttransplantation proteinuria: an approach to diagnosis and management. Clin J Am Soc Nephrol 6: 1786–1793, 2011

in proteinuria was significant (weighted mean difference −0.47 g/day; 95 % CI −0.86 to 0.08; $P = 0.02$). This analysis, however, showed that patients on an ACE-inhibitor or ARB for at least 12 months had a reduced GFR compared to those not taking these medications (weighted mean difference −5.8 mL/min; 95 % CI −10.60 to −0.99; $P = 0.02$). There was insufficient data from this review to comment on the effect of these medications on patient or allograft survival.

In 2009, the Cochrane Renal Group published a systematic review of all antihypertensive agents in kidney transplantation ($n = 60$ trials). In this review, the use of an ACE-inhibitor or ARB did not result in a significant reduction in proteinuria (mean difference −0.08 g/day; 95 % CI −0.23 to 0.06). ACE-inhibitor or ARB use resulted in a significant reduction in GFR when compared to calcium channel blockers (mean difference −11.5 mL/min; 95 % CI −7.2 to −15.8) and a no-significant reduction when compared to placebo (mean difference −8.1 mL/min; 95 % CI −18.6 to 2.4). Again, because of the small number of trials ascertaining important clinical outcomes and heterogeneity in the data, no conclusion could be made about the effect of ACE-inhibitor or ARB on patient or graft survival.

In the nontransplant CKD population sodium restriction has been shown to reduce proteinuria over and above that achieved with blockade of the renin–angiotensin system. In a randomized crossover trial, 52 patients (currently on lisinopril 40 mg/day) were treated consecutively for 6 weeks with an ARB (valsartan 320 mg/day) and a low sodium diet (target 50 mmol Na^+/day). As expected, the addition of valsartan significantly decreased mean proteinuria from 1.68 to 1.44 g/day ($P = 0.003$). However, the addition of a low sodium diet decreased residual proteinuria to an even greater extent (from 1.68 to 0.85 g/day ($P < 0.001$)). The reduction of proteinuria by the addition of a low sodium diet to ACE inhibition (51 %; 95 % CI 43–58 %) was significantly larger ($P < 0.001$) than the reduction of proteinuria by the addition of an ARB to ACE inhibition (21 %; 95 % CI 8–32 %). These data suggest that the simple, inexpensive intervention of dietary salt restriction could significantly enhance proteinuria reduction.

Although it might be assumed that ACE-inhibitor and ARB use in renal transplant patients would have the same beneficial effect on major clinical outcomes as in the non-transplant CKD population, this is not supported by the published data to date. An ACE-inhibitor or ARB can be used to lower proteinuria in an effort to prevent or reduce proteinuria-related complications (e.g., edema, hyperlipidemia) but should not be used with the specific intent to delay the progression of CKD or improve survival. The choice of using these agents must be weighed against the known adverse events such as anemia and hyperkalemia as well as the documented reduction in GFR shown in the systematic reviews.

References

1. Akbari A, White CA, Shahbazi N, Booth RA, Hiremath S, Knoll GA. Spot urine protein measurements: are these accurate in kidney transplant recipients? Transplantation. 2012;94(4):389–95.
2. Amer H, Cosio FG. Significance and management of proteinuria in kidney transplant recipients. J Am Soc Nephrol. 2009;20:2490–2.
3. Amer H, Fidler ME, Myslak M, Morales P, Kremers WK, Larson TS, et al. Proteinuria after kidney transplantation, relationship to allograft histology and survival. Am J Transplant. 2007;7(12): 2748–56.
4. Biesenbach G, Zazgornik J, Janko O, Hubmann R, Syre G. Effect of mild dietary protein restriction on urinary protein excretion in patients with renal transplant fibrosis. Wien Med Wochenschr. 1996;146(4):75–8.
5. Chung J, Park SK, Park JS, Kim SC, Han DJ, Yu E. Glomerulonephritis is the major cause of proteinuria in renal transplant recipients: histopathologic findings of renal allografts with proteinuria. Clin Transplant. 2000;14(5):499–504.
6. Cross NB, Webster AC, Masson P, O'Connell PJ, Craig JC. Antihypertensive treatment for kidney transplant recipients. Transplantation. 2009;88:7–18.
7. D'Cunha PT, Parasuraman R, Venkat KK. Rapid resolution of proteinuria of native kidney origin following live donor renal transplantation. Am J Transplant. 2005;5(2):351–5.
8. Fernandez-Fresnedo G, Escallada R, Rodrigo E, De Francisco AL, Cotorruelo JG, Sanz DC, et al. The risk of cardiovascular disease associated with proteinuria in renal transplant patients. Transplantation. 2002;73(8):1345–8.
9. Fernandez-Fresnedo G, Plaza JJ, Sanchez-Plumed J, Sanz-Guajardo A, Palomar-Fontanet R, Arias M. Proteinuria: a new marker of long-term graft and patient survival in kidney transplantation. Nephrol Dial Transplant. 2004;19(3):47–51.
10. First MR, Vaidya PN, Maryniak RK, Weiss MA, Munda R, Fidler JP, et al. Proteinuria following transplantation. Correlation with histopathology and outcome. Transplantation. 1984;38(6):607–12.
11. Halimi JM, Laouad I, Buchler M, Al Najjar A, Chatelet V, Houssaini TS, et al. Early low-grade proteinuria: causes, short-term evolution and long-term consequences in renal transplantation. Am J Transplant. 2005;5(9):2281–8.
12. Halimi JM, Buchler M, Al Najjar A, Laouad I, Chatelet V, Marliere JF, et al. Urinary albumin excretion and the risk of graft loss and death in proteinuric and non-proteinuric renal transplant recipients. Am J Transplant. 2007;7(3):618–25.
13. Hiremath S, Fergusson D, Doucette S, Mulay AV, Knoll GA. Renin angiotensin system blockade in kidney transplantation: a systematic review of the evidence. Am J Transplant. 2007;7(10):2350–60.
14. Ibis A, Altunoglu A, Akgul A, Usluogullari CA, Arat Z, Ozdemir FN, et al. Early onset proteinuria after renal transplantation: a marker for allograft dysfunction. Transplant Proc. 2007;39(4):938–40.
15. Karthikeyan V, Karpinski J, Nair RC, Knoll G. The burden of chronic kidney disease in renal transplant recipients. Am J Transplant. 2004;4(2):262–9.
16. Kidney Disease: Improving Global Outcomes (KDIGO) Blood Pressure Work Group. KDIGO clinical practice guideline for the management of blood pressure in chronic kidney disease. Kidney Int Suppl. 2012;2:337–414.
17. Kidney Disease: Improving Global Outcomes (KDIGO) Transplant Work Group. KDIGO clinical practice guideline for the care of kidney transplant recipients. Am J Transplant. 2009;9 Suppl 3:S1–157.
18. Kim HC, Park SB, Lee SH, Park KK, Park CH, Cho WH. Proteinuria in renal transplant recipients: incidence, cause, and prognostic importance. Transplant Proc. 1994;26(4):2134–5.
19. Knoll GA. Proteinuria in kidney transplant recipients: prevalence, prognosis, and evidence-based management. Am J Kidney Dis. 2009;54:1131–44.
20. Letavernier E, Legendre C. mToR inhibitors-induced proteinuria: mechanisms, significance, and management. Transplant Rev. 2008;22(2):125–30.
21. Myslak M, Amer H, Morales P, Fidler ME, Gloor JM, Larson TS, et al. Interpreting post-transplant proteinuria in patients with proteinuria pre-transplant. Am J Transplant. 2006;6(7):1660–5.
22. Panek R, Lawen T, Kiberd BA. Screening for proteinuria in kidney transplant recipients. Nephrol Dial Transplant. 2011;26:1385–7.
23. Park JH, Park JH, Bok HJ, Kim BS, Yang CW, Kim YS, et al. Persistent proteinuria as a prognostic factor for determining long-term graft survival in renal transplant recipients. Transplant Proc. 1924;32(7):2000.
24. Rodrigo E, Pinera C, Ruiz JC, Fernandez-Fresnedo G, Escallada R, Herraez I, et al. Quantitation of 24-hour urine protein excretion in kidney transplant patients by the use of protein to creatinine ratio. Transplant Proc. 2003;35(2):702.
25. Roodnat JI, Mulder PG, Rischen-Vos J, van Riemsdijk IC, van Gelder T, Zietse R, et al. Proteinuria after renal transplantation affects not only graft survival but also patient survival. Transplantation. 2001;72(3):438–44.
26. Salahudeen AK, Hostetter TH, Raatz SK, Rosenberg ME. Effects of dietary protein in patients with chronic renal transplant rejection. Kidney Int. 1992;41(1):183–90.
27. Sancho A, Gavela E, Avila A, Morales A, Fernandez-Najera JE, Crespo JF, et al. Risk factors and prognosis for proteinuria in renal transplant recipients. Transplant Proc. 2007;39(7):2145–7.
28. Shamseddin MK, Knoll GA. Posttransplantation proteinuria: an approach to diagnosis and management. Clin J Am Soc Nephrol. 2011;6:1786–93.
29. Slagman MC, Waanders F, Hemmelder MH, Woittiez AJ, Janssen WM, Heerspink HJ, Navis G, Laverman GD. Moderate dietary sodium restriction added to angiotensin converting enzyme inhibition compared with dual blockade in lowering proteinuria and blood pressure: randomised controlled trial. BMJ. 2011;343:d4366. doi:10.1136/bmj.d4366.
30. Steinhauslin F, Wauters JP. Quantitation of proteinuria in kidney transplant patients: accuracy of the urinary protein/creatinine ratio. Clin Nephrol. 1995;43(2):110–5.
31. Torng S, Rigatto C, Rush DN, Nickerson P, Jeffery JR. The urine protein to creatinine ratio (P/C) as a predictor of 24-hour urine protein excretion in renal transplant patients. Transplantation. 2001;72(8): 1453–6.
32. Vathsala A, Verani R, Schoenberg L, Lewis RM, Van Buren CT, Kerman RH, et al. Proteinuria in cyclosporine-treated renal transplant recipients. Transplantation. 1990;49(1):35–41.
33. Yakupoglu U, Baranowska-Daca E, Rosen D, Barrios R, Suki WN, Truong LD. Post-transplant nephrotic syndrome: a comprehensive clinicopathologic study. Kidney Int. 2004;65(6):2360–70.

Urologic Issues in the Renal Transplant Patient

30

Michael Phelan, Andrew Kramer, and Richard Bryson

Erectile Dysfunction

Epidemiology

Erectile dysfunction (ED) in the renal transplant population is a common and important problem. The causes are multifactorial and often associated with underlying medical comorbidities. The prevalence of ED associated with renal insufficiency and failure is high, especially with concomitant diabetes mellitus, and likely compounded by the physical and psychological toll of dialysis [1]. Indeed, the prevalence of ED in dialysis patients has remained elevated throughout the years, with some estimates as high as 70 % in those undergoing dialysis [2, 3]. Other studies have placed this estimate even higher, with 81.4 % of patients on hemodialysis having moderate to severe ED [4, 5], with patients reporting significantly decreased or complete absence of erections with this comorbidity.

Pathophysiology of Erectile Dysfunction

Sexual stimuli can be varied, ranging from tactile to visual, and these are processed by the brain and then carried to the penis via parasympathetic neural pathways. Ultimately, this sexual stimulation induces release of neurotransmitters from the nerves in the corpus cavernosum, with resultant smooth muscle dilatation. As blood rushes into the corpora due to vasodilatation of arterioles, there is trapping of blood in the expanding sinusoids, stretching of the tunica, and temporary blockage of the emissary veins that drain the penis [6].

Age is an independent risk factor for ED, thus putting the transplant population at a higher risk based on this demographic alone [7]. Additionally, the ED that develops may be caused by endothelial dysfunction, vascular issues, endocrine and hormonal axis, and structural/anatomic damage from trauma to the corporal smooth muscle [8].

The hypothalamic-pituitary axis must be considered in the transplant patient presenting with ED, so that hypogonadism can be diagnosed and treated when appropriate. Pulsatile release of gonadotropin-releasing hormone (GnRH) is required for the hormonal axis to work properly. When patients are in a state of chronic uremia, this pulsatile release is altered, causing suppression of the normal mechanism involved in the stimulation of the pituitary. Ultimately, a combination of other hormonal imbalances ensues, including lowered plasma testosterone, increase in luteinizing hormone and follicle-stimulating hormone, increased testosterone elimination, and impaired Leydig cell function [9]. There may also be impaired Sertoli cell function, further raising levels of FSH. Because LH and FSH are artificially elevated, and the hypothalamus is not in pulsatile mode, the result is inhibition of the pituitary and decreased testosterone. Lastly, hyperprolactinemia is increased in patients with renal dysfunction, resulting in ED and exacerbating hypogonadism. While the mechanism of how hyperprolactinemia causes ED remains unclear, it may also act to lower testosterone levels through feedback inhibition of the hypothalamic-pituitary axis.

Neurologic and vascular pathways are altered in the renal failure and transplant patient, resulting in ED at a higher rate than the background population [10, 11]. ED has been identified as a heralding sign of diabetic neuropathy, though even in the absence of diabetes, patients with renal insufficiency can develop neuropathy from the uremia alone. The parasympathetic pathway must be intact to allow for smooth muscle relaxation of the corpus cavernosum. When autonomic neuropathy develops, ED often ensues and is indeed often an early manifestation of systemic neurologic disease. In considering ED and the relationship to renal dysfunction, the cause is multifactorial rather than stemming from a single source. Endothelial dysfunction and atherosclerosis are felt to be paramount in the causation of ED as well [12, 13].

M. Phelan, M.D. • A. Kramer, M.D. (✉) • R. Bryson, M.D.
University of Maryland School of Medicine, 29 South Greene Street, Suite 500, Baltimore, MD 21201, USA
e-mail: akramer@smail.umaryland.edu

M.R. Weir and E.V. Lerma (eds.), *Kidney Transplantation: Practical Guide to Management*,
DOI 10.1007/978-1-4939-0342-9_30, © Springer Science+Business Media New York 2014

Treatment

Assessment begins with a full history and physical examination and a close partnership with a nephrologist or internist who is helping to manage the patient. Once erectile dysfunction has been diagnosed, and it is felt to be primarily organic in nature, then medical optimization should occur as an initial therapeutic measure. Not only does this lead to better outcomes from a renal insufficiency standpoint, but the ED often improves as the metabolic issues associated with the underlying disease are ameliorated. Hemoglobin levels, hormone levels, electrolyte disturbances, and plasma lipid and glucose levels can be assessed as a useful first approach to improving sexual function. An appointment with a psychiatrist to treat underlying depression or a meeting with a sex therapist to manage psychological issues associated with the chronic disease state can be helpful in repairing ED. Prior to an appointment, a patient may fill out a validated questionnaire such as an IIEF or an SHIM (sexual health inventory for men) score. Operative reports from a transplant, if done, may be reviewed as well. It has been documented that utilization of the internal iliac artery in revascularization may reduce the blood flow to the cavernosal arteries of the penis, but this did not cause ED if unilateral. If contralateral iliac arteries have been used for revascularization of a graft, then there may be a significant vascular component to the ED.

For diagnosis, an adequate history and examination may be enough to proceed with treatment. However, objective testing can prove to be helpful in directing treatment and assuring patients that the correct etiology has been identified. As previously described, hormone testing can identify hypogonadism if present and can be replaced if low. If vascular etiologies are suspected, then Doppler studies and dynamic intracavernosal cavernosometry and cavernosography (DICC) may be useful.

Oral therapy is a first-line treatment for ED, provided there are no contraindications such as use of or possible need for use of nitrates for cardiac disease or severely debilitated medical status whereby sexual activity would be dangerous [14, 15]. The first phosphodiesterase-5 inhibitor (PDE-5 inhibitor), sildenafil, was introduced in 1998. The mechanism is to reduce the breakdown of the active cGMP to the inactive noncyclic GMP. The active form, cGMP, causes smooth muscle dilatation of the arterioles in the male genitalia, inducing vasodilatation in the corpus cavernosa, thus causing tumescence. This class of drugs has been proven to be safe and efficacious in a broad number of patients, and there are now three distinct drugs available with a similar mechanism. Cyclosporine, tacrolimus, and sildenafil are all metabolized by cytochrome p450 enzymes, so medications such as ketoconazole that inhibit this process could increase the concentrations of all three [16].

Sildenafil has demonstrated significant efficacy in the dialysis patient in several studies. There have not been additional side effects noted in this subpopulation with the use of PDE-5 inhibitors, though the most common issues encountered are nasal congestion, headache, and slight visual disturbances. The starting dose is 50 mg of sildenafil or tadalafil and 10 mg of vardenafil. For renal dosing in patients with creatinine clearances of less than 30 mL/min, the recommending starting dose is half of this, or 25 mg of sildenafil. These PDE-5 inhibitors function best when taken 30–60 min prior to sexual activity.

Intraurethral suppositories also exist and are safe and effective means of treating ED in the dialysis or transplant population. This is known as MUSE (medicated intraurethral suppository for erection) and contains prostaglandin E-1 [17]. This medication is pushed into the lubricated urethra, and the pellet dissolves and induces an erection within minutes. Success rates have been favorable with this therapy, though not studied specifically in the transplant patient. A common but often well-tolerated side effect is penile pain.

Intracavernosal injections can be administered into the base of the penis, causing vasodilatation within minutes of self-administration. The medications typically given are phentolamine, papaverine, and prostaglandin E-1, in varying doses depending on individual patient response [18]. This is an on-demand treatment, with minimal systemic effects, that can be titrated up or down depending on patient preference or response to therapy. Onset of response is rapid, and duration must be monitored and discussed with a physician to maintain an adequate response while avoiding priapism, the most serious risk associated with this form of therapy. Other risks include scarring and damage to the corpus cavernosa, bleeding and hematoma, and pain with injection. The discontinuation rate of injectable therapies for ED is high, perhaps due to the cumbersome nature of the treatment and the discomfort of injection.

Vacuum devices with constriction bands are another viable option for managing the ED in the renal insufficiency and transplant patient. With this therapy, a cylinder is placed over the phallus, and negative pressure applied to draw blood in. Then to maintain this erection, a constrictive ring can be applied to the base of the penis to maintain the erection. While the systemic effects of this are negligible, and the success rates in producing a usable erection have exceeded 90 % in many studies, the side effects have caused high levels of discontinuation in many series. These include a dusky and cool-feeling penis, lack of sensation, and local discomfort.

Finally, penile implant or penile prosthesis surgery has been in existence since 1973 [19]. As a general rule, clinicians should wait until renal transplantation has been completed if this process is being considered. Once transplantation is complete, ED may improve and be amenable to medical therapy, thus avoiding surgery. Prosthetic devices range from semirigid, which are the most simple and can be bent up or down depending on patient preference, to inflatable containing a pump and a reservoir. A surgical consideration in transplant patients is if a graft is located in the pelvis, the reservoir must be carefully placed or positioned on the contralateral side of the pelvis to avoid injury to the transplanted organ.

Penile prostheses have been studied specifically in the transplant patient population, with generally very favorable results [20]. A concern of infection due to immunosuppression has been raised and remains a viable concern, but an increased incidence of infection in the post-transplant patient has not been seen. Some surgeons have noted increased difficulty in placing prostheses in this population, due to corporal fibrosis and scarring of the corpora, which may be a sequela of the underlying disease state and microvascular disease [21].

Bladder Cancer

Bladder cancer management in the transplant patient is a difficult urological issue in that the clinical course seems more complex and the cancer more aggressive in this population. The immunosuppressed status of the individual renders the screening, treatment options, and outcomes different from the general population. However, with the increase in renal transplantation and the longevity of this cohort of patients, this is a problem that is likely to become more common. It is believed that the susceptibility to malignancies is increased due to the immunosuppression and the neoplastic effects of the drugs used in these patients [22].

Epidemiology

Many have sought to determine if the incidence and natural history of bladder cancer in the transplant population are different from that of the general population. A large study from the University of Wisconsin demonstrated a 3.31 relative risk of developing bladder cancer as a result of renal transplantation, highlighting the need to completely evaluate hematuria in this population [23].

Another large study from Taiwan also highlighted the increased incidence in this population, with a cumulative incidence of transitional cell carcinoma of the urinary tract of 3.0 % at 3 years, 7.2 % at 6 years, and 17.5 % at 10 years of graft survival [24]. Studies have demonstrated more extensive disease at presentation as well. Therefore, the signs (hematuria) and symptoms (urgency, frequency) of urothelial carcinoma of the urinary tract must be aggressively pursued.

Evaluation

Hematuria, particularly painless gross hematuria, is concerning for malignancy of the bladder. When discovered, the diagnostic tests required include a CT or MRI of the upper tracts, a cystoscopy or panendoscopy of the urethra and bladder, and urine cytology. Once a transplant has been performed, the remaining urothelium, including the native kidneys and ureters, must be inspected periodically for epithelial carcinomas arising due to the field effect of this disease [25]. At time of cystoscopy, it is standard to do retrograde pyelograms and selective urine cytology from the native ureters, perhaps with ureteroscopy of these ureters and renal pelvises to rule out disease in the native upper tracts [26].

BCG in Transplant Patients

Bacillus Calmette–Guérin (BCG) is offered as the treatment of choice as a preventative measure in patients with CIS (carcinoma in situ) of the bladder or recurrent bouts of superficial bladder cancer with numerous disease sites in the bladder. Historically, BCG was contraindicated in renal transplant patients due to the risk of complications and morbidity, namely BCG sepsis. However, there is a small series of immunosuppressed patients in whom BCG was given with no added morbidity [27]. This is encouraging, as BCG has been shown to reduce the recurrence of bladder cancer in the general population; in the transplant population, this BCG option was historically restricted or avoided because BCG was once considered a contraindication in the immunosuppressed.

Invasive Bladder Cancer and Choice of Urinary Diversion

Invasive bladder cancer represents about 15 % of all cases, defined by invasion into the muscularis propria, or T2 disease. Once diagnosed with high-risk bladder cancer, a choice of withdrawing or reducing immunosuppression should be strongly considered. The surgical treatment of these patients differs from the management of superficial disease, because the disease progression is much more aggressive, and local therapy and resection are felt to not be curative. For T2 disease or beyond, options include cystectomy with urinary diversion or aggressive local resection with chemotherapy and radiotherapy.

The medical comorbidities that coexist in the renal transplant population drive some of the thought behind choosing a particular type of urinary diversion. One issue is electrolyte disturbances, which with larger bowel segments can be exacerbated due to prolonged urinary dwelling in these segments. Some patients who are awaiting or have received a kidney transplant may have marginal renal function, and some with good function after transplant would certainly be at risk for future renal insufficiency where the graft gets compromised due to a myriad of factors. Given this, the simpler diversion may be considered first, such as an ileal conduit, since there is little to no capacity for urinary storage, so the absorption of electrolytes and issues with electrolyte derangement would be considerably mitigated. Furthermore, with less risk of short gut syndrome and the sequelae of using longer segments of small or large intestine, patients with simpler diversions have less electrolyte and digestive issues owing to the simpler reconstruction with less bowel removed [28]. Since transplant patients have often had major abdominal surgery, maintaining a more straightforward approach to urinary diversion allows for a simpler recovery with less need for intra-abdominal adhesions and complications, also favorable in this population. However, several studies point to successful results in transplant recipients who received orthotopic bladder substitutes such as Studer pouches [29].

Another consideration in transplant recipients who undergo urinary diversion is the choice of ureteroneocystostomy. There are risks and benefits to creation of different types of anastomosis between ureter and intestinal segment in cases of cystectomy for invasive bladder cancer [30]. A non-refluxing ureteral anastomosis has benefits in protecting the graft from refluxed urine, especially that which may be mixed with mucous and possibly contaminated [31]. However, an increased stricture rate in a non-refluxing anastomosis can potentially be more prone to anastomotic stricture, and in this case, this would be especially costly because graft compromise could lead directly to renal insufficiency and failure.

Complete urinary tract extirpation in the setting of bladder cancer in the renal transplant recipient or candidate is a consideration that has been explored by several groups who have done this procedure successfully [32]. This is an attractive consideration, given that if the native kidneys and ureters could be removed at the time of cystectomy and urinary diversion, it would eliminate the need for surveillance of this urothelium in the future. Clearly the additional surgery involved and the associated risks present a significant downside. A group at the University of Maryland published a series of nine patients who underwent this procedure, and the survival rate was 86 % at 31 months. In this series, simultaneous bilateral nephroureterectomy, cystectomy or cystoprostatectomy, and creation of urinary diversion were done [32]. Three of these patients had not yet received a renal transplant yet, but could not be considered for a donor until they met certain guidelines regarding their cancer-free status. Dialysis was resumed postprocedure.

Prostate Cancer: Considerations in Renal Transplant Candidates and Renal Transplant Recipients

Prostate cancer is the most commonly diagnosed non-cutaneous malignancy among men in the United States and is the second leading cause of cancer death in men, accounting for nearly 10 % of cancer deaths in the United States [33]. Prostate-specific antigen (PSA)-based screening has resulted in the majority of patients being diagnosed with clinically localized disease that is amenable to definitive surgery or radiation with curative intent [34]. Despite advances in the diagnosis and treatment of prostate cancer, there are aspects of this disease that remain controversial. Additionally the United States Preventive Task Force has recommended against screening for prostate cancer due to the side effects of diagnosis and treatment. This controversial recommendation is not endorsed by the American Urological Association (AUA) or the American Cancer Society [35]. Urology consultation for prostate cancer screening and treatment is frequently sought for patients with end stage renal disease (ESRD) where renal transplantation is the ideal treatment. There are currently no established guidelines for prostate cancer screening and treatment specific for men with ESRD who are candidates for renal transplantation or for men who are renal transplant recipients [36]. Prostate cancer screening practices in renal transplant recipients have been extrapolated from the general population. Aspects of prostate cancer screening and management that apply to renal transplant candidates and recipients will be reviewed.

Prostate Cancer Screening

Screening for malignancy is a component of the medical evaluation that is performed on potential renal transplant candidates. The presence of malignancy, such as prostate cancer, can disqualify a patient from renal transplantation candidacy [37]. Prostate cancer screening involves yearly PSA measurement and digital rectal examination in men 50 years old or older, with earlier screening performed in those at higher risk based on ethnicity and/or family history. Studies have shown no difference in PSA before and after HD and before and after renal transplantation. PSA therefore remains a useful marker for prostate disease in patients with ESRD [36]. The diagnosis of prostate cancer ultimately requires prostate biopsy. Transrectal ultrasound-guided prostate biopsies are typically performed under local anesthesia and can be performed on an immunosuppressed patient without an increased risk of complications when compared to a nontransplant population [38].

Screening for prostate cancer can potentially create a dilemma for patients with ESRD who require renal replacement therapy to decrease their mortality risk. Renal transplantation is the ideal form of renal replacement therapy; however, the presence of prostate cancer detected through screening is a contraindication to transplantation. Traditional policy requires that men with ESRD and prostate cancer have a 5-year PSA recurrence-free period prior to being considered for renal transplantation. The overall survival, however, for patients on HD at 5 years is approximately 41 % compared with an overall 7-year all-cause survival rate of 90 % among patients with localized prostate cancer treated with radical prostatectomy. Patients with ESRD and prostate cancer clearly face a greater risk of mortality on HD than as a result of localized prostate cancer [39].

The concept of a 5-year waiting period is based on a study that reported an 18 % prostate cancer recurrence rate among 33 renal transplant patients, most of whom had been treated for their prostate cancer 2–5 years prior to transplantation [40]. The patients in this study, however, had largely been diagnosed and treated prior to the PSA screening era at which time prostate cancer tended to be more advanced at the time of diagnosis. Additionally, this study did not evaluate the relationship between cancer recurrence and factors such as PSA level, Gleason score, and stage, all of which have since been shown to be predictive of prostate cancer recurrence. Nomograms have since been developed which incorporate various patient-specific factors in order to generate an individual's risk of prostate cancer recurrence after definitive management. The standard 5-year wait between treatment of prostate cancer and renal transplantation has more recently been challenged in light of the following facts: (a) nomograms are capable of predicting an individual's risk of disease recurrence, (b) there is no evidence that ESRD or HD increases the risk of developing prostate cancer, and (c) it is unclear whether the pathophysiology of prostate cancer is affected by immunosuppression [39]. Renal transplantation is therefore believed to provide significant gains in life expectancy even among patients with ESRD and prostate cancer [36].

Prostate Cancer in ESRD and After Transplantation

ESRD has been associated with increased risk for various malignancies including skin cancer, lymphoma, Kaposi's sarcoma, and renal cell carcinoma. The standardized incidence ratio for prostate cancer in an ESRD population has been reported between 0.7 and 1.2 [36].

A long-recognized relationship exists between malignancy and transplantation. The increased incidence of malignancy in transplant recipients has been attributed to decreased immunosurveillance, activation of oncogenic viruses, and chronic inflammation. The United States Renal Data System (USRDS) has reported that genitourinary malignancies are the second most common tumors in transplant recipients after skin cancers [38]. The effects of renal transplantation and chronic immunosuppression on the natural history of prostate cancer remain unclear. Some studies have reported that transplant patients are at increased risk for prostate cancer whereas others have reported a risk equal to that of the general population [36, 41]. Comparison of cancer risk after transplantation to that in the general population has been difficult for several reasons. Generally, transplant recipients undergo more diligent screening and follow-up than the general population and therefore prostate cancer is diagnosed more frequently in this cohort of patients. In addition, recent trends favor an older cohort of patients in whom prostate cancer is of particular concern regardless of transplantation status. Indeed, the average age of transplant recipients has been increasing and improved immunosuppressive agents have resulted in longer allograft survival, both of which result in an older cohort of patients in which prostate cancer must be considered [36].

Immunosuppression has been clearly associated with the development of malignancy in renal transplant patients; however, the effect on prostate cancer is not clear. Azathioprine, which inhibits DNA repair mechanisms, has been associated with squamous cell cancer development but does not appear to affect prostate cancer. Calcineurin inhibitors (CNIs) such as cyclosporine inhibit interleukin-2 production and T-cell growth [36]. CNIs have been associated with post-transplant malignancies, and in an experimental model of prostate cancer in rats, cyclosporine was shown to increase the incidence of metastatic forms of this malignancy [42]. Mycophenolate mofetil (MMF) blocks purine biosynthesis and appears to have protective effects against the development of skin cancer in transplant patients and may also have antiproliferative properties in prostate cancer cell lines. Sirolimus, which blocks G1 to S-phase cell cycle progression, is known to have anticarcinogenic properties, but its effect on prostate cancer is currently unknown [36].

A relationship between prostate cancer and immunosuppression is suggested by findings in men with human immunodeficiency virus (HIV). Prostate cancer not only occurs earlier in HIV-infected patients than in control populations but also has a detection rate that is associated with the duration of viral infection (or duration of immunosuppression). Interestingly, a recent study of 62 renal transplant patients reported a high rate of locally advanced disease (36 % T3/T4) and metastatic disease (19.3 %) at presentation. In contrast, the European Randomized Study of Screening for Prostate Cancer showed a rate of locally advanced and metastatic disease of 15.5 % and 1.3 %, respectively, in the screened group versus 23 % and 11.6 % in the non-screened group [41]. According to this study, transplant recipients appear to have a higher rate of locally advanced and metastatic prostate cancer compared to rates in the general population regardless of whether or not screening was performed [41]. One possible explanation for this finding is that patients with ESRD have low testosterone levels which have been associated with more advanced pathological stage. A second explanation, which is supported by the same study that reported a higher rate of locally advanced prostate cancer in renal transplant recipients, is that immunosuppression affects prostate cancer progression. Kleinclauss et al. reported that maintenance immunosuppressive therapy with CNI and AZA with or without steroids was associated with a significant higher rate of locally advanced or metastatic disease compared with protocols including CNI with or without steroids. In fact, CNI and AZA maintenance therapy was found to be the only risk factor for locally advanced prostate cancer in this study [41]. In summary, prostate cancer in the population of renal transplant recipients appears to occur with a higher rate of locally advanced disease which is associated with combined use of AZA and CNI.

Prostate Cancer Treatment

The majority of prostate cancers diagnosed in the era of PSA screening, in both general and transplant populations, represent low-volume, localized disease (PSA < 10, Gleason score 6 or less). The standard management options for localized prostate cancer in the nontransplant population include radical prostatectomy, radiation therapy, and active surveillance [38]. Controversy exists regarding the ideal management of localized prostate cancer in the general population, and naturally, this controversy extends to the transplant population as well. The discussion that follows will focus on the management of localized prostate cancer in men who are transplant candidates or prior renal transplant recipients.

As alluded to previously, the primary issue associated with managing prostate cancer in men who are transplant candidates is determining the appropriate timing of transplantation after a man has underwent definitive curative therapy for his prostate cancer. A 5-year PSA recurrence-free period has traditionally been used; however, more current data suggest that recurrence risk can be accurately determined based on clinical data and that prostate cancer recurrence or progression does not appear to be significantly altered by immunosuppression [39]. In light of these findings, the amount of time a patient must wait before undergoing renal transplantation after receiving primary therapy for localized prostate cancer should be based on an individualized risk assessment rather than a generalized 5-year period.

Consideration must also be given to choosing a treatment modality for renal transplant candidates with localized prostate cancer. Radiation therapy (external beam radiation and brachytherapy) and radical prostatectomy (perineal, retropubic, laparoscopic) are both potentially curative treatment options. The fact that serum PSA level is utilized to measure response to treatment and monitor for recurrence, both of which are important factors that will determine a patient's candidacy for transplantation, could influence one's choice between radiation and prostatectomy in the pre-transplant population. Whereas serum PSA level quickly becomes undetectable after successful treatment with radical prostatectomy, the response to radiotherapy is considerably slower and may not be evident for 24–30 months. Additionally, monitoring for recurrence in patients after radiation therapy is difficult because many patients maintain a detectable serum PSA level. Surgical management also allows for pathologic analysis of the tissue specimen and accurate assessment of recurrence risk through the use of nomograms. As such, some practitioners preferentially utilize radical prostatectomy for the treatment of localized prostate cancer in patients who are renal transplant candidates [39].

When prostate cancer is diagnosed in a transplant patient, there are no randomized controlled trials to guide treatment [36]. Most of the information regarding prostate cancer treatment in this select population is limited to case reports pertaining to open radical retropubic prostatectomy [43]. Prostatectomy offers several advantages, including pathological staging and simpler postoperative PSA monitoring. There are surgical risks, however, that are specific to patients having had a renal transplant. Such patients are at increased risk for impaired wound healing and postoperative wound infection. Surgical dissection, including lymphadenectomy, may be made more difficult by the presence of scar tissue and a graft in the iliac fossa with the associated risk of injuring the ureteroneocystostomy. A transperitoneal approach with robot-assisted radical prostatectomy (RARP) may be made more difficult by prior peritoneal dialysis which could result in peritoneal adhesions. A perineal approach for prostatectomy has been utilized both in renal transplant candidates and recipients with the potential advantage of avoiding the iliac fossa and any injuries to the graft that may occur with retraction.

Despite these complicating factors, outcomes for transplanted patients treated with open prostatectomy appear to be equivalent to the general population [44]. Although more challenging in patients with a previous renal transplant, RARP can be performed in such patients with outcomes similar to the general population [45]. As with radical surgery, the presence of a renal transplant also presents challenges to the application of radiation therapy for treating prostate cancer in this patient population. Despite techniques such as intensity-modulated radiation therapy (IMRT) and 3D conformal therapy which aim to limit exposure to surrounding tissues, the exit dose alone can still exceed the toxicity limits of the kidney allograft and ureter [38]. Radiation-induced allograft ureteral injury is of primary concern and is a limiting factor in the application of external beam radiation therapy for prostate cancer in renal transplant patients [36]. In contrast to external beam radiation therapy, brachytherapy has been utilized with reported success in renal transplant patients. The direct placement of radioactive seeds into the prostate results in minimal exposure to surrounding pelvic structures and therefore makes this form of radiation therapy a reasonable option for renal transplant patients [38]. Current data suggests that transplant patients undergoing brachytherapy for low-risk, localized prostate cancer achieve outcomes similar to those reported in the general population [43]. Potential drawbacks of radiotherapy include the absence of pathological staging and unpredictable postoperative PSA kinetics.

Summary

Prostate cancer screening and management in the renal transplant population largely follow practices applied to the general population. Total serum PSA testing can be applied in ESRD patients before and after transplantation. Whether there is an increased risk of prostate cancer in transplant patients remains unclear. At the time of diagnosis, however, more recent data suggests that renal transplant patients are at increased risk for locally advanced prostate cancer when treated with a CNI and AZA maintenance immunosuppressive therapy.

Hematuria

Preoperative Evaluation

Hematuria is classified as gross hematuria or microscopic hematuria. Gross hematuria is visible on a voided specimen. Microscopic hematuria is not visible and usually is detected on screening urine analysis. Microscopic hematuria cannot be confirmed on urine dipstick and requires formal microscopic examination. Microscopic hematuria is defined by greater than 3 red blood cells per high-powered field. Microscopic hematuria is very common in the renal failure population. The most common etiology of hematuria in this patient population is medical renal disease. Hematuria in the setting of ESRD is often associated with cellular casts. It may also be the result of inflammation or infection. However, hematuria can be the result of more serious unrecognized urologic problems. Hematuria may result from urologic malignancy, benign prostatic hyperplasia, and kidney stones. Distinguishing between benign hematuria and hematuria that will require further investigation and/or surgery is therefore important in the pre-transplant work-up.

The formal work-up for hematuria involves investigation of the urine, bladder, and upper tracts. A urine culture is typically where the investigation begins. In the absence of a documented urinary tract infection, cystoscopy and upper tract studies follow. A flexible cystoscopy can be performed in the office setting under local anesthesia. The flexible cystoscopy is required to rule out bladder pathology such as urothelial carcinoma. If a urine cytology was obtained, a negative urine cytology does not preclude the need for cystoscopy as low-grade tumors are not typically detected on cytology [46]. The most accepted upper tract study is a three-phase contrast-enhanced computer tomography. The intravenous contrast is nephrotoxic and therefore cannot be used in the pre-dialysis end stage renal failure patient. In the pre-dialysis patient, upper tracts should be investigated with a combination of renal ultrasound or magnetic resonance urography and a retrograde pyelogram. The retrograde pyelogram can be performed at the time of cystoscopy but will require fluoroscopic equipment. However, if the patient is already on dialysis, a CT urogram is the standard investigation of the upper tracts. Utilizing urine studies, cystoscopy, and CT urogram, benign hematuria can be defined and distinguished from the concerning causes of hematuria such as bladder cancer, kidney cancer, and kidney stones.

Given the high prevalence of microscopic hematuria in the renal failure population, the clinical challenge is to determine who requires a formal hematuria work-up [47]. There are no absolute guidelines for hematuria work-up in the ESRD population. In the setting of gross hematuria, a formal work-up is required. In the setting of microscopic hematuria and ESRD, a great deal of clinical judgment is necessary to determine which patients should proceed with a formal work-up. The AUA Guidelines: Diagnosis, Evaluation and Follow-up of Asymptomatic Microhematuria in Adults is an excellent resource. These guidelines state that the presence of cellular casts does not eliminate the potential requirement for a formal hematuria work-up. With such a challenging population, how does a clinician decide when to proceed with the formal work-up? The presence of risk factors for urologic malignancy may help guide the clinician (Table 30.1). The presence of one or more of these risk factors should trigger a consult for a formal hematuria work-up.

Table 30.1 Risk factors for malignancy in patients with hematuria

Male gender
Age (>35 years)
Smoking history
Chemical exposure (benzenes or aromatic amines)
History of gross hematuria
History of other urologic disease
Irritative voiding symptoms
History of pelvic irradiation
Chronic urinary tract infection
Carcinogenic exposures: chemotherapy/alkylating agents
Chronic indwelling catheter or foreign body

Adapted from AUA Asymptomatic Microhematuria Guideline 2012

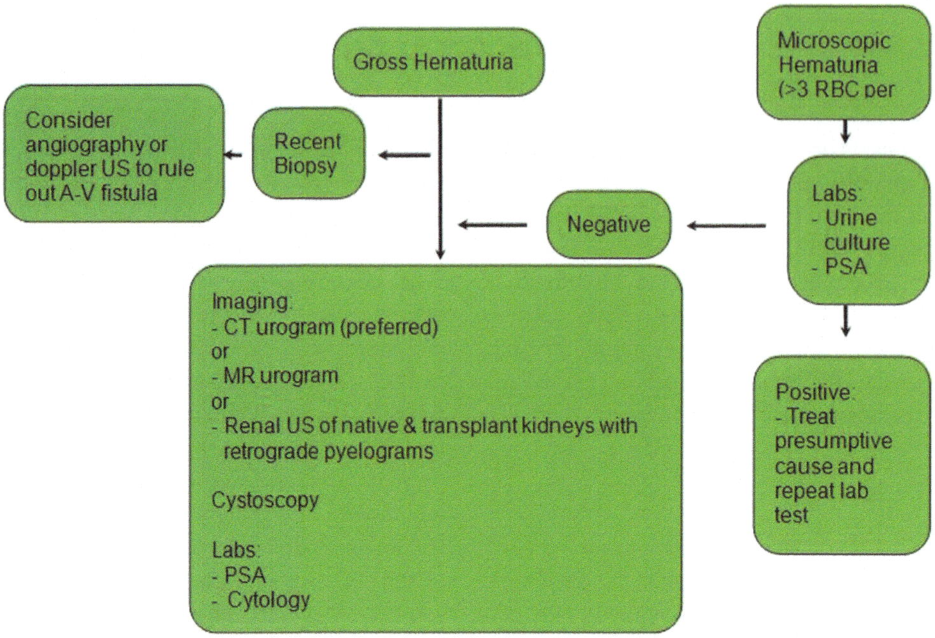

Fig. 30.1 Hematuria evaluation (Adapted from AUA Asymptomatic Microhematuria Guideline 2012)

Postoperative Hematuria

Immediate post-kidney transplant hematuria can be classified as surgical or pathological. Surgical hematuria is bloody urine that has resulted from or during the surgical procedure. Hematuria in this setting may result from bleeding at the site of the ureteral anastomosis or from Foley catheter trauma. In most cases surgical hematuria is self-limiting and requires no intervention. However, if the hematuria results in clinical instability, intervention may be required. A cystoscopic examination provides the diagnosis and if necessary the ability to fulgurate a bleeding surgical site.

Remote hematuria in the transplant recipient may be the result of kidney biopsy, rejection, or other pathologic entities. Immediate hematuria following a percutaneous renal biopsy is usually self-limiting. However, persistent hematuria following a kidney transplant biopsy may signify the formation of a pseudoaneurysm or an arterial venous malformation. These vascular injuries are best managed with angiography and embolization [48].

In the absence of surgical hematuria, infection and rejection merit consideration. Rejection may be associated with a decline of renal function. The diagnosis of rejection is determined with clinical judgment and/or renal biopsy. A urine culture is helpful to determine the presence of a bacterial or viral infection [49]. Urine cytology has historically played a role in the hematuria work-up. However, in the most recent AUA guidelines for hematuria work-up, urine cytology is not recommended as a necessary diagnostic test (Fig. 30.1). A formal hematuria work-up should be performed for transplant patients with risk factors for malignancy (Table 30.1).

Renal Cell Carcinoma

Renal cancer is the third most common urologic cancer. In 2008 there were about 54,000 new cases of kidney cancer. There are about 13,000 deaths per year secondary to kidney cancer [50]. Patients with renal failure, especially those with acquired cystic renal disease (ACKD), are at greater risk of developing renal cancer [51]. The number of people developing renal failure and requiring a kidney transplant increases each year [50]. With the increasing population of renal failure patients and the elevated risk of developing renal cancer in this patient population, one would project that renal cancer will be a growing problem. Furthermore, with the increased number of kidney transplants [52] and the associated survival benefit, there will likely be an increase in the rate of kidney cancer seen in this select population.

Preoperative Diagnosis of a Renal Mass

A suspicious renal mass can be detected as an incidental finding or as the result of a screening process. Many pretransplant patients undergo abdominal imaging for a variety of reasons. The imaging studies frequently reveal an abnormal mass that is suspicious for renal cancer. The most definitive studies to characterize a renal mass are as follows: CT scan with and without IV contrast or MRI with and without IV contrast. In the pre-dialysis renal failure patient, these studies are not possible because of the contraindication to administrating IV dye due to nephrotoxicity or nephrogenic systemic fibrosis, respectively [53–55]. In this patient population, a renal ultrasound with Doppler flow is the best alternative. In the setting of a suspicious mass, the clinical management should be individualized. If the patient has already undergone a successful transplant, a native nephrectomy should be performed. The native nephrectomy can be performed with laparoscopic or open techniques. In most cases, the native kidney is small and laparoscopic technique is the preferred approach. Fortunately, renal cell carcinoma does not seem to flourish while under immunosuppression and therefore the immunosuppression does not need to be reduced [56]. However, urothelial carcinoma, which may develop in the renal pelvis, ureter, or bladder, can proliferate more rapidly and may require immunosuppressive adjustment as well as aggressive removal of the entire urothelial surface and creation of a urinary diversion with a bowel segment [32].

If a small, suspicious renal mass occurs in a patient who is not on dialysis, the renal mass can be observed with serial radiographic studies. Removal of the kidney prior to the initiation of dialysis may result in dialysis. In most cases renal cell carcinoma is a slow-growing tumor and close observation does not greatly increase the risk of metastasis. In this patient population, a nephrectomy is preformed upon the initiation of dialysis.

In the clinical scenario of a newly diagnosed renal cancer, the question of when it is safe to transplant often arises. In our institution, it has been our practice to proceed with transplantation without delay if the pathology of the native kidney is low grade and low stage. These "fast-track" clearance patients have recently been reviewed. Ten patients were transplanted following a recent nephrectomy for a renal cancer. The mean interval from the diagnosis of kidney cancer to transplant was 5 months. There were no recurrences or development of metastatic disease at a mean of 29 months (manuscript in preparation). If the patient has high-grade or high-stage renal cell carcinoma, we will typically wait for 18 months to rule out the development of metastatic disease or local recurrence.

Renal Mass in the Allograft

There are three clinical settings in which an allograft is identified with renal cancer. The most common scenario is when a renal mass develops in the allograft sometime following the renal transplant. The treatment options are allograft nephrectomy or a nephron-sparing procedure such as ablation or a partial nephrectomy. Partial nephrectomy remains a technically challenging procedure. Typically in a partial nephrectomy procedure, the renal hilum is occluded with vascular clamps. This allows the renal cancer to be excised in a bloodless fashion. In the transplanted kidney, access to the renal hilum is often impossible due to extensive scaring and adhesions. Partial nephrectomy procedures in allografts have been reported but are technically challenging [57, 58]. Renal tumor ablation with either radiofrequency or cryosurgery has been reported; however, the long-term outcomes of these techniques are pending [57]. The allograft nephrectomy should be reserved for large tumors or in patients in whom the graft has failed. The goal in managing the renal transplant patient with an allograft renal mass is twofold: adequate cancer control and preservation of a functioning transplant.

There are two other more controversial clinical scenarios in which an allograft renal mass or cancer occurs. The first is the discovery of a renal mass in a cadaveric kidney and the second is an incidental renal mass found on work-up of a live donor. Such allografts are typically rejected. However, with the ever-expanding gap between supply and demand of kidney allografts, there has been some initial successful experience with use of these organs that challenges this practice. In a cadaveric kidney, the renal mass is detected in the process of a back table bench preparation or on a CT scan. The partial nephrectomy is performed on a back table and the remaining unaffected kidney is used for transplantation [59, 60]. An incidental renal mass found on a live donor provides a challenge. This donor now must be faced with the issues of a diagnosis of a cancer and whether or not to proceed with the donation. Extensive informed consent is paramount for both the donor and recipient. Clearly, these are difficult issues and the use of an allograft with a renal mass probably should be reserved for high-risk recipients who may not survive an extended waiting period. For this patient population, the risks of a cancer recurrence are likely lower than the risk of dialysis.

Autosomal Dominant Polycystic Kidney Disease

Autosomal dominant polycystic kidney disease (ADPKD) is a common cause of renal failure [61]. Nearly 10 % of the ESRD population is composed of ADPKD patients [62]. In addition to renal failure, many ADPKD patients have clinical problems directly related to the kidneys themselves. Renal colic, nephrolithiasis, and pyelonephritis are common. The mass effect of these kidneys may result in early satiety and shortness of breath. Moreover, the mass effect of some ADPKD kidneys is so great that there is no room in the patient to accommodate a renal allograft (Fig. 30.2). In these

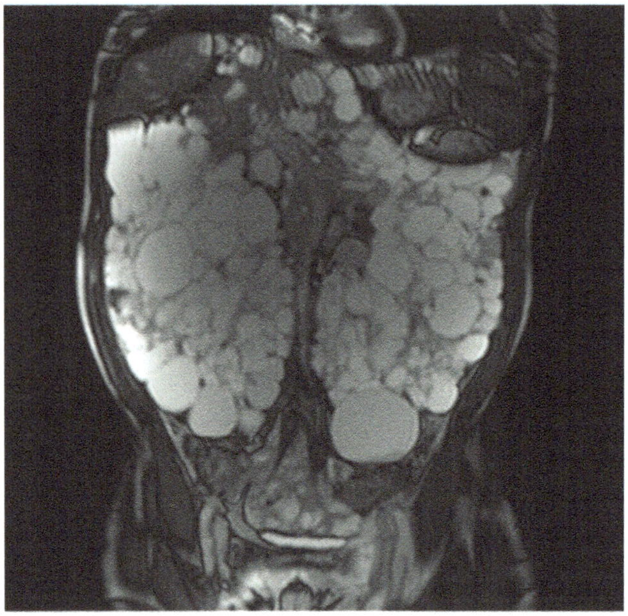

Fig. 30.2 MRI: polycystic kidneys

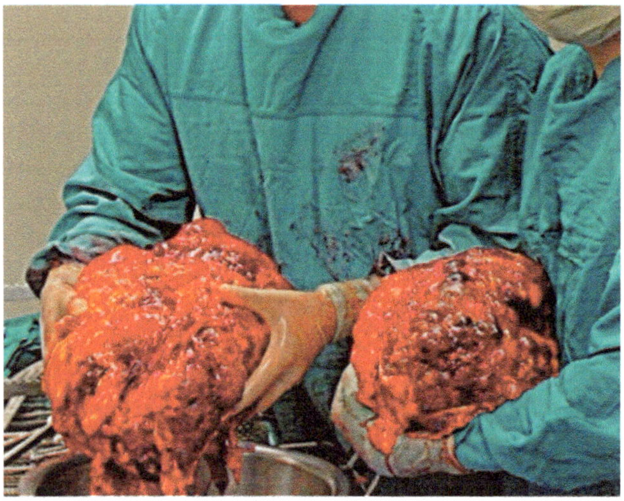

Fig. 30.3 Surgically removed polycystic kidneys

patients, bilateral nephrectomy may be required (Fig. 30.3). The bilateral nephrectomy can be performed in a staged fashion (before or after the transplant) or in a simultaneous fashion under the same anesthesia as the kidney transplant procedure. In pre-transplant patients, a staged pre-transplant nephrectomy will require a dialysis bridge until the patient is successfully transplanted. For many patients, a dialysis bridge is a major inconvenience. If a living donor is available, many patients would be eligible for a simultaneous bilateral nephrectomy and living donor transplant. This simultaneous approach has historically been avoided as it has been associated with risks and complications [63, 64]. Concomitant bilateral nephrectomy may be associated with longer operative times, increased blood loss, transfusions, and the potential of having the transplant cancelled if there is a surgical complication during the transplant. However, there is now a growing clinical experience with bilateral nephrectomy and simultaneous transplant with successful outcomes [65, 66]. The recent success may be associated with refinement in technique and improved surgical technology. The surgery is associated with large fluid shifts and hypotension and these may have detrimental effects on the transplant outcome if not managed appropriately. An experienced anesthesia team is therefore essential to the success of a simultaneous bilateral nephrectomy and renal transplant.

Renal Calculi

Renal calculi can occur in the native kidneys or the allograft. Incidental, asymptomatic stones in the native kidney do not require any intervention. However, if the burden in the native kidney is significant, it may present with pain or urinary tract infections. Pain in a native, atrophic kidney is rare; however, if the stone is obstructing a kidney that still produces urine, pain may develop. The surgical management of an obstructing stone is determined by the location and size of the stone. Proximal ureteral stones can be treated with extracorporeal shock wave lithotripsy (ESWL) or ureteroscopy and laser lithotripsy. Large native kidney stones associated with recurrent urinary tract infections (struvite stones) must be removed in order to successfully eliminate the infection. Removing the stone with endoscopic technique is an option; however, for stones >2 cm, endoscopic therapy may require multiple surgeries. In this particular scenario, one should consider a laparoscopic nephrectomy as an alternative approach.

Renal calculi may form de novo in the allograft or, alternatively, renal calculi may be transplanted and subsequently detected on radiographic studies. The incidence of allograft stones is about 0.4–1 % [67, 68]. The clinical management of asymptomatic calculi detected in a renal allograft should be individualized. For tiny asymptomatic stones, the best management may be observation. For stones that result in symptoms of obstruction, hematuria, or infection, urologic intervention is usually required. Allograft stones can be treated with ESWL [69, 70], ureteroscopy and laser lithotripsy [71], or percutaneous nephrolithotomy [68, 72, 73]. The goal of therapy is to eradicate the stone without injury to the transplant and/or native urinary tract. Surgical intervention in the transplanted kidney is challenging. ESWL is challenging as the pelvic bones shield the allograft from shock waves. Retrograde ureteroscopy is challenging because that transplant ureteral length is short and the neoureteral orifice is often difficult to access. The percutaneous approach is invasive and associated with risks including bleeding, vascular complications, and injury to overlying bowel. Nonetheless, the percutaneous approach is our preferred surgical approach in the setting of symptomatic allograft stones. In our experience, an interventional radiologist establishes the initial access which is then serially dilated over a short period of time to 16 Fr. A flexible cystoscope is then used in an antegrade fashion and the stone is obliterated with a holmium laser. If a ureteral stone is present, a flexible ureteroscope is used in an antegrade fashion to access the transplant ureter. From our experience with allograft nephrectomies, we have learned that the allograft is much more fragile than a native kidney. We therefore avoid active balloon dilation of an allograft for fear of bleeding or renal rupture.

Hydronephrosis

Hydronephrosis is a description indicating fullness in the renal pelvis and/or ureter that is frequently visualized on ultrasound examination of the transplanted kidney. Ultrasound of the allograft is a common diagnostic tool that is often used to evaluate elevated creatinine, blood flow, and renal anatomy during biopsy. A diagnosis of hydronephrosis of the transplant is not unusual and is not equivalent to a diagnosis of obstruction. A renal ultrasound is not a physiologic test and therefore the presence of obstruction cannot be established with ultrasound. In fact, an incidental diagnosis of hydronephrosis in the setting of a normal, stable creatinine probably does not require any further work-up. However, hydronephrosis in the setting of an elevated creatinine merits further investigation.

Vesicoureteral reflux, which is common in transplanted kidneys, may lead to the development of hydronephrosis. The simplest initial diagnostic step is to repeat the renal ultrasound with an empty bladder. An empty bladder can be established by Foley catheter or voiding immediately before the ultrasound. Dissipation of the hydronephrosis with these techniques rules out obstruction and further medical evaluation is required to determine the cause of the elevated creatinine.

Persistent hydronephrosis and elevated creatinine with an empty bladder suggest the possibility of a ureteral obstruction. Ureteral obstruction may result from ischemia or inflammation. Ureteral obstruction occurs in 2–10 % of cases making it one of the most common complications of renal transplant [74–76]. Seventy one percent of ureteral strictures occur within 3 months of the transplant [76, 77]. The majority occurs at the ureteral-vesical junction. Ureteral obstruction can be diagnosed with a MAG-3 lasix renogram. This is a physiologic study and provides information regarding uptake, excretion, and drainage. The patient should be well hydrated and the urinary bladder should be drained with a Foley catheter [78, 79]. The Foley catheter allows constant drainage and a more accurate assessment of the transplanted ureter which is very often difficult to interpret.

Ureteral obstruction secondary to inflammation or edema may be managed with a ureteral stent or a nephrostomy tube. These tubes can be removed when the inflammation or edema has resolved. The advantage of a nephrostomy tube is twofold. First, it relieves the obstruction and preserves renal function. Second, it also allows a diagnosis and anatomic evaluation of the level of obstruction. A nephrostogram is an excellent study to evaluate the anatomy of the obstruction. If the obstruction does not resolve within a reasonable time frame, the obstruction is likely secondary to stricture rather than edema.

Ureteral strictures often require surgical intervention. The surgical remedy depends on the length and location of the stricture. Ureteral reconstruction may require neoureteral anastomosis, pyelovesical anastomosis, or ureteroureteral (transplant ureter to native ureter) anastomosis. Reconstruction technique and strategy are individualized as the etiologies and location of the stricture may vary. For short ureteral strictures (2 cm) located at the ureteral vesical junction, an attempt at a minimally invasive repair is a reasonable first step. These strictures can be balloon dilated; however, the long-term success of balloon dilation ranges from 55 to 60 % [75, 80–84]. Given the high failure rate, modifications of the endoscopic balloon dilation have been implemented. Short ureteral strictures have been successfully incised with a holmium:YAG laser and balloon dilation [85].

References

1. Saenz de Tejada I, Goldstein I, Azadzoi K, Krane R, Cohen RA. Impaired neurogenic and endothelium-mediated relaxation of penile smooth muscle from diabetic men with impotence. N Engl J Med. 1989;320:1025–30.
2. Procci WR, Goldstein DA, Adelstein J, Massry SG. Sexual dysfunction in the male patient with uremia: a reappraisal. Kidney Int. 1981;19:317–23.
3. Ayub W, Fletcher S. End stage renal disease and erectile dysfunction: is there any hope? Nephrol Dial Transplant. 2000;15:1525–8.
4. Ahmad M, Rafiuddin Q, Hassan U, Ahmad A, Husain S. Impact of renal transplantation on erectile dysfunction due to chronic renal failure in male patients. J Ayub Med Coll Abbottabad. 2009;21:69–71.
5. Zamd M, Gharibi MB, Ramadni B, Zaid D. Sexual dysfunction in male patients undergoing HD in Morocco. Saudi J Kidney Dis Transpl. 2005;16:33–9.
6. Dean R, Lue T. Physiology of penile erection and pathophysiology of erectile dysfunction. Urol Clin North Am. 2005;21:279–81.
7. Selvin E, Burnett AL, Platz EA. Prevalence and risk factors for erectile dysfunction in the US. Am J Med. 2007;120:151–7.
8. Mallick HN, Manchanda SK, Kumar VM. Sensory modulation of the medial preoptic area neuronal activity by dorsal penile nerve stimulation in rats. J Urol. 1994;151:759.
9. Lim V, Fang V. Gonadal dysfunction in uremic men. A study of the hypothalamo-pituitary testicular axis before and after renal transplantation. Am J Med. 1975;58:655–62.

10. McCulloch DK, Young RJ, Prescott RJ, Campbell IW, Clarke BF. The natural history of impotence in diabetic men. Diabetologia. 1984;26:437–40.
11. Cartledge JJ, Eardley I, Morrison JF. Advanced glycation end-products are responsible for the impairment of corpus cavernosal smooth muscle relaxation seen in diabetes. BJU Int. 2001;87: 402–7.
12. Gazzaruso C, Solerte SB, Pujia A. Erectile dysfunction as a predictor of cardiovascular events and death in diabetic patients with angiographically proven asymptomatic coronary artery disease: a potential protective role for statins and 5-phosphodiesterase inhibitors. J Am Coll Cardiol. 2008;51:2040–4.
13. Ma RCW, SO WY, Yang X. Erectile dysfunction predicts coronary heart disease in Type 2 diabetes. J Am Coll Cardiol. 2008;51: 2045–50.
14. Fagelman E, Fagelman A, Shabsigh R. Efficacy, safety, and use of sildenafil in urologic practice. Urology. 2001;57:1141–4.
15. El-Galley R, Rutland H, Talic R, Keane T, Clark H. Long-term efficacy of sildenafil and tachyphylaxis effect. J Urol. 2001; 166:927–31.
16. Niwa T, Yamamoto S, Saito M, Shiraga T, Takagi A. Effect of cyclosporine and tacrolimus on cytochrome p450 activities in human liver microsomes. Yakugaku Zasshi. 2007;127:209–16.
17. Raina R, Agarwal A, Ausmundson S, Mansour D, Zippe CD. Long-term efficacy and compliance of MUSE for erectile dysfunction following radical prostatectomy: SHIM analysis. Int J Impot Res. 2005;17:86–90.
18. McMahon CG. Comparison of the response to the intracavernosal injection of a combination of papaverine and phentolamine, prostaglandin E1 alone and a combination of all three in the management of impotence. Int J Impot Res. 1991;3:133–42.
19. Scott FB, Bradley WE, Timm GW. Management of erectile impotence. Use of implantable inflatable prosthesis. Urology. 1974; 2:80–2.
20. Rowe SJ, Montague DK, Steinmuller DR, Lakin MM, Novick AC. Treatment of organic impotence with penile prosthesis in renal transplant patients. Urology. 1993;41:16–20.
21. Cuellar DC, Sklar GN. Penile prosthesis in the organ transplant recipient. Urology. 2001;57:138–41.
22. Gallagher M, Kelly P, Jardine M, Perkovic V, Cass A, Craig J, Eris J, Webster A. Long-term cancer risk of immunosuppressive regimens after kidney transplantation. J Am Soc Nephrol. 2010; 21:852–8.
23. Buzzeo BD, Heisey DM, Messsing EM. Bladder cancer in renal transplant recipients. Urology. 1997;50:525–8.
24. Wu MJ, Lian JD, Yang CR, Cheng CH, Chen CH, Lee WC, Shu KH, Tang MJ. High cumulative incidence of urinary tract transitional cell carcinoma after kidney transplantation in Taiwan. Am J Kidney Dis. 2004;43:1091–7.
25. Briggs JD. Causes of death after renal transplantation. Nephrol Dial Transplant. 2001;16:1545.
26. Doublet JD, Peraldi MN, Gattegno B. Renal cell carcinoma of native kidneys: prospective study of 129 renal transplant patients. J Urol. 1997;158:42–4.
27. Palou J, Angerri O, Segarra J, et al. Intravesical bacillus Calmette-Guèrin for the treatment of superficial bladder cancer in renal transplant patients. Transplantation. 2003;76:1514–6.
28. Lang H, Petriconi R, Wenderoth U, Volkmer B, Hautmann R, Gschwend J. Orthotopic ileal neobladder reconstruction in patients with bladder cancer following renal transplantation. J Urol. 2005;173:881–4.
29. Giessing M, Türk I, Schoenberger B, Loening S. Orthotopic neobladder after kidney transplantation in a male patient with recurring urothelial carcinoma and renal cancer. J Urol. 2001;166:1383.
30. Karam G, Hétet JF, Maillet F. Late ureteral stenosis following renal transplantation: risk factors and impact on patient and graft survival. Am J Transplant. 2006;6:352.
31. Masahiko H, Kazunari T, Tokumoto T, et al. Comparative study of urosurgical complications in renal transplantation: intravesical versus extravesical ureterocystoneostomy. Transplant Proc. 2000;32: 1844.
32. Holton MR, Van Zijl PS, Oberle WT, Jacobs SC, Sklar GN. Complete urinary tract extirpation: the University of Maryland experience. Urology. 2006;68:65–9.
33. Jemal A, Siegel R, Xu J, et al. Cancer statistics, 2010. CA Cancer J Clin. 2010;60:277.
34. Loeb S, Carter HB. Early detection, diagnosis, and staging of prostate cancer. In: Wein AJ et al., editors. Campbell-Walsh urology. 10th ed. Philadelphia, PA: Elsevier Saunders; 2012. p. 2763–70.
35. Moyer VA. Screening of prostate cancer: US Preventive Task force recommendation statement. Ann Intern Med. 2012;157:120–34.
36. Breyer BN, Whitson JM, Freise CE, Meng MV. Prostate cancer screening and treatment in the transplant population: current status and recommendations. J Urol. 2009;181:2018–26.
37. Chen CJ, Heldt JP, Anderson KM, et al. Prostate specific antigen levels and prostate cancer detection rates in patients with end stage renal disease. J Urol. 2012;187:2061–7.
38. Muruve NA, Shoskes DA. Genitourinary malignancies in solid organ transplant recipients. Transplantation. 2005;80:709–16.
39. Secin FP, Carver B, Kattan MW, Eastham JA. Current recommendations for delaying renal transplantation after localized prostate cancer treatment: are they still appropriate? Transplantation. 2004;78:710–2.
40. Penn I. Evaluation of transplant candidates with pre-existing malignancies. Ann Transplant. 1997;2:14–7.
41. Kleinclauss F, Gigante M, Neuzillet Y, et al. Prostate cancer in renal transplant recipients. Nephrol Dial Transplant. 2008;23:2374–80.
42. Pollard M. Enhancement of metastasis of prostate adenocarcinoma cells by immune-suppressive cyclosporine A. Cancer Lett. 1997; 111:221–4.
43. Coombs CC, Hertzfeld K, Barrett W. Outcomes in transplant patients undergoing brachytherapy for prostate cancer. Am J Clin Oncol. 2012;35:40–4.
44. Antonopoulos IM, Nahas WC, Piovesan AC, et al. Radical retropubic prostatectomy for localized prostate cancer in renal transplant patients. Urology. 2008;72:1362–5.
45. Smith DL, Jellison FC, Heldt JP, et al. Robot-assisted radical prostatectomy in patients with previous renal transplantation. J Endourol. 2011;10:1643–7.
46. Parker J, Spiess PE. Current and emerging bladder cancer urinary biomarkers. ScientificWorldJournal. 2011;11:1103–12.
47. Moreno JA, Martin-Cleary C, Gutierrez E, et al. Haematuria: the forgotten CKD factor? Nephrol Dial Transplant. 2012;27:28–34.
48. Sharma AK, Sunil S, Rowlands P, Bakran A. Pseudoaneurysm with severe haematuria in renal allograft after renal biopsy treated by percutaneous embolization. Nephrol Dial Transplant. 2002;17: 934–5.
49. Hirsch HH, Brennan DC, Drachenberg CB, et al. Polyomavirus-associated nephropathy in renal transplantation: interdisciplinary analyses and recommendations. Transplantation. 2005;10:1277–86.
50. Jemal A, Siegel R, Ward E, et al. Cancer statistics, 2008. CA Cancer J Clin. 2008;58:71.
51. Matson MA, Cohen EP. Acquired cystic kidney disease: occurrence, prevalence and renal cancers. Medicine. 1990;69:217.
52. United Stated Renal Data System. USRDS 2007 annual data report. Bethesda, MD: National Institute of Health (NIH), US Department of Health and Human Services (DHHS); 2007.
53. Marckmann P, Skov L, Rossen K, et al. Nephrogenic systemic fibrosis: suspected etiological role of gadodiamide used for contrast-enhanced magnetic resonance imaging. J Am Soc Nephrol. 2006;17:2359–62.
54. Grobner T. Gadolinium—a specific trigger for the development of nephrogenic fibrosing dermopathy and nephrogenic systemic fibrosis? Nephrol Dial Transplant. 2006;21:1104–8.

55. Thomsen H. Nephrogenic systemic fibrosis: a serious late adverse reaction to gadodiamide. Eur Radiol. 2006;16:2619–21.
56. Suson K, Sausville J, Sense A, Phelan M. Native nephrectomy for renal cell carcinoma in transplant recipients. Transplantation. 2011;91:1376–9.
57. Leveridge M, Musquera M, Evans A, et al. Renal cell carcinoma in the native and allograft kidneys of renal transplant recipients. J Urol. 2011;196:219–23.
58. Sankari B, Chueh S. Simultaneous laparoendoscopic single-site radical nephrectomy for native kidney and open nonischemic partial nephrectomy to treat concomitant renal cell carcinoma in native and transplant kidneys and to preserve allograft function. Urology. 2012;79:139–44.
59. Barama A, St-Louis G, Nicolet V, et al. Renal cell carcinoma in kidney allografts: a case series from a single center. Am J Transplant. 2005;5:3015–8.
60. Cox A, Nguan C, Luke P. Partial nephrectomy for renal cell carcinoma in long term renal allografts: operative and post-operative considerations. Can J Urol. 2005;12:2887–90.
61. Gabow P. Autosomal dominant polycystic kidney disease. N Engl J Med. 1993;329:332.
62. Parfrey P, Bear J, Morgan J, et al. The diagnosis and prognosis of autosomal dominant polycystic kidney disease. N Engl J Med. 1990;323:1085.
63. Fuller T, Brennan T, Feng S, Kang SM, et al. End stage polycystic kidney disease: indications and timing of native nephrectomy relative to kidney transplantation. J Urol. 2005;174:2284.
64. Ismail H, Fletcher S, Kaouk J, Derweesh I, et al. Simultaneous vs. sequential laparoscopic bilateral nephrectomy and renal transplantation. Transplantation. 2005;80:1124.
65. Glassman D, Nipkow L, Bartlett S, Jacob S. Bilateral nephrectomy with concomitant renal graft transplantation for autosomal dominant polycystic kidney disease. J Urol. 2000;164:661.
66. Kramer A, Sausville J, Haririan A, Bartlett S, et al. Simultaneous bilateral native nephrectomy and living donor renal transplantation are successful for polycystic kidney disease: The University of Maryland experience. Urology. 2009;181:724–8.
67. Klingler H, Kramer G, Lodde M, Marberger M. Urolithiasis in allograft kidneys. Urology. 2002;59:344–8.
68. Stavodimos K, Adamis S, Tyritis S, Georgios Z, Constantinides C. Renal transplant lithiasis: analysis of our series and review of the literature. J Endourol. 2012;26:38–44.
69. Li S, Wang Q, Chen W. Treatment of urinary lithiasis following kidney transplantation with extracorporeal shock-wave lithotripsy. Chin Med J. 2011;124:1431–4.
70. Markic D, Valencic M, Grskovic A, et al. Extracorporeal shock-wave lithotripsy of ureteral stone in a patient with en bloc kidney transplantation: a case report. Transplant Proc. 2011;43:2110–2.
71. Hyams E, Marien T, Quirouet A, Andonian S, Shah O, Matlaga B. Ureteroscopy for transplant lithiasis. J Endourol. 2012;7:819–22.
72. Krambeck A, LeRoy A, Patterson D, Gettman MT. Percutaneous nephrolithotomy success in the transplanted kidney. J Urol. 2009;180:2545–9.
73. Wyatt J, Kolettis P, Burns J. Treatment outcomes for percutaneous nephrolithotomy in renal allografts. J Endourol. 2009;11:1821–4.
74. Jones JW, Hunter DW, Matas AJ. Percutaneous treatment of ureteral strictures after renal transplant. Transplantation. 1993;55:1193–4.
75. Liberman SF, Keller FS, Barry JM, et al. Percutaneous antegrade transluminal ureteroplasty for renal allograft ureteral stenosis. J Urol. 1982;128:122–4.
76. Shoskes D, Hanbury D, Cranston D, et al. Urological complications in 1,000 consecutive renal transplants. J Urol. 1995;153:18–21.
77. Schwartz BF, Chatman JR, Bretan P, et al. Treatment of refractory kidney transplant ureteral strictures using balloon cautery endoureterotomy. Urology. 2001;58:536–9.
78. Dubovsky EV, Russel CD, Bischof-Delaloye A, et al. Report of the radionuclides in nephrourology committee for evaluation of transplanted kidney (review of techniques). Semin Nucl Med. 1999; 29:175–88.
79. Jaskowski A, Jones RM, Murie JA, et al. Urological complications in 600 consecutive renal transplant. Br J Surg. 1987;74:922–5.
80. Collado A, Camparros J, Guirado L, et al. Balloon dilation in the treatment of ureteral stenosis in kidney transplant recipients. Eur Urol. 1989;34:339–403.
81. Streem SB, Novick AC, Steinmuller DR, et al. Long-term efficacy of ureteral dilation for ureteral stenosis. J Urol. 1988;140:32–5.
82. Voegeli DR, Crummy AB, McDermott JC, et al. Percutaneous dilation of ureteral strictures in renal transplant patients. Radiology. 1986;169:185–8.
83. Benoit G, Icard P, Bensadoun H, et al. Value of antegrade ureteral dilation for later ureteral obstruction in renal transplants. Transpl Int. 1989;2:33–5.
84. Kim JC, Banner MP, Ramchandani P, et al. Balloon dilation of ureteral strictures after renal transplantation. Radiology. 1993;186: 717–22.
85. Kristo B, Phelan M, Gritsch HA, Schulam P. Treatment of renal transplant ureterovesical anastomotic strictures using antegrade balloon dilation with or without holmium: YAG laser. Urology. 2003;62:631–4.

Practical Renal Allograft Pathology

31

Cinthia B. Drachenberg and John C. Papadimitriou

Abbreviations

AIN	Allergic interstitial nephritis
AMR	Antibody-mediated rejection
ATN	Acute tubular necrosis
C4d	C4d complement fragment
CD3	Stain for T-cells
CD68	Stain for macrophages
CMR	T-cell-mediated rejection
CMV	Cytomegalovirus
CNI	Calcineurin inhibitor
DGF	Delayed graft function
DSA	Donor-specific antibody
EBV	Epstein–Barr virus
EM	Electron microscopy
FSGS	Focal segmental glomerulosclerosis
GBM	Glomerular basement membranes
H&E	Hematoxylin and eosin
HUS	Hemolytic uremic syndrome
IF	Immunofluorescence stains
IF/TA	Interstitial fibrosis/tubular atrophy of no specific etiology
KTxBx	Kidney transplant biopsies
MAPI	Maryland aggregate pathology index for donor biopsies
MPGN	Membranoproliferative glomerulonephritis
MT	Masson's trichrome stain
PAMS	Periodic acid methenamine silver stain (Jones stain)
PAS	Periodic acid stain
PTC	Peritubular capillaries
PTLD	Post-transplant lymphoproliferative disorder
PV	Polyomavirus
PVN	Polyomavirus allograft nephropathy
SV40	Simian virus 40 stain for polyomavirus
TG	Transplant glomerulopathy
TMA	Thrombotic microangiopathy

Renal Allograft Biopsy: Generalities

Routine evaluation of kidney transplant biopsies (KTxBx) has been essential for the continuous clinical, surgical, and pharmacological advances in renal transplantation. Most therapeutic decisions, including the selection of immunosuppression protocols to be tailored to the individual patient, are primarily based on KTxBx findings [1].

The current chapter has been prepared for the non-pathologists involved in the treatment of renal transplant patients, to help them become familiar with the main histopathological concepts in this field.

Clinicopathological Integration

A few histological findings are pathognomonic of specific pathological processes leading to unambiguous morphological diagnoses (e.g., intimal arteritis for rejection, CMV inclusions). In practice, however, most KTxBx can and need to be interpreted only in the context of the clinical presentation and other laboratory data. Close communication between the pathologist and the treating clinical team results in the best diagnostic yield from KTxBx examination. Pertinent clinical information should therefore be made available to the pathologist at the time of biopsy interpretation (see Table 31.1).

C.B. Drachenberg, M.D. (✉) • J.C. Papadimitriou, M.D., Ph.D.
Department of Pathology, University of Maryland School of Medicine, 22 South Greene Street, NBW43, Baltimore, MD 20201, USA
e-mail: cdrac001@umaryland.edu; jpapa001@umaryland.edu

M.R. Weir and E.V. Lerma (eds.), *Kidney Transplantation: Practical Guide to Management*,
DOI 10.1007/978-1-4939-0342-9_31, © Springer Science+Business Media New York 2014

Table 31.1 Clinical information

Time post-transplant
Type of transplant: living donor or cadaveric
Donor history if pertinent
Infection including history of HIV, hepatitis C, etc.
Peritransplantation surgical complications
Indication for biopsy
Increase in serum creatinine (rapid, slow)
Type of immunosuppression
Changes in immunosuppression
Use of nephrotoxic drugs
Urine culture results
Proteinuria
Dehydration
Renal artery stenosis
Abnormal imaging studies (i.e., hydronephrosis)

Prevention, diagnosis, and treatment of antibody-mediated rejection (AMR) require monitoring for the presence of circulating *donor-specific antibodies* (DSAs) at regular intervals after transplantation, as well as at the time of biopsy and whenever rejection is suspected [2–4]. As discussed in detail below, accurate classification of rejection according to the Banff schema requires correlation between the biopsy findings and DSA studies [2].

Biopsy Adequacy

According to the Banff schema a specimen must contain ten or more glomeruli and at least two arteries to be considered adequate [5].

Due to the fact that many pathological processes involve the allograft in a patchy, random manner, the sensitivity of the biopsy depends on the amount of tissue available for evaluation. To diagnose or rule out acute allograft rejection with some degree of certainty, it is necessary to evaluate a sample of renal cortex containing sufficient number of glomeruli and arteries. Evaluation of two tissue needle cores is desirable to achieve a sensitivity of 99 % for the diagnosis of acute rejection. This is in contrast to a sensitivity of 90 % for a single core [6, 7]. Biopsies containing only medulla are in general considered inadequate because in those samples, acute allograft rejection will be missed or underestimated in half of the cases [8]. On the other hand, examination of renal medulla may be sufficient to diagnose other pathological entities (i.e., acute pyelonephritis, polyomavirus nephropathy) (PVN) [9].

The amount of tissue required also depends on the biopsy indication. There are clinical situations in which enough tissue material must be obtained to allow for the performance of ancillary studies such as immunofluorescence and electron microscopy (EM). This is particularly important if the biopsy is performed for a possible glomerular disease.

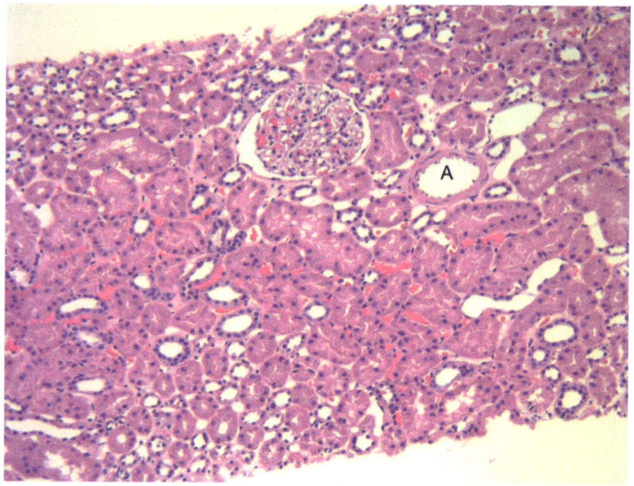

Fig. 31.1 H&E-stained biopsy from a graft with excellent function (protocol biopsy at 12 months). There is no inflammation. The tubules are "back to back" with no significant intervening connective tissue. *A* normal arteriole. Note the thin wall and the widely open lumen

Routine Histological Studies

Light microscopic evaluation of renal biopsies includes the performance of hematoxylin and eosin (H&E)-stained sections (Fig. 31.1), as well as a set of routinely used special stains (periodic acid stain [PAS], periodic acid methenamine silver stain (Jones stain) [PAMS], Masson's trichrome stain [MT], and C4d complement fragment [C4d] stain) [4, 5]. Table 31.2 summarizes the main morphological features and diagnostic associations identified with each of these stains (Fig. 31.2). The *C4d stain* is required for the identification of an important subset of AMRs [4, 10, 11]. C4d is a complement split product that remains covalently bound to target structures after complement activation has occurred, allowing for its recognition in tissue sections. This is in contrast to most products of complement activation that are immediately degraded and cannot be detected on standard tissue processing. Deposition of C4d in peritubular capillaries (PTC) identifies ongoing humoral rejection that may otherwise escape identification. The C4d stain can be performed in fresh-frozen as well as formalin-fixed tissue with comparable results [4].

Although not considered part of the routine biopsy work-up, immunohistochemical stains for macrophages (i.e., CD68) and T-cells (i.e., CD3) can highlight the subtle forms of microvascular inflammation that characterize early AMR [12, 13].

Main Ancillary Studies

Infectious Processes

In addition to standard serological studies for infectious processes (i.e., CMV, hepatitis C, HIV), *immunohistochemical*

Table 31.2 Routinely* used special stains: main diagnostic value

PAS*
Tubules: Tubulitis, destruction of tubular basement membranes, thickening of basement membranes (atrophy)
Glomeruli: Glomerulitis (mononuclear cells in capillaries), reduplication of basement membranes (transplant glomerulopathy), increase in mesangial matrix, hyalinosis
Vessels: Hyalinosis
Other: Identification of fungal organisms
Silver stain (PAMS, Jones stain)*
Tubules: Tubulitis, destruction of tubular basement membranes, thickening of basement membranes (atrophy)
Glomeruli: Glomerulitis (mononuclear cells in capillaries), reduplication of basement membranes (transplant glomerulopathy), increase in mesangial matrix
Trichrome stain*
Collagen deposition: Interstitial fibrosis, arterial sclerosis, glomerular sclerosis, fibrin thrombi, fibrinoid necrosis
C4d stain*
Staining of peritubular capillaries in AMR (also see ref. [10])
Immunohistochemical stains for viral infections
Cytomegalovirus
SV40 (cross reacts with BK virus and JC virus)
EBV latent membrane protein (LMP-1)
EBER—Epstein–Barr-encoded RNA (in situ Hybridization)
Adenovirus

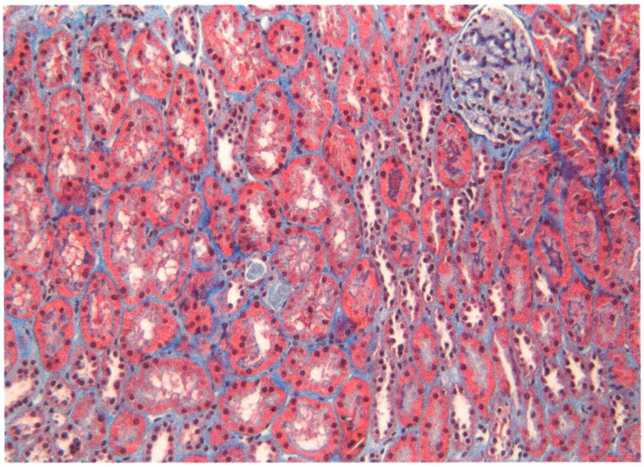

Fig. 31.2 Masson's trichrome-stained biopsy from a well functioning graft. Stain for collagen highlights minimal connective tissue between tubules. There is no evidence of tubular atrophy or interstitial fibrosis

stains and in situ hybridization are used for the identification of a variety of infectious organisms in tissue: SV40 (simian virus 40 stain for BK and JC polyomaviruses), CMV (for cytomegalovirus), EBV (for Epstein–Barr virus/post-transplant lymphoproliferative disorder [PTLD]), immunostains for adenovirus, etc. Stains for acid-fast bacilli and fungi are performed in biopsies with granulomatous inflammation or if these infections are suspected [1]. *Molecular studies*, particularly PCR, are also useful to demonstrate the presence of infectious organisms in tissue samples although these studies are not routinely used for diagnostic purposes.

Routine determination of polyomavirus *BK viral loads* in plasma and urine is essential for prevention and monitoring of polyomavirus allograft nephropathy (PVN). Evaluation of routine urine cytology with identification of the PV-infected "decoy cells" is an inexpensive and simple tool to determine if a patient has significant PV replication in the urinary tract. Persistent PV BK urinary shedding is associated with PVN and has markedly increased risk of graft loss [14, 15].

Electron microscopy studies and *immunofluorescence* stains (IF; for immunoglobulins and complement components) are required for the evaluation of post-transplant glomerular processes in the same manner as it is done in native kidney biopsies. Furthermore, ultrastructural studies of glomeruli and PTC are essential for the diagnosis of early AMR in order to demonstrate the characteristic basement membrane abnormalities.

It is important to remember that the immunofluorescence technique can be applied only to tissues that are fresh-frozen (i.e., not fixed in formaldehyde).

Pretransplant Biopsy

Deceased Donor Evaluation (Harvest Biopsies)

Routine use of kidneys from less than ideal donors requires pretransplant histological evaluation for determination of organ quality. Pretransplant assessment is indicated for kidneys from older donors, or from those with history of hypertension, diabetes, or renal dysfunction (extended criteria donors) [16].

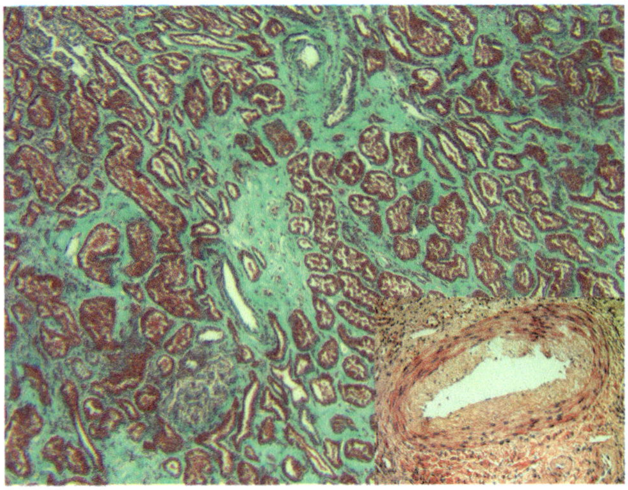

Fig. 31.3 Masson's trichrome-stained biopsy from a donor with chronic hypertensive disease (extended criteria donor). The tubules are separated by an abnormal amount of connective tissue which is highlighted by the collagen stain. An arteriole with a thick wall and narrowed rounded lumen is noted in the *top center*. The H&E-stained insert demonstrates an interlobular artery with fibrointimal sclerosis (arteriosclerosis)

Hypertensive Disease

The most common donor-related histological abnormalities are secondary to long-standing arterial hypertension [17]. The large and small arteries show sclerosis and sclerosis with hyalinosis, respectively, leading to various degrees of luminal narrowing (Fig. 31.3). The interstitium shows increased fibrosis and there is corresponding atrophy of the tubular components. Subcapsular ischemic scars as well as a significant number of scattered obsolescent glomeruli are also indicative of chronic hypertension (nephrosclerosis). The Maryland aggregate pathology index (MAPI) is a histological scoring system based on the presence or absence of five morphological features associated with hypertensive/chronic ischemic renal parenchymal injury (hyalinosis of glomerular-size arterioles, >15 % global glomerulosclerosis, significant arterial sclerosis, periglomerular fibrosis, and cortical scar) which are assigned scores according to their relative significance. The MAPI has been shown to be predictive of post-transplant graft survival or failure [16].

Donor Diabetes

Approximately 4 % of all kidney transplants in the United States are derived from diabetic donors [17, 18]. Identification of fully developed nodular diabetic glomerulosclerosis in a donor kidney biopsy is a contraindication for transplantation; however, milder diabetic glomerular involvement is compatible with acceptable outcomes [18, 19].

Renal Cell Carcinoma

With the increased utilization of organs from older donors there has been an increase in the identification of renal cell carcinomas both in deceased and living donors (≈1 %). Organs with small, completely resected, low grade tumors are now routinely utilized for transplantation with excellent outcomes [20]. Frozen section evaluation is required for rapid histological characterization diagnosis of any donor mass. In this setting, the two most common lesions are small renal cell carcinomas and angiomyolipomas. The latter are benign connective tissue tumors that do not pose any risk to the recipient irrespective of their size [21].

Other Donor-Related Issues

A variety of other processes can be identified in pretransplant donor biopsies, one of the most common being mesangial IgA deposition and membranous nephropathy, both of which appear not to have a negative post-transplantation impact. Similarly, other forms of mild glomerulonephritis can resolve after transplantation [22]. In addition, we have seen successful outcomes after transplantation of kidneys with mild sarcoidosis and eclampsia-related glomerular injury. The decision about transplanting organs with known pathological processes is made after careful consideration, on a case-by-case basis.

Living Donor Evaluation

Living donors may present with potentially significant renal disease requiring careful evaluation before donation. The risk factors for renal disease associated with living-donation have been characterized [23]. Kidney biopsies are more often performed for hematuria in otherwise healthy living donors. In this context the identification of thin basement membrane disease is common; in general terms this process is not considered per se a contraindication for donation.

Post-implantation Biopsies: Time 0 Biopsy

Similar to donor harvest biopsies, baseline graft biopsies performed before or after reperfusion provide essential information about the status of the organ at the time of transplantation, in particular regarding the presence of underlying chronic vascular disease (donor hypertensive disease) [22]. Microvascular and/or glomerular thrombosis in implantation biopsies correlates with ischemic injury and was associated with higher risk of rejection in one study [24].

Biopsies for Graft Dysfunction in the Early Post-transplant Period

Delayed Graft Function

Acute Tubular Necrosis

Biopsies from patients with delayed graft function (DGF) in the early post-transplant period usually show acute tubular necrosis (ATN). This injury is presumed to be ischemic in nature as a result of the organ procurement procedures and

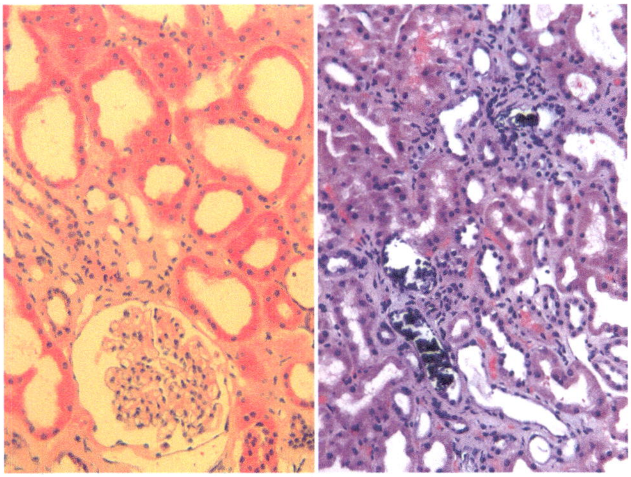

Fig. 31.4 Acute tubular necrosis. Marked dilatation of the tubular lumina and flattening (simplification) of the tubular epithelium are noted on the *left image*. Compare with Fig. 31.1 where the normal tubular cells are tall and fill most of the luminal space. The image on the *right* shows features of tubular injury and scattered tubular microcalcifications, which tend to develop in areas of tubular necrosis

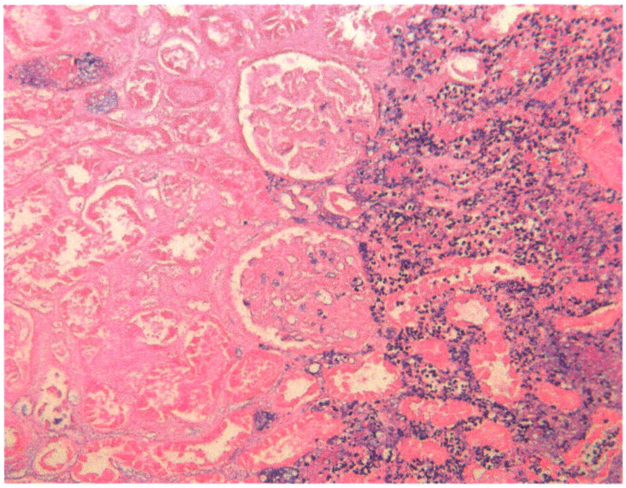

Fig. 31.5 Cortical infarct. Ischemic necrosis of the renal cortex is appreciated on the *left side* of the image (loss of nuclear profiles). On the *right* a band of neutrophilic infiltrates demarcates the edge of the infarct

reperfusion injury. Tubular injury can be subtle, consisting only of cytoplasmic vacuolization, loss of brush border, and isolated cell necrosis or apoptosis. In more pronounced cases there is frank disintegration and sloughing of the tubular cells that can accumulate as debris in the tubular lumina. When there is pronounced tubular cell loss there is flattening of the remaining tubular lining and partial denudation of the basement membranes. Tubular calcifications are common in areas of previous tubular injury (Fig. 31.4). Interstitial edema and mild interstitial inflammation, often including some eosinophils, can be present in ATN. If the inflammation is significant and there is tubulitis, a concurrent acute cellular rejection should be suspected. The presence of multifocal neutrophilic capillaritis and/or microscopic thrombi requires correlation with the C4d stain and DSA studies to rule out ATN associated with early acute AMR.

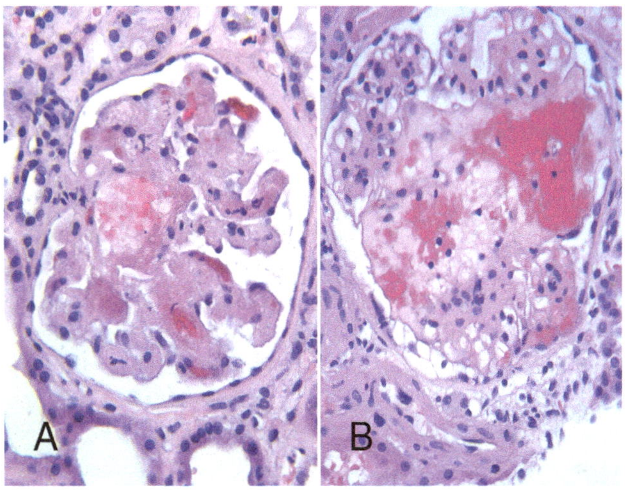

Fig. 31.6 Thrombotic microangiopathy (TMA) leading to glomerular necrosis in a pre-sensitized patient with early acute AMR (**a**), and similar changes due to ischemic endothelial injury in a patient with prolonged cold ischemia time (**b**)

Coagulation Necrosis: Infarction

Severe ischemic injury often secondary to hemodynamic issues or surgical complications may result in focal of diffuse parenchymal necrosis. Localized infarcts are often unsuspected clinically and may become evident only in a needle biopsy for evaluation of DGF. Identification of infarction in core biopsies is usually associated with significant ischemic injury and always leads to subsequent fibrous scarring of the infarcted areas (Fig. 31.5). Therefore, depending on the extent of parenchyma involved, infarcts may be associated with poor graft function or primary non-function.

Ischemic Endothelial Injury

In patients with DGF, glomerular endothelial cell swelling and microthrombi that may mimic early acute AMR may result from ischemic injury to endothelial cells [25, 26] (Fig. 31.6). These changes are usually reversible unless the ischemic process has also led to multifocal areas of infarction. In patients with microvascular changes suspected to represent ischemic endothelial injury, examination of a C4d stain and serological studies to document the absence of DSA are necessary to confirm the purely ischemic nature of the injury.

Preexisting Donor Hypertensive Vascular Disease

Prolonged DGF or poor renal function may be the result of suboptimal perfusion of the graft due to preexisting vascular sclerosis (narrowing) [16]. In addition to the donor-related vascular sclerosis these biopsies may show frank ATN or milder forms of tubular injury (Fig. 31.4).

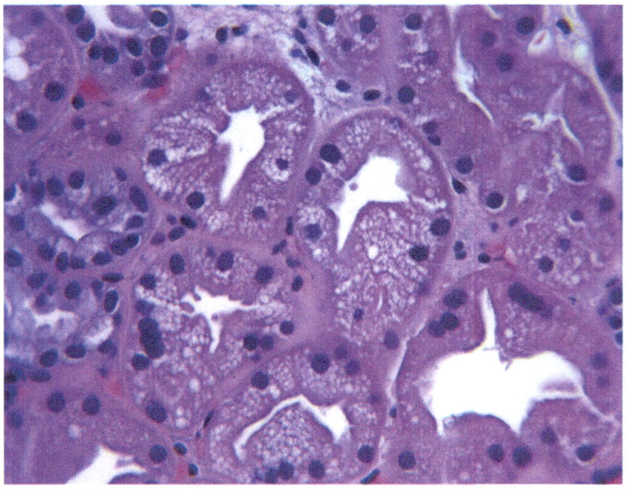

Fig. 31.7 Isometric tubular vacuolization. The tubular cells have a "foamy," clear cytoplasm with accumulation of multiple vacuoles. Tubular injury secondary to multiple etiologies (i.e., calcineurin inhibitor [CNI] toxicity, ischemia, osmotic nephrosis) can manifest with this change

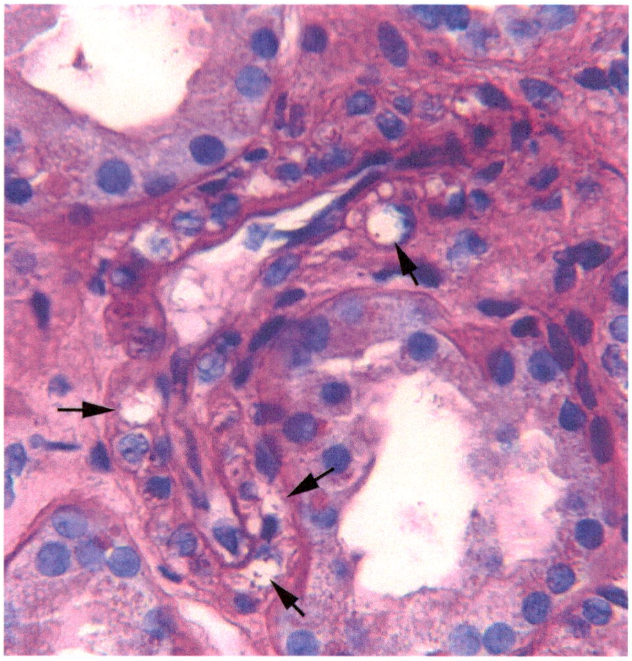

Fig. 31.8 Myocyte injury due to CNI toxicity. High power view of a pre-glomerular arteriole shows marked vacuolization of some myocytes (*arrows*). Some of the clear spaces represent myocyte cell necrosis (drop-out); note scattered granular structures consistent with nuclear fragments/apoptotic bodies

Suboptimal Graft Function

Suboptimal or slow graft function is a common indication for early KTxBx in patients that do not require dialysis but that continue to have poorer than expected renal function. The most common pathological findings in these patients are tubular injury (i.e., tubular cell vacuolization, ATN-like changes, etc.), and donor-related issues, particularly related to chronic hypertensive donor disease (e.g., patches of cortical scarring, vascular sclerosis, and arteriolar hyalinosis) or less commonly related to preexisting conditions such as donor diabetes. In patients with persistent tubular injury, ongoing ischemia (i.e., stenosis of the renal artery anastomosis), urinary obstruction, and drug toxicity should be ruled out clinically.

Acute calcineurin inhibitor (CNI) toxicity can be the cause of suboptimal graft function in the early post-transplant period. Isometric tubular vacuolization (finely vacuolated cytoplasmic droplets), a feature typically associated with acute CNI toxicity, is not specific and can be observed in most other forms of tubular injury including ischemic injury and in osmotic nephrosis (Fig. 31.7). A more specific lesion associated with high levels of CNI consists of ballooning, apoptosis or necrosis, and drop-out of arteriolar myocytes. These uncommon changes are dose related and are typically reversible with dose adjustments [27] (Fig. 31.8).

Thrombotic microangiopathy (TMA), most commonly idiopathic, or considered to be secondary to CNI or rapamycin toxicity, may be associated with early graft dysfunction. TMA is discussed in detail in section "Thrombotic microangiopathy" [28, 29].

Acute Allograft Rejection

Early Acute AMR

The most characteristic lesions of early acute AMR result from lytic endothelial cell graft injury due to damage by alloantibodies (i.e., anti-HLA DSA).

Specifically, circulating DSA in conjunction with complement activation leads to endothelial cell swelling and necrosis with superimposed formation of microthrombi. Accumulation of inflammatory cells (neutrophils and macrophages) in glomerular and PTC appearing as glomerulitis and capillaritis is also a common feature of acute AMR [4].

Early acute AMR develops in a proportion of presensitized patients despite conditioning protocols and may also occur in the early post-transplantation period in patients with no apparent risk for AMR [30].

In contrast to milder forms of early acute AMR which are characterized by attenuated endothelial injury that may even resemble bland ATN, in hyperacute rejection, the most severe form of AMR, there are abundant preformed circulating antibodies leading to diffuse arterial and venous necrosis with secondary thrombosis and parenchymal infarction [4]. A diagnosis of pure acute AMR requires exclusion of features of T-cell-mediated rejection (CMR).

The current Banff classification of acute AMR is based on the combination of (1) *C4d+*, (2) the *presence of circulating*

Table 31.3 Banff 97 diagnostic categories for renal allograft biopsies—Banff '09 update

1. Normal
2. Antibody-mediated changes (may coincide with categories 3, 4 and 5 and 6)
Due to documentation of circulating antidonor antibody, C4d[a], and allograft pathology
C4d deposition without morphologic evidence of active rejection
C4d+, the presence of circulating antidonor antibodies, no signs of acute or chronic CMR or AMR (i.e., g0, cg0, ptc0, no ptc lamination (<5 layers by electron microscopy), no ATN-like minimal inflammation). Cases with simultaneous borderline changes are considered as indeterminate
Acute antibody-mediated rejection[b]
C4d+, the presence of circulating antidonor antibodies, morphologic evidence of acute tissue injury, such as (type/grade)
I. ATN-like minimal inflammation
II. Capillary and/or glomerular inflammation (ptc/g >0) and/or thromboses
III. Arterial—v3
Chronic active antibody-mediated rejection[b]
C4d+, the presence of circulating antidonor antibodies, morphologic evidence of chronic tissue injury, such as glomerular double contours and/or peritubular capillary basement membrane multilayering and/or interstitial fibrosis/tubular atrophy and/or fibrous intimal thickening in arteries
3. Borderline changes: "Suspicious" for acute T-cell-mediated rejection (may coincide with categories 2 and 5, and 6)
This category is used when no intimal arteritis is present, but there are foci of tubulitis (t1, t2, or t3) with minor interstitial infiltration (i0 or i1) or interstitial infiltration (i2, i3) with mild (t1) tubulitis
4. T-cell-mediated rejection (CMR, may coincide with categories 2 and 5 and 6)
Acute T-cell-mediated rejection (*type/grade*):
IA. Cases with significant interstitial infiltration (>25 % of parenchyma affected, i2 or i3) and foci of moderate tubulitis (t2)
IB. Cases with significant interstitial infiltration (>25 % of parenchyma affected, i2 or i3) and foci of severe tubulitis (t3)
IIA. Cases with mild to moderate intimal arteritis (v1)
IIB. Cases with severe intimal arteritis comprising >25 % of the luminal area (v2)
III. Cases with "transmural" arteritis and/or arterial fibrinoid change and necrosis of medial smooth muscle cells with accompanying lymphocytic inflammation (v3)
Chronic active T-cell-mediated rejection
"Chronic allograft arteriopathy" (arterial intimal fibrosis with mononuclear cell infiltration in fibrosis, formation of neo-intima)
5. Interstitial fibrosis and tubular atrophy, no evidence of any specific etiology (may include nonspecific vascular and glomerular sclerosis, but severity graded by tubulointerstitial features)
Grade
I. Mild interstitial fibrosis and tubular atrophy (<25 % of cortical area)
II. Moderate interstitial fibrosis and tubular atrophy (26–50 % of cortical area)
III. Severe interstitial fibrosis and tubular atrophy/loss (>50 % of cortical area)
6. Other: Changes not considered to be due to rejection—acute and/or chronic (for diagnoses see table 14 in [49]; may include isolated g, cg, or cv lesions and coincide with categories 2, 3, 4, and 5)

Modified from ref. [4]

The 2009 updates are underlined. All existing scoring categories (*g* glomerulitis, *t* tubulitis, *v* intimal arteritis, *i* mononuclear interstitial inflammation, *ptc* peritubular capillaritis, *cg* allograft glomerulopathy/double contours, *ct* tubular atrophy, *ci* interstitial fibrosis, *cv* vascular fibrointimal thickening) remain unchanged [5, 31]

ATN acute tubular necrosis

[a]Please refer to Banff 2007 classification paper [31]

[b]Suspicious for antibody-mediated rejection if C4d (in the presence of antibody) or alloantibody (C4d+) not demonstrated in the presence of morphologic evidence of tissue injury

antidonor antibodies, and (3) *morphologic evidence of acute tissue injury* (see Table 31.3 [4, 31]). Acute AMR is categorized in types or grades I, II, or III (I. ATN-like minimal inflammation, II. capillary and or glomerular inflammation and/or thromboses, and III. arterial necrosis). In essence, the Banff Category I (C4d+ and ATN-like changes only) represents a milder form of Category II (characterized additionally by microvascular inflammation and microthrombi). Category III is defined by arterial fibrinoid necrosis resembling lesions seen in hyperacute rejection and therefore represents a more severe form of AMR in comparison to Categories I and II.

Differential diagnosis of acute AMR: The most important differential diagnosis of early acute AMR is ischemic injury leading to microvascular thrombosis [25, 26] (Fig. 31.6). History of prolonged cold ischemia time and/or surgical complications may support the impression of ischemic graft injury; however, evaluation of C4d staining and DSA studies are essential to rule out a concurrent component of acute AMR. In our experience some degree of C4d staining may be present in early biopsies with ischemic injury, but this typically resolves in subsequent biopsies. Renal function recovers in most patients with ischemic endothelial injury, unless

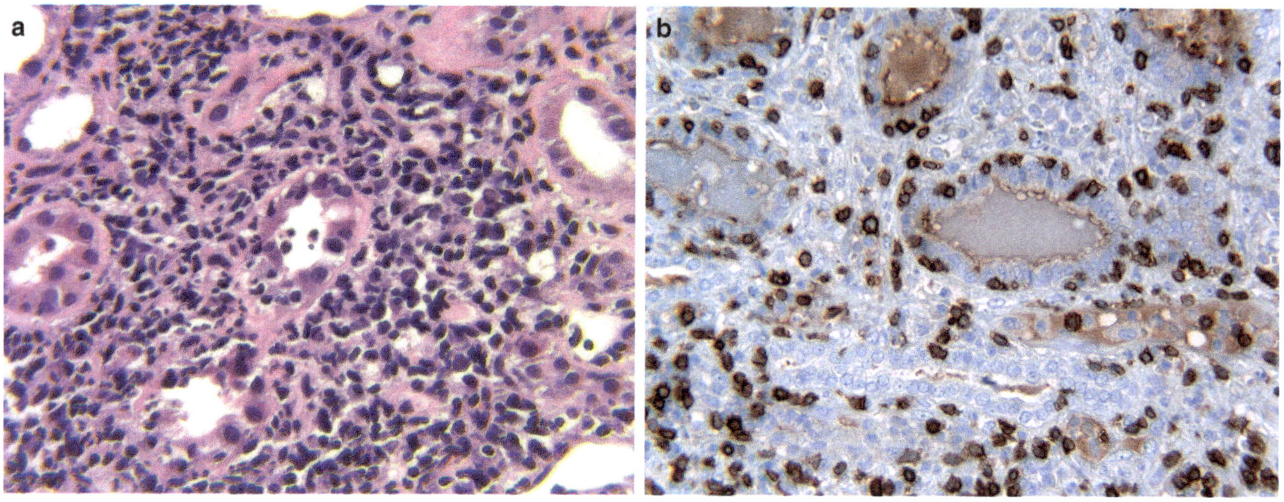

Fig. 31.9 (**a**) Acute CMR (Type I). The interstitium contains dense, active inflammatory infiltrates. The tubule in the center is partially destroyed by severe tubulitis. (**b**) Acute CMR with severe tubulitis (Type 1B). CD3 demonstrates numerous T-lymphocytes that have permeated the tubular basement membranes

there is very extensive microvascular thrombosis or infarcts which would eventually lead to diffuse glomerular sclerosis and formation of scars. TMA of other etiologies—including CNI toxicity—may also require differentiation from acute AMR (see section "Thrombotic Microangiopathy").

Acute CMR

Acute CMR is characterized by interstitial T-cell and macrophage infiltrates, tubular inflammation (tubulitis), and inflammation of the arterial endothelium (intimal arteritis). A diagnosis of pure acute CMR requires exclusion of AMR (evaluation of C4d stain and negative DSA studies).

The current Banff classification of acute CMR uses the following categories: Borderline—suspicious, Type I (A and B), Type II (A and B), and Type III (see Table 31.3).

Borderline changes: "Suspicious" for acute CMR is used when no intimal arteritis is present, but there are foci of tubulitis with minor interstitial infiltration or interstitial infiltration with only mild tubulitis.

On the other hand, Types I–III are considered diagnostic of acute CMR. In essence, Type I rejection is defined by tubulitis (Fig. 31.9), Type II is defined by arterial inflammation without necrosis (intimal arteritis, endarteritis) (Fig. 31.10), and Type III is characterized by arterial necrosis and accompanying lymphocytic inflammation (Fig. 31.11). Whereas Type II CMR (intimal arteritis) is the most diagnostic form, Type I requires differentiation from other causes of graft inflammation (i.e., PVN, infections, nonspecific inflammation) and Type III requires differentiation from AMR due to overlap of necrotizing vascular lesions in the severe forms of CMR and AMR.

Differential diagnosis of CMR: In the early post-transplantation period when most transplants lack significant nonspecific changes acute rejection reactions can be diagnosed with relative ease. In the late post-transplant period,

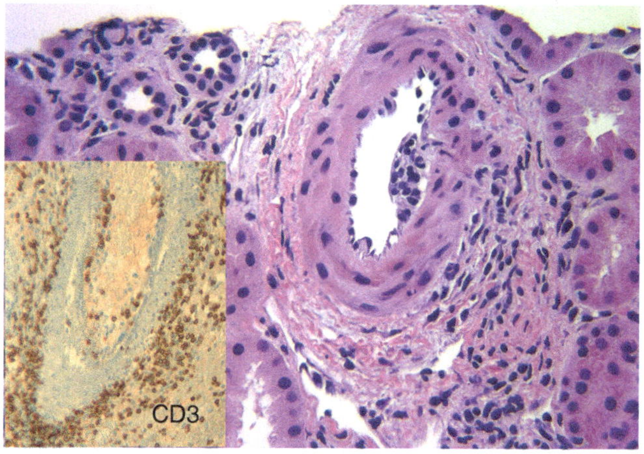

Fig. 31.10 Acute CMR (Type II). Interlobular artery with intimal arteritis characterized by subintimal accumulation of lymphocytes and associated endothelial cell damage. *Inset*: CD3 stain highlights T-lymphocytes in the intimal arteritis. Interstitial perivascular inflammation is also prominent

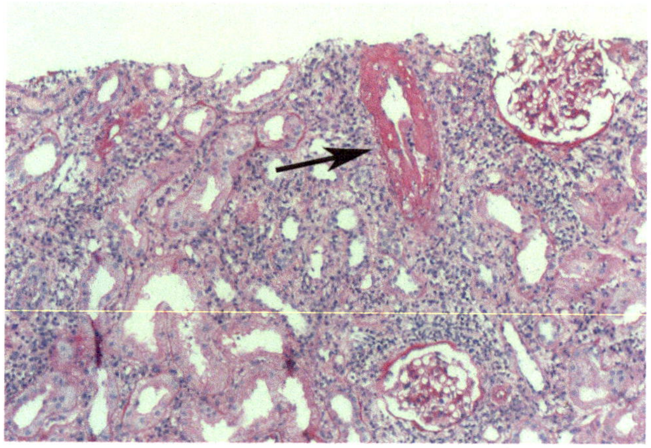

Fig. 31.11 Acute CMR with arterial necrosis (Type III). In addition to prominent interstitial infiltrates and tubulitis, an artery shows transmural necrosis (*arrow*). Note scattered lymphoid cells in the vascular wall and an area of intimal arteritis

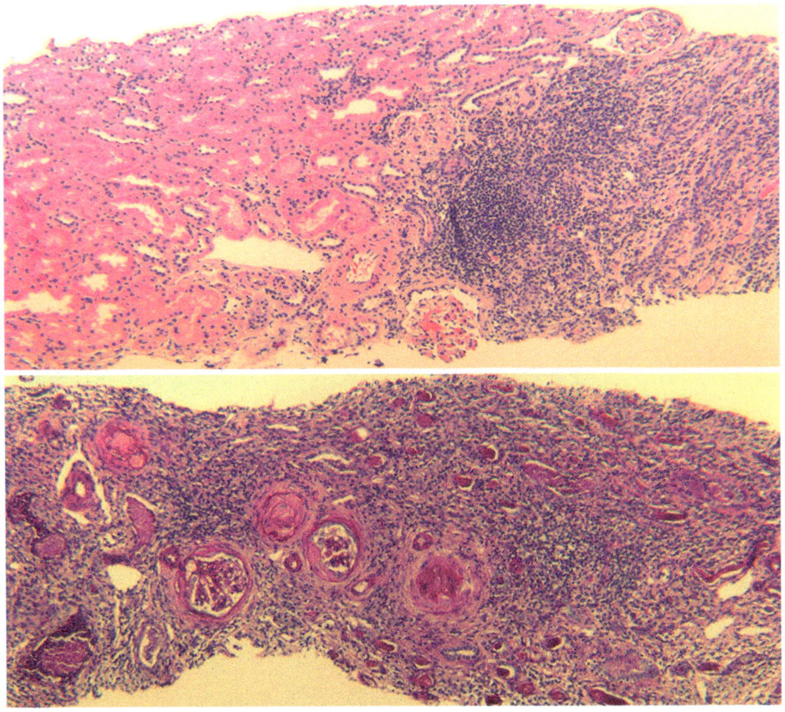

Fig. 31.12 Cortical scarring. A focal scar with prominent chronic inflammation is noted in the right area of the *top image*. Extensive, diffuse scarring is noted in the *lower image*, also associated with marked chronic inflammation

nonspecific features of chronicity secondary to multiple immunological and non-immunological insults greatly complicate pathological interpretations. In particular, scarred areas often show interstitial inflammation with some degree of tubulitis in atrophying tubules.

Intimal arteritis is indicative of alloimmune injury and is considered one of the most important features of acute CMR (see section "Spectrum of Arterial Changes"). Biopsies with atypical features should always raise the suspicion for a combined process (i.e., mixed AMR and CMR).

In the absence of arterial involvement, tubulointerstitial inflammation alone may also be secondary to infections (section "Infections"), obstruction, scarring from previous injury, etc.

Inflammation identified in scars is typically considered nonspecific and unresponsive to treatment, therefore of little diagnostic value (Fig. 31.12). Two issues, however, should be considered in biopsies with extensive scarring: (1) it is important to assess if the specimen is representative of the clinical presentation and of the kidney in general (i.e., a repeat biopsy is indicated if only inflamed scars are sampled in a kidney with ideal function because the specimen is likely not representative) and (2) inflamed scars may hold the clue to a specific diagnosis (i.e., evolving PV allograft nephropathy, evolving obstructive nephropathy); evaluation of SV40 stain, correlation with ultrasound findings, etc. will provide important information in these cases.

In rare transplant patients biopsied for acute graft dysfunction there are clinical features suggesting the possibility of allergic interstitial nephritis (AIN) (e.g., exposure to allergenic drug(s), peripheral eosinophilia, rash). Because AIN and acute CMR Type I (tubulointerstitial inflammation) cannot be differentiated on morphological grounds, a diagnosis of AIN rests mainly on the clinicopathological correlations and subsequent follow-up [32].

Early Recurrence of Primary Glomerular Disease (Also See Section "Biopsies for Graft Dysfunction in the Late Post-transplant Period")

In the early post-transplantation period, recurrent focal segmental glomerulosclerosis (FSGS) may manifest within hours or days with increasing proteinuria. Graft dysfunction, including anuria, may also be present in the most severe cases. The earliest morphological evidence of recurrent FSGS requires electron microscopic studies in order to demonstrate effacement of the foot processes of podocytes. Progression of the FSGS is associated with appearance of fully developed segmental sclerotic lesions (Fig. 31.13). Recurrence of hemolytic uremic syndrome (HUS) may also manifest in early biopsies with the typical thrombotic microangiopathic features [33].

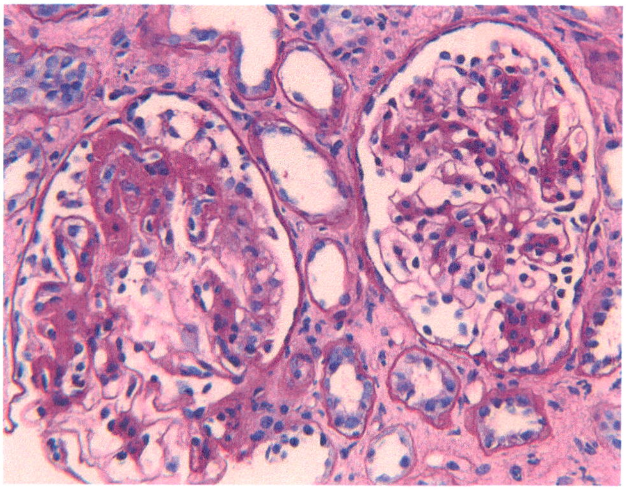

Fig. 31.13 Recurrent focal segmental glomerulosclerosis (FSGS). Periodic acid stain (PAS)-stained section of a biopsy performed 3 weeks post-transplantation shows development of segmental sclerotic lesions (glomerulus on the *right*) in a patient who presented with recurrence of FSGS within days of transplantation

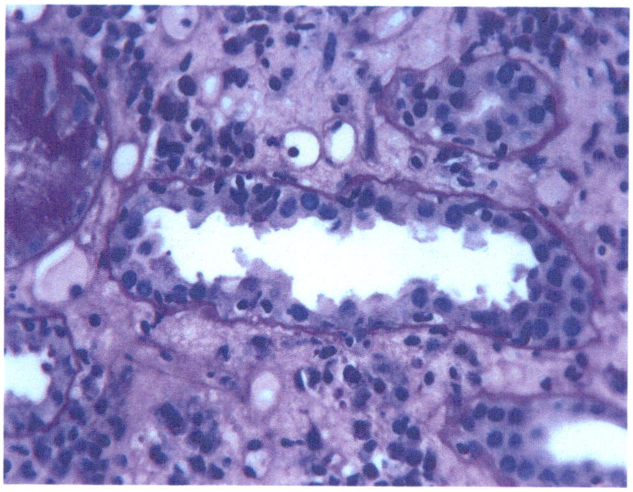

Fig. 31.14 Protocol biopsy with interstitial infiltrates and tubulitis: subclinical acute CMR. PAS highlights the outline of the tubular basement membranes. Several lymphocytes have gone through the basement membrane and are located amidst the tubular epithelial cells. Lymphocytes are differentiated from the epithelial cells by their darkly stained nuclei with condensed chromatin

Protocol Biopsies

Protocol or surveillance biopsies are performed electively in normally functioning grafts for the purpose of early recognition and treatment of pathological processes. Subclinical acute allograft rejection, either CMR or AMR, can be found in a significant proportion of protocol biopsies [34, 35] (Figs. 31.14 and 31.15). The findings in subclinical AMR have been emphasized in a recent study that demonstrated a wide spectrum of lesions ranging from pure microvascular inflammation (glomerulitis, capillaritis) to well-developed chronic lesions (transplant glomerulopathy [TG]) [35].

Biopsies for Graft Dysfunction in the Late Post-transplant Period

Chronic Active AMR

Two broad categories of late-chronic AMR can be identified: (1) chronic microvascular injury developing in approximately 40 % of highly sensitized patients with or without history of early acute AMR and (2) chronic microvascular injury developing in approximately 20 % of non-sensitized patients who develop de novo DSA. In both settings most patients experience eventual progression to graft failure, but the rate of progression and the histological manifestations vary considerably from one patient to another and in serial biopsies from the same patient [11, 26, 30, 35–37].

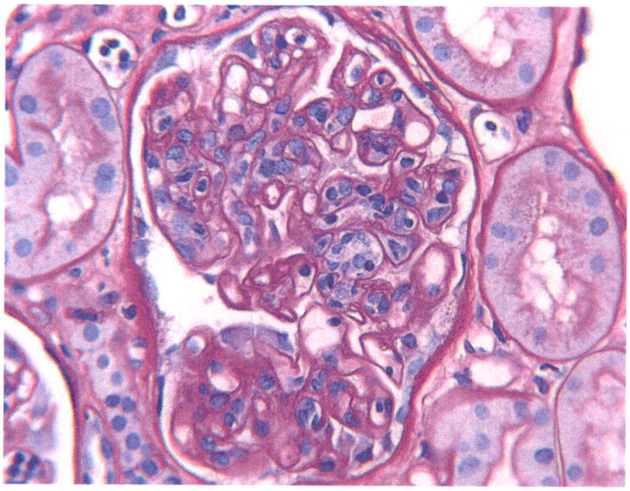

Fig. 31.15 Subclinical AMR. Protocol biopsy at 12 months post-transplantation in a 62-year-old woman found to have multiple anti-HLA donor-specific antibody (DSA) at the time of the biopsy. There is glomerulitis characterized by narrowing of the glomerular capillary lumina due to endocapillary hypercellularity and swelling of endothelial cells. Also note development of transplant glomerulopathy (duplication of glomerular basement membranes [GBM] at 11 o'clock)

The current Banff schema (Tables 31.3 and 31.4) defines *chronic active AMR* as follows: (1) C4d+, (2) the presence of circulating antidonor antibodies, and (3) morphologic evidence of chronic tissue injury, such as glomerular double contours and/or PTC basement membrane multilayering and/or interstitial fibrosis/tubular atrophy (IF/TA) and/or fibrous

Table 31.4 Revised [62] classification of antibody-mediated rejection (ABMR) in renal allografts

Acute/Active ABMR; all three features must be present for diagnosis[a,b]
1. Histologic evidence of acute tissue injury, including one or more of the following
– Microvascular inflammation (g>0 and/or ptc>0)
– Intimal or transmural arteritis (v>0)
– Acute thrombotic microangiopathy, in the absence of any other cause
– Acute tubular injury, in the absence of any other apparent cause
2. Evidence of current/recent antibody interaction with vascular endothelium, *including at least one of the following*
– Linear C4d staining in peritubular capillaries
– At least moderate microvascular inflammation ([g+ptc] ≥ 2)
– Increased expression of gene transcripts in the biopsy tissue indicative of endothelial injury
3. Serologic evidence of donor-specific antibodies (HLA or other antigens)
Chronic, Active ABMR; all three features must be present for diagnosis[a,c]
1. Morphologic evidence of chronic tissue injury, including one or more of the following
– Transplant glomerulopathy (cg>0), if no evidence of chronic TMA
– Severe peritubular capillary basement membrane multilayering (requires EM)
– Arterial intimal fibrosis of new onset, excluding other causes[j]
2. Evidence of current/recurrent antibody interaction with vascular endothelium, *including at least one of the following*
– Linear C4d staining in peritubular capillaries (C4d2 or C4d3 by IF on frozen sections or C4d>0 by IHC on paraffin sections)
– At least moderate microvascular inflammation ([g+ptc] ≥ 2)
– Increased expression of gene transcripts in the biopsy tissue indicative of endothelial injury, if thoroughly validated
3. Serologic evidence of donor-specific antibodies (HLA or other antigens)
C4d Staining without Evidence of Rejection; all three features must be present for diagnosis[d]
1. Linear C4d staining in peritubular capillaries (C4d 2 or C4d3 by IF on frozen sections, or C4d>0 by IHC on paraffin sections)
2. g=0, ptc=0, cg=0 (by LM and by EM if available), v=0, no TMA, no peritubular capillary basement membrane multilayering, no acute tubular injury (in the absence of another apparent cause for this)
3. No acute cell-mediated rejection (Banff 97 type 1A or greater) or borderline changes

Adapted from Hass M., et al. Am J Transpl 2014 (in press)
g, cg, ptc, v, C4d correspond to Banff scores described on the Banff 97 schema (Racusen, LC et al. Kidney Int 1999 Feb;55(2):713–23)
LM light microscopy, *EM* electron microscopy, *TMA* thrombotic microangiopathy, *IF* immunofluorescence, *IHC* Immunohistochemistry
[a]For all ABMR diagnosis, it should be specified in the report whether the lesion is C4d-positive (C4d2 or C4d3 by IF on frozen sections; C4d> by IHC on paraffin sections) or without evident C4d deposition (C4d0 or C4d1 by IF on frozen sections; C4d0 by IHC on paraffin sections
[b]These lesions may be clinically acute, smoldering or subclinical. Biopsies showing two of the three features, except those with DSA and C4d without histologic abnormalities potentially related to ABMR or TCMR (C4d staining without evidence of rejection may be designated as "suspicious" for acute active ABMR
[c]In the absence of evidence of current/recent antibody interaction with the endothelium (those features in section 2), the term active should be omitted
[d]The clinical significance of these findings may be quite different in grafts exposed to anti-blood-group antibodies (ABO-incompatible allografts)

intimal thickening in arteries. Although all the morphological elements listed are known to be associated with chronic AMR, only the ones pertaining to the microvasculature are specific enough of AMR.

Transplant glomerulopathy, characterized by extensive remodeling of the glomerular microvasculature with duplication of the glomerular basement membranes (GBM), is the most characteristic, albeit advanced, feature of chronic AMR (Figs. 31.16 and 31.17).

Microvascular inflammation (glomerulitis, capillaritis) typically precedes the advanced chronic changes and has been demonstrated to correlate with graft outcome in several studies [12, 13, 35, 38].

Early remodeling of the glomerular microvasculature (development of double contours in the GBM) can only be appreciated on electron microscopic studies. More advanced duplication is appreciated by light microcopy with special stains for basement membranes (PAS, PAMS). Multilamellation of the basal lamina of PTC correlates with transplant glomerulopathy and also indicates chronic microvascular injury and remodeling. This hallmark feature of chronic AMR can only be appreciated on electron microscopy (Fig. 31.18). The 2013 Banff schema update (Table 31.4) provides detailed guidelines for the diagnosis of AMR, including acute/active and chronic forms of the disease.

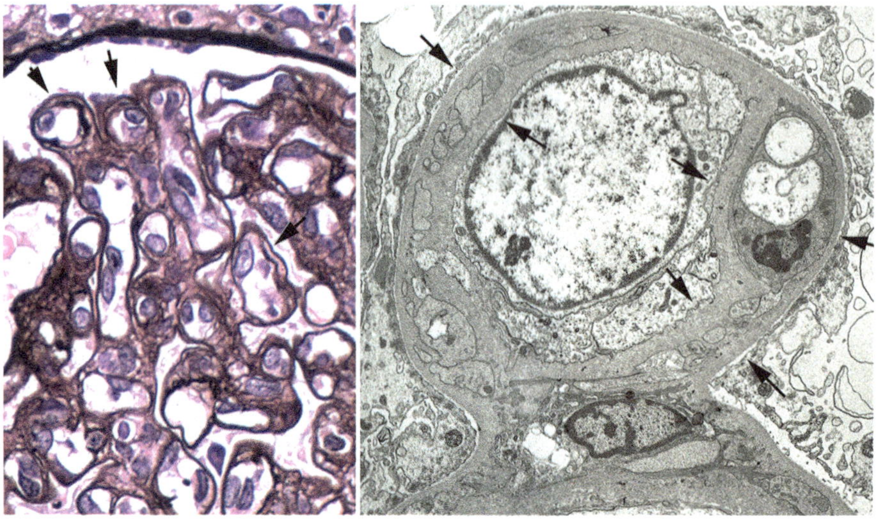

Fig. 31.16 Transplant glomerulopathy. PAMS (silver stain) demonstrates duplication of GBM in multiple glomerular loops. On the *right*, an electron micrograph demonstrates transplant glomerulopathy, characterized by GBM duplication with interposition of cellular components and matrix, between the two layers of basement membrane. The capillary lumen is occluded by a markedly swollen endothelial cell

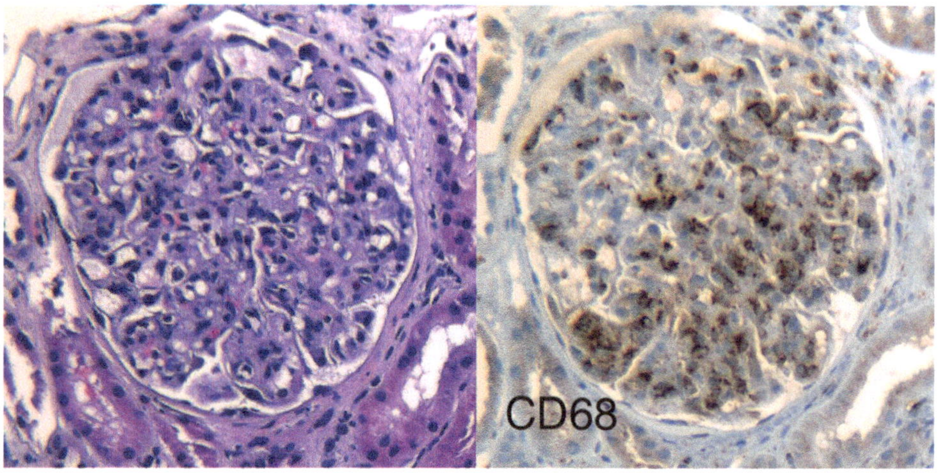

Fig. 31.17 Global involvement by glomerulitis, leading to occlusion of most capillary lumina. On the *right*, the same glomerulus stained with CD68 stain demonstrates large numbers of macrophages which typically accumulate in the microvasculature in patients with chronic AMR

Chronic CMR

The 2013 Banff schema update (Table 31.4) provides detailed guidelines for the diagnosis of AMR, including acute/active and chronic forms of the disease. Typical acute CMR promptly responds to treatment [5] and leaves significant sequelae only in cases with very extensive or protracted tubulitis (results in tubular atrophy) or severe multifocal intimal arteritis (leads to arterial sclerosis). The current Banff schema defines the category of *chronic active CMR* as "chronic allograft arteriopathy" if there is identification of arterial intimal fibrosis with mononuclear cell infiltration in fibrosis or formation of neo-intima [39, 40] (Fig. 31.19). This category, which is likely to be modified in the near future as allograft arteriopathy, can also be associated with AMR.

IF/TA and arteriosclerosis can result from other etiologies and are not specific for chronic CMR (Fig. 31.20) (see sections "Chronic Changes: Graft Sclerosis" and "Spectrum of Arterial Changes").

Biopsy Findings in the Setting of Noncompliance

Acute CMR in the late transplant period is most commonly associated with decrease in immunosuppression, either medically indicated (i.e., severe infections, tumors) or due to patient noncompliance.

In many cases the typical features of acute CMR are partially obscured by evolving chronic injury (parenchymal scarring, dense inflammatory infiltrates in scarred areas,

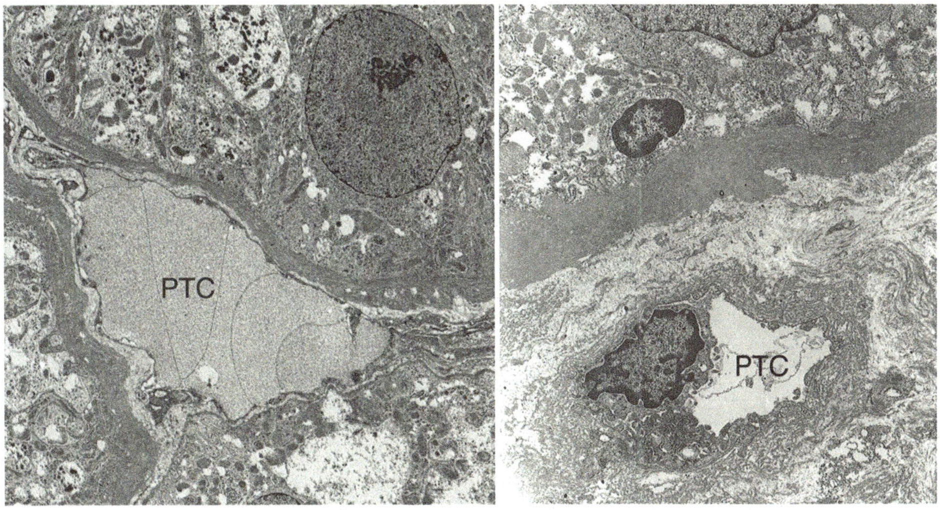

Fig. 31.18 Electron micrographs of peritubular capillaries (PTC). On the *left*, a normal PTC with a delicate basal lamina, closely apposed to the corresponding tubular basement membranes. On the *right*, PTC with extensive remodeling (multilamellation of the basal lamina), typical of biopsies with chronic AMR. There is increase in interstitial connective tissue leading to an abnormal separation of the PTC from its corresponding tubule

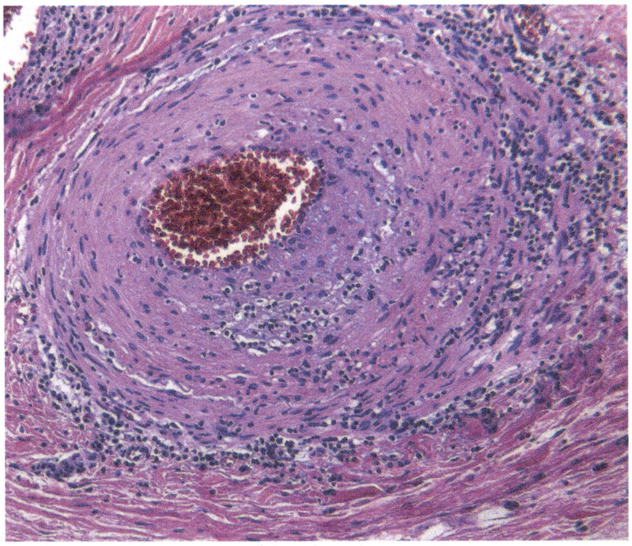

Fig. 31.19 Active transplant arteriopathy. Artery with severe fibrointimal thickening and transmural accumulation of inflammatory cells

nonspecific tubulitis in atrophying tubules, etc.). Clinicopathological correlations, comparison with previous biopsies, etc. are necessary in order to arrive at the best diagnosis in these cases.

In patients that have interrupted immunosuppression (noncompliance), it is common to see combined features of acute CMR and acute AMR including C4d positivity in PTC due to appearance of circulating DSA [41] (Fig. 31.21).

Glomerular Diseases

In addition to transplant glomerulopathy, there are numerous glomerular diseases that affect the allografts at various time points after transplantation. Specifically, FSGS, membranoproliferative glomerulonephritis (MPGN) type 1, dense deposit disease, membranous glomerulopathy, and HUS are all known to recur after transplantation and in most cases their identification portends poor prognosis for the graft.

Hepatitis C infection negatively impacts patient and graft outcomes overall; however, hepatitis C-related GN is a rare cause of graft failure per se [42]. It is important nevertheless to emphasize the significant morphological similarities between hepatitis C GN and transplant glomerulopathy, the latter being most commonly secondary to chronic AMR in patients with documented DSA [43].

Recurrent or de novo diabetic glomerulosclerosis is a common finding in long-term KTxBx and less commonly can also be seen within the first years after transplantation [44].

De novo FSGS is common in long-term transplants, appearing in approximately a third of patients with allograft scarring (interstitial fibrosis and tubular atrophy). FSGS in this context is typically secondary (adaptive) to nephron loss and glomerular hyperfiltration [45, 46].

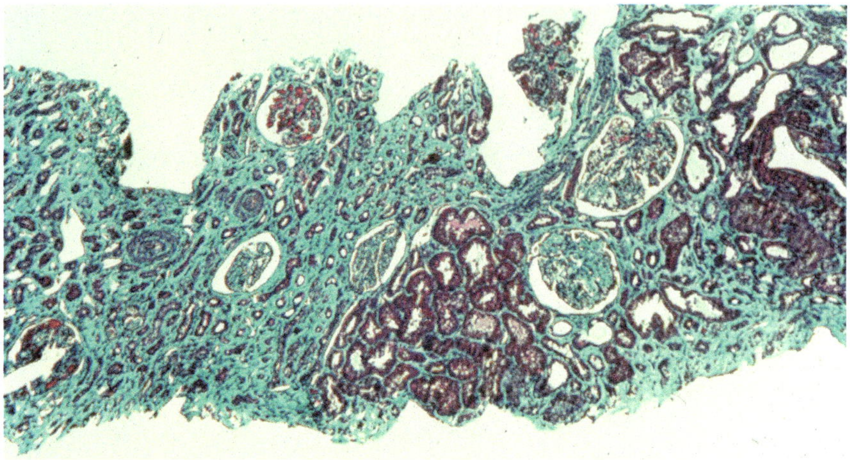

Fig. 31.20 Masson's trichrome-stained biopsy from a graft with moderate IF/TA. Note patches of preserved cortical parenchyma in which clusters of proximal tubules can be recognized in contrast to the areas with extensive tubular atrophy/fibrosis

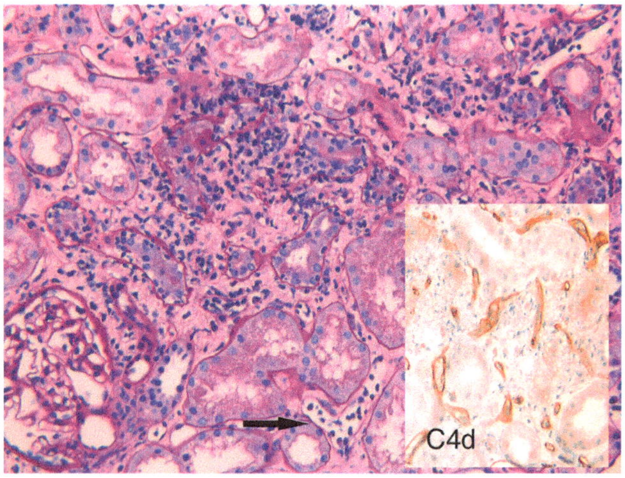

Fig. 31.21 Mixed acute CMR and AMR. Biopsy from a patient who voluntarily interrupted all immunosuppression medications 4 weeks earlier. There is tubulitis indicating acute CMR, as well as capillaritis (*arrow*) and diffuse C4d positivity in PTC (*inset*)

Infections

PV-associated allograft nephropathy (PVN) is caused by the BK virus in most instances and is characterized by the presence of viral cytopathic changes in tubular cells. The nuclei of the infected cells are large, hyperchromatic, and contain a large basophilic, "gelatinous" inclusion (Fig. 31.22). Immunohistochemical stains or in situ hybridization for SV40 are necessary to confirm the presence of polyoma virus in the intranuclear inclusions. In the early stages of PVN the viral cytopathic changes are associated with minimal or no inflammation. PVN is a multifocal process that can be missed in the early stages due to sampling. As the disease progresses, patches of dense mononuclear inflammation, sometimes granulomatoid in nature, develop associated with ongoing virally induced tubular damage and evolving tubular atrophy/loss. Viral inclusions are very sparse or may be absent in the late stages of PVN [9].

Concurrent evaluation of urine cytology for the presence of "decoy cells" or determination of BK viruria is a useful adjuvant in the diagnosis but cannot replace viremia as the most significant marker of parenchymal involvement in PVN. Persistent BK viremia of >10,000 viral copies/mL (for several weeks) is indicative of PVN, even if an allograft biopsy is negative for SV40-infected cells (presumptive PVN). Patients with uncontrolled PVN have increasing amounts of BK viral DNA in blood. Serial quantitation of BK viral load in plasma is critical for diagnosis, and is used to monitor the response to treatment [47].

Other manifestations of BK virus infections in kidney transplant patients include symptomatic PV cystitis, ureteritis leading to ureteral obstruction, and polyomavirus-associated neoplasms [48].

JC PVN, a rare complication of immunosuppression, has similar morphological and clinicopathological features as BK PVN. Although the same diagnostic algorithm applies to JC PVN viremia is typically low, in comparison [49].

Patients with long-standing polyomavirus replication are at higher risk of developing carcinomas of the urinary tract [50] (Fig. 31.22).

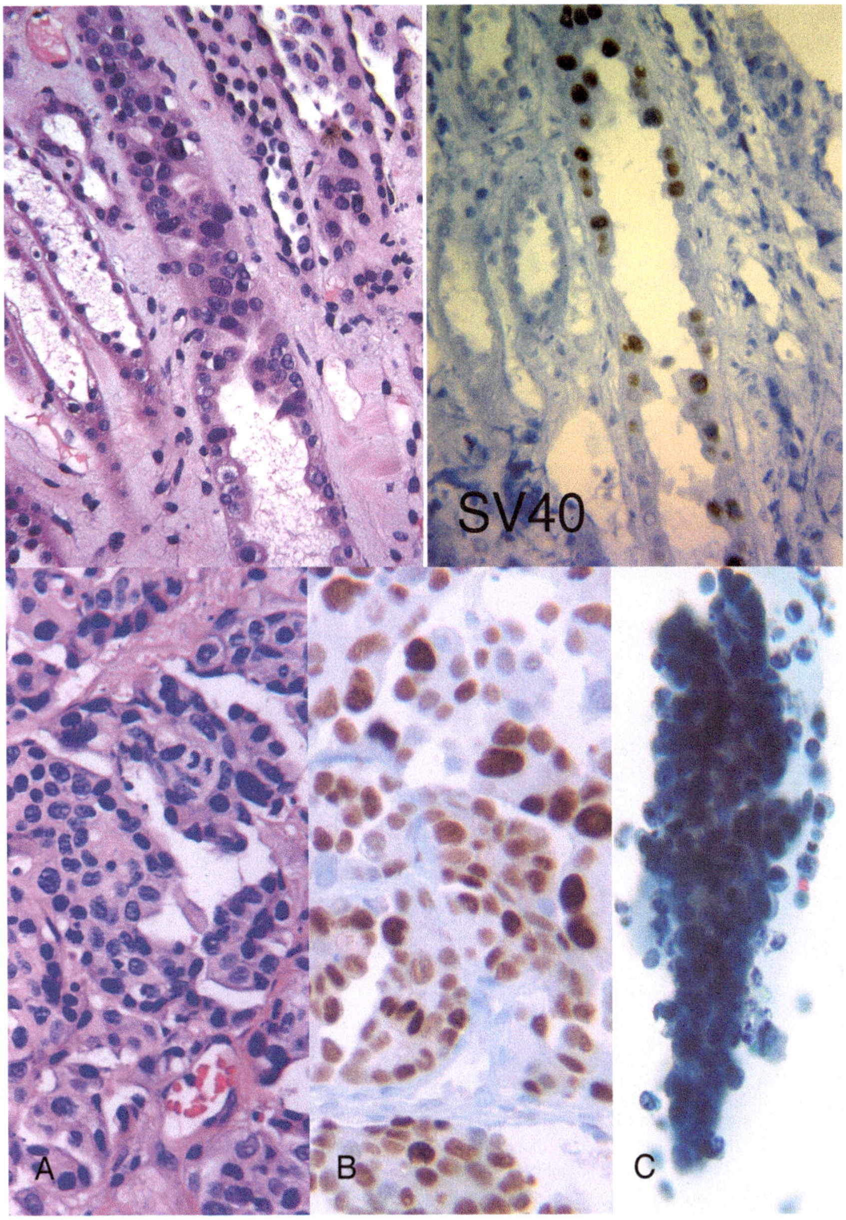

Fig. 31.22 (**a**) Polyomavirus allograft nephropathy (PVN). On the *left*, H&E stain demonstrates a tubule lined by cells with dark, enlarged nuclei strongly suggestive of viral cytopathic changes. On the *right*, SV40 stain demonstrates numerous nuclei of PV-infected cells. (**b**) Polyomavirus-associated bladder tumor in a patient with long-standing BK infection. (*a*) H&E stain; (*b*) SV40 stain with diffuse staining of the tumor cells; and (*c*) Papanicolaou stain of urine cytology with tumor fragment. The abnormal urine cytology findings lead to the diagnosis of the tumor

CMV

CMV infection is currently very rare. The diagnosis is made by the identification of enlarged cells with the typical cytopathic changes. In these cells the large nucleus contains a prominent eosinophilic inclusion often separated by the nuclear membrane by a halo ("owl's eye" appearance) and the abundant enlarged cytoplasm contains smaller granular reddish inclusions. The cytopathic effects of CMV infection can be observed most often in the glomerular endothelial cells leading to CMV glomerulitis in which the enlarged infected endothelial cells together with reactive changes in adjacent endocapillary cells lead to occlusion of the glomerular capillary lumina (Fig. 31.23). In contrast, in CMV tubulointerstitial nephritis there are enlarged infected tubular cells with associated tubulointerstitial mononuclear inflammation. Immunohistochemical stains for CMV confirm the presence of the virus in the cells with cytopathic changes [51] (Fig. 31.23).

Adenovirus allograft infection should also be considered in the morphological differential diagnosis of viral cytopathic changes in KTxBx. Renal manifestations of this infection

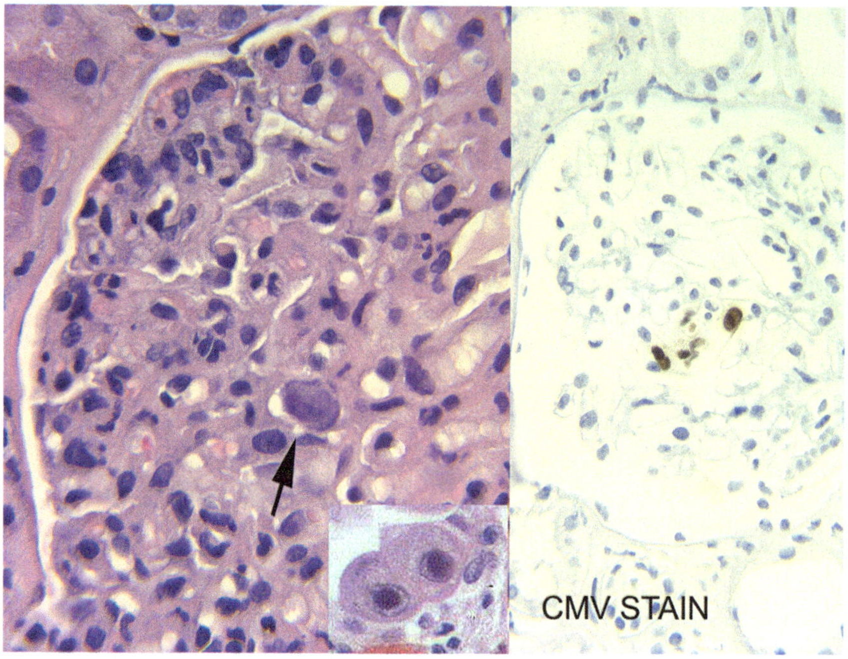

Fig. 31.23 Cytomegalovirus (CMV) nephritis. H&E-stained glomerulus on the *left* contains a CMV-infected cell (*arrow*) and prominent glomerulitis. *Inset* shows tubular cells with typical nuclear and cytoplasmic CMV inclusions. On the *left*, immunostain for CMV in a glomerulus with minimal glomerulitis highlights a cluster of CMV-infected cells

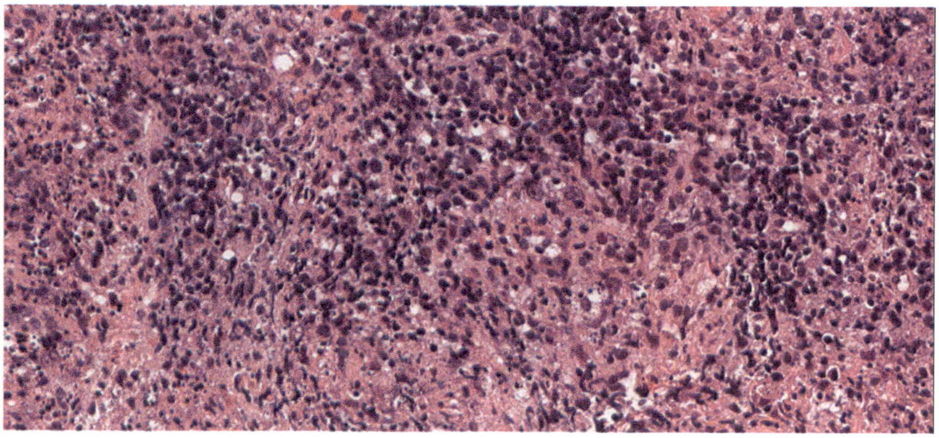

Fig. 31.24 Post-transplant lymphoproliferative disorder is characterized by extensive, confluent inflammatory infiltrates that show more cytological atypia and more destructive growth in comparison to the infiltrates in acute rejection

are very rare and are typically associated with systemic symptoms. Adenovirus graft nephropathy presents with prominent tubulointerstitial inflammation which may be granulomatous and is often destructive. The diagnosis is confirmed with adenovirus immunohistochemical stains or in situ hybridization [52].

EBV

EBV-related PTLD is characterized by polymorphic (mixed cellularity) or monomorphic predominantly B-cell inflammatory infiltrates. PTLD involves the renal parenchyma forming nodular, expansile, and sometimes destructive lesions. This is in contrast to the predominantly T-cell infiltrates in typical acute rejection. The presence of necrosis and cytological atypia are very helpful for the diagnosis [53] (Fig. 31.24). Immunohistochemical stains for EBV-related proteins to identify expression on the B-lymphocytes composing the PTLD are routinely done to confirm the diagnosis. Monomorphic PTLD is evaluated with the tools used to characterize lymphomas.

Bacterial and Fungal Pyelonephritis

Acute pyelonephritis. In bacterial infections the tubulointerstitial inflammation may be associated with necrosis and neutrophils are the predominant cell type [54] (Fig. 31.25). Clusters of neutrophils in the tubular lumina (purulent casts) are typical of acute pyelonephritis. Fungal infections have overlapping features with bacterial infections but may show

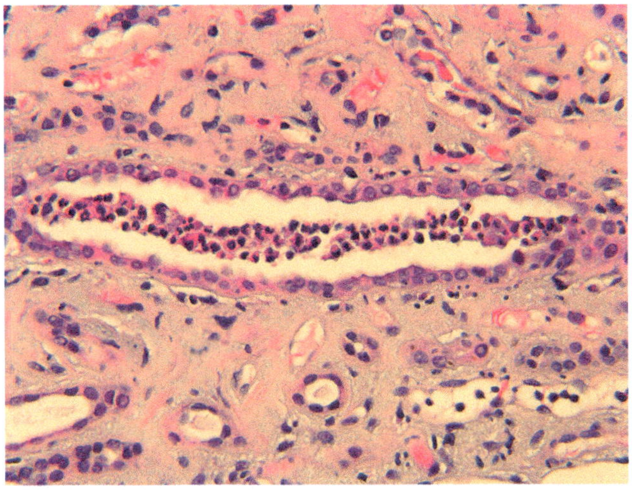

Fig. 31.25 Acute bacterial pyelonephritis is characterized by a predominance of neutrophilic infiltrates in the interstitium and in the tubules. A large purulent cast is noted in this image

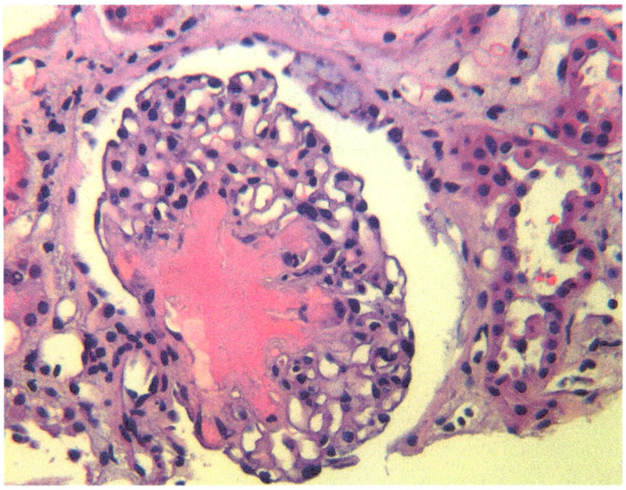

Fig. 31.27 De novo TMA in a patient with CNI toxicity. The hilum of this glomerulus is distended and occluded by a thrombus

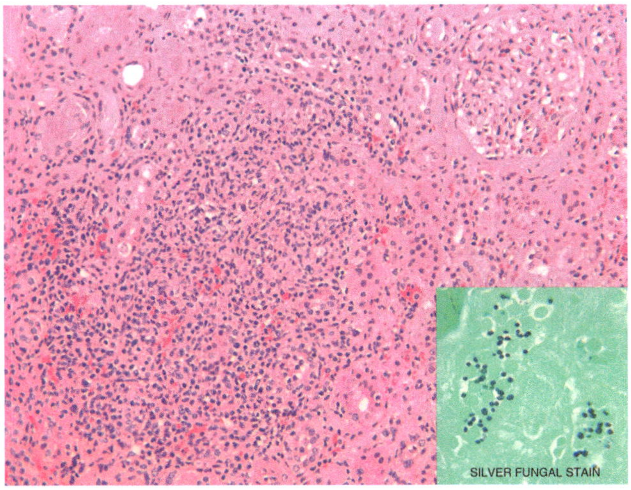

Fig. 31.26 Fungal pyelonephritis is characterized by prominent lymphocytic and macrophage infiltrates, sometimes forming granulomas. *Inset*, silver stain demonstrates clusters of fungal spores within the inflamed area

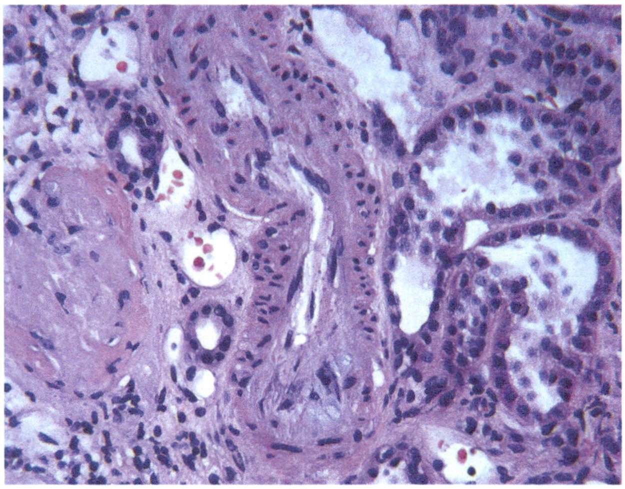

Fig. 31.28 Chronic TMA is characterized by thickening of the arterial walls, mostly secondary to edematous (myxoid) fibrointimal proliferation

a predominance of mononuclear inflammation and granulomas (Fig. 31.26). Although sometimes special stains (e.g., PAS for fungi) can identify the organism in question, microbiology studies and clinical correlation are essential for the diagnosis.

Thrombotic Microangiopathy

Morphological Definition

Acute TMA (early findings) is characterized by fibrin thrombi in glomerular capillaries and/or arterioles (Fig. 31.27). The glomerular tufts show various changes related to endothelial injury with swelling, associated with dissolution of the mesangium (mesangiolysis) and fragmented endothelial cells. The arteriolar walls may show fibrinoid necrosis.

Chronic TMA (late findings) results from organization of acute lesions and appears with areas of segmental glomerular sclerosis, mesangial expansion, and duplication of the capillary basement membranes (double contours). Chronic TMA manifests in interlobular size arteries with mucoid intimal hyperplasia (accumulation of edematous paucicellular amorphous material in the intima) which leads to marked narrowing of the lumen (Fig. 31.28). Generalized chronic ischemic parenchymal changes are often present.

In KTxBx TMA Is Associated with Various Clinical Settings

TMA in the context of DGF may have the following etiologies: (a) early acute AMR which is typically associated with neutrophilic peritubular capillaritis, diffuse C4d positivity, and DSA (Fig. 31.6); (b) ischemic endothelial injury which often presents with heterogeneous parenchymal involvement (normal appearing glomeruli alternating with extensive thrombotic glomerular capillary injury) (Fig. 31.6); (c) CNI toxicity often associated with high drug levels; and (d) recurrence of primary HUS [33].

TMA in patients with DSA is important at all times post-transplantation, often leading to accelerated graft failure. Acute TMA lesions predominate in early acute AMR; however, acute and chronic lesions typically coexist in patients with late-chronic AMR. C4d positivity is variable in the latter setting [13, 26, 30].

"Idiopathic" *or de novo TMA* is often attributed to CNI or rapamycin drug toxicity. This diagnosis can be made with relative certainty in patients with toxic levels of CNI agents or if the lesions disappear after discontinuation of the drug; however, all other etiologies (in particular AMR) need to be excluded [27, 28, 55].

Recurrence of primary HUS is high in patients with genetic abnormalities of the complement system. Genetic abnormalities of complement factors H and I have been associated with de novo TMA. It has been suggested that genetic complement abnormalities may represent an important risk factor for drug toxicity-related TMA [33].

Chronic Changes: Graft Sclerosis

Variable degrees of parenchymal fibrous scarring (interstitial fibrosis, tubular atrophy, arterial sclerosis, arteriolar hyalinosis, etc.) are universally observed in long-term renal allografts, even in patients that never had clinically evident episodes of acute rejection or acute graft dysfunction. With careful clinicopathological correlations, however, allograft failure can be attributed to a specific etiology in the vast majority of patients [56].

The Banff schema provides the descriptive diagnosis of IF/TA to be applied when there is no evidence of any specific etiology. IF/TA is graded as follows: I. mild interstitial fibrosis and tubular atrophy (<25 % of cortical area), II. moderate interstitial fibrosis and tubular atrophy (26–50 % of cortical area), and III. severe interstitial fibrosis and tubular atrophy/loss (>50 % of cortical area).

Chronic CNI Toxicity

Interstitial fibrosis, tubular atrophy, glomerulosclerosis (focal segmental and global), and arteriolar hyalinosis are considered features of chronic CNI toxicity [57] (Fig. 31.29). In part because these pathological features are nonspecific, it has been suggested that the prevalence of CNI toxicity has been overestimated [58, 59]. In the appropriate clinical setting, newly developing nodular arteriolar hyalinosis and striped fibrosis are often considered an indication of CNI toxicity (Fig. 31.30).

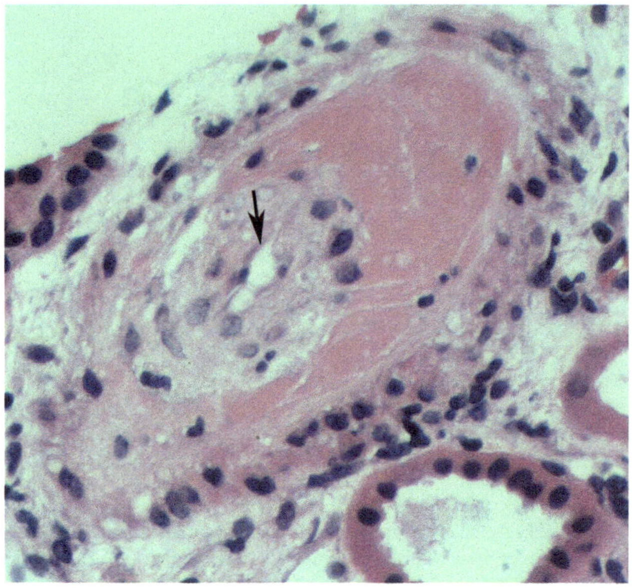

Fig. 31.29 Severe arteriolar hyalinosis. There is very marked thickening of the wall due to extensive accumulation of amorphous extracellular material (hyalin). The lumen is markedly narrowed (*arrow*)

Spectrum of Arterial Changes

The arterial branches in KTxBx provide important information about the status of the graft and their lesions correlate with a variety of diagnostic entities.

Inflammation of the arterial endothelium (*intimal arteritis, endarteritis*) used to be considered the most specific diagnostic feature of acute T-cell-mediated allograft rejection. More recently it is widely accepted that this lesion is also associated with the presence of DSA and AMR in which case the presence of arterial inflammation denotes a worse prognosis. From the practical point of view, the dual implication of intimal arteritis (for both CMR and AMR) highlights the importance of correlating the KTxBx findings with concurrent DSA studies [39, 40].

When arteriosclerosis is identified in very early KTxBx it most likely represents hypertensive or age-related donor vascular changes (Fig. 31.3).

Arteriosclerosis is a common finding in long-term KTxBx and it is related to both nonimmune injury (e.g., recipient's hypertensive disease) and alloimmune injury, including chronic CMR and chronic exposure to DSA (Fig. 31.31).

In its active phase, vascular rejection is easily recognizable by the presence of cellular inflammatory lesions involving the

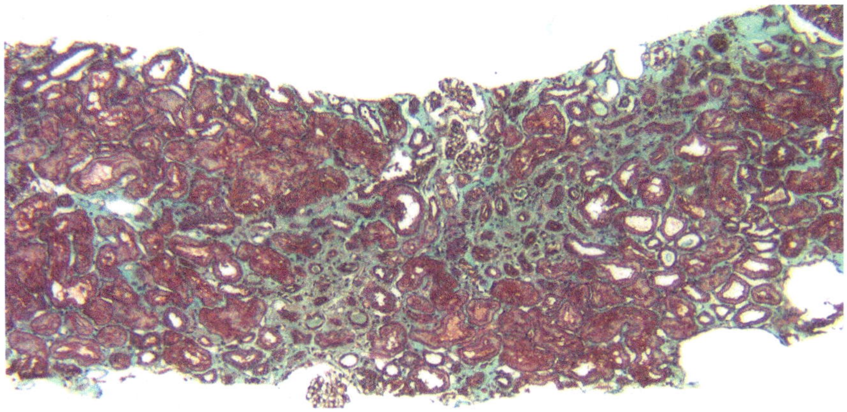

Fig. 31.30 Striped fibrosis. Masson's trichrome-stained biopsy shows areas of interstitial fibrosis/tubular atrophy, alternating with areas of better preserved (less fibrotic) cortical parenchyma

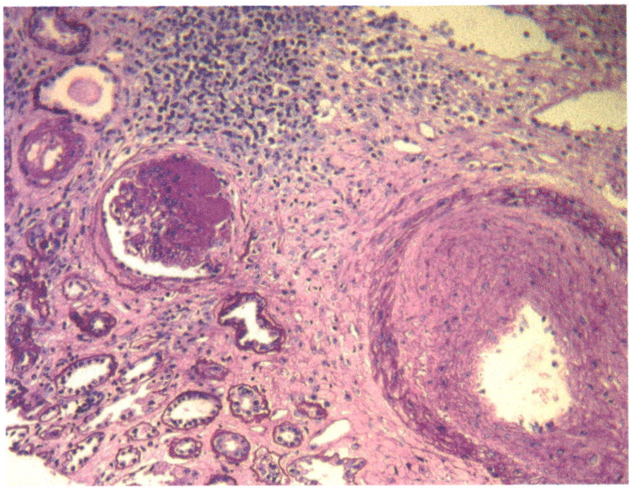

Fig. 31.31 Severe arteriosclerosis in a 10-year-old transplant associated with generalized ischemic changes including interstitial fibrosis, tubular atrophy, and glomerular sclerosis. The etiology of arteriosclerosis in allografts is often multifactorial

intimal layer (intimal arteritis, endarteritis) predominantly composed of T-cells and macrophages, typically in association with endothelial injury and activation.

The term transplant arteriopathy applies to the chronic arterial lesions resulting from acute or ongoing alloimmune injury (previous endarteritic/vaculitis lesions), but identification of chronic lesions is complicated by the fact that these lesions are paucicellular or acellular (fibrotic, sclerotic lesions), strongly resembling other forms of arteriosclerosis (Fig. 31.31).

Since old, inactive, transplant arteriopathy may be morphologically indistinguishable from simple hypertensive arteriosclerosis, evaluation of previous KTxBx from the same patient and performance of immunostains for T-lymphocytes in the paucicellular lesions can help support a diagnosis of transplant arteriopathy.

Further complicating the issue, chronic exposure to DSA appears to be associated with rapid development of vascular sclerosis evolving without clearly evident cellular/endarteritic lesions, therefore resembling non-alloimmune arteriosclerosis. It has been proposed that accelerated arteriosclerosis that occurs in the presence of circulating DSA (particularly Class II HLA) should be considered another variant of transplant arteriopathy [39].

Clinicopathological Discrepancies

Polyomavirus Allograft Nephropathy

A diagnosis of "presumptive PVN" is considered in a patient with a biopsy without significant pathology and negative SV40 stain, but sustained BK viremia (>10,000 copies/mL for 3 weeks) [47].

In rare instances, false-negative BK viremia has been reported in patients with BK PVN due to infection with viral genotypes for which the currently used diagnostic tests have low sensitivity [60]. A discrepancy of this type, or the possibility of JC PVN, should be considered in patients with histological evidence of PVN—SV40-positive-infected cells, but negative BK viremia.

AMR

The *absence of C4d staining* does not preclude a diagnosis of AMR, particularly in late-chronic AMR if the other diagnostic elements are present. Specifically, microvascular inflammation is considered to be strongly suggestive of AMR and has important prognostic implications [11, 61].

Negative DSA with histological evidence of AMR may be related to fluctuating DSA levels, technical inability to demonstrate anti-HLA DSA that is actually present, and non-anti-HLA antibodies (i.e., anti-endothelial antibodies, etc.).

Lack of correlation between transplant glomerulopathy and proteinuria is not uncommon. Although extensive transplant glomerulopathy in patients with chronic active AMR is typically associated with proteinuria, there is no linear correlation between proteinuria and the extent of transplant glomerulopathy, particularly in earlier stages.

Other

Diffuse parenchymal scarring in protocol KTxBx is clinically problematic and requires careful clinicopathological correlations. The main processes leading to this situation are multifocal infarcts in the peritransplantation period leading to cortical scars or ongoing ischemic injury, ongoing or repeated infections (chronic pyelonephritis), evolving PVN, and history of previous CMR episodes. A small number of patients have prominent scarring that cannot be explained. Evaluation of previous biopsies (pretransplant and post-transplant if available) may help explain the fibrosing process.

References

1. Williams WW, Taheri D, Tolkoff-Rubin N, Colvin RB. Clinical role of the renal transplant biopsy. Nat Rev Nephrol. 2012;8(2):110–21 [Research Support, N.I.H., Extramural Research Support, Non--U.S. Gov't Review].
2. Gaston RS, Cecka JM, Kasiske BL, Fieberg AM, Leduc R, Cosio FC, et al. Evidence for antibody-mediated injury as a major determinant of late kidney allograft failure. Transplantation. 2010;90(1):68–74.
3. Howell WM, Harmer A, Briggs D, Dyer P, Fuggle SV, Martin S, et al. British Society for Histocompatibility & Immunogenetics and British Transplantation Society guidelines for the detection and characterisation of clinically relevant antibodies in allotransplantation. Int J Immunogenet. 2010;37(6):435–7.
4. Sis B, Mengel M, Haas M, Colvin RB, Halloran PF, Racusen LC, et al. Banff '09 meeting report: antibody mediated graft deterioration and implementation of Banff working groups. Am J Transplant. 2010;10(3):464–71 [Clinical Conference Research Support, Non--U.S. Gov't].
5. Racusen LC, Solez K, Colvin RB, Bonsib SM, Castro MC, Cavallo T, et al. The Banff 97 working classification of renal allograft pathology. Kidney Int. 1999;55(2):713–23.
6. Colvin RB, Cohen AH, Saiontz C, Bonsib S, Buick M, Burke B, et al. Evaluation of pathologic criteria for acute renal allograft rejection: reproducibility, sensitivity, and clinical correlation. J Am Soc Nephrol. 1997;8(12):1930–41 [Comparative Study Multicenter Study Research Support, U.S. Gov't, P.H.S.].
7. Sorof JM, Vartanian RK, Olson JL, Tomlanovich SJ, Vincenti FG, Amend WJ. Histopathological concordance of paired renal allograft biopsy cores. Effect on the diagnosis and management of acute rejection. Transplantation. 1995;60(11):1215–9.
8. Bonsib SM, Reznicek MJ, Wright FH. Renal medulla in the diagnosis of acute cellular rejection. Transplantation. 1989;48(4):690–2.
9. Drachenberg CB, Papadimitriou JC, Hirsch HH, Wali R, Crowder C, Nogueira J, et al. Histological patterns of polyomavirus nephropathy: correlation with graft outcome and viral load. Am J Transplant. 2004;4(12):2082–92.
10. Batal I, Girnita A, Zeevi A, Saab BA, Stockhausen S, Shapiro R, et al. Clinical significance of the distribution of C4d deposits in different anatomic compartments of the allograft kidney. Mod Pathol. 2008;21(12):1490–8 [Research Support, N.I.H., Extramural].
11. Haas M. Pathologic features of antibody-mediated rejection in renal allografts: an expanding spectrum. Curr Opin Nephrol Hypertens. 2012;21(3):264–71.
12. de Kort H, Willicombe M, Brookes P, Dominy KM, Santos-Nunez E, Galliford JW, et al. Microcirculation inflammation associates with outcome in renal transplant patients with de novo donor-specific antibodies. Am J Transplant. 2013;13(2):485–92.
13. Papadimitriou JC, Drachenberg CB, Munivenkatappa R, Ramos E, Nogueira J, Sailey C, et al. Glomerular inflammation in renal allografts biopsies after the first year: cell types and relationship with antibody-mediated rejection and graft outcome. Transplantation. 2010;90(12):1478–85.
14. Drachenberg CB, Papadimitriou JC. Polyomavirus-associated nephropathy: update in diagnosis. Transpl Infect Dis. 2006;8(2):68–75 [Review].
15. Randhawa P, Ho A, Shapiro R, Vats A, Swalsky P, Finkelstein S, et al. Correlates of quantitative measurement of BK polyomavirus (BKV) DNA with clinical course of BKV infection in renal transplant patients. J Clin Microbiol. 2004;42(3):1176–80 [Comparative Study Research Support, Non-U.S. Gov't Research Support, U.S. Gov't, P.H.S.].
16. Munivenkatappa RB, Schweitzer EJ, Papadimitriou JC, Drachenberg CB, Thom KA, Perencevich EN, et al. The Maryland aggregate pathology index: a deceased donor kidney biopsy scoring system for predicting graft failure. Am J Transplant. 2008;8(11):2316–24 [Research Support, Non-U.S. Gov't].
17. Ojo AO, Leichtman AB, Punch JD, Hanson JA, Dickinson DM, Wolfe RA, et al. Impact of pre-existing donor hypertension and diabetes mellitus on cadaveric renal transplant outcomes. Am J Kidney Dis. 2000;36(1):153–9.
18. Ahmad M, Cole EH, Cardella CJ, Cattran DC, Schiff J, Tinckam KJ, et al. Impact of deceased donor diabetes mellitus on kidney transplant outcomes: a propensity score-matched study. Transplantation. 2009;88(2):251–60 [Research Support, Non-U.S. Gov't].
19. Huebner TA, Papadimitriou JC, Drachenberg CB, Gonzalez A, Philosophe B, Munivenkatappa R. Frozen section evaluation of pre-implantation donor kidneys: application of the Maryland Aggregate Pathology Index. Pathol Case Rev. 2010;15(5):174–9 [Case report].
20. Valente M, Furian L, Rigotti P. Organ donors with small renal cancer: report of 3 cases. Transplant Proc. 2012;44(7):1846–7.
21. Lappin DW, Hutchison AJ, Pearson RC, O'Donoghue DJ, Roberts IS. Angiomyolipoma in a transplanted kidney. Nephrol Dial Transplant. 1999;14(6):1574–5 [Case Reports].
22. Nickeleit V. The pathology of kidney transplantation. In: Ruiz P, editor. Transplantation pathology. New York: Cambridge University Press; 2009. p. 45–110.
23. Reese PP, Caplan AL, Kesselheim AS, Bloom RD. Creating a medical, ethical, and legal framework for complex living kidney donors. Clin J Am Soc Nephrol. 2006;1(6):1148–53 [Research Support, N.I.H., Extramural].
24. Gaber LW, Gaber AO, Tolley EA, Hathaway DK. Prediction by postrevascularization biopsies of cadaveric kidney allografts of rejection, graft loss, and preservation nephropathy. Transplantation. 1992;53(6):1219–25 [Research Support, Non-U.S. Gov't].
25. Liptak P, Kemeny E, Morvay Z, Szederkenyi E, Szenohradszky P, Marofka F, et al. Peritubular capillary damage in acute humoral rejection: an ultrastructural study on human renal allografts. Am J Transplant. 2005;5(12):2870–6 [Research Support, Non-U.S. Gov't].
26. Drachenberg CB, Papadimitriou JC. Endothelial injury in renal antibody mediated allograft rejection: a schematic view based on pathogenesis. Transplantation. 2013;95(9):1073–83.
27. Naesens M, Kuypers DR, Sarwal M. Calcineurin inhibitor nephrotoxicity. Clin J Am Soc Nephrol. 2009;4(2):481–508 [Review].
28. Barone GW, Gurley BJ, Abul-Ezz SR, Gokden N. Sirolimus-induced thrombotic microangiopathy in a renal transplant recipient. Am J Kidney Dis. 2003;42(1):202–6 [Case Reports].
29. Saikali JA, Truong LD, Suki WN. Sirolimus may promote thrombotic microangiopathy. Am J Transplant. 2003;3(2):229–30 [Case Reports].

30. Stegall MD, Gloor JM. Deciphering antibody-mediated rejection: new insights into mechanisms and treatment. Curr Opin Organ Transplant. 2010;15(1):8–10 [Review].
31. Solez K, Colvin RB, Racusen LC, Haas M, Sis B, Mengel M, et al. Banff 07 classification of renal allograft pathology: updates and future directions. Am J Transplant. 2008;8(4):753–60.
32. Josephson MA, Chiu MY, Woodle ES, Thistlethwaite JR, Haas M. Drug-induced acute interstitial nephritis in renal allografts: histopathologic features and clinical course in six patients. Am J Kidney Dis. 1999;34(3):540–8.
33. Noris M, Remuzzi G. Thrombotic microangiopathy after kidney transplantation. Am J Transplant. 2010;10(7):1517–23 [Research Support, Non-U.S. Gov't].
34. Buchmann TN, Wolff T, Bachmann A, Guerke L, Steiger J, Mihatsch MJ, et al. Repeat true surveillance biopsies in kidney transplantation. Transplantation. 2012;93(9):908–13 [Comparative Study].
35. Papadimitriou JC, Drachenberg CB, Ramos E, Kukuruga D, Klassen DK, Ugarte R, et al. Antibody-mediated allograft rejection: morphologic spectrum and serologic correlations in surveillance and for cause biopsies. Transplantation. 2013;95(1):128–36.
36. Issa N, Cosio FG, Gloor JM, Sethi S, Dean PG, Moore SB, et al. Transplant glomerulopathy: risk and prognosis related to anti-human leukocyte antigen class II antibody levels. Transplantation. 2008;86(5):681–5 [Research Support, Non-U.S. Gov't].
37. Wiebe C, Gibson IW, Blydt-Hansen TD, Karpinski M, Ho J, Storsley LJ, et al. Evolution and clinical pathologic correlations of de novo donor-specific HLA antibody post kidney transplant. Am J Transplant. 2012;12(5):1157–67 [Research Support, Non-U.S. Gov't].
38. Einecke G, Sis B, Reeve J, Mengel M, Campbell PM, Hidalgo LG, et al. Antibody-mediated microcirculation injury is the major cause of late kidney transplant failure. Am J Transplant. 2009;9(11):2520–31 [Research Support, Non-U.S. Gov't].
39. Lefaucheur C, Loupy A, Vernerey D, Duong-Van-Huyen JP, Suberbielle C, Anglicheau D, et al. Antibody-mediated vascular rejection of kidney allografts: a population-based study. Lancet. 2013;381(9863):313–9.
40. Nankivell BJ. Antibody-mediated vascular rejection: relation to causation. Lancet. 2013;381(9863):275–7.
41. Sellares J, de Freitas DG, Mengel M, Reeve J, Einecke G, Sis B, et al. Understanding the causes of kidney transplant failure: the dominant role of antibody-mediated rejection and nonadherence. Am J Transplant. 2012;12(2):388–99 [Comparative Study Multicenter Study Research Support, Non-U.S. Gov't].
42. Kasiske BL, Snyder JJ, Gilbertson D, Matas AJ. Diabetes mellitus after kidney transplantation in the United States. Am J Transplant. 2003;3(2):178–85.
43. Baid-Agrawal S, Farris III AB, Pascual M, Mauiyyedi S, Farrell ML, Tolkoff-Rubin N, et al. Overlapping pathways to transplant glomerulopathy: chronic humoral rejection, hepatitis C infection, and thrombotic microangiopathy. Kidney Int. 2011;80(8):879–85.
44. Hariharan S, Smith RD, Viero R, First MR. Diabetic nephropathy after renal transplantation. Clinical and pathologic features. Transplantation. 1996;62(5):632–5.
45. Cosio FG, Frankel WL, Pelletier RP, Pesavento TE, Henry ML, Ferguson RM. Focal segmental glomerulosclerosis in renal allografts with chronic nephropathy: implications for graft survival. Am J Kidney Dis. 1999;34(4):731–8 [Research Support, U.S. Gov't, P.H.S.].
46. Nankivell BJ, Borrows RJ, Fung CL, O'Connell PJ, Allen RD, Chapman JR. Evolution and pathophysiology of renal-transplant glomerulosclerosis. Transplantation. 2004;78(3):461–8 [Research Support, Non-U.S. Gov't].
47. Hirsch HH, Randhawa P. BK virus in solid organ transplant recipients. Am J Transplant. 2009;9 Suppl 4:S136–46 [Research Support, N.I.H., Extramural Research Support, Non-U.S. Gov't].
48. Drachenberg CB, Hirsch HH, Ramos E, Papadimitriou JC. Polyomavirus disease in renal transplantation: review of pathological findings and diagnostic methods. Hum Pathol. 2005; 36(12):1245–55 [Review].
49. Drachenberg CB, Hirsch HH, Papadimitriou JC, Gosert R, Wali RK, Munivenkatappa R, et al. Polyomavirus BK versus JC replication and nephropathy in renal transplant recipients: a prospective evaluation. Transplantation. 2007;84(3):323–30 [Comparative Study].
50. Alexiev BA, Randhawa P, Vazquez Martul E, Zeng G, Luo C, Ramos E, et al. BK virus-associated urinary bladder carcinoma in transplant recipients: report of 2 cases, review of the literature, and proposed pathogenetic model. Hum Pathol. 2013;44(5):908–17.
51. Onuigbo M, Haririan A, Ramos E, Klassen D, Wali R, Drachenberg C. Cytomegalovirus-induced glomerular vasculopathy in renal allografts: a report of two cases. Am J Transplant. 2002;2(7):684–8 [Case Reports].
52. Storsley L, Gibson IW. Adenovirus interstitial nephritis and rejection in an allograft. J Am Soc Nephrol. 2011;22(8):1423–7 [Case Reports].
53. Randhawa PS, Magnone M, Jordan M, Shapiro R, Demetris AJ, Nalesnik M. Renal allograft involvement by Epstein-Barr virus associated post-transplant lymphoproliferative disease. Am J Surg Pathol. 1996;20(5):563–71 [Research Support, Non-U.S. Gov't].
54. Fonseca Jr LE, Shapiro R, Randhawa PS. Occurrence of urinary tract infection in patients with renal allograft biopsies showing neutrophilic tubulitis. Mod Pathol. 2003;16(4):281–5 [Comparative Study].
55. Laftavi MR, Weber-Shrikant E, Kohli R, Patel S, Feng L, Said M, et al. Sirolimus-induced isometric tubular vacuolization: a new sirolimus histopathologic manifestation. Transplant Proc. 2010;42(7):2547–50 [Case Reports].
56. El-Zoghby ZM, Stegall MD, Lager DJ, Kremers WK, Amer H, Gloor JM, et al. Identifying specific causes of kidney allograft loss. Am J Transplant. 2009;9(3):527–35 [Research Support, Non-U.S. Gov't].
57. Chapman JR. Chronic calcineurin inhibitor nephrotoxicity-lest we forget. Am J Transplant. 2011;11(4):693–7.
58. Ekberg H, Johansson ME. Challenges and considerations in diagnosing the kidney disease in deteriorating graft function. Transpl Int. 2012;25(11):1119–28 [Research Support, Non-U.S. Gov't].
59. Matas AJ. Calcineurin inhibitors: short-term friend, long-term foe? Clin Pharmacol Ther. 2011;90(2):209–11.
60. Randhawa P, Kant J, Shapiro R, Tan H, Basu A, Luo C. Impact of genomic sequence variability on quantitative PCR assays for diagnosis of polyomavirus BK infection. J Clin Microbiol. 2011;49(12):4072–6 [Evaluation Studies Research Support, N.I.H., Extramural].
61. Haas M. C4d-negative antibody-mediated rejection in renal allografts: evidence for its existence and effect on graft survival. Clin Nephrol. 2011;75(4):271–8 [Review].
62. Haas M, Sis B, Racusen LC, Solez K et al. Banff 2013 meeting report: inclusion of c4d-negative antibodymediated rejection and antibody-associated arterial lesions. Am J Transplant. 2014; 14(2):272–83.

Imaging of the Renal Transplant Recipient

32

Maria Manning and Jade Wong-You-Cheong

Ultrasound

Ultrasound (US) is the most frequently used imaging technique in renal transplantation. The superficial location of the renal transplant in the iliac fossa allows access for high-resolution ultrasound imaging. Gray scale evaluation of renal transplant morphology includes evaluation of the size, corticomedullary differentiation, and echotexture of the allograft, as well as detection of hydronephrosis, stone or mass, and postoperative complications such as fluid collections or hematomas. Morphologically, the transplanted kidney has similar imaging characteristics as the native kidney (Fig. 32.1a), though corticomedullary differentiation and vasculature are better seen in most patients. Once transplanted, there is compensatory hypertrophy of the allograft, which grows by approximately 40 % within 6 months following transplantation [1]. The collecting system of the normal transplant may be mildly dilated due to increased volume of urine produced by the sole functioning kidney and possibly due to minor reflux at the ureterovesical anastomosis [2]. The bladder is also evaluated.

Morphologic evaluation is supplemented by color/power and duplex Doppler evaluation for parenchymal blood flow and patency of the renal arteries (single or multiple) and veins (Fig. 32.1b–d). Doppler ultrasound is an ideal initial modality for the detection and evaluation of vascular complications such as thrombosis, stenosis, or arteriovenous fistulae. Pediatric en bloc transplants are technically more challenging because of the smaller size of the renal arteries and veins (Fig. 32.2a, b). Normal Doppler arterial waveforms consist of continuous antegrade flow throughout the cardiac cycle with low resistance diastolic flow (Fig. 32.3). Abnormal intrarenal arterial resistance can be quantified by calculation of indices such as the resistive index (RI) and the pulsatility index (Fig. 32.3). While both indices reflect altered hemodynamics, the resistive index (RI) is the most commonly used. Normal resistive index ranges from 0.65 to 0.70 [3, 4]. RI values depend on local vascular status rather than renal function, and measurements are neither very sensitive nor specific [5, 6]. Causes of increased intrarenal resistive index include rejection, acute tubular necrosis (ATN), hydronephrosis, and vascular thrombosis. Though nonspecific for diagnosis, elevated RI values after transplantation have been shown to be associated with poor allograft and patient survival [7].

Research is ongoing in the evaluation of contrast-enhanced ultrasound using microbubble contrast agents, which is performed regularly outside of the United States, and has shown promise in the evaluation of renal transplant perfusion [8], specifically as a potential noninvasive means in the differentiation of acute rejection versus ATN as the cause of delayed graft function [9]. However, at this time, ultrasound cannot distinguish the causes of graft dysfunction, and biopsy remains the standard for diagnosis.

Ultrasound is a real-time, rapidly performed modality that is widely available and relatively cheap. It can be performed at the bedside, as is often required, and does not use ionizing radiation or nephrotoxic contrast. Limitations include suboptimal visualization in patients with large body habitus and extensive intestinal gas. Additionally, the quality of ultrasound examinations is dependent upon the technical skills and experience of the operator. Ultrasound is highly sensitive in the detection of hydronephrosis, fluid collections, and vascular complications. It is also an excellent modality for guidance during interventional procedures, such as biopsy (Fig. 32.4), aspiration or drainage of fluid collections, and access for antegrade pyelography or percutaneous nephrostomy placement.

M. Manning, M.D. • J. Wong-You-Cheong, M.D. (✉)
Department of Diagnostic Radiology, University of Maryland School of Medicine, 22 S. Greene Street, Baltimore, MD 21201-1595, USA
e-mail: MManning@umm.edu; JWong@umm.edu

M.R. Weir and E.V. Lerma (eds.), *Kidney Transplantation: Practical Guide to Management*, DOI 10.1007/978-1-4939-0342-9_32, © Springer Science+Business Media New York 2014

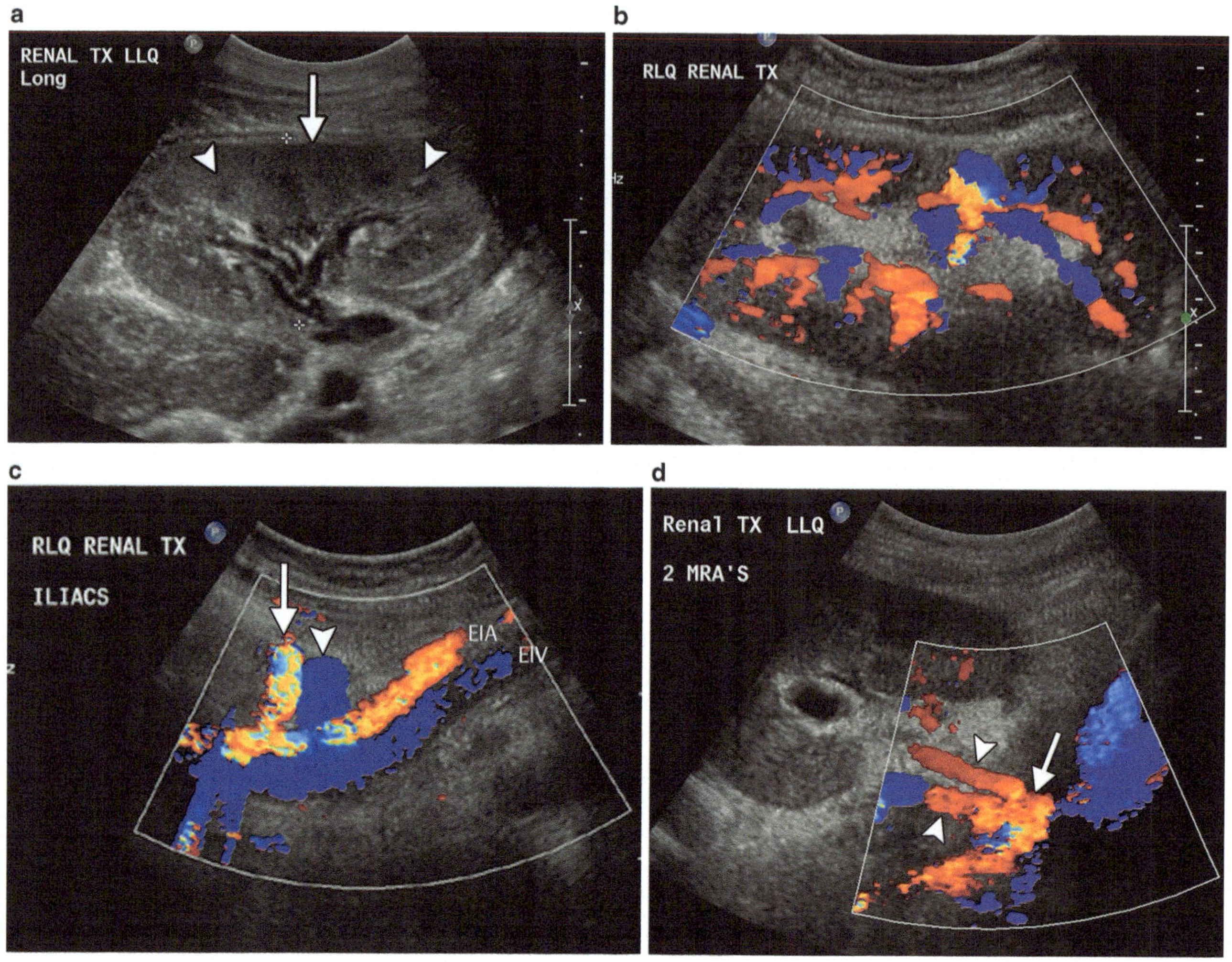

Fig. 32.1 Normal ultrasound. (**a**) Normal gray scale ultrasound obtained in the long axis through the renal transplant. The renal sinus is the bright central echo containing vessels and renal pelvis. It is surrounded by the gray hypoechoic cortex (*arrow*) with darker pyramids (*arrowheads*) at the corticomedullary junction. (**b**) Longitudinal color Doppler image shows flow throughout the allograft. (**c**) Longitudinal color Doppler along the course of the external iliac vasculature shows patency of the arterial (*arrow*) and venous (*arrowhead*) anastomoses to the external iliac artery (*EIA*) and vein (*EIV*). (**d**) Color Doppler image through the renal hilum shows an arterial patch (*arrow*) anastomosed to the iliac artery with two patent renal arteries (*arrowheads*)

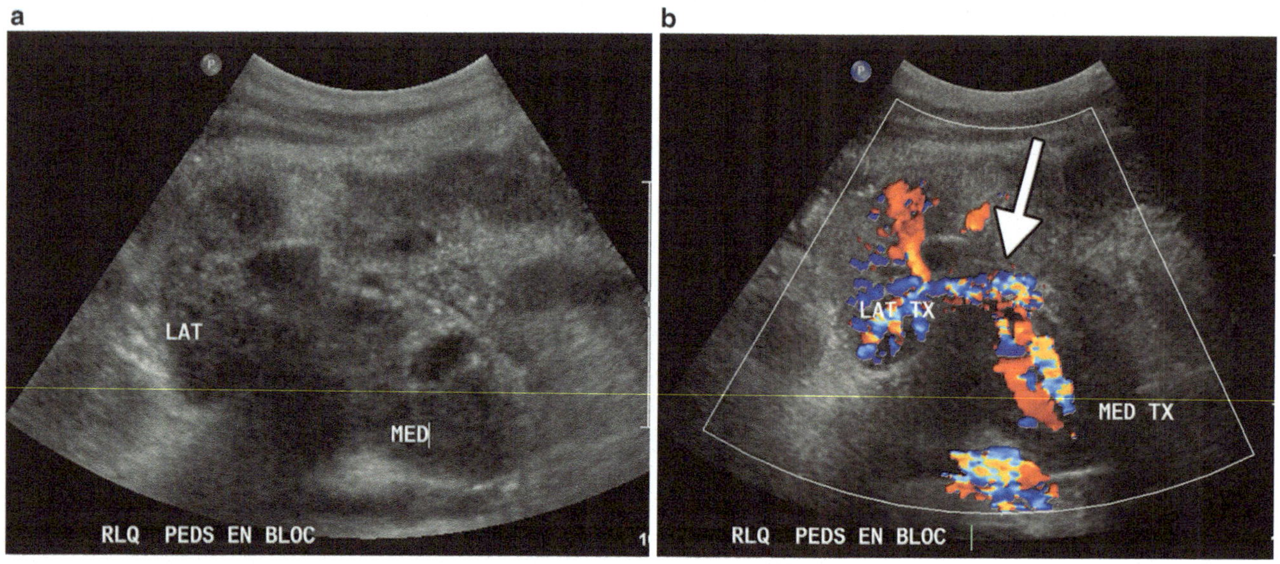

Fig. 32.2 Pediatric en bloc renal transplants. (**a**) Gray scale image of the two renal transplants (*LAT*, *MED*) shows the hila facing each other. (**b**) Color Doppler image shows the vascular anatomy with donor aorta and vena cava (*arrow*)

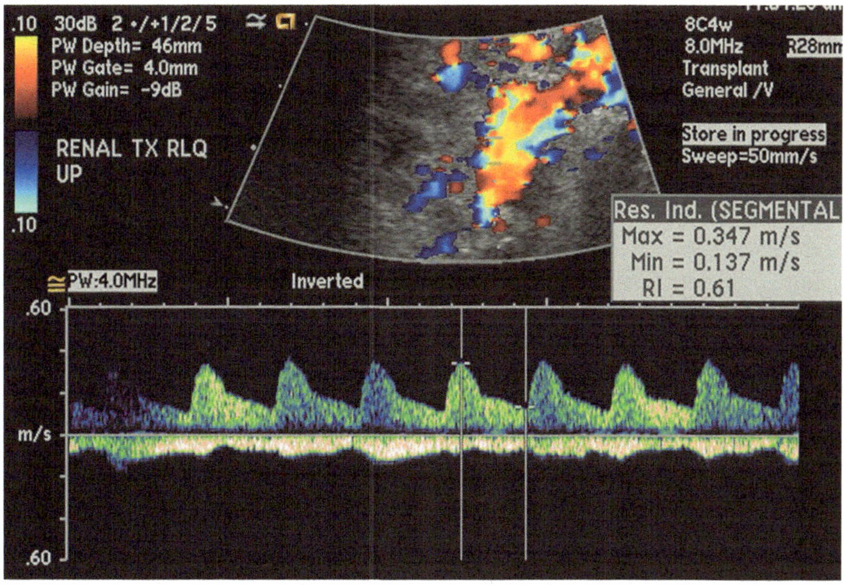

Fig. 32.3 Resistive index. Duplex Doppler tracing of an intrarenal artery demonstrates continuous antegrade, low resistance arterial flow throughout the cardiac cycle. The resistive index has been measured at 0.61

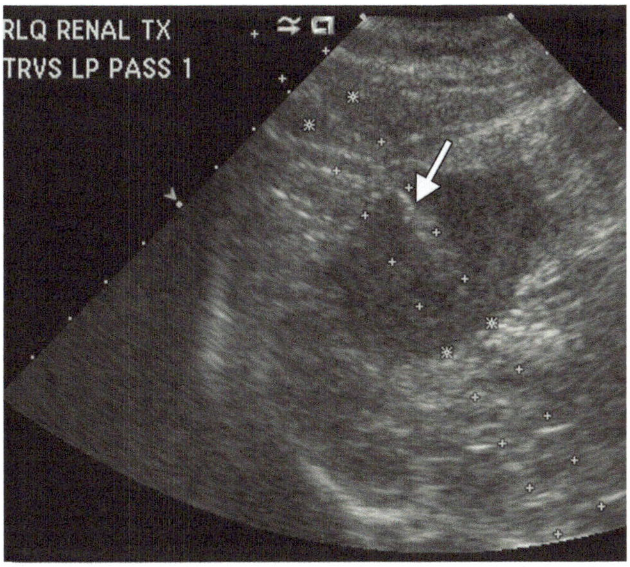

Fig. 32.4 Ultrasound-guided biopsy. The trajectory of the core needle biopsy can be seen in the lower pole peripheral cortex (*arrow*)

Computed Tomography

Computed tomography (CT) utilizes ionizing radiation to produce cross-sectional images with high spatial resolution. In general, computed tomography can be performed in the preoperative assessment of potential recipients and postoperatively for symptoms and signs outside of the renal transplant, e.g., fever, leukocytosis, or gastrointestinal complaints. An optimal CT examination requires iodinated contrast administered orally and intravenously. However, iodinated intravascular contrast may cause contrast-induced nephropathy (CIN) in patients with preexisting renal impairment and diabetes, and its use should be judicious in renal transplant recipients [10, 11]. Elevation in serum creatinine after the use of contrast agents within the early postoperative period is likely multifactorial, with contributory causes including ATN, rejection, cyclosporine toxicity, and dehydration. Prehydration prior to the CT study decreases the risk of contrast nephrotoxicity but does not eliminate it [10]. Although never specifically or adequately evaluated in the renal transplant population, other prophylactic measures such as administration of the antioxidant acetylcysteine are employed by many clinicians in hopes of preventing or reducing the nephrotoxicity of contrast agents.

In the immediate postoperative period, restoration of renal function may be delayed and it is therefore our practice to withhold intravenous contrast until renal function is adequate, or the use of vascular contrast considered absolutely necessary. A stable serum creatinine below 1.5–2.0 mmol/mL [1.5–2.0 mg/dL] or eGFR above 60 mL/min is a general cutoff for administering intravenous contrast media unless clinical urgency dictates the need for contrast-enhanced studies. When indicated, a reduced dose of iodinated contrast may be used. For most postoperative indications such as fever, pain, and diarrhea, an adequate CT study can be obtained without intravenous contrast but preferably with oral contrast. Alternatively, a magnetic resonance study may be substituted, as is discussed later.

CT is excellent for detection and anatomic localization of fluid collections and for guidance of interventional procedures. Transplant biopsies may also be performed using CT guidance instead of ultrasound for deep or less accessible allografts.

A non-contrast CT scan may be useful in evaluating for stones in the native kidney or renal allograft and ureters.

Multidetector CT cystography has become the standard technique for evaluation of traumatic bladder injuries and is now standard at our institution for evaluation of bladder leaks after renal transplantation [12–14]. After a pre-contrast image acquisition, approximately 250–300 mL of diluted iodinated contrast is infused through a Foley catheter and another series of images is obtained when the bladder is distended. CT cystography is highly sensitive to small leaks and 3D multiplanar reformations increase diagnostic confidence. In parallel, CT nephrostography is extremely useful for the diagnosis of ureteral leaks and strictures but requires the prior placement of a percutaneous nephrostomy tube.

Magnetic Resonance Imaging

Magnetic resonance imaging (MRI) is a very versatile modality. MRI can be performed in multiple planes, does not use ionizing radiation, and has high contrast resolution, making it more sensitive than CT to pathologic change within tissues. The use of varying pulse sequences enables tissue characterization (such as fluid, fat, and hematoma) and differentiation of fluid collections. Masses in the allograft and native kidneys or other sites are readily evaluated. MR can detect flowing blood in major vessels without the use of iodinated contrast. In the past, gadolinium-based contrast agents (GBCAs) were considered preferential to iodinated intravascular contrast material in the evaluation of patients with renal failure. GBCAs increased image resolution and improved detection of small vessels allowing the acquisition of high quality angiographic images noninvasively, with a lack of nephrotoxicity [15]. However, current awareness of the association of GBCAs with nephrogenic systemic fibrosis (NSF) in patients with reduced renal function has significantly impacted the use of GBCAs, requiring careful screening of patients at risk and tailoring of examinations to maximize useful information while minimizing exposure.

Non-contrast-dependent angiographic techniques based on fast spin-echo, gradient-echo, phase-contrast, and inversion-recovery principles have been developed or maximized to assess the renal transplant vasculature, including ECG-gated 3D non-enhanced magnetic resonance angiography (MRA) performed with selective inversion-prepared fast imaging with steady state free-precession (TrueFISP). This has been shown to depict the renal transplant arteries comparable to contrast-enhanced MRA [16, 17], and is used most commonly at our institution. When contrast-enhanced MRI is unavoidable, the dose and type of GBCA should be carefully selected to minimize risk, as recent studies have shown that when restrictive GBCA administration guidelines based on glomerular filtration rate (GFR) are followed, the incidence of developing NSF significantly decreases [18].

Functional MRI of renal allografts is a field of active research. MR techniques such as contrast-enhanced perfusion imaging, diffusion-weighted imaging, BOLD (blood oxygen level-dependent) imaging, and arterial spin labeling are available to measure perfusion, blood oxygen level, and GFR [19–22]. This has great potential in the noninvasive diagnosis of transplant dysfunction. Newer techniques such as MR elastography which measures tissue stiffness may in future play a role in the detection and quantification of fibrosis [23]. Diffusion-weighted imaging has become increasingly useful in the detection and staging of cancer with future potential in tissue characterization and grading of neoplasms and lymphadenopathy [24].

MRI is contraindicated in patients with most pacemakers and some metallic implants such as intracranial aneurysm clips and heart valves. Patients with claustrophobia may be unable to tolerate MRI despite sedation. Other disadvantages of MRI include the cost, availability, and relative length of the studies. Many of the newer sequences are breath held and require patient cooperation. Artifacts from surgical clips and stents may degrade image quality and cause spurious stenoses [25, 26].

Nuclear Scintigraphy

Nuclear scintigraphic renal studies are of value for the assessment of renal allograft function. For many years, technetium 99m pentetate (DTPA) was the most frequently used radiopharmaceutical for evaluation of renal allografts. In the last decade, this agent has been replaced by technetium 99m mertiatide (MAG3). Technetium 99m MAG3 is an agent that undergoes predominantly tubular secretion, and is a more efficient imaging agent than technetium DTPA. Images are obtained over the kidney immediately after the intravenous injection of technetium MAG3 to assess perfusion of the transplant, with development of perfusion parameters for quantitative evaluation [27]. Normal, decreased, or absent allograft renal blood flow may be calculated by comparison of the intensity of radiotracer activity over the kidney with the adjacent aorta or iliac blood vessels. GFR and effective renal plasma flow (ERPF) may be calculated. However, serial studies are often necessary in the determination of abnormal renal perfusion and ideally, a baseline MAG3 study is obtained within several days of the transplantation. Study quality may be compromised by poor hydration, and evaluation of the transplant may also be limited by uptake and secretion of MAG3 within the native kidneys if these remain partially functional.

Renal transplant vascular complications may be identified during the perfusion phase of technetium MAG3 studies although these abnormalities are more optimally evaluated and detected with Doppler ultrasound techniques.

Delayed scintigraphic imaging of the renal transplant is obtained after 30 min. The secretion of MAG3 into the renal collecting system, ureter, and bladder is measured and imaged. MAG3 studies remain very helpful for the detection of urinary leak and ureteral obstruction that most often occur at the anastomosis of the transplant ureter to the recipient bladder. MAG3 studies may also be helpful in the detection of vesico-ureteric reflux. This complication is frequently seen in transplanted kidneys due to the absence of a sphincter at the ureterovesical junction. Radiotracer intensity over the ureter and kidney may alternate over time due to periodic reflux of radiotracer-labeled urine from the bladder into the ureter and renal pelvis.

Isotope renography can be used to investigate renal dysfunction. In ATN, perfusion is normal but excretion is delayed and decreased. With rejection both perfusion and excretion are abnormal. However since other causes of graft dysfunction may have a similar picture, isotope renography is not of major value for the detection of rejection in transplant kidneys.

Interventional Radiology

While conventional catheter-based angiography remains the gold standard for the diagnosis of arteriovenous fistulae, pseudoaneurysms, and renal artery or vein stenosis, in practice, vascular abnormalities are usually initially detected by Doppler ultrasound and may be confirmed by MR or CT angiography. Instead, conventional angiography with digital subtraction techniques is reserved for confirmation of suspected abnormalities immediately prior to percutaneous transcatheter interventions such as angioplasty and stent placement in transplant artery stenosis or embolization of a fistula [28, 29]. Allograft arterial and venous thrombosis is usually diagnosed by ultrasound and the role of interventional radiology is limited to mechanical thrombectomy and catheter-directed thrombolysis in select cases [30, 31].

The limitations of conventional angiography include the relative invasiveness and the required use of nephrotoxic iodinated intravascular contrast media. To limit the nephrotoxicity of administered iodinated contrast, catheter-based angiography can be performed using low doses of low- or iso-osmolar contrast material [32], possibly in conjunction with carbon dioxide gas, which has been used as a sole intravascular agent but has poor image contrast [33, 34]. Although GBCAs have historically been used as intra-arterial angiographic contrast agents, given the emergence of NSF and the relatively high doses needed for equivalent radio-opacity, they are no longer acceptable in patients with renal dysfunction [32].

Interventional radiologists play an invaluable role in the postoperative management of transplant-related complications by performing endovascular treatment, percutaneous urinary intervention, and abscess or fluid drainage [32, 35–37], as will be addressed later under the specific complication.

Radiography

There is a limited role for abdominal radiography, limited to evaluation of stents, foreign bodies, renal calculi, and bowel complications. Chest radiography is widely used postoperatively.

Pre-transplant Work-up

Patients with long-standing renal disease often have many comorbidities which can affect graft and patient survival. Given the high demand for, and shortage of, donated kidneys, pre-transplant screening plays an important role in detecting coexisting illnesses and to evaluate feasibility of transplantation. This evaluation typically includes complete history and physical examination, with appropriate laboratory testing and up-to-date preventative health measures including colonoscopy and/or mammograms [38]. Basic radiologic imaging, including chest radiograph and abdominal ultrasound, is usually performed with more advanced imaging dictated by historical or clinical factors.

In many centers, preoperative contrast-enhanced CT arteriography (CTA) of the abdomen and pelvis is obtained in potential recipients. Selection criteria include age >50, chronic renal disease caused by diabetes and hypertension, known history of atherosclerosis or identification of atherosclerotic calcifications on radiography, or prior transplantation [39]. Important considerations include potential need for pre-transplant nephrectomy; evaluation for preexisting renal cell carcinoma or other malignancy, particularly in the dialysis population; and evaluation for sufficient atherosclerotic plaque-free patent vasculature for vascular anastomoses. In patients already on dialysis, normal dose contrast-enhanced CTA is performed. For patients who are predialysis, the risk of CIN can be lessened by hydration, before and after contrast administration [11, 40–42]. A recent study using 50–60 % of the standard dose of contrast for CTA with pre- and post-procedural hydration did not result in development of CIN in patients not yet on dialysis [43]. Additionally, at our institution, we are evaluating the potential of low kV (80 kV) CT scanning to potentiate lower doses of intravenous contrast (less than half the standard dose of 100 cc). Oral contrast is not administered as the high density interferes with volume rendering and creation of 3D reconstructions used for evaluation and presurgical mapping of vascular calcification.

Additionally, using CT, the native urinary tract can be assessed to determine need for concurrent nephrectomy (i.e., polycystic kidneys) or the presence of malignancy, given increased risk of renal cell carcinoma in the long-term dialysis-dependent patient [44].

Post-transplant Imaging Evaluation

The use of routine postoperative imaging is institution dependent. Common indications for imaging are absent or decreased urine output, delayed graft function, rising or persistently elevated creatinine, fever, pain over the allograft, or drop in hematocrit. Hypertension or hematuria may also prompt imaging evaluation. Patients with delayed graft function may have baseline imaging studies prior to discharge, which can be useful for comparison when follow-up studies are obtained. Ultrasound is the most commonly performed modality due to its unique advantages previously described. However CT, scintigraphy, and MR are complementary modalities in the radiologic armamentarium.

Complications After Renal Transplantation

Immediate complications, occurring in the first week, are mostly related to the surgical procedure and include renal artery or vein thrombosis, hemorrhage, and ureteral edema. Nonsurgical complications consist mainly of ATN and acute rejection. Early complications occur between 1 week and 1 month and include acute rejection, urinary leak, infection, fluid collections, and vascular thrombosis. After 1 month, lymphoceles, acute or chronic rejection, ureteral strictures, renal artery stenosis, infection, cyclosporine toxicity, recurrence of renal pathology, and neoplasms form the bulk of problems likely to be encountered. Overall, the most common complications are perinephric fluid collections which occur in up to 50 % of recipients [45, 46]. General complications relating to abdominal surgery are also encountered and include postoperative ileus, bowel obstruction, venous thromboembolic disease, and infections (systemic, pulmonary, renal, or bowel in origin). CT is the most useful imaging study when searching for infection or in patients with nonspecific chest or abdominal symptoms. Ultrasound is the study of choice for extremity deep venous thrombosis but is limited in the upper mediastinum or pelvis. For suspected thoracic, pelvic, or inferior vena cava thrombus, CT with contrast or MRI is the preferred modality. Multidetector CT pulmonary arteriography is the study of choice for pulmonary embolism.

Parenchymal Complications

Parenchymal complications include rejection, acute or chronic, delayed graft function, and calcineurin inhibitor toxicity. Time of onset of graft dysfunction and measurement of calcineurin inhibitor levels may be diagnostically helpful in distinguishing these complications. However in the majority of cases with elevation of serum creatinine or decreased urine output, ultrasound with Doppler is essential to exclude vascular and urologic complications.

Rejection

Since the development of more effective perioperative multidrug immunosuppressive therapies as well as the essential elimination of hyperacute rejection with modern cross matching techniques, rejection occurs less often in the first week after surgery. However, rejection remains a frequent cause of allograft dysfunction after that time and has a cardinal impact on patient and graft survival.

Despite early claims that altered transplant echogenicity, increased corticomedullary differentiation, and other subtle gray scale changes were predictive of acute rejection, it is now generally agreed that there are no specific gray scale sonographic characteristics of acute rejection [47, 48]. Allograft swelling and elevated resistive index (RI values > 0.8) or absent diastolic flow on Doppler arterial evaluation may be observed at sonography (Fig. 32.5a, b), but these findings are neither sensitive nor specific in the acute setting [49–52]. In one study, more than 50 % of allografts with biopsy-proven rejection had normal RIs of 0.7 or less [52]. The problem is that the RI is calculated in larger arteries, such as the interlobar or arcuate artery, and is interpreted as indirect evidence of disease at the capillary level. Unfortunately, there is susceptibility to error resulting from the effect of systemic disease, such as atherosclerosis, and renal artery stenosis [53]. Since acute rejection of a kidney graft primarily involves the subcapsular capillaries, early and detailed evaluation of blood flow in this area is highly desirable [54].

Continued technical developments in US imaging and the introduction of ultrasound-specific contrast medium (microbubbles) have shown promise for the assessment and quantification of microvascular perfusion. Several studies have shown direct correlation of delayed parenchymal perfusion with pathologically proven rejection, compared to perfusion dynamics seen in patients with normal function or ATN [53–55]. However, more research needs to be done, and until ultrasound contrast medium is approved for use in the US, this work remains "in progress" [8, 9]. Therefore, at this time, the main value of ultrasound in acute transplant dysfunction is to identify ureteric obstruction or vascular complications such as ischemia or thrombosis as the underlying cause. If these potential causes of allograft dysfunction have been excluded, percutaneous biopsy with sonographic guidance is usually performed to determine the specific etiology (Fig. 32.4). Nuclear scintigraphy, CT, and MRI are not of value in this setting.

Chronic Rejection

Chronic rejection is one of the most common causes of renal allograft failure [56]. It may present after a few months, and usually is detected because of elevated serum creatinine, often with proteinuria. Ultrasound is performed to exclude

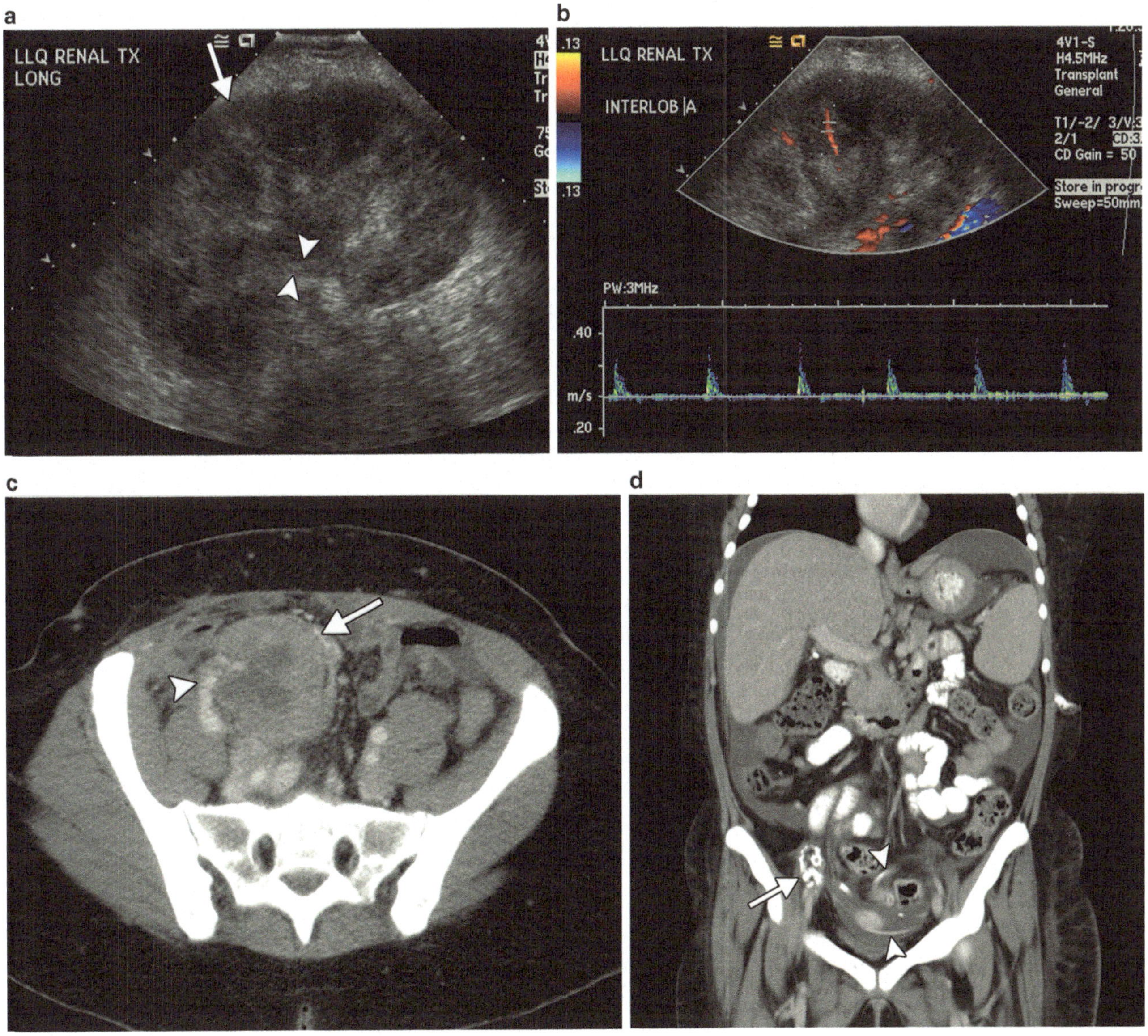

Fig. 32.5 Failed renal transplants. (**a**) Longitudinal gray scale ultrasound shows an enlarged, globular renal transplant with increased parenchymal echogenicity (*arrow*) and urothelial thickening (*arrowheads*). (**b**) Color and spectral Doppler imaging shows poor color flow and high resistance arterial waveforms with no diastolic flow. (**c**) Axial contrast enhanced CT through the pelvis shows an enlarged renal transplant (*arrow*) with patchy enhancement and patent vasculature (*arrowhead*), nonspecific imaging findings in a patient with biopsy proven acute on chronic rejection. (**d**) Coronal maximum projection-reconstructed CT image shows an atrophic calcified renal transplant (*arrow*) in the right lower quadrant. Also noted is a peritoneal dialysis catheter in the pelvis (*arrowheads*) and associated abdominopelvic ascites

structural causes of dysfunction. The allograft may be normal in size on ultrasound, but over time is likely to become progressively atrophic. A thin hyperechoic cortex with sparing of the medullary pyramids may be seen in advanced cases. As with acute rejection, Doppler arterial waveforms may be normal. However in a recent study, Doppler arterial resistive index measurements above 0.8 in a segmental branch on a single occasion more than 3 months after transplantation have been shown to be predictive of eventual graft failure [7]. Chronic rejection may be difficult to differentiate from acute rejection and cyclosporine toxicity on the basis of ultrasound findings, and unless the allograft is atrophic and calcified (Fig. 32.5d), with decreased color flow, percutaneous biopsy using sonographic guidance is usually performed to determine the cause.

Delayed Graft Function/Acute Tubular Necrosis

ATN is the most common cause of delayed graft function in the first week after surgery. Imaging is generally performed to exclude other causes of poor graft function as there are no specific imaging characteristics of ATN. Allograft swelling and elevated resistive index may be observed at sonography, but are nonspecific. As mentioned previously in the rejection section, contrast-enhanced ultrasound allows for assessment of the allograft microperfusion, and several studies have shown abnormal perfusion dynamics in patients with biopsy-proven ATN, compared to normal early graft function and acute rejection [9, 53]. Although the early results are interesting, more research is required, and biopsy remains the diagnostic gold standard [8]. At nuclear scintigraphy, relative preservation of perfusion with impaired clearance of tracer is noted [57, 58].

Severe acute rejection can increase intrarenal resistance resulting in elevated high peak systolic velocity and reversal or loss of diastolic flow [2, 45, 66]. This may culminate in thrombosis.

Vascular Complications

Up to 3 % of renal transplant recipients develop vascular complications [59, 60] with 66 % occurring within 1 month of transplantation. Early complications include renal artery or vein thrombosis, renal artery kinking or compression by collections, and hemorrhage. Renal artery thrombosis is the most common vascular cause of graft loss. After 1 month, the most common complication is renal artery stenosis. While not uncommon, biopsy-related complications such as arteriovenous fistulae are likely to resolve spontaneously and are not as clinically significant. Less common complications are renal vein stenosis and renal torsion [61].

Renal Vascular Thrombosis

Renal vein and renal artery thrombosis present with acute deterioration in graft function and urine output. Doppler ultrasound is the study of choice. An infarcted allograft will be swollen without evidence of parenchymal flow at color or spectral Doppler (Fig. 32.6a). With complete arterial thrombosis, there will be no detectable arterial flow in the allograft but a spiked preocclusive waveform may be detected in the renal artery proximal to the clot [2, 45, 62]. When there is more than one renal artery, accessory renal artery thrombosis may be suspected by failure to detect flow in all the arteries and by segmental absence or decrease of color flow in the renal parenchyma (Fig. 32.6b). Segmental infarcts may be wedge shaped and hypoechoic.

In early stage venous thrombosis, the renal artery may still be patent with Doppler showing an abnormally high resistance waveform and reversal of flow in diastole (Fig. 32.7) [63, 64]. Confirmation of renal artery or vein thrombosis with other imaging modalities is rarely required and delays surgical management. There is rarely a role for interventional radiologic thrombolysis.

Dissection of the main renal artery is rare. It is usually associated with technical intraoperative difficulties. The dissection flap will not usually be detected by ultrasound; however, decreased color flow and decreased peak velocities are indirect signs (Fig. 32.8a). CTA, MRA, or conventional angiography is superior for diagnosis (Fig. 32.8b) [65]. Treatment may be attempted by angioplasty and percutaneous stent placement (Fig. 32.8c) [65].

Renal Artery Stenosis

It is not uncommon to have mild to moderate vessel narrowing at the arterial anastomosis in early postoperative period [67]. Close follow-up is recommended rather than intervention. Later, renal artery stenosis is the most common vascular complication of renal transplantation, occurring in 0.51–12 % of recipients and usually within 1 year [29, 59, 60, 68, 69]. Typical presenting features are hypertension and graft dysfunction, and occasionally a bruit. A hemodynamically significant stenosis is one which narrows the lumen by 50 %. The site of the stenosis can be at the anastomosis (in 50 %), in the donor artery, or on the recipient side. Etiology is multifactorial with contributory factors including atherosclerosis, surgical trauma and technique (e.g., torsion or angulation at the vascular anastomosis), rejection, and infection.

Ultrasound is very useful as a noninvasive screening tool. The iliac artery, renal artery anastomosis, and entire renal artery are evaluated with color Doppler for areas of altered color flow and aliasing (disturbance of color signal because of elevated velocity). Peak systolic velocity is measured at multiple sites to determine the highest peak systolic velocity. The most commonly used Doppler criteria for renal artery stenosis include an elevation of peak systolic velocity to 2–2.5 m/s (Fig. 32.9a), a velocity gradient between the stenotic and non-stenotic segments greater than 2:1, or a ratio of peak systolic velocity in the renal artery to external iliac artery (EIA) of 1.8–2 [70, 71]. In a high-risk population, these criteria achieve a sensitivity of 87–94 % and specificity of 86–100 % [45, 70, 72, 73]. However in a low risk population, the false-positive rate is high when a threshold of 2.5 m/s is used and follow-up rather than angiography should be considered [74]. Kinking and tortuosity may cause a spurious elevation of peak systolic velocity (Fig. 32.10).

Due to technical difficulty in evaluating the renal artery anastomosis in some patients, indirect evaluation of renal artery stenosis can also be performed. Intrarenal arterial waveforms are evaluated for a delayed acceleration time (pulsus tardus) and slow rise to peak (pulsus parvus) (Fig. 32.9b). Threshold values in common use include a resistive index below 0.55 [45, 71], an acceleration time greater than 0.07–0.1 s [75]. Of note, these criteria are not applicable to pediatric transplants [76].

Catheter contrast angiography (with digital subtraction) is the reference standard for diagnosis and grading of renal artery stenosis (Fig. 32.9c). Pressure measurements can be performed to determine the significance of areas of narrowing and treatment can be performed at the same time. However angiography is invasive and requires contrast medium.

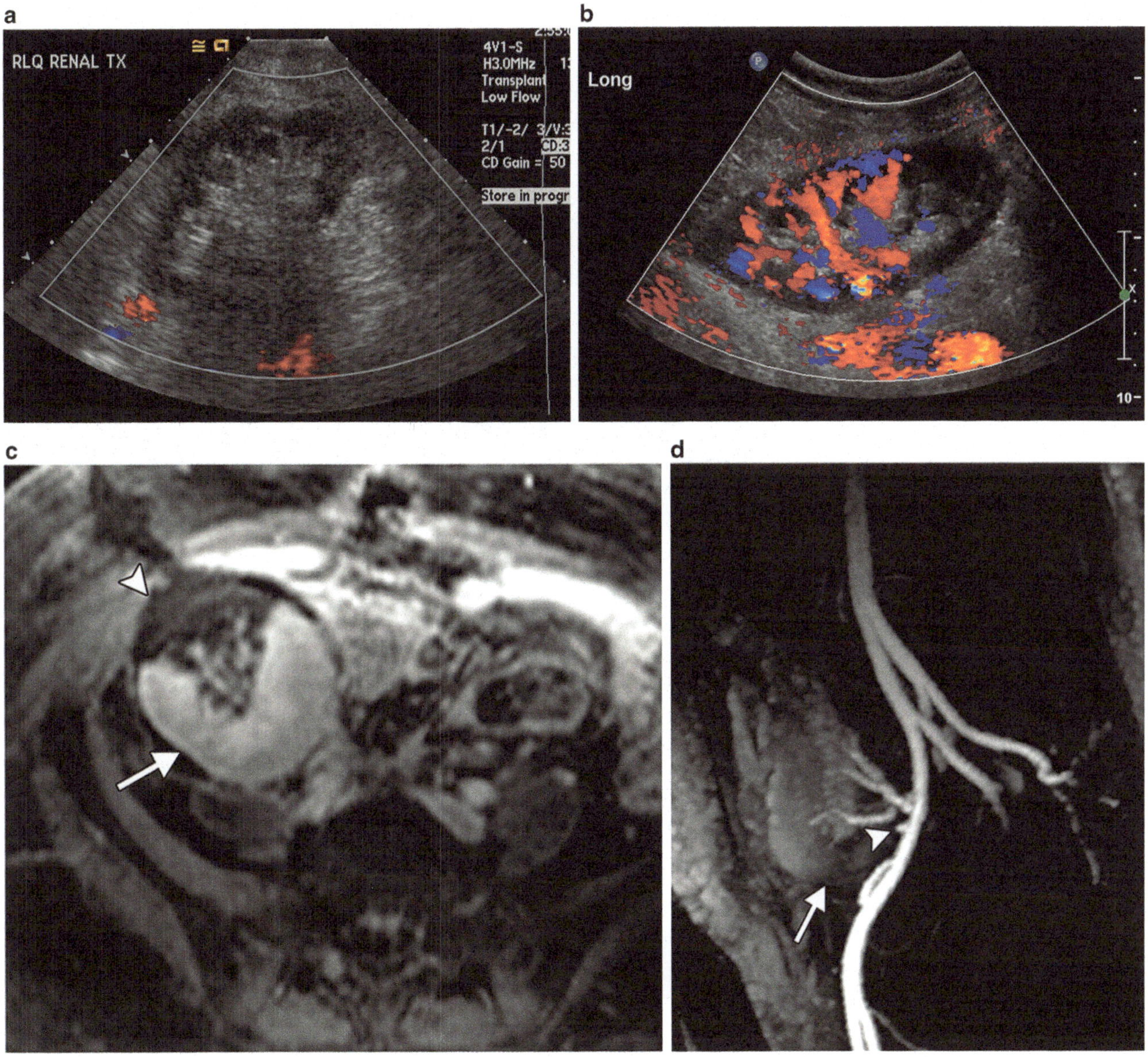

Fig. 32.6 Renal artery thrombosis. (**a**) Longitudinal color Doppler image shows the absence of color flow throughout the renal transplant. (**b**) Longitudinal color Doppler image shows segmental lower pole ischemia secondary to thrombosis of one renal artery in a patient with two renal arteries. (**c**) Fat suppressed, post-contrast T1 weighted MR image shows a wedge-shaped area of non-perfusion (*arrowhead*), with normal enhancement of the remainder of the transplant (*arrow*). (**d**) MRA shows occlusion of the inferior renal artery (*arrowhead*), with no enhancement of the lower pole (*arrow*)

Furthermore multiple injections and projections are necessary to analyze the aortoiliac segments and for tortuous or overlapping vasculature.

CT or MR contrast angiography may be performed prior to catheter angiography, in cases of non-diagnostic ultrasound or as a screening test. These modalities have the advantage of a wider field of imaging to include the entire aortoiliac and pelvic vasculature (after a single bolus of intravenous contrast) with the ability to manipulate the data in three dimensions. They are accurate in the diagnosis of transplant renal artery stenosis. Contrast-enhanced MRA is reported to have a sensitivity of 93.7 %, specificity of 80 %, accuracy of 88.5 %, positive predictive value of 88.2 %, and a negative predictive value of 88.9 % when compared to angiography (Fig. 32.11a) [15]. Pseudorenal artery stenosis from iliac stenosis and diffuse atherosclerotic disease may be detected, as well as perfusion defects and infarcts [26]. MRA may be limited by artifacts caused by certain arterial stents and metallic surgical clips. These cause signal loss and may prevent evaluation of vascular patency (Fig. 32.11b) [26]. Additionally MIP reconstruction techniques may overestimate degree of stenosis [26]. In allograft recipients with poor renal function, non-contrast MRA may be extremely helpful (Fig. 32.11c) [77–79].

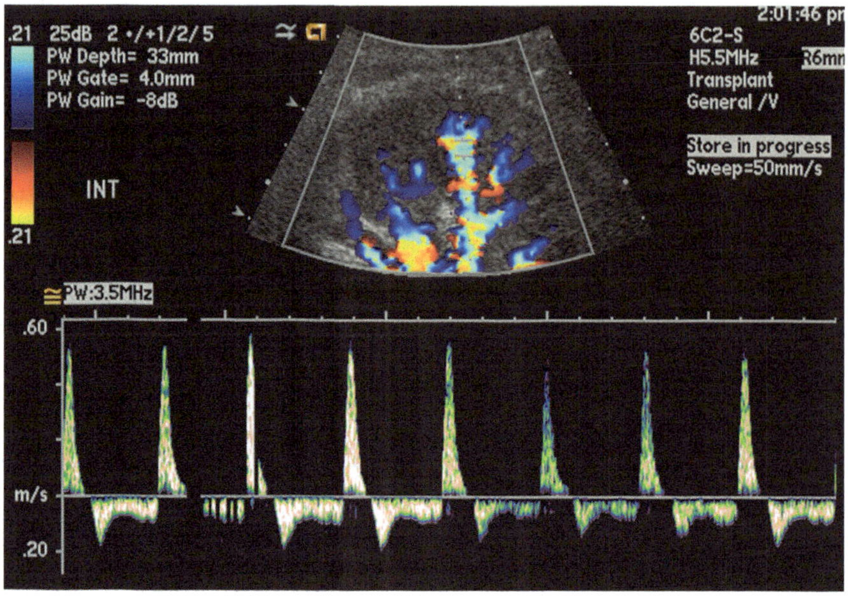

Fig. 32.7 Renal vein thrombosis. Duplex Doppler waveform shows high systolic arterial peaks with reversal of flow in diastole

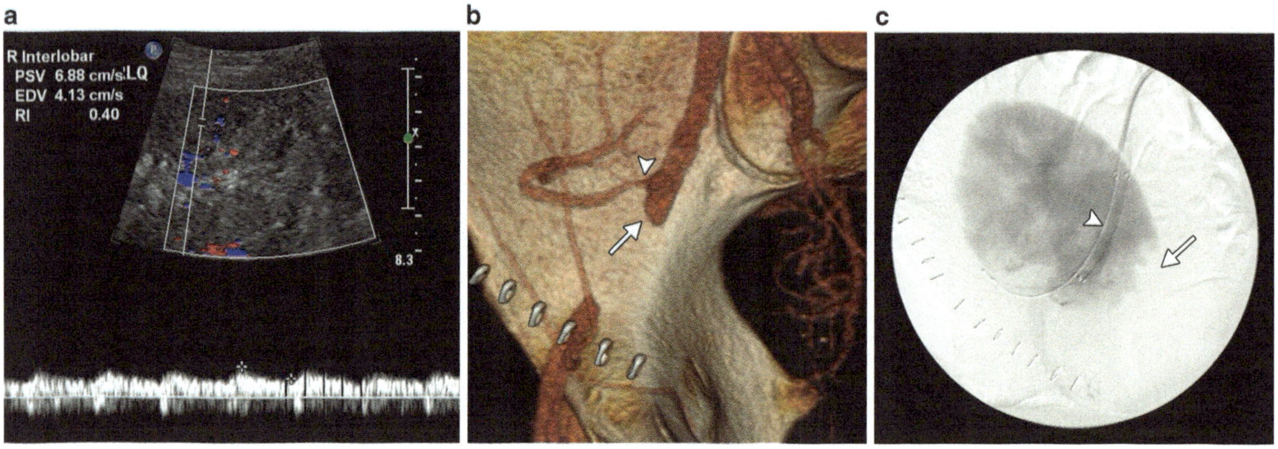

Fig. 32.8 Renal and iliac artery dissection. Doppler ultrasound shows a dampened intrarenal arterial waveform with a low resistive index of 0.40 (**a**). CT arteriogram shows occlusion of the EIA (*arrow*). There is stenosis of the transplant renal artery (*arrowhead*) (**b**). Digital subtraction image confirmed the findings which were treated with stents. Note the stent (*arrowhead*) and the lower pole infarct (*arrows*) (**c**)

Renal artery stenosis is initially treated by percutaneous transluminal angioplasty (PTA) with a success rate of 85–93 % and a complication rate of 4 % [32]. Complications include dissection, arterial rupture, and thrombosis. Restenosis occurs in 5–30 %, and may be treated by repeat PTA with or without stenting. Stenoses which are not amenable to or have failed endovascular approaches are managed surgically. Arterial kinks do not respond to endovascular techniques and typically require surgery [60]. Stenosis in the iliac artery above the main renal artery may impair graft function, and can also be treated with PTLA or stent.

The findings at radionuclide scintigraphy are not specific, and captopril renography is of limited diagnostic value in this setting.

Compartment Syndrome

An uncommon cause of early graft dysfunction is the renal compartment syndrome [80, 81]. Compression of the allograft in the pelvic cavity results in abnormal perfusion with reversed or absent diastolic flow and venous outflow obstruction (Fig. 32.12). Early diagnosis permits graft salvage.

Arteriovenous Fistulae and Pseudoaneurysm

Intrarenal arteriovenous fistulae are not uncommon after percutaneous biopsy, reportedly occurring in 1–18 % of biopsies [32, 60]. Pseudoaneurysms are less common. Both may be clinically silent and discovered incidentally by Doppler ultrasound. Typical presentation is gross hematuria after a biopsy.

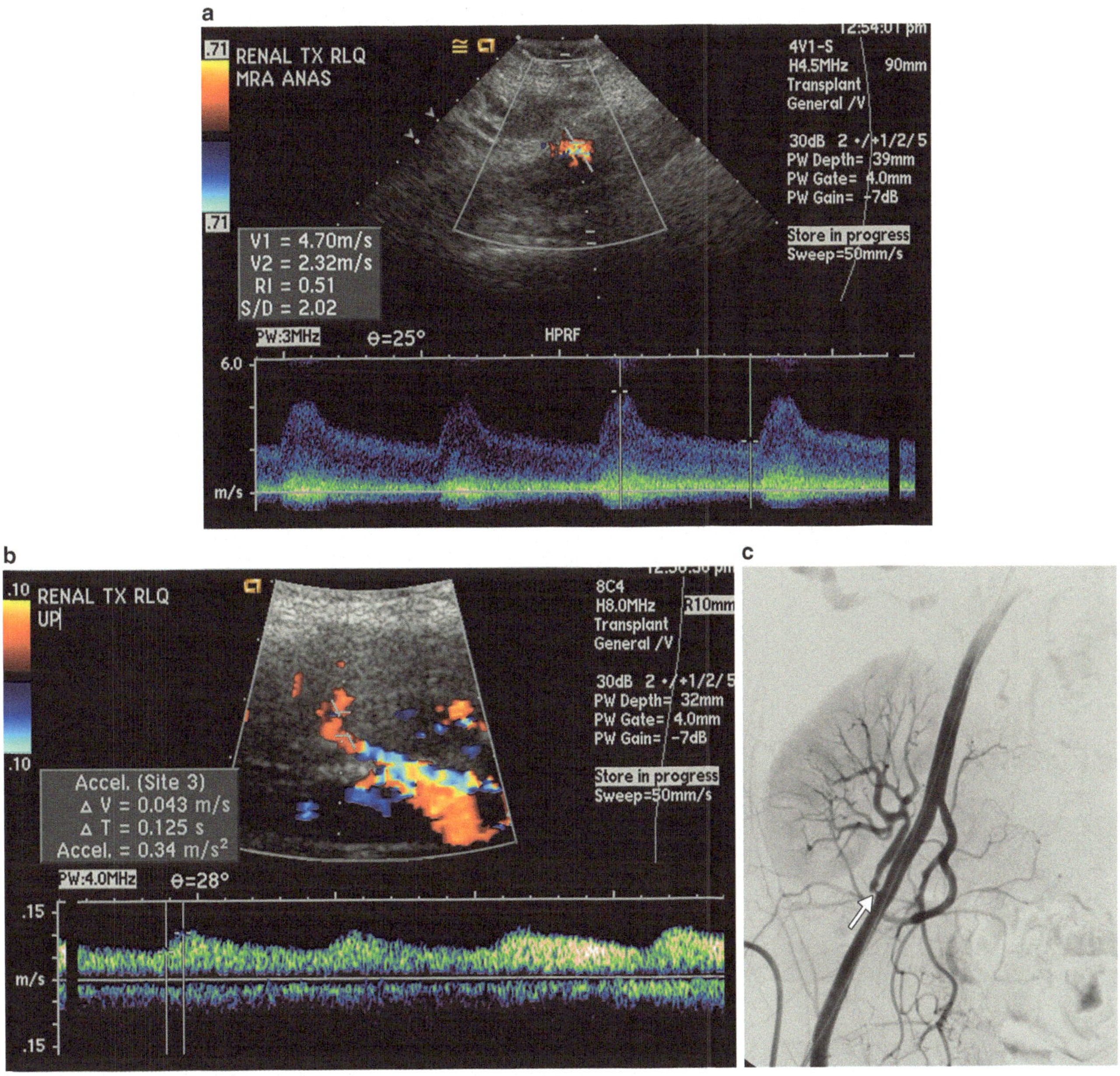

Fig. 32.9 Renal artery stenosis. (**a**) Duplex waveform at the renal artery anastomosis shows elevation of peak velocity, measuring 4.7 m/s. (**b**) Intrarenal waveform has a tardus–parvus pattern with decreased acceleration index and increased acceleration time of 0.125 s. (**c**) Catheter angiography confirming stenosis (*arrow*)

Rarely, hemorrhage, shunting, and graft dysfunction may occur. Extrarenal arteriovenous fistulae and pseudoaneurysms are secondary to surgical technique and are very rare.

On gray scale sonography, arteriovenous fistulae are usually invisible unless large when they appear as anechoic tubular or round structures. Color Doppler characteristics include a focal area of color aliasing with high velocities and perivascular turbulence manifest as a color "flurry" which may be transmitted to the surrounding tissues (Fig. 32.13a). Doppler waveforms show a characteristic high velocity, low resistance arterial waveform in the feeding artery and an arterialized venous waveform (Fig. 32.13b) [2, 45, 82]. The feeding artery and vein are generally not resolved with Doppler sonography, unless large. As many arteriovenous fistulae resolve spontaneously, management is initially conservative. Large or symptomatic arteriovenous fistulae can be treated by transcatheter embolization with metallic coils. Selective arteriography is initially performed to determine the road map (Fig. 32.13c). Success rates are high with minimal loss of parenchyma and few procedural complications [32, 83].

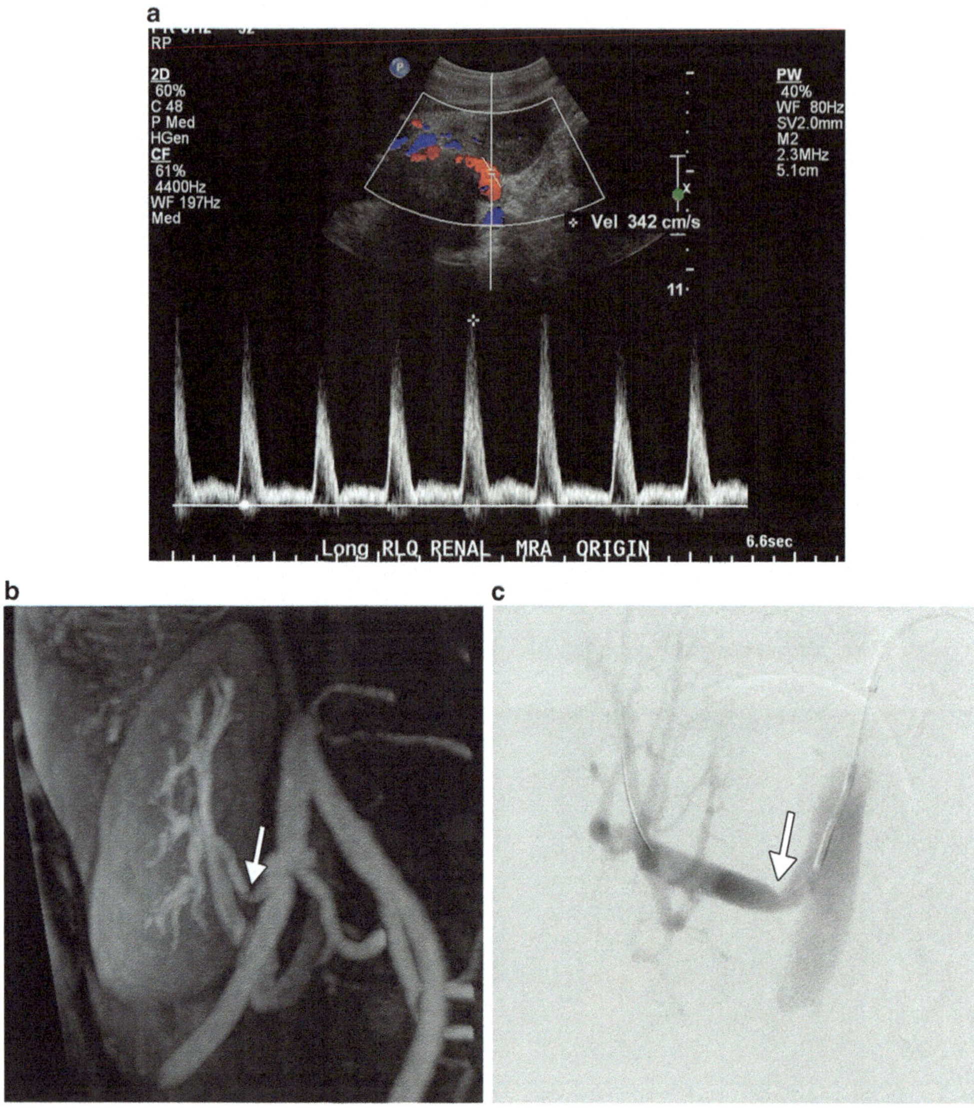

Fig. 32.10 Renal artery kink. (**a**) Duplex waveform shows elevation in peak velocity in the proximal renal artery, measuring 342 cm/s. (**b**) MRA performed without contrast shows angulation of the proximal renal artery (*arrow*) which was proven to be a kink (*arrow*) at angiography (**c**)

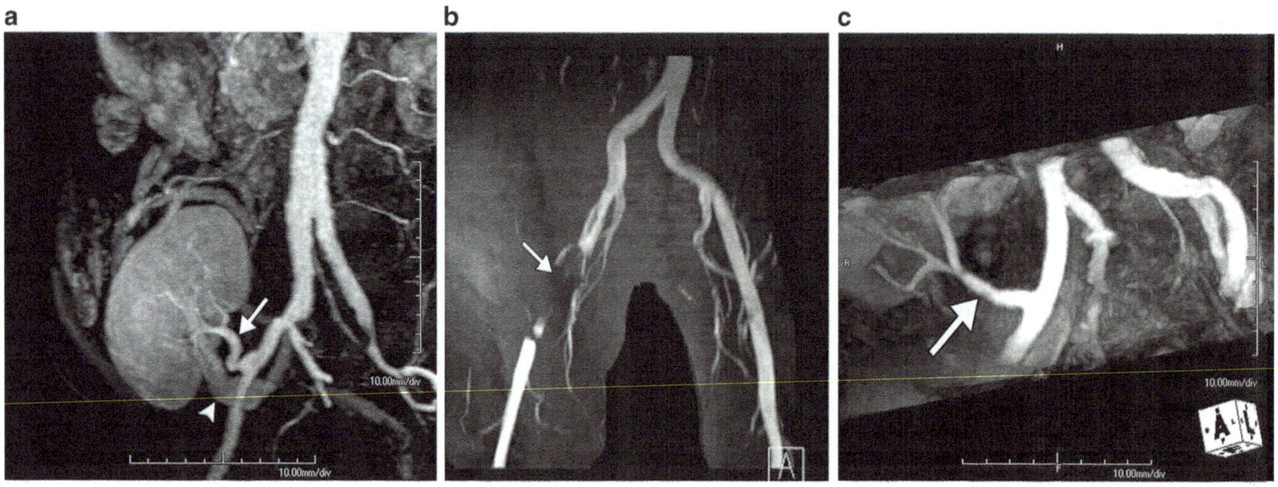

Fig. 32.11 MRA. (**a**) Oblique reconstruction of contrast-enhanced MRA of the pelvic arterial supply demonstrates a normal renal artery (*arrow*) with minimal aortoiliac atherosclerosis. Incidentally noted is opacification of the main renal vein (*arrowhead*). (**b**) Contrast-enhanced MRA performed after stenting of iliac artery dissection. Loss of signal is noted at the level of the stent (*arrow*), precluding evaluation of the lumen. (**c**) Oblique reconstruction of non-contrast MRA of the pelvic arterial supply demonstrates a normal renal artery (*arrow*)

Fig. 32.12 Compartment syndrome. There is global decrease in color flow throughout the renal transplant. The arterial waveforms (*arrow*) show loss of diastolic flow but there is elevation of the velocity in the segmental vein (*arrowhead*)

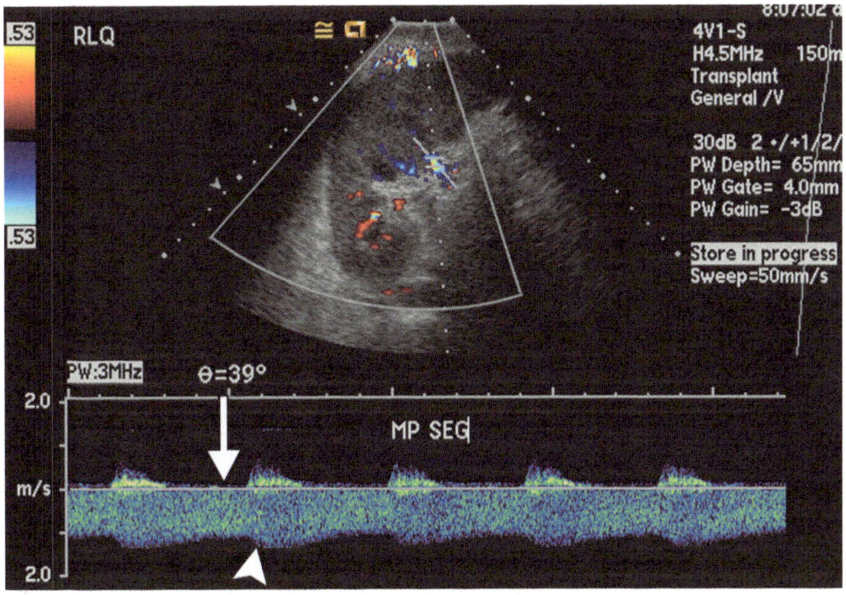

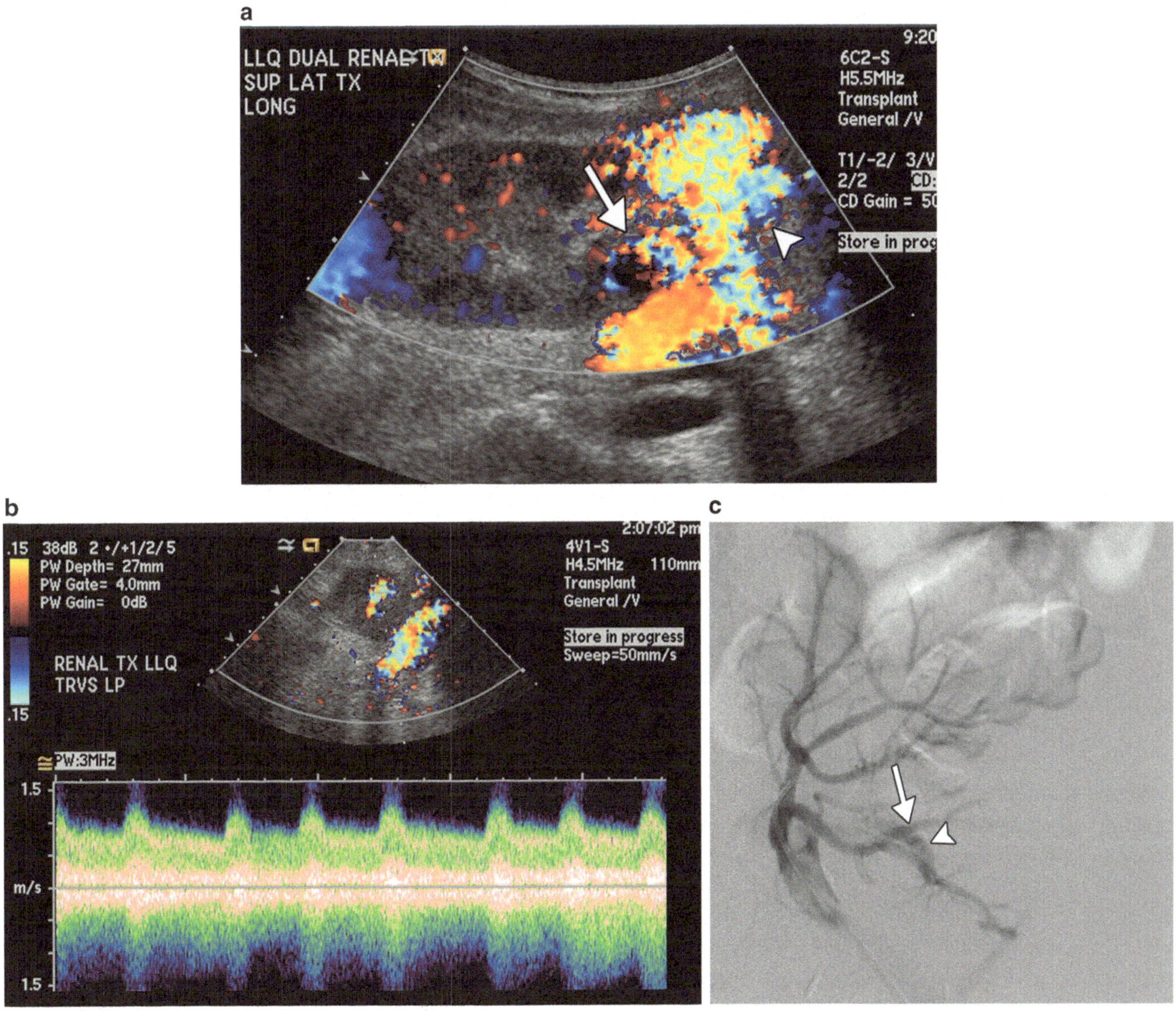

Fig. 32.13 Arteriovenous fistula. (**a**) Longitudinal color Doppler image shows a large lower pole arteriovenous fistula (*arrow*) with perivascular color flurry (*arrowhead*). (**b**) Duplex Doppler shows high velocity, low resistance arterial flow. (**c**) Digital subtraction selective renal artery angiogram showing an abnormal communication between an interlobular artery (*white arrow*) and early filling of an adjacent renal vein (*arrowhead*)

Pseudoaneurysms may appear as a simple or complex cyst on gray scale ultrasound (Fig. 32.14a). Specific Doppler characteristics are "yin yang" swirling flow within the pseudoaneurysm sac and to and fro flow on Doppler interrogation of the neck of the pseudoaneurysm (Fig. 32.14b, c) [2, 45]. Pseudoaneurysms may coexist with arteriovenous fistulae. Extrarenal pseudoaneurysms tend to occur at the arterial anastomosis either from surgical technique or from surrounding infection. They are more prone to rupture. Pseudoaneurysms of both types may be treated by embolization although large extrarenal pseudoaneurysms are difficult to treat and may require surgery (Fig. 32.14d, e).

Renal Vein Stenosis

This is a rare complication, usually resulting from perivascular fibrosis or compression by fluid collections. Fibrosis is difficult to treat by venous angioplasty as recoil is a problem. Primary stenting may be better [29, 84]. Gray scale findings include luminal narrowing or venous compression by a fluid collection. Doppler findings are more specific, and consist of aliasing on color Doppler and a focal velocity increase at the venous stenosis. To be significant, the velocity at the stenosis must be three to four times higher than in the normal venous segment [66]. Collateral veins may suggest the diagnosis. Arterial perfusion and diastolic flow may also be reduced.

Urologic Complications

Urologic complications occur in up to 6 % of recipients. The most common are ureteral stricture and leak which may be secondary to surgical technique, ischemia, and necrosis [59, 85, 86]. Other complications include ureteral or bladder stones and bladder outlet obstruction [85].

Hydronephrosis develops in 3–6.5 % of patients [87, 88] and may be early or late. In the early postoperative period, hydronephrosis may be secondary to edema, clot, calculus, or extrinsic compression by collections, hematoma, or an overdistended bladder. Later, ureteral strictures from ischemia, fibrosis, rejection, or infection (including BK virus (BKV) infection) predominate [28, 88]. Ureteral obstruction is caused by an ischemic stricture of the ureter in 90 % [89].

Ureteral strictures can be asymptomatic until graft dysfunction is discovered, or may be discovered by routine imaging. Hydronephrosis is most readily diagnosed by ultrasound but can be seen at CT, nuclear scintigraphy, and MRI. Ultrasound is excellent for the diagnosis of hydronephrosis where the dilated urine filled renal pelvis and calyces displace the echogenic sinus fat (Fig. 32.15a). Branching dilated calyces help to distinguish this entity from sinus cysts. The normal transplant ureter is not usually visible; when dilated, it will appear as a fluid-filled tubular structure between the renal pelvis and the bladder (Fig. 32.15b). Infection or rejection may cause thickening of the uroepithelium. Dilatation does not always signify obstruction however and may be secondary to vesico-ureteral reflux, a flaccid collecting system, an extrarenal pelvis, or a persistently dilated system post-obstruction or infection. Measurement of renovascular impedance using the resistive or pulsatility index has not proven useful in distinguishing obstruction from non-obstructive dilatation [2, 90]. Correlation with serum creatinine and urine output is valuable. Confirmation of obstruction can be achieved with technetium 99m MAG3 studies and a diuretic challenge; however, poor renal function will affect study validity [27]. Ureteral strictures are confirmed with CT or fluoroscopic nephrostography after obtaining catheter access to the collecting system (Fig. 32.15c, d). Confirmed ureteral obstruction can be drained by a percutaneous nephrostomy pending definitive management with balloon angioplasty, stent, or surgery (Fig. 32.15e).

Echoes and debris within the collecting system may represent blood clot, fungus, proteinaceous material, or infected debris. Gas may reflux into the collecting system from Foley catheterization of the bladder. Rarely, emphysematous pyelonephritis may produce gas throughout the renal parenchyma.

Urinary leak is an early complication occurring in 2 % [59]. Presenting features include rising creatinine, decreasing urine output, pain and swelling over the allograft or in the ipsilateral lower limb, increasing ascites, and fluid leakage from wound. Imaging will show a nonspecific fluid collection which can be aspirated for confirmation. Other than needle sampling, confirmation of a urine leak can be achieved with an isotope renogram, water-soluble contrast fluoroscopic cystogram or CT cystogram. The latter two have the advantage of directly demonstrating the location of the leak (Fig. 32.16a–c). Leaks are treated promptly because of risk of infection in the immunosuppressed host. Management depends upon the location of the leak [32]. Bladder or distal ureteral leaks may be managed by prolonged bladder catheter drainage or surgical repair whereas more proximal leaks may be treated by percutaneous nephrostomy or ureteral stenting pending definitive open repair [28, 32].

Urinary calculi are uncommon, occurring in 0.17–3 % of renal transplants [87]. These may occur de novo or be transplanted with the allograft and may present with acute obstruction, elevated creatinine, or infection. Stones in the native kidneys may also be a source of problems such as renal colic and infection after transplantation. Preoperative or intraoperative imaging can detect stones and prevent accidental stone transplantation. Calculi are readily diagnosed by ultrasound or CT, although small stones may be occult at ultrasound (Fig. 32.17a, b). Management depends on stone size.

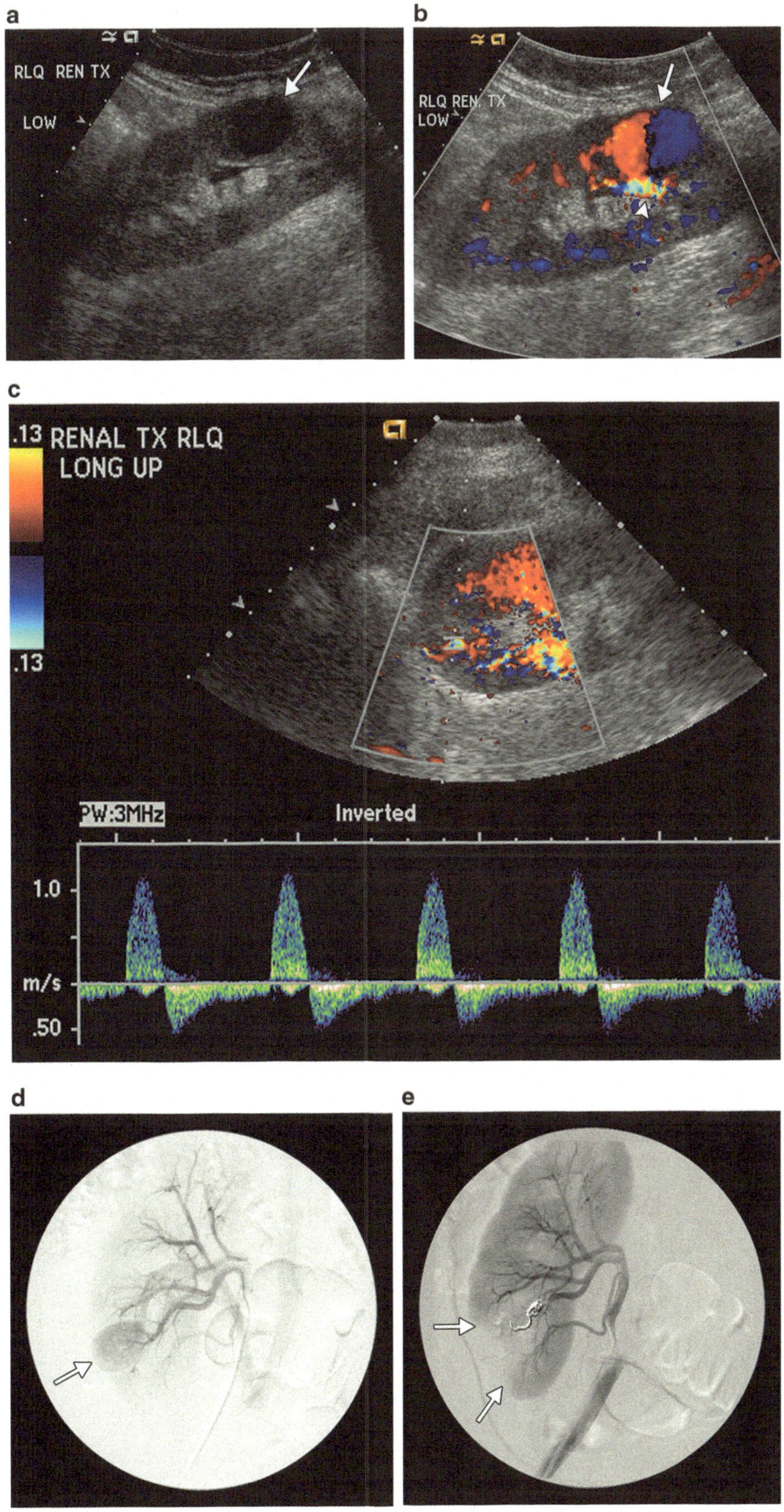

Fig. 32.14 Pseudoaneurysm. (**a**) Gray scale ultrasound shows an anechoic round structure in the lower pole (*arrow*). (**b**) Color Doppler reveals the vascular nature with internal yin yang swirling flow (*arrow*) and aliasing at the neck (*arrowhead*). (**c**) Duplex Doppler of the neck of a pseudoaneurysm demonstrating to and fro flow. (**d**) Selective digital subtraction catheter angiography shows opacification of a larger lower pole pseudoaneurysm (*arrow*). (**e**) Catheter angiography shows successful embolization with coils, with wedge-shaped perfusion defect (*arrows*)

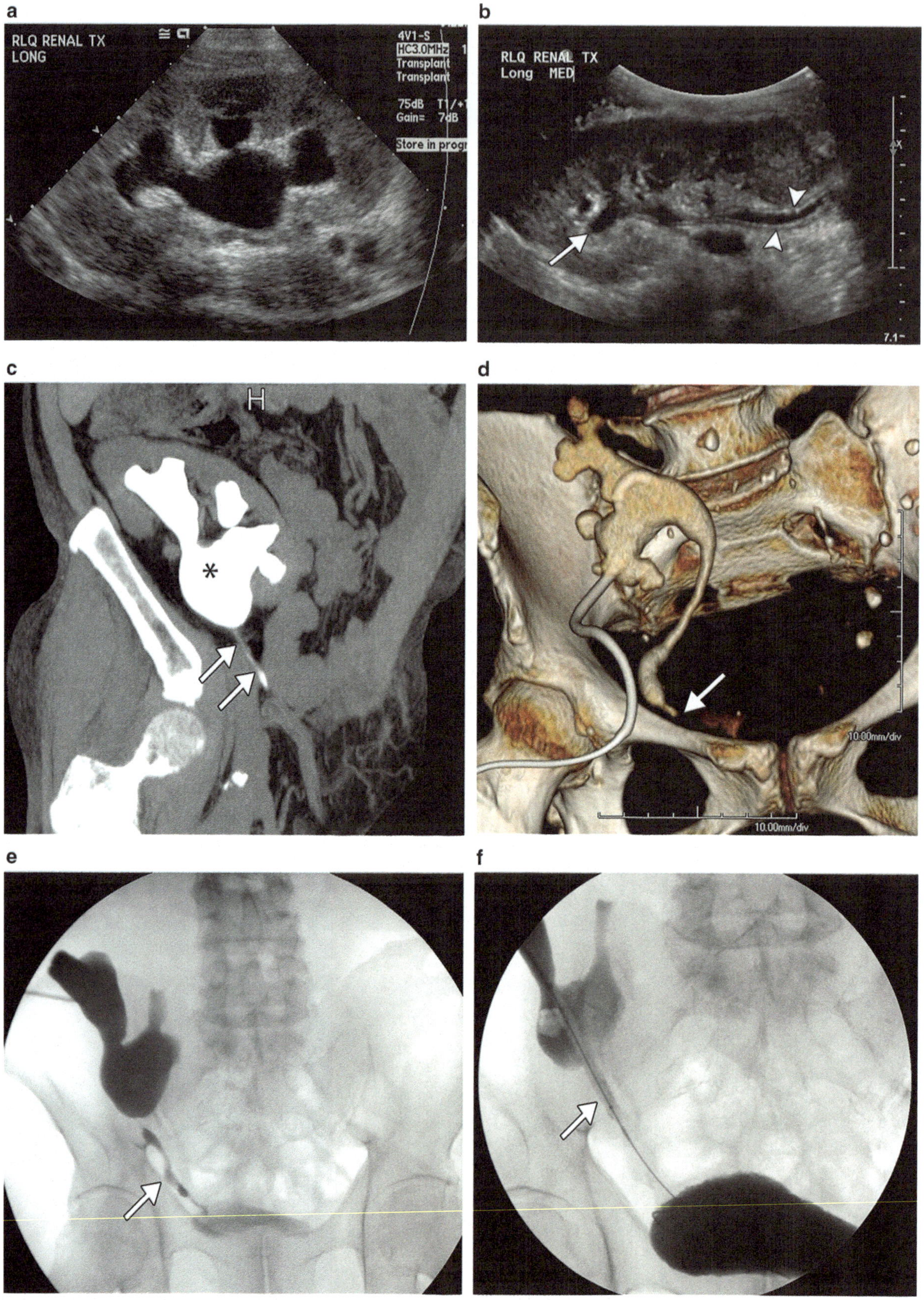

Fig. 32.15 (**a**) Gray scale ultrasound shows fluid within dilated calyces and renal pelvis. (**b**) Longitudinal gray scale image along the course of a ureter shows hydroureter with wall thickening (*arrowheads*) and mild hydronephrosis (*arrow*). (**c**) CT nephrostogram showing diffuse ureteral narrowing (*arrow*) and severe hydronephrosis (*asterisk*) (**d**) 3D volume rendered reconstruction shows the obstructed ureter (*arrow*) (**e/f**) Conventional nephrostogram performed before (**d**) and during (**e**) balloon dilatation (*arrow*) of the ureteral stricture

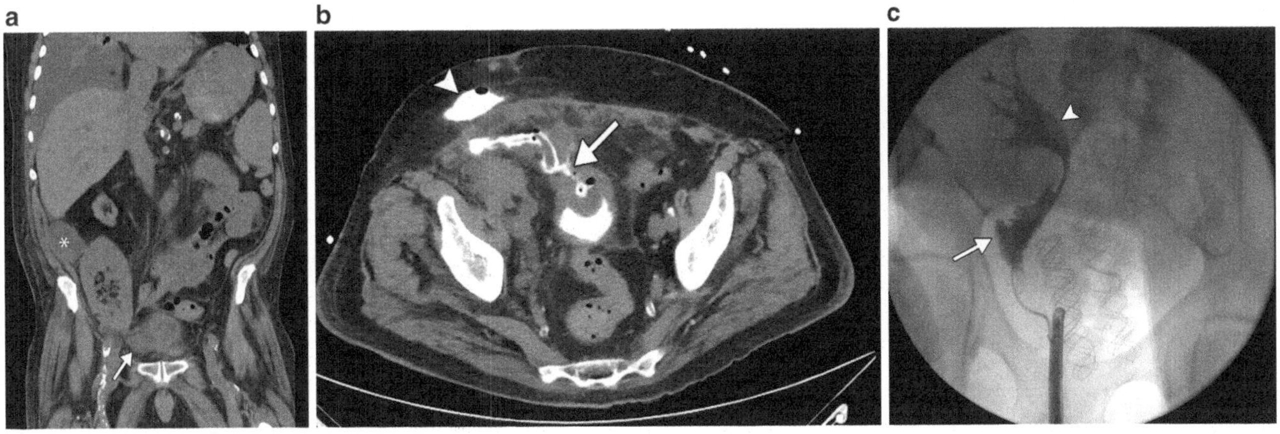

Fig. 32.16 Urinary leak. (**a**) Unenhanced coronal CT shows a fluid collection superolateral (*asterisk*) and a smaller collection medial (*arrow*) to the renal transplant. (**b**) Axial image during CT cystogram shows leakage of contrast from the bladder (*arrow*) into the right pelvis and anterior abdominal wall (*arrowhead*). (**c**) Conventional cystogram/retrograde ureterogram shows a leak (*arrow*). The transplant collecting system (*arrowhead*) is not dilated

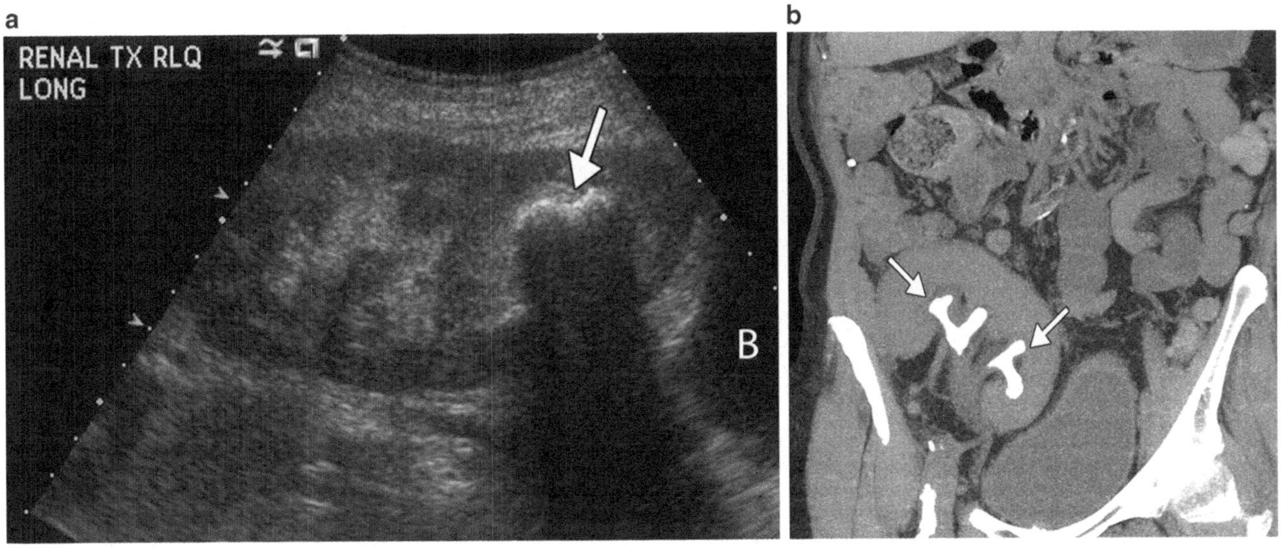

Fig. 32.17 Calculus. (**a**) Longitudinal gray scale ultrasound showing a lower pole calculus (*arrow*). The calculus is echogenic and causes posterior acoustic shadowing. Bladder (*B*). (**b**) Coronal CT shows a branched calculus in the upper and lower calyces of a right lower quadrant transplant (*arrows*)

Fluid Collections

Perigraft fluid collections may represent seromas, hematomas, lymphoceles, abscesses, and urinomas. Seromas, hematomas, and urinomas develop earlier than lymphoceles. Lymphoceles occur in 0.6–20 % of recipients overall, typically after 4 weeks, and are centered around the vascular pedicle of the allograft [59, 91]. Most fluid collections are asymptomatic but large collections can exert mass effect on the ureter, kidney, and vasculature with impairment of renal function. Infected collections may cause fever and pain. Fluid collections are easily detected by imaging with ultrasound, CT, and MRI (Fig. 32.18a, b). While time of onset and location may be diagnostically helpful, the appearance of the various collections (excluding hematoma) is similar. Imaging cannot diagnose an infected fluid collection unless it contains gas. Percutaneous aspiration (usually ultrasound guided) is necessary for microbiological evaluation and measurement of creatinine. Symptomatic lymphoceles can be managed by percutaneous drainage but they frequently recur. Further management options include percutaneous sclerotherapy and open or laparoscopic marsupialization [32]. Abscesses may be managed by percutaneous drains and antibiotics.

Most periallograft hematomas are contained in the pelvis, the appearance of hematoma varying depending on its age. Acute hematomas are hyperechoic and even solid appearing, potentially mistaken for pelvic fat or even bowel (Fig. 32.19a).

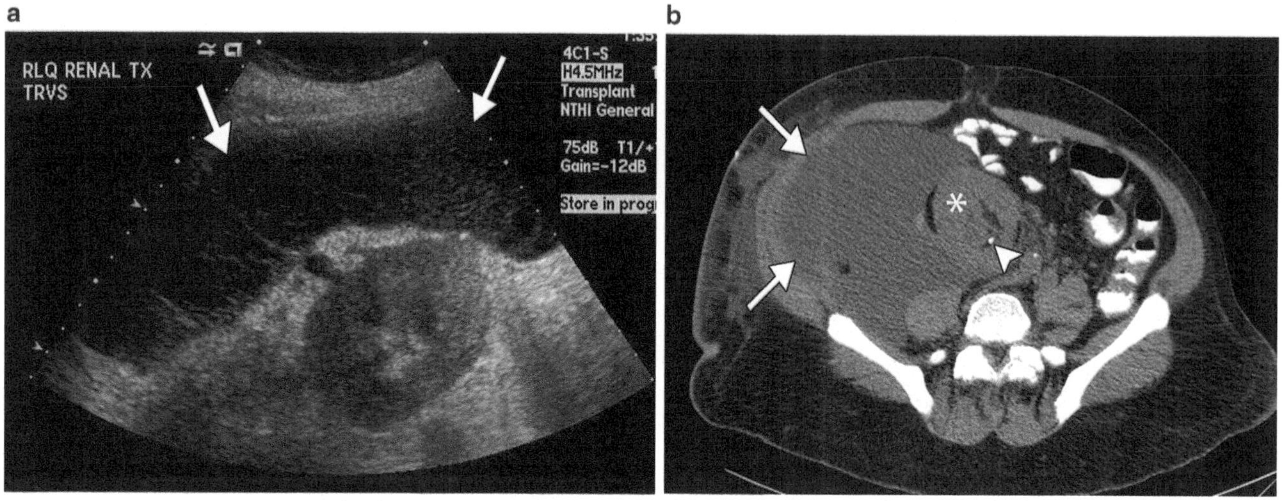

Fig. 32.18 Lymphocele. (**a**) Ultrasound shows a large complex fluid collection (*arrows*) displacing the transplant. (**b**) Computed tomography performed with oral contrast only. There is a large fluid collection (*arrows*) displacing the renal transplant (*asterisk*). A stent is seen within the renal pelvis (*arrowhead*)

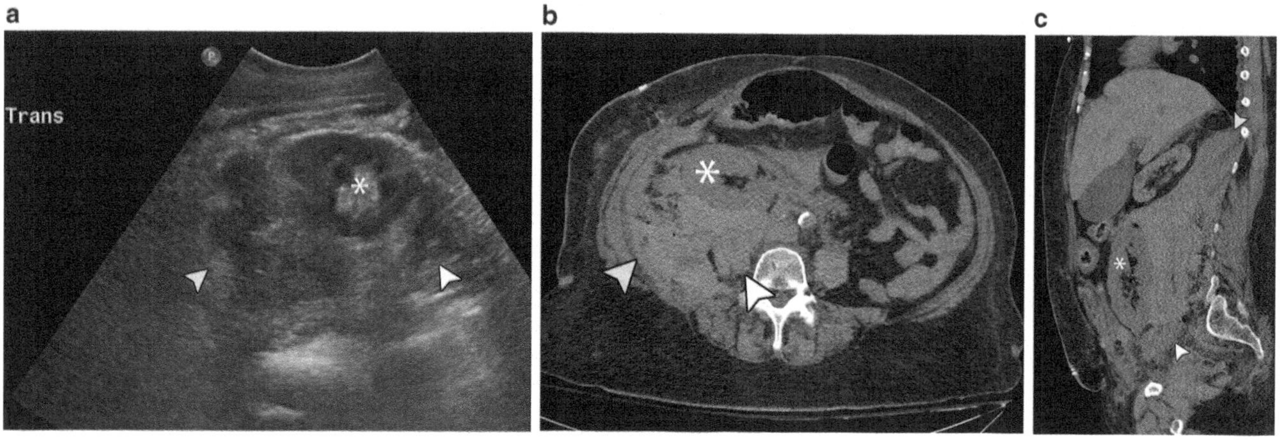

Fig. 32.19 Hematoma. (**a**) Ultrasound shows a complex perinephric hematoma (*arrowheads*) surrounding the transplant (*asterisk*). Axial (**b**) and sagittal (**c**) CT performed without oral or intravenous contrast shows higher density hematoma (*arrowhead*) in the retroperitoneum, displacing the renal transplant (*asterisk*) anteriorly

With degradation of blood products, hematomas become more cystic with internal fine septations or may be entirely anechoic. Free intraperitoneal hemorrhage is less common but readily detectable by sonography. Deep retroperitoneal or pelvic hematomas however may be missed by ultrasound. CT is a more sensitive imaging modality and can be performed immediately without any oral contrast. Acute hemorrhage is hyperattenuating on unenhanced CT (Fig. 32.19b, c). While MR is not indicated for hemorrhage, acute hematoma has high signal intensity on T1-weighted images and is more variable on T2-weighted images.

Infection

Infection in the allograft is diagnosed by urine and blood cultures. Imaging findings are nonspecific and include graft swelling, urothelial thickening, altered perfusion, and hydronephrosis with debris. Parenchymal abscesses are rounded fluid collections with a thick wall and internal debris. They may be aspirated under ultrasound guidance for diagnosis and treatment.

BKV infection is now recognized as a serious cause of graft loss [92–94]. Up to 8 % of recipients develop BKV-associated nephropathy with a graft loss rate of up to 40–50 % [93, 94]. BKV infection can be detected and monitored with serum and urine viral DNA. Imaging has a limited role in the diagnosis of BKV nephropathy. However ureteral stricture and hydronephrosis have been reported [95]. Ultrasound may be used to guide allograft biopsy for histologic confirmation.

The role of imaging in other infections depends on the target organ. CT is useful for screening the patient with fever and leukocytosis. Gastrointestinal or infectious disease such as colitis, diverticulitis, pneumonia, or intra-abdominal

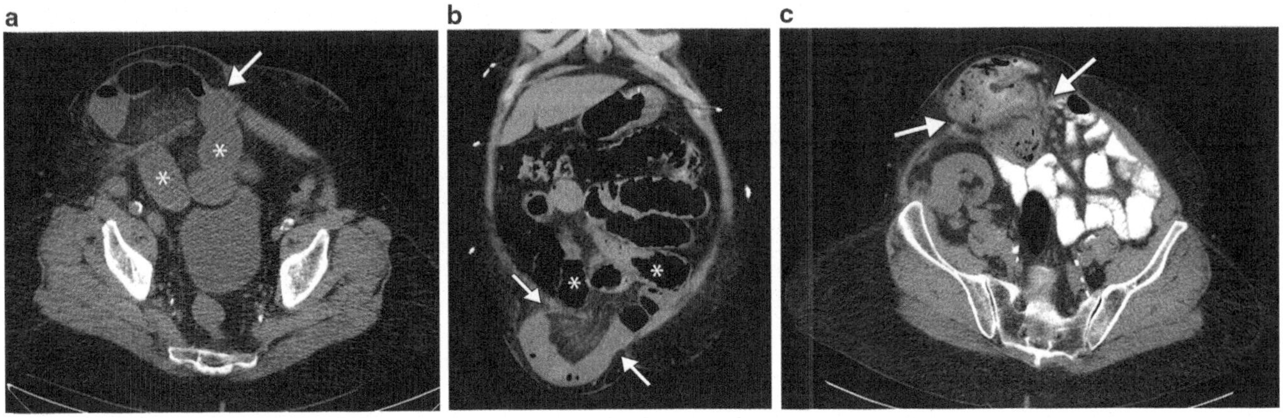

Fig. 32.20 Incisional hernia. Axial CT shows dilated small bowel (*asterisk*) secondary to an incisional hernia (*arrow*). (**a/b**) Axial (**a**) and coronal (**b**) CT without oral contrast shows dilated small bowel loops (*asterisk*) secondary to an incisional hernia (*arrows*). (**c**) Axial CT with oral contrast shows small bowel loops herniating through the incisional defect (*arrows*), without causing small bowel obstruction

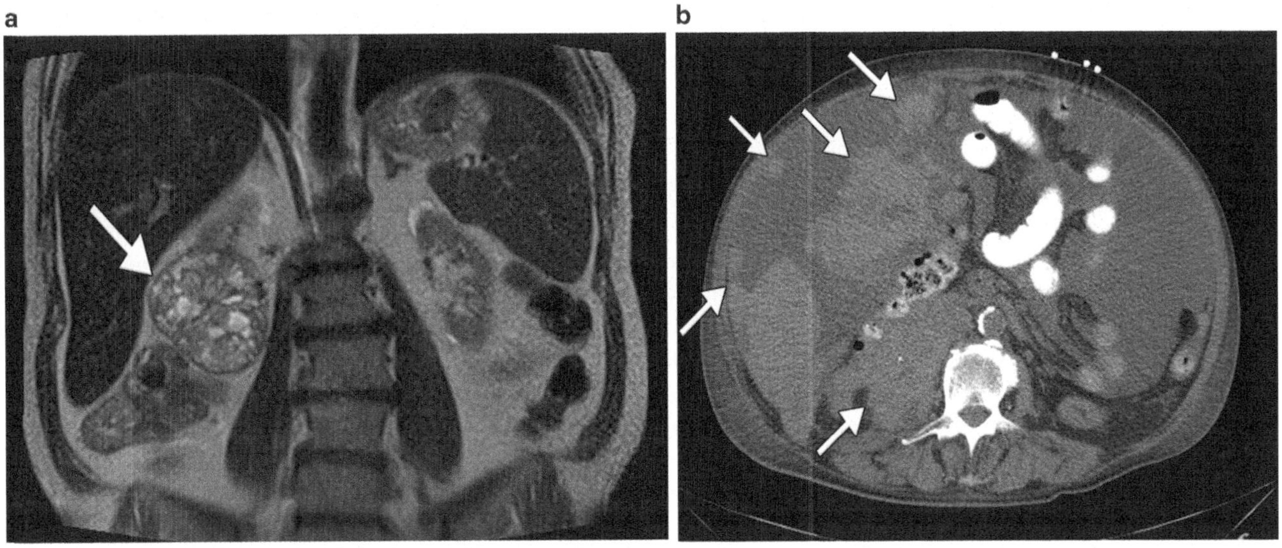

Fig. 32.21 Renal cell carcinoma. (**a**) Coronal T2-weighted MR shows a mixed solid and cystic mass in the lower pole of the native right kidney (*arrow*). Note the atrophic left kidney. (**b**) Following right nephrectomy, the patient developed extensive metastatic disease throughout the peritoneal cavity and right renal fossa (*arrows*) demonstrated by CT

infection may be found. Wound-related complications such as infection (1 %) and hernia or dehiscence (1.5 %) can be diagnosed with CT or US (Fig. 32.20) [59].

Post-transplant Malignancy

Between 6 and 20 % of recipients develop cancer after 10 years, the most common being skin (95 % are nonmelanoma, mainly squamous cell). There is also a twofold increased risk of non-skin malignancy after solid organ transplantation due to immunosuppression [96–98]. Mortality is high (up to 50 %) [96, 99]. Cancers may arise de novo in the recipient, may be recurrent in the recipient, or may be transmitted from the donor. Virus-induced malignancies such as lymphoma, Kaposi sarcoma, and anogenital and liver cancer are increased 3–50 times [99, 100]. Imaging findings may not be specific but image-guided biopsy may provide the diagnosis.

Renal cell carcinoma is more common in native kidneys of renal transplant recipients and the second most common malignancy after transplantation (Fig. 32.21) [98]. Early cases may result from malignant transformation in cysts associated with end stage kidneys and hemodialysis [99]. However renal carcinoma in native kidneys may develop in the absence of acquired cystic disease [101]. Clear cell subtype is slightly more common than papillary carcinoma and the prognosis is good [102]. Native renal cell carcinoma tends to be bilateral, multifocal, and less aggressive and can be treated with partial or total nephrectomy [103]. Renal carcinoma can also occur in the allograft, with papillary carcinoma being more common [102].

Many of these tumors are detected incidentally at imaging. Ultrasound is generally the first-line modality for the allograft but is less sensitive in the evaluation of the native kidneys which may be atrophic and/or replaced by cysts.

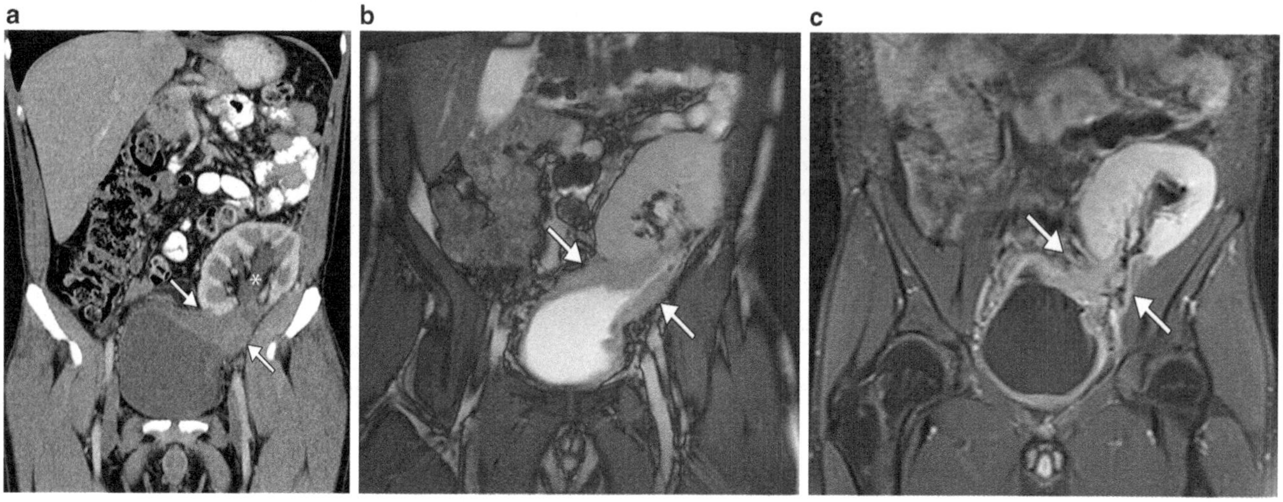

Fig. 32.22 Urothelial carcinoma in a 37-year-old man with a history of reflux nephropathy presenting with hematuria 6 years after cadaveric renal transplant. (**a**) Enhanced CT shows infiltrating tumor (*arrows*) at the bladder dome extending superiorly and encasing the ureter. There is hydronephrosis (*asterisk*). (**b**) Coronal T2-weighted image better shows the irregular bladder wall thickening extending superiorly to encase the transplanted ureter (*arrows*). (**c**) Enhanced MR shows avid enhancement of the tumor, with infiltration of the surrounding fat (*arrows*)

More comprehensive evaluation and staging is provided by CT or MR performed with intravenous contrast (Fig. 32.21). Renal carcinoma is typically a mass with no fatty component in which enhancement (a surrogate for neovascularity) occurs after intravenous contrast, imaged by CT, MRI, or contrast-enhanced ultrasound [104–107]. Necrosis, calcification, hemorrhage, and cystic components all contribute to tumor heterogeneity at imaging. In contrast to clear cell RCC, papillary renal carcinoma is typically smaller, more homogenous, and enhances less [108]. However cystic variants may occur. Comprehensive staging is multimodality based and includes MRI and PET–CT.

Urothelial bladder cancer may be as common as renal carcinoma in some series. It occurs in younger patients and has a more aggressive course [109] (Fig. 32.22).

Post-transplant Lymphoproliferative Disorder

Post-transplant lymphoproliferative disorder (PTLD) is a spectrum of disease related to transmission of Epstein–Barr virus (EBV) in 90 % of cases. Around 1 % of renal recipients develop PTLD, usually within the first year [110]. However PTLD can occur at any time, with a median time of onset of 5 years [110]. PTLD may be nodal or extra-nodal. In renal transplant recipients, extra-nodal disease is more common and the allograft is involved in 10 % [110]. Any solid or hollow viscera (liver, spleen, lung, bowel, bone marrow) can be involved by single or multiple masses [110]. Presenting features are nonspecific, and can include fever, weight loss, lymphadenopathy, or declining renal function. Incidental discovery at imaging is not unusual. Imaging findings are not specific, and can mimic lymphoma, metastasis, or infection. There may be focal or diffuse involvement of organs and bowel. Soft tissue masses at the renal transplant hilum are very suggestive [111, 112]. These tend to be hypoechoic at ultrasound with internal vascularity and causing hydronephrosis. At MRI, the low T2 signal intensity of the renal hilar mass and poor enhancement is characteristic [111]. Pathological diagnosis is necessary and can be achieved with ultrasound or CT-guided biopsy depending upon location. CT and FDG PET/CT are useful for diagnosis, staging, and follow-up (Fig. 32.23).

Summary

This chapter has attempted to familiarize the renal physician or surgeon with the role of imaging in the management of renal transplantation. The wide range of post-transplant complications is difficult to evaluate and distinguish on clinical and laboratory examination. This review provides guidance regarding the role of various radiologic modalities in early and accurate diagnosis and the contribution of percutaneous interventional techniques to patient management. While imaging is currently of limited value in the diagnosis of parenchymal disorders such as acute rejection, the ability to exclude other causes of transplant dysfunction is still valuable. In the future, noninvasive imaging tools may reduce the need for transplant biopsy.

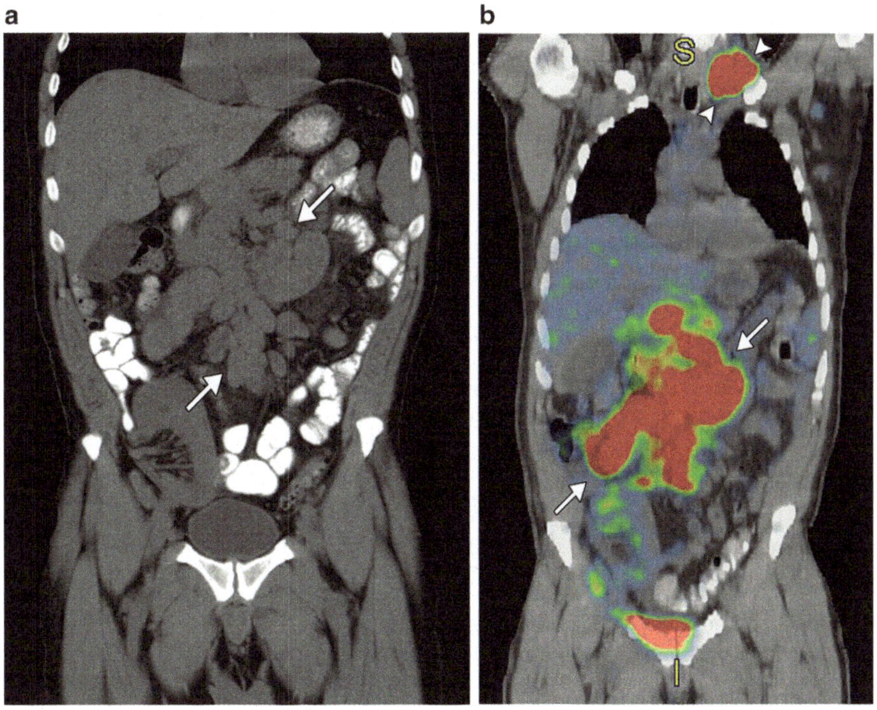

Fig. 32.23 B cell lymphoma in a 65-year-old, 5 years after renal transplant. (**a**) Unenhanced coronal CT shows multiple enlarged lymph nodes (*arrows*) in the mesentery. The renal transplant is not involved. (**b**) CT/PET fusion shows abnormal metabolic activity in the mesenteric lymph nodes (*arrows*) as well as left cervical lymph nodes (*arrowheads*)

Key Points

1. Imaging plays a key role in the pre- and postoperative evaluation of renal transplantation.
2. Ultrasound imaging is most useful in the diagnosis of hydronephrosis, fluid collections, and vascular complications.
3. Imaging findings of rejection are nonspecific.
4. CTA and MRA are useful for confirmation of vascular complications prior to intervention.

References

1. Khosroshahi HT, Tarzamni M, Oskuii RA. Doppler ultrasonography before and 6 to 12 months after kidney transplantation. Transplant Proc. 2005;37(7):2976–81. PubMed PMID: 16213279.
2. Cosgrove DO, Chan KE. Renal transplants: what ultrasound can and cannot do. Ultrasound Q. 2008;24(2):77–87; quiz 141–2. PubMed PMID: 18528243.
3. Baxter GM. Ultrasound of renal transplantation. Clin Radiol. 2001;56:802–18.
4. Khosroshahi HT, Heris HK, Makhdami N, Habibzadeh A, Badrogli N, Oskoii R, Jahannavard N. Time-dependent Doppler ultrasonographic findings in transplanted kidneys from living donors: a 5-year follow-up study. Transplant Proc. 2011;43(2):482–4. PubMed PMID: 21440739.
5. Quarto Di Palo F, Rivolta R, Elli A, et al. Relevance of resistive index ultrasonographic measurement in renal transplantation. Nepron. 1996;73:195–200.
6. Gao J, Rubin JM, Xiang DY, He W, Auh YH, Wang J, Ng A, Min R. Doppler parameters in renal transplant dysfunction: correlations with histopathologic changes. J Ultrasound Med. 2011;30(2):169–75. PubMed PMID: 21266554.
7. Radermacher J, Mengel M, Ellis S, et al. The renal arterial resistance index and renal allograft survival. N Engl J Med. 2003;349:115–24.
8. McArthur C, Baxter GM. Current potential renal applications of contrast-enhanced ultrasound. Clin Radiol. 2012;67(9):909–22. Epub 2012 Mar 30.
9. Grzelak P, Szymczyk K, Strzelczyk J, et al. Perfusion of kidney graft pyramids and cortex in contrast-enhanced ultrasonography in the determination of the cause of delayed graft function. Ann Transplant. 2011;23(16):48–53.
10. Ahuja TS, Niaz N, Agraharkar M. Contrast-induced nephrotoxicity in renal allograft recipients. Clin Nephrol. 2000;54: 11–4.
11. Katzberg RW, Newhouse JH. Intravenous contrast medium-induced nephrotoxicity: is the medical risk really as great as we have come to believe? Radiology. 2010;256(1):21–8. PubMed PMID: 20574082.
12. Tonolini M, Bianco R. Multidetector CT cystography for imaging colovesical fistulas and iatrogenic bladder leaks. Insights Imaging. 2012;3(2):181–7. Epub 2012 Feb 4. PubMed PMID: 22696044; PubMed Central PMCID: PMC3314733.
13. Chan DP, Abujudeh HH, Cushing Jr GL, Novelline RA. CT cystography with multiplanar reformation for suspected bladder rupture: experience in 234 cases. AJR Am J Roentgenol. 2006;187(5): 1296–302. PubMed PMID: 17056919.

14. Titton RL, Gervais DA, Hahn PF, Harisinghani MG, Arellano RS, Mueller PR. Urine leaks and urinomas: diagnosis and imaging-guided intervention. Radiographics. 2003;23(5):1133–47. PubMed PMID: 12975505.
15. Ismaeel MM, Abdel-Hamid A. Role of high resolution contrast-enhanced magnetic resonance angiography (HR CeMRA) in management of arterial complications of the renal transplant. Eur J Radiol. 2011;79(2):e122–7. Epub 2011 May 20. PubMed PMID: 21601400.
16. Lanzman RS, Voiculescu A, Walther C, Ringelstein A, Bi X, Schmitt P, Freitag SM, Won S, Scherer A, Blondin D. ECG-gated nonenhanced 3D steady-state free precession MR angiography in assessment of transplant renal arteries: comparison with DSA. Radiology. 2009;252(3):914–21. PubMed PMID: 19635833.
17. Liu X, Berg N, Sheehan J, Bi X, Weale P, Jerecic R, Carr J. Renal transplant: nonenhanced renal MR angiography with magnetization-prepared steady-state free precession. Radiology. 2009;251(2): 535–42. Epub 2009 Mar 4. PubMed PMID: 19261926.
18. Wang Y, Alkasab TK, Narin O, Nazarian RM, Kaewlai R, Kay J, Abujudeh HH. Incidence of nephrogenic systemic fibrosis after adoption of restrictive gadolinium-based contrast agent guidelines. Radiology. 2011;260(1):105–11. Epub 2011 May 17. PubMed PMID: 21586680.
19. Michaely HJ, Herrmann KA, Nael K, Oesingmann N, Reiser MF, Schoenberg SO. Functional renal imaging: nonvascular renal disease. Abdom Imaging. 2007;32(1):1–16. Epub 2006 Jan 30. PubMed PMID: 16447077.
20. Sadowski EA, Djamali A, Wentland AL, Muehrer R, Becker BN, Grist TM, Fain SB. Blood oxygen level-dependent and perfusion magnetic resonance imaging: detecting differences in oxygen bioavailability and blood flow in transplanted kidneys. Magn Reson Imaging. 2010;28(1):56–64. Epub 2009 Jul 3. PubMed PMID: 19577402; PubMed Central PMCID: PMC2891158.
21. Palmucci S, Mauro LA, Veroux P, Failla G, Milone P, Ettorre GC, Sinagra N, Giuffrida G, Zerbo D, Veroux M. Magnetic resonance with diffusion-weighted imaging in the evaluation of transplanted kidneys: preliminary findings. Transplant Proc. 2011;43(4):960–6. PubMed PMID: 21620026.
22. Artz NS, Sadowski EA, Wentland AL, Grist TM, Seo S, Djamali A, Fain SB. Arterial spin labeling MRI for assessment of perfusion in native and transplanted kidneys. Magn Reson Imaging. 2011;29(1):74–82. Epub 2010 Sep 17. PubMed PMID: 20850241; PubMed Central PMCID: PMC3005910.
23. Lee CU, Glockner JF, Glaser KJ, Yin M, Chen J, Kawashima A, Kim B, Kremers WK, Ehman RL, Gloor JM. MR elastography in renal transplant patients and correlation with renal allograft biopsy: a feasibility study. Acad Radiol. 2012;19(7):834–41. Epub 2012 Apr 13. PubMed PMID: 22503893; PubMed Central PMCID: PMC3377786.
24. Bonekamp S, Corona-Villalobos CP, Kamel IR. Oncologic applications of diffusion-weighted MRI in the body. J Magn Reson Imaging. 2012;35(2):257–79. doi:10.1002/jmri.22786. PubMed PMID: 22271274.
25. Hohenwalter MD, Skowlund CJ, Erickson SJ, et al. Renal transplant evaluation with MR angiography and MR imaging. Radiographics. 2001;21:1505–17.
26. Jain R, Sawhney S. Contrast-enhanced MR angiography (CE-MRA) in the evaluation of vascular complications of renal transplantation. Clin Radiol. 2005;60(11):1171–81. PubMed PMID: 16223613.
27. El-Maghraby TA, de Fijter JW, van Eck-Smit BL, Zwinderman AH, El-Haddad SI, Pauwels EK. Renographic indices for evaluation of changes in graft function. Eur J Nucl Med. 1998; 25(11):1575–86. PubMed PMID: 9799356.
28. Hobart MG, Streem SB, Gill IS. Renal transplant complications: minimally invasive management. Urol Clin North Am. 2000;27: 787–98.
29. Sandhu C, Patel U. Renal transplant dysfunction: the role of interventional radiology. Clin Radiol. 2002;57:772–83.
30. Kim HS, Fine DM, Atta MG. Catheter-directed thrombectomy and thrombolysis for acute renal vein thrombosis. J Vasc Interv Radiol. 2006;17(5):815–22. PubMed PMID: 16687747.
31. Melamed ML, Kim HS, Jaar BG, Molmenti E, Atta MG, Samaniego MD. Combined percutaneous mechanical and chemical thrombectomy for renal vein thrombosis in kidney transplant recipients. Am J Transplant. 2005;5(3):621–6. PubMed PMID: 15707419.
32. Kobayashi K, Censullo ML, Rossman LL, Kyriakides PN, Kahan BD, Cohen AM. Interventional radiologic management of renal transplant dysfunction: indications, limitations, and technical considerations. Radiographics. 2007;27(4):1109–30. PubMed PMID: 17620470.
33. Nicolini A, Ferraresso M, Lovaria M, et al. Carbon dioxide subtraction angiography for management of kidney transplant vascular complications. Transplant Proc. 2001;33:3388–9.
34. Moresco KP, Patel NH, Namyslowski Y, et al. Carbon dioxide angiography of the transplanted kidney: technical considerations and imaging findings. Am J Roentgenol. 1998;171:1271–6.
35. Beecroft JR, Rajan DK, Clark TW, Robinette M, Stavropoulos SW. Transplant renal artery stenosis: outcome after percutaneous intervention. J Vasc Interv Radiol. 2004;15(12):1407–13. PubMed PMID: 15590798.
36. Valpreda S, Messina M, Rabbia C. Stenting of transplant renal artery stenosis: outcome in a single center study. J Cardiovasc Surg (Torino). 2008;49(5):565–70. PubMed PMID: 18670375.
37. Marini M, Fernandez-Rivera C, Cao I, Gulias D, Alonso A, Lopez-Muñiz A, Gómez-Martínez P. Treatment of transplant renal artery stenosis by percutaneous transluminal angioplasty and/or stenting: study in 63 patients in a single institution. Transplant Proc. 2011;43(6):2205–7. PubMed PMID: 21839234.
38. Pham PT, Pham PA, Pham PC, Parikh S, Danovitch G. Evaluation of adult kidney transplant candidates. Semin Dial. 2010;23(6):595–605. doi:10.1111/j.1525-139X.2010.00809.x. PubMed PMID: 21175834.
39. Catalá V, Martí T, Diaz JM, Cordeiro E, Samaniego J, Rosales A, De La Torre P. Use of multidetector CT in presurgical evaluation of potential kidney transplant recipients. Radiographics. 2010;30(2):517–31. PubMed PMID: 20228332.
40. Koc F, Ozdemir K, Kaya MG, Dogdu O, Vatankulu MA, Ayhan S, Erkorkmaz U, Sonmez O, Aygul MU, Kalay N, Kayrak M, Karabag T, Alihanoglu Y, Gunebakmaz O. Intravenous N-acetylcysteine plus high-dose hydration versus high-dose hydration and standard hydration for the prevention of contrast-induced nephropathy: CASIS–a multicenter prospective controlled trial. Int J Cardiol. 2012;155(3):418–23. Epub 2010 Nov 23. PubMed PMID: 21106264.
41. Calabrò P, Bianchi R, Crisci M, Caprile M, Bigazzi MC, Palmieri R, Golia E, De Vita A, Romano IJ, Limongelli G, Russo MG, Calabrò R. Use and efficacy of saline hydration and N-acetyl cysteine to prevent contrast-induced nephropathy in low-risk populations undergoing coronary artery angiography. Intern Emerg Med. 2011;6(6):503–7. Epub 2011 Jan 29. PubMed PMID: 21279477.
42. Bader BD, Berger ED, Heede MB, Silberbaur I, Duda S, Risler T, Erley CM. What is the best hydration regimen to prevent contrast media-induced nephrotoxicity? Clin Nephrol. 2004;62(1):1–7. PubMed PMID: 15267006.
43. Smith D, Chudgar A, Daly B, Cooper M. Evaluation of potential renal transplant recipients with computed tomography angiography. Arch Surg. 2012;147(12):1114–22. doi:10.1001/archsurg.2012.1466. PubMed PMID: 23248013.
44. Maisonneuve P, Agodoa L, Gellert R, Stewart JH, Buccianti G, Lowenfels AB, Wolfe RA, Jones E, Disney AP, Briggs D, McCredie M, Boyle P. Cancer in patients on dialysis for end-stage renal disease: an international collaborative study. Lancet. 1999;354(9173):93–9. PubMed PMID: 10408483.

45. Park SB, Kim JK, Cho KS. Complications of renal transplantation: ultrasonographic evaluation. J Ultrasound Med. 2007;26(5):615–33. PubMed PMID: 17460004.
46. Jones JW, Hunter DW, Matas AJ. Post transplant lymphoceles: a critical look into the risk factors, pathophysiology and management. J Urol. 1993;150:22–6.
47. Linkowski GD, Warvariv V, Filly RA, et al. Sonography in the diagnosis of acute renal allograft rejection and cyclosporin toxicity. Am J Roentgenol. 1987;148:291–5.
48. Kelcz F, Pozniak MA, Pirsch JD, Oberly TD. Pyramidal appearance and resistive index: insensitive and nonspecific sonographic indicators of renal transplant rejection. Am J Roentgenol. 1990;155:531–5.
49. Don S, Kopecky KK, Filo RS, et al. Duplex Doppler US of renal allografts: causes of elevated resistive index. Radiology. 1989; 171:709–12.
50. Genkins SM, Sanfillippo FP, Carroll BA. Duplex Doppler sonography of renal transplants: lack of sensitivity and specificity in establishing pathologic diagnosis. Am J Roentgenol. 1989;152:535–9.
51. Grant EG, Perrella RR. Wishing won't make it so: duplex Doppler sonography in the evaluation of renal transplant dysfunction. Am J Roentgenol. 1990;155:538–9.
52. Perchik JE, Baumgartner BR, Bernardino ME. Renal transplant rejection. Limited value of duplex Doppler sonography. Invest Radiol. 1991;26:422–6.
53. Fischer T, Filimonow S, Dieckhöfer J, et al. Improved diagnosis of early kidney allograft dysfunction by ultrasound with echo enhancer–a new method for the diagnosis of renal perfusion. Nephrol Dial Transplant. 2006;21(10):2921–9. Epub 2006 Jul 5. PMID: 16822787.
54. Fischer T, Dieckhofer J, Muhler M, et al. The use of contrast-enhanced US in renal transplant: first results and potential clinical benefit. Eur Radiol. 2005;15 Suppl 5:E109–16. PMID: 18637238.
55. Clevert DA, D'Anastasi M, Jung EM. Contrast-enhanced ultrasound and microcirculation: efficiency through dynamics—current developments. Clin Hemorheol Microcirc. 2013;53:171–86. Epub ahead of print. PMID: 22986755.
56. Howard RJ, Patton PR, Reed AI, et al. The changing causes of graft loss and death after kidney transplantation. Transplantation. 2002;73:1923–8.
57. Shah A. Radionuclide imaging in organ transplantation. Radiol Clin North Am. 1995;33:473–96.
58. Kim EE, Pjura G, Lowry P, et al. Cyclosporin-A nephrotoxicity and acute cellular rejection in renal transplant recipients: correlation between radionuclide and histologic findings. Radiology. 1986;159:443–6.
59. Eufrásio P, Parada B, Moreira P, Nunes P, Bollini S, Figueiredo A, Mota A. Surgical complications in 2000 renal transplants. Transplant Proc. 2011;43(1):142–4.
60. Aktas S, Boyvat F, Sevmis S, Moray G, Karakayali H, Haberal M. Analysis of vascular complications after renal transplantation. Transplant Proc. 2011;43(2):557–61. PubMed PMID: 21440760.
61. Wong-You-Cheong JJ, Grumbach K, Krebs TL, Pace ME, Daly BD, Chow CC, Johnson LB, Bartlett ST. Torsion of intraperitoneal renal transplants: imaging appearances. Am J Roentgenol. 1998;171:1355–9.
62. Rouviere O, Berger P, Beziat C, et al. Acute thrombosis of renal transplant artery: graft salvage by means of intra-arterial fibrinolysis. Transplantation. 2002;73:403–9.
63. Reuther G, Wanjura D, Bauer H. Acute renal vein thrombosis in renal allografts: detection with duplex Doppler US. Radiology. 1989;170:557–8.
64. Kaveggia LP, Parrella RR, Grant EG, et al. Duplex Doppler sonography in renal allografts: the significance of reversed flow in diastole. Am J Roentgenol. 1990;155:295–8.
65. Takahashi M, Humke U, Girndt M, et al. Early posttransplantation renal allograft perfusion failure due to dissection: diagnosis and interventional treatment. Am J Roentgenol. 2003;180:759–63.
66. Tublin ME, Dodd III GD. Sonography of renal transplantation. Radiol Clin North Am. 1995;33:447–59.
67. Gufler H, Weimer W, Neu K, Wagner S, Rau WS. Contrast enhanced MR angiography with parallel imaging in the early period after renal transplantation. J Magn Reson Imaging. 2009;29(4):909–16. PubMed PMID: 19306426.
68. Jakobsen JA, Brabrand K, Egge TS, et al. Doppler examination of the allografted kidney. Acta Radiol. 2003;44:3–12.
69. Hurst FP, Abbott KC, Neff RT, Elster EA, Falta EM, Lentine KL, Agodoa LY, Jindal RM. Incidence, predictors and outcomes of transplant renal artery stenosis after kidney transplantation: analysis of USRDS. Am J Nephrol. 2009;30(5):459–67. Epub 2009 Sep 24. PubMed PMID: 19776559.
70. de Morais RH, Muglia V, Mamere AE, et al. Duplex Doppler sonography of transplant renal artery stenosis. J Clin Ultrasound. 2003;31:135–41.
71. Ardalan MR, Tarzamani MK, Shoja MM. A correlation between direct and indirect Doppler ultrasonographic measures in transplant renal artery stenosis. Transplant Proc. 2007;39(5):1436–8. PubMed PMID: 17580156.
72. Baxter GM, Ireland H, Moss JG, Harden PN, Junor BJ, Rodger RS, Briggs JD. Colour Doppler ultrasound in renal transplant artery stenosis: which Doppler index? Clin Radiol. 1995;50(9):618–22. PubMed PMID: 7554736.
73. Snider JF, Hunter DW, Muradian GP, et al. Transplant renal artery stenosis: evaluation with duplex sonography. Radiology. 1989;172:1027–30.
74. Patel U, Khaw KK, Hughes NC. Doppler ultrasound for detection of renal transplant artery stenosis-threshold peak systolic velocity needs to be higher in a low-risk or surveillance population. Clin Radiol. 2003;58(10):772–7. PubMed PMID: 14521886.
75. Gottlieb RH, Lieberman JL, Pabico RC, Waldman DL. Diagnosis of renal artery stenosis in transplanted kidneys: value of Doppler waveform analysis of the intrarenal arteries. AJR Am J Roentgenol. 1995;165(6):1441–6. PubMed PMID: 7484582.
76. Cook A, Khoury A, Kader K, Hebert D, Navarro O, Pippi-Salle J, Farhat W. Does peak systolic velocity correlate with renal artery stenosis in a pediatric renal transplant population? Pediatr Transplant. 2006;10(5):608–12. PubMed PMID:16856998.
77. Glockner JF, Takahashi N, Kawashima A, Woodrum DA, Stanley DW, Takei N, Miyoshi M, Sun W. Non-contrast renal artery MRA using an inflow inversion recovery steady state free precession technique (Inhance): comparison with 3D contrast-enhanced MRA. J Magn Reson Imaging. 2010;31(6):1411–8. PubMed PMID: 20512894.
78. Utsunomiya D, Miyazaki M, Nomitsu Y, Komeda Y, Okigawa T, Urata J, Yamashita Y. Clinical role of non-contrast magnetic resonance angiography for evaluation of renal artery stenosis. Circ J. 2008;72(10):1627–30. Epub 2008 Aug 27. PubMed PMID: 18728334.
79. Serai S, Towbin AJ, Podberesky DJ. Non-contrast MRA using an inflow-enhanced, inversion recovery SSFP technique in pediatric abdominal imaging. Pediatr Radiol. 2012;42(3):364–8. Epub 2011 Nov 10. PubMed PMID: 22072071.
80. Heer MK, Trevillian PR, Hardy DB, Hibberd AD. Salvaging kidneys with renal allograft compartment syndrome. Transpl Int. 2012;25(4):e47–9. doi:10.1111/j.1432-2277.2012.01442.x. Epub 2012 Feb 6. PubMed PMID: 22309228.
81. Ball CG, Kirkpatrick AW, Yilmaz S, Monroy M, Nicolaou S, Salazar A. Renal allograft compartment syndrome: an underappreciated postoperative complication. Am J Surg. 2006;191(5):619–24. PubMed PMID: 16647348.
82. Middleton WDE, Bellman GM, Melon GL, et al. Post-biopsy renal transplant arteriovenous fistulas: color Doppler ultrasound characteristics. Radiology. 1989;171:253–7.
83. Loffroy R, Guiu B, Lambert A, Mousson C, Tanter Y, Martin L, Cercueil JP, Krausé D. Management of post-biopsy renal allograft arteriovenous fistulas with selective arterial embolization: immediate

and long-term outcomes. Clin Radiol. 2008;63(6):657–65. Epub 2008 Feb 20. PubMed PMID: 18455557.
84. Pine J, Rajaganeshan R, Baker R, Lewington A, Patel J, Menon K, Kessel D, Ahmad N. Early postoperative renal vein stenosis after renal transplantation: a report of two cases. J Vasc Interv Radiol. 2010;21(2):303–4. PubMed PMID: 20123217.
85. Streeter EH, Little DM, Cranston DW, et al. The urological complications of renal transplantation: a series of 1535 patients. BJU Int. 2002;90:627–34.
86. Fayek SA, Keenan J, Haririan A, Cooper M, Barth RN, Schweitzer E, Bromberg JS, Bartlett ST, Philosophe B. Ureteral stents are associated with reduced risk of ureteral complications after kidney transplantation: a large single center experience. Transplantation. 2012;93(3):304–8. PubMed PMID: 22179401.
87. Sackett DD, Singh P, Lallas CD. Urological involvement in renal transplantation. Int J Urol. 2011;18(3):185–93.
88. Faenza A, Nardo B, Catena F, et al. Ureteral stenosis after kidney transplantation. Transpl Int. 1999;12:334–40.
89. Berger PM, Diamond JR. Ureteral obstruction as complication of renal transplantation: a review. J Nephrol. 1998;11:20–3.
90. Salgado OJ, Martin MG, Urdaneta B, et al. Serial pulsatility index measurements in renal grafts before, during and after episodes of urinary obstruction. J Ultrasound Med. 1999;18:827–30.
91. Zagdoun E, Ficheux M, Lobbedez T, Chatelet V, Thuillier-Lecouf A, Bensadoun H, Ryckelynck JP, Hurault de Ligny B. Complicated lymphoceles after kidney transplantation. Transplant Proc. 2010;42(10):4322–5. PubMed PMID: 21168691.
92. Ramos E, Drachenberg CB, Papadimitriou JC, et al. Clinical course of polyoma virus nephropathy in 67 renal transplant patients. J Am Soc Nephrol. 2002;13:2145–51.
93. Cannon RM, Ouseph R, Jones CM, Hughes MG, Eng M, Marvin MR. BK viral disease in renal transplantation. Curr Opin Organ Transplant. 2011;16(6):576–9.
94. Dall A, Hariharan S. BK virus nephritis after renal transplantation. Clin J Am Soc Nephrol. 2008;3 Suppl 2:S68–75. PubMed PMID: 18309005; PubMed Central PMCID: PMC3152275.
95. Gupta M, Miller F, Nord EP, Wadhwa NK. Delayed renal allograft dysfunction and cystitis associated with human polyomavirus (BK) infection in a renal transplant recipient: a case report and review of literature. Clin Nephrol. 2003;60:405–14.
96. Tremblay F, Fernandes M, Habbab F, deB Edwardes MD, Loertscher R, Meterissian S. Malignancy after renal transplantation: incidence and role of type of immunosuppression. Ann Surg Oncol. 2002;9(8):785–8. PubMed PMID: 12374662.
97. Lutz J, Heemann U. Tumours after kidney transplantation. Curr Opin Urol. 2003;13(2):105–9. PubMed PMID: 12584469.
98. Végsö G, Toronyi E, Hajdu M, Piros L, Görög D, Deák PA, Doros A, Péter A, Langer RM. Renal cell carcinoma of the native kidney: a frequent tumor after kidney transplantation with favorable prognosis in case of early diagnosis. Transplant Proc. 2011;43(4):1261–3. PubMed PMID: 21620106.
99. Engels EA, Pfeiffer RM, Fraumeni Jr JF, Kasiske BL, Israni AK, Snyder JJ, Wolfe RA, Goodrich NP, Bayakly AR, Clarke CA, Copeland G, Finch JL, Fleissner ML, Goodman MT, Kahn A, Koch L, Lynch CF, Madeleine MM, Pawlish K, Rao C, Williams MA, Castenson D, Curry M, Parsons R, Fant G, Lin M. Spectrum of cancer risk among US solid organ transplant recipients. JAMA. 2011;306(17):1891–901.
100. Kasiske BL, Snyder JJ, Gilbertson DT, Wang C. Cancer after kidney transplantation in the United States. Am J Transplant. 2004;4(6):905–13. PubMed PMID: 15147424.
101. Szmidt J, Durlik M, Gałazka Z, Nazarewski S, Górnicka B, Ziarkiewicz-Wróblewska B, Bojakowski K, Nowacka-Cieciura E, Lao M. Low-stage renal carcinoma of the native kidneys in renal transplant recipients. Transplant Proc. 2002;34(2):583–4. PubMed PMID: 12009631.
102. Leveridge M, Musquera M, Evans A, Cardella C, Pei Y, Jewett M, Robinette M, Finelli A. Renal cell carcinoma in the native and allograft kidneys of renal transplant recipients. J Urol. 2011;186(1):219–23.
103. Klatte T, Marberger M. Renal cell carcinoma of native kidneys in renal transplant patients. Curr Opin Urol. 2011;21(5): 376–9.
104. Prando A, Prando D, Prando P. Renal cell carcinoma: unusual imaging manifestations. Radiographics. 2006;26(1):233–44.
105. Israel GM, Silverman SG. The incidental renal mass. Radiol Clin North Am. 2011;49:369–83.
106. Gerst S, Hann LE, Li D, Gonen M, Tickoo S, Sohn MJ, Russo P. Evaluation of renal masses with contrast-enhanced ultrasound: initial experience. Am J Roentgenol. 2011;197(4):897–906.
107. Fan L, Lianfang D, Jinfang X, Yijin S, Ying W. Diagnostic efficacy of contrast-enhanced ultrasonography in solid renal parenchymal lesions with maximum diameters of 5 cm. J Ultrasound Med. 2008;27(6):875–85.
108. Vikram R, Ng CS, Tamboli P, Tannir NM, Jonasch E, Matin SF, Wood CG, Sandler CM. Papillary renal cell carcinoma: radiologic-pathologic correlation and spectrum of disease. Radiographics. 2009;29(3):741–54.
109. Cox J, Colli JL. Urothelial cancers after renal transplantation. Int Urol Nephrol. 2011;43(3):681–6.
110. Borhani AA, Hosseinzadeh K, Almusa O, Furlan A, Nalesnik M. Imaging of posttransplantation lymphoproliferative disorder after solid organ transplantation. Radiographics. 2009;29(4): 981–1000.
111. Ali MG, Coakley FV, Hricak H, Bretan PN. Complex posttransplantation abnormalities of renal allografts: evaluation with MR imaging. Radiology. 1999;211(1):95–100. PubMed PMID: 10189458.
112. Lopez-Ben R, Smith JK, Kew 2nd CE, Kenney PJ, Julian BA, Robbin ML. Focal posttransplantation lymphoproliferative disorder at the renal allograft hilum. AJR Am J Roentgenol. 2000;175(5):1417–22. PubMed PMID: 11044055.

Kidney and Pancreas Transplantation

33

David K. Klassen

Historical Background

Pancreas transplantation was first performed by Kelly and Lillehei at the University of Minnesota in 1966 [1]. This was done in conjunction with a kidney transplant from the same donor. This first case was a partial pancreatic graft with ligation of the pancreatic duct. The pancreas allograft worked for 6 days and then developed complications of pancreatitis and a pancreatic fistula, necessitating removal of the graft. This was the first of a series of 14 patients done at the University of Minnesota extending to 1973. In a report of ten of these cases, nine received pancreas transplants in conjunction with a renal allograft from the same deceased donor [2]. Only one graft functioned for more than a year. Among these early patients, patient survival at 1 year was 42 % and graft survival was 7 %. Because of these results, relatively few procedures were performed until the late 1970s. Since that time, evolution of surgical techniques and medical management as well as the development of more effective immunosuppressive medications has produced significant improvements in outcomes. More than 30,000 simultaneous kidney-pancreas transplants (SPK) and over 9,000 pancreas after kidney (PAK) or pancreas transplant-alone (PTA) procedures have now been done worldwide [2]. In the United States pancreas transplantation steadily increased peaking at 1,484 procedures in 2004, but since that time there has been a gradual decrease in the numbers of transplants performed [3].

Following the initial Minnesota experience, subsequent pancreas transplant procedures saw the evolution of pancreatic graft duct management techniques. These included free intraperitoneal drainage [4] duct occlusion with synthetic polymers [5], bladder drainage [5, 6], and enteric drainage [7]. The concept of bladder drainage was introduced by Gliedman with a ureter-pancreatic duct anastomosis [5]. This was further extended by Sollinger [6] when a pancreaticocystostomy was performed by anastomosing the pancreatic duct to the bladder mucosa. A modification to this technique was the inclusion of a duodenal button with pancreatic graft [8]. Corry further modified the bladder technique with the duodenal segment technique [9]. This became popular as the difficult separation of the duodenum from the pancreatic head was avoided, thus minimizing the potential for bleeding and injury to accessory ducts. An advantage of this technique was the ability to monitor pancreatic graft rejection by urinary amylase levels. This facilitated an earlier diagnosis and potentially more effective treatment of rejection episodes, improving graft survival rates. The introduction of triple immunosuppression with cyclosporine, azathioprine, and corticosteroids in the 1980s resulted in continued improvement in graft survival rates with the University of Minnesota reporting graft survival rates to 70 %.

From the late 1980s until 1995, the systemic venous delivery of insulin with bladder drainage of exocrine secretions was the most popular technique and was used in more than 90 % of pancreas transplants. This technique was well-tolerated in the majority of patients. Metabolic and urologic complications, however, resulted from the obligatory fluid and bicarbonate losses and the exposure of the usually acidic and enzyme-free lower genitourinary tract to pancreatic enzymes. These complications included urinary tract infections, hematuria, acute or chronic urinary retention due to cystitis, leaks, and episodes of urethritis. Metabolic acidosis resulted from obligatory bicarbonate losses. These complications required the conversion of bladder drainage to enteric drainage in as many as 10–25 % of patients [10–12]. As a result, there was a resurgence of the enteric drainage technique to correct intractable complications of the bladder drainage procedure. Additionally the development and application of percutaneous pancreas allograft biopsy techniques [13, 14] allowed the direct histologic assessment of the pancreas using serum amylase and lipase levels to screen for rejection. This made the monitoring of urinary enzyme levels unnecessary. Further innovations to

D.K. Klassen, M.D. (✉)
Division of Nephrology, Department of Medicine,
University of Maryland School of Medicine,
22 South Greene Street, Baltimore, MD 21201, USA
e-mail: dklassen@medicine.umaryland.edu

M.R. Weir and E.V. Lerma (eds.), *Kidney Transplantation: Practical Guide to Management*,
DOI 10.1007/978-1-4939-0342-9_33, © Springer Science+Business Media New York 2014

the surgical technique included venous drainage of the pancreas allograft into the portal venous system. Direct delivery of insulin to the liver abrogated the hyperinsulinemia associated with systemic drainage. The rationale was to improve the metabolism of lipids and glucose by the liver and accurately reproduce the physiology of the native pancreas.

Options for Therapy and Patient Selection

Pancreas transplantation restores a euglycemic state, improves quality of life by freeing the patient from exogenous insulin, and to a varying extent prevents the progression of neuropathy and permits the reversal of micro- and macrovascular complications of long-standing diabetes mellitus.

Pancreas transplantation can be performed simultaneously with or subsequent to a kidney transplant. This is done in diabetic patients with established renal disease who plan to have or have had a kidney transplant. The patients must meet criteria for kidney transplantation and not have excessive surgical risks for the dual transplant procedure. Pancreas graft survival may be better when transplantation is done simultaneously with a kidney transplant.

Pancreas transplantation can also be done in patients without indications for kidney transplantation. These patients typically have a history of brittle diabetes, frequent acute and severe episodes of hypoglycemia or hyperglycemia, ketoacidosis requiring medical intervention, and consistent failure of insulin-based management to prevent these acute complications. Pancreas transplantation alone is restricted to patients whose diabetic complications are or will be worse than the potential effects of the required long-term immunosuppression.

A patient with type 1 diabetes and kidney failure is thus faced with a number of options for kidney replacement therapy. There is consensus that chronic dialysis is the poorest option because of the higher mortality associated with this modality compared to kidney transplantation [15]. For acceptable kidney transplant candidates, there are several options: kidney transplantation alone, either living donor or cadaveric donor, SPK transplantation, or sequential kidney transplantation followed by pancreas transplantation. Living donor transplantation is associated with the best long-term patient and graft survival, but lacks the benefit of a pancreas transplant with improvement in quality of life from euglycemia. Simultaneous kidney-pancreas transplantation has the next best long-term survival but requires a period of waiting time for suitable organs. Kidney transplantation alone followed by a pancreas transplant is another option with acceptable patient and pancreas graft survival. Finally, patients who are not candidates for pancreas transplantation or do not have a suitable living donor may undergo cadaveric kidney transplantation. Cadaveric renal transplantation alone has the worst long-term survival, but selection bias may be an important factor in reported outcomes because patients selected for pancreas transplantation may have fewer comorbidities. Several studies have compared the outcomes between type 1 diabetic patients receiving cadaveric transplantation alone versus simultaneous kidney transplant procedures [16–19]. Long-term survival may be improved with combined kidney transplant procedures, but such recipients tend to be younger and receive transplants from younger donors, which may account for the difference in survival.

The SRTR database [3] shows that pancreas allograft survival in SPK recipients is distinctly better than either PTA or PAK allograft survival. This is true both in the short term and in the long term. One-year pancreas graft survival was 96 % and 10-year pancreas graft survival was 67 % for SPK recipients compared to 82 % and 42 %, respectively, for PAK recipients and 81 % and 40 %, respectively, for PTA recipients. Kidney allograft survivals are very good for SPK recipients with 1- and 10-year survivals of 95 % and 69 %, respectively. This compares to 92 and 44 % 1- and 10-year survivals for deceased donor renal transplants. Living donor kidney transplants had 1- and 10-year graft survivals of 96 and 60 %.

Many recipients with a suitable living donor may prefer to proceed with kidney transplantation than wait on dialysis for an SPK transplant. If the transplant is successful, then pancreas transplantation can be performed.

Knoll et al. [20] examined the optimal strategy for type 1 diabetic recipients with ESRD using a decision model. Outcome measures were life expectancy and quality-adjusted life expectancy. In this analysis, LRT recipients alone had the best long-term life expectancy and quality of life. PAK and SPK recipients had the next best outcome. Worst was cadaveric transplantation and dialysis. When LRT transplants were removed from the analysis, SPK had the greatest life expectancy compared to PAK.

For a type 1 diabetic with ESRD, preemptive transplantation with a living donor or deceased donor or SPK is optimal. Avoidance of dialysis and the attendant complications should be the goal. For patients with a living donor, consideration should be given to proceeding with the transplant rather than wait for an SPK transplant. A PAK can then follow after a period of stability. Recipients without a living donor and who are acceptable candidates should be listed for SPK, deceased donor transplantation, or both. Deceased donor transplant recipients alone can then be considered for PAK.

The relative benefits of PAK or PTA transplantation must be weighed against the potential for increased morbidity and mortality of the procedure. An analysis of the SRTR data indicated increased mortality for patients undergoing these procedures compared to patients on the waiting list treated with conventional therapy alone [21]. The relative risk for death over a 4-year follow-up for PTA and PAK was 1.57 and 1.42. Patients undergoing an SPK transplant had a 60 % reduction in mortality compared to patients on the waiting list.

One hundred eleven PTA procedures were performed in the United States in 2011. This procedure is considered in type 1 diabetics with severe secondary complications of diabetes or life-threatening hypoglycemic unawareness. A major additional consideration for these patients is the presence of renal insufficiency or proteinuria. Recipients with a creatinine clearance of less than 60 mL/min may develop significant renal insufficiency when transplanted and treated with a calcineurin inhibitor. Such patients may be best served by waiting for an SPK transplant when the need for renal replacement therapy approaches. This consideration also applies to patients with long-standing existing kidney transplants looking to receive pancreas transplants.

The study noted above [20] found a trend toward an increased risk of death extending out to 4 years after PTA compared to patients who remain on the waiting list with conventional therapy. Analysis of longer-term data may provide further insights into the risks and benefits of the PTA procedure.

There has been a gradual decline in the number of pancreas transplants done in the United States since 2004. This decline has been most notable in pancreas transplant-alone procedures (PTA and PAK). In the most recent 2011 SRTR report, there were 791 SPK, 149 PAK, and 111 PTA procedures performed. The reasons for this decline are not clear but likely relate to the continued significant morbidity associated with pancreas transplantation and the lower graft survivals relative to other solid organ transplants. In the most recent SRTR data [3], solitary pancreas transplantation had a 1-year graft survival which was the lowest of all solid organs. Improvements in the medical management of diabetes may also be a factor. What in the past was considered intensive medical therapy for type 1 diabetes, and shown to be associated with improved long-term outcomes by the Diabetes Control and Complications Trial [22], is now standard of care and has been associated with improved long-term outcomes compared to past medical therapy.

Absolute contraindications to pancreas transplantation include significant non-correctable or intractable coronary artery disease demonstrated by coronary angiography or recent myocardial infarction. Because of the significant risk of underlying coronary heart disease in patients with advanced diabetes, all pancreas transplant candidates should undergo a careful cardiac risk evaluation. Many centers require a cardiac catheterization. Additional contraindications include active infection and history of malignancy treated in the past 3 years (excluding nonmelanoma skin cancer). Other contraindications include hepatitis B surface antigen positivity, active untreated peptic ulcer disease or substance abuse, major untreated psychiatric illness, inability to provide consent, and recent history of medical noncompliance. Systemic illness that limits life expectancy or compromises survival, or irreversible hepatic or pulmonary dysfunction, may preclude consideration for transplantation. Successful kidney-pancreas transplantation has been reported for HIV-infected patients who are well controlled on combined antiretroviral therapy [23]. Relative contraindications include advanced age, morbid obesity (BMI greater than 35), peripheral vascular disease, and severe aortoiliac disease. Some centers do not consider patients with type 2 diabetes, but in the most recent SRTR registry report from 2011, 8 % of reported cases were classified as type 2 diabetes [3]. Data suggests that pancreas transplantation may confer benefits for selected patients with type 2 diabetes [24] although this has been suggested to be related bias from differences in patient selection and donor organ quality [25]. Older recipient age is a risk factor for all transplant procedures. Despite this concern, the overall trend in pancreas transplantation has been the transplantation of older recipients [3]. The proportion of recipients greater than 45 years of age in 1992 was 9 %. In 2011 24 % of pancreas transplant recipients were over 50 years of age.

Surgical Technique

Currently the large majority of pancreas transplants in the United States are performed with primary enteric drainage. An ongoing debate is the venous drainage of the pancreas. Initially because of anatomic location required by the bladder drainage technique, most pancreas transplants were drained into the systemic venous circulation via the iliac vein. The venous drainage of the native pancreas is into the portal vein.

The hepatic first-pass uptake and metabolism of insulin is from 50 to 90 % in normal individuals. Drainage into the systemic circulation results in hyperinsulinemia, and this could have significant long-term metabolic consequences, such as accelerated atherosclerosis, hypertension, and hyperlipidemia. Since 1996, the number of SPK and PAK procedures utilizing portal venous drainage has been increasing. Despite the increased use of portal venous drainage, there has been no significant improvement in graft survival or metabolic outcomes in recipients attributed to this technique.

The procurement and back table preparation of the pancreas are beyond the scope of this review. Pancreas transplantation can be performed through a midline incision or lower quadrant extraperitoneal incisions. In general, the pancreas transplant is performed on the right side of the abdomen due to a more favorable venous anatomy of the right iliac system. Because the liver is often procured with the pancreas, the celiac axis remains with the liver. This requires surgical reconstruction of the arterial anatomy of the pancreas. This is accomplished with a donor Y graft that is used to reconstruct the superior mesenteric artery and the splenic artery. The arterial revascularization is usually performed by anastomosis of the Y graft to the right common iliac or external iliac artery. Venous drainage of the pancreas is then accomplished using the iliac vein for systemic drainage or the superior mesenteric vein for portal drainage. During back table preparation, the duodenal segment is prepared by suturing the proximal and distal ends of the duodenum. The duodenum is then opened along its antimesenteric border and sutured to the small bowel. In some case, a Roux-en-Y limb is utilized for the enteric pancreas drainage to isolate the anastomosis from the bowel contents and minimize the risks of an enteric leak.

Surgical Complications of Pancreas Transplantation

Pancreas graft thrombosis or leaks from the duodenal anastomosis are the most significant complications immediately following pancreas transplantation. Although the incidence of early vascular thrombosis is decreasing, registry data shows that the current rate of early pancreas graft loss due to thrombosis is 7.7 % [3]. Graft thrombosis is more common in solitary pancreas transplantation. A number of factors contribute to this problem, including the low microvascular blood flow in the pancreas allograft and the complex arterial reconstruction required for pancreas transplantation. Pancreatitis related to reperfusion injury may increase resistance to blood flow in the pancreas allograft, resulting in secondary thrombosis. Pancreas graft thrombosis is usually an early event, with a peak incidence in the first 2 weeks post-transplant. This usually presents as a sudden onset of hyperglycemia. There may be associated abdominal pain and allograft tenderness. Duplex ultrasonography will rapidly confirm this diagnosis. It is unusual that thrombectomy of the allograft is successful. Most allografts will require removal. Intra-abdominal hemorrhage is a relatively common complication following transplantation. This has been reported to occur in up to 15 % of cases [26]. The use of anticoagulation as a strategy to avoid early pancreas allograft thrombosis is associated with an increased incidence of intra-abdominal bleeding. Minor bleeding is treated conservatively with correction of anticoagulation and transfusion. However, significant intra-abdominal hemorrhage requires a laparotomy. Occasionally the distal portion of the ligated splenic vein will undergo thrombosis; however, this is generally not of great clinical significance.

Intra-abdominal Infections

Intra-abdominal infections after pancreas transplantation are one of the most serious complications. This complication is associated with high morbidity and also results in significant decreases in patient and allograft survival. The incidence of intra-abdominal infections following pancreas transplantation has been decreasing. Registry data from the early 1990s showed an approximate 20 % rate of intra-abdominal infection. More recent data has shown that intra-abdominal infections have decreased significantly [27]. This has been attributed to improved surgical technique, reduced rates of rejection with newer immunosuppressive medications, improvements in antibiotic prophylaxis, and improved donor and recipient selection.

Intra-abdominal infection usually occurs within the first 1–2 months following pancreas transplantation. Patients commonly present with fever, abdominal pain, distention, and ileus. Commonly abdominal exploration and drainage of intra-abdominal collections are required. Less commonly intra-abdominal infections can be treated conservatively with CT-guided percutaneous drainage of fluid collections and long-term antibiotics. In many cases multiple laparotomies may be needed to control the infection. Allografts with pancreatitis may be at increased risk for infection. Anastomotic leaks and partial allograft necrosis have been identified as risk factors. Intra-abdominal fungal infections are associated with high morbidity and mortality.

Graft Pancreatitis

Following the initial transplant procedure, allograft pancreatitis, defined by prolonged elevation of the serum amylase and lipase, is not uncommon [28]. Normally the serum amylase and lipase decline to normal levels during the first week following the transplant procedure. Prolonged elevated amylase and lipase may be related to procurement and reperfusion injury. The treatment of allograft pancreatitis is conservative. It must, however, be distinguished from early acute rejection, which will have the same biochemical findings. This may require a percutaneous or CT-guided allograft biopsy. In bladder-drained pancreas transplants, urinary retention, commonly due to neurogenic bladder, may cause reflux pancreatitis. This presents later than graft pancreatitis associated with the initial surgical procedure. Reflux pancreatitis may also be confused with acute rejection. Placement of a Foley catheter to decompress the bladder usually results in a rapid normalization of the biochemical abnormalities.

Survival

The 1-, 5-, and 10-year probability of graft failure or death reported to the Scientific Registry of Transplant Recipients [3] at the end of 2011 are shown in Table 33.1. Cohorts for the report include transplants performed during 2010 for the 1-year, 2006 for 5-year, and 2001 for 10-year survival. Pancreas allograft survival rates have improved over the past decade, with the greatest improvement seen in the PAK and the PTA 1-year graft survival rates. In the most recent 2011 data the probability of death or pancreas graft loss at 1 year was 0.04. This is in stark contrast to earlier eras, when 1-year pancreas graft survival for SPK was 75 % and graft survival for PTA and PAK was 50 %. Improved 1-year survival has translated into improved long-term survival, with 10-year probability of death or pancreas graft loss being 0.33 for SPK recipients. Results for PAK and PTA allografts have lagged behind those for SPK but have also shown significant improvement. Gruesner et al. [29] reported long-term pancreas graft survival from transplants done between 1978 and 2005 reported to the International Pancreas Transplant Registry. Ten-year pancreas allograft survival was 68 %, 46 %, and 39 % for SPK, PAK, and PTA transplants, respectively, and the 20-year graft survival rates were 45 %, 16 %, and 12 %, respectively.

PAK transplantation may improve the kidney allograft outcomes compared to diabetic kidney transplant recipients who do not receive a pancreas transplant. A recent study looked at all PAK recipients in the United States between 1989 and 2007 and compared their risk of kidney failure to a well-matched group of diabetic kidney only transplant recipients. In over 2,700 cases the PAK recipients had a decreased long-term risk of kidney allograft failure. An association with pre-PAK glomerular filtration rate with kidney survival was not evident until 3 years after pancreas transplantation, and patients with a pre-PAK GFR of 30–39 mL/min still attained a 10-year post-PAK survival of 69 % [26].

Death due to cardiovascular disease remains the number one cause of death for all categories of pancreas transplantation. Risk factors for patient survival for SPK transplants include kidney graft loss, age greater than 45 years, technical or immunologic loss of the pancreas transplant, and diabetes for greater than 25 years. The most important risk factor for death with a PAK or PTA was either technical loss of the pancreas or rejection. This confers a three- to fourfold higher risk of death in these categories.

Immunosuppression for Kidney and Pancreas Transplantation

The significant improvements in the results of kidney and pancreas transplantation have been due in large part to advances in immunosuppression [30]. The impact of newer immunosuppressive agents has been most notable in PAK and PTA transplants. The basic approach to immunosuppression for kidney and pancreas transplant recipients is similar to that for kidney transplant recipients. The incidence of acute rejection for patients receiving a pancreas transplants (Table 33.2) is significantly higher than a kidney transplant alone. The 1-year incidence of acute rejection is 17 % for SPK transplants, 20 % for PAK transplants, and 24 % for PTA transplants [3]. This is approximately double the rates of rejection seen in kidney transplants. With cyclosporine-, azathioprine-, and prednisone-based immunosuppression, the 1-year incidence of rejection in SPK and PAK recipients was as high as 80 %. The increased immunogenicity of the pancreas transplant has resulted in more intensive induction and maintenance immunosuppression being used for pancreas transplantation. The early and generally vigorous acute rejection associated with pancreas transplantation under conventional immunosuppression resulted in the nearly universal application of antibody-based induction therapy. With the introduction of tacrolimus and mycophenolate mofetil in the mid-1990s, the 1-year incidence of acute rejection in pancreas transplant recipients was reduced to approximately 30 %. Current agents available for induction include the polyclonal T-cell-depleting antibodies, such as Thymoglobulin or Campath. Interleukin-2 receptor blockade such as basiliximab is less commonly used for pancreas transplantation. Maintenance immunosuppression is generally based on the calcineurin inhibitors, tacrolimus, or cyclosporine. These are commonly used in conjunction with mycophenolate mofetil or mycophenolic acid. Corticosteroids are commonly used as a third agent in maintenance immunosuppression.

Table 33.1 Probability of pancreas graft failure or death

	1 year	5 years	10 years
SPK	0.039	0.161	0.329
PAK	0.178	0.462	0.577
PTA	0.198	0.460	0.605

Data is from the SRTR 2011 Annual Report. 1-year data is from patients transplanted in 2010, 5-year data is from patients transplanted in 2006, and 10-year data is from patients transplanted in 2001

Table 33.2 Incidence of first acute rejection among patients receiving a pancreas transplant in 2005–2009

	1 year (%)	3 years (%)	5 years (%)
SPK	16	24	29
PAK	18	28	33
PTA	24	33	41

Data is from the SRTR Annual Report. For SPK recipients, acute rejection may be either pancreas or kidney

Corticosteroid avoidance or withdrawal protocols have been successful and have been increasingly employed [31, 32]. Registry data now suggests that up to 40 % of transplant patients are not maintained on corticosteroids [3].

Most kidney and pancreas transplant programs currently use a quadruple induction protocol. Immunosuppression is achieved by induction with rabbit antithymocyte globulin and alemtuzumab which have been reported to provide equivalent results [31, 33]. These agents are generally infused for 7 days beginning on the first postoperative day for antithymocyte globulin or intraoperatively in the case of alemtuzumab. The response to antithymocyte globulin is monitored by measuring CD3-positive lymphocytes and adjusting the dose of the induction agent accordingly. Since the mid-1990s, the majority of pancreas transplant programs have used tacrolimus as the basis of immunosuppression. This is begun immediately post-transplant unless there is delayed graft function of the kidney. Tacrolimus levels are generally targeted to the 8–12 ng/mL range in the early stages of transplantation and are generally tapered to lower levels over the first few months. Mycophenolate preparations are a commonly used additional agent. This is commonly begun with a dose in the range of 1,000 mg twice a day of mycophenolate mofetil or the equivalent dose of mycophenolic acid. This dose is generally maintained unless reduction for bone marrow suppression or gastrointestinal side effects is required.

Infection prophylaxis generally is similar to that employed in kidney transplantation with oral antifungal medication for prevention of thrush, antibiotic prophylaxis for urinary tract infection, and antiviral prophylaxis with valganciclovir to prevent reactivation of cytomegalovirus. Additionally pancreas transplant recipients have been reported to develop BK virus infections either in the transplanted kidney or in the native kidney in the case of PTA recipients [34–36] and screening for evidence of polyomavirus reactivation with serum PCR or urine cytology is recommended.

There are a variety of new approaches to immunosuppression in kidney and pancreas transplant recipients that are being evaluated such as the use of calcineurin-free or minimization regimens with sirolimus [37]. Giancio et al. [38] have reported improved rejection rates and equivalent patient and allograft survival rates with the combination of tacrolimus and sirolimus and steroids compared to tacrolimus with mycophenolate mofetil and steroids. The role of co-stimulatory blockade with agents such as belatacept remains to be defined.

Diagnosis and Treatment of Pancreas Rejection

An accurate and timely diagnosis of acute rejection has historically been one of the most difficult clinical problems in transplantation. This has been a limiting factor in the clinical success of pancreas transplantation, especially in PAK or PTA transplants. SPK transplantation has had the distinct advantage of allowing the assessment of renal function to be a surrogate marker for pancreas rejection, since in the large majority of such cases, acute rejection occurs simultaneously in both the kidney and pancreas allograft. Isolated pancreas allograft rejection has been reported to occur in probably less than 10 % of rejections in kidney and pancreas transplant recipients [39]. Assessment of the kidney for rejection using a simple needle biopsy in most cases allowed the accurate and relatively timely diagnosis of acute rejection of the pancreas. Rejection in the kidney can be identified in some cases even if the serum creatinine is unchanged from baseline values. This approach could not be applied to solitary pancreas transplantation, and this limitation was felt to be one of the major reasons for the inferior success of solitary pancreas transplantation.

Pancreas allograft function is generally monitored through serial measurements of serum amylase and lipase. Other serum and urinary markers for the diagnosis of rejection have not proven to be superior to serum amylase and lipase values. In the occasionally encountered bladder-drained pancreas transplants, the urinary amylase can be monitored to assess pancreas function. In this situation, acute rejection is associated with a decrease in urine amylase. Serum levels of amylase and lipase are significantly increased in acute rejection; however, occasional cases of histologically proven pancreas rejection have been seen in patients with no abnormalities of serum amylase or lipase. Serum enzymes are, however, nonspecific for the diagnosis of pancreas rejection. Serum amylase is considered to have an approximate 90 % sensitivity and a significantly lower specificity for the diagnosis of acute rejection.

Pancreas allograft rejection is difficult to diagnose by clinical findings. In most cases of pancreas allograft rejection, the clinical symptoms are nonexistent. In 5–20 % of patients with pancreas allograft rejection, there is associated abdominal pain and discomfort. This is likely related to peritoneal irritation from an acutely inflamed allograft. Fever may occasionally be present, but is not uniform. Inflammation of the surrounding bowel may result in an ileus and symptoms of abdominal obstruction. It is important to note that hyperglycemia is a very late finding in acute allograft rejection due to the large beta cell reserve inherent in the pancreas allograft. Patients presenting with hyperglycemia related to rejection represent advanced aggressive rejection and generally have a poor outcome with respect to reversal of the acute rejection episode.

In the pancreas allograft as in other solid organ transplants, histologic assessment of rejection is the gold standard by which the diagnosis of rejection is made. Most programs have adopted percutaneous pancreas allograft biopsy as the procedure of choice for the diagnosis of pancreas allograft rejection. This technique is very similar to that employed in kidney allograft biopsies. The pancreas is localized within the abdomen using real-time ultrasonography. The major vascular structures are identified, and a core needle biopsy using an 18-gauge automated biopsy needle is obtained for histologic assessment. This technique has a complication rate similar to that of kidney allograft biopsies. The most common complication is bleeding from the allograft. This occurs in less than 5 % of cases. In cases where there is bowel overlying the pancreas allograft, a CT-guided percutaneous biopsy can sometimes be successfully employed or, failing this, a laparoscopic biopsy can be obtained.

A standard histologic grading scheme for pancreas allograft biopsies has been developed [40]. This grading scheme has been shown to correlate with outcome following treatment of identified acute rejection episodes. Core needle biopsies have also been utilized to diagnose post-transplant lymphoma presenting in the pancreas allograft, CMV pancreatitis, and islet cell toxicity associated with calcineurin inhibitors. Pancreas biopsies also allow the assessment of chronic rejection within the pancreas allograft. This is manifested by allograft fibrosis and vascular changes similar to that seen in other solid organs. An approach to histologic grading of chronic rejection has also been described [41] and this, too, correlates with the clinical outcome of the graft. Chronically rejecting pancreas allografts with advancing fibrosis gradually decrease in size and may sometimes be difficult to identify either by ultrasound or by CT scan. A patient presenting with significant hyperglycemia, a normal serum amylase and lipase, and an unidentifiable pancreas allograft almost invariably has end-stage chronic pancreas allograft rejection and will need to resume exogenous insulin. Confusion resulting form the development of type 2 diabetes can usually be resolved by checking the serum c-peptide level. The c-peptide level is low in a chronically rejected pancreas allograft but is elevated in type 2 diabetes.

Pancreas allografts are subject to antibody-mediated rejection. The histologic criteria for diagnosis of antibody-mediated rejection have been defined by Drachenberg et al. [42] as part of the Banff transplant pathology process. Successful treatment of acute antibody-mediated pancreas allograft rejection using plasmapheresis and intravenous immunoglobulin has been reported [43]. The significance of donor-specific antibodies in the outcomes of pancreas transplantation has not been well defined. Early development of donor-specific antibody has been observed in approximately 15–20 % of pancreas transplant recipients with no impact on early outcomes in a small study [44]. Longer follow-up of donor-specific antibody-positive pancreas transplant recipients has suggested a negative impact on graft survival [45].

Acute cellular rejection is generally treated with agents similar to those used for acute kidney allograft rejection. Traditionally, pancreas allograft rejection has been felt to be poorly responsive to pulse steroids. Anti-T-cell antibody therapy is the mainstay of pancreas allograft rejection therapy. In recent years, however, the use of more potent maintenance immunosuppressive agents and the use of biopsy to diagnose acute rejection at earlier clinical stages have allowed corticosteroids to be used more successfully for the treatment of pancreas rejection. Treatment with a daily dose of 500 mg of methylprednisolone for 3 days followed by tapering doses over 2 weeks is commonly the first-line therapy and is effective in the majority of cases. Initial treatment of severe rejection or rejection resistant to therapy with corticosteroids requires the use of antilymphocyte antibody therapy. Polyclonal antilymphocyte globulin is the most commonly used preparation. This is usually given for up to 7 days. The dose is adjusted to maintain low levels of CD3-positive lymphocytes. These antilymphocyte antibody therapies are highly effective and result in reversal of the pancreas allograft rejection in over 90 % of cases.

Effects of Pancreas Transplantation on Secondary Complications of Diabetes

One of the most debilitating secondary complications of diabetes is hypoglycemic unawareness. Patients with long-standing diabetes become desensitized to the symptoms of hypoglycemia that would normally serve as a warning to dangerously low levels of glucose. The normal defense mechanism includes secretion of both glucagon and epinephrine. Both of these responses may be impaired in some diabetics. Successful pancreas transplantation is able to largely abrogate this problem. Hypoglycemic clamp studies in pancreas transplant recipients have shown that both glucagon and epinephrine responses are substantially improved, although they may remain somewhat less than matched control subjects [46–48]. This freedom from hypoglycemic unawareness is one of the major benefits of successful pancreas transplantation for many recipients.

It has been more difficult to document a significant effect of pancreas transplantation on diabetic retinopathy [49–53]. The majority of patients studied have had advanced retinopathy at the time of transplantation. Although retinopathy may be stabilized, it may require longer-term follow-up to document significant benefits on progression of retinopathy.

There is evidence that diabetic nephropathy may be stabilized and even improved following successful pancreas transplantation [54–56]. Most studies involving this issue have been relatively small, and long-term follow-up of up to 10 years has been required to demonstrate a positive benefit. Shorter-term studies have shown no benefit [57]. Studies have shown that patients receiving a pancreas transplant may have improvements in glomerular basement membrane thickness and mesangial volume and glomerular structure when long-term follow-up is available. This benefit has been observed in the native kidneys of patients who have received a solitary pancreas transplant, as well as in the transplanted kidney in patients receiving both kidney and pancreas transplants.

Numerous reports have examined the effect of pancreas transplantation on diabetic neuropathy [46, 58–64]. Improvements in autonomic function have been documented. There may be substantial improvement in orthostatic hypotension. Life expectancy in patients with autonomic insufficiency has been reported to be significantly increased [62]. Sensory nerve conduction velocities have also been shown to significantly increase following pancreas transplantation. It has been suggested that early transplantation before the onset of severe neuropathy may maximize the degree of recovery possible after pancreas transplantation.

Little data is available on the effects of pancreas transplantation on macrovascular disease. Studies examining the effects of pancreas transplantation on the progression of macrovascular and coronary heart disease or on the progression of peripheral vascular disease have been inconclusive. Serum lipid profiles and blood pressure do improve following successful pancreas transplantation which might be expected to improve macrovascular risk. It has been reported that the carotid intima-medial thickness decreases following pancreas transplantation [65, 66].

The effects on end-stage renal disease and long-standing diabetes have a significant impact on the patient's perceived quality of life. Numerous studies have attempted to examine quality of life following pancreas transplantation, as well as kidney transplantation. These studies attempt to assess an individual's perception of health, well-being, and happiness, as well as their physical and social functions. Although it may be difficult to select a truly appropriate control for quality of life studies, a number of studies have shown that successful pancreas transplantation and simultaneous kidney-pancreas transplantation result in improved physical functioning, activities of daily living, energy levels, and social and vocational rehabilitation. Freedom from daily insulin injections and blood glucose monitoring is an important result of successful pancreas transplantation. The trade-offs with respect to the side effects of immunosuppression are perceived by most patients to be less burdensome than the demands of ongoing management of insulin-dependent diabetes. Despite the limitations of study design, the improvement in quality of life and possible prevention of progression of secondary complications of diabetes make pancreas transplantation a valuable therapeutic option for selected patients with insulin-dependent or type 2 diabetes.

References

1. Kelly WD, Lillehei RC, Merkel FK, Idezuki Y, Goetz FC. Allotransplantation of the pancreas and duodenum along with the kidney in diabetic nephropathy. Surgery. 1967;61(6):827–37.
2. Lillehei RC, Simmons RL, Najarian JS, et al. Pancreatico-duodenal allotransplantation: experimental and clinical experience. Ann Surg. 1970;172(3):405–36.
3. Scientific Registry of Transplant Recipients: 2011 annual data report; 2013. http://srtr.transplant.hrsa.gov/annual_reports/2011/
4. Sutherland DE, Goetz FC, Najarian JS. Intraperitoneal transplantation of immediately vascularized segmental pancreatic grafts without duct ligation. A clinical trial. Transplantation. 1979;28(6):485–91.
5. Gliedman ML, Gold M, Whittaker J, et al. Clinical segmental pancreatic transplantation with ureter-pancreatic duct anastomosis for exocrine drainage. Surgery. 1973;74(2):171–80.
6. Sollinger HW, Cook K, Kamps D, Glass NR, Belzer FO. Clinical and experimental experience with pancreaticocystostomy for exocrine pancreatic drainage in pancreas transplantation. Transplant Proc. 1984;16(3):749–51.
7. Sutherland DE, Goetz FC, Najarian JS. One hundred pancreas transplants at a single institution. Ann Surg. 1984;200(4):414–40.
8. Sollinger HW, Stratta RJ, Kalayoglu M, Pirsch JD, Belzer FO. Pancreas transplantation with pancreaticocystostomy and quadruple immunosuppression. Surgery. 1987;102(4):674–9.
9. Nghiem DD, Corry RJ. Technique of simultaneous renal pancreatoduodenal transplantation with urinary drainage of pancreatic secretion. Am J Surg. 1987;153(4):405–6.
10. Burke GW, Gruessner R, Dunn DL, Sutherland DE. Conversion of whole pancreaticoduodenal transplants from bladder to enteric drainage for metabolic acidosis or dysuria. Transplant Proc. 1990;22(2):651–2.
11. Sollinger HW, Odorico JS, Knechtle SJ, D'Alessandro AM, Kalayoglu M, Pirsch JD. Experience with 500 simultaneous pancreas-kidney transplants. Ann Surg. 1998;228(3):284–96.
12. West M, Gruessner AC, Metrakos P, Sutherland DE, Gruessner RW. Conversion from bladder to enteric drainage after pancreaticoduodenal transplantations. Surgery. 1998;124(5):883–93.
13. Allen RD, Wilson TG, Grierson JM, et al. Percutaneous biopsy of bladder-drained pancreas transplants. Transplantation. 1991;51(6):1213–6.
14. Klassen DK, Weir MR, Cangro CB, Bartlett ST, Papadimitriou JC, Drachenberg CB. Pancreas allograft biopsy: safety of percutaneous biopsy-results of a large experience. Transplantation. 2002;73(4):553–5.
15. Wolfe RA, Ashby VB, Milford EL, et al. Comparison of mortality in all patients on dialysis, patients on dialysis awaiting transplantation, and recipients of a first cadaveric transplant. N Engl J Med. 1999;341(23):1725–30.
16. Becker BN, Brazy PC, Becker YT, et al. Simultaneous pancreas-kidney transplantation reduces excess mortality in type 1 diabetic patients with end-stage renal disease. Kidney Int. 2000;57(5):2129–35.
17. Bunnapradist S, Cho YW, Cecka JM, Wilkinson A, Danovitch GM. Kidney allograft and patient survival in type I diabetic recipients of cadaveric kidney alone versus simultaneous pancreas kidney transplants: a multivariate analysis of the UNOS database. J Am Soc Nephrol. 2003;14(1):208–13.
18. Ojo AO, Meier-Kriesche HU, Hanson JA, et al. The impact of simultaneous pancreas-kidney transplantation on long-term patient survival. Transplantation. 2001;71(1):82–90.

19. Reddy KS, Stablein D, Taranto S, et al. Long-term survival following simultaneous kidney-pancreas transplantation versus kidney transplantation alone in patients with type 1 diabetes mellitus and renal failure. Am J Kidney Dis. 2003;41(2):464–70.
20. Knoll GA, Nichol G. Dialysis, kidney transplantation, or pancreas transplantation for patients with diabetes mellitus and renal failure: a decision analysis of treatment options. J Am Soc Nephrol. 2003;14(2):500–15.
21. Venstrom JM, McBride MA, Rother KI, Hirshberg B, Orchard TJ, Harlan DM. Survival after pancreas transplantation in patients with diabetes and preserved kidney function. JAMA. 2003;290(21): 2817–23.
22. The effect of intensive treatment of diabetes on the development and progression of long-term complications in insulin-dependent diabetes mellitus. The Diabetes Control and Complications Trial Research Group. N Engl J Med. 1993;329(14):977–86.
23. Grossi PA, Righi E, Gasperina DD, et al. Report of four simultaneous pancreas-kidney transplants in HIV-positive recipients with favorable outcomes. Am J Transplant. 2012;12(4):1039–45.
24. Osei K, Henry ML, O'Dorisio TM, Tesi RJ, Sommer BG, Ferguson RM. Physiological and pharmacological stimulation of pancreatic islet hormone secretion in type I diabetic pancreas allograft recipients. Diabetes. 1990;39(10):1235–42.
25. Wiseman AC, Gralla J. Simultaneous pancreas kidney transplant versus other kidney transplant options in patients with type 2 diabetes. Clin J Am Soc Nephrol. 2012;7(4):656–64.
26. Singh PK, Kumar R, Sharma A, et al. Role of apoptotic proteins in REC-2006 mediated radiation protection in hepatoma cell lines. Evid Based Complement Alternat Med. 2011;2011:758326.
27. Gruessner RW, Burke GW, Stratta R, et al. A multicenter analysis of the first experience with FK506 for induction and rescue therapy after pancreas transplantation. Transplantation. 1996;61(2): 261–73.
28. Stratta RJ, Taylor RJ, Lowell JA, et al. Selective use of Sandostatin in vascularized pancreas transplantation. Am J Surg. 1993;166(6): 598–604.
29. Gruessner AC, Sutherland DE, Gruessner RW. Long-term outcome after pancreas transplantation. Curr Opin Organ Transplant. 2012;17(1):100–5.
30. Demartines N, Schiesser M, Clavien PA. An evidence-based analysis of simultaneous pancreas-kidney and pancreas transplantation alone. Am J Transplant. 2005;5(11):2688–97.
31. Reddy KS, Devarapalli Y, Mazur M, et al. Alemtuzumab with rapid steroid taper in simultaneous kidney and pancreas transplantation: comparison to induction with antithymocyte globulin. Transplant Proc. 2010;42(6):2006–8.
32. Vessal G, Wiland AM, Philosophe B, Fink JC, Weir MR, Klassen DK. Early steroid withdrawal in solitary pancreas transplantation results in equivalent graft and patient survival compared with maintenance steroid therapy. Clin Transplant. 2007;21(4): 491–7.
33. Uemura T, Ramprasad V, Matsushima K, et al. Single dose of alemtuzumab induction with steroid-free maintenance immunosuppression in pancreas transplantation. Transplantation. 2011;92(6): 678–85.
34. Haririan A, Hamze O, Drachenberg CB, Ramos E, Weir MR, Klassen DK. Polyomavirus reactivation in native kidneys of pancreas alone allograft recipients. Transplantation. 2003;75(8): 1186–90.
35. Kroth LV, Henkin CS, Peres LD, et al. Prevalence of urinary decoy cells and associated risk factors in a Brazilian kidney, pancreas, and kidney-pancreas transplant population. Transplant Proc. 2012; s44(8):2394–6.
36. Valette G. [Not Available]. Rev Hist Pharm (Paris). 1974;62(220): 24–34.
37. Yamazoe T, Fujimoto A, Yamazaki M, et al. [Clinical efficacy of the novel antiepileptic agent levetiracetam: evaluation in patients with localization-related epilepsy]. Brain Nerve. 2012;64(10): 1169–74.
38. Ciancio G, Sageshima J, Chen L, et al. Advantage of rapamycin over mycophenolate mofetil when used with tacrolimus for simultaneous pancreas kidney transplants: randomized, single-center trial at 10 years. Am J Transplant. 2012;12(12):3363–76.
39. Klassen DK, Hoen-Saric EW, Weir MR, et al. Isolated pancreas rejection in combined kidney pancreas transplantation. Transplantation. 1996;61(6):974–7.
40. Drachenberg CB, Odorico J, Demetris AJ, et al. Banff schema for grading pancreas allograft rejection: working proposal by a multi-disciplinary international consensus panel. Am J Transplant. 2008;8(6):1237–49.
41. Papadimitriou JC, Drachenberg CB, Klassen DK, et al. Histological grading of chronic pancreas allograft rejection/graft sclerosis. Am J Transplant. 2003;3(5):599–605.
42. Drachenberg CB, Torrealba JR, Nankivell BJ, et al. Guidelines for the diagnosis of antibody-mediated rejection in pancreas allografts-updated Banff grading schema. Am J Transplant. 2011;11(9):1792–802.
43. Melcher ML, Olson JL, Baxter-Lowe LA, Stock PG, Posselt AM. Antibody-mediated rejection of a pancreas allograft. Am J Transplant. 2006;6(2):423–8.
44. Mujtaba MA, Fridell JA, Higgins N, et al. Early findings of prospective anti-HLA donor specific antibodies monitoring study in pancreas transplantation: Indiana University Health Experience. Clin Transplant. 2012;26(5):E492–9.
45. Cantarovich D, De AS, Akl A, et al. Posttransplant donor-specific anti-HLA antibodies negatively impact pancreas transplantation outcome. Am J Transplant. 2011;11(12):2737–46.
46. Barrou Z, Seaquist ER, Robertson RP. Pancreas transplantation in diabetic humans normalizes hepatic glucose production during hypoglycemia. Diabetes. 1994;43(5):661–6.
47. Diem P, Redmon JB, Abid M, et al. Glucagon, catecholamine and pancreatic polypeptide secretion in type I diabetic recipients of pancreas allografts. J Clin Invest. 1990;86(6):2008–13.
48. Kendall DM, Rooney DP, Smets YF, Salazar BL, Robertson RP. Pancreas transplantation restores epinephrine response and symptom recognition during hypoglycemia in patients with long-standing type I diabetes and autonomic neuropathy. Diabetes. 1997;46(2):249–57.
49. Koznarova R, Saudek F, Sosna T, et al. Beneficial effect of pancreas and kidney transplantation on advanced diabetic retinopathy. Cell Transplant. 2000;9(6):903–8.
50. Petersen MR, Vine AK. Progression of diabetic retinopathy after pancreas transplantation. The University of Michigan Pancreas Transplant Evaluation Committee. Ophthalmology. 1990;97(4):496–500.
51. Ramsay RC, Goetz FC, Sutherland DE, et al. Progression of diabetic retinopathy after pancreas transplantation for insulin-dependent diabetes mellitus. N Engl J Med. 1988;318(4): 208–14.
52. Scheider A, Meyer-Schwickerath E, Nusser J, Land W, Landgraf R. Diabetic retinopathy and pancreas transplantation: a 3-year follow-up. Diabetologia. 1991;34 Suppl 1:S95–9.
53. Wang Q, Klein R, Moss SE, et al. The influence of combined kidney-pancreas transplantation on the progression of diabetic retinopathy. A case series. Ophthalmology. 1994;101(6):1071–6.
54. Bilous RW, Mauer SM, Sutherland DE, Najarian JS, Goetz FC, Steffes MW. The effects of pancreas transplantation on the glomerular structure of renal allografts in patients with insulin-dependent diabetes. N Engl J Med. 1989;321(2):80–5.
55. Bohman SO, Tyden G, Wilczek H, et al. Prevention of kidney graft diabetic nephropathy by pancreas transplantation in man. Diabetes. 1985;34(3):306–8.

56. Fioretto P, Steffes MW, Sutherland DE, Goetz FC, Mauer M. Reversal of lesions of diabetic nephropathy after pancreas transplantation. N Engl J Med. 1998;339(2):69–75.
57. Le DH, Deroover A, Coimbra C, et al. Evolution of native kidney function after pancreas transplantation alone. Transplant Proc. 2012;44(9):2829–33.
58. Allen RD, Al-Harbi IS, Morris JG, et al. Diabetic neuropathy after pancreas transplantation: determinants of recovery. Transplantation. 1997;63(6):830–8.
59. Aridge D, Reese J, Niehoff M, et al. Effect of successful renal and segmental pancreatic transplantation on peripheral and autonomic neuropathy. Transplant Proc. 1991;23(1 Pt 2): 1670–1.
60. Gaber AO, Cardoso S, Pearson S, et al. Improvement in autonomic function following combined pancreas-kidney transplantation. Transplant Proc. 1991;23(1 Pt 2):1660–2.
61. Navarro X, Kennedy WR, Loewenson RB, Sutherland DE. Influence of pancreas transplantation on cardiorespiratory reflexes, nerve conduction, and mortality in diabetes mellitus. Diabetes. 1990;39(7):802–6.
62. Navarro X, Kennedy WR, Sutherland DE. Autonomic neuropathy and survival in diabetes mellitus: effects of pancreas transplantation. Diabetologia. 1991;34 Suppl 1:S108–12.
63. Navarro X, Sutherland DE, Kennedy WR. Long-term effects of pancreatic transplantation on diabetic neuropathy. Ann Neurol. 1997;42(5):727–36.
64. Secchi A, Martinenghi S, Galardi G, Comi G, Canal N, Pozza G. Effects of pancreatic transplantation on diabetic polyneuropathy. Transplant Proc. 1991;23(1 Pt 2):1658–9.
65. Jukema JW, Smets YF, van der Pijl JW, et al. Impact of simultaneous pancreas and kidney transplantation on progression of coronary atherosclerosis in patients with end-stage renal failure due to type 1 diabetes. Diabetes Care. 2002;25(5):906–11.
66. Larsen JL, Colling CW, Ratanasuwan T, et al. Pancreas transplantation improves vascular disease in patients with type 1 diabetes. Diabetes Care. 2004;27(7):1706–11.

Drug Interactions in Solid Organ Transplant Recipients

34

Wana Manitpisitkul, Nikita S. Wilson, Sabrina Lee, and Matthew R. Weir

Introduction

Multiple advancements in immunosuppressive regimens have occurred since the first use of azathioprine in combination with corticosteroids in the early 1960s [1–3]. However, a major breakthrough came in the 1980s with the introduction of the first calcineurin inhibitor, cyclosporine. Cyclosporine, which interferes with IL-2 gene transcription that is essential for activation and proliferation of cytotoxic T cells, improved 1-year graft survival rates to greater than 80 % and reduced the use of corticosteroids for treatment of a cute rejection. The combination of cyclosporine, azathioprine, and corticosteroids became the cornerstone of maintenance therapy. In 1994, tacrolimus, which inhibits the activity of calcineurin by forming a complex with FK-binding protein, was approved by the FDA for prevention of allograft rejection in liver transplant recipients and subsequently for use in renal transplantation. Early studies in renal transplant recipients found tacrolimus to be effective for prevention of acute allograft rejection [4–7]. Mycophenolate mofetil (MMF; CellCept®), a reversible inhibitor of inosine monophosphate dehydrogenase (IMPDH), a critical rate-limiting enzyme in the de novo purine synthesis, was also approved during the same period. Clinical studies have shown MMF to be more effective in prevention of acute rejection compared to azathioprine, when used in combination with cyclosporine and corticosteroids [8–10]. Mycophenolic acid (MPA; Myfortic®), an enteric-coated form of the active metabolite of MMF, was introduced to the market in 2004. Sirolimus and everolimus, macrolide antibiotics that diminish lymphocyte responses to costimulatory signal 2 by binding to mammalian target of rapamycin (mTOR) receptor, were added to the list of immunosuppressive agents in 1999 and 2010, respectively. Belatacept, a fusion protein which acts as a selective T-cell costimulation blocker, was the latest addition to the immunosuppressant regime.

Immunosuppressive regimens continue to broaden and become more complex with the introduction of newer, more potent immunosuppressive agents. Because of their narrow therapeutic index and significant inter- and intra-patient variability due to genetic polymorphisms in P-glycoprotein and cytochrome P450 (CYP) enzyme systems, close therapeutic drug monitoring has become an important part of post-transplant care to reduce the incidence of pharmacokinetic and pharmacodynamic drug–drug interactions. With the improvement in allograft and patient survival, other comorbidities, such as opportunistic infections, post-transplant diabetes, hypertension, osteoporosis, dyslipidemia, and psychiatric diseases, have also emerged as important issues in transplant recipients. A combination of the increasing use of medications for the treatment of these comorbidities and the narrow therapeutic index of immunosuppressants can lead to potentially significant drug–drug interactions.

The purpose of this review is to provide an overview of common drug–drug interactions in transplant recipients.

Drug–Drug Interactions

Drug–drug interactions can be divided into two categories: pharmacokinetic or pharmacodynamic interactions. In a pharmacokinetic drug interaction, the administration of one drug may alter the pharmacokinetic parameters, such as

W. Manitpisitkul, Pharm.D.
Department of Pharmacy, University of Maryland Medical Center, Baltimore, MD, USA

N.S. Wilson, Pharm.D.
Vanderbilt Transplant Center, Vanderbilt University Medical Center, Nashville, TN 37232, USA

S. Lee, Pharm. D.
Department of Transplant, Keck Medical Center of USC, Los Angeles, CA 90033, USA

M.R. Weir, M.D. (✉)
Division of Nephrology, Department of Medicine, University of Maryland School of Medicine, 22 South Greene Street, N3W143, Baltimore, MD 21201, USA
e-mail: mweir@medicine.umaryland.edu

M.R. Weir and E.V. Lerma (eds.), *Kidney Transplantation: Practical Guide to Management*, DOI 10.1007/978-1-4939-0342-9_34, © Springer Science+Business Media New York 2014

absorption, distribution, metabolism, and elimination, of another drug. Pharmacodynamic interactions refer to drug–drug interactions that occur when one drug alters the toxicity or decreases the efficacy of another agent.

Pharmacokinetic Drug Interactions

The gastrointestinal tract, enterohepatic recirculation, tissue- and protein-binding sites, biliary excretion, drug metabolism enzymes, and drug transporter system are considered potential sites of pharmacokinetic interactions [11].

Several factors, including drug delivery to the intestine (presence of food, gastric pH, and gastric emptying time), intestinal lumen absorption, intestinal metabolism, and hepatic first-pass extraction, affect drug absorption after an oral administration [12]. Studies have shown that the rate of MMF absorption is delayed by food, but without significant effect on the extent of absorption [13, 14]. Due to significant gastrointestinal side effects and a clinically insignificant decrease in the rate of absorption, MMF is recommended to be taken with food. In contrast to MMF, the rate and extent of absorption of tacrolimus is significantly affected by the presence and composition of food. A study in healthy volunteers found that when administered with high fat meal, tacrolimus mean area under the curve (AUC) and maximum blood concentration (C_{max}) were decreased by 37 % and 77 %, respectively [15]. It is recommended that tacrolimus be taken on an empty stomach. Since drug absorption commonly occurs in the intestinal area, prokinetic agents have been shown to increase the rate and extent of absorption. When administered with metoclopramide, the bioavailability of cyclosporine and tacrolimus has been shown to increase by approximately 30 % and 20 %, respectively [16].

Since cyclosporine, tacrolimus, sirolimus, and everolimus are metabolized through the CYP450 enzyme system, inhibition and induction of CYP450-mediated metabolism is generally regarded as the most significant drug–drug interaction. Although the liver has been considered the main site of pharmacokinetic interaction, high levels of CYP450 3A expression has also been found in the small intestine [17]. Inhibition of CYP450 enzymes leads to a decrease in metabolism, which results in an increase in drug exposure and risk of drug-specific toxicity. Induction of CYP450 enzymes increases the amount of enzymes due to either an increase in gene transcription or decrease in enzyme degradation [18]. Enzyme inhibition occurs almost immediately after administration of an inhibitor drug, while enzyme induction, a slower and time-dependent process, is achieved over approximately a 2-week period [19–22].

In addition to CYP450 enzyme systems, active transporters, such as P-glycoprotein and organic anion-transporting polypeptides, also play an important role in pharmacokinetic drug interactions. Because of their geographical proximity and shared substrates, P-glycoprotein and CYP3A4 form a cooperative barrier against xenobiotics and drugs such as immunosuppressants [23, 24].

Calcineurin Inhibitors: Cyclosporine and Tacrolimus

Cyclosporine is a small cyclic polypeptide consisting of 11 amino acids isolated from *Beauveria nivea* while tacrolimus is a macrolide antibiotic isolated from *Streptomyces tsukubaensis*. Tacrolimus is often still referred to as FK which derived from its original molecular designation of FK506. The immunosuppressive effect of calcineurin inhibitors is dependent upon the formation of a complex with cytoplasmic receptor proteins, cyclophilin for cyclosporine and FK binding protein for tacrolimus. Calcineurin acts as a phosphatase that dephosphorylates nuclear factor of activated T cells leading to its passage through the nuclear membrane and thus initiation of gene transcription. The cyclosporine or tacrolimus complex inhibits calcineurin activity and thereby impairs the expression of several cytokine genes that promote T-cell activation, including those for IL-2, IL-4, interferon-γ, and tumor necrosis factor-α.

The original formulation of cyclosporine, the oil-based Sandimmune®, has largely been replaced by the microemulsion formulations, Neoral® and Gengraf®. Following oral administration, absorption of Sandimmune® is incomplete and variable. Time to peak concentration (T_{max}) is achieved after an average of approximately 4 h. Neoral® has an increased and more reliable bioavailability compared to Sandimmune®, resulting in less variability in the pharmacokinetics. Peak cyclosporine levels (C_{max}) of Neoral® are higher, and the trough concentrations are better correlated with systemic exposure, as reflected by the area under the concentration-time curve (AUC).

The immunosuppressive activities of cyclosporine and tacrolimus are primarily due to the parent drugs. Since both drugs are extensively metabolized by the CYP enzyme system, substances known to inhibit or induce these systems may result in increased metabolism or a decrease in bioavailability.

Calcineurin Inhibitor Drug–Drug Interactions (Table 34.1)

Anti-infectives

Infection continues to be a major cause of morbidity and mortality in transplant recipients. Risk factors for the development of infection include T- and B-cell depletion by induction agents, T- and B-cell dysfunction caused by the use of calcineurin inhibitors, and neutropenia

Table 34.1 Clinically relevant drug interactions with immunosuppressive medications

Immunosuppressive agent	Interacting agent	Effect of interacting agent	Recommendations/monitoring
Calcineurin inhibitors			
	Antifungals		
	Anidulafungin	No significant effect	
	Amphotericin B	Increased risk of nephrotoxicity	Appropriate hydration; monitor renal function closely
	Caspofungin	Increased hepatic enzymes with cyclosporine	Monitor transaminases closely; consider alternatives if elevation in hepatic enzymes occurs
	Fluconazole	Inhibits metabolism	Monitor CNI levels closely
	Ketoconazole	Inhibits metabolism	Monitor levels closely
			Decrease CNI dose by 50–75 %
	Micafungin	No significant effect	
	Posaconazole	Inhibits metabolism	Monitor CNI levels closely
			Decrease cyclosporine by 25 % and tacrolimus by 66 %
	Voriconazole	Inhibits metabolism	Monitor levels closely
			Decrease CNI dose by 50–75 %
	Antibiotics		
	Azithromycin	Little effect	
	Clarithromycin	Inhibits metabolism	Empiric dose reduction; monitor CNI levels closely
	Erythromycin	Inhibits metabolism	Empiric dose reduction; monitor CNI levels closely
	Rifampin	Induces metabolism	Increase in dose; monitor CNI levels closely
	Antiretrovirals		
	Protease inhibitors	Inhibits metabolism	Dose reduction; monitor CNI levels closely
	Anticonvulsants		
	Barbiturates	Induces metabolism	Increase in dose; monitor CNI levels closely
	Benzodiazepines	No effect	
	Carbamazepine and Oxcarbazepine	May induce metabolism	Monitor CNI levels; may require increase in dose
	Levetiracetam	No effect	
	Modafinil	Induces metabolism	Dose reduction; monitor CNI levels
	Phenytoin	Induces metabolism	Dose reduction; monitor CNI levels closely
	Valproic acid	No direct effect	Monitor levels
	Antihypertensives		
	ACEIs/ARBs	May increase risk of hyperkalemia	Monitor potassium
	Beta-blockers	Carvedilol may inhibit metabolism	Monitor CNI levels
	Diltiazem, verapamil, and nifedipine	Inhibit metabolism	Decrease CNI dose by 25 %; monitor CNI levels closely
	Dihydropyridine calcium channel blockers	No effect	
	Colchicine and NSAIDs		
	Colchicine	Inhibition of colchicine metabolism; competitive inhibition of cyclosporine metabolism	Dose adjustment of colchicine per package labeling required
	NSAIDs	Increased risk of nephrotoxicity	Avoid if possible; use for short period of time if necessary with close monitoring
	Lipid-lowering agents		
	HMG-CoA reductase inhibitors	Increased statin exposure with cyclosporine	Significant dose reduction of statin; monitor CPK
		No effect with tacrolimus	
	Psychiatric drugs		
	Citalopram	No reports	Monitor CNI levels
	Desvenlafaxine	No reports	Caution due to CYP 3A4 metabolism of desvenlafaxine
	Duloxetine	No reports	Monitor CNI levels
	Fluvoxamine	Inhibits metabolism	Monitor CNI levels closely; dose reductions may be necessary
	Fluoxetine, paroxetine, and citalopram	Little effect	Monitor CNI levels
	Haloperidol	QT prolongation	Monitor QTc interval
	Lithium	Increased risk of nephrotoxicity	Monitor renal function closely
	Nefazodone	Inhibits metabolism	Avoid if possible
	Quetiapine and olanzapine	QT prolongation	Monitor QTc interval
	Sertraline	May inhibit metabolism	Conflicting reports—monitor levels closely
	Venlafaxine	Little effect	Monitor CNI levels

(continued)

Table 34.1 (continued)

Immunosuppressive agent	Interacting agent	Effect of interacting agent	Recommendations/monitoring
Antimetabolites			
MMF and MPA			
	Calcineurin inhibitors		
	Cyclosporine	Reduction in MPA AUC	Dose adjustment may be necessary
	Antivirals		
	Acyclovir	Possible increase in AUC	Monitor for adverse events
	Ganciclovir	Decreased clearance of ganciclovir	Monitor for adverse events
	Gastrointestinal drugs		
	Antacids	Decrease in AUC and C_{max}	Avoid concomitant administration if possible
	Proton pump inhibitors	MMF decrease in C_{max} and T_{max} MPA—no effect	Caution with MMF
	Phosphate binders		
	Calcium-free phosphate binders	Decrease in AUC and C_{max}	Administer 2 h after MMF
	Miscellaneous drugs		
	Cholestyramine	Decrease in AUC	Concomitant use not recommended
	Oral contraceptives	Decrease in levonorgestrel AUC	Caution with levonorgestrel
	Anti-infectives		
	Ciprofloxacin and amoxicillin/clavulanic acid	Decrease in trough levels	Caution
	Norfloxacin and metronidazole	Decrease in AUC	Concomitant use not recommended with combination
	Trimethoprim/sulfamethoxazole	Small reduction in AUC	Does not appear clinically significant
	Rifampin	Increase in exposure	Monitor for adverse events
Azathioprine			
	Xanthine oxidase inhibitors		
	Allopurinol	Increase in 6-mercaptopurine	Avoid concomitant use
Mammalian target of rapamycin inhibitors			
	Calcineurin inhibitors		
	Cyclosporine	Increase in sirolimus AUC	Monitor levels; if given concomitantly, give sirolimus 4 h after cyclosporine
		Increase in everolimus AUC	Monitor levels; dose adjustment may be necessary
	Antifungals		
	Ketoconazole	Increase in C_{max}, T_{max}, and AUC	Monitor levels; significant dose reduction required
	Voriconazole	Increase in C_{max} and AUC	Monitor levels; significant dose reduction required
	Calcium channel blockers		
	Non-dihydropyridine calcium channel blockers	Increase in C_{max} and AUC	Monitor levels; dose reduction may be required
	Antibiotics		
	Erythromycin	Increase in C_{max} and AUC	Monitor levels; consider azithromycin as an alternative
	Rifampin	Decrease in C_{max} and AUC	Monitor levels; significant dose increase required
	Antiretrovirals		
	HIV protease inhibitors	Increase in AUC	Monitor levels; dose reduction may be required

associated with purine antagonists [25]. Infections due to T cell-mediated defects include cytomegalovirus, herpes simplex virus, *Pneumocystis jiroveci* pneumonia, mucosal candidiasis, cryptococcus, and mucormycosis. Neutropenia-related infections include gram-positive and gram-negative bacterial infections, aspergillosis, and disseminated candidiasis [26–28].

Antifungals

The incidence of invasive fungal infections has become increasingly common in organ transplant recipients, ranging from 11 to 42 %, with the highest incidence reported in liver transplant patients [29–31]. Current options for the treatment of fungal infections include azole antifungals, amphotericin B, and the newest class of antifungals, echinocandins.

The azole antifungals have been extensively used in transplant recipients. All the azole antifungals have varying CYP3A4 inhibitory potencies, with ketoconazole being the most potent followed by itraconazole, posaconazole, voriconazole, and lastly fluconazole. Ketoconazole has been shown to increase the AUC of cyclosporine by almost threefold, requiring up to an 80 % reduction in cyclosporine dose [32]. Because of this interaction, clinicians have combined ketoconazole with a calcineurin inhibitor-based regimen for cost reduction benefit [32–35]. In a 10-year follow-up study by El-Agroudy and colleagues, the long-term use of ketoconazole for cyclosporine dose reduction was found to be safe, cost sparing, and associated with a significantly lower incidence of chronic allograft nephropathy [36]. Newer triazole antifungals, voriconazole and posaconazole, have an extended spectrum of activity against the *Candida* species, including *C. krusei* and *C. glabrata*, *Aspergillus*, and *Cryptococcus*. A randomized, double-blind, cross-over study in kidney transplant recipients found that the addition of voriconazole increased the mean cyclosporine AUC by 1.7-fold [37, 38]. It is recommended that the dose of cyclosporine be cut in half when voriconazole is added to the regimen. Voriconazole has also been shown to inhibit the metabolism of tacrolimus. In healthy volunteers, the addition of voriconazole has been shown to triple the AUC of tacrolimus, thus leading to the recommended 66 % dose reduction of tacrolimus when voriconazole is added to the regimen [38]. A retrospective study, which examined the impact on tacrolimus trough concentration after switching from fluconazole to voriconazole in allogenic hematopoietic stem cell transplant recipients, showed that the mean concentration/dose ratio of tacrolimus was increased 4.5-fold, prompting a 75 % dose reduction of tacrolimus [39]. Posaconazole has also been shown to significantly increase tacrolimus maximum blood concentration and area under concentration-time curve by 121 % and 358 %, respectively [40]. A study in four adult heart transplant recipients found that concomitant administration of posaconazole with cyclosporine increased cyclosporine exposure, requiring a 14–29 % cyclosporine dose reduction [40]. The manufacturer recommends reducing the cyclosporine dose by 25 % and tacrolimus dose by 66 % at the initiation of posaconazole treatment [41]. At the initiation and discontinuation of azole antifungals, dosage adjustment and close monitoring of calcineurin inhibitor concentration are recommended.

The echinocandins, caspofungin, micafungin, and anidulafungin, have good in vitro and in vivo activities against *Aspergillus* and *Candida species*. Data from in vitro and clinical studies indicate that caspofungin is not an inhibitor or inducer of the CYP450 enzyme system [42]. However, in a phase 1 clinical study, concomitant administration of caspofungin with cyclosporine resulted in an abnormal elevation of alanine aminotransferase (ALT) [42]. A limited number of subsequent studies examined this potential drug–drug interaction [43–47]. Marr et al. reported the hepatic safety profile in 40 patients concomitantly treated with caspofungin and cyclosporine. Transaminase elevation, >5 times the upper limit of normal or >3 times baseline, occurred in 14 patients (35 %) receiving concomitant therapy during a 14-day follow-up period [44]. Five patients had aspartate aminotransferase (AST) elevations that were considered possibly related to concomitant therapy, although no clinical evidence of hepatotoxicity or serious hepatic events was reported. In a retrospective study, Saner et al. reported the safety profile of concomitant administration of caspofungin in 12 liver transplant recipients receiving cyclosporine ($N=7$) or tacrolimus ($N=5$) [43]. No hepatotoxicity or liver enzyme elevation was reported. Due to the limitation of the size of these studies, when considering adding caspofungin to a cyclosporine regimen, the potential risk and benefit should be considered and hepatic function should be closely monitored. Early studies evaluating drug interactions found no effect of single or multiple doses of micafungin on the pharmacokinetic parameters of cyclosporine or tacrolimus [48]. An in vitro study did not find anidulafungin to be a CYP450 inhibitor or inducer and was not metabolized by the CYP450 enzyme system. In clinical studies, co-administration of anidulafungin did not significantly alter the pharmacokinetics of cyclosporine or tacrolimus [49, 50].

Amphotericin B remains an important antifungal, especially in the treatment of invasive mycoses [51]. Amphotericin B-induced nephrotoxicity, due to reduced renal blood flow and renal tubular dysfunction, continues to be an important dose-limiting side effect, especially in transplant recipients that may have some degree of renal dysfunction. Calcineurin inhibitors may also increase the nephrotoxicity of amphotericin B. Several lipid-based formulations of amphotericin B have been introduced to the market. Among these formulations, liposomal amphotericin B (Ambisome®) was reported as the least nephrotoxic [52]. To prevent nephrotoxicity, patients should be hydrated with 200–500 mL of 0.9 % normal saline before and after administration of amphotericin B [52].

Antibiotics

The macrolide antibiotics are frequently used in the treatment of various infections, including atypical bacteria such as *Legionella pneumophila* and *Mycoplasma pneumoniae*. Erythromycin and clarithromycin share a 14-membered macrocyclic lactone ring structure. These macrolides form inactive complexes with CYP3A enzymes and thus inhibit the metabolism of drugs requiring this enzyme, including tacrolimus and cyclosporine. In contrast, azithromycin has a 15-membered ring structure that does not complex with CYP3A enzymes and is thought to have little effect on the metabolism of the calcineurin inhibitors [53]. Therefore, when plausible, it may be beneficial to use azithromycin as the macrolide of choice to avoid this interaction. Concomitant use of calcineurin inhibitors and erythromycin or clarithromycin requires empiric dose reduction and close monitoring of calcineurin inhibitor plasma concentrations.

Rifampin is a potent CYP3A4 enzyme inducer, increasing hepatic and intestinal metabolism of CYP3A4 substrates, including the calcineurin inhibitors. Rifampin has been found to decrease cyclosporine trough concentrations by 73 % after administration of a single dose [54]. Kim et al. investigated the pharmacokinetic profile of cyclosporine in kidney transplant recipients before and after the administration of rifampin and found a significant decrease in cyclosporine concentration. A dose increase of 2.5–3 times was needed in order to maintain optimal cyclosporine trough concentrations [55]. Other studies also confirmed that, in addition to an increase in dosing frequency, a 3–5-fold increase in cyclosporine dose is required when using rifampin in order to achieve satisfactory trough concentrations [56, 57]. Similar findings were observed in heart transplant recipients when rifampin was co-administered with cyclosporine [58]. The same interaction is also seen when rifampin was administered with tacrolimus in kidney transplant recipients. A tacrolimus dose increase of up to tenfold is often needed [59, 60].

Antiretroviral Therapy

HIV protease inhibitors are known to cause significant drug interactions through inhibition of the CYP3A4 enzyme and P-glycoprotein efflux pump, leading to an increase in systemic blood levels of CYP3A4 or P-glycoprotein substrates. Pharmacokinetic studies have consistently shown that when administered in conjunction with HIV protease inhibitors, calcineurin inhibitor doses need to be reduced significantly to maintain similar trough concentrations. When co-administered, the lopinavir/ritonavir combination significantly increases tacrolimus exposure, with a tenfold increase in half-life. This pronounced effect results in the need for significant tacrolimus dose and administration frequency reduction [61–63]. Case reports in kidney transplant patients have shown that the combination of saquinavir or darunavir with tacrolimus resulted in an increase in tacrolimus trough concentrations, necessitating a 96.5 % reduction in dose to maintain stable trough levels [64, 65]. In liver transplant patients, the addition of nelfinavir to a tacrolimus-based regimen required a 16–70-fold decrease in tacrolimus dose to maintain similar trough concentrations [66, 67]. Similarly, in kidney transplant patients, an 85 % dose reduction of cyclosporine was required when cyclosporine and nelfinavir and indinavir were concomitantly administered [68]. Vogel et al. observed a need for a 5–20 % cyclosporine dose reduction when lopinavir/ritonavir was administered in liver transplant patients receiving cyclosporine [69]. To avoid drug-induced toxicity, close therapeutic drug monitoring and dose adjustment are necessary when immunosuppressants are co-administered with protease inhibitors.

Anticonvulsant Medications

Seizures are common in both the pre- and post-transplant population. Calcineurin inhibitors have been associated with lowering the seizure threshold.

Barbiturates markedly reduce cyclosporine and tacrolimus levels. Doses up to two or three times the previous regimen may be required to maintain adequate levels. Carbamazepine may also decrease cyclosporine or tacrolimus levels, but the effect is less pronounced. Similarly, oxcarbazepine may decrease levels as well. Benzodiazepines and valproic acid do not affect drug levels, but valproic acid has been associated with hepatotoxicity, which may result in alterations in metabolism. Modafinil can cause a reduction in calcineurin inhibitor levels up to 50 %. Phenytoin, a common first-line therapy used in the treatment of many types of seizures, causes CYP 3A4 enzyme induction [70, 71]. Due to the upregulation of metabolism, calcineurin inhibitor therapeutic drug concentrations are difficult to maintain [72, 73]. On average, two times the previous dose of cyclosporine or tacrolimus is required for patients receiving phenytoin. Levetiracetam, a newer anticonvulsant, does not undergo hepatic metabolism. Due to negligible effects on CYP450 system, levetiracetam is a safe option for transplant patients receiving calcineurin inhibitors.

Antihypertensive Medications

Cardiovascular disease is the leading cause of mortality in the kidney transplant population. Patients with kidney disease often have hypertension pre-transplant that is worsened by maintenance immunosuppression regimens [74]. Calcineurin inhibitors induce hypertension through endothelin-mediated vasoconstriction, decreased nitric oxide production, and increased renal tubular sodium reabsorption [74]. To confound the situation, corticosteroids also increase blood pressure primarily through increased sodium retention [75]. Non-dihydropyridine calcium channel blockers, diltiazem and verapamil, are effective in treating hypertension and maintaining normal sinus rhythm in the setting of atrial fibrillation. However, these agents are potent CYP3A4 inhibitors, thereby increasing calcineurin inhibitor concentrations [76–78]. Cautious monitoring is required when initiating these agents, with a suggested empiric calcineurin inhibitor dose decrease of 25 % [76]. The dihydropyridine calcium channel blockers are relatively devoid of this interaction with the exception of nifedipine, which undergoes similar enzymatic metabolism [79].

Angiotensin converting enzyme inhibitors (ACEIs) and angiotensin receptor blockers (ARBs) are effective in decreasing both blood pressure and proteinuria. However, hyperkalemia may be a dangerous consequence when calcineurin inhibitors and ACEIs or ARBs are used concomitantly with sulfamethoxazole/trimethoprim, a common post-transplant prophylactic medication [80].

Despite exacerbation of comorbid diseases such as depression and erectile dysfunction, beta-blockers have been generally regarded as safe and effective for the treatment of hypertension in the post-transplantation setting. Notably, a retrospective study showed a significant increase in cyclosporine trough concentrations with the addition of carvedilol [81]. However, this interaction was absent when cyclosporine was co-administered with metoprolol. Carvedilol administration with cyclosporine increased the cyclosporine bioavailability by 40 % in one laboratory study [82]. As more data is needed regarding the effects of P-glycoprotein on cyclosporine and tacrolimus levels, caution should be taken when initiating carvedilol. Ultimately, the risk and side effects must be balanced with the management of hypertension and decreased mortality rates when choosing an appropriate agent.

Drugs That May Exaggerate Calcineurin Inhibitor Nephrotoxicity

Gout is a common condition that plagues not only the general population but solid organ transplant recipients as well. The calcineurin inhibitors, especially cyclosporine, have been associated with hyperuricemia [83]. Colchicine, commonly used in gout prophylaxis and acute attacks, must be used cautiously when administered concomitantly with the calcineurin inhibitors. Cyclosporine is thought to decrease the metabolism of colchicine through inhibition of P-glycoprotein, resulting in an increase in colchicine plasma concentrations and the potential for serious toxicity. In addition, concomitant use may result in increased cyclosporine plasma concentration and subsequent nephrotoxicity through competition for CYP3A4 metabolism. Appropriate dosage adjustments per colchicine package labeling must be followed to use this combination safely [84].

Nonsteroidal anti-inflammatory drugs (NSAIDs) have also been associated with nephrotoxicity and should be avoided with calcineurin inhibitors if possible. However, NSAIDs can be given for short periods under close observation.

Any drug with the potential to cause nephrotoxicity should be used with caution in combination with calcineurin inhibitors because the vasoconstrictive effect of calcineurin inhibitors tends to potentiate other nephrotoxic mechanisms.

Lipid-Lowering Agents

HMG-CoA reductase inhibitors are the most commonly used agents for the treatment of dyslipidemia in transplant recipients. Studies have shown that administration of cyclosporine, in combination with an HMG-CoA reductase inhibitor, can increase the systemic exposure to statins leading to an increase in incidence of rhabdomyolysis [85–93]. This interaction was initially thought to be due to competitive inhibition of CYP3A4-mediated drug metabolism by cyclosporine, increasing exposure of fluvastatin and pravastatin. However, interactions with the non-CYP3A4-dependent statins have also been reported, indicating a more complex interaction. It is recommended that when used in combination with cyclosporine, the statin dose should be significantly reduced to prevent serious adverse reactions. In contrast to cyclosporine, Lemahieu et al. reported no significant impact on the pharmacokinetics of atorvastatin and its metabolites when used in combination with tacrolimus [94]. Further studies are necessary to evaluate if this lack of interaction can be applied to the other HMG-CoA reductase inhibitors. When statins are co-administered with calcineurin inhibitors, patients should be closely monitored for any signs and symptoms of myopathy and/or rhabdomyolysis.

Psychiatric Drugs

Depression is common in both the pre-transplant and post-transplant periods. Factors such as chronic illness, lethargy, anxiety associated with waiting for transplant, medications, including post-transplant immunosuppressive agents, as well as post-transplant complications have been associated with the development of depression [95]. Selective serotonin reuptake inhibitors (SSRI) are the most commonly prescribed class of medications used to treat depression. Nefazodone and fluvoxamine are known CYP3A4 inhibitors. While case reports of significant drug interactions with fluvoxamine are lacking, nefazodone has been shown to increase both cyclosporine and tacrolimus trough levels tenfold after initiation [96–100]. Based on the in vitro potential for CYP3A4 inhibition, sertraline should exhibit the least effects, followed by fluoxetine and citalopram [101]. While conflicting reports have been published regarding sertraline's effects on cyclosporine concentrations, fluoxetine, paroxetine, and citalopram do not alter cyclosporine trough concentrations, which may in part be due to their diminished effects on CYP3A4 [100, 102–105]. Ultimately, nefazodone should be avoided in the transplant population and vigilant therapeutic drug monitoring should be considered when a new SSRI is initiated. Venlafaxine, the serotonin–norepinephrine reuptake inhibitor, is an attractive alternative to SSRI. It has been proven to have little effect on the CYP3A4 enzyme system and is metabolized through the CYP2D6 pathway [106]. To date, desvenlafaxine and duloxetine have not been reported to interact with the calcineurin inhibitors. However, desvenlafaxine has been shown to undergo CYP3A4 metabolism; therefore, caution should be taken since safety data is lacking surrounding this class of medications.

In addition to the pharmacokinetic interactions, the potential for toxicity of antidepressants and antipsychotics must be considered when choosing appropriate therapy. Lithium, a known cause of renal failure, may have its nephrotoxic effects potentiated by calcineurin inhibitors. Drugs that may cause QT prolongation, such as haloperidol, quetiapine, and olanzapine, may be potentiated in the setting of high calcineurin inhibitor trough concentrations.

Antimetabolites: Mycophenolate Mofetil (MMF), Mycophenolic Acid (MPA), and Azathioprine

MPA, a fermentation product of *Penicillium brevicompactum*, is a noncompetitive, reversible inhibitor of IMPDH and therefore inhibits the de novo pathway of guanosine nucleotide synthesis without incorporation to DNA [107, 108]. After oral or intravenous administration, mycophenolate mofetil is rapidly absorbed and converted to MPA [109]. MPA is eliminated through glucuronidation via uridine diphosphate glucuronosyltransferases (UGT) to the pharmacologically inactive 7-*O*-MPA-glucuronide (MPAG) in the gastrointestinal tract, liver, and kidney [110, 111]. After the first peak (C_{max}), intra-intestinal bacterial breakdown of MPAG to MPA and enterohepatic recirculation resulted in a second plasma concentration peak observed 8–12 h post dose [14, 109].

MMF and MPA Drug–Drug Interactions (Table 34.1)

Cyclosporine

Cyclosporine has been shown to reduce the AUC of MPA by inhibiting MPAG excretion into the bile via the bile-mediated multidrug resistance protein 2 (MRP-2) transporter. This reduces systemic MPA availability by decreasing the enterohepatic recirculation leading to an elimination of the second MPA plasma concentration peak [112–118]. Limited data has been reported on the MMF and tacrolimus drug interaction. In vitro data showed that tacrolimus may increase MPA plasma concentrations due to inhibition of UGT [119]. However MPA AUC and MPAG levels were not statistically affected in rats treated with tacrolimus, when compared to the control group treated with MMF alone [113]. Kagaya et al. reported that in 71 Japanese renal transplant patients, the pharmacokinetics of MPA and MPAG were unaffected by higher tacrolimus blood concentrations [120]. Thus, fixed-dose MPA therapy in combination with different CNI regimens may lead to different MPA exposure. The differences of MPA exposure due to interaction with different CNIs could have significant clinical consequences. Clinical studies have reported a clear association between the risk of acute rejection and total MPA AUC (0–12 h). The relationship between adverse effects of MPA, such as anemia, leukopenia, GI symptoms, and infection, and the AUC 0–12 h is less well established. Some studies have shown better correlation between the incidence of infection or leukopenia with free rather than total MPA levels. Others have suggested that adverse events are better predicted by MMF dose, rather than blood concentration. Although there are no clear recommendations, close monitoring of MMF-related toxicity and MMF dosage adjustment may be necessary when patients are switched from cyclosporine- to tacrolimus-based therapy.

Antivirals

Acyclovir

Acyclovir is commonly used post-transplant and exerts its antiviral effects via inhibition of DNA polymerase. Acyclovir is converted to acyclovir monophosphate by virally encoded thymidine kinase which is then converted to acyclovir triphosphate by cellular enzymes. Acyclovir triphosphate competitively inhibits viral DNA polymerase by acting as an analog to deoxyguanosine triphosphate. Incorporation of acyclovir triphosphate into DNA results in chain termination.

Pharmacokinetic studies between mycophenolate mofetil and acyclovir have reported conflicting results. In a study involving 12 healthy subjects, no differences in MPA or acyclovir pharmacokinetic parameters were reported when a single dose of MMF 1 g and acyclovir 800 mg were co-administered. However, a slight increase in MPAG AUB was observed [121]. In another study of 12 healthy volunteers who were also co-administered MMF 1 g and acyclovir 800 mg, no significant changes in MPA AUC and C_{max} were observed [107]. However, MPAG and acyclovir AUCs were increased 10.6 % and 21.9 %, respectively. Furthermore, a different study in healthy volunteers did not demonstrate differences in MPA or MPAG pharmacokinetic parameters following co-administration of MMF 1 g and acyclovir 800 mg [122]. However, significant increases in acyclovir C_{max}, T_{max}, and AUC and a significant decrease in acyclovir half-life and renal clearance were reported when co-administered with MMF.

Ganciclovir

Ganciclovir is commonly used following solid organ transplant to prevent as well as treat cytomegalovirus infections. Ganciclovir is phosphorylated intracellularly to its active metabolite, which competitively inhibits binding of deoxyguanosine triphosphate to DNA polymerase resulting in inhibition of viral DNA synthesis. In a single-dose crossover study, Wolfe et al. demonstrated that mean AUC, C_{max}, and T_{max} of MPA, MPAG, and ganciclovir were not significantly altered when the MMF mofetil 1 g and ganciclovir 5 mg/kg were co-administered [123]. However, it was observed that renal clearance of ganciclovir was decreased by approximately 12 % when it was co-administered with MMF mofetil. This was thought to be secondary to the competition for renal tubular secretion between ganciclovir and MPAG. Caution should be exercised in the setting of renal dysfunction where plasma concentrations of both MPAG and ganciclovir are known to be elevated. The competitive tubular secretion may lead to further increases in drug concentrations and result in unwanted adverse events.

Antacids with Magnesium and Aluminum Hydroxides

Antacids are commonly used following transplant as many of the drugs used post-transplant have the potential to cause gastrointestinal side effects. The first report of a potential interaction between antacids and MMF occurred in rheumatoid arthritis patients. Bullingham et al. performed a crossover study investigating the effect of 10 mL of Maalox® TC (1,200 mg aluminum hydroxide and magnesium hydroxide) on the pharmacokinetic parameters of MPA and MPAG after administration of a single 2 g dose of MMF [124]. The study reported a decrease in MPA AUC and C_{max} by approximately 17 % and 37 %, respectively, compared to MPA pharmacokinetic parameters in the fasting state. A decrease in MPAG AUC and C_{max} was also observed following co-administration with antacids. As such, it is recommended that MPA products not be co-administered with antacids in order to maintain optimal dosing in transplant patients.

Proton Pump Inhibitors (CellCept® vs. Myfortic®)

Similarly, proton pump inhibitors (PPIs) are often used to prevent gastrointestinal side effects common to many of the medications necessary after transplant. A few studies have shown that PPIs have an effect on the pharmacokinetics of CellCept®. In a retrospective study in renal transplant recipients, Van Gelder et al. found the MPA AUC to be unaffected by the concomitant use of PPIs; however, the authors did notice a delayed MPA C_{max} from postoperative day 7 onward [125]. Miura et al. investigated the effect of co-administration of lansoprazole or rabeprazole on the pharmacokinetics of MPA in renal transplant recipients [126]. Lansoprazole was found to decrease MPA C_{max} and T_{max} while rabeprazole appeared to have no effect on MPA kinetics. This difference was thought to be due to the higher stomach pH that is induced by lansoprazole compared to rabeprazole. In heart transplant recipients, pantoprazole was found to significantly decrease MPA C_{max} and AUCs and is associated with increased acute rejection and transplant vasculopathy [127].

However, there is no evidence to suggest that PPIs have the same effect on Myfortic®, the enteric-coated formulation of MPA. In an open, block-wise randomized, crossover study with a 1-week washout period between phases A (CellCept®) and B (Myfortic®) performed in 12 healthy volunteers, use of pantoprazole resulted in a significant decrease in MPA C_{max} and AUC and MPAG AUC. However, pharmacokinetic parameters were unaffected when pantoprazole was co-administered with Myfortic® [128]. A similarly designed study using omeprazole in 12 healthy volunteers verified the previous results where MPA C_{max} and AUC and MPAG AUC were reduced by omeprazole but Myfortic® parameters were unchanged [129]. The difference was attributed to reduced dissolution of MMF in a high-pH environment resulting in reduced absorption of MPA.

Sevelamer

The effect of sevelamer on the pharmacokinetics of MMF was studied in ten adult and eight pediatric renal transplant recipients with stable graft function [130]. Mean MPA AUC was reduced by 23 % after only a single dose of sevelamer and by 26 % after 4 days of sevelamer treatment. This reduction was thought to be secondary to a decrease in C_{max} by 32 % and 36 % after a single dose and after 4 days of treatment, respectively, suggesting that sevelamer and other calcium-free phosphate binders should not be co-administered with MMF. Therefore, it is recommended that calcium-free phosphate binders be administered 2 h after MMF in order to minimize the decrease in MPA absorption.

Cholestyramine

As with many medications, an interaction exists between cholestyramine and MMF. Twelve healthy volunteers were given cholestyramine 4 g TID for 24 h prior and 3 days following administration of single-dose MMF 1.5 g in a crossover study. MPA AUC was found to be reduced by 37 %, which was almost entirely attributable to the reduction of MPA concentration from 6 h onward. This is consistent with interruption of enterohepatic recirculation thought to be via binding of recirculating MPAG with cholestyramine. Therefore, concomitant use of MMF and cholestyramine is not recommended [107].

Oral Contraceptives

Eighteen women with psoriasis were given MMF 1 g BID along with combined oral contraceptives containing ethinylestradiol and levonorgestrel, desogestrel, or gestodene [107]. The AUCs of ethinylestradiol and 3-keto desogestrel appeared to be unaffected, but levonorgestrel AUC was significantly decreased by 15 % following administration of MMF. Mean serum levels of LH, FSH, and progesterone were not significantly affected. Therefore, it is recommended to use caution when using MMF and hormonal contraceptives concomitantly and additional barrier contraceptive methods must be used.

Antibiotics

Norfloxacin and Metronidazole

Eleven healthy volunteers received a single dose of MMF 1 g on day 4 of a 5-day course of either norfloxacin, metronidazole, or a combination of the two [107]. Mean MPA AUC was significantly decreased in the combination group of norfloxacin and metronidazole compared to mycophenolate mofetil alone. However, neither antibiotic alone had the same effect on MPA AUC as the combination. Thus, MMF is not recommended when norfloxacin and metronidazole are used in combination.

Ciprofloxacin and Amoxicillin/Clavulanic Acid

In a prospective study of 64 renal transplant recipients, clinically indicated treatment with either ciprofloxacin or amoxicillin/clavulanic acid was administered for 7–14 days [131]. Pharmacokinetic evaluation of MPA demonstrated a 46 % decrease in median MPA trough levels with both antibiotics within 3 days of antibiotic initiation. MPA trough levels recovered spontaneously to 79 % of baseline 14 days after antibiotic initiation, and trough levels normalized within 3 days of antibiotic cessation. This was thought to be due to antibiotic-induced reduction of B-glucuronidase-producing bacteria which leads to decreased enterohepatic recirculation of MPA. However, caution should be exercised when interpreting these findings as a formal pharmacokinetic study measuring a full AUC was not performed, and thus the impact on overall MPA exposure is unknown.

Trimethoprim/Sulfamethoxazole

Trimethoprim/sulfamethoxazole is the first-line agent for prevention of PCP and thus use is common in transplant recipients. In a crossover study, healthy volunteers were co-administered a single dose of MMF 1.5 g on day 8 of a 10-day course of trimethoprim 160 mg/sulfamethoxazole 800 mg BID. MPA AUC was reduced by 7 % and C_{max} was comparable [107]. No changes were observed in the MPAG C_{max} and AUC with the administration of trimethoprim/sulfamethoxazole.

Rifampin

An increase in MMF exposure of more than twofold has been reported in a heart–lung transplant recipient when rifampin was co-administered [132]. The interaction between MMF and rifampin is hypothesized to be through induction of UGT and does not involve the CYP system.

Azathioprine Drug–Drug Interactions (Table 34.1)

Azathioprine is an imidazolyl derivative of mercaptopurine. After oral administration, azathioprine is metabolized to 6-mercaptopurine (6-MP). Allopurinol inhibits the conversion of 6-mercaptopurine to an inactive metabolite by inhibiting xanthine oxidase. The addition of allopurinol to azathioprine leads to higher blood concentrations of 6-mercaptopurine and results in serious life-threatening myelosuppression. The combination should be avoided. If necessary, when administered concomitantly with allopurinol, the azathioprine dose should be reduced by 67–75 % [133].

Mammalian Target of Rapamycin Inhibitors

The mammalian target of rapamycin inhibitors (mTORi), sirolimus and everolimus, inhibit T-lymphocyte activation and proliferation by binding to cytoplasmic protein, FK506 binding protein-12, to form a complex that binds to and inhibits the regulatory kinase, mTOR. This inhibition suppresses cytokine-mediated T-cell proliferation, halting progression from the G1 to S phase of the cell cycle. Sirolimus (Rapamune®), also known as rapamycin, is a macrolide antibiotic compound that is structurally related to tacrolimus. Everolimus (Zortress®), also known as *RAD*, is a similar compound with a shorter half-life.

mTOR inhibitors are extensively metabolized in the liver by CYP3A4 isoenzymes and to some extent in the intestinal wall. They are also substrates for the multidrug efflux pump, P-glycoprotein. Therefore, absorption and subsequent elimination may be influenced by drugs that affect CYP3A4 and/or P-glycoprotein. Concurrent treatment with strong inhibitors (e.g., ketoconazole, itraconazole, voriconazole, clarithromycin, ritonavir) and inducers (e.g., rifampin, rifbutin) should be used with caution. Inhibitors of P-glycoprotein (e.g., digoxin, cyclosporine) may decrease the efflux of everolimus from intestinal cells and increase everolimus blood concentrations.

mTORi Drug–Drug Interactions (Table 34.1)

Cyclosporine

Cyclosporine is both a substrate and inhibitor of CYP3A4 and P-glycoprotein. Studies have shown that concomitant administration of sirolimus with cyclosporine could result in a 50–80 % increase in sirolimus AUC [134]. In a single-dose drug–drug interaction study, concomitant use of sirolimus and cyclosporine resulted in an increase in the C_{max} and AUC of sirolimus. However, when given 4 h after cyclosporine administration, sirolimus C_{max} and AUC were both increased by only 33 %. Because of this, sirolimus is recommended to be taken 4 h after cyclosporine administration.

Similarly, cyclosporine significantly increased everolimus steady-state C_{max} (82 %; range: 25–158%) and AUC (168 %; range: 46–365 %) when compared to administration of everolimus alone [135]. Dose adjustment of everolimus may be necessary if the cyclosporine dose is altered.

Antifungals

Ketoconazole is a strong inhibitor of CYP3A4 and P-glycoprotein. In a multi-dose study, ketoconazole administration significantly affected the rate and extent of absorption of sirolimus. Sirolimus C_{max}, T_{max}, and AUC were increased by 4.3-fold, 38 %, and 10.9-fold, respectively [134]. Similarly, multiple-dose administration of ketoconazole 200 mg twice daily for 5 days to 12 healthy volunteers increased everolimus C_{max}, AUC, and half-life by 3.9-, 15-fold, and 89 %, respectively [135]. Voriconazole also has a significant effect on sirolimus pharmacokinetics. A single-blinded, randomized, placebo-controlled study in healthy male subjects found an average increase in C_{max} and AUC of sirolimus of 7- and 11-fold, respectively, when sirolimus was administered concomitantly with voriconazole [39]. However, a case series evaluating allogeneic hematopoietic stem cell transplant recipients, receiving both sirolimus and voriconazole, found no clinically significant toxicity and significant change in sirolimus trough concentrations when sirolimus dose was decreased by 90 % after the addition of voriconazole [136]. A pilot study, assessing the safety of concurrent administration of sirolimus and voriconazole, also found that sirolimus trough concentrations remained stable in patients with baseline sirolimus concentration of 12 ng/mL or lower when sirolimus dose was reduced by 50 % before administration of voriconazole [137].

Non-dihydropyridine Calcium Channel Blockers

Verapamil and diltiazem are substrates and inhibitors of CYP3A4 and P-glycoprotein. Concomitant administration of sirolimus 2 mg daily and verapamil 180 mg every 12 h to 26 healthy volunteers significantly affected the bioavailabilty of sirolumus and verapamil. Sirolimus C_{max} and AUC were increased 2.3- and 2.2-fold, respectively [134]. The C_{max} and AUC of the pharmacologically active *S*(−) enantiomer of verapamil were both increased 1.5-fold and T_{max} was decreased by 1.2 h. Similarly, multiple-dose administration of verapamil three times daily for 5 days to 16 healthy volunteers significantly increased everolimus C_{max} and AUC by 2.3- and 3.5-fold, respectively [135]. Simultaneous oral administration of diltiazem with sirolimus has been shown to increase C_{max}, T_{max}, and AUC of sirolimus by 1.4-, 1.3-, and 1.6-fold, respectively.

Erythromycin

Erythromycin is a substrate and inhibitor of CYP3A4 and P-glycoprotein. In a multi-dose study in healthy subjects, erythromycin significantly affected the bioavailability of sirolimus. Sirolimus C_{max}, AUC, and T_{max} were increased by 4.4-, 4.2-fold, and 0.4 h, respectively [134]. Similarly, administration of erythromycin three times daily for 5 days to 16 healthy volunteers significantly increased everolimus C_{max} and AUC by 2- and 4.4-fold, respectively, and half-life was increased by 39 % [135].

Rifampin

Rifampin is a potent inducer of CYP3A4 and P-glycoprotein. In a multi-dose study, rifampin decreased sirolimus AUC and C_{max} by 82 % and 71 %, respectively [134]. Similarly, pretreatment of 12 healthy subjects with multiple doses of rifampin followed by a single dose of everolimus increased everolimus clearance by nearly threefold and decreased everolimus C_{max} and AUC by 58 % and 63 %, respectively [135].

HIV Protease Inhibitor

Interactions have also been observed with concurrent use of sirolimus and HIV protease inhibitors in a case series. Low-dose nelfinavir was found to increase sirolimus concentrations, AUC, and half-life [138].

Conclusion

Drug–drug interaction continues to be a clinically significant problem affecting transplant recipients. Immunosuppression regimens continue to broaden and become more complex because of their narrow therapeutic index and significant inter- and intra-patient variability due to genetic polymorphisms in P-glycoprotein and CYP enzyme systems. The narrow therapeutic index of immunosuppressants combined with the use of medications for the treatment of comorbidities, including post-transplant diabetes, hypertension, osteoporosis, dyslipidemia, and psychiatric diseases, can lead to significant drug–drug interactions. Close therapeutic drug monitoring remains an important part of post-transplant care.

References

1. Hume DM, Magee JH, Kauffman HM, et al. Renal homotransplantation in man in modified recipients. Ann Surg. 1963; 158:608–44.
2. Murray JE, Merrill JP, Harrison JH, et al. Prolonged survival of human kidney homografts by immunosuppressive drug therapy. N Engl J Med. 1963;268:1315–23.
3. Woodruff MF, Robson JS, Nolan B, et al. Homotransplantation of kidney in patients treated by preoperative local radiation and postoperative administration of an antimetabolite (Imuran). Lancet. 1963;2:675–82.
4. Pirsch JD, Miller J, Dierhoi MH, et al. A comparison of tacrolimus (FK506) and cyclosporine for immunosuppression after cadaveric renal transplantation. FK506 Kidney Transplant Study Group. Transplantation. 1997;63:977–83.
5. Mayer AD, Dmitrewski J, Squifflet JP, et al. Multicenter randomized trial comparing tacrolimus (FK506) and cyclosporine in the prevention in the prevention of renal allograft rejection: a report of

the European Tacrolimus Multicenter Renal Study Group. Transplantation. 1997;64:436–43.
6. Jensik SC; and the FK 506 Kidney Transplant Study Group. Tacrolimus (FK 506) in kidney transplantation: three-year survival results of the US multicenter, randomized, comparative trial. Transplant Proc. 1998;30:1216–8.
7. Neylan JF; for the FK 506 Kidney Transplant Study Group. Racial differences in renal transplantation after immunosuppression with tacrolimus versus cyclosporine. Transplantation. 1998;65:515–23.
8. European Mycophenolate Mofetil Cooperative Study Group. Placebo-controlled study of mycophenolate mofetil combined with cyclosporin and corticosteroids for prevention of acute rejection. Lancet. 1995;345:1321–5.
9. Sollinger HW; for the U.S. Renal Transplant Mycophenolate Mofetil Study Group. Mycophenolate mofetil for the prevention of acute rejection in primary cadaveric renal allograft recipients. Transplantation. 1995;60:225–32.
10. The Tricontinental Mycophenolate Mofetil Renal Transplantation Study Group. A blinded, randomized clinical trial of mycophenolate mofetil for the prevention of acute rejection in cadaveric renal transplantation. Transplantation. 1996;61:1029–37.
11. Pond SM. Pharmacokinetic drug interactions. In: Benet LZ, Massoud N, Gambertoglio JG, editors. Pharmacokinetic basis for drug treatment. New York: Raven; 1984. p. 1995–220.
12. Wacher VJ, Salphati L, Benet LZ. Active secretion and enterocytic drug metabolism barriers to drug absorption. Adv Drug Deliv Rev. 1996;20:99–112.
13. Kelly PA, Burckar GJ, Venkataramanan R. Tacrolimus: a new immunosuppressive agent. Am J Health Syst Pharm. 1995; 50:1521–35.
14. CellCept [package insert]. Nutley, NJ: Roche Laboratories; 2008.
15. Prograf [package insert]. Deerfield, IL: Astellas Pharma US, Inc; 2009.
16. Campana C, Regazzi MB, Buggia I, Molinaro M. Clinically significant drug interaction with cyclosporin. An update. Clin Pharmacokinet. 1996;30:141–79.
17. Wacher VJ, Silverman JA, Zhang Y, et al. Role of p-glycoprotein and cytochrome P450 3A in limiting oral absorption of peptides and peptidomimetics. J Pharm Sci. 1998;87:1322–30.
18. Whitelock JP, Denison MS. Induction of cytochrome P450 enzymes that metabolize xenobiotics. In: Ortiz de Montellano PR, editor. Cytochrome P450: structure, mechanism and biochemistry. 2nd ed. New York: Plenum Press; 1995. p. 367–90.
19. Venkatakrishnan K, Von Moltke LL, Greenblatt DJ. Human drug metabolism and the cytochromes P450: application and relevance of in vitro models. J Clin Pharmacol. 2001;41:1149–79.
20. Zhang Y, Benet LZ. The gut as a barrier to drug absorption: combine role of cytochrome P450 3A and P-glycoprotein. Clin Pharmacokinet. 2001;40:159–68.
21. Davidson MH. Dose differing metabolism by cytochrome P450 have clinical importance? Curr Atheroscler Rep. 2002;2:14–9.
22. Lin JH, Lu AYH. Inhibition and induction of cytochrome P450 and the clinical applications. Clin Pharmacokinet. 1998; 35:361–90.
23. Wacher J, Wu CY, Benet LZ. Overlapping substrate specificities and tissue distribution of cytochrome P4503A and P-glycoprotein: implications for drug delivery and cancer chemotherapy. Mol Carcinog. 1995;13:129–34.
24. Hall SD, Thummel KE, Watkins PB, et al. Molecular and physical mechanisms of first-pass extraction. Drug Metab Dispos. 1999;27:161–6.
25. Fischer SA. Infections in the transplant recipient. Med Health R I. 2002;85:125–7.
26. Patel R. Infections in recipients of kidney transplant. Infect Dis Clin North Am. 2001;15:901–52.
27. Cavallo R, Merlino C, Re D, et al. B19 virus infection in renal transplant recipients. J Clin Virol. 2003;26:361–8.
28. Lin SJ, Schranz J, Teutsch SM. Aspergillosis case-fatality rate: systematic review of literature. Clin Infect Dis. 2001; 32(3):358–66.
29. Nucci M. Emerging moulds: Fusarium, Scedosporium and Zygomycetes in transplant recipients. Curr Opin Infect Dis. 2003;16(6):607–12.
30. Singh N. Fungal infections in recipients of solid organ transplantation. Infect Dis Clin North Am. 2003;17:113–34.
31. Hagerty JA, Ortiz J, Reich D, et al. Fungal infections in solid organ transplant patients. Surg Infect. 2003;4:263–71.
32. Abraham MA, Thomas PP, John GT, Job V, Shankar V, Jacob CK. Efficacy and safety of low-dose ketoconazole (50mg) to reduce the cost of cyclosporine in renal allograft recipients. Transplant Proc. 2003;35:215–6.
33. Butman SM, Wild JC, Nolan PE, et al. Prospective study of safety and financial benefit of ketoconazole as adjunctive therapy to cyclosporine after heart transplantation. J Heart Lung Transplant. 1991;10:351–8.
34. First MR, Schroeder TJ, Alexander JW, et al. Cyclosporine dose reduction by ketoconazole administration in real transplant recipients. Transplantation. 1991;51(2):365–70.
35. Sobh MA, Hamdy AF, El-Agroudy AE, et al. Coadministration of ketoconazole and cyclosporine for kidney transplant recipients: long-term evaluation and study of metabolic consequences. Am J Kidney Dis. 2001;37(3):510–7.
36. El-Agroudy A, Sobh M, Hamdy A, ghoneim M. A prospective, randomized study of coadministration of ketoconazole and cyclosporine A in kidney transplant recipients: ten-year follow-up. Transplantation. 2004;77:1371–6.
37. Romero M, Latorre A, Manzanares C, et al. Effect of fluconazole on the pharmacokinetics of cyclosporine in renal transplant patients. Clin Pharmacol Ther. 2002;71:226–34.
38. Vfend [package insert]. New York, NY: Pfizer; 2008.
39. Kowazoe H, Takiguchi Y, Tanaka H, et al. Change of the blood concentration of tacrolimus after the switch from fluconazole to voriconazole in patients receiving allogenic hematopoietic stem cell transplantation. Biol Pharm Bull. 2006;29(12):2528–31.
40. Sansone-Parsons A, Krishna G, Martinho M, et al. Effect of oral posaconazole on the pharmacokinetics of cyclosporine and tacrolimus. Pharmacotherapy. 2007;27(6):825–34.
41. Noxafil [package insert]. Kenilworth, NJ: Schering-Plough Corp; 2006.
42. Cancidas [package insert]. Whitehouse Station, NJ: Merck & Co.; 2008.
43. Saner F, Gensicke J, Rath P, et al. Safety profile of concomitant use of caspofungin and cyclosporine or tacrolimus in liver transplant patients. Infection. 2006;34(6):328–32.
44. Marr KA, Hachem R, Papanicolaou G, et al. Retrospective study of hepatic safety profile of patients concomitantly treated with caspofungin and cyclosporine A. Transpl Infect Dis. 2004;6:110–6.
45. Sanz-Rodriguez C, Lopez-Duarte M, Jurado M, et al. Safety of the concomitant use of caspofungin and cyclosporin A in patients with invasive fungal infections. Bone Marrow Transplant. 2004;34:13–20.
46. Christopeit M, Eikam M, Bhre G. Comedication of caspofungin acetate and cyclosporine A after allogeneic haematopoietic stem cell transplantation leads to negligible hepatotoxicity. Mycoses. 2008;51 Suppl 1:19–24.
47. Morrissey CO, Slavin MA, O'Reilly MA, et al. Caspofungin as salvage monotherapy for invasive aspergillosis in patients with haematological malignancies or following allogeneic stem cell transplantation: efficacy and concomitant cyclosporin A. Mycoses. 2007;50 Suppl 1:24–7.

48. Mycamine [package insert]. Deerfield, IL: Astellas Pharma US, Inc; 2008.
49. Dowell JA, Stogniew M, Krause D, Henkel T, Weston IE. Assessment of safety and pharmacokinetics of anidulafungin when administered with cyclosporine. J Clin Pharmacol. 2005;45:227–33.
50. Dowell JA, Stogniew M, Krause D, et al. Lack of pharmacokinetic interaction between anidulafungin and tacrolimus. J Clin Pharmacol. 2007;47:305–14.
51. Perfect JR. New antifungal agents. Transpl Infect Dis. 2002;4 Suppl 3:52–61.
52. Cagnoni PJ. Liposomal amphotericin B versus conventional amphotericin B in the empirical treatment of persistently febrile neutropenic patients. J Antimicrob Chemother. 2002;49 Suppl 1:81–6.
53. Paterson DL, Singh N. Interactions between tacrolimus and antimicrobial agents. Clin Infect Dis. 1997;25:1430–40.
54. Wandel C, Bohrer H, Bocker R. Rifampicin and cyclosporine dosing in heart transplant recipients. J Cardiothorac Vasc Anesth. 1995;9(5):621–2.
55. Kim YH, Yoon YR, Kim YW, et al. Effects of rifampin on cyclosporine disposition in kidney recipients with tuberculosis. Transplant Proc. 1998;30:3570–2.
56. Al-Sulaiman MG, Dhar JM, al-Khader AA. Successful use of rifampicin in the treatment of tuberculosis in renal transplant patients immunosuppressed with cyclosporine. Transplantation. 1990;50(4):597–8.
57. Hebert MF, Roberts JP, Prueksaritanont T, et al. Bioavailability of cyclosporine with concomitant rifampin administration is markedly less than predicted by hepatic enzyme induction. Clin Pharmacol Ther. 1992;52(5):453–7.
58. Freitag V, Skiftono RD, Lake KD. Effect of short-term rifampin on stable cyclosporine concentrations. Ann Pharmacother. 1999;33:871–2.
59. Moreno M, Latorre A, Manzanares C, et al. Clinical management of tacrolimus drug interactions in renal transplant patients. Transplant Proc. 1999;31:2252–3.
60. Chenhsu R, Loong C, Chou M, et al. Renal allograft dysfunction associated with rifampin-tacrolimus interaction. Ann Pharmacother. 2000;34:27–31.
61. Teichner E, Vincent I, Bonhomme-Faivre L, et al. Effect of highly active antiretroviral therapy on tacrolimus pharmacokinetics in hepatitis C virus and HIV co-infected liver transplant recipients in the ANRS HC-08 study. Clin Pharmacokinet. 2007;46(11):941–52.
62. Jain AB, Venkataramanan R, Eghtesad B, et al. Effect of coadministered lopinavir and ritonavir (Kaletra) on tacrolimus blood concentration transplantation patients. Liver Transpl. 2003;9:954–60.
63. Schonder KS, Shullo MA, Okusanya O. Tacrolimus and lopinavir/ritonavir interaction in liver transplantation. Ann Pharmacother. 2003;37:1793–6.
64. Mertz D, Battegay M, Marzolini C, et al. Drug-drug interaction in a kidney transplant recipient receiving HIV salvage therapy and tacrolimus. Am J Kidney Dis. 2009;54:e1–4.
65. Hardy G, Stanke-Labesque F, Contamin C, et al. Protease inhibitors and diltiazem increase tacrolimus blood concentration in a patient with renal transplantation: a case report. Eur J Clin Pharmacol. 2004;60:603–5.
66. Schvarcz R, Rudbeck G, Soderdahl G, et al. Interaction between nelfinavir and tacrolimus after orthoptic liver transplantation in a patient coinfected with HIV and hepatitis C virus (HCV). Transplantation. 2000;69(10):2194–5.
67. Jain A, Venkataramanan R, Shapiro R, et al. The interaction between antiretroviral agents and tacrolimus in liver and kidney transplant patients. Liver Transpl. 2002;8:841–5.
68. Franssetto L, Baluom M, Jacobsen W, et al. Cyclosporine pharmacokinetics and dosing modifications in human immunodeficiency virus-infected liver and kidney transplant recipients. Transplantation. 2005;80:13–7.
69. Vogel M, Voigt E, Michaelis H, et al. Management of drug-to-drug interactions between cyclosporine a and the protease-inhibitor lopinavir/ritonavir in liver-transplanted HIV-infected patients. Liver Transpl. 2004;10:939–44.
70. Wang PW, Ketter TA. Pharmacokinetics of mood stabilizers and new anticonvulsants. Psychopharmacol Bull. 2002;36:44–66.
71. Willmore LJ. Clinical pharmacology of new antiepileptic drugs. Neurology. 2000;55:S17–24.
72. Thompson PA, Mosley CA. Tacrolimus-phenytoin interaction. Ann Pharmacother. 1996;30:544.
73. Fridell JA, Jain K, Patel K, et al. Phenytoin decreases the blood concentrations of sirolimus in a liver transplant recipient: case report. Ther Drug Monit. 2004;25:117–9.
74. Koomans HA, Ligtenberg G. Mechanisms and consequences of arterial hypertension after renal transplantation. Transplantation. 2001;27:S9–12.
75. Olyaei AJ, deMattos AM, Bennett WM. A practical guide to the management of hypertension in renal transplant recipients. Drugs. 1999;58:1011–27.
76. Bunnag S, Vareesangthip K, Ong-ajyooth L. Effect of diltiazem on the pharmacokinetics of microemulsion cyclosporine A in renal transplantation. J Med Assoc Thai. 2006;89 Suppl 2: S228–34.
77. Jones TE, Morris RG. Pharmacokinetic interaction between tacrolimus and diltiazem: dose-response relationship in kidney and liver transplant recipients. Clin Pharmacokinet. 2002;41:381–8.
78. Bottiger Y, Sawe J, Brattstrom C, et al. Pharmacokinetic interaction between single oral doses of diltiazem and sirolimus in healthy volunteers. Clin Pharmacol Ther. 2001;69:32–40.
79. Seifeldin RA, Marcos-Alvarez A, Gordon FD, et al. Nifedipine interaction with tacrolimus in liver transplant recipient. Ann Pharmacother. 1997;31:571–5.
80. Lewis JB, Heldermann JH. Is it time for ACE inhibitors in chronic allograft nephropathy? Am J Kidney Dis. 2000;35:154–6.
81. Bader FM, Hagan ME, Crompton JA, et al. The effect of beta-blocker use on cyclosporine level in cardiac transplant recipients. J Heart Lung Transplant. 2005;24:2144–7.
82. Amioka K, Kuzuya T, Kushihara H, et al. Carvedilol increases ciclosporin bioavailability by inhibiting P-glycoprotein-mediated transplant. J Pharm Pharmacol. 2007;59:1383–7.
83. Kidney Disease: Improving Global Outcomes (KDIGO) Transplant Work Group. KDIGO clinical practice guideline for the care of kidney transplant recipients. Am J Transplant. 2009;9 Suppl 3:S1–155.
84. Colcrys [package insert]. Deerfield, IL: Takeda Pharmaceuticals America, Inc.; 2012.
85. Olbricht C, Wanner C, Eisenhauer T, et al. Accumulation of lovastatin, but not pravastatin, in the blood of cyclosporine treated kidney graft patients after multiple doses. Clin Pharmacol Ther. 1997;65:311–21.
86. Christians U, Jacobsen W, Floren LC. Metabolism and drug interactions of 3-hydroxy-3methylglutaryl coenzyme A reductase inhibitors in transplant patients: are the statins mechanistically similar? Pharmacol Ther. 1998;80:1–34.
87. Gruer PJ, Vega JM, Mercuri MF, et al. Concomitant use of cytochrome P4503A inhibitors and simvastatin. Am J Cardiol. 1999;84:811–5.
88. Dunn CJ, Wagstaff AJ, Perry CM, Plosker GL, Goa KL. Cyclosporin: an updated review of the pharmacokinetic properties, clinical efficacy and tolerability of microemulsion-based formulation (neural) in organ transplantation. Drugs. 2001;61:1957–2016.

89. Gullestad L, Nordal KP, Berg KJ, et al. Interaction between lovastatin and cyclosporine A after heart and kidney transplantation. Transplant Proc. 1999;31(5):2163–5.
90. Arnadottir M, Eriksson LO, Thysell H, et al. Plasma concentration profiles of simvastatin 3-hydroxy-3-methyl-glutaryl-coenzyme A reductase inhibitory activity in kidney transplant recipients with and without cyclosporine. Nephron. 1993;62(3):410–3.
91. Regazzi MB, Iacona I, Campana C, et al. Clinical efficacy and pharmacokinetics of HMG-CoA reductase inhibitors in heart transplant patients treated with cyclosporin A. Transplant Proc. 1994;26(5):2644–5.
92. Park JW, siekmeier R, Merz M, et al. Pharmacokinetics of pravastatin in heart-transplant patients taking cyclosporine A. Int J Clin Pharmacol Ther. 2002;10(10):439–50.
93. Åsberg A. Interaction between cyclosporine and lipid-lowering drugs: implications for organ transplant recipients. Drugs. 2003; 63:367–78.
94. Lemahieu WPD, Hermann M, Asberg A, et al. Combined therapy with atorvastatin and calcineurin inhibitors: no interaction with tacrolimus. Am J Transplant. 2005;5:2236–43.
95. Rocha G, Figueiredo CE, d'Avila D, et al. Depressive symptoms and kidney transplant outcome. Transplant Proc. 2001;33:3424.
96. Wright DH, Lake KD, Bruhn PS, et al. Nefazodone and cyclosporine drug-drug interaction. J Heart Lung Transplant. 1999;18: 913–5.
97. Helms-Smith KM, Curtis SL, Hatton RC. Apparent interaction between nefazodone and cyclosporine. Ann Intern Med. 1996; 125:424.
98. Garton T. Nefazodone and CYP 3A4 interactions with cyclosporine and tacrolimus. Transplantation. 2002;74:745.
99. Olyaei AJ, DeMattos A, Norman DJ, et al. Interaction between tacrolimus and nefazodone in a stable renal transplant recipient. Pharmacotherapy. 1998;18:1356–9.
100. Campo JV. Tacrolimus toxic reaction associated with the use of nefazodone: paroxetine as an alternative agent. Arch Gen Psychiatry. 1998;55:1050–2.
101. Richelson E. Pharmacokinetic interactions of new antidepressants: a review of the effects on the metabolism of other drugs. Mayo Clin Proc. 1997;72:835–47.
102. Lill J, Bauer L, Horn J, et al. Cyclosporine-drug interactions and the influence of patient age. Am J Health Syst Pharm. 2000; 57:1579–84.
103. Markowitz JS, Gill HS, Hunt NM, et al. Lack of antidepressant-cyclosporine pharmacokinetics interactions. J Clin Psychopharmacol. 1998;18:91–3.
104. Liston HL, Markowitz JS, Hunt N, et al. Lack of citalopram effect on the pharmacokinetics of cyclosporine. Psychosomatics. 2001; 42:370–2.
105. Strouse TB, Fairbanks LA, Skotzko CE, et al. Fluoxetine and cyclosporine in organ transplantation. Psychosomatics. 1996;37:23–30.
106. Ereshefsky K, Dugan D. Review of the pharmacokinetics, pharmacogenetics, and drug interaction potential of antidepressants: focus on venlafaxine. Depress Anxiety. 2000;12:30–44.
107. Cellcept [package insert]. South San Francisco, CA: Genentech USA, Inc.; 2012.
108. Myfortic [package insert]. East Hanover, NJ: Novartis Pharmaceutical Corporation; 2012.
109. Bullingham R, Monroe S, Nichols A, et al. Pharmacokinetics and bioavailability of mycophenolate mofetil in healthy subjects after single-dose oral and intravenous administration. J Clin Pharmacol. 1996;36:315–24.
110. Picard N, Ratanasavanh D, Premaud A, et al. Identification of the UDP-glucuronosyltransferase isoforms involved in mycophenolic acid phase II metabolism. Drug Metab Dispos. 2005;33: 139–46.
111. Bowalgaha K, Miners JO. The glucuronidation of mycophenolic acid by human liver, kidney, and jejunum microsomes. Br J Clin Pharmacol. 2001;52:605–9.
112. Hesselink DA, van Hest RM, Mathot RAA, et al. Cyclosporine interacts with mycophenolic acid by inhibiting the multidrug resistance-associated protein 2. Am J Transplant. 2005;5:987–95.
113. Van Gelder T, Klupp J, Barten MJ, et al. Comparison of the effects of tacrolimus and cyclosporine on the pharmacokinetics of mycophenolic acid. Ther Drug Monit. 2001;23:119–28.
114. Naesens M, Kuypers DR, Verbeke K, Vanrenterghem Y. Multidrug resistance protein 2 genetic polymorphisms influence mycophenolic acid exposure in renal allograft recipients. Transplantation. 2006;82:1074–84.
115. Zucker K, Rosen A, Tsaroucha A, et al. Unexpected augmentation of mycophenolic acid pharmacokinetics in renal transplant patients receiving tacrolimus and mycophenolate mofetil in combination therapy, and analogous in vitro findings. Transpl Immunol. 1997;5:225–32.
116. Kobayashi M, Saitoh H, Tadano K, et al. Cyclosporin A, but not tacrolimus, inhibits the biliary excretion of mycophenolic acid glucuronide possibly mediated by multidrug resistance associated protein 2 in rats. J Pharmacol Exp Ther. 2004;309:1029–35.
117. Westley IS, Brogan LR, Morris RC, et al. Role of MRP2 in the hepatic disposition of mycophenolic acid: effect of cyclosporine. Drug Metab Dispos. 2006;34:261–6.
118. Naderer OJ, Dupuis RE, Heinzen EL, et al. The influence of norfloxacin and metronidazole on the disposition of mycophenolate mofetil. J Clin Pharmacol. 2005;45:219–26.
119. Zucker K, Tsaroucha A, Olson L, et al. Evidence that tacrolimus augments the bioavailability of mycophenolate mofetil through the inhibition of mycophenolic acid glucuronidation. Ther Drug Monit. 1999;21:35–43.
120. Kagaya H, Miura M, Satoh S, et al. No pharmacokinetic interaction between mycophenolic acid and tacrolimus in renal transplant recipients. J Clin Pharmacol Ther. 2008;33:193–201.
121. Shah J, Juan D, Bullingham R. A single dose drug interaction study of mycophenolate mofetil and acyclovir in normal subjects [abstract]. J Clin Pharmacol. 1994;34:1029.
122. Gimenez F, Foeillet E, Bourdon O, Weller S, Garret C, Roselyne B, et al. Evaluation of pharmacokinetic interactions after oral administration of mycophenolate mofetil and valaciclovir or acyclovir to healthy subjects. Clin Pharmacokinet. 2004; 43(10):685–92.
123. Wolfe EJ, Mathur V, Tomlanovich S, Jung D, Wong R, Griffy K, et al. Pharmacokinetics of mycophenolate mofetil and intravenous ganciclovir alone and in combination in renal transplant recipients. Pharmacotherapy. 1997;17(3):591–8.
124. Bullingham R, Shah J, Goldblum R, Schiff M. Effects of food and antacid on the pharmacokinetics of single doses of mycophenolate mofetil in rheumatoid arthritis patients. Br J Clin Pharmacol. 1996;41:513–6.
125. Van Gelder T, Pescovitz MD, Elzein H, Hamzeh F. The effect of gastric pH modulators on the pharmacokinetics of mycophenolate mofetil (MMF) in de novo renal transplant recipients (abstract 230). Presented at international congress on transplantation, Vienna, Austria; 2004.
126. Miura M, Satoh S, Inoue K, et al. Influence of lansoprazole and rabeprazole on mycophenolic acid pharmacokinetics one year after renal transplantation. Ther Drug Monit. 2008;30:46–51.
127. Kofler S, Deutsch MA, Bigdeli AK, et al. Proton pump inhibitor co-medication reduces mycophenolate acid drug exposure in heart transplant recipients. J Heart Lung Transplant. 2009;28:605–11.
128. Rupprecht K, Schmidt C, Raspe A, et al. Bioavailability of mycophenolate mofetil and enteric-coated mycophenolate sodium is differentially affected by pantoprazole in healthy volunteers. J Clin Pharmacol. 2009;49:1196–201.

129. Kees MG, Steinke T, Moritz S, et al. Omeprazole impairs the absorption of mycophenolate mofetil but not of enteric-coated mycophenolate sodium in healthy volunteers. J Clin Pharmacol. 2012;52:1265–72.
130. Pieper A, Buhle F, Bauer S, Mai I, Budde K, Haffner D, et al. The effect of sevelamer on the pharmacokinetics of cyclosporine A and mycophenolate mofetil after renal transplantation. Nephrol Dial Transplant. 2004;19:2630–3.
131. Borrows R, Chusney G, Loucaido M, James A, Van Tromp J, Cairns T, et al. The magnitude and time course of changes in mycophenolic acid 12-hour predose levels during antibiotic therapy in mycophenolate mofetil-based renal transplantation. Ther Drug Monit. 2007;29:126.
132. Kuypers D, Verleden G, Naesens M, et al. Drug interaction between mycophenolate mofetil and rifampin: possible induction of uridine diphosphate-glucuronosyltransferase. Clin Pharmacol Ther. 2008;78(1):81–8.
133. Imuran [package insert]. Greenville, NC: Prometheus Lab Inc; 2008.
134. Rapamune [package insert]. Philadelphia, PA: Wyeth Pharmaceuticals Inc.; 1999.
135. Zortress [package insert]. East Hanover, NJ: Novartis Pharma Stein AG; 2013.
136. Marty FM, Lowry CM, Cutler CS, et al. Voriconazole and sirolimus coadministration after allogeneic hematopoietic stem cell transplantation. Biol Blood Marrow Transplant. 2006; 12(5):552–9.
137. Saad A, Depestel D, Carver P. Factors influencing the magnitude and clinical significance of drug interactions between azole antifungals and select immunosuppressants. Pharmacotherapy. 2006;26(12):1730–44.
138. Jain A, Venkataramanan R, Fridell JA, et al. Nelfinavir, a protease inhibitor, increases sirolimus levels in liver transplantation patient: a case report. Liver Transpl. 2002;8:838–40.

Index

M.R. Weir and E.V. Lerma (eds.), *Kidney Transplantation: Practical Guide to Management*,
DOI 10.1007/978-1-4939-0342-9, © Springer Science+Business Media New York 2014

Q

R

S